S0-BZJ-985

The Art and Science of Diabetes Self-Management Education

A Desk Reference for Healthcare Professionals

Editor in Chief
Carolé Mensing, RN, MA, CDE

Section Editors
Marjorie Cypress, MSN, C-ANP, CDE
Cindy Halstenson, RD, LD, CDE
Sue McLaughlin, BS, RD, CDE
Elizabeth A. Walker, DNSc, RN, CDE

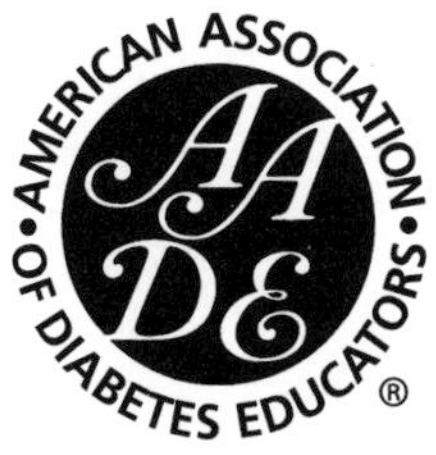

A Core Knowledge Publication of the
American Association of Diabetes Educators

A Core Knowledge Publication of the
American Association of Diabetes Educators

The Art and Science of Diabetes Self-Management Education
A Desk Reference for Healthcare Professionals

Published by the American Association of Diabetes Educators

ISBN 1-881876-21-7

Printed and bound in the United States of America

Library of Congress Cataloging-in-Publication Data

The art and science of diabetes self-management education : a desk reference for healthcare professionals / editor, Carolé Mensing ; section editors, Elizabeth Walker . . . [et al.] ; medical editor, Nancy Williams.
p. ; cm.
Includes bibliographic references and index.
ISBN 1-881876-21-7 (hardcover)
1. Diabetes. 2. Self-care, Health. 3. Patient education.
I. Mensing, Carolé. II. American Association of Diabetes Educators.
[DNLM: 1. Diabetes Mellitus—therapy. 2. Self Care—methods.
3. Patient Education—methods. WK 850 A784 2006]
RC660.4.A78 2006
616.4'62—dc22 2006008818

TABLE OF CONTENTS

SECTION 3
Facilitating Successful Self-Management

INTRODUCTION

Diabetes has reached epidemic levels and continues to grow. The harsh reality is that seven percent of all Americans (nearly 21 million people) have the disease, and a staggering 1.3 million adults are newly diagnosed each year. Poorly controlled diabetes inflicts devastating complications that diminishes the quality and length of life of patients. Diabetes is the leading cause of blindness, end stage kidney disease, and non-traumatic amputations in the US. Also, it is disturbing to observe that the disease is occurring at younger ages than ever before in our history.

One of the biggest challenges facing people with diabetes is learning how to live with, and manage, their condition on a daily basis. A key health care professional who can help them with this critical task is the diabetes educator.

I'm a great supporter of diabetes educators because they possess the ability to interweave all the elements of proper diabetes management together and work with patients to develop an achievable blueprint for living a healthier life with their diabetes.

Richard H. Carmona, MD, MPH
Surgeon General

PREFACE

Keymakers

Some people see a closed door,
And turn away.

Others see a closed door,
Try the knob
And if it doesn't open . . .
They turn away.

Still others see a closed door,
Try the knob,
If it doesn't open,
They find a key,
If the key doesn't fit . . .
They turn away.

A rare few see a closed door,
Try the knob,
If it doesn't open,
They find a key,
If the key doesn't fit. . .

They make one.

—Author unknown

If you are reading this book, chances are that you have the gift of being a keymaker. Readers will find that this reference book is a key that opens the door of change—change in how educators view the science of diabetes and change in how we deliver information to enable more effective diabetes self-management. *The Art and Science of Diabetes Self-Management Education: A Desk Reference for Healthcare Professionals* represents a timely, new vision in communications and publications from the American Association of Diabetes Educators (AADE). The book serves as a resource for all health professionals, community professionals, and individuals who fulfill roles as a keymaker in providing education to individuals with diabetes.

This major publication has been in the works for more than two and a half years. Before this *Desk Reference*, the AADE was well known for its multivolume set entitled *A CORE Curriculum for Diabetes Education.* The *CORE*, as the publication came to be known, was a well-received textbook that evolved and gained credibility with each of its 5 editions. The *CORE* became the major text published by the AADE and paved the way for this more broadly useful reference book.

The *Desk Reference*, as the name implies, is intended to be an authoritative and accessible resource on applying the concepts of diabetes self-management and effective use of educational principles. The book aligns with the AADE's strategic mission and vision and is intended to impact practice, enhancing the contribution of skilled diabetes educators to the care team and improving the lives of those affected by diabetes. The AADE considers this new book a Core Knowledge Publication and sees it as paving the way for an array of specialized publications.

As a book on diabetes education, this publication is unique among desk references, in particular because it weaves the art of the educator's professional practice through the complex, multidisciplinary science of diabetes and its chronic complications. The book takes its focus and direction from several notable trends: the growing recognition that management of diabetes and its chronic complications requires significant and appropriate self-care; the increasing body of evidence that diabetes education makes an important difference in the lives of individuals affected by diabetes and the adequacy of their health care; and the shift from acute care medical management to the chronic care model,[1] an approach appropriately reflective of the chronic and progressive disease that is diabetes.

Content development has been guided by several important and widely accepted documents: the National Standards for Diabetes Self-Management Education,[2] the National Standards for Outcome Measurement,[3] the AADE's most recent Strategic Plan,[4] the Scope and Standards of Practice and Standards of Professional Performance developed by the AADE,[5] and the Clinical

Practice Standards of the American Diabetes Association.[6] Our focus in writing this book has been to provide rigorously developed, evidence-based technical content.

Progressing from science to art

Within this book, a wealth of material is presented in 3 distinct and intentionally organized sections.

- *Understanding the Individual's Health Behaviors and Choices* is Section 1. This set of 6 chapters presents background and theoretical foundations essential to providing effective self-management education.
- *Translating Science to Art: Understanding the Disease and its Treatment* is Section 2. Progressing through 18 content-rich chapters discussing various aspects of the disease, its therapies, and chronic complications, readers come to understand and appreciate the technical information essential for contributing most effectively to successful diabetes education.
- *Facilitating Successful Self-Management* is Section 3. Here, in 11 chapters, the authors have set out the new "Core" of knowledge for well-designed diabetes education. The first 4 chapters discuss "process" issues regarding the delivery of diabetes self-management education. The AADE 7 Self-Care Behaviors™ are the organizing principle for the final 7 chapters. Readers of this section receive a state-of-the-art education.

To familiarize yourself with the resources and contents of this book, first read the overviews for each of the 3 sections. They will guide you to chapters discussing issues of most immediate concern to your work and expand your horizons as well. Next, you may wish to review the back of the chapters, to find the "pearls for practice" that have been summarized there from the body of the chapter. Throughout the book, each chapter concludes with educational "pearls," which can be thought of as outcomes available to the reader for professional and personal growth and development. The pearls synthesize a chapter's content into educational strategies appropriate for use with people with diabetes, professional peers, volunteers, and others involved in the diabetes self-management education effort. Some pearls highlight salient "take home" points—ideas that the person with diabetes can take away from the teaching/educational experience and apply to daily life. Other pearls highlight what is most important to teach and what is important to learn.

As readers explore the book, doors will be opened in their professional development and understanding. Readers gain insight into principles of teaching and learning that help educators make their interventions more effective. The book encompasses both group and individual learning. It delineates teaching strategies and tools appropriate for children and those best for adults and older adults. Factors that enhance the educator's effectiveness are addressed—for example, cultural competence, the ability to employ strategies to teach persons with low literacy levels, assessing readiness to learn, and unique aspects of working with physically and mentally handicapped individuals. Considerations for those with special needs and in special settings have been addressed because education must be customized to the needs of the individual. Focusing on the individual is a theme woven throughout the text. Another recurring theme is the book's practical focus; eventually, all information is synthesized into keys of value in diabetes education, keys that open doors for those with diabetes and keys that enhance the role of the educator as a keymaker.

The diabetes educator profession is moving toward the ideal of having all persons with diabetes be successful self-managers, providing *them* with the key for opening doors of hope and health. Positively impacting the lives of people with diabetes is the ultimate goal of this book and of the endeavors of the AADE. A timely and unique publication, this reference book will advance the profession's ability to work toward this goal.

The overall goal for the *Desk Reference* was to develop an excellent and comprehensive resource for any healthcare professional or community professional involved in the clinical management of diabetes and the education of people affected by the disease. Distinctively, though, this book communicates the unique body of knowledge developed and applied by diabetes educators—an increasingly important subject for which the AADE and its members are viewed as a leading authority. The AADE perceives, as the key guiding principle for all its work and support of those in the profession, that the unique and valued outcome of diabetes education is behavior change. This unique and valued education is, of course, delivered by the diabetes educator, the ultimate keymaker!

Encompassing the whole

My intention, as editor-in-chief guiding this new publication, was to ensure that we provided a resource, laid the groundwork, and continued to promote all educators in their work and in their awesome role as keymakers.

I want to thank each of the authors for their expertise and willingness to write for this book. Each has made a significant and unique contribution. My heartfelt thank you also to the reviewers and consultants whose knowledge and attention to detail was essential to ensuring coverage and quality in our publication.

I am especially grateful to my dear co-editors, Elizabeth, Marjorie, Cindy, and Sue, without whom this reference book would not be the quality product it is. Their expertise, caring, and diligence for accuracy were unending—their mark is in every chapter. They not only offered their all-consuming commitment of time to this project, because they believed in the worth of the effort, but also offered counsel, support, and guidance to me. The medical editor—technical editor, wordsmith, maker of "magic"—appropriately placed each chapter's material in its best light to, as one author described it, "make us read better than we write." I extend my deep thanks to the staff at the AADE, who held our feet to the fire of deadlines, offered advice, and worked hard to keep us on task. I offer sincere thanks also to my many educator friends—in particular, Marion Franz, Lois Book, my coworkers, and diabetes educators across the country, who are my role models. Finally, I have a special thank you for my educator friend, who advised me to think about being part of this project, because we both have the keymaker vision.

I thank you all for this professional and personal growth opportunity. What an inspiring, door-opening experience it has been for me and the entire reference book team. This project has been an excellent example of the benefits of involvement in the work of your professional association. Those willing to make the sacrifices of their time, through their unique contributions, advanced the profession while building personal skills and a more extensive professional network that will serve them for years to come.

Readers, you will want to keep this resource book handy: it is a shiny, new key in your hands. Turn the knob, turn the page, open the door to the opportunities we have unlocked and present to you between the covers of this new book!

Carolé Mensing, RN, MA, CDE
Editor in Chief (Primary Keymaker)

References

1. Wagner EH, Austin BT, Von Korff M. Improving outcomes in chronic illness. Managed Care Quarterly. 1996;4:12-25.

2. Mensing C, Boucher J, Cypress M, et al. National standards for diabetes self-management education. Diabetes Care. 2006;29suppl 1:S78-85.

3. Mulcahy K, Maryniuk M, Peeples M, et al. Diabetes self-management education core outcome measures (technical review). Diabetes Educ. 2003;29:768-98.

4. AADE Mission Statement, Vision Statement, Code of Ethics, Goals, Value Statement. Diabetes Educ. 2006;32:25.

5. American Association of Diabetes Educators. The scope of practice, standards of practice, and standards of professional performance for diabetes educators. Diabetes Educ. 2005;31:487-513.

6. American Diabetes Association. Summary of revisions for the 2006 Clinical Practice Recommendations. Diabetes Care. 2006;29suppl 1:S3.

ACKNOWLEDGMENTS

In 2005, AADE adopted a new mission with the key phrase "driving professional practice". To further this mission, AADE is proud to present this premier desk reference for diabetes self-management education. It contains the combined insights, experience, and research of many of our colleagues who represent excellence in diabetes education and clinical care. As president of AADE, I would like to take this opportunity to thank all those individuals who have willingly contributed their time and expertise in developing this incredible resource for the practice of diabetes education. The AADE leadership is grateful for your dedication, your hard work, and most of all for your commitment to our profession.

Many people have contributed to the success of this book and I would especially like to thank the Editor in Chief, Carolé Mensing. Her perseverance and vision have been a guiding force as she coordinated the work of the editors who worked with over 60 authors to produce the 35 chapters. This book is a testament to her dedication to diabetes education and to diabetes educators.

I want to thank the Publications Steering Group who developed the vision of the publication and planned its course for completion. AADE is fortunate to have such a group of committed, knowledgeable members.

I also would like to express gratitude to all the authors and reviewers who volunteered their time and to our dedicated AADE staff who supported them. Truly the success of this publication will be due to their contributions.

On behalf of AADE , I would like to thank all of you who contributed to this unique and timely reference. The benefits of your work will be demonstrated through the impact it will have on the practice of current and future colleagues.

Malinda Peeples, RN, MA, CDE
President, American Association of Diabetes Educators

Editors and Editorial Staff

Editor in Chief

Carolé Mensing, RN, MA, CDE, is the coordinator of the ADA recognized Diabetes Self-Management Program at the University of Connecticut, Farmington. She provides education and clinical follow up with diabetes clients, insulin management, case management, etc. She participates in the medical/dental school program and is a guest lecturer at U Conn and at the University of Hartford.

Carolé has played an integral part in the establishment of a number of Diabetes Education programs throughout the county, and chaired the Task Force which published the National Standards for Diabetes Self-Management Education (Washington, DC, May 2000). She is a nationally known speaker and leader in the field of diabetes care and education. She is currently a diabetes clinical nurse specialist and has been a certified diabetes educator (CDE) since 1986. She has served as her local AADE/CADE chapter president and is a Past President, Health Care and Education, of the American Diabetes Association.

Section 1 Editor

Elizabeth A. Walker, DNSc, RN, CDE, Professor of Medicine and Professor of Epidemiology and Population Health, is the director of the Prevention and Control Division for the Diabetes Research and Training Center at the Albert Einstein College of Medicine, Bronx, New York. Dr. Walker does behavioral intervention studies in minority diabetes populations to promote medication adherence and lifestyle change. She is also a behavioral scientist focusing on medication adherence in the Diabetes Prevention Program Outcomes Study. Elizabeth has been a diabetes nurse specialist in both inpatient and community settings and a certified diabetes educator since 1986. In 2000, she served as President, Health Care & Education, of the American Diabetes Association.

Section 2 Editors

Marjorie Cypress, MSN, C-ANP, CDE, is an adult nurse practitioner specializing in diabetes in Albuquerque, New Mexico. She has worked in diabetes management and in education of patients and healthcare professionals for over 20 years in New York and New Mexico. She has authored numerous articles and has lectured nationally on diabetes management and promotion of self-care behaviors. She is a past chair of the National Certification Board for Diabetes Educators, and has served on many national committees for the American Diabetes Association and the American Association of Diabetes Educators. Marjorie is currently a doctoral candidate at the University of New Mexico, College of Nursing.

Cindy Halstenson, RD, LD, CDE, is the Diabetes Clinical Program Manager for Ovations, a United Health Group company in Minnetonka, Minnesota. Cindy has specialized in diabetes care and education over the past 15 years, including clinical care, population healthcare improvement, and clinical program management. She has served as Chair or President for the American Diabetes Association, Minnesota area, the Minneapolis-St. Paul Diabetes Educators, the Minnesota Dietetic Association, and the Diabetes Care and Education dietetic practice group of the American Dietetic Association. She currently serves on the National Certification Board for Diabetes Educators Board of Directors.

Section 3 Editor

Sue McLaughlin, BS, RD, CDE, has worked in diabetes care and education for over 20 years, in a variety of settings. Current practice is at The Nebraska Medical Center in Omaha, Nebraska, where she works in pediatric and adult endocrinology, and as an instructor and lifestyle coach for the Ho-Chunk Hope Grant, SDPI Diabetes Prevention Program with the Winnebago, Nebraska tribe. She has served on the American Diabetes Association Board of Directors, the Nominating Committee and Chair of the Council Chairs Committee and the Council on Nutritional Science and Metabolism. She is a past president of the Heartland Association of Diabetes Educators and a past chair of the Diabetes Care and Education dietetic practice group of the American Dietetic Association.

Medical Editor

Nancy Williams, MS
BioText Communications
Arlington Heights, Illinois

Executive Liaison

Mary M. Austin, MA, RD, CDE
Immediate Past President, American Association of Diabetes Educators
Nutrition and Diabetes Specialist
Principle, The Austin Group LLC
Shelby Township, Michigan

AADE Staff

Lana Vukovljak, MA, MS
Chief Learning Officer

Mary E. Sears
Director of Educational Content Delivery

Rebecca Seflow Hartzell
Project Manager

Contributors

Ann L. Albright, PhD, RD
University of California
San Francisco, California

Bob Anderson, EdD
University of Michigan
Ann Arbor, Michigan

Marilynn S. Arnold, MS, RD, LD, CDE
The Children's Medical Center
Dayton, Ohio

Rodolfo M. Banda, MD
Valley Retina Institute
McAllen, Texas

Carolyn Banion, RN, MN, CPNP, CDE
The Children's Hospital
University of Colorado Health Sciences Center
Barbara Davis Center
Aurora, Colorado

Joan K. Bardsley, RN, MBA, CDE
MedStar Research Institute
Hyattsville, Maryland

Jackie L. Boucher, MS, RD, BC-ADM, CDE
HealthPartners
Minneapolis, Minnesota

Carol A. Brownson, MSPH
Washington University
School of Medicine in St. Louis and National Program Office
Diabetes Initiative of The Robert Wood Johnson Foundation
St. Louis, Missouri

Dorothy Burns, PhD, RN
Hampton University
Hampton, Virginia

Laura D. Byham-Gray, PhD, RD, CNSD
University of Medicine and Dentistry of New Jersey
Stratford, New Jersey

Kiralee K. Camp, MS
Health Education
Park Nicollet Institute
St. Louis Park, Minnesota

Belinda P. Childs, ARNP, BC-ADM, CDE
Mid America Diabetes Associates
Wichita, Kansas

Susan Cornell, BS, PharmD, CDE, CDM
Midwestern University Chicago
College of Pharmacy
Downers Grove, Illinois

Devra K. Dang, PharmD, BCPS
University of Connecticut
School of Pharmacy
Storrs, Connecticut

Mary de Groot, PhD
Ohio University
Department of Psychology
Athens, Ohio

Linda M. Delahanty, MS, RD
Massachusetts General Hospital
Boston, Massachusetts

Michael M. Engelgau, MD, MS
Division of Dibetes Translation
National Center for Chronic Disease Prevention and Health Promotion
Centers for Disease Control and Prevention
Atlanta, Georgia

Edwin B. Fisher, PhD
University of North Carolina at Chapel Hill and National Program Office
Diabetes Initiative of The Robert Wood Johnson Foundation
Chapel Hill, North Carolina

Marion J. Franz, MS, RD, LD, CDE
Nutrition Concepts by Franz, Inc.
Minneapolis, Minnesota

Janine Freeman, RD, LD, CDE
Diabetes Nutrition Consultant
Atlanta, Georgia

Martha M. Funnell, MS, RN, CDE
University of Michigan
Ann Arbor, Michigan

Patti B. Geil, MS, RD, FADA, CDE
Diabetes Care & Communications
Lexington, Kentucky

Victor H. Gonzalez, MD
Valley Retina Institute PA
McAllen, Texas

Diana W. Guthrie, PhD, ARNP, CDE
Mid America Diabetes Associates
Wichita, Kansas

Richard A. Guthrie, MD, FAAP, FACE, CDE
Mid America Diabetes Associates
Wichita, Kansas

Felicia Hill-Briggs, PhD ABPP
Johns Hopkins University
School of Medicine
Baltimore, Maryland

Debbie A. Hinnen, ARNP, BC-ADM, CDE, FAAN
Mid America Diabetes Associates
Wichita, Kansas

Tommy Johnson, PharmD, CDE
University of Georgia
College of Pharmacy
Athens, Georgia

Edna G. Johnson-Gutierrez, RN, MSN, ANP-BC, CDE
Clovis Family Healthcare
Clovis, New Mexico

Karmeen Kulkarni, MS, RD, BC-ADM, CDE
Diabetes Center
St. Marks Hospital
Salt Lake City, Utah

Daniel Lorber, MD, FACP, CDE
Diabetes Care and Information Center of New York
New York, New York

Gayle M. Lorenzi, RN, CDE
University of California
Amylin Pharmaceuticals, Inc.
San Diego, California

Sarah L. Lovegreen, MPH
Saint Louis University
School of Public Health
St. Louis, Missouri

Susan D. Martin, RD, LD, CDE
Mid America Diabetes Associates
Wichita, Kansas

Melinda D. Maryniuk, MEd, RD, CDE, FADA
Joslin Diabetes Center
Boston, Massachusetts

Gail D'Eramo Melkus, EdD, C-ANP, FAAN
Yale School of Nursing
New Haven, Connecticut

Cathy A. Mullooly, MS, RCEP, CDE
Joslin Clinic
Boston, Massachusetts

Dara L. Murphy, MPH
Division of Dibetes Translation
National Center for Chronic Disease Prevention and Health Promotion
Centers for Disease Control and Prevention
Atlanta, Georgia

K.M. Venkat Narayan, MD, MPH
Division of Diabetes Translation
National Center for Chronic Disease Prevention and Health Promotion
Centers for Disease Control and Prevention
Atlanta, Georgia

James W. Pichert, PhD
Vanderbilt Diabetes Research and Training Center
Nashville, Tenessee

Robert E. Ratner, MD, FACP, FACE
MedStar Research Institute
Hyattsville, Maryland

Diane M. Reader, RD, CDE
International Diabetes Center
Minneapolis, Minnesota

Laurie Ruggiero, PhD
University of Illinois at Chicago
Chicago, Illinois

David G. Schlundt, PhD
Vanderbilt Diabetes Research and Training Center
Nashville, Tenessee

Laura Shane-McWhorter, PharmD, BCPS, FASCP, BC-ADM, CDE
University of Utah
College of Pharmacy
Salt Lake City, Utah

Anne H. Skelly, PhD, RN, CS, ANP
University of North Carolina
School of Nursing
Chapel Hill, North Carolina

Geralyn R. Spollett, MSN, ANP, CDE
Yale University
Department of Endocrinology and Metabolism
New Haven, Connecticut

Condit F. Steil, PharmD, FAPhA, CDE
Samford University
McWhorter School of Pharmacy
Birmingham, Alabama

Tricia S. Tang, PhD
University of Michigan
Ann Arbor, Michigan

Alyce M. Thomas, RD
St. Joseph's Regional Medical Center
Paterson, New Jersey

Donna M. Tomky, MSN, APRN, C-ANP, CDE
Lovelace Health Systems
Department of Endocrinology Diabetes
Albuquerque, New Mexico

Dace L. Trence, MD, FACE
University of Washington Medical Center
Seattle, Washington

Virginia Valentine, CNS, BC-ADM, CDE
Diabetes Network Inc.
Albuquerque, New Mexico

Jeffrey J. VanWormer, MS
HealthPartners Health Behavior Group
Minneapolis, Minnesota

Frank Vinicor, MD, MPH
Division of Dibetes Translation
National Center for Chronic Disease Prevention and Health Promotion
Centers for Disease Control and Prevention
Atlanta, Georgia

Aaron I. Vinik, MD, PhD, FCP, MACP
The Strelitz Diabetes Institutes
Eastern Virginia Medical School
Norfolk, Virginia

Etta J. Vinik, MA (Ed)
The Strelitz Diabetes Institutes
Eastern Virginia Medical School
Norfolk, Virginia

Christopher J. Vito, PharmD
Forum Extended Care Pharmacy
Chicago, Illinois

Julie Wagner, PhD
University of Connecticut Health Center
Division of Behavior Sciences and Community Health
Farmington, Connecticut

Judith Wylie-Rosett, EdD, RD
Albert Einstein College of Medicine
Bronx, New York

Reviewers

Roger P. Austin, MS, RPh, CDE
Henry Ford Health System
Detroit, Michigan

Susan L. Barlow, RD, CDE
Amylin Pharmaceuticals
Carmel, Indiana

Lois J. Book, EdD, MS, BSN, RN
Columbia, Maryland

Jennifer Brindisi, MA
University of Connecticut Health Center
Farmington, Connecticut

Thomas E. Buckley, RPh, MPH
University of Connecticut
School of Pharmacy
Storrs, Connecticut

Ronald J. DeVizia, PharmD
Kerr Drug, Inc.
Zebulon, North Carolina

Patti L. Duprey, ARNP, MSN, CDE
The Diabetes Center at MDW
North Conway, New Hampshire

Kristina Ernst, BSN, RN, CDE
Division of Diabetes Translation
Centers for Disease Control and Prevention
Atlanta, Georgia

Alison B. Evert, RD, CDE
University of Washington Medical Center
Seattle, Washington

James A. Fain, PhD, RN, BC-ADM, FAAN
University of Massachusetts Dartmouth
College of Nursing
Dartmouth, Massachusetts

Linda B. Haas, PhC, RN, CDE
VA Suget Sound Heatlth Care System
University of Washington
School of Nursing
Seattle, Washington

Carol J. Homko, RN, PhD, CDE
Temple University
Philadelphia, Pennsylvania

Barb A. Kocurek, PharmD, BCPS, CDE
Baylor Health Care System
Irving, Texas

Kaye M. Kramer, BSN, MPH
University of Pittsburgh
Pittsburgh, Pennsylvania

Davida F. Kruger, MSN, APRN-BC, BC-ADM
Henry Ford Health Systems
Division of Endocrinology and Metabolism
Detroit, Michigan

Wendy Kusion, RN, MSN, APRN-BC, CDE
Sparrow Regional Diabetes Center
Lansing, Michigan

Carolyn J. Leontos, MS, RD, CDE
University of Nevada Cooperative Extension
Las Vegas, Nevada

Charles D. Ponte, PharmD, CDE, BCPS, BC-ADM, FASHP, FCCP, FAPhA
West Virginia University
Robert C. Byrd Health Sciences Center
Morgantown, West Virginia

Dawn Satterfield, RN, MSN, PhD
Centers for Disease Control
Native Diabetes Wellness Program
Atlanta, Georgia

Jane J. Seley, MPH, MSN, GNP, CDE
New York Presbyterian/WC
New York, New York

Mike Taylor, RN, MHA, CDE
Integral Life Solutions
Columbia, Maryland

Dace L. Trence, MD, FACE
University of Washington Medical Center
Seattle, Washington

Patti Urbanski, MEd, RD, LD, CDE
Duluth Family Practice Residency Program
Duluth, Minnesota

Hope S. Warshaw, MMSc, RD, CDE, BC-ADM
Hope Warshaw Associates, LLC
Alexandria, Virginia

Katie Weinger, EdD, RN
Joslin Diabetes Center
Boston, Massachusetts

Anne E. Whittington, MBA, MSN, RN, CDE
Navy Medical Center San Diego
San Diego, California

Joel Zonszein, MD, CDE, FACP, FACE
Albert Einstein College of Medicine
Bronx, New York

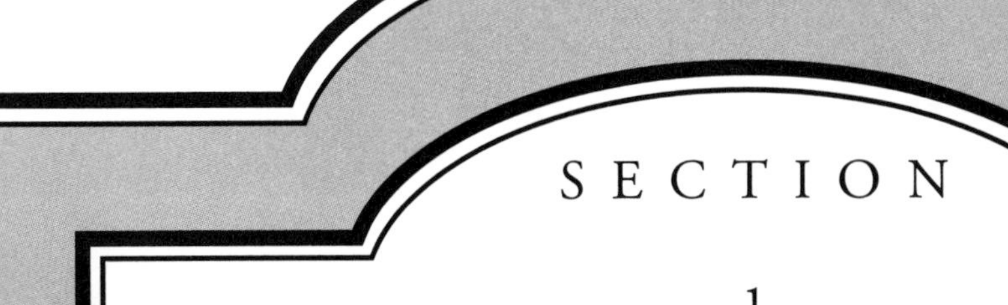

SECTION

1

Understanding the Individual's Health Behaviors and Choices

Section Editor

Elizabeth A. Walker, DNSc, RN, CDE

Within you lies abundant power to help you make it through any challenge you encounter.

—Catherine Feste

SECTION 1 OVERVIEW

Elizabeth A. Walker, DNSc, RN, CDE

> ***Within you lies abundant power to help you make it through any challenge you encounter.***
>
> **—Catherine Feste[1]**

When an individual with a chronic disease assumes self-management responsibilities, the person gains the opportunity to better control the disease and retain the highest possible quality of life. In so doing, the person takes on a lifetime of self-management tasks. On any given day, and even during any period of life, the individual can choose to perform these self-management tasks well, partially, or not at all.[2] Although this activated and knowledgeable individual has significant responsibility and greater control, his self-management is not intended to be performed in isolation. Healthcare providers, families, and communities create an important environmental support system that can work in concert with self-management. Catherine Festes's words of empowerment, above, are encouragement to those who daily cope with this disease, and to those who care for them. Cathy has lived well with type 1 diabetes since 1957 and has devoted her life's work to motivation for health. Her philosophy is that the best possible quality of life is attainable and prevention of physical and psychosocial complications should be the focus of self-management support.[1]

When planning and implementing diabetes self-management education (DSME), the health behaviors, relationships, and interactions of the affected individual are essential factors to consider. The educator must take into account how the individual performs health behaviors and makes lifestyle and medical care choices. Fundamental to the delivery of effective DSME is the educator's understanding of the psychological and sociological factors that influence individual health behaviors and choices. These factors, both internal and external, have a profound effect on the person's satisfaction and success in self-management. Members of the diabetes care team, whether in primary care or specialty practice settings, are asked to think more broadly about the person within the environment in order to maximize the control of diabetes and minimize its complications. This is a new way of thinking for many providers.

Diabetes self-management is, by its nature, personal; however, when a chronic disease such as diabetes is so prevalent within a society, the consequences of each individual's actions and choices exacerbate the public health challenges of disease prevention and control. When primary prevention is a possibility, as with type 2 diabetes, the domain of self-management education is widened to encompass both prediabetes and diabetes. In each case, behavior change for self-management is integral to positive health outcomes. The chapters in Section 1 of this book have value for those involved in individual patient care, educational endeavors, and public health programs. Understanding what factors influence the individuals' health choices and behaviors helps the professional facilitate and support important behavior changes—changes that lower the risk of diabetes and its complications and lessen their effect on individuals and society.

Theoretical models or frameworks are tools used in this book to assist healthcare professionals in making the conceptual leaps that enable better support for self-management. Several models are used as heuristics or guides throughout the book. Carolé Mensing's introduction framed the overarching perspective of this book, focusing attention on diabetes self-management through the lens of the Chronic Care Model.[3] This model places responsibility for self-management with the affected individual while emphasizing the importance of structured self-management support activities and systems within communities to facilitate healthy behavior changes. The Chronic Care Model also places self-management support into the broad healthcare delivery system. Two other models will be introduced in this section overview to help guide the reader's thinking about health behavior and choices: a social-ecological model or approach and a health program planning model.

An ecological approach aids in understanding individual health behaviors and choices. A social-ecological approach or model, focusing on the levels of interaction and influence between the individual and the larger community and environment, is an important tool to widen clinicians' thinking and actions related to diabetes self-management.[4-5] Many ecological approaches have been cited in the literature,[6] and ecological models have been used to give guidance for primary and secondary prevention of various health problems. The ecological model has value because it is broad, practical, and intuitive. This approach illustrates how environmental influences affect individual behavior and the performance of self-management tasks. Shown in Figure 1, the social-ecological approach highlights the levels of interaction and influence between the individual and the larger community and environment. The model helps those on the diabetes care team see the relevance of adopting a more holistic approach—we see the individual within the family or small group, functioning within the larger system, group, or culture, which in turn is functioning within the circle of the broad community and the policies it sets.[5]

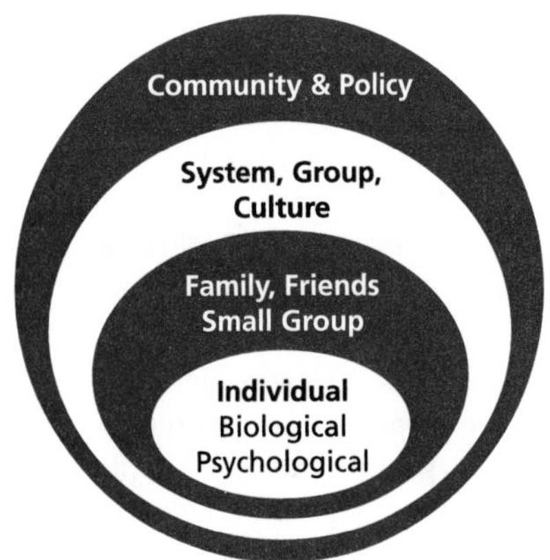

FIGURE 1 An Ecological Model

Source: Reprinted with permission from the American Diabetes Association. Diabetes Care. 2002;25:599-606. © Copyright 2002, American Diabetes Association.

An understanding of the social-ecological approach, and how it differs from the more customary behavioral change models often used in diabetes care and self-management education, must encompass not only the individual and environmental aspects of health promotion, but also cultural, bio-psychosocial, and sociological perspectives.[4] Thus, to understand how to best implement diabetes self-management education, the educator must assess not only individual needs, but also environmental needs and organizational, community, cultural, and sociologic needs. Not surprisingly, multidisciplinary collaboration is important when taking a social-ecological approach.

Behavior change—the goal in both public health and patient care

Section 1 begins with the public health approach and primary, secondary, and tertiary prevention in order to pull together these important elements and resources. Throughout this section, the focus is on the individual and how that person adapts, adopts, and maintains health behaviors and makes lifestyle and medical care choices. Chapters 1 through 6 develop these topics in detail. Discussion moves from crucial issues in public health to aspects more pertinent to individual patient care and education. Regardless of whether the goal is sweeping changes in the health of a nation or tailored efforts to prevent or control diabetes in a single individual or at the community level, the goals include informed decisions and healthy behavior change leading to improved quality of life—the desired outcome.

Because it is now known that the most prevalent type of diabetes, type 2 diabetes mellitus, can be prevented or significantly delayed in onset, this first section of the book begins with an important chapter on public health and primary prevention of diabetes, written by experts from the Centers for Disease Control and Prevention. Chapter 1 presents the epidemiology of diabetes and its complications and the public health issues and national programs related to prevention and control of diabetes. The chapter provides a basic understanding of why public health approaches must be implemented at each level of prevention.

Next, we look at the integral role of behavior change in prevention. The chapter 2 authors are nutrition and lifestyle experts who helped shape the successful Diabetes Prevention Program (DPP) lifestyle intervention.[7] They summarize the evidence for using lifestyle behaviors, such as healthy eating and increased physical activity, to prevent type 2 diabetes. The DPP and several other type 2 diabetes prevention studies provide ample evidence for primary prevention of diabetes through lifestyle changes. The challenges of translating the DPP lifestyle intervention into other real-world settings are discussed.

Moving from public health to matters more pertinent to individual patient care, chapters 3 through 6 examine various issues of self-management and health through the lens of the individual's behavior. What influences individuals and their knowledge, beliefs, skills, decisions, and previous and current behavior patterns?

Chapter 3 explores and highlights how health behavior theories can illuminate the challenges of behavior change. The authors, experts in educational psychology and self-management education, offer the reader evidence-based models that focus on the individual and self-management and how people make health decisions and initiate actions. Consistent with the ecological approach, environmental influences are a consideration in most models.

Psychosocial and emotional issues related to self-management and care are the foci of chapter 4. The authors, 3 psychologists in diabetes behavioral research, present background literature on diabetes self-management and the effects of depression, anxiety, eating disorders, stress, and other psychosocial issues. Understanding underlying psychological issues helps clinicians and educators assess barriers to health and self-management and discern ways of preventing them from occurring or coping with these challenges once they are identified. Each of these mental health issues must also be understood within the context of the individual's demographics, including age, ethnicity, race, and gender.

Social support is the topic of chapter 5. As portrayed in the ecological approach, family, friends, coworkers, places of worship, institutions, and communities can provide various types and levels of social support. The authors, 2 nurse researchers, explain how social support can be measured and evaluated as a mediating or moderating variable for behavior change and self-management. Among the chapter highlights are a presentation and critique of the research on the impact of social support in diabetes care and self-management.

Finally, chapter 6 explores the outer ring in the social-ecological approach—how aspects of community and society either facilitate or become barriers to individual or group success in self-management. The authors, experts in community programs for diabetes and other chronic diseases, introduce an innovative ecological approach to explain what tools are useful at the community level to support an individual in diabetes self-management.

The content of chapters in this section of the book will be better understood within the context of the PRECEDE-PROCEED model for health planning,[8] because this model takes the very broad perspective of planning for health from the individual to the population and policy level. PRECEDE is an acronym for predisposing, reinforcing and enabling constructs in educational/ecological diagnosis and evaluation. (PROCEED stands for policy, regulatory, and organizational constructs in educational and environmental development, and this aspect , while beyond the scope of this book, can be explored in more detail in the recent text by Green and Kreuter.[8]) Section 1 uses the PRECEDE part of the model, as it positions the individual within the context of the complex internal and external environment surrounding and influencing him or her.

Figure 2 is a generic representation of Green and Kreuter's model.[8] The model can guide the reader (reading from right to left) from the individual factors to group or public health issues, ie, from quality of life concerns, to health, and to the genetic, behavioral, and environmental impacts on an individual or community. It includes factors, such as knowledge, attitudes, and resources, that influence individuals—these are described throughout Section 1. This model also uses an ecological approach for various assessments, plans, and evaluations for primary prevention of disease as well as secondary prevention of complications related to diseases.

That the PRECEDE-PROCEED model has quality of life as the ultimate outcome is not without significance. When educators and providers focus on the individual, family, or community, as opposed to the system of care, then what is truly of concern is the person's mental and social well-being, and not only the absence of disease or complications.[9] Chapters in Section 1 and throughout this book contribute to the health professional's knowledge base to support this goal.

Learning to provide diabetes care and education from a broader perspective, such as with the approaches and models described in this overview and the set of chapters that follow it, will open up opportunities for more effective interventions by healthcare providers and provide individuals living with diabetes with more options for self-management support.

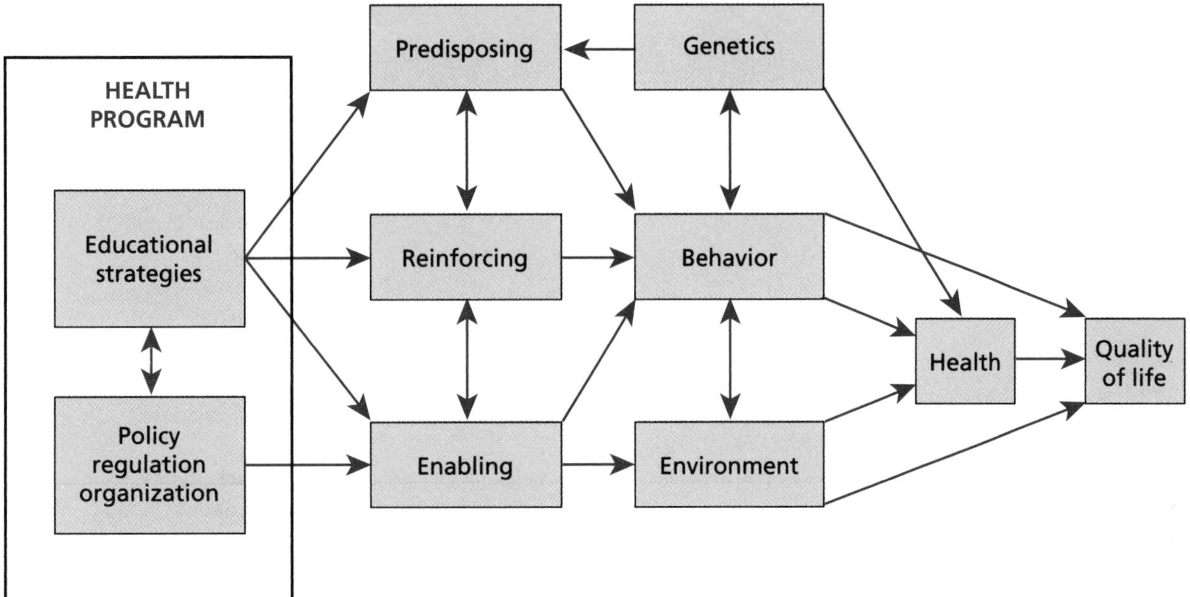

FIGURE 2 PRECEDE-PROCEED Model for Health Program Planning

Source: Adapted with permission from Green LW, Kreuter MW. Health Program Planning: An Educational and Ecological Approach, 4th ed. Boston, Mass: McGraw-Hill; 2005:10.

References

1. Feste C. The Physician Within, 2nd ed. New York: Henry Holt and Company; 1993:196.
2. Lorig KR, Holman H. Self management education: history, definition, outcomes, and mechanisms. Ann Behav Med. 2003;26:1-7.
3. Wagner EH. Chronic disease management: what will it take to improve care for chronic illness? Effec Clin Pract. 1998;1:2-4.
4. Stokols D. Translating social ecological theory into guidelines for community health promotion. Am J Health Promot. 1996;10:282-98.
5. Fisher EB, Walker EA, Bostrum A, Fischhoff B, Haire-Joshu D, Bennett Johnson S. Behavioral science research in the prevention of diabetes. Diabetes Care. 2002;25:599-606.
6. Sallis JF, Owen N. Ecological models of health behavior. In: Health Behavior and Health Education: Theory, Research and Practice, 3rd ed. Glanz K, Lewis FM, Rimer BK, eds. San Francisco, Calif: Jossey-Bass; 2002:462-84.
7. The Diabetes Prevention Program Research Group. The Diabetes Prevention Program: description of the lifestyle intervention. Diabetes Care. 2002;25:2165-71.
8. Green LW, Kreuter MW. Health Program Planning: An Educational and Ecological Approach, 4th ed. Boston, Mass: McGraw-Hill; 2005.
9. Norris SL. Health–related quality of life among adults with diabetes. Curr Diab Rep. 2005;5:124-30.

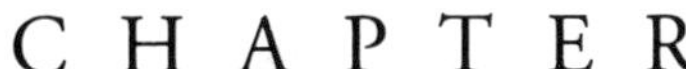

CHAPTER

1

Diabetes and the Public Health Perspective

Authors

Michael M. Engelgau, MD, MS
Dara L. Murphy, MPH
K.M. Venkat Narayan, MD, MPH
Frank Vinicor, MD, MPH

Key Concepts

- Diabetes is a growing public health problem requiring a multilevel system response.
- The burden of diabetes encompasses serious chronic and acute complications and lifelong management.
- National diabetes programs provide structure for regional and local responses to the diabetes epidemic.
- Translation research attempts to take the best scientific knowledge and translate it into effective practices for clinical care and self-management education.

Introduction

The diabetes epidemic that emerged during the twentieth century is a major public health problem. Diabetes already has taken an extraordinary toll on the US population through its acute and chronic complications, which can lead to disability and premature death. Additional efforts to prevent or delay diabetes complications, or better yet, prevent or delay the development of diabetes itself, are badly needed. In 1975, the congressionally appointed National Commission on Diabetes recommended that the Centers for Disease Control and Prevention (CDC) establish a program in diabetes education and control.[1] This was the first time that diabetes was clearly recognized as a public health problem because (*1*) much of diabetes self-care occurs outside the clinic and in the home and community, (*2*) the entire diabetic population needs attention (not just those who attend clinics), (*3*) effective public policy is needed to increase awareness and to make available effective interventions, and, finally, (*4*) success in controlling the diabetes burden requires efforts at the individual, provider, healthcare system, and community level.

This chapter describes the public health burden of diabetes and then discusses efforts by the public health community to translate clinical research findings into strategies that can be broadly implemented in real-world settings. The chapter describes the activities of the National Diabetes Education Program (NDEP) and the CDC's National Diabetes Prevention and Control Program (NDPCP), both of which use public health-based strategies to prevent and control diabetes on a population level.

The Language of Public Health

- **Translation research** refers to comprehensive efforts to translate the best-available scientific knowledge on health-related topics into effective clinical and public health practices.

Diabetes Prevention

There are 3 levels of diabetes prevention: primary, secondary, and tertiary.

- **Primary prevention** refers to preventing or delaying the onset of diabetes, such as was the goal for intensive lifestyle interventions from several recent clinical trials, including the Diabetes Prevention Program in the United States.
- **Secondary prevention** refers to preventing or delaying the progression of microvascular complications (eg, retinopathy). An intervention such as intensive glycemic control with near-normalization of the A1C value is an example.
- **Tertiary prevention** refers to preventing disability from diabetes complications. An example is timely detection of proliferative retinopathy and early laser therapy to prevent vision loss or blindness.

Burden of Disease

Descriptions of the burden of diabetes can also use several measures. This chapter focuses on the following:

- **Total number** refers to the number of people affected in the population.
- **Prevalence** refers to the proportion of the population at any point in time who are affected.
- **Incidence** refers to the number of new cases during a defined time interval (eg, 1 year) divided by the total population at risk for becoming a case.

Public Health Burden

Prevalence and Incidence

As of 2005, 20.8 million Americans (7% of the US population) of all ages were estimated to have diabetes (all types of diabetes including type 1 and type 2),[2] and about 30% (6.2 million) of them were unaware they had the disease. Although diabetes affects all segments of the US population, the disease disproportionately affects certain demographic groups, as the following data show:

- *Age.* Almost 50% of all cases of diagnosed diabetes in the United States are among people aged 60 years or older, and the prevalence rate among people in this age group is more than 10 times that of Americans younger than age 40.[3]
- *Race/Ethnicity.* Minority populations also are disproportionately affected, with the prevalence of diagnosed diabetes being 2 to 4 times higher in most racial/ethnic minority populations (eg, African Americans, Hispanic Americans, American Indians/Alaska Natives, and Asian/Pacific Islanders) than among the non-Hispanic white population.[3,4] The highest reported diabetes prevalence in the world (over 50%) is among the Pima Indians of the southwestern United States.[5]
- *Educational Level.* Educational level is also associated with diabetes prevalence. The results of 1 study showed that the prevalence of diagnosed diabetes among US adults with less than a high school education was more than twice that of college graduates.[6]
- *State by State.* Rates of diagnosed diabetes among US adults also vary substantially by state, with 2001 prevalence rates ranging from 5.0% in Minnesota to 10.5% in Alabama.[6]

Since 1958, the number of Americans with diagnosed diabetes has increased eightfold, while the prevalence of diagnosed diabetes in the United States has increased fourfold (Figure 1.1).[3,4] Increases occurred across all demographic categories, including gender, race/ethnicity, and age.[3] The prevalence of diagnosed diabetes also increased by at least 33% during the 1990s in all adult age groups, with the largest relative increases in the age groups of 30 to 39 and 40 to 49 years of age (95% and 83%, respectively).[6] Many factors have contributed to these increases in the prevalence of diagnosed diabetes, including changes in diagnostic criteria, enhanced detection, lower mortality rates among diabetes patients, changes in population demographics (eg, aging and relatively greater increases in minority populations who experience higher prevalence rates), and an increase in diabetes incidence.

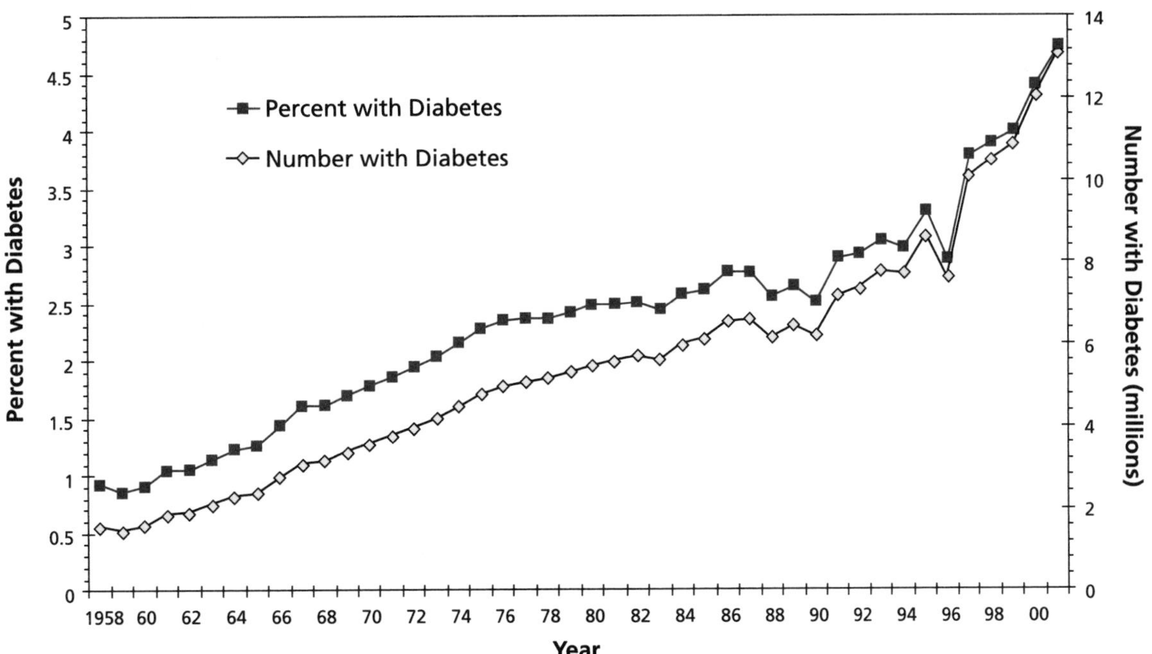

FIGURE 1.1 Time Trend in the Percent of Population and Number of Persons with Diabetes in the United States,* 1958-2002

*Based on single-year National Health Information Survey

Children and Adolescents. Diabetes trends among children and adolescents are also disturbing. Type 2 diabetes among children was first reported among Pima Indian children in 1979, but has since been reported among US children of most racial and ethnic groups.[7] Because of sparse data, estimates of changes in the overall incidence of type 1 diabetes among children in the United States have varied, with some study results showing rates to have increased and some showing rates to have decreased.[8] However, worldwide type 1 diabetes registries suggest that the overall incidence of type 1 diabetes is increasing.[8]

In 2005, new cases of diabetes were diagnosed among approximately 1.5 million US adults aged 20 years or older.[2] Results from several US community-based cohort studies have shown increases in diabetes incidence in specific populations; for example, data from the San Antonio Heart Study showed that between 1980 and 1988 the incidence of diabetes roughly tripled among both non-Hispanic whites and Mexican Americans (2.6% to 9.4% and 5.7% to 15.7%, respectively).[9]

Diabetes Complications

Cardiovascular, Eye, Kidney, and Lower Extremity Diseases

Cardiovascular Disease. In a 2000 study, 37.2% of Americans with diabetes who were aged 35 years or older reported having been diagnosed with a cardiovascular condition, and the percentage increased with age.[3] Other studies have shown that although the absolute rate of cardiovascular disease among people with diabetes was higher among men than women (as in the general population), the range in increased risk for cardiovascular disease attributable to diabetes was higher among women than men (from 2 to 4 times higher for women and from 1.5 to 2.5 times higher for men).[10]

Retinopathy. Diabetic retinopathy, the leading cause of blindness (defined as a best-corrected visual acuity of less than 20/200) among people 20 to 64 years of age, has been estimated to cause 12,000 to 24,000 new cases of blindness each year in the United States, approximately 12% of all new cases.[11] Although devastating, blindness is actually a relatively rare complication. Significant visual impairment (defined as a best-corrected visual acuity of less than 20/40) among people with diabetes is much more common and can reduce the functional status of those affected. Results from a national population-based survey showed that 25% of Americans with diabetes had significant visual impairment, approximately double the proportion among those without diabetes, and that both cataracts and cataract surgery were more common among people with diabetes.[12] A higher rate of open-angle glaucoma among people with diabetes has been found in most but not all studies.[13]

Nephropathy. Diabetes is the leading cause of kidney failure. In the United States in 2001, diabetic nephropathy accounted for approximately 40% of new cases of end-stage renal disease (ESRD) (ie, kidney failure requiring dialyses or transplantation) that year.[3] Indeed, diabetes patients are the fastest-growing group of dialysis and transplantation recipients. New cases of ESRD attributed to diabetes increased from an estimated 7000 in 1984 to over 41,000 in 2000.[3]

Lower Extremity Diseases. Because people with diabetes are at increased risk for lower extremity diseases, including peripheral neuropathy and peripheral arterial disease (PAD), they have substantially higher rates of lower extremity amputations (LEAs) than members of the general population. An estimated 15% of people with diabetes will have a diabetic foot ulcer during their lifetime;[14] of these, projections indicate that 6% to 43% will ultimately undergo an LEA.[15] Among people in the United States with diabetes who have had an amputation, as many as 85% may have had a preceding foot ulcer.[15] Currently, more than half of all nontrauma-related LEAs in the United States were estimated to be among people with diagnosed diabetes.[3]

Currently, 8.1% of the US diabetic population over 40 years of age were estimated to have PAD (defined as an ankle-to-brachial artery blood pressure index of less than 0.90) versus 4.0% among those without diabetes.[16] Those with diabetes were also found to have roughly 2 to 3 times the prevalence of peripheral neuropathy symptoms (29.9% versus 10.2%), insensate feet (based on monofilament testing, 26.4% versus 14.0%), and either peripheral neuropathy or insensate feet (45.3% versus 20.7%). All told, 47.4% of people in the United States with diabetes had at least 1 lower extremity condition (PAD, peripheral neuropathy, insensate feet, ulcer, or LEA).[16]

Acute Metabolic Complications

Diabetic ketoacidosis (DKA) and hypoglycemia both are important metabolic complications of diabetes. In population-based studies, DKA was found to be the initial manifestation of diabetes in 15% to 26% of the cases. Although population-based data are scant on the occurrence of hypoglycemia, 2 major clinical trials of interventions aimed at glycemic control did assess the correlation between exposure to such interventions and the incidence of significant hypoglycemic episodes (defined as episodes requiring attention from someone other than the patient). In the UK Prospective Diabetes Study (UKPDS), people with type 2 diabetes who were treated intensively were found to have a significantly higher rate of such episodes during the study period than those who received conventional care (1.8% versus 0.7%; P <.0001). In the other study, the Diabetes Control and Complications Trial (DCCT), conducted in the United States, the rate of significant hypoglycemic episodes among younger people with type 1 diabetes was 3 times higher among those who received intensive treatment than among those who received conventional treatment (62 episodes versus 19 episodes per 100 patient-years; P <.001).[18,19]

Disability

The results of 1 study showed that people in the United States with diabetes were much more likely to have physical limitations than those without diabetes (66% versus 29%, P <.001).[20] In another study among people in the United States 60 years of age or older, 32% of the women and 15% of the men with diabetes were unable to either walk one-quarter of a mile, climb stairs, or do housework, whereas only 14% of the women and 8% of the men without diabetes were unable to perform at least 1 of these activities.[21] In addition, results from several prospective studies using repeated neuropsychological tests and diagnostic protocols have shown that diabetes is significantly related to the risk for cognitive impairment or dementia among the elderly.[22]

Unemployment and reduced productivity may also be manifestations of disability. When adjusted for demographic variables, the work disability rate was estimated to be more than 3 times higher among persons with diabetes than among those without the disease (26% versus 8%).[23] In another study in the United States, having diabetes without complications was not significantly associated with the number of workdays lost over a 2-week period, but having diabetes with complications was associated with an average increase of 3.2 lost workdays, and people with diabetes were in jobs that tended to earn about one-third less than those without diabetes.[24]

Diabetes During Pregnancy

Gestational diabetes mellitus (GDM) affects up to 14% of pregnant women in the United States, about 135,000 women per year.[25] Women at highest risk for developing GDM are those who are older than 25 years, obese, or members of racial/ethnic groups with a high prevalence of diabetes; those who have a history of abnormal glucose tolerance; and those with first-degree relatives with diabetes.[26] Macrosomia (fetal weight >90th percentile for age) may occur in up to 40% of the offspring of women with GDM.[27] Children born to mothers with GDM have been found to be at a higher-than-normal risk of developing obesity, impaired glucose tolerance, or diabetes at an early age; these elevated risks appear to be the result of exposure to intrauterine hyperglycemia from the mother.[27,28] In addition, mothers who had GDM have been found to be at increased risk of developing type 2 diabetes within a decade of the pregnancy.[29]

Type 1 or type 2 diabetes in the mother can also adversely affect fetal development and cause the fetus to be at higher-than-normal risk for malformations, macrosomia, and altered beta-cell and islet development.[30] In addition, the US rate of perinatal death, which has fallen in recent years, and the rate of stillbirths were both found to be about 4 times higher among infants of women with diabetes.[30]

Diabetes-Related Deaths

The annual age-adjusted mortality rate among US adults with diabetes is about twice that of those who do not have diabetes. Results from a large meta-analysis of 10 prospective studies showed that men with diabetes were 1.9 times more likely to die during the study periods than were those without diabetes and that women with diabetes were 2.6 times more likely to do so than the women without diabetes.[31] Among middle-aged people with diabetes, life expectancy is reduced by 5 to 10 years, and for the entire population with diabetes, an estimated 13 years is lost by both men and women.[32] The increased risk of death associated with diabetes is greater for younger people (ratio of 3.6:1 for people aged 25 to 44 years and 1.5:1 for those aged 65 to 74 years).[32]

In 1999, diabetes was estimated to be the sixth-leading cause of death in United States, and it has remained at that ranking since.[33] Diabetes was listed as the underlying cause of death on 68,399 death certificates[3] and as a contributing cause of death on an additional 141,265 death certificates.[15] However, diabetes was listed on the death certificate of only about 35% to 40% of decedents with diabetes and as the underlying cause of death on the certificates of only about 10% to 15%.[34] These death certificate findings suggest that estimates of the annual US diabetes-related mortality rate based on death certificate data may be substantially lower than the true rate. Cardiovascular disease has been found to be the reported underlying or contributing cause of up to 65% of all deaths among Americans with diabetes and of up to 80% of the deaths among some subpopulations of diabetics.[35]

The Future

Based on current trends, projections of the future impact of diabetes are not comforting. Age-, sex-, and race-specific prevalence rates for diagnosed diabetes (of all types) and census projection estimates from 1 study indicated that the number of Americans with diagnosed diabetes would increase 165% between 2000 and 2050 (from 11 to 29 million) and that the overall prevalence of diagnosed diabetes in the United States would increase from 4.0% to 7.2%.[36] The prevalence is expected to increase the most among those more than 75 years old (271% among women and 437% among men), and it is expected to increase substantially more among the black population (363% among men and 217% among women) than among the white population (148% among men and 107% among women).

The overall projected increase in the US diabetes prevalence rate is attributable to 3 factors:

- Projected demographic changes in the population (37%)
- A projected increase in the US diabetes prevalence rate (36%)
- Projected population growth (27%)

Unfortunately, increasing prevalence rates among younger age groups and the emergence of type 2 diabetes in children may worsen these projections.

Public Health Response

In 1975, the National Commission on Diabetes recommended that the CDC establish a program in diabetes education and control.[1] Ultimately, this resulted in establishment of the Division of Diabetes Translation (DDT) within the CDC's National Center for Chronic Disease Prevention and Health Promotion. The goal of the DDT is to facilitate improvements in the diabetes-related health status of Americans in 2 ways:

- By developing and maintaining national and state-based diabetes surveillance systems and monitoring population-level diabetes prevention practices
- By moving (or "translating") diabetes research findings into widespread clinical and public health practices

National and State-Based Diabetes Surveillance Systems

The DDT has developed and is maintaining the National Diabetes Surveillance System.[3] This system uses data from several national surveys as well as vital records data to assess the past and current burden of diabetes in the US population and to project future US diabetes trends. Much of the diabetes data cited earlier in this chapter were from studies based on data from the system. A list of the surveillance system's major data sources and of the diabetes-related health parameters it assesses can be found in Table 1.1.

TABLE 1.1 National Diabetes Surveillance System: Major Data Sources and Categories

Major Data Sources
Behavioral Risk Factor Surveillance System
National Health and Nutritional Examination Survey
National Health Interview Survey
National Underlying Cause-of-Death Data and Multiple Cause-of-Death Data
National Hospital Discharge Survey
National Inpatient Survey
National Ambulatory Care Survey
National Hospital Ambulatory Medical Care Survey
US Renal Data System
Bureau of Census
Major Categories of Diabetes Data Collected
Incidence
Prevalence
Major Complications
Death
Lower extremity amputations
End-stage renal failure
Blindness
Diabetic ketoacidosis
Cardiovascular disease
Disability
Use of Health Services
Hospital admissions
Outpatient visits
Emergency room visits
Costs
Preventive Healthcare Practices and Behaviors
People at risk for diabetes
People with diabetes
Diabetes Among Pregnant Women
Gestational diabetes
Existing type 1 and type 2 diabetes
Secular Trends in All Categories of Diabetes Data

Monitoring Health-Related Behaviors. Monitoring the health-related behaviors of a population is now recognized as another important dimension of diabetes surveillance, not only to identify who might be at risk for diabetes, but also to determine how people who already have diabetes can best maintain their health. To monitor the health-related behaviors of the US population, the CDC developed and implemented the state-based Behavioral Risk Factor Surveillance System (BRFSS). The BRFSS collects extensive information on health-related behaviors important to chronic diseases through annual population-based telephone surveys conducted by health departments in all 50 states and the District of Columbia.

Epidemiological Studies. Epidemiological studies to better understand the reasons behind various health trends usually focus on the absolute population risk for a health outcome and on the difference in risk across groups. The results of such studies reflect the total burden of a particular outcome on a particular group better than relative risk determinations. Epidemiological studies can also be used to better understand the economic burden posed by diabetes; however, to determine the various economic implications of diabetes, researchers need data from several perspectives, including that of persons with diabetes, healthcare providers, healthcare systems (eg, managed care organizations), governments, and society in general. Regardless of the perspective from which it is assessed, the economic burden of diabetes is substantial.

Translation Research

The term "translation research" refers to comprehensive efforts to translate the best-available scientific knowledge on health-related topics into effective clinical and public health practices.[37] Translation research also aims to assess the extent to which recommended standards of care have been implemented, to understand the barriers to their implementation, and to intervene throughout all levels of healthcare delivery and public health to improve both the quality of care and the health outcomes for those whom the care is designed to reach. These outcomes also include the quality of life for those individuals.

The need for translation research becomes obvious if we consider that several efficacious and cost-effective strategies to prevent or delay diabetes complications have emerged during the past decade, but have yet to be widely implemented.

In the United States, there has been a considerable gap between the care recommended for diabetes patients and the care that many of these patients actually receive.[38] In 1988 to 1995, for example, among US diabetes patients 18 to 75 years of age, 18% had an A1C >9.5%, 34.3% were hypertensive (blood pressure ≥140/90 mm Hg), and 58% had a low-density lipoprotein cholesterol level ≥130 mg/dL. In addition, during the previous year, only 63% had had a dilated eye examination, only 55% had had a foot examination, just 38% were self-monitoring their blood glucose level, only 46% had received an influenza vaccination, and only 27% had received a pneumococcal vaccination.[38] More recent data indicate encouraging increases in the percentage of Americans with diabetes who had received an eye examination (up 7%), foot examination (6%), influenza vaccination (5%), and pneumococcal vaccination (15%) in the previous year and in the percentage who self-monitored their blood glucose level (15%); however, optimal care is still not being widely achieved.[39]

Translation research may be viewed as an extension of effectiveness research, but in its evolution it has encompassed new dimensions (Figure 1.2). The purpose of translation research is to devise solutions to real-world healthcare delivery problems, as opposed to basic science,

> **Closing the Gap**
>
> In the United States, there has been a considerable gap between diabetes care that has been recommended and the care that has been received.

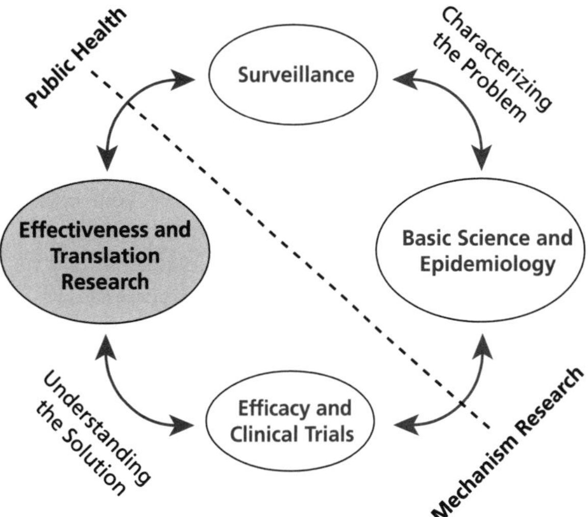

FIGURE 1.2 Translation Research in the Context of Other Types of Research and Public Health Assessments

Source: Narayan KM, Benjamin E, Gregg EW, Norris SL, Engelgau MM. Diabetes Translation Research: where are we and where do we want to be. Ann Intern Med. 2004;140:959. Reprinted with permission.

epidemiology, and public health surveillance, whose primary purpose is to characterize those problems.

Translation research targets real-world problems in healthcare delivery

Translation research is concerned with the impact, generalizability, and transferability of healthcare solutions. It focuses on assessing the effectiveness of those solutions and their long-term sustainability in real-world settings, with an emphasis on efficiency (ie, the relative value of a healthcare solution under conditions of finite resources), equity (ie, fair distribution of resources), and the provision of optimal health care for as many people as possible.

Although considerable progress has been made in translation research, several new avenues will need to be pursued to meet the challenges of chronic disease control in the twenty-first century. Beginning with studies aimed at documenting quality of care using nonstandard measures, translation research has evolved toward better and more standardized methods of characterizing quality of care, and these improved methods have allowed researchers to better understand barriers to improving quality of care. Numerous small studies have tested simple care-improvement interventions at the level of the provider, the healthcare system, and the patient, while others have assessed the feasibility of implementing system-wide reengineering and the effects of such reengineering on diabetes care.[40] One ongoing study, Translating Research Into Action for Diabetes (TRIAD),[41] a multicenter observational study sponsored by the CDC and National Institutes of Health, is examining the association between the quality of diabetes care received by patients and the organizational structure of the healthcare delivery system used by those patients.

Several interventions at the patient, provider, or system level have shown promise for improving diabetes care in small, single-site studies. In addition, results of a systematic review by Renders and colleagues showed that the management of diabetes care can be improved through multifaceted interventions aimed at healthcare providers and through organizational interventions designed to increase patient monitoring (eg, centralized computer tracking systems or the use of nurses to regularly contact patients).[42] The review also showed that patient-oriented interventions can lead to improved patient outcomes and that nurses can play an important role in patient-oriented interventions, by educating patients or helping them adhere to their treatment regimen.

Over the past century, the system of healthcare in the United States has evolved to manage acute diseases rather than chronic disorders such as diabetes. Recently, the Institute of Medicine argued that newer systems of care and ways of thinking about delivering health care are needed to tackle complex diseases such as diabetes.[43] According to their argument, rather than address the healthcare system as a set of individual component parts, translation research needs to address the healthcare system as a complex, interactive, interconnected, and adaptive system. Thus, to obtain better health outcomes, the healthcare system needs translation research that is sufficiently multidisciplinary to include new scientific fields—fields such as complexity, leadership, and the management of change. At the same time, our problem solving must draw on epidemiology, health service research, sociology, policy science, economics, operational research, and other fields. The opportunities offered by translation research are tremendous, and we need to seize them to stop the onrushing tide of diabetes both in the United States and around the world.

National Public Health Diabetes Programs

While translation research is shedding light on *how* to improve diabetes care, as well as on how to improve the quality of life and other health outcomes of diabetes patients, broadly implementing the interventions identified by such research remains a challenge. As the Institute of Medicine noted, public health programs at all levels have an important role in ensuring that effective interventions are broadly implemented.[43] In addition to helping meet population-level public health goals, such as sufficient numbers of qualified healthcare providers, the work of public health agencies includes building and maintaining partnerships and relationships with private healthcare organizations and other sectors of society that can contribute to public health at the population and community levels. The complexity of this effort requires an organized response through an efficient, strategic, and synergistic use of the limited public health funds dedicated to diabetes.

The CDC supports 2 national public health programs that address diabetes:

- The National Diabetes Education Program (NDEP)
- The National Diabetes Prevention and Control Program (NDPCP)

National Diabetes Education Program. The NDEP, which is also supported by the NIH, was created in the mid-1990s to disseminate the findings of the DCCT: that people can substantially reduce their risk for diabetes complications through improved glycemic control. Established in 1998, this program currently includes a network of more than 200 public and private organizations that work to increase awareness about diabetes and its control among healthcare providers and people at risk for diabetes. Working in partnership with these organizations, the NDEP develops and adapts health communication campaigns, community interventions, and tools to improve diabetes care and prevention, especially for communities with a high burden of diabetes. The NDEP is currently conducting 3 overarching national public campaigns, each in response to findings from specific scientific studies:

- *Control Your Diabetes. For Life.*
- *Be Smart About Your Heart. Control the ABCs of Diabetes.*
- *Small Steps, Big Rewards. Prevent Type 2 Diabetes.*

The focus of each is described in the sidebar.

US Public Health Campaigns Targeting Diabetes

Control Your Diabetes. For Life.
This, the first and oldest NDEP campaign, focuses on the benefits of improving glycemic control that were found in the DCCT.

Be Smart About Your Heart. Control the ABCs of Diabetes.
The ABCs to be controlled are these: A1C, blood pressure, and cholesterol. This campaign incorporates several strategies to prevent or delay diabetes complications that have emerged during the past decade, including strategies to control blood pressure, lipid levels, and glycemia that emerged from the UKPDS and other landmark studies. During the development of the campaign, focus group discussions showed that people with diabetes were generally not aware of the strong relationship between diabetes and cardiovascular disease.

Small Steps, Big Rewards. Prevent Type 2 Diabetes.
This, the NDEP's most recent campaign, incorporates the Diabetes Prevention Program findings that modest lifestyle changes can prevent or delay the onset of type 2 diabetes among people at high risk for the disease.

The NDEP campaigns, products, and tools are all in the public domain and available to all organizations throughout the country. Because many local organizations may not have the resources and expertise to develop, design, and test health communication messages and processes, the resources of the NDEP are critical to our national effort to reduce the diabetes burden.

Reducing the Burden

National public health resources are critical to efforts to reduce the burden of diabetes in the United States.

National Diabetes Prevention and Control Program. The CDC's NDPCP is a mature diabetes public health program that was started in 1977. Currently, the NDPCP supports health department programs in all 50 states, the District of Columbia, and 8 US-affiliated jurisdictions. These programs are part of the NDEP partnership network and offer an important mechanism for targeting, tailoring, and timing activities to support NDEP campaigns and the use of NDEP tools. However, the NDPCP's efforts also include conducting population-based diabetes surveillance, developing and maintaining strategic partnerships, supporting the implementation of translation research findings, and using a public health framework to evaluate the effectiveness of various interventions.

The approach adopted by the NDPCP and implemented by state-based program participants has evolved through 3 distinct historical phases (Figure 1.3).[44] Each phase was a response to findings from major new studies and built upon the efforts of the prior phase. The program expansions that occurred during each phase were driven by the belief that the public health institution has an ethical responsibility to ensure that people will benefit as quickly as possible from new health-related knowledge.[45,46]

Current NDPCP program objectives, which include increasing US rates of eye exams, foot exams, vaccinations, and A1C testing to levels recommended in *Healthy People 2010*, provide a benchmark against which public health and healthcare systems can measure their success. Although these objectives do not cover all of the important areas in diabetes prevention and control, they do provide reference points that can be useful to health officials attempting to design or modify state-based programs. As noted, these programs must continually incorporate new scientific findings if they are to be as effective as possible in reducing the future diabetes burden.

Conclusions

The diabetes epidemic has already taken an extraordinary toll on the US population, but the disease and its chronic complications will exact a far larger toll in the future if current trends continue. Urgent efforts are needed to stem this tide. Fortunately, we now have effective tools with which to prevent or delay the development of diabetes complications, and better yet, to prevent or delay the development of diabetes itself.[46]

This chapter has described the public health burden of diabetes in the United States and the role of public health organizations and initiatives in stemming the tide of the diabetes epidemic. In this endeavor, public health provides the following much-needed assistance:

- Development of national surveillance systems to describe the magnitude of the epidemic
- Support of epidemiological studies to elucidate why the diabetes burden has been increasing
- Support of translation research to assess implementation of standards of care, understand the barriers to their implementation, and intervene throughout all levels of healthcare delivery and public health systems to improve quality of care

Finally, we have described how 2 national diabetes programs, the NDEP and the NDPCP, have progressed toward developing strong national and state-level public health capacities to implement and evaluate the effectiveness of diabetes prevention and control interventions.

The current challenge to public heath in the face of limited resources is to mobilize and help coordinate the efforts of the diverse public and private organizations that are concerned with controlling and reducing the diabetes burden. Slowing this complex and devastating chronic disease will require effective synergistic action at many levels—and public health has a major role in coordinating this effort.

Acknowledgments

The authors acknowledge the *Annals of Internal Medicine* for allowing extensive use of material published in a supplement entitled *Diabetes Translation and Public Health: 25 Years of CDC Research and Programs* (2004 supplement, volume 40, number 11), edited by K.M. Venkat Narayan, L. Jack, and C. Laine.

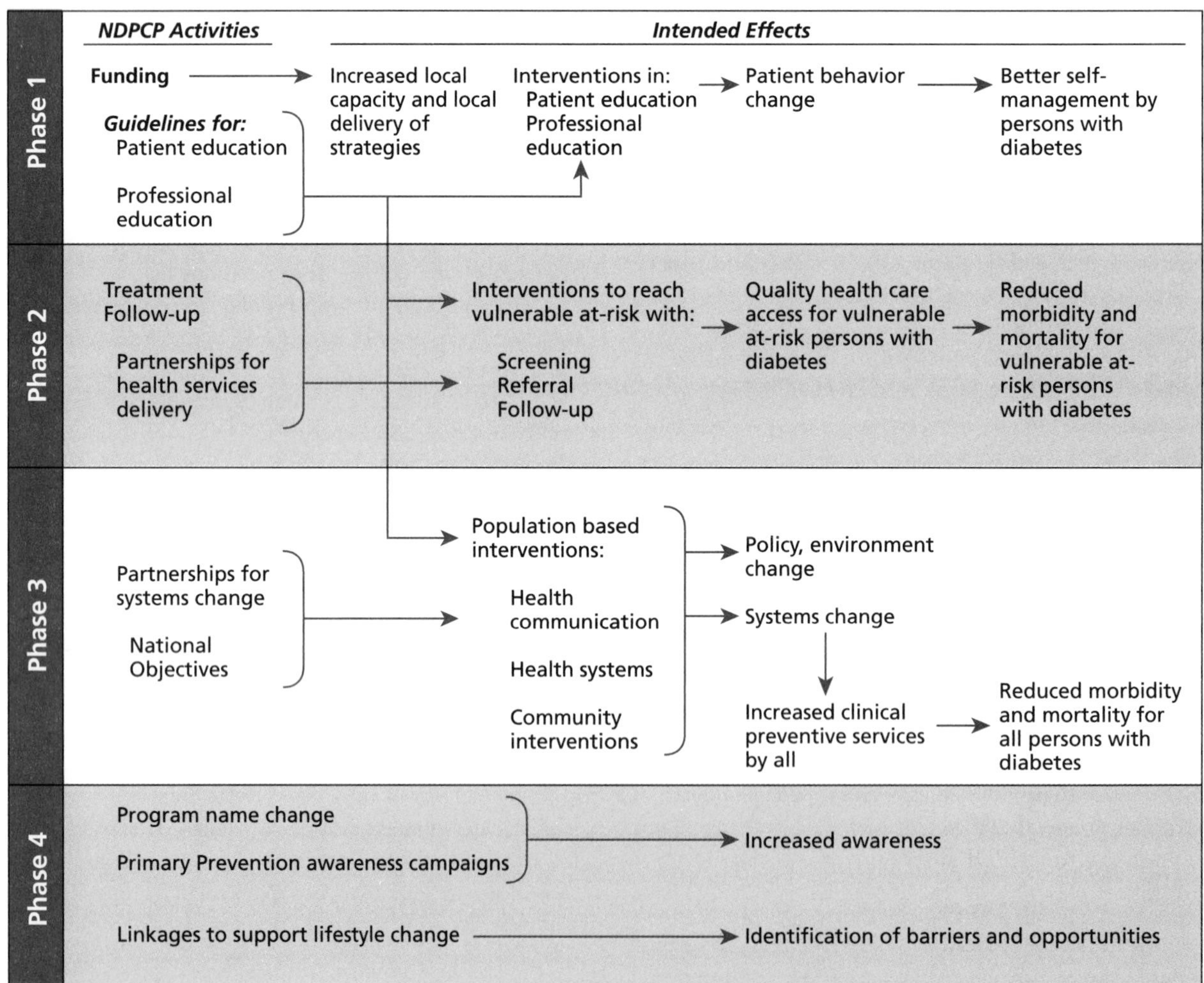

FIGURE 1.3 The Phases of Development for the National Diabetes Prevention and Control Program (NDPCP)

Source: Murphy D, Chapel T, Clark C. Moving diabetes care from science to practice: the evolution of the National Diabetes Prevention and Control Program. Ann Intern Med. 2004;140(11):980. Reprinted with permission.

Focus on Education: Pearls for Practice

Teaching Strategies

The epidemic of diabetes. In 1975, diabetes first surfaced as a public health issue. Since then, prevalence has increased in every state, and, based on current projections, it will continue to increase at a rapid rate. When teaching and making presentations, present graphics and information that clearly show the rapid growth projection and then accentuate the importance of public health interventions aimed at lifestyle changes that can alter this projection.

From research to translation. Resources such as the CDC and local public health departments provide projects and programs (such as "Control your Diabetes. For Life.") to reach out and promote changes and to bring new insights that can change long-held habits by creating public awareness. Contact these resources through their Web sites or through local directories and access their materials. Slides, handouts, and teaching tools are available just for the asking.

Messages for Patients

Be familiar with resources and participate. Make an effort to learn about the diabetes research and programs available through national, state, and local agencies. Use information from these sources to make personal changes. Participate in community-sponsored diabetes activities and programs. Offer to be a part of research or surveillance projects to assist others in benefiting from the information gained.

Internet Resources

www.cdc.gov/diabetes/ndep/index.htm
National Diabetes Education Program of the US Centers for Disease Control and Prevention

www.cdc.gov/diabetes
Division of Diabetes Translation of the US Centers for Disease Control and Prevention

http://diabetes.niddk.nih.gov/dm/pubs/america
Diabetes in America, 2nd edition (chapters of this book are available as separate PDF files)

http://betterdiabetescare.nih.gov/MAINintroduction.htm
National Institutes of Health "Making Systems Change for Better Diabetes Care"

http://diabetes.niddk.nih.gov
National Diabetes Information Clearinghouse of the National Institute of Diabetes and Digestive and Kidney Diseases

References

1. National Institutes of Health. Report of the National Commission on Diabetes to the Congress of the United States. Washington, DC: US Government Printing Office; 1976. NIH Publication 76-1018.
2. Centers for Disease Control and Prevention (CDC). National Diabetes Fact Sheet: general information and national estimates on diabetes in the United States, 2005. Atlanta, Ga: CDC, 2005. On the Internet at: www.cdc.gov/diabetes/pubs/factsheet05.htm. Accessed 20 Dec 2005.
3. Centers for Disease Control and Prevention. Diabetes Surveillance System. Atlanta, Ga: US Department of Health and Human Services. Available at www.cdc.gov/diabetes/statistics/index.htm. Accessed 20 Dec 2005.
4. Kenny SJ, Aubert RE, Geiss LS. Prevalence and incidence of non-insulin-dependent diabetes. In: Diabetes

in America, 2nd ed. Harris MI, Cowie CC, Stern MP, Boyko EJ, Reiber GE, Bennett PH, eds. Bethesda, Md: The National Institutes of Health; 1995:47-68.

5. Knowler WC, Saad MF, Pettitt DJ, Nelson RG, Bennett PH. Determinants of diabetes mellitus in the Pima Indians. Diabetes Care. 1993;16:216-27.

6. Mokdad AH, Ford ES, Bowman BA, et al. Prevalence of obesity, diabetes, and obesity-related health risk factors, 2001. JAMA. 2003;289:76-9.

7. Fagot-Campagna A, Pettitt DJ, Engelgau MM, et al. Type 2 diabetes among North American children and adolescents: an epidemiologic review and a public health perspective. J Pediatr. 2000;136:664-72.

8. Onkamo P, Vaananen S, Karvonen M, Tuomilehto J. Worldwide increase in incidence of type I diabetes: an analysis of the data on published incidence trends. Diabetologia. 1999;42:1395-403.

9. Burke JP, Williams K, Gaskill SP, Hazuda HP, Haffner SM, Stern MP. Rapid rise in the incidence of type 2 diabetes from 1987 to 1996: results from the San Antonio Heart Study. Arch Intern Med. 1999; 159:1450-6.

10. Barzilay JI, Spiekerman CF, Kuller LH, et al. Prevalence of clinical and isolated subclinical cardiovascular disease in older adults with glucose disorders: the Cardiovascular Health Study. Diabetes Care. 2001;24:1233-9.

11. Will JC, Geiss LS, Wetterhall SF. Diabetic retinopathy (letter). N Engl J Med. 1990;323:613.

12. Saaddine JB, Narayan KMV, Engelgau MM, Aubert RE, Klein R, Beckles GLA. Prevalence of self-rated visual impairment among adults with diabetes. Am J Public Health. 1999;89:1200-5.

13. Klein BE, Klein R, Jensen SC. Open-angle glaucoma and older-onset diabetes: The Beaver Dam Eye Study. Ophthalmology. 1994;101:1173-7.

14. Palumbo PJ, Melton LJ. Peripheral vascular disease and diabetes. In: Diabetes in America. Harris MI, Hamman RF eds. Washington DC: US Government Printing Office; 1985. NIH publication 85-1468.

15. Apelqvist J, Castenfors J, Larsson J, Stenstrom A, Agardh CD. Wound classification is more important than the site of ulceration in the outcome of diabetic foot ulcers. Diabet Med. 1989;6:526-30.

16. Gregg EW, Sorlie P, Paulose-Ram R, et al. Prevalence of lower extremity disease in the U.S. population. Diabetes Care. 2004;27:1591-7.

17. Johnson DD, Palumbo PJ, Chu CP. Diabetic ketoacidosis in a community-based population. Mayo Clinic Proc. 1980:55:83-8.

18. UK Prospective Diabetes Study (UKPDS) Group. Intensive blood glucose control with sulphonylureas or insulin compared with conventional treatment and risk of complications in patients with type 2 diabetes (UKPDS 33). Lancet. 1998;352:837-53.

19. The Diabetes Control and Complications Trial Research Group. The effect of intensive treatment of diabetes on the development and progression of long-term complications in insulin-dependent diabetes mellitus. N Engl J Med. 1993;329:977-86.

20. Ryerson B, Tierney EF, Thompson TJ, et al. Excess physical limitations among adults with diabetes in the US population, 1997-1999. Diabetes Care. 2003;26:206-10.

21. Gregg EW, Beckles GLB, Williamson DF, et al. Diabetes and physical disability among older US adults. Diabetes Care. 2000;23:1272-7.

22. Gregg EW, Engelgau MM, Narayan V. Complications of diabetes in elderly people: underappreciated problems include cognitive decline and physical disability. BMJ. 2002;325:916-7.

23. Mayfield JA, Deb P, Whitecotton L. Work disability and diabetes. Diabetes Care. 1999;22:1105-9.

24. Ng YC, Jacobs P, Johnson JA. Productivity losses associated with diabetes in the US Diabetes Care. 2001;24:257-61.

25. Coustan DR. Gestational diabetes. In: Diabetes in America, 2nd ed. Harris MI, Cowie CC, Stern MP, Boyko EJ, Reiber GE, Bennett PH, eds. Bethesda, Md: National Institutes of Health; 1995:703-17.

26. Jovanovic L, Pettitt DJ. Gestational diabetes mellitus. JAMA. 2001;286:2516-8.

27. Kjos SL, Buchanan TA. Gestational diabetes mellitus. N Engl J Med. 1999;341:1749-56.

28. Pettitt DJ, Aleck KA, Baird HR, Carraher MJ, Bennett PH, Knowler WC. Congenital susceptibility to NIDDM: role of intrauterine environments. Diabetes. 1998;37:622-8.

29. Dabelea D, Hanson RK, Lindsay RS, et al. Intrauterine exposure to diabetes conveys risks for type 2 diabetes and obesity: a study of discordant sibships. Diabetes. 2000;49;2208-11.

30. Girling JC, Dornhorst A. Pregnancy and diabetes mellitus. In: Textbook of Diabetes. Pickup J, Williams G, eds. London, England: Blackwell Science; 1997:72.1.

31. Lee WL, Cheung AM, Cape D, Zinman B. Impact of diabetes on coronary artery disease in women and men: a meta-analysis of prospective studies. Diabetes Care. 2000;23:962-8.

32. Manuel DG, Schultz SE. Diabetes health status and risk factors. In: Diabetes in Ontario. An ICES Practice Atlas. Hux J, Booth G, Slaughter PM, Laupacis A, eds. 2003. On the Internet at: www.ices.on.ca. Accessed 22 May 2003.

33. Anderson RN, Minino AM, Hoyert DL, Rosenberg HM. Comparability of cause of death between ICD-9 and ICD-10: preliminary estimates. Nat Vital Stat Rep. 2001;49(2):1-32.

34. Bild DE, Stevenson JM. Frequency of recording diabetes on US death certificates: analysis of the 1986 National Mortality Followback Survey. J Clin Epidemiol. 1992;45:275-81.

35. Haffner SM, Lehto S, Ronnemaa T, Pyorala K, Laakso M. Mortality from coronary heart disease in subjects with type 2 diabetes and in nondiabetic subjects with and without prior myocardial infarction. N Engl J Med. 1998;339:229-34.

36. Boyle JP, Honeycutt AA, Narayan KMV, et al. Projection of diabetes burden through 2050: impact of changing demography and disease prevalence in the US. Diabetes Care. 2001;24:1936-40.

37. Narayan KM, Gregg EW, Engelgau MM, et al. Translation research for chronic disease: the case of diabetes. Diabetes Care. 2000;23:1794-8.

38. Saaddine JB, Engelgau MM, Beckles GL, Gregg EW, Thompson TJ, Narayan KM. A diabetes report card for the United States: quality of care in the 1990s. Ann Intern Med. 2002;136:565-74.

39. Centers for Disease Control and Prevention. Preventive care practices among people with diabetes mellitus, US, 1995 and 2001. MMWR Morb Mortal Wkly Rep. 2002;51:965-69.

40. Jha AK, Perlin JB, Kizer KW, Dudley RA. Effect of the transformation of the Veterans Affairs Health Care System on the quality of care. N Engl J Med. 2003;348:2218-27.

41. The TRIAD Study Group. The Translating Research Into Action for Diabetes (TRIAD) study: a multicenter study of diabetes in managed care. Diabetes Care. 2002;25:386-9.

42. Renders CM, Valk GD, Griffin SJ, Wagner EH, Eijk Van JT, Assendelft W. Interventions to improve the management of diabetes in primary care, outpatient, and community settings. Diabetes Care. 2001;24:1821-33.

43. Institute of Medicine Committee on Quality of Health Care in America. Crossing the Quality Chasm: A New Health System for the 21st Century. Washington, DC: National Academy Press; 2001.

44. Murphy D, Chapel T, Clark C. Moving diabetes care from science to practice: the evolution of the National Diabetes Prevention and Control Program. Ann Intern Med. 2004;140:978-84.

45. Kass N. An Ethics Framework for Public Health. Am J Public Health. 2001;91:1776-82.

46. Bowman B, Gregg E, Williams D. Translating the science of primary, secondary, and tertiary prevention to inform the public health response to diabetes. J Public Health Manag Pract. 2003; Suppl Nov:S8-14.

CHAPTER

2

Lifestyle for Prevention: Choices, Changes, Challenges

Authors

Linda Delahanty, MS, RD
Judith Wylie-Rosett, EdD, RD

Key Concepts

- Developing greater familiarity with the risk factors most linked to development of type 2 diabetes
- Examining more closely the complex interaction between environmental and genetic variables associated with increased risk for developing type 2 diabetes
- Recognizing the importance of overweight, obesity, and central obesity in development of type 2 diabetes
- Assessing prediabetes and planning interventions for those with this diagnosis
- Translating lessons from landmark studies into prevention education and interventions
- Developing familiarity with interventions of value in preventing type 2 diabetes, particularly lifestyle interventions
- Recognizing food intake and physical activity as key factors in successful lifestyle intervention: with emphasis placed on moderate weight loss through a low-fat, hypocaloric diet; regular physical activity; and programs that provide regular participant contact and education
- Becoming aware of intervention-related predictors of success in weight loss and weight management
- Viewing the diabetes educator's role outside traditional clinical settings; examining public health as well as clinical approaches to prevention
- Focusing clinical approaches on high-risk individuals
- Preparing for the impact of Medicare legislation allowing medical nutrition therapy for prediabetes and obesity

Introduction

The world has seen a dramatic rise in the incidence of type 2 diabetes. The prevention and delay of diabetes and the chronic complications associated with it have thus become urgently important in both public health and patient care. Information on the prevention and delay of type 2 diabetes, particularly in high-risk individuals, is presented first in this book so that prevention will not be viewed as an afterthought or secondary interest of diabetes educators, and so that diabetes educators will not be viewed as minor players in prevention. Education plays a large role in preventing and delaying the onset of this disease as well as in preventing and controlling its devastating complications.

Applying the Evidence

A large part of this chapter is devoted to examining research considering lifestyle interventions in the prevention and delay of the development of type 2 diabetes. Both the conclusions that can be drawn from major studies and the research emerging on the role of the community environment are discussed. Evidence from landmark clinical trials is examined, and findings are translated into information of value to diabetes educators and others involved in patient education and public health intervention. A highlight of this chapter is its comparison of intervention techniques and outcomes of 4 major adult diabetes prevention trials that have significantly contributed to this evidence base.

Sources of evidence considered in this chapter include observational as well as clinical trial data. The data cited here have also been used to form the evidence base for the statement by the AADE[1] on prevention of type 2 diabetes and the role of the diabetes educator. The AADE's white paper emphasizes intervention opportunities during the identifiable prediabetic phase, with the aim of halting or slowing the natural history of diabetes pathophysiology. Prediabetes is also a topic of this chapter.

The chapter's review of the clinical trial evidence underscores the effectiveness of lifestyle interventions in diabetes prevention. In particular, readers see how moderate weight loss—through a low-fat, hypocaloric diet; regular physical activity; and programs that provide regular participant contact and education—can markedly reduce the incidence of type 2 diabetes.[2-5] As this chapter translates the research findings, readers see how the AADE 7 Self-Care Behaviors™ apply in diabetes prevention.

Understanding the Risk Factors

Risk factors are a topic of keen interest in prevention of type 2 diabetes. Focusing on what diabetes educators need to know and can contribute, this chapter provides information about the following topics:

- The complex interactions between environmental and genetic variables that so often affect an individual's risk[6]
- Research directions for further exploration of the interaction of genetics and environment in diabetes prevention
- Prevention across the age spectrum and among diverse populations and settings
- Personal lifestyle factors that regulate energy balance (food intake and physical activity, in particular)—in diabetes prevention, these are recognized as essential elements to address in interventions

Emphasizing Weight Management

Significant emphasis is being placed on controlling body weight to prevent and delay the development of type 2 diabetes in individuals. Existing obesity guidelines, presented here, provide categories for classifying weight and weight distribution. The list below summarizes intervention-related predictors of weight loss and maintenance:[7]

- Attending intervention sessions
- Self-monitoring (usually, a diary of food intake or eating behavior)
- Planning behavioral strategies and problem-solving activities
- Engaging in physical activity
- Achieving a sense of success, usually weight loss, soon after starting

Public Health and Clinical Approaches

Both clinical and public health approaches to diabetes prevention are included in this chapter. The importance of partnering with community agencies has been emphasized by the National Diabetes Education Program (NDEP), as a joint effort of the Centers for Disease Control and Prevention (CDC) and the National Institutes of Health (NIH). Readers gain insight into how these governmental agencies are striving to develop community participation in diabetes prevention.[8]

The chapter concludes by addressing future directions for diabetes prevention and research. Throughout the chapter, the focus is on the role of lifestyle interventions in preventing type 2 diabetes. Because prevention of type 1 diabetes primarily involves medications to reduce autoimmunity, type 1 diabetes is not discussed here; readers interested in that aspect are referred to chapter 8. For information on prevention of the chronic complications associated with diabetes, readers are encouraged to review chapter 20.

Risk Factors and Their Interactions

This section discusses risk factors that are useful to consider and watch. Interaction of these factors can further increase the risk of developing type 2 diabetes.

- Lifestyle variables—these are particularly important in concert with other risk factors
- Genes and family factors
- Risk increasing with age and factors that become significant with aging
- Risk, and opportunities, after gestational diabetes mellitus
- Ethnic predispositions, including some reasons for them
- Overweight and obesity, particularly a large waist circumference
- Prediabetes

Lifestyle Variables

Lifestyle variables that appear to lower the risk of diabetes are consistent with current dietary recommendations for the general public.[8] They include attaining a higher level of physical activity; higher intake of fiber from whole grains, legumes, and vegetables; and lower fat intake.

Lifestyle Variables of Particular Importance in Preventing Type 2 Diabetes
• Physical activity levels
• Food intake
• Amount of dietary fat

Family and Genetic Influences

The risk for developing type 2 diabetes involves a complex interaction of lifestyle and genetic factors. Individuals with a positive family history of type 2 diabetes have an increased risk of type 2 diabetes. The occurrence of multiple cases of diabetes within a family can be the result of genetic susceptibility, shared environment, or lifestyles that increase the risk of diabetes; most likely, a combination of genetic and behavioral influences are at work.[9]

Age-Related Risk

The incidence of diabetes increases rapidly with age. Factors that predispose the older adult to diabetes include the following:

- Age-related decreases in insulin and insulin sensitivity
- Adiposity
- Decreased physical activity

- Multiple prescription medications
- Coexisting illnesses

Risk After Gestational Diabetes

Gestational diabetes mellitus (GDM) is a major risk factor for developing type 2 diabetes. The prevalence of GDM varies from 1% to 14% based on the risk factors of the population being assessed and the diagnostic criteria used.[10] Women with a diagnosis of GDM have a 40% to 60% chance of developing subsequent type 2 diabetes.[11] The prevalence rate can be reduced to 25% by combining the following approaches:

- Controlling body weight
- Increasing physical activity

Chapter 12 provides more information on gestational diabetes and how women who have GDM have the opportunity to intervene and lower their chances of developing type 2 diabetes.

Ethnic Differences: Diabetes Prevalence and Relative Risk[12]

- *Non-Hispanic Whites:* 13.1 million, or 8.7%, of all non-Hispanic whites age 20 years or older have diabetes. Data for high-risk population subgroups are compared to non-Hispanic whites, taking into account population age differences.
- *Non-Hispanic Blacks:* Non-Hispanic blacks are 1.8 times as likely to have diabetes as non-Hispanic whites. An estimated 3.2 million, or 13.3%, of all non-Hispanic blacks age 20 years or older have diabetes.
- *Hispanic/Latino Americans:* Mexican Americans, the largest Hispanic/Latino subgroup, are 1.7 times as likely to have diabetes as non-Hispanic whites. Residents of Puerto Rico are 1.8 times as likely to have diagnosed diabetes as US non-Hispanic whites. An estimated 2.5 million, or 9.5%, of the total Hispanic/Latino population age 20 years or older have diabetes.
- *American Indians and Alaska Natives:* American Indians and Alaska Natives are 2.2 times as likely to have diabetes as non-Hispanic whites. Among individuals receiving care from the Indian Health Service, 15.1%, or 118,000, American Indians and Alaska Natives age 20 years or older have diabetes (both diagnosed and undiagnosed diabetes), with rates varying from 8.1% among Alaska Natives to 26.7% in the southern United States and 27.6% in southern Arizona.
- *Asian Americans and Pacific Islanders*: In Hawaii and California, compared to whites, Native Hawaiians and other Pacific Islanders age 20 years or older are more than 2 times and 1.5 times as likely to have diagnosed diabetes in Hawaii and California, respectively. The total prevalence of diabetes (both diagnosed and undiagnosed diabetes) is not available for Asian Americans and Pacific Islanders.

Role of the Thrifty Genotype. A genetic adaptation termed the "thrifty genotype" may partially explain ethnic and racial differences in the risk for developing diabetes (for example, why Asian populations are more likely to develop diabetes at relatively lower body weights than other populations).[13] Examining the thrifty genotype involves consideration of genetic and environmental interactions and the concept of thrifty phenotype. The premise of the thrifty genotype/phenotype theory is that individuals who are genetically predisposed to energy efficiency are more likely to survive famine, and population groups historically exposed to frequent famines have more individuals who are energy efficient.[9] When food is more plentiful, however, having genotypes predisposed to energy efficiency could increase the likelihood to gain weight, accumulate intra-abdominal fat around vital organs, and develop insulin resistance; thus, the risk for developing type 2 diabetes increases. Advances in genetic research will provide a more in-depth understanding of genetic polymorphisms and how lifestyle and diet may affect the expression of a single gene with several variants of the DNA base pairs.

Risks Related to Overweight and Obesity

Individuals who are overweight or obese may be at high risk for type 2 diabetes. Overweight and obesity classifications, based on body mass index (BMI, weight/height^2), are given below (in kg/m^2); central obesity guidelines are also given.

National Institutes of Health (NIH) adult classification:[7]

- *Underweight*: BMI <18.5
- *Normal:* BMI 18.5 to 24.9
- *Overweight:* BMI 25.0 to 29.9
- *Obese:* BMI ≥30.0

World Health Organization (WHO) classification for different Asian populations:[15]

- *Observed risk cutoff point:* BMI varies from 22 to 25 kg/m^2
- *High-risk cutoff point:* BMI varies from 26 to 31 kg/m^2

Central obesity increases risk:

Variability in risk is associated with differences in intra-abdominal fat deposition, which, independent of total adiposity, is linked to insulin resistance and the risk of cardiovascular disease. Hence, body fat distribution must be assessed along with body weight.

Central Obesity. Individuals who have increased visceral fat, which refers to fat deposited around abdominal organs, appear to have a greater risk for type 2 diabetes than those with subcutaneous fat. Intra-abdominal obesity has a greater supply of capillaries, making it more metabolically active than subcutaneous fat or fat in the hips and thighs. As a result, there is a greater flux or turnover of free fatty acids (FFA). In the liver, these FFA contribute to insulin resistance (lipotoxicity).[16] Furthermore, FFA may be used as a fuel source instead of glucose and, thus, contribute to hyperglycemia.

Currently, there is a universal standard for assessing central obesity for the diverse population in the United States, although the WHO standards[15] should be considered in assessing Asian Americans.

NIH guideline on central obesity:[7]

- *Men:* Waist circumference >102 cm (>40 in)
- *Women:* Waist circumference >88 cm (>35 in)

Most individuals who meet the current criteria for central obesity are also overweight or obese and, as such, would be candidates for diabetes prevention strategies to reduce body weight. There is insufficient research to address the potential effects of interventions that uniquely target central obesity, independent of overall obesity. Thus, the focus for diabetes prevention in individuals with central adiposity is as follows:

- Reduce overall fat mass (including visceral fat deposits) with lifestyle changes to decrease energy intake by lowering dietary fat, following a healthy dietary pattern, and increasing energy expenditure through physical activity

Interacting Risk Factors

Of particular interest is how obesity and lifestyle relate to developing insulin resistance and visceral fat accumulation. Figure 2.1 depicts interactions between lifestyle factors (physical activity and dietary intake) and genetic factors.

Traditionally, family history (genetics) and aging have been identified as the nonmodifiable risk factors for diabetes and lifestyle and weight as the modifiable risk factors. However, interactions between genetics and lifestyle determine diabetes risk through their interactive roles in regulating body fat accumulation (the number, size, distribution, and hormonal signals from fat cells). In turn, the cytokines (hormones) secreted by fat cells appear to increase inflammation, insulin resistance and, ultimately, the risk of developing diabetes. Aging can also increase body fat accumulation, insulin resistance, and risk of diabetes.

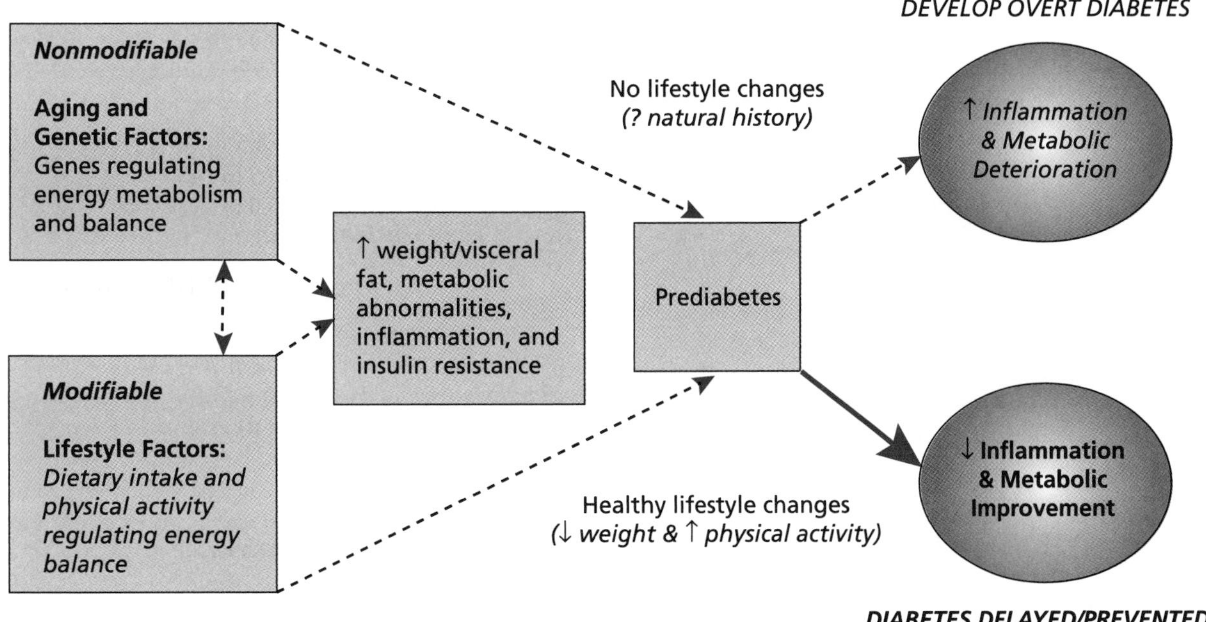

FIGURE 2.1 Developing or Preventing Diabetes—Interactions Between Genetic and Lifestyle Factors

Weight and physical activity are critical facets of intervention:

Weight gain and physical inactivity foster the natural history of diabetes development (insulin resistance and metabolic pathways leading to overt diabetes). In contrast, lifestyle changes that reduce body weight and increase physical activity decrease the risk of developing diabetes.

Genetic factors are important determinates of type 2 diabetes and the predisposing risk factors, but lifestyle largely regulates gene expression in determining diabetes development. There is emerging evidence that genes affecting energy metabolism and the risk of developing type 2 diabetes have several variant forms (genetic polymorphisms). Research advances also indicate that cytokines are associated with inflammation and appear to increase risk of developing diabetes and cardiovascular disease. Variant forms of a gene can affect responsiveness to lifestyle intervention in reducing the risk of developing diabetes.

Longitudinal cohort studies have provided insights about how distribution of body weight, weight history, and lifestyle are related to the risk of developing diabetes. The Newcastle Thousand Families study, for example, prospectively collected data on 412 study participants that included birth weight and nutrition during childhood and adult lifestyle and body composition at age 50 years. The study found that compared to early life, adult lifestyle and body composition (higher body fat and higher waist-to-hip ratio) are the greatest risk factors for type 2 diabetes.[14]

Prediabetes

Individuals with either impaired fasting glucose (IFG) or impaired glucose tolerance (IGT) are at high risk for type 2 diabetes.[17] The recommended terminology for this condition is prediabetes. Over a 5-year period, approximately 30% to 40% of individuals with IGT or IFG develop type 2 diabetes. Current American Diabetes Association (ADA) guidelines for each are as follows:

- *IFG:* Fasting glucose level between 100 and 125 mg/dL (5.6 and 6.9 mmol/L).
- *IGT:* 2-hour post-75-g glucose load glucose concentration of between 140 and 199 mg/dL (7.8 and 11.0 mmol/L)

There are no standards for using A1C tests to screen for prediabetes, but individuals with an A1C above the population mean (often considered 5.5%) are at increased risk for developing diabetes.[18]

Use of Medical Record Data. Using medical record data from national registries of the Finnish adult population, Lindstrom and Tuomilehto developed a Diabetes Risk Score and evaluated its sensitivity and specificity for predicting the development of having diabetes treated by medication in 5 to 10 years.[19] The Diabetes Risk Score had sensitivity of 0.78 to 0.81 and specificity of 0.76 to 0.77.[19] The Finnish population is less ethnically and racially diverse than the US population, but medical record data holds promise for easily and accurately identifying individuals at high risk for developing diabetes.

Effectiveness of Lifestyle Intervention in Diabetes Prevention

A systematic review by Norris et al examined clinical trials in diabetes prevention.[20] There have been 4 landmark clinical trials that have demonstrated the effectiveness of lifestyle intervention in the prevention of type 2 diabetes in the United States and abroad. These clinical trials and their results are described below. The descriptions that follow emphasize the diet, activity, and weight-loss components of the lifestyle interventions.

Malmo, Sweden

The first of these clinical trials was a 6-year feasibility study in Malmo, Sweden, that prospectively studied 181 men 47 to 49 years of age with impaired glucose tolerance (IGT) who received a diet and activity intervention and a reference group of 79 men who received no intervention.[2] The 79 men in the reference group were informed about their condition by letter or at the clinic. Although they received no specific diabetes prevention treatment at the clinic, most of them received intervention in some form (for example, to treat hypertension or evaluate alcohol consumption).

Lifestyle Intervention

At the outset, a physician and a dietitian met with the men and their wives to review the condition of impaired glucose tolerance and provide dietary information and advice. Participants who were overweight were asked to lose weight; however, no specific weight-loss goal was recommended. Thus, the diet goals were to reduce calories if overweight, reduce saturated fat by substituting polyunsaturated fat whenever possible, reduce simple sugars, and increase complex carbohydrates. The physical activity goal was to complete two 45- to 60-minute sessions of moderate-intensity activity per week.

After the initial instruction, participants could opt to follow the diet and exercise program on their own or in organized groups of 10 to 15 once per month for 6 months at a time. Sixty-eight participants (38%) followed the protocol as organized groups, with a 6-month period of supervised physical training followed by a 6-month period of dietary treatment, or vice versa. After 12 months, participants could either follow the protocol on their own, together with previous group partners, or in local sports clubs for the next 5 years of the study.[2,21]

Results

Specific changes in diet were not reported. The estimated maximal oxygen uptake averaged over the entire study period was significantly higher for the intervention group (P <.001) compared with the reference group. At 1 year, the mean weight loss was >6 kg (7% weight loss) and at 6-year follow-up, the mean weight loss was 3.3 kg (2.3 ± 5.4%). After the 5-year intervention, only 10.6% of men in the intervention group developed diabetes compared with 28.6% of men in the reference group.[2]

Diabetes Risk. The relative risk of developing type 2 diabetes in the intervention group compared to the reference group was 0.37 (95% confidence interval, 0.20-0.68; P <.003).[2]

Incidence of Diabetes. Overall, this study found a 63% reduction in the incidence of diabetes in these men with IGT compared to the reference group.[2]

Blood Pressure. Blood pressure was reduced in both the intervention and reference groups with IGT; however, the prevalence of medication for hypertension was lower in the intervention group than the reference group.[2]

Lipids. The IGT intervention group also had a substantial reduction in serum triglycerides that was still evident after 6 years.[2]

Limitations

There were 2 major limitations to this study. First, the men were not randomly assigned to the treatment groups. Second, the 2 treatment groups differed by medical condition at baseline. Also, because there was no detailed description of the intervention, assessing the frequency of contact for the intervention is difficult; participants could have had a minimum of 1 initial instruction and opted to follow the program on their own, or they could have attended a maximum of monthly groups for the 5-year treatment period.

Da Qing, China

The first randomized diabetes prevention clinical trial was a 6-year study among 577 Chinese men and women with impaired glucose tolerance who were 25 years of age and older.[3,22] The study participants were identified via a citywide health screening from 33 area health clinics and randomized by clinic into 1 of 4 groups: diet only, physical activity only, diet plus physical activity, or a control group. Participants in the control group received general information about diabetes and IGT and informational brochures with general instructions about diet and increased leisure activities.

Lifestyle Intervention

A physician and team provided individual counseling on diet and weight goals for the diet-only intervention. Diet and weight-loss goals were based on each participant's initial BMI. Participants with a BMI <25 had no weight-loss goal. Their diet goals were to consume 25 to 30 kcal/kg, 55% to 65% carbohydrate, 10% to 15% protein, and 25% to 30% fat, with a focus on more vegetables, less simple sugars; and control of alcohol intake. Participants who had a BMI ≥25 had a goal to lose 0.5 to 1 kg per month until a BMI of 23 was achieved; they also received individualized calorie targets based on initial weight and an exchange-type diet specifying the recommended number of servings to consume from cereals, vegetables, meat, milk, and oils each day. Participants in the activity-only group were instructed to increase leisure physical activity by a minimum of 1 unit per day (1 unit was either 5 minutes of very strenuous activity, 10 minutes of strenuous activity, 20 minutes of moderate activity equivalent to brisk walking, or 30 minutes of mild activity such as slow walking). Participants in the diet-plus-activity group were instructed to focus on the diet, exercise, and weight goals mentioned above.

After initial instruction, compliance was assessed every 3 months, and physicians repeated individual counseling instructions. In addition, counseling sessions in small groups were conducted weekly for 1 month, then monthly for 3 months, and then once every 3 months for the remainder of the study.[3,22]

Results

At baseline, the calorie intake and diet composition of the 4 treatment groups was similar. The diet intervention group was consuming an average of 2485 calories per day, consisting of 60% carbohydrate, 11% protein, 26% fat, and 3 g of alcohol per day. After 6 years, the diet group and the diet-plus-activity group appeared to have lower calorie intakes and a diet composition that was slightly lower in percentage of carbohydrate and protein and slightly higher in percentage of fat; however, these differences were not statistically significant. Both the physical activity and diet-plus-activity groups significantly increased their reported units of leisure activity, but the 2 groups not using exercise did not. The participants with a BMI <25 in the diet-only intervention did not lose weight and did not experience a lower incidence of diabetes compared to the control group;

however, the overweight participants in the diet-only and diet-plus-exercise groups did lose weight and experience lower diabetes incidence rates than the overweight control group. There was also significant reduction in the incidence of diabetes in both activity arms for both lean and overweight participants.

Diabetes Risk. After adjustment for baseline BMI and fasting glucose, there was a diabetes risk reduction of 31% for diet-only ($P < .03$), 46% for activity-only ($P < .0005$), and 42% for diet and physical activity ($P < .005$) compared to the control group.

Blood Pressure and Lipids. The impact of the lifestyle intervention on blood pressure and lipid levels was not reported.

Limitations

This study randomly assigned participants by clinic groups rather than individual random assignment. The dietary assessment methods were not capable of thoroughly assessing dietary changes, and the interviewers conducting the assessments were not masked to the intervention. The baseline diet for the diet-only treated group with a BMI <25 was already consistent with the diet goals for the intervention; therefore, a significant change in diet for that subgroup was unlikely to occur.

Finnish Diabetes Prevention Study

In the Finnish Diabetes Prevention Study, 522 overweight men and women (BMI ≥25 kg/m^2) with impaired glucose tolerance, 40 to 64 years of age, were randomly assigned to an intensive lifestyle or control group.[4,23-25] Each subject in the control group was given general information about diet and exercise, either in an individual session or in a group session lasting 30 to 60 minutes.

Lifestyle Intervention

Each subject in the intervention group received detailed counseling by nutritionists. Lifestyle goals were to reduce weight by 5% or more, reduce intake of total fat to <30% of calories and saturated fat to <10% of calories, increase intake of fiber to at least 15 g per 1000 calories, and increase physical activity to at least 30 minutes per day. Dietary advice was tailored to each participant based on 3-day food records completed 4 times per year.[23]

Each participant received 7 sessions lasting 30 to 60 minutes with a nutritionist during the first year and 1 session every 3 months thereafter. The first-year sessions had planned topics such as diabetes risk factors, saturated fat, fiber, physical activity, and problem solving; however, discussions were individualized. In addition, there were voluntary group sessions, expert lectures, low-fat cooking lessons, supermarket tours, and between-visit phone calls and letters.

Participants also received individual guidance on increasing the level of physical activity. Supervised, progressive, individually tailored, circuit-type resistance training sessions were offered to participants to improve functional capacity and strength of large muscle groups. Voluntary group walking and hiking activities were also organized. In addition, an exercise competition among the 5 study centers was organized twice during the study to enhance motivation.

Results

The mean duration of follow-up was 3.2 years. At 1 year, 43% achieved a weight loss of >5%, 47% achieved the target of <30% of calories from fat, 26% achieved the target of <10% saturated fat, 25% achieved the fiber intake goal, and 86% achieved the exercise goal of >4 hours of activity per week. Mean weight loss by the end of year 1 was 4.2 kg (4.7%). At year 2, the intervention group lost 3.5 kg and the control group lost 0.8 kg.

Diabetes Risks. The risk of developing diabetes was reduced by 58% in the intervention group.

Incidence of Diabetes. The cumulative incidence of diabetes was 11% in the lifestyle intervention group and 23% in the control group.

Lipids and Other Measures. Significantly greater improvements were seen in weight, BMI, waist circumference, A1C, the ratio of serum total cholesterol to high-density lipoprotein cholesterol (HDL-C), and serum triglycerides in the intervention group compared with the control group at both 1 year and 3 years.

The reduction in the incidence of diabetes was directly associated with changes in lifestyle. Thirteen subjects in the intervention group and 48 in the control group did not achieve any of the lifestyle goals; diabetes developed in 38% and 31% of these subjects, respectively. Diabetes did not develop in any of the 49 subjects in the intervention group or in the 15 subjects in the control group who achieved 4 or 5 of the lifestyle goals.

Limitations

There are no major limitations to this study; however, there are some limitations to generalizing the findings due, first, to the homogeneous population of Finns that were studied and, second, to cultural differences in diet, activity, and environmental variables involved with lifestyle change. The number of contacts provided to deliver the lifestyle intervention also must not be underestimated; there were many extra group activities and phone and mail communications offered to enhance adherence to the diet and activity goals, and the frequency of these additional contacts was not reported.

Diabetes Prevention Program

The Diabetes Prevention Program (DPP) was designed to determine the safest and most effective approaches to preventing or delaying development of type 2 diabetes among an ethnically diverse group of individuals with IGT. The study compared a lifestyle intervention and a pharmacologic intervention (metformin) with a placebo.[5,26-32] This randomized, controlled clinical trial was conducted in 27 centers across the United States and enrolled 3234 men and women with impaired glucose tolerance who ranged in age from 25 to 85 years old. Approximately 45% of the participants were from minority ethnic groups (eg, African American and Hispanic) and 20% were 60 years of age or older. Subjects in the placebo and metformin arms received written information regarding lifestyle recommendations and an annual 20- to 30-minute individual session.

Lifestyle Intervention

The lifestyle intervention had 2 goals: first, to achieve a weight loss of ≥7% of initial body weight by decreasing daily caloric intake by 500 to 1000 calories and eating <25% of total calories from fat, and second, to increase physical activity to at least 150 minutes per week.

Participants were given calorie and fat gram goals based on initial body weight. Participants in the lifestyle arm met with a lifestyle coach 16 times in the first 24 weeks to review a 16-lesson curriculum that focused on diet, physical activity, and behavioral modification strategies. The minimum frequency of follow-up was at least once every 2 months in person, with alternate monthly contact via phone or e-mail; however, participants could be seen as often as weekly if needed. If participants were not meeting lifestyle goals for weight loss or activity, lifestyle coaches used a variety of tool-box strategies to address specific barriers to adherence. In addition, participants were offered group classes and motivational campaigns lasting 4 to 6 weeks 3 times per year to provide peer support and friendly competition and help sustain progress with lifestyle changes.

Results

At week 24, 50% of the participants in the lifestyle arm achieved the weight-loss goal of ≥7% of body weight; at study end, 38% achieved this goal. At week 24, 74% of the participants in the lifestyle arm exercised at least 150 minutes a week; at study end, 58% did. After 1 year, the lifestyle intervention group had reduced fat intake by 6.6% and reduced their calorie intake by an average of 450 calories per day. In contrast, the groups taking the medication or placebo had reduced fat intake by 0.8% and reduced calorie intake by 296 and 249 calories per day, respectively. The average weight loss in the lifestyle intervention group was 7% at 24 weeks and 5.6 kg (5%) at study end; in comparison, the groups taking the medication or placebo lost 2.1 and 0.1 kg respectively (P <.001).[5,31]

Due to the tremendous success of both intervention groups, the study ended 1 year early; average follow-up was 2.8 years.

Diabetes Risk. Among individuals randomized to the lifestyle intervention group, there was a 58% reduction in risk of developing type 2 diabetes over a 3-year period. Among individuals randomized to the metformin intervention, risk was reduced by 31%.

Other Important Findings. Other important findings include the following:

- Treatment effects did not differ according to sex, race, or ethnic group
- The lifestyle intervention was highly effective in all groups
- Metformin was nearly ineffective in older individuals (>60 years of age) and in those with lower BMI (BMI <30). Metformin was as effective as lifestyle in individuals 24 to 44 years of age or in those with a BMI >35.
- To delay or prevent diabetes during a period of 3 years, 14 persons would need to be treated with metformin to prevent 1 case, whereas only 7 persons would need to be treated with lifestyle intervention to prevent 1 case.

Blood Pressure and Lipids. At baseline, 30% of study participants had hypertension; however, the presence of hypertension increased in the groups taking the medication or placebo. In contrast, there was no significant change in the prevalence of hypertension in the lifestyle intervention group. The lifestyle intervention resulted in significantly greater reductions in systolic and diastolic blood pressure and triglycerides compared to groups taking the medication or placebo. The lifestyle intervention also significantly increased the HDL-C and reduced the incidence of proatherogenic LDL phenotype B.[28]

Moreover, at 3-year follow-up, the lifestyle intervention reduced the use of drug therapy for control of lipids by 25% and blood pressure by 27% to 28% compared with the groups taking the medication or placebo.[28] The lifestyle intervention also reduced the incidence of metabolic syndrome by 41% (P <.001) compared to a 17% risk reduction with metformin (P <.03).[29] Lifestyle intervention also had a positive impact on nontraditional markers of cardiovascular disease by reducing subclinical inflammation and improving fibrinolysis. Compared to placebo, the lifestyle intervention significantly decreased C-reactive protein (CRP) and fibrinogen levels, while metformin produced smaller but still significant changes in CRP and fibrinogen levels. In the intensive lifestyle group, change in weight was the strongest predictor of reduction in CRP for both men and women.[30]

Limitations

There are no major limitations to this study; however, there are some limitations to generalizing the findings. First, the DPP participants were highly screened based on physiological study criteria and ability to complete behavioral tasks during a run-in period. Also, although the DPP study population was ethnically diverse, they were a highly educated group compared to the average education level found in the National Health and Nutrition Examination Survey (NHANES) study population, which is considered more representative of the US population.[8] Translation of this intensive lifestyle intervention into the clinical practice setting is still needed.

Conclusive evidence on effectiveness of lifestyle intervention for IGT:

The results of these 4 landmark clinical trials provide conclusive evidence about the effectiveness of a lifestyle intervention in preventing or delaying diabetes in those with impaired glucose tolerance.

Table 2.1 shows the characteristics of the populations in each of these clinical trials and shows that lifestyle interventions for diabetes prevention have been successful in large numbers of men and women of diverse racial and ethnic backgrounds. The lifestyle interventions have also been implemented with people age 25 to 85 years old and with BMIs ranging from as low as 22 kg/m^2 in the Da Qing and the DPP studies (for Asian Americans) to greater than 40 kg/m^2 in the DPP. Even more importantly, the lifestyle interventions have been implemented long-term (as long as 6 years) with very little attrition of participants. The DPP studied the largest, most ethnically diverse sample of people with IGT and was able to demonstrate that lifestyle intervention is effective regardless of age, ethnicity, or BMI.

Table 2.2 compares the diet, activity, and weight-loss goals for the 4 clinical trials.[33] The diets in these studies typically focused on calorie targets based on initial body weight and a diet composition that was low in fat (<30% of calories from fat), saturated fat, and simple sugars; high in vegetables and fiber; and moderate in alcohol. The activity goals were similar as well, with a focus on aerobic activity ranging from a minimum of 20 to 30 minutes per day to 60 minutes or more spread over 3 or more days per week, ideally at least 5 days per week.

TABLE 2.1 Characteristics of Participants in the Landmark Studies

Clinical Trial	*Sample Size*	*Gender (% female)*	*Race/ Ethnicity*	*Age (years)**	*BMI (kg/m^2)**	*Length of Follow-up (years)*	*Attrition (%)*
Malmo Study	181	0	Swedes	48 ± 0.7 (range: 47-49)	26.6 ± 3.1	6	11
Da Qing Study	577	47	Chinese	45.0 ± 9.1 (range: 25 or older)	25.8 ± 3.8	6	8
Finnish Diabetes Prevention Study	522	67	Finns	55 ± 7.0 (range: 40-65)	31.1± 4.6	Mean 3.2 (range: 1.6-6.0)	8
Diabetes Prevention Program	3234	67.7	White: 55% African American: 20% Hispanic: 16% American Indian: 5% Asian: 4%	50.6 ± 10.7 (range: 25 or older)	34.0 ± 6.7	Mean 2.8 (range: 1.8-4.6)	8

*Mean ± S.D. at baseline

TABLE 2.2 Description of the Weight Loss, Nutrition, and Physical Activity Interventions Used in Type 2 Diabetes Clinical Trials

Clinical Trial	*Weight-Loss Goal*	*Diet Goals*	*Activity Goal (type)*	*Activity Goal (F/I/T)*	*Change in Weight Loss*	*Change in Diet, Activity*	*RR*
Malmo Study 181 men 0 women	WL suggested, but no specific goal set	Reduce calories, saturated fat, and simple sugars; increase complex carbohydrates	Aerobic (walk), jog, soccer, calisthenics, and badminton	Moderate (more intensive activity performed late in training) 2 weekly 60-min sessions	*WL:* confirmed WL >6 kg at 1 y and 3.3 kg at 5 y	*Diet:* not reported *Activity:* significant increase in mean oxygen uptake values based on submaximal bicycle ergometer test	63%
Da Qing Study 210 men 187 women	*If BMI <25:* no WL goal *If BMI ≥25:* lose 0.5 to 1.0 kg/mo to BMI of 23	*If BMI <25:* 25–30 kcal/kg, 55% to 65% carbohydrates, 10% to 14% protein, 25% to 30% fat, more vegetables, less simple sugars, control alcohol *If BMI ≥25:* individualized calorie targets, exchange-type diet	Aerobic (ranging from slow walking to running), swimming, and basketball	Mild to strenuous intensity; 1 unit/day, time dependent on intensity Most individuals brisk-walked 20 min/day	*WL:* inconclusive WL varied by intervention group and DM status *Diet only:* +0.93 kg (no DM); -2.43 (DM) *Exercise only:* +0.71 kg (no DM); -1.93 kg (DM) *Diet and exercise:* -1.77 kg (no DM); -3.33 kg (DM)	*Diet:* no significant change in calories/ macronutrient profile *Activity:* significant increase in reported average units per day of exercise	*Diet:* 31% *Activity:* 46% *Diet and activity:* 42%
Finnish Diabetes Prevention Study 91 men 174 women	≥5% of initial weight	Decrease total calories to achieve weight goal, <30% fat, <10% saturated fat, ≥15 g of fiber/1000 kcal	Aerobic (also some resistance training)	Moderate to somewhat vigorous intensity 30 min/day	*WL:* confirmed WL 4.2 kg at 1 y and 3.5 kg at 2 y	*Diet:* not reported *Activity:* significant increase in reported physical activity levels	58%

(continued)

TABLE 2.2 Description of the Weight Loss, Nutrition, and Physical Activity Interventions Used in Type 2 Diabetes Clinical Trials

Clinical Trial	*Weight-Loss Goal*	*Diet Goals*	*Activity Goal (type)*	*Activity Goal (F/I/T)*	*Change in Weight Loss*	*Change in Diet, Activity*	*RR*
Diabetes Prevention Program 345 men 734 women	≥7% of initial weight	Individualized calorie targets to achieve a 1–2 lb/wk WL, <25% fat	Aerobic (brisk walking)	Moderate intensity; 150 min, minimum of 10 min per time Spread over 3 days or more per week	*WL:* confirmed WL. 7% WL at 6 mo and 5.6 kg (5%WL) at study end	*Diet:* calories decreased by 450 ± 26 kcal/day and fat decreased by 6.6% at 1 yr *Activity:* 74% met goal of 150 min at 6 mo and 58% at 2.8 yr; significant increase in reported activity levels	58%

Key: BMI = body mass index; DM = diabetes mellitus; F/I/T = frequency/intensity/time; RR = risk reduction; WL = weight loss

Reprinted with permission: Kriska AM, Delahanty LM, and Pettee KK. Lifestyle intervention for the prevention of type 2 diabetes: translation and future recommendations. Current Diabetes Reports. 2004;4:113-8.

Most of the lifestyle interventions focused on weight loss; however, in the Da Qing study, BMI was not a criterion for eligibility and if BMI was <25, a weight-loss goal was not prescribed. The lean participants in the diet intervention did not appear to make any significant changes in the macronutrient composition of their diets, did not lose weight, and did not experience a reduction in diabetes incidence compared to the control group. Alternatively, in the DPP, eligible participants had to have a BMI of at least 24 kg/m^2, except for Asian Americans (descendants from Japanese, Chinese, other East Asian groups, East Indians, and Pacific Rim Australian populations) who were eligible with a BMI ≥22, as this has been demonstrated to be a relevant obesity cut-point representing increased risk of type 2 diabetes among Asian American individuals.[4,15,21,34] The DPP lifestyle intervention, which aimed for 7% weight loss regardless of initial BMI, was effective in all ethnic groups and at all levels of BMI.

Lifestyle Intervention: Effectiveness in 4 Landmark Studies

- *Weight Loss:* Weight losses ranged from 5% to 7% of initial body weight.
- *Diabetes Risk.* Risk reduction for developing diabetes ranged from 31% to as high as 63%.
- *Other Measures.* Most of the studies documented improvements in other clinical outcomes such as blood pressure, triglyceride levels, and cholesterol-to-HDL ratios as well as reductions in the amounts of medications needed to control blood pressure and lipids.[28]

The DPP also documented improvements in other nontraditional markers of cardiovascular disease—decreased tissue plasminogen activator (tPA), CRP, and fibrinogen levels—with lifestyle intervention.[30]

Table 2.3 summarizes and compares elements of the lifestyle intervention processes used in the studies.

TABLE 2.3 Lifestyle Intervention: Process Characteristics from Landmark Studies

Clinical Trial	*Intervention Frequency*	*Intervention Duration (years)*	*Number of Contacts*	*Format*	*Intervention Staff*	*Incidence/100 Person-Years (95% CI)*	*Number Needed to Treat**
Malmo Study	Initial mtg. and follow-up on own or in groups of 10-15 once per mo.; 6 mo. of diet treatment and then 6 mo. supervised physical training or vice versa	5	1-60†	Initial individual instruction with follow-up on own or in group	Nurse, dietitian and physiotherapist physician	NR	NR
Da Qing Study	Initial mtg. and individual counseling by physician every 3 mo.; counseling sessions in groups weekly for 1 mo., monthly for 3 mo., and once each 3 mo. thereafter	6	30	Individual and group	Physician and team	*Diet + PA:* 8.0 *Diet only:* 10.1 *PA only:* 10.7 *Control:* 15.2	13.9 19.1 22.2
Finnish Diabetes Prevention Study	7 sessions in 1st year with nutritionist and 1 session every 3 mo. thereafter	Avg. 3.2 (range: 1.6-6.0)	15	Individual sessions; exercise groups offered	Dietitian, other unclear	*Lifestyle:* 3.2 *Control:* 7.8	21.7
Diabetes Prevention Program	16 individual sessions with coach in 24 weeks, at least once per mo. contact thereafter; 4-8 week group classes; 3 campaigns per year	Avg. 2.8 (range: 1.8-4.6)	40	Individual lessons with group classes	Lifestyle coach (usually dietitian)	*Lifestyle:* 4.8 *Pharma:* 7.8 *Placebo:* 11.0	6.9 13.9

*Calculated from the incidence per 100 person-years
†Range of contacts possible based on intervention description
NR = not reported, PA = physical activity

In each study, the lifestyle intervention process was not always described in detail; however, all 4 trials described a process of setting goals, tailoring the intervention to the individual, opportunities for group sessions in addition to individual sessions, and frequent follow-up contacts to provide accountability and reinforce goals. The lifestyle intervention process for the Finnish Diabetes Prevention Study and the DPP have been described in the most detail. Similarities between the interventions in these 2 studies are summarized in the sidebar.

Interventions to Prevent Diabetes:
Similarities from the Finnish Diabetes Prevention Study and the Diabetes Prevention Program

- Participants received education on preplanned topics and skill training on practical goal setting and problem solving to address specific individual barriers
- Voluntary group sessions, expert lectures, and phone and mail follow-up were used to supplement individual sessions with a goal toward facilitating gradual, step-wise, long-term behavioral changes.
- Weight charts or graphs were used to show participants progress over time
- Participants were offered the option of meal replacements for 1 to 2 meals per week to boost weight loss
- Participants were offered supervised activity sessions and exercise competitions/campaigns to increase motivation and provide peer support
- Participants were asked to self-monitor food intake

Both the DPP and Finnish programs asked participants to self-monitor food intake. In the Finnish study, participants were asked to complete 3-day food records 4 times per year. In the DPP, participants were asked to self-monitor activity, food intake, calories, and fat grams daily during the first 24 weeks and then at least 1 week per month thereafter. In the DPP, frequency of dietary self-monitoring was related to success at achieving both the physical activity goal and the weight-loss goal.[32] Moreover, participants who were 65 years of age or older were more likely to complete self-monitoring records, report a lower percentage of calories from fat, and meet the activity and weight-loss goals than those who were less than 45 years old. Not surprisingly then, older participants had a greater (71%) risk reduction in the development of diabetes with lifestyle intervention. Lifestyle coaches in the DPP taught participants to use a problem-solving approach to manage high-risk situations (stress, vacations, and eating out, for example) and used a tool-box approach to deal with barriers to lifestyle change.

Although data on the number of cases per 100 person-years needed to treat to prevent a single case of diabetes is not typically used by diabetes care providers in patient care, managed care organizations and policy makers consider this information important in determining diabetes prevention services.

Self-Care Behaviors

Relationship to Diabetes Prevention

Successful lifestyle intervention to prevent diabetes in the 4 landmark studies required participants to manage their self-care behaviors in relation to each of the self-care behaviors listed below.

- Healthy eating
- Increased physical activity
- Self-monitoring of food and activity
- Medication taking, with adherence to pharmacologic treatment in the DPP
- Problem solving, to deal with barriers to reaching weight loss and activity goals
- Healthy coping, to deal with stress and other emotions that trigger overeating and inactivity
- Reducing risks, by adhering to a frequent follow-up schedule to reassess health outcomes

Thus, one can see that the AADE 7 Self-Care Behaviors™ model is also of value to diabetes educators in efforts to prevent diabetes.

Translating Prevention Research for Diverse Populations and Settings

Both clinical and public health approaches are being used to delay or prevent type 2 diabetes.[35-38] Screening with blood tests to identify high-risk individuals is only recommended in clinical settings to assure that follow-up is available, although diabetes risk assessment with questionnaires may help identify individuals who need referral to a clinical setting for further evaluation. Table 2.4 provides an overview of clinical and public health strategies for preventing diabetes in various age groups.

Clinical Strategies

Diabetes educators can incorporate clinical strategies into guidelines and practice protocols to address the needs of individuals at risk for diabetes. The interface between primary care and diabetes practices provides opportunities for identifying high-risk adults; however, diabetes

TABLE 2.4 Strategies to Prevent Type 2 Diabetes Across the Life Span*

	Public Health Strategies	*Clinical Strategies*
Prenatal	• Increase awareness of link between gestational diabetes and future type 2 diabetes risk • Increase awareness of prenatal weight gain, physical activity, and nutrition recommendations	• Screen for gestational diabetes • Provide tailored counseling regarding prenatal weight gain • Link prenatal gestational diabetes care to follow-up assessment of family diabetes risk and family weight management
Infant and toddlers	• Promote healthy lifestyles for families using day care and other settings • Integrate discussion of family lifestyle into well-care visit	• Monitor weight for those above and below the weight curves; discuss weight trends with parents • Refer families for weight management as needed
Young children	• Develop school-based interventions to promote healthy body weight (walking to school, school foods, physical activity during school routine) • Develop community recreational resources • Promote community healthier food options	• Refer at-risk children and their families to weight programs • Increase availability of weigh- management programs to meet the needs of families with overweight children
Preteen and teenage youth	• Promote lifelong physical activity in school and community • Engage youth in cooking and planning healthy food options in school and community • Promote healthy lifestyle and coping techniques to reduce risk • Target reduction on sources of excess calories (sugary beverages, fried foods, energy-dense snacks, supersize portions)	• Offer weight management programs that focus on needs for independence while providing support • Address the complex behavioral and psychosocial needs of overweight adolescents
Young adults	• Promote healthier lifestyle at worksites • Promote family-based physical activity and eating • Increase awareness of central adiposity in relation to diabetes risk	• Provide weight-management programs that can fit into the schedule of overweight young adults • Screen for and address lifestyle issues related to metabolic syndrome
Adults in midlife	• Increase awareness of midlife weight gain • Promote integration of walking into lifestyle	• Integrate weight management into programs targeting metabolic changes associated with menopause • Address subclinical metabolic abnormalities
Older adults	• Promote physical activity in senior centers • Offer healthier food options in senior feeding programs • Promote group walks in community that accommodate pace of older adults	• Provide comprehensive weight-control programs that meet the needs of older adults with weight-related metabolic and physical abnormalities
All ages	• Develop community resources to promote greater activity (safe/attractive options for walking, biking, etc) • Make healthier food options readily available • Address barriers to healthier lifestyle at community level	• Expand third-party coverage for medical nutrition therapy for prediabetes and weight management • Link medical nutrition therapy and weight management to primary care systems

*All strategies in the table need further evaluation because of the limited research addressing diabetes prevention across the age spectrum.

educators need to consider how to build an appropriate interface to address the needs of high-risk infants and children.

Public Health Strategies

The public health strategies involve focusing on the population as a whole and focusing on environmental factors that may increase or decrease diabetes risk. Expanding the practice settings as well as the scope of practice for diabetes educators offers opportunities for preventing diabetes. Diabetes educators should consider settings in which the populations targeted for diabetes prevention gather at least once a week. The type of intervention can address environmental changes (for example, with regard to food served in cafeterias or vending machines) or promote physical activity (for example, with exercise breaks). Diabetes educators may also play a role in considering how to develop or expand onsite recreational offerings. Even promoting use of staircases as an alternative to the elevator is a strategy for increasing physical activity that can be considered.

Practice Settings

Collaborations need to include developing a range of programs to promote healthy body weight in settings that are natural gathering places for the population groups at risk for diabetes and for the public in general.

- *For Children and Youth.* Practice settings may include day care centers and schools. Diabetes educators can be involved in collaborating with school personnel about a curriculum that promotes a healthy body weight and diabetes prevention or in developing programs for high-risk youth who are overweight or at risk for becoming overweight.
- *For Adults.* Worksite settings and senior adult facilities are good venues for promoting diabetes prevention.
- *Within the Community.* Diabetes educators can also seek collaborations to develop diabetes prevention activities with faith-based and other community organizations that offer programs across the age span. Such organizations are good sites for providing weight-control programs for individuals or families and developing food purchasing co-ops to increase access to wholesome foods.

Creative collaborations are needed to provide a concerted effort in reducing the increasing public health burden of diabetes. Preventing diabetes requires "thinking outside the box" of the traditional clinical setting and environment; the traditional setting was established to address diabetes self-management training for individuals with established diabetes.

Clinical Approach for High-Risk Individuals

Lifestyle interventions to prevent diabetes can target high-risk individuals with prediabetes based on having IFG of 100 to 125 mg/dL or being diagnosed as having IGT after an oral glucose tolerance test. Since many diabetes educators have contact with individuals in a traditional clinical setting, they are likely to focus on high-risk individuals using a medical nutrition therapy approach. There are increasing efforts to identify and treat high-risk individuals in both pediatric and adult medical care settings.

Complementary Therapies

Nutraceuticals (also known as supplements or dietary supplements) that have been promoted to prevent diabetes include natural agents that may slow carbohydrate absorption such as soluble fiber (most notably, glucomannan and chlorogenic acid) and legume-derived alpha-amylase inhibitors. Vitamin and mineral supplements promoted to prevent diabetes include the following:[37]

- *Biotin,* which, theoretically, in large doses may exert effects on beta cells, the liver, and skeletal muscle
- *Magnesium,* which is epidemiologically associated with reduced diabetes risk and greater insulin sensitivity
- *Chromium picolinate,* which appears to promote insulin sensitivity in individuals who may be chromium deficient
- *Calcium/vitamin D,* which could help preserve insulin sensitivity by preventing secondary hyperparathyroidism
- *Other suggested supplements,* such as extracts of bitter melon and of cinnamon

The American Diabetes Association has not, however, found sufficient evidence to warrant recommending any of these dietary supplements to individuals with prediabetes.[35] Chapter 19 discusses bitter melon, cinnamon, and chromium (although not specifically for use in prediabetes), provides a context for considering complementary therapies, and recommends resources for more information.

Weight Management in Children and Teens

The increasing prevalence of overweight youth in the United States and the associated increase in medical comorbidities has created a growing need for effective weight-management interventions.[39] The recommended treatment for an overweight child to achieve a more healthful weight uses 4 primary behavioral strategies:

- Reduce energy intake while maintaining optimal nutrient intake to protect growth and development
- Increase energy expenditure by promoting more physical movement and less sedentary activity
- Actively engage parents and primary caretakers as agents of change
- Facilitate a supportive family environment

Although general lifestyle guidelines for youth have empirical support, the global impact of these guidelines on the pediatric obesity epidemic has been limited, particularly for adolescents with more severe obesity and for African American, Native American, and Hispanic and Latino children. This has prompted efforts to adapt strategies that have been effective in adult weight management for use in pediatric behavioral intervention programs. These include the following:

- Using Motivational Interviewing to increase readiness for health behavior changes (see chapter 3)
- Modifying the carbohydrate content of children's diets
- Using culturally appropriate messages and materials
- Improving cultural competency of healthcare providers
- Using computer-based strategies

Randomized, controlled clinical trials are needed to test the safety and efficacy of these approaches before they can be recommended for clinical practice. The lifestyle interventions actively being implemented in the Studies to Treat Or Prevent Pediatric Type 2 Diabetes (STOPP-T2D) may provide some of these answers.

Medicare Medical Nutrition Therapy Act of 2005

Therapy for Prediabetes and Obesity

The Medicare Medical Nutrition Therapy Act of 2005 may, if passed, help Medicare beneficiaries receive medical nutrition therapy for prediabetes and obesity. The Act amends the Medicare Part B provision for medical nutrition therapy of the Benefits Improvement and Protection Act, which was passed in December 2000.[40] The broader language of the 2005 Act is designed to include all Medicare beneficiaries who have diseases, conditions, or disorders that the Secretary of the Department of Health and Human Services determines to require medical nutrition therapy (MNT), rather than just those who have diabetes and renal disease, as the previous Act allowed. The 2005 Act also grants the Secretary discretion to determine to what extent that therapy is allowed.

In and of itself, the 2005 Act does not extend MNT benefits. The Medicare Medical Nutrition Therapy Act of 2005 is expected to eventually extend Medicare MNT coverage, through the Center for Medicare and Medicaid Services, to include treating the following conditions when medically reasonable and necessary:

- Prediabetes
- Obesity
- Dyslipidemia
- Hypertension and prehypertension
- HIV/AIDS
- Cancer

This legislation may open the door to private insurers covering MNT. Historically, when Medicare begins coverage for a particular service or procedure, private insurers follow suit.

Public Health

A Community Approach to Diabetes Prevention

Community-based prevention activities may reduce the risk of diabetes. Understanding the community and healthcare facility allows better implementation of risk-reduction activities on a community level. A joint statement from the American Cancer Society, American Diabetes Association, and American Heart Association calls for public health approaches to obesity prevention to reduce the risks of developing cancer and heart disease as well as diabetes.[36]

Disparate rates of diabetes are related to environmental factors at the individual, family, and community level. Community differences in diabetes prevalence can be evaluated using a sociological framework. For example, social capital can be assessed to evaluate environmental quality. Statistical models can be used to assess the reciprocal relationship between civic engagement and health or other outcomes. With respect to diabetes risk, key variables appear to include the following:

- Level of engagement with local establishments, such as businesses, churches, hospitals, schools, health departments, and parks and recreation departments
- Interactions with neighbors for community improvement
- Food selection, including the ability to make choices based on health or other values
- Recreational opportunities
- Perceived safety

Subjective impressions of community members are more important than objective measurement by external groups. Community evaluation involves assessing the availability and quality of food and physical activity resources (eg, food markets, ability to use nonmotorized transportation, and recreational facilities).

The National Diabetes Education Program (NDEP) has tailored its diabetes prevention effort based on ongoing collaborations and input from representatives of high-risk population groups.[9] Community-based participatory research to help tailor diabetes prevention efforts requires the following:

- Integrating residents and representatives of the community and researchers as equal partners in every phase of the project
- Structurally and functionally integrating the intervention and evaluation research components
- Having a flexible agenda responsive to demands from the broader environment
- Creating a project that represents learning opportunities for all those involved

The emerging implementation model for community interventions is defined through an ongoing negotiation process.[41]

Conclusions and Future Directions

There is evidence-based support for a lifestyle intervention to prevent type 2 diabetes that focuses on weight loss of at least 5% to 7% of initial body weight and a diet low in fat (<30% of calories from fat, <10% saturated fat) and high in vegetables and fiber. Lifestyle intervention for individuals with IGT should target a BMI ≥24; however, for Asian Americans and possibly others, there appear to be benefits from weight loss and increased activity at lower levels of BMI (BMI ≥22).

Maintaining Weight Loss and Physical Activity

Whether the benefits of initial weight loss endure despite some regain is unclear. Possibly losing weight and regaining some back is more important than never losing any. The major clinical trials have not yet published papers examining this issue; however, a study by Swindburn et al[42] provides some preliminary data.

This 1-year, randomized, controlled trial of a reduced-fat diet versus a usual diet in 136 participants with IGT resulted in a 3.3-kg weight loss at 1 year in the intervention group and a significant improvement in glucose tolerance status compared to the control group, which gained 0.6 kg. The intervention group had no follow-up after the 1-year intervention and proceeded to regain weight with a weight loss of 3.15 kg at 2 years and 1.6 kg at 3 years and a gain of 1.06 kg at 5-year follow-up. At 5 years, the weight status of the intervention group and the control group were not significantly different, and there was no intervention effect on glucose tolerance at 2, 3, or 5 years. In this study, participants were not instructed to or expecting to lose weight; they were told they were in a study to test the effect of fat intake on blood sugar levels. In addition, the attrition rate was 24% at 2 years, 27% at 3 years, and 24% at 5-year follow-up.

A longer term follow-up of the DPP cohort will come from the Diabetes Prevention Program Outcomes study (DPPOS). With this study's large sample size and low attrition rates to date, more definitive answers and perspective on these issues may be obtained. The DPPOS will specifically address the following questions:

- How well can the weight loss and activity goals be maintained?
- What are the 5- to 10-year effects of lifestyle and metformin treatments on diabetes onset?
- Does delay in diabetes onset result in delay in diabetes complications?

Finding ways to help individuals sustain motivation and focus on lifestyle changes is important so these individuals are successful in keeping weight off and preventing diabetes for as long as possible. Within the DPPOS, all participants receive a quarterly lifestyle class, those in the metformin group continue on their prescribed medication, and the original lifestyle participants are offered 2 motivational campaigns per year.

Sociological Approaches

More translation research is necessary to facilitate efficient and cost-effective implementation of effective lifestyle interventions in various healthcare settings and population subgroups. Community-based research offers promise to examine environmental factors. New concepts include measuring social capital, which involves assessing social and behavioral determinants of health and well-being.[43] Recent analyses of state health and sociological data suggest that social capital may account for much of the relationship of the effects of poverty on obesity and diabetes. Multilevel, multimethod statistical analyses also provide opportunities to evaluate the effects of policy and environmental changes on the rates of obesity and diabetes.[44]

Genetics

Future research will provide valuable insights regarding the interaction of genes and diet in relation to the prevention of type 2 diabetes.[12] Lifestyle intervention trials of diabetes prevention with relatively few study participants and large observation cohort studies can help determine who may be genetically susceptible or resistant to the desired effects of a lifestyle intervention (weight loss and prevention of diabetes).

To date, the Finnish Diabetes Study has examined over 40 genes that have 1 or more single nucleotide polymorphisms (SNPs) that are involved in obesity, lipid metabolism, energy expenditure, body composition, insulin sensitivity, and insulin secretion. Variability in the nucleotides on the DNA strands appears to affect the double bonds and how genes function in regulating the complex interaction of physiological variables that determine diabetes risk. For example, individuals with a certain variant of a particular gene may lose less weight than those with a different variant of the same gene in response to a weight-loss dietary intervention.

Studies are underway to examine the roles of ghrelin (a hormone secreted by the stomach), which stimulates appetite, and adiponectin (a hormone secreted by fat cells that may reduce the inflammation). Adiponectin may potentially counteract the inflammatory effects of the cytokines, which fat cells also secrete. Research is likely to discover how genes and lifestyle interact in regulating the secretion and function of countless other factors involved in obesity and diabetes.

Focus on Education: Pearls for Practice

Teaching Strategies

- **Cohort studies.** Longitudinal, prospective cohort studies have provided important insights about how distribution of body weight, weight history, and lifestyle are related to the risk of developing diabetes. Presenting this information in language that is age- and intellectually appropriate offers the proof people need to begin to understand and contemplate what lifestyle changes need to take place to lower risk and diminish complications.

- **Landmark clinical trials.** The 4 landmark clinical trials that have contributed to the evidence base demonstrating the effectiveness of lifestyle interventions in preventing diabetes have common features, including diet, activity, and weight-loss goals; the process and duration of intervention; retention of participants in lifestyle treatment; and results in terms of diabetes risk reduction.

- **Genetics research.** Lifestyle interventions may, in the future, be tailored to the individual based on knowledge of how genotype variations affect response to lifestyle interventions.

- **Instructional tips.** Prepare handouts with tips to begin or support behaviors for losing weight, maintaining exercise as a daily activity, and meal planning options and references. Provide hands-on examples of snacks during class, and incorporate other elements in support of weight management and physical activity. Role-model healthy choices.

Messages for Patients

- **Know your risk factors.** Lifestyle and body composition (higher body fat and higher waist-to-hip ratio) are the greatest risk factors in adulthood. Modest lifestyle changes to reduce weight and decrease fat intake make a difference.

- **Implement important lifestyle changes.** Weight, activity, food intake, and meal planning are lifestyle elements that can be changed, especially with support and information from providers and educators.

- **Science is bringing hope for better solutions.** Research is discovering how genes and lifestyle interact in regulating countless factors involved in obesity and diabetes.

Suggested Readings

Diabetes Prevention Program Study Repository. For further information regarding the Diabetes Prevention Program lifestyle session, materials, and learning objectives. On the Internet: http://www.bsc.gwu.edu/dpp/manuals.htmlvdoc. Accessed 25 Jan 2006.

Knowler WC, Barrett-Connor E, Fowler SE, et al, for the Diabetes Prevention Research Group. Reduction in the evidence of type 2 diabetes with lifestyle intervention or metformin. N Engl J Med. 2001; 346:393-403.

Norris SL, Zhang X, Avenall A, et al. Long-term effectiveness of weight loss interventions in adults with prediabetes: a review. Am J Prev Med. 2005;28:126-39.

The Diabetes Prevention Program Research Group. The Diabetes Prevention Program (DPP): description of lifestyle intervention. Diabetes Care. 2002, 25:2165-71.

Tuomilehto J, Lindstrom J, Eriksson JG, et al. Prevention of type 2 diabetes mellitus by changes in lifestyle among subjects with impaired glucose tolerance. N Engl J Med. 2001;344:1342-50.

Wing RR, Hamman RF, Bray GA, et al; the Diabetes Prevention Program Research Group. Achieving weight and activity goals among diabetes prevention program lifestyle participants. Obes Res. 2004;12:1426-34.

References

1. American Association of Diabetes Educators. White paper on the prevention of type 2 diabetes and the role of the diabetes educator. Diabetes Educ. 2002;28:964-71.
2. Eriksson KF, Lindgarde F. Prevention of type 2 (non-insulin-dependent) diabetes mellitus by diet and exercise: the 6-year Malmo feasibility study. Diabetologia. 1991;34:891-8.
3. Pan XR, Li GW, Hu YH, et al. Effects of diet and exercise in preventing NIDDM in people with impaired glucose tolerance: the DaQing IGT and Diabetes Study. Diabetes Care. 1997;20:537-44.
4. Tuomilehto J, Lindstrom J, Eriksson JG, et al. Prevention of type 2 diabetes mellitus by changes in lifestyle among subjects with impaired glucose tolerance. N Engl J Med. 2001;344:1342-50.
5. Knowler WC, Barrett-Connor E, Fowler SE, et al, for the Diabetes Prevention Research Group. Reduction in the evidence of type 2 diabetes with lifestyle intervention or metformin. N Engl J Med. 2001; 346:393-403.
6. Wild S, Roglic G, Green A, Sicree R, King H. Global prevalence of diabetes: estimates for the year 2000 and projections for 2030. Diabetes Care. 2004;27:1047-53.
7. National Heart, Lung, and Blood Institute. Clinical Guidelines on the Identification, Evaluation, and Treatment of Overweight and Obesity in Adults. Bethesda, Md: National Heart, Lung, and Blood Institute; 1998.
8. National Diabetes Education Program. Diabetes Prevention. www.ndep.nih.gov/diabetes/prev/prevention.htm. Accessed 21 Nov 2005.
9. Roche HM, Phillips C, Gibney MJ. The metabolic syndrome: the crossroads of diet and genetics. Proc Nutr Soc. 2005;64:371-7.
10. Kim C, Newton KM, Knopp RH. Gestational diabetes and the incidence of type 2 diabetes. a systematic review. Diabetes Care. 2002;25:1862-8.
11. American Diabetes Association. Gestational diabetes mellitus (position statement). Diabetes Care. 2003;26 Suppl 1:S103-5.
12. Centers for Disease Control. National diabetes fact sheet 2005. http://www.cdc.gov/diabetes/pubs/factsheet05.htm. Accessed 27 Nov 2005.
13. Prentice AM, Rayco-Solon P, Moore SE. Insights from the developing world: thrifty genotypes and thrifty phenotypes. Proc Nutr Soc. 2005;64:153-61.
14. Pearce MS, Unwin NC, Relton CL, Alberti KG, Parker L. Lifecourse determinants of fasting and post-challenge glucose at age 50 years: the Newcastle Thousand Families Study. Eur J Epidemiol. 2005;20:915-23.
15. World Health Organization Consultation. Appropriate body-mass index for Asian populations and its implications for policy and intervention strategies. Lancet. 2004;363:157-63.
16. Salmenniemi U, Ruotsalainen E, Pihlajamaki J, et al. Multiple abnormalities in glucose and energy metabolism and coordinated changes in levels of adiponectin, cytokines, and adhesion molecules in subjects with metabolic syndrome. Circulation. 2004;110:3842-8.
17. American Diabetes Association. Diagnosis and classification of diabetes mellitus (position statement). Diabetes Care. 2006;29:S3-48.

18. Edelman D, Olsen MK, Dudley TK, Harris AC, Oddone EZ. Utility of hemoglobin A1c in predicting diabetes risk. J Gen Intern Med. 2004;19:1175-80.

19. Lindstrom J, Toumilehto J. The Diabetes Risk Score: a practical tool to predict diabetes risk. Diabetes Care. 2003; 26:725-31.

20. Norris SL, Zhang X, Avenall A, et al. Long-term effectiveness of weight loss interventions in adults with pre-diabetes: a review. Am J Prev Med. 2005;28:126-39.

21. Lindgarde F, Eriksson KF, Lithell H, Saltin B. Coupling between dietary changes, reduced body weight, muscle fiber size and improved glucose tolerance in middle-aged men with impaired glucose tolerance. Acta Medica Scandinavica. 1982;212:99-106.

22. Li G, Hu Y, Yang W, et al. Effects of insulin resistance and insulin secretion on the efficacy of interventions to retard development of type 2 diabetes mellitus: the DA Qing IGT and Diabetes Study. Diabetes Res Clin Pract. 2002;58:193-200.

23. Lindström J, Louheranta A, Mannelin M, et al. The Finnish Diabetes Prevention Study (DPS): lifestyle intervention and 3-year results on diet and physical activity. Diabetes Care. 2003;26:3230-6.

24. Uusitupa M, Lindi V, Louheranta A, et al. Long-term improvement in insulin sensitivity by changing lifestyles of people with impaired glucose tolerance: 4-year results from the Finnish Diabetes Prevention Study. Diabetes. 2003;52:2532-8.

25. Uusitipa M. Gene-diet interaction in relation to the prevention of obesity and diabetes; evidence from the Finnish Diabetes Prevention Study. Nutr Metab Cardiovasc Dis. 2005;15:225-33.

26. The Diabetes Prevention Program Research Group. The Diabetes Prevention Program (DPP): description of the lifestyle intervention. Diabetes Care. 2002;25:2165-71.

27. Wylie-Rosett J, Delahanty L. An integral role of the dietitian: implications of the Diabetes Prevention Program. J Am Diet Assoc. 2002;102(8):1065-8.

28. The Diabetes Prevention Program Research Group. Impact of intensive lifestyle and metformin therapy on cardiovascular disease risk factors in the Diabetes Prevention Program. Diabetes Care. 2005;28(4):888-94.

29. The Diabetes Prevention Program Research Group. The effect of metformin and intensive lifestyle intervention on the metabolic syndrome: The Diabetes Prevention Program randomized trial. Ann Intern Med. 2005;142:611-9.

30. The Diabetes Prevention Program Research Group. Intensive lifestyle intervention or metformin on inflammation and coagulation in participants with impaired glucose tolerance. Diabetes. 2005;54:1566-72.

31. Mayer-Davis EJ, Sparks KC, Hirsh K, et al, for the Diabetes Prevention Research Group. Dietary intake in the Diabetes Prevention Program cohort: baseline and 1-year post randomization. Ann Epidemiol. 2004;14:763-72.

32. Wing RR, Hamman RF, Bray GA, et al. The Diabetes Prevention Program Research Group. achieving weight and activity goals among diabetes prevention program lifestyle participants. Obes Res. 2004;12:1426-34.

33. Kriska AM, Delahanty LM, Pettee KK. Lifestyle intervention for the prevention of type 2 diabetes: translation and future recommendations. Cur Diab Rep. 2004;4:113-8.

34. Newell-Morris LI, Treder RP, Shurman WP, et al. Fatness, fat distribution and glucose intolerance in second generation Japanese-American (Nesi) men. Am J Clin Nutr. 1989;50:9-18.

35. American Diabetes Association. Standards of medical care (position statement). Diabetes Care. 2006;29 Suppl 1:S4-42.

36. Eyre H, Kahn R, Robertson RM, American Cancer Society, the American Diabetes Association and the American Heart Association Collaborative Writing Group. Preventing cancer, cardiovascular disease and diabetes: a common agenda for the American Cancer Society, American Diabetes Association and American Heart Association. Diabetes Care. 2004;27:1812-24.

37. Mc Carty MF. Nutraceutical resources for diabetes prevention: an update. Med Hypothesis. 2005;64:151-8.

38. Glasgow RE, Wagner EH, Kaplan RM, et al. If diabetes is a public health problem, why not treat it as one? a population-based approach to chronic illness. Ann Behav Med. 1999;21:159-70.

39. Kirk S, Scott BJ, Daniels SR Pediatric obesity epidemic: treatment options. J Am Diet Assoc. 2005;105(5 Suppl 1):S44-51.

40. American Medical Directors Association. AMDA Fact Sheet on S. 604 and H.R. 1582 Medicare Medical Nutrition Therapy Act of 2005. On the Internet: www.amda.com/federalaffairs/factsheets/congress109/s604.htm. Accessed 25 Nov 2005.

41. Potvin L, Cargo M, McComber AM, Delorimer T, Macaulay AC. Implementing participatory intervention and research in communities: lessons from the Kahnawake Schools Diabetes Prevention Project in Canada. Soc Sci Med. 2003;56:1295-1305.

42. Swinburn BA, Metcalf PA, Ley SJ. Long-term (5-year) effects of a reduced-fat diet intervention in individuals with glucose intolerance. Diabetes Care. 2001;24(4):619-24.

43. Holtgrave DR, Crosby R. Is social capital a protective factor against obesity and diabetes? findings from an exploratory study. Ann Epidemiol. In press, corrected proof: available online 24 Oct 2005.

44. Windle M, Grunbaum JA, Elliott M, et al. Healthy passages: a multilevel, multimethod longitudinal study of adolescent health. Am J Prev Med. 2004;27:164-72.

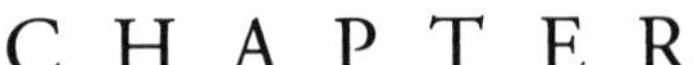

CHAPTER

3

Self-Management of Health

Authors

Bob Anderson, EdD
Martha M. Funnell, MS, RN, CDE
Tricia S. Tang, PhD

Key Concepts

- Be familiar with behavioral and educational theories that support self-management of health. These include Patient Empowerment, the Health Belief Model, Social Cognitive Theory, the Theory of Reasoned Action and Theory of Planned Behavior, and the Transtheoretical Model with its construct of Stages of Change.
- Be aware that some models also support patient-centered communication techniques useful for stimulating behavior change, such as Motivational Interviewing.
- Learn to assess whether a theory will assist in understanding the intended goals and purpose in a specific application, whether that will be in program design or individual practice. Will the theory describe, explain, predict, or control or influence outcomes as desired?
- Think critically about the appropriateness of a theory for a specific application: Does the theory resonate within this context? Does it extend thinking? Is the approach useful in this situation? Can its main attributes be measured in this application?
- Recognize the compatibility or incompatibility of theories used in combination within an educational program.

Introduction

The mission of diabetes self-management education (DSME) is to help individuals with diabetes acquire the knowledge, skills, attitudes, and behaviors needed to optimize both their self-management of diabetes and their quality of life. The field of diabetes education has advanced substantially over the past 25 years. The profession has learned that a knowledge-based approach to DSME is not enough to accomplish the mission. Knowledge may be a necessary component of DMSE, but acquiring information is not enough to ensure that the individual has learned all he or she needs to know to live well with a lifelong chronic illness.

Modern diabetes education programs focus on helping people with diabetes identify and adopt the behaviors that will optimize their diabetes self-management and overall well-being. These education programs address knowledge and skill acquisition, but they include much more. For example, they teach problem solving and goal setting, they address the psychosocial aspects of diabetes along with the clinical aspects, they help the person with diabetes define and acquire social support, and they teach the coping skills necessary for managing diabetes in challenging social situations and personal relationships.

The purpose of this introduction is not to list all the attributes of modern DSME, but to illustrate how complex and sophisticated this specialty has become. In addition to having clinical and teaching skills, today's diabetes educator needs to understand and be able to apply theoretical approaches to facilitating the self-directed behavior changes of their patients (or clients). Moreover, those involved in this educational effort need to be able to distinguish and even combine evidence-based theoretical approaches to behavior change that have proved efficacious in DSME. The purpose of this chapter is to help educators gain the knowledge necessary to develop and apply a sound theory-based approach to DSME.

Before presenting the major theoretical approaches for influencing the self-management behavior of those with diabetes, this chapter outlines considerations pertinent to choosing theories appropriately for application in diabetes education. After discussing how to choose theories to apply to a program or individual practice, the chapter describes 5 theories that are of value in understanding an individual's health behavior and seeking to influence it. A patient-centered communication technique is also presented. A summary is given of each approach, including a look at the body of evidence regarding its use in diabetes education:

- Patient Empowerment
- Health Belief Model
- Social Cognitive Theory
- Theory of Reasoned Action and Theory of Planned Behavior
- Transtheoretical Model, incorporating the construct of Stages of Change
- Motivational Interviewing

Applying Theory in Diabetes Education

The word theory was used several times in the introduction. Before an educator selects specific theoretical approaches to behavior change to apply in program design or individual practice, time must be spent thinking about the usefulness of the theory, or theories, in the intended application. Educators and other clinicians need to carefully choose the behavioral and educational theories they will apply—both for individual practice and in the design, conduct, and evaluation of education programs.[1] Chosen wisely, the theories help members of the diabetes care team understand and influence the behavior of the individuals with diabetes whom they serve. With a clear conception of what theories are and how they can be used, the educator can best compare the relative merits of specific theoretical approaches to facilitating health-related behavior change. Material in this section provides the information necessary for such comparisons.

Matching Theory With Purpose

Behavioral and educational theories are usually selected for use in educational program design and individual practice based on how well they meet 1 or more of the 4 purposes detailed below: describing, explaining, predicting, and controlling/influencing.[2-4]

Describing. The first purpose of a theory is describing the phenomena of interest. The theory tells us the way things are, but not why they are the way they are or how they are likely to change. The value of descriptive theory is largely dependent on how coherent and thorough it is. For example, suppose we had noticed that patients graduating from the diabetes education program on the east side of town got consistently higher scores on the same knowledge test than patients graduating from another program on the west side of town. We could begin our theory building by developing a thorough description about what we observed. How many observations were involved? Was the difference in test scores always in the same direction and similar in magnitude? Were the patients in both programs similar (eg, age, gender, socioeconomic status) Were the educators in both programs Certified Diabetes Educators? The answers to these and similar questions would constitute our descriptive theory.

Explaining. The second purpose of theory is explanation. Our descriptive theory has answered the question, "What is happening?" Now attention turns to the question, "Why is it happening?" We want to know what caused the differences in the knowledge test scores. We might examine the programs to see if we could develop a theory to explain what we had observed. If the only significant difference we could find between the 2 programs was that the program on the east side of town provided 60% more instructional time than the other, we might theorize that increasing the amount of time spent on instruction accounted for the better test results.

Predicting. The third purpose of a theory is prediction. Using the example above, our new educational theory would be considered robust if it proved to be true in other settings (ie, other diabetes programs). Consistent correlations, in the expected direction between instructional time and educational achievement, derived from data found in other studies would support a prediction of similar results based on these factors.

Controlling or Influencing. Our new education theory would be viewed as even more robust and useful if we conducted experiments that demonstrated we could manipulate instructional time to produce (influence) better educational outcomes. The ability of our theory to influence educational achievement in this example could be contrasted with a theory that is less useful (for our purposes) because it cannot be manipulated to produce better outcomes (eg, a theory about IQ and learning).

Choosing a Theory That Fits

When choosing a theory to apply to a program design or for individual practice, 3 areas of inquiry are important to consider: how well it resonates with us, how it extends our thinking, and how useful it appears to be.

Does It Resonate? The first area of inquiry addresses the compatibility between the theory and our sense of how people learn and behave. Questions to ask are, "Does this theory fit with my experience of how I learn and change?" and/or "Does it resonate with my approach to diabetes education?" Those working in diabetes education are unlikely to make effective use of a theory unless they feel an affinity for the vision or worldview embedded in it.

Does It Extend Thinking? The second area of inquiry considers whether the theory helps organize and expand our ideas and observations into a coherent pattern. Does this theory provide a thorough description of the phenomena of interest? Does this theory offer a plausible explanation for why things happen the way they do? Does the theory challenge us to reflect on aspects of our practice or program design that we may not have considered fully? In other words, is the theory not only consistent with our perspective on learning and behaving, but does it help enhance and expand our perspective?

Is This Approach Useful? The third area of inquiry should address the utility of the theory. Can this theory be translated into specific practice behaviors or strategies that will enhance our effectiveness? Does this theory help us design and evaluate our education programs?

Choosing an Approach That Can Be Measured

A theory's usefulness is also very much related to the user's ability to measure its main attributes. For example, from the earlier example on using multiple theories, we would need to answer the following types of questions: What measures of Patient Empowerment and the Health Belief Model exist? Have these measures/instruments been shown to be valid and reliable?

Ensure the theory is appropriate to the specific practice or program:

- Is there a convincing evidence base indicating that this theory can be used to facilitate learning and behavior change effectively?
- Is it a good fit with the kind of diabetes care and education I provide?
- Can this theory help guide my practice and program design in one or more of these ways: Can I visualize how I would apply this theory in one-to-one interactions with patients? Can I visualize how I would apply this theory when group teaching? Can I incorporate this theory into the design of my program?
- After conducting some sessions (or programs), will it be apparent whether or not this theory improved my practice (or programs)?

Using Multiple Theories

Educators can and often do use more than one theory in individual practice and in developing education programs. When using a combination of theories, compatibility is important; the theories must embody the same worldview. Also, each theory must make an independent contribution to the user's effectiveness. For example:

- *The Patient Empowerment approach posits this:* Individuals will carry out self-management tasks more consistently and over a longer period of time if those tasks were freely chosen by patients to help them reach their own goals.[5]
- *The Health Belief Model posits this:* The health-related choices people make are a function of their beliefs about their susceptibility to the disease (diabetes, in this instance) and its complications, the severity of diabetes and its complications, the efficacy of available treatments, and the ability to carry out those treatment options.[6]
- *In combination:* These two frameworks for understanding could be combined and incorporated into the design of a patient education program. Patient Empowerment could be used as the program's overall approach to facilitating behavior change, and the Health Belief Model could be used to order and sequence the educational content of the program.

Both at the individual practitioner and program levels, theories can be important tools for the design, understanding, and conduct of diabetes patient education. Theory-based practice and evaluation add to professionals' understanding of how to be effective educators and enhance the credibility of the profession.

Theoretical Approaches to Behavior Change

Five major approaches to influencing the health behavior of persons with diabetes are described in this section:

- Patient Empowerment
- Health Belief Model
- Social Cognitive Theory
- Theory of Reasoned Action and Theory of Planned Behavior
- Transtheoretical Model

In addition, this section looks at a patient-centered communication technique, aimed at stimulating behavior change, that has been used to improve diabetes self-management:

- Motivational Interviewing

For each approach to behavior change, this chapter describes the theory and its primary components, applies the theory to diabetes-related behavior, and summarizes the research to date that has used the theory in understanding and promoting diabetes self-management. The "Case in Point" shows how the concepts of each approach can be applied to a diabetes-specific patient example. Tables throughout the chapter summarize information on each approach and then address issues pertinent to the case so readers can see the differences and similarities among the components of each model.

Patient Empowerment

Patient Empowerment was introduced in 1991 to the diabetes literature[7] and has been incorporated into a variety of educational and care programs since then.[8,9] Patient Empowerment is more of a philosophical approach than a theory. Although it has all the elements necessary for

Case in Point: Applying Behavioral Models in Diabetes Care and Education

MG is a 48-year-old woman who was diagnosed with type 2 diabetes 5 years ago. She is a mother of 2 children, ages 13 and 16. For the past 12 months, MG has been working as a receptionist at the internal medicine outpatient clinic affiliated with a teaching hospital in the greater Detroit area. Prior to this position, she worked as an office assistant at a small advertising agency. Her current job provides healthcare benefits, and her previous position did not.

- MG does not check her blood glucose regularly during her work day because she feels self-conscious about coworkers discovering she has diabetes
- She encounters difficulty when making nutritional choices because her husband and children prefer high-fat and high-sugar foods for snacks and mealtimes
- Until several months ago, she had not been involved in any regular exercise

robust theory that were described in the first part of this chapter, Patient Empowerment goes beyond theory in that it speaks to values and vision of the educator. Empowerment grew out of the traditions of community psychology, adult education, and counseling psychology. Empowerment is defined as helping patients discover and develop their inherent capacity to be responsible for their own lives and gain mastery over their diabetes.[7] The Empowerment approach is based on 3 characteristics of diabetes that differentiate this disease from an acute illness:[5]

- The choices that have the greatest effect on metabolic and other outcomes are made by patients, not health professionals
- Patients are in control of their self-management
- The consequences of self-management decisions accrue first and foremost to patients; thus, it is both their right and responsibility to be the primary decision-makers

Within the Empowerment approach, the purpose of education is to enable participants to gain more power over their lives, increase the number of choices available to them, and enhance their ability to influence the individuals and organizations around them.[7] A 5-step behavior change model is a fundamental component for applying this approach to diabetes self-management education. The purpose of the model is to assist patients in identifying behaviors they wish to address and then create a self-directed behavior change plan. The role of the diabetes educator is to ask questions and actively listen to the patients' responses so that patients learn through hearing themselves and through reflection prompted by the educator's questions. Table 3.1 illustrates the 5-step model used in Patient Empowerment.

Evidence Base. Patient Empowerment has been used as the theoretical basis for patient education among both individuals[10,11] and groups of patients.[12-15] A study conducted to evaluate an education program designed specifically to teach patients the skills of Empowerment resulted in significant improvements in self-efficacy and metabolic outcomes, although diabetes clinical content was not part of the program.[16,17]

In a more recent study among African Americans, the Empowerment approach was used to develop a problem-based, culturally tailored diabetes self-management education program offered at a variety of community-based settings in a large urban area.[18-20] Using a wait-listed control group design, the intervention was provided over 6 weeks for a total of 10 hours of education. The sessions were led by a nurse and dietitian, both of whom were Certified Diabetes Educators. The mean number of sessions attended was 5.2, and all participants showed a broad array of small-to-modest positive metabolic and other changes that were maintained or improved during the 1-year follow-up period.[18]

Strategies implemented in this program that embodied the Empowerment approach included the following:

- Affirming that the person with diabetes is responsible for and in control of the daily self-management of diabetes
- Educating patient to promote informed decision-making rather than adherence/compliance
- Teaching how to set goals and providing weekly experience in setting goals
- Integrating clinical, psychosocial, and behavioral aspects of diabetes into education
- Affirming participants as experts in their own learning needs

TABLE 3.1 Empowerment-Based, Self-Directed Behavior Change Model

Step	*Questions*	*Case in Point*
Define problem	What is your greatest concern about diabetes? What is hardest for you? What is causing you the most distress?	MG has struggled with her weight and making changes in her eating habits since her diabetes was diagnosed. She identifies the "real" issue as her family and their lack of support for her efforts.
Identify feelings	What are your thoughts or feelings about this concern?	MG is very afraid that if she does not lower her blood glucose levels she will go blind or lose a leg. She also feels angry at her family that they do not seem concerned about her future health. She does not feel she can be open about her diabetes at work because she is worried the staff in the clinic will judge her food and other choices. During the discussion, she recognizes that feeling alone in managing diabetes is the hardest thing for her.
Identify long-term goals	What do you want? What are your options? What barriers will you face? How important is it for you to address this issue? What are the costs and benefits of addressing this problem? Of not addressing this problem?	MG believes that to truly take charge of her diabetes she needs to gain support for her efforts, primarily from her family.
Identify short-term behavior change plan	Are you willing to take steps to solve this problem? What are some steps you could take? What are you going to do? When? How will you evaluate it?	MG feels that the first step is to write down exactly how she feels and what she wants so that she can better ask her family for their help. She will complete this during the next week.
Implement and evaluate plan	How did it go? What did you learn? What would you do differently next time? What will you do when you leave here today?	Upon reading back what she had written, MG recognizes that while she cannot force her family to change, she also has not asked for their support or told them what she needs. She decides to speak with her husband privately next week. In addition, she will attend a weight-loss support group with a friend to see if she finds this helpful.

- Affirming the ability of participants to determine an approach to diabetes self-management that will work for them
- Affirming the innate capacity of patients to identify and learn to solve their own problems
- Creating opportunities for social support
- Providing ongoing self-management support following diabetes self-management education

Using this same approach in a pilot study providing weekly support groups for African Americans yielded significant improvements in body mass index, cholesterol levels, and self-care behavior.[19] Although the sessions were offered weekly for 24 weeks, participants were encouraged to attend only as often as they felt the need. Ninety percent of the subjects attended at least 1 session and 40% attended at least 12 sessions. Five components were identified as the basis for this program:

1. **Reflecting** on diabetes self-management experiments: Sessions began with a discussion of participant's experiences over the past week
2. **Discussing** the emotional impact of living with diabetes: Discussion of psychosocial aspects of diabetes was integrated with clinical content discussion
3. **Solving problems** systematically in the group: Primary focus of program was participant-driven; based on their problems and concerns
4. **Responding** to diabetes self-management questions: Clinical content typically provided by lecture was instead given in response to questions raised by participants
5. **Choosing** a diabetes self-management experiment: Participants were encouraged to select a self-management goal as a behavioral experiment for the next week

Health Belief Model

The Health Belief Model (HBM) has been widely used as a theoretical framework to understand health behavior change and maintenance.[21] The model was first introduced in the 1950s when behavioral scientists at the US Public Health Service sought to understand the low participation rates in government-sponsored, cost-free, and easily accessible screening, detection, and immunization programs.[21,22] Under this model, a patient's decision to perform a "target" health behavior is influenced by the following factors:[21]

- Level of personal vulnerability the patient feels about developing the illness
- Seriousness the patient believes the illness is or has the potential to be
- Efficacy of the behavior, in patient's view, in preventing the development or minimizing consequences of the illness
- Costs or deterrents associated with performing the behavior relative to the benefits achieved as a result

This Health Belief Model was expanded, later, to include 2 additional constructs:[21]

- Cues to action
- Self-efficacy

Table 3.2 provides definitions of the expanded model's constructs and examples of these constructs in relation to diabetes self-management.

Evidence Base. A large and growing body of research has utilized the Health Belief Model in explaining diabetes self-care behaviors.[22-29] Among a sample of 31 African American women diagnosed with type 2 diabetes, Koch investigated differences between women who engaged in regular physical activity and those who did not.[23] He found significant group differences in the perceived benefits and perceived barriers: the physical activity group reported greater perceived benefits and less perceived barriers than their counterparts. Another study conducted by Aljasem and colleagues examined the role of barriers and self-efficacy in self-management behaviors in 309 patients diagnosed with type 2 diabetes.[24] The data revealed that the more barriers patients perceived to performing self-care behaviors, the less likely they were to follow a healthy diet or engage in physical activity. Additionally, patients who reported a greater level of self-efficacy were more likely to test their blood glucose frequently and less likely to forget taking their medication or engage in binge-eating behavior.

The HBM has also been applied to diabetes self-management research conducted outside the United States.[30-33] In a sample of 128 Chinese men and women diagnosed with type 2 diabetes, Tan et al reported that subjects who felt

TABLE 3.2 Health Belief Model: Constructs and Application to Diabetes Self-Management

Construct	*Definition*	*Case in Point*
Perceived susceptibility	Estimate of personal vulnerability to developing an illness	MG's diabetes has been poorly controlled for 5 years, and her father had gone blind as a result of diabetes. Therefore, she believes her risk level for developing diabetes-related complication is high.
Perceived severity	Perception of how serious an illness is and can be if diagnosed	MG thinks that if she does not get her blood glucoses under control she will go blind or lose a leg because of her diabetes.
Perceived benefits	Perception of how a specific action will lead to a positive outcome	MG believes that checking her blood glucose frequently and taking her diabetes medication as prescribed will substantially minimize the chances of her going blind or having her leg amputated in the long-term.
Perceived barriers	Perception of the deterrents to engaging in a behavior or the costs associated with a behavior	MG feels that checking her blood glucose several times a day can be a burden. She also does not want her coworkers to find out she has diabetes because she is worried they will start monitoring what she eats throughout the day.
Self-efficacy	Level of confidence one has in engaging in the identified health behavior	MG feels fairly confident that she can find a private place to check her blood glucoses during the work day.
Cues to action	External stimulus used to activate health behavior	MG sees TV commercials about the latest blood glucose monitors and remembers to check her own blood glucose.

a greater vulnerability to developing diabetes-related complications, who believed diabetes to be a very serious condition, and who reported fewer deterrents to engaging in self-care behaviors were more likely to engage in diabetes-related preventive care behaviors.[30] Similarly, a study conducted with 34 aboriginal subjects with type 2 diabetes living in British Columbia found perceived severity and perceived barriers to be predictors of A1C improvement over a period of 18 months.[31] Moreover, subjects who believed diabetes to be a serious condition and reported fewer barriers to self-management at 18 months were more likely to have reduced their A1C between baseline and an 18-month follow-up.

Given the research supporting the HBM in explaining and predicting diabetes self-management behaviors, it is not surprising that many researchers have used it as the framework in designing self-management interventions. For instance, using this model as a framework, Wdowik et al conducted focus groups and interviews with college students diagnosed with type 1 diabetes to explore factors associated with diabetes self-management practices.[33] Results identified prominent barriers to self-care in this group, including such things as economic constraints, stress, fear of hypoglycemic events, and dietary restrictions. Findings from this qualitative study were used to design an intervention called "Control on Campus." The researchers found that students assigned to the intervention group demonstrated greater improvements in diabetes-related knowledge, attitudes, and behaviors than the control group. Specifically, they found at the end of the study that the intervention students reported reduced anxiety around glucose testing, greater frequency of glucose testing, and greater likelihood of glucose testing when experiencing symptoms.

Based on constructs of the Health Belief Model, Scollan-Koliopoulos developed and implemented a church-based educational intervention aimed at improving foot care among African Americans diagnosed with type 2 diabetes.[34] Prior to the intervention, participants completed self-report surveys assessing their perceived risk for diabetes-related amputation as well as beliefs and behaviors related to amputation. The intervention consisted of 3 parts: viewing a video on how to perform foot care, observing a foot care demonstration by a healthcare provider, and developing the skills to use a monofilament. In addition, participants were given educational materials on diabetes and foot care. Following this intervention, several participants served as outreach educators and disseminated information to 27 other African Americans, distributed 36 pamphlets, and demonstrated foot care to 12 others.

Social Cognitive Theory

Social Cognitive Theory (SCT) evolved from Bandura's Social Learning Theory (SLT), which stated that individuals learn not only from their own personal experiences, but also from observing the behaviors and behavioral consequences of others.[21] Adding further complexity, SCT examines health behavior as a constantly changing and evolving interaction between the individual and his/her environment. Social Cognitive Theory contains multiple constructs that can be used to understand health behavior change. This section describes the major constructs and applies them to diabetes self-management. Social Cognitive Theory addresses 2 areas:[21]

- Psychosocial factors that influence health behavior
- Methods of stimulating behavior change

Table 3.3 presents and defines the concepts of Social Cognitive Theory and applies them to an example of diabetes self-management.

Evidence Base. Social Cognitive Theory has been widely used in understanding diabetes care practices and designing diabetes intervention programs. The theory has been applied for patients with type 1 and type 2 diabetes and used across different age groups, including adolescents and adults.[35-39] Self-management interventions have focused on the following:

- Increasing physical activity
- Improving dietary choices and patterns
- Promoting frequent blood glucose testing

A literature review conducted by Allen examined the research, from 1985 to 2002, on the role of SCT, specifically the construct of self-efficacy, in explaining and predicting physical activity and the long-term maintenance of activity over time among patients with diabetes.[35] Of the 13 studies reviewed that met preestablished criteria, all studies with a correlational design found a significant positive association between self-efficacy and physical activity, and all studies with a predictive design found self-efficacy to be a significant predictor for physical activity. The studies that specifically examined physical activity maintenance found that self-efficacy predicted patient ability to sustain physical activity over the study follow-up period.

Other self-management studies using SCT as a framework have focused exclusively on improving dietary habits. For instance, Miller et al applied the SCT principles of expectations and self-efficacy in developing a 10-week intervention aimed at increasing food label knowledge and skills among 93 older patients with a recent diagnosis of type 2 diabetes.[37] Compared to the control group, subjects in the experimental group demonstrated a greater knowledge of food labels and a greater number of positive outcome expectations. The experimental groups also reported a greater confidence in engaging in behaviors that facilitated self-management and avoiding behaviors that deterred self-management.

TABLE 3.3 Social Cognitive Theory: Concepts, Definitions, and Application to Diabetes Self-Management

Concept	*Definition*	*Case in Point*
Reciprocal determinism	The constant interaction of the individual, behavior, and environment	MG wants to take care of her diabetes better, so she starts to cook lower fat dinners. Her family complains these meals do not taste good. Fresh produce is also very costly at the local grocery. Given all these issues, after 2 weeks MG returns to cooking as she had previously.
Environment	The external factors and surroundings of an individual	The climate and atmosphere at MG's home/family, work, community, neighborhood, social circle, etc.
Behavioral capability	The knowledge and skills required to perform a specific behavior	MG recently attended a diabetes self-management educational program. In this program, she learned how to check her blood glucose in a way that does not invite attention or cause disruption in her work day. As a result, her capability in performing this behavior is high.
Expectations	The result that an individual anticipates as a result of performing a specific behavior	MG believes that if she starts exercising and playing tennis regularly, her A1C will probably be lower at the next physician visit.
Observational learning	Utilizing the experiences of others' performance of a behavior as a way to acquire that specific behavior	MG has seen her father's health deteriorate as a result of not taking care of his diabetes. He also did not receive annual retinopathy screenings. At the age of 64, her father had gone blind. Due to this experience, MG has received annual eye exams.
Reinforcements	The responses an individual receives that facilitate or deter the future performance of a specific behavior	Three weeks after starting tennis, MG noticed her clothes were fitting better. This weight loss served as a positive reinforcement for her to continue playing tennis 3 times per week.
Self-efficacy	The level of confidence an individual has with regard to performing a behavior successfully	Given that MG enjoys playing tennis and uses it as a time to socialize with her girlfriends, she has a high level of confidence that this will remain a permanent part of her lifestyle.

Finally, some studies have developed SCT-guided interventions to improve multiple diabetes care-related behaviors. Toobert and colleagues utilized SCT principles in developing the Mediterranean Lifestyle Trial, an intervention aimed at preventing coronary heart disease among high-risk women diagnosed with type 2 diabetes.[39] These authors hypothesize that self-efficacy along with other concepts are key mechanisms in improving and maintaining self-care behaviors such as healthy nutritional choices, physical activity, and emotional coping.

Theory of Reasoned Action and Theory of Planned Behavior

The Theory of Reasoned Action (TRA) developed by Fishbein is extended by Azjen in the Theory of Planned Behavior (TPB). This combined model (TRA-TPB) of behavior change operates through 3 major constructs:

- Attitudes and beliefs the individual has toward the target health behavior
- How the individual thinks others in the general public or community view the health behavior (subjective norm)
- Extent to which the individual is equipped with the knowledge and skills to perform the behavior (perceived behavioral control)

These 3 constructs work together to determine how strong an individual's intention is related to performing the health behavior, which, consequently, leads to the likelihood that individual will demonstrate the health behavior.[21] Table 3.4 lists the elements of the TRA-TPB model and applies them to a diabetes-specific example.

Evidence Base. A study conducted by Syrala and colleagues utilized the TRA-TPB to examine the relationship between dental care practices and diabetes self-management among patients diagnosed with type 1

TABLE 3.4 Theory of Reasoned Action and Theory of Planned Behavior—Concepts and Application to Diabetes Self-Management

Concept	*Case in Point*
Attitude and belief about behavior	MG believes that physical activity is an effective method of managing her blood glucose levels
Subjective norm	MG values the opinion of her healthcare team (physician, nurse educator, and dietitian) who have all recommended that engaging in some type of physical activity will help manage her diabetes.
Perceived behavioral control	MG would like to play tennis as her physical activity. She took tennis lessons in the past, knows there are tennis courts near her house, and has two friends who have offered to play with her.
Behavioral intention	Based on the factors above, MG's intention to start playing tennis as one way of managing her diabetes is fairly strong.
Behavior	MG incorporates physical activity into her schedule 3 times a week for 60 minutes.

diabetes.[40] In a sample of 149 patients ages 16 to 72 attending a diabetes clinic affiliated with a teaching institution in Finland, these researchers found a significant positive relationship between attitudes toward and normative beliefs related to tooth brushing and tooth brushing intentions and behavior. Additionally, individuals who expressed a greater intention to brush their teeth were more likely to report more frequent brushing behavior. Finally, individuals with better attitudes and greater intentions to brush demonstrated better diabetes self-management and had lower A1C levels, respectively.

Components of the TRA-TPB have been integrated in a proposed prevention program targeting minority children at risk for developing type 2 diabetes. Specifically, Burnet et al outlined the TRA-TPB-related constructs including beliefs and knowledge, attitudes, normative beliefs, and behavioral intention as critical aspects of prevention behavior.[41] Burnet et al theorize that a child's beliefs and knowledge about an illness or associated health behaviors influence the child's attitudes about the health behavior. In turn, attitudes in combination with a child's belief about the public perception of the health behavior (normative beliefs) factor into the child's intention to perform the behavior. Finally, a child's level of intention to take action will ultimately determine the actual occurrence of the health behavior.

Transtheoretical Model

The Transtheoretical Model (TTM) was first introduced by DiClemente and Prochaska as a framework for understanding smoking cessation behavior.[21] A major construct within this model is Stages of Change. The behavior change process is marked by 6 distinct stages.[21]

Precontemplation → Contemplation →
Preparation → Action → Maintenance → Termination

The model focuses on an individual's "readiness" to make a behavior change. Behavior change, viewed in a temporal perspective, is seen as an ongoing process, rather than as a specific outcome. During the process, an individual will have different levels of motivation to change behavior. Table 3.5 lists and defines the stages of change in the Transtheoretical Model and applies them to a diabetes-specific example.

Evidence Base. The Transtheoretical Model has been used for the following in diabetes management:

- To understand diabetes self-management behaviors
- To customize self-care interventions aimed at promoting physical activity,[42-46] healthy dietary habits,[47,48] and blood glucose testing[49] (see chapter 30, Being Active, for example)

Kirk and colleagues conducted a randomized controlled trial of 70 patients with type 2 diabetes comparing usual exercise information plus an exercise consultation to usual exercise information.[43] Guided by the TTM, the exercise consultation was tailored to the stage of physical activity readiness in which subjects were classified. The intervention group received the stage-matched consultation at the start of the study and 6 months later. Follow-up telephone consultations were also conducted at 1-month and 3-months postintervention. The experimental group significantly increased the number of minutes of moderate activity per week and the number of times per week they engaged in physical activity, while the control group showed no changes in either indicator. A greater number of participants from the intervention group advanced across a stage of change. Similar to the study of Kirk et al,[43] Kim and colleagues developed a stage-matched intervention to promote physical activity among Korean

TABLE 3.5 Transtheoretical Model: Stages of Change and Application to Diabetes Self-Management

Stage	*Definition*	*Case in Point*
Precontemplation	Individual is not aware of the problem and has no intentions of changing his/her health behavior	MG was diagnosed with type 2 diabetes 5 years ago. At that time, she was not aware of the long-term health-related complications and, therefore, did nothing to lower her blood glucose.
Contemplation	Individual is aware of the problem and intends to change his/her behavior; knows the benefits associated with the health behavior change, but also is acutely aware of the drawbacks; can be in a state of ambivalence	Last year, MG started to understand that if she did not take care of her diabetes, she could eventually develop kidney or eye problems. She also knew that self-management involved a set of responsibilities including regularly checking her blood glucose.
Preparation	Individual makes plans that will facilitate the health behavior change	Three months ago, MG started looking for diabetes education or support groups. She also looked into joining tennis clubs so she could actively start playing tennis.
Action	Individual actively engages in the behavior change	MG checks her blood glucose before and 2 hours after every meal. She also plays tennis 3 times a week.
Maintenance	Individual demonstrates the ability to sustain the behavior change	MG has continued checking her blood glucose prior to and following meals and continues to play tennis 3 times per week.

patients with type 2 diabetes.[45] The intervention consisted of 3 components: a counseling technique based on TTM-related constructs, physical activity training customized to the participant, and telephone counseling. Following the 12-week intervention, compared to the control group, the intervention group progressed to a more advanced change stage, increased physical activity levels, decreased fasting blood glucose, and decreased A1C.

The usefulness of the TTM for understanding readiness to change dietary behaviors has also been supported in the literature. In a sample of 768 overweight patients enrolled in a diabetes self-management trial, Vallis et al identified patient-specific factors associated with different stages of changing dietary behavior.[48] Among those subjects diagnosed with type 2 diabetes, the subjects classified in the action stage were significantly more likely to be female, report a higher quality of life, and engage in healthy dietary habits than those in other stages.

A study conducted by Jones and colleagues compared a TTM-based intervention (Pathways to Change) to usual care in improving 3 self-care behaviors: blood glucose testing, dietary habits, and smoking cessation.[49] The intervention was delivered via mail and telephone counseling over a 12-month period. Distinct components of the intervention targeted readiness to change for the 3 self-management behaviors. Compared to the usual care group, the intervention group demonstrated significant improvements in frequency of blood glucose testing, percentage of calorie intake from fat, and fruit and vegetable consumption per day. With regard to smoking cessation behavior, a greater proportion of the intervention group than the control group advanced to the action-oriented stage.

Motivational Interviewing

Motivational Interviewing (MI) is a communication technique consistent with several health behavior change theories, including the Transtheoretical Model (Stages of Change) and Social Cognitive Theory. MI is a patient-centered approach that aims to identify and resolve ambivalence toward behavior change, and, subsequently, stimulate motivation to take action.[21] MI consists of the 4 guiding principles listed and described below.[21] Table 3.6 gives examples of how these principles can be applied in diabetes care.

Evidence Base. Motivational Interviewing has gained increasing attention as a counseling technique to incorporate in diabetes self-management interventions.[50-58] Smith et al investigated the unique benefit that MI might add to standard behavioral intervention aimed at improving self-care practices and promoting weight loss.[56] Twenty-two women with type 2 diabetes who were over the age of 50 were randomly assigned to either a standard

TABLE 3.6 Motivational Interviewing—Principles and Application to Diabetes Care

Expressing Empathy. "It seems like cooking healthy meals and developing better diet habits are stressful for you because your husband and kids prefer more high-fat, high-carbohydrate foods such as pizza, fast food, and potato chips. It is common for patients who have families to struggle with this issue. Are there times when following a healthy diet is more difficult?"
Developing Discrepancy. "So, it sounds like it is difficult for you to maintain healthy eating habits because your husband and children prefer high-fat foods such as pizza, cheeseburgers, and macaroni and cheese. They also like to have sugary snacks around the house for when they come home from school. However, I also hear you saying that you really want to change your eating habits, that you feel good when you eat more vegetables and high-fiber foods and avoid soda and junk food. Do you think your dietary choices affect your blood glucose levels?"
Rolling With Resistance. "It is completely understandable why you feel overwhelmed by needing to take care of your own health as well as making sure your husband and children are happy. Changes in eating choices and habits are one of the biggest challenges for families. Other people have dealt with these same issues. Would you like to talk about some of the different solutions others have tried?"
Supporting Self-Efficacy. "It sounds like you have been quite successful with increasing your physical activity by taking up tennis again. I can see that changing your eating habits has been a little bit more challenging. Are there any strategies you used for increasing your physical activity that you could also use for improving your eating choices and patterns? Sometimes, we need to tackle one behavior at a time since these are really big changes. After you feel confident about your physical activity program, you might be better able to really focus on your diet goals.

Motivational Interviewing: Guiding Principles

Expressing Empathy

Emphasizes active listening as well as creating a safe and accepting environment in which the patient can express personal thoughts, feelings, and experiences. The counselor's primary role is to identify ambivalence, provide support, and relay facts. Giving advice and direct teaching are avoided. Should some level of persuasion be beneficial, this process is conducted in a nurturing manner. Ultimately, the patient, not the counselor, determines the pace and direction of the conversation and makes the decision to embark on behavior change.

Developing Discrepancies

Involves identifying the core values of the patient, what the patient deems important in his or her life, and whether the patient's current behavior is consistent with or runs counter to those values. The counselor attempts to uncover and expose discrepancies between the patient's current behavior and values and future aspirations. The counselor assists the patient in exploring the negative outcomes related to current behavior, experiencing a sense of discontent and discomfort, and ideally fostering an increasing motivation to change. The counselor provides any relevant factual information and highlights inconsistencies between goals and current health behavior. The patient serves as the active agent of change, responsible for integrating the facts, resolving discrepancies, and building the necessary motivation to take action.

Rolling With Resistance

Encourages the counselor to work in tandem with the patient when the patient is exhibiting reluctance to take action, rather than to directly confront the patient. The counselor's job is not to coerce or lead, but instead to facilitate the process of developing greater motivation. The counselor fosters new ways of thinking about the situation, but avoids making any specific recommendations or expressing any bias. The patient is in charge of generating solutions that are feasible and workable given personal priorities, goals, and circumstances.

Supporting Self-Efficacy

Reinforces the patient's confidence in taking action and making behavior changes. The counselor promotes an atmosphere of optimism that helps solidify patients' beliefs that they can perform the specific tasks they set out to accomplish.

16-week group weight-control program (instruction in diet, exercise, and behavior modification) versus the standard program plus 3 personal MI sessions. Compared to the control groups, the MI group performed significantly better with regard to maintaining food diaries and documenting blood glucose. While there were not differences in the amount of weight lost between the 2 groups, the mean A1C for the MI group was significantly lower than for their counterparts.

MI has also been used in programs targeting adolescents with diabetes. In a group of 22 patients ages 14 to 18 years, Channon and colleagues examined the health impact of a MI-based counseling intervention on blood glucose control, quality of life, and psychological functioning.[58] Preintervention and postintervention results revealed a significant reduction in A1C, fear of hypoglycemia, and perceived difficulty of living with diabetes.

Conclusion

The self-management of diabetes is the primary determinant of diabetes-related health outcomes, in the short and long term. With each passing year, diabetes self-management is becoming more complex. In response to the combination of this increasing complexity and the growing body of knowledge about health-related behavior change, diabetes self-management education must become increasingly sophisticated to be effective. These programs can only be as sophisticated as the diabetes educators who design and conduct them. This chapter has outlined the resources necessary to help educators develop the sophistication to incorporate evidence-based approaches to facilitating self-directed behavior change into their programs and practices.

Questions and Controversies

While there are a variety of self-management theories, some theories are more consistent with a compliance/adherence approach, while others are more consistent with an empowerment or patient-centered approach. Healthcare professionals involved in the design of diabetes self-management education programs as well as educators considering their individual practice must consider the following questions when selecting and applying theories:

- Based on their own views of and values related to self-management education, which theories are most compelling for their situation?
- Do the specific teaching methods and strategies used within the practice reflect this approach?

Theories can be implemented in different ways, based on the philosophy of the educator. For example, Stages of Change can be used by educators to categorize patients or as a way for patients to reflect on their own readiness to change. Motivational interviewing can be used to help patients reflect on their own level of motivation or to try to motivate patients toward a particular behavior the educator believes is in the patient's best self-management interest. The professional must consider the following:

- How have these theories been used in this practice?
- Are the theories employed consistent with the purpose and philosophy of that practice?

Focus on Education: Pearls for Practice

Teaching Strategies

- **Select and employ the theories that will guide the practice.** Establish a framework, define an approach and purpose, and provide a common language for the healthcare team and their patients. Educators then reflect this philosophy in the program design. Instructors agree on this and build programs designed to fit the theory.

- **Base outcomes on evidence.** Initiate use of tools to measure change, success, and progress, and then compare results with expectations.

Messages for Patients

- **Making decisions.** Learn as much information as is available. Learn the skills necessary to make decisions. Identify options and discuss them with the healthcare team, family, and educators before making a final decision.

- **Be involved in planning your self-care.** Be clear on what you plan to do and the criteria upon which you will judge your success. Know that the plan can be altered.

References

1. Fain J, Nettles A, Charron-Prochownik D. Diabetes patient education research: an integrative literature review. Diabetes Educ. 1999;25 Suppl:7-15.
2. Meleis A. Theoretical Nursing: Development and Progress. Philadelphia, Pa: Lippincott; 1997.
3. Fawcett J, Downs F. The Relationship Between Theory and Research, 2nd ed. Philadelphia, Pa: FA Davis; 1992.
4. Polit DF, Beck CT, Hungler BP. Essentials of Nursing Research: Methods, Appraisal, and Utilization, 5th ed. Philadelphia, Pa: Lippincott; 2001.
5. Anderson RM, Funnell MM. The Art of Empowerment: Stories and Strategies for Diabetes Educators, 2nd ed. Alexandria, Va: American Diabetes Association; 2005.
6. Wdowik MJ, Kendall PA, Harris MA, Auld G. Expanded health belief model predicts diabetes self-management in college students. J Nutr Educ. 2001; 33:17-23.
7. Funnell MM, Anderson RM, Arnold MS, et al. Empowerment: an idea whose time has come in diabetes education. Diabetes Educ. 1991;17:37-41.
8. Funnell MM, Anderson RM. Patient empowerment: a look back, a look ahead. Diabetes Educ. 2003;9:454-64.
9. Norris SL, Lau J, Smith SJ, Schmid CH, Engelgau MM. Self-management education for adults with type 2 diabetes: a meta-analysis on the effect on glycemic control. Diabetes Care. 2002;25:1159-71.
10. Davis ED, Vander Meer JM, Yarborough PC, Roth SM. Using solution-focused therapy strategies in empowerment-based education. Diabetes Educ. 1999; 25:249-57.
11. Dijkstra R, Braspenning J, Grol R. Empowering patients: how to implement a diabetes passport in hospital care. Patient Educ Couns. 2002;47:173-7.
12. Deakin TA, Cade JE, Williams DDR, Greenwood DC. Empowered patients: better diabetes control, greater freedom to eat, no weight gain. Diabetologia. 2003;46 Suppl 2:A90.
13. Gillard ML, Nwankwo R, Fitzgerald JT, et al. Informal diabetes education: impact on self-management and blood glucose control. Diabetes Educ. 2004;30:136-42.
14. Pibernik-Okanovic M, Prasek M, Poljicanin-Filipovic T, Pavlic-Renar I, Metelko Z. Effects of an empowerment-

based psychosocial intervention on quality of life and metabolic control in type 2 diabetic patients. Patient Educ Couns. 2004;52:193-9.

15. Skinner TC, Cradock S, Arundel F, Graham W. Lifestyle and behavior: four theories and a philosophy: self-management education for individuals newly diagnosed with type 2 diabetes. Diabetes Spectrum. 2003;16:75-80.

16. Anderson RM, Funnell MM, Butler PM, Arnold MS, Feste CC. Patient empowerment: results of a randomized controlled trial. Diabetes Care. 1995;18:943-9.

17. Arnold MS, Butler PM, Anderson RM, Funnell MM, Feste C. Guidelines for facilitating a patient empowerment program. Diabetes Educ. 1995;21:308-12.

18. Anderson RM, Funnell MM, Nwankwo R, Gillard ML, Oh MS, Fitzgerald JT. Evaluation of a problem-based empowerment program for African Americans with diabetes. Results of a randomized controlled trial. Ethn Dis. 2005;15:671-8.

19. Tang TS, Gillard ML, Funnell MM, et al. Developing a new generation of ongoing diabetes self-management support interventions: a preliminary report. Diabetes Educ. 2005;31:91-7.

20. Funnell MM, Nwankwo R, Gillard ML, Anderson RM, Tang TS. Implementing an empowerment-based diabetes self-management education program. Diabetes Educ. 2005; 31:53-61.

21. Glanz K, Rimer BK, Marcus Lewis F, eds. Health Behavior & Health Education: Theory, Research & Practice, 3rd ed. San Francisco, Calif: Jossey-Bass; 2002.

22. Rosenstock IM. Historical origins of the health belief model. Health Educ Monogr. 1974;2:328-35.

23. Koch J. The role of exercise in the African-American woman with type 2 diabetes mellitus: application of the health belief model. J Amer Acad Nurse Pract. 2002;14:126-9.

24. Aljasem LI, Peyrot M, Wissow L, Rubin RR. The impact of barriers and self-efficacy on self-care behaviors in type 2 diabetes. Diabetes Educ. 2001;27:393-404.

25. Pham DT, Fortin F, Thibaudeau MF. The role of the health belief model in amputees' self-evaluation of adherence to diabetes self-care behaviors. Diabetes Educ. 1996;22:126-32.

26. Swift CS, Armstrong JE, Beerman KA, Campbell RK, Pond-Smith D. Attitudes and beliefs about exercise among persons with non-insulin-dependent diabetes. Diabetes Educ. 1995;21:533-40.

27. Polly RK. Diabetes health beliefs, self-care behaviors, and glycemic control among older adults with non-insulin-dependent diabetes mellitus. Diabetes Educ. 1992;18:321-7.

28. Bond GG, Aiken LS, Somerville SC. The health belief model and adolescents with insulin-dependent diabetes mellitus. Health Psychol. 1992;11:190-8.

29. Kurtz SM. Adherence to diabetes regimens: empirical status and clinical applications (review). Diabetes Educ. 1990;16:50-9.

30. Tan MY. The relationship of health beliefs and complication prevention behaviors of Chinese individuals with type 2 diabetes mellitus. Diabetes Res Clin Pract. 2004;66:71-7.

31. Daniel M, Messer LC. Perceptions of disease severity and barriers to self-care predict glycemic control in Aboriginal persons with type 2 diabetes mellitus. Chronic Dis Can. 2002;23:130-8.

32. Spikmans FJ, Brug J, Doven MM, Kruizenga HM, Hofsteenge GH, van Bokhorst-van der Schueren MA. Why do diabetic patients not attend appointments with their dietitians? J Hum Nutr Diet. 2003;16:151-8.

33. Wdowik MJ, Kendall PA, Harris MA, Keim KS. Development and evaluation of an intervention program: "Control on Campus." Diabetes Educ. 2000;26:95-104.

34. Scollan-Koliopoulos M. Theory-guided intervention for preventing diabetes-related amputations in African Americans. J Vascular Nurs. 2004;22:126-33.

35. Allen NA. Social cognitive theory in diabetes exercise research: an integrative literature review. Diabetes Educ. 2004;30:805-19.

36. Hays LM, Clark DO. Correlates of physical activity in a sample of older adults with type 2 diabetes. Diabetes Care. 1999;22:706-12.

37. Miller CK, Edwards L, Kissling G, Sanville L. Evaluation of a theory-based nutrition intervention for older adults with diabetes mellitus. J Amer Diet Assoc. 2002;102:1069-81.

38. Miller CK, Edwards L, Kissling G, Sanville L. Nutrition education improves metabolic outcomes among older adults with diabetes mellitus: results from a randomized controlled trial. Prev Med. 2002;34:252-9.

39. Toobert DJ, Strycker LA, Glasgow RE, Barrera M, Bagdade JD. Enhancing support for health behavior change among women at risk for heart disease: the Mediterranean lifestyle trial. Health Educ Res. 2002;17:574-85.

40. Syrajala AH, Niskanen MC, Knuuttila ML. The theory of reasoned action in describing tooth brushing, dental caries and diabetes adherence among diabetic patients. J Clin Periodontol. 2002;29:427-32.

41. Burnet D, Plaut A, Courtney R, Chin MH. A practical model for preventing type 2 diabetes in minority youth (review). Diabetes Educ. 2002;28:778-95.

42. Kirk AF, Higgins LA, Hughes AR, et al. A randomized, controlled trial to study the effect of exercise consultation on the promotion of physical activity in people with type 2 diabetes: a pilot study. Diabetic Med. 2001;18:877-82.

43. Kirk A, Mutrie N, MacIntyre P, Fisher M. Increasing physical activity in people with type 2 diabetes. Diabetes Care. 2003;26:1186-92.

44. Kirk AF, Mutrie N, MacIntyre PD, Fisher MB. Promoting and maintaining physical activity in people with type 2 diabetes. Amer J Prev Med. 2004;27:289-96.

45. Kim CJ, Hwang AR, Yoo JS. The impact of a stage-matched intervention to promote exercise behavior in participants with type 2 diabetes. Int J Nurs Studies. 2004;41:833-41.

46. Yoo JS, Hwang AR, Lee HC, Kim CJ. Development and validation of a computerized exercise intervention program for patients with type 2 diabetes mellitus in Korea. Yonsei Med J. 2003;44:892-904.

47. Kasila K, Poskiparta M, Karhila P, Kettunen T. Patients' readiness for dietary change at the beginning of counseling: a transtheoretical model-based assessment. J Hum Nutr Diet. 2003;16:159-66.

48. Vallis M, Ruggiero L, Greene G, et al. Stages of change for healthy eating in diabetes: relation to demographic, eating-related, health care utilization, and psychosocial factors. Diabetes Care. 2003;26:1468-74.

49. Jones H, Edwards L, Vallis TM, et al. Changes in diabetes self-care behaviors make a difference in glycemic control: the diabetes stages of change (DiSC) study. Diabetes Care. 2003;26:732-7.

50. Carino JL, Coke L, Gulanick M. Using motivational interviewing to reduce diabetes risk (review). Prog Cardiovascular Nurs. 2004;19:149-54.

51. VanWormer JJ, Boucher JL. Motivational interviewing and diet modification: a review of the evidence. Diabetes Educ. 2004;30:404-6, 408-10, 414-6.

52. Doherty Y, Hall D, James PT, Roberts SH, Simpson J. Change counselling in diabetes: the development of a training programme for the diabetes team. Patient Educ Couns. 2000;40:263-78.

53. Trigwell P, Grant PJ, House A. Motivation and glycemic control in diabetes mellitus. J Psychosom Res. 1997;43:307-15.

54. Stott NC, Rees M, Rollnick S, Pill RM, Hackett P. Professional responses to innovation in clinical method: diabetes care and negotiating skills. Patient Educ Couns. 1996;29:67-73.

55. Stott NC, Rollnick S, Rees MR, Pill RM. Innovation in clinical method: diabetes care and negotiating skills. Fam Pract. 1995;12:413-8.

56. Smith DE, Heckemeyer CM, Kratt PP, Mason DA. Motivational interviewing to improve adherence to a behavior weight-control program for older obese women in NIDDM. A pilot study. Diabetes Care. 1997;20:52-4.

57. Clark M, Hampson SE. Implementing a psychological intervention to improve lifestyle self-management in patients with type 2 diabetes. Patient Educ Couns. 2001;42:247-56.

58. Channon S, Smith VJ, Gregory JW. A pilot study of motivational interviewing in adolescents with diabetes. Arch Dis Childhood. 2003;88:680-3.

CHAPTER

4

Understanding the Individual: Emotional and Psychological Challenges

Authors

Laurie Ruggiero, PhD
Julie Wagner, PhD
Mary de Groot, PhD

Key Concepts

- Recognize that persons with diabetes are at risk for mental health problems, such as depression, eating disorders, and anxiety
- Understand the signs and symptoms, prevalence, and risk factors for mental health problems in persons with diabetes
- Choose mental health screening strategies appropriate to the practice setting
- Be familiar with the treatment options for the most common mental health problems
- Appreciate the important role of diabetes educators in recognizing mental health problems and coordinating appropriate treatment
- Coordinate diabetes self-management education with mental health treatment

Introduction

Diabetes is a lifelong disease that impacts the person's life in many ways each day. Experiencing negative feelings about diabetes, its treatment, and one's own situation is normal. There are many experiences during the onset and course of diabetes that may make people vulnerable to negative emotions. In particular, this includes the initial diagnosis, whether that occurs in youth, adulthood, or pregnancy, and transition periods, which occur with normal development (eg, adolescence), disease progression (eg, end of honeymoon period, onset of complications), and treatment (eg, initiation of insulin). In addition, throughout the course of diabetes, the person is faced with the complex behavioral demands of this disease that may further compound the emotional responses. These emotional responses cover the range of negative affect, such as denial, fear, frustration, sadness, overwhelmed, guilt, anger, and burnout.

Feeling these negative emotions is not a problem in itself. These negative emotions become problematic and need intervention when they meet 1 or more of these criteria:[1]

- Emotion lasts for an extended duration of time
- Emotion is severe in intensity
- Emotion interferes in the person's life

In addition, there are specific symptoms that, in and of themselves, require further attention:

- Intentional insulin omission
- Suicidal ideation or intent
- Fasting or purging for weight loss

Diabetes educators need to help people with diabetes understand that having negative feelings about diabetes, its treatment, and their own situation is normal. Educators need to understand when these emotions are problematic and require evaluation and intervention.

This chapter focuses primarily on adults because the majority of people with diabetes are adults; however, consistent with an overall theme of the book, aspects of mental health problems at various ages and stages in life are considered. Specifically, information on youth, women with diabetes during pregnancy, and older adults is briefly highlighted in areas where appropriate. (Children, teens, and older adults are further discussed in chapters 9 and 10, on type 1 and type 2 diabetes, and pregnancy is addressed more fully in chapters 11 and 12.) The focus in this chapter is on 3 of the more common emotional or psychological problems found in people with diabetes: depression, anxiety, and eating disorders. Two other vulnerable situations for people with diabetes are also briefly discussed: stress and adjustment in pregnant women with diabetes.

Common Challenges for Those With Diabetes

Emotional/Psychological Problems

- Depression
- Anxiety
- Eating disorders

Vulnerable Situations

- Stress
- Adjustment in pregnant women with diabetes

The individual sections on depression, anxiety, and eating disorders each provide an overall description of the condition and the symptoms and major subtypes, prevalence rates of the condition, risk factors, unique aspects for people with diabetes, treatment options, and screening strategies for diabetes educators. The chapter closes with a section providing practice-based strategies to support diabetes educators in working with people regarding emotional or psychological challenges.

Depression

Key questions this section addresses:

- What is depression?
- How common is it in people with diabetes?
- Who is most at risk?
- What treatment options are available?
- What is the diabetes educator's role in detecting depression in people with diabetes?

What is depression?

Depression is defined as a spectrum of mood disorders characterized by persistent periods of sadness or lack of interest in usual activities. Depression diagnoses differ by the level of severity and impairment associated with the symptoms and the degree to which environmental stressors may have preceded the period of depressed mood. Three depressive disorder diagnoses will be reviewed:

- Major Depressive Disorder
- Dysthymic Disorder
- Adjustment Disorder with Depressed Mood

Major Depressive Disorder

Major Depressive Disorder (MDD) has been defined by the American Psychiatric Association[1] as a period lasting *2 weeks or longer* in which the individual has experienced 5 of these 9 symptoms most of the day, nearly every day:

- Depressed or sad mood
- Lack of interest or pleasure
- Unintentional changes in weight or appetite
- Difficulty falling asleep, staying asleep, or early awakening
- Fatigue
- Difficulty with concentration or decision-making
- Psychomotor retardation or agitation (ie, moving slowly or feeling fidgety or restless)
- Feelings of worthlessness or excessive or inappropriate guilt
- Suicidal ideation or plan

Individuals experiencing MDD will show significant impairment in social or occupational functioning. Persons with comorbid medical diagnoses (eg, hypothyroidism) and medications that may induce similar symptoms should not be considered to have a primary diagnosis of MDD.

Dysthymic Disorder

Individuals may experience prolonged periods of depressive symptoms that result in impairment to social or occupational functioning.[1] Dysthymic Disorder may be diagnosed if individuals meet criteria for the following symptoms over a *2-year period*:

- Depressed mood, most of the day, more days than not
- Unintentional changes in appetite
- Sleep disturbance (ie, hypersomnia, insomnia)
- Low energy or fatigue
- Low self-esteem
- Poor concentration or difficulty making decisions
- Feelings of hopelessness

A diagnosis of Dysthymic Disorder would be contraindicated in the presence of manic symptoms (eg, excessive euphoric or irritable mood), medical conditions that may mimic these symptoms (eg, hypothyroidism), or medication side effects.

Adjustment Disorder With Depressed Mood

Adjustment Disorder with Depressed Mood is defined by the American Psychiatric Association[1] as the development of depressive symptoms within a 3-month period of time following a stressor (eg, divorce). Symptoms are characterized as follows:

- Symptoms causing impairment in social, occupational, or other areas of important functioning, *or*
- Symptoms in excess of what would be expected from exposure to the stressor

Symptoms in this diagnostic category present as a lower level of severity compared to those in MDD. Symptoms associated with Adjustment Disorder with Depressed Mood are expected to remit within 6 months of the time of onset.

Cultural Manifestations of Depression Presentations

Depressive symptoms should be evaluated in the context of the individual's cultural frame of reference. Individual presentations of depressive symptoms may vary:

- Expressions of depressed affect, sadness, or tearfulness may predominate, *or*
- Symptoms of boredom or of loss of interest or pleasure may predominate (the individual does not identify with symptoms of sadness or tearfulness), *or*

- Somatic symptoms such as sleep disturbance, changes in appetite or weight, increased pain distress, or gastrointestinal symptoms may predominate[2]

Diabetes educators should also be aware that culture-bound syndromes may also be present for individuals who identify with a minority cultural group or who are bicultural.[1] These syndromes are expressions of distinct periods of emotional distress that are understood within a specific cultural context (eg, *nervios*). Such expressions of emotional distress may not conform to Western medicine's standardized definitions of mental disorders, but nonetheless should alert the diabetes educator to the need for further assessment and potential referral.

How common is depression in people with diabetes?

Depression in Adults

> ***Depression is twice as common in persons with diabetes:***

In recent years, accumulating evidence has found that depression is twice as common in patients with type 1 and type 2 diabetes than in the general population.[3] Approximately 1 in 4 persons with diabetes will have experience with depression in their lifetime.[3]

In a review of 42 studies examining rates of depression in various populations, average rates of self-reported depression were found to be 21.3% in those with type 1 diabetes and 27.0% in those with type 2 diabetes.[3] Rates of depression varied by type of depression measurement. Studies using diagnostic interviews showed lower rates of clinically significant depression (11.4%) than those using self-report questionnaires (31.0%).[3]

Gender. Women with diabetes have 1.6 times the risk of depression compared to their male counterparts, with 28.2% of women and 18% of men reporting significant depressive symptoms.[3]

Ethnicity/Race. Documentation of self-reported depression in communities of color has been limited, but emerging evidence suggests that the rates of depression among African Americans,[4] Latinos,[5] Native Hawaiians,[6] and other communities of color[7] are comparable to or exceed those of the white population with diabetes.

Duration. The duration of depressive episodes in persons with diabetes may be longer and more persistent than those documented in the general population.[8] One study of persons enrolled in a diabetes education program found that 34% of participants continued to report clinically significant depressive symptoms 6 months after initial evaluation.[8]

Depression in Children and Adolescents

The prevalence of depression in children and adolescents with type 1 diabetes appears to be 2 to 3 times greater than in children without diabetes.[9]

Comorbid depression and diabetes appear to be associated with a 10-fold increase in suicide and suicidal ideation, increased severity and risk of depression recurrence, and longer duration of each episode compared to children without diabetes.[9] Correlates of depression in children and adolescents are the following:[9]

- Older age
- Maternal depression
- Family dysfunction or stress
- Health status

Gender. Evidence suggests that females may be more prone than males to the development of comorbid depression as children and adults, but rates of depression among males are higher than those found in the nondiabetes population.[9,10]

Type 2 Diabetes. Limited data is currently available on rates of depression among children and adolescents with type 2 diabetes in youth. One study has suggested that 20% of pediatric patients presenting with type 2 diabetes were positive for the presence of comorbid depression, attention-deficit hyperactivity disorder, bipolar disorder, and schizophrenia.[11] Females (63%) were more represented in the comorbid sample than males (37%). Further research is needed to establish definitive rates of comorbid depression in this emerging population.

Who is most at risk for depression?

Correlates of depression in adults with type 1 and type 2 diabetes appear to be the following:[12]

- Female
- Younger age
- Lower levels of education
- Not married
- Smoking
- BMI ≥30
- Higher glycosylated hemoglobin values
- Treatment with insulin
- Presence of diabetes complications (men only)

What are the unique aspects of the combination of depression and diabetes?

Increased Risk of Depression in People With Diabetes

The underlying mechanisms that govern the relationship between diabetes and depression are not yet well understood. Environmental, genetic, and hormonal factors have been noted to have commonalities between depression and diabetes. Environmental factors, such as poverty, appear to increase the risk of developing comorbid diabetes and depression.[13] Genetic heritability may also play a role. There is some evidence to suggest that a history of depression may double the risk of developing type 2 diabetes in later life.[14] There is increasing evidence that both depression and diabetic hypoglycemia result in alterations of brain structures, including grey matter and within the hippocampus.[15] Research in animal models has noted possible hormonal mechanisms that may account for the relationship between depression and diabetes, including the role of cortisol in both counterregulatory hormonal mechanisms in diabetes and depression.[16]

Children and Adolescents. Among children and adolescents with type 1 diabetes, a relationship between immune functioning (glutamic acid decarboxylase, GAD) and the production of gamma-aminobutyric acid (GABA) neurotransmitters has been proposed.[9] Counterregulatory hormones, such as cortisol, may also play a role in the development of comorbid depression and diabetes.[9]

More research is needed to fully determine the multiple, complex interrelationships of these comorbid disorders.

Negative Consequences of Depression in Adults With Diabetes

Although the mechanisms underlying diabetes and depression are not well understood, the impact of comorbid depression on persons with type 1 and type 2 diabetes has been well-documented.

Effect on Diabetes and Its Complications. Examination across studies has shown that depression has a small but significant negative impact on glycemic control in persons with type 1 and type 2 diabetes.[17] Depression has also been shown to have a moderate relationship with worsened diabetes complications, including retinopathy, neuropathy, macrovascular, and microvascular complications.[18]

Effect on Diabetes Self-Care. Persons with comorbid depression and diabetes have been noted to show significant decrements in adherence to multiple components of the diabetes self-care regimen, including worsened adherence to medication and dietary recommendations.[19]

Higher Costs. The costs associated with comorbid diabetes and depression are considerable.[20] Depression has been associated with increased overall costs of health care, higher rates of ambulatory care, and greater prescription use.[19] In one study, patients with depression and diabetes had healthcare costs 4.5 times greater than diabetes patients without depression.[19] As severity of depression increased, so did the costs. Patients with the greatest depression severity had 51% higher costs of primary care services, 75% higher costs of ambulatory care services, and 86% overall healthcare costs compared to those without depression.[19]

> **_Depression is Costly_**
>
> Diabetes and depression can add significantly to personal financial costs.

Disability and Mortality Risk. Comorbid depression has also been found to be associated with increased functional disability[21] and increased risk for mortality.[22]

Quality of Life. Studies of quality of life (QOL) have demonstrated lower overall functional health scores and lower diabetes-specific QOL scores among patients with diabetes and major depression.[23] Evidence suggests that depression appears to amplify the negative effects of chronic illness on health-related QOL.[24]

Negative Consequences of Depression in Youth With Diabetes

Among children and adolescents, the impact of comorbid depression is also significant.

Effect on Self-Care, Diabetes, and Its Complications. Depression has been found to be associated with decreased adherence to self-management behaviors and poorer metabolic control, potentially leading to increased risk of long-term diabetes complications.[9]

Hospitalizations. Recent evidence suggests that the presence of depression and other internalizing disorders in diabetic adolescents ages 13 to 18 years may significantly increase the risk of hospital readmission.[25] This trend was not observed in children ages 5 to 12 years with diabetes and depression or other internalizing disorders.[25]

Psychosocial Difficulties. Children and adolescents with diabetes and depression have been found to have greater psychosocial difficulties, such as family stress or dysfunction.[9]

Taken together, this evidence on children and adults points to the significant physical, fiscal, and emotional impacts depression may have on an individual with either type 1 or type 2 diabetes. Although diabetes educators are not responsible for the diagnosis and treatment of depression or other mental disorders, diabetes educators can play a vital role in identifying and facilitating treatment for depression in their patients.

What treatment options are available for people with diabetes and depression?

In light of the substantial impact depression may have on the person with diabetes, there is encouraging evidence that depression can be effectively treated using standard treatment strategies.

Two primary treatment strategies for those with diabetes and depressive symptoms:

- Psychotherapy—specifically, use of cognitive behavioral therapy (CBT)
- Pharmacotherapy

Psychotherapy

Psychotherapy may be conducted with individuals, couples, or families or within a group setting. Although there are a variety of psychotherapy orientations (eg, psychodynamic, interpersonal, client-centered, family systems, CBT), psychotherapy seeks to work with patients to promote emotional and behavioral coping through emotional catharsis, understanding of family and behavioral patterns, and/or adoption of coping skills to manage mood and behavior. No efficacy trials have been conducted to treat depression in children with type 1 or type 2 diabetes,[9] but a variety of therapeutic approaches have been used to treat depression in adult patients with diabetes.[26-32] One such approach has been the use of CBT. This approach emphasizes the adoption of coping skills through an understanding of the thoughts, feelings, and behaviors that promote or prevent depressed mood.

Cognitive Behavioral Therapy. CBT has been shown to be efficacious in patients with depression and diabetes.[26] In a randomized controlled trial, 52 subjects with major depression and type 2 diabetes were randomly assigned to general diabetes education or 10 sessions of CBT with a psychologist. Participants receiving psychotherapy showed significant improvements in depressive symptoms immediately following therapy and at a 6-month follow-up evaluation.[26] Those in the CBT group also showed improvement in glycemic control 6 months following the end of therapy.[26]

Collaborative Care. Recent therapeutic trials have involved a collaborative approach between primary care providers, nurses, and mental health professionals to provide depression treatment to patients with diabetes.[27] In the Pathways Study, a stepped-care approach was used by trained nurses within a primary care setting. Persons enrolled in the intervention arm received the option of receiving antidepressant medication or the problem-solving therapy during the first 10 to 12 weeks. Participants received an initial 1-hour evaluation appointment followed by half-hour follow-up appointments (face-to-face) twice per month. Participants whose depressive symptoms did not show improvement at this level of care were referred to a psychiatrist.[27] The trial demonstrated that this approach to depression treatment was effective in improving short- and long-term depression outcomes for those with diabetes and depression.[27] Similar results were found for older adults with type 2 diabetes and comorbid depression.[28] Results from these recent trials point to the effectiveness of collaborative care for adult and elderly patients with comorbid depression and diabetes.

Pharmacotherapy

A variety of medication approaches to the management of depressive symptoms have been shown to be efficacious in persons with type 1 and type 2 diabetes. Antidepressant medication options have greatly increased for persons in the general population, with decreasing levels of side effects. Common antidepressant medications are listed in Table 4.1. These medications may also be used to treat pain from diabetic neuropathy at lower doses.[29]

Tricyclic antidepressants (TCAs) predominantly affect norepinephrine neurotransmitters.[29] Efficacy studies of the treatment of depression in persons with type 1 and type 2 diabetes have demonstrated that nortriptyline (25 to 50 mg daily) is effective in reducing depression symptoms with hyperglycemic effects.[30]

TABLE 4.1 Psychotropic Medications by Class for Treatment of Depression

Selective Serotonin Reuptake Inhibitors (SSRIs)		*Other Antidepressants*		*Tricyclics (TCAs)*	
Generic name	*Brand name*	*Generic name*	*Brand name*	*Generic name*	*Brand name*
Escitalopram	Lexapro	Venlafaxine	Effexor	Amitriptyline	Elavil
Citalopram	Celexa	Nefazodone	Serzone	Desipramine	Norpramin
Fluoxetine	Prozac	Bupropion	Wellbutrin	Imipramine	Tofranil
Paroxetine	Paxil	Mirtazapine	Remeron	Nortriptyline	Aventyl, Pamelor
Sertraline	Zoloft	Trazodone	Desyrel	Doxepin	Sinequan
		Duloxetine	Cymbalta		

Selective-serotonin reuptake inhibitors (SSRIs) alleviate depressive symptoms by blocking the absorption of naturally produced serotonin in the brain. As serotonin levels elevate over time, depressive symptoms are reduced. Two SSRIs—fluoxetine (Prozac, 40 mg daily) and sertraline (Zoloft, 50 mg daily)—have been shown to be efficacious in the treatment of depression with the additional benefit of improvement in glycemic control.[31,32]

Although other TCA and SSRI medications have been shown to be efficacious in the treatment of depression in the general population, further research is needed to establish the efficacy of these medications for the treatment of depression in adults and children with type 1 and type 2 diabetes.[9] Further research is also needed to investigate the potential impact of these medications on glycemic control. Research on the specific mechanisms of these medications suggests that other SSRIs may reduce glycemic levels in persons with diabetes.[29] However, clinical trials specific to persons with diabetes and depression are needed to confirm these models in humans.

Those who are prescribed antidepressant medications by their primary care or mental health provider will be advised to take these medications daily. Depression symptom reduction generally occurs within 3 to 6 weeks following the initiation of medication, due to the titrating effects of increased neurotransmitter levels in the brain. Medication side effects vary and may be more prominent at the initiation of medication. Patients should be advised by the prescribing provider to discontinue medication in a stepwise fashion when indicated. Immediate discontinuation of antidepressant medications may result in flu-like symptoms such as headache and nausea. Long-term treatment courses of antidepressant medications have been shown to be effective in reducing depression recurrence in the general population.

What is the diabetes educator's role in detecting depression in people with diabetes?

Although the diagnosis and treatment of comorbid depression is beyond the scope of diabetes education, diabetes educators can play a crucial role in the detection of depression:

- Providing education on the impact of depression on diabetes outcomes
- Screening for depression
- Providing education on effectiveness of treatment
- Facilitating treatment
- Fostering healthy coping as a preventive measure

Screening for Depression

Diabetes educators can play an important role in screening their patients for depression. Depression screening can range from the use of formal questionnaires to informal clinical questions that may be posed during a routine interview. Table 4.2 lists questionnaires that may be used

TABLE 4.2 Depression in Persons With Diabetes: Tools for Assessment

Measure	*Contact Information*
PRIME MD/Patient Health Questionnaire (PHQ) Measures depression Kroenke K, Spitzer RL, Williams JBW. The PHQ-9: validity of a brief depression severity measure. J Gen Intern Med. 2001;16:606-13.	In the public domain; available at the Web site of the Health Resources and Services Administration, Bureau of Primary Health Care, US Department of Health and Human Services: www.healthdisparities.net/hdc/html/tools.aspx (choose "Tools posted by the Health Disparities Community")
Beck Depression Inventory (BDI) Measures depression Beck AT, Steer RA, Garbin MG. Psychometric properties of the Beck Depression Inventory: twenty-five years of evaluation. Clin Psycho Rev. 1988;8:77-100.	The Psychological Corporation. Web page describes the Beck Depression Inventory–II, which is available for purchase from The Psychological Corporation: www.psychcorpcenter.com/bdi-II.htm
Symptom Checklist—Revised (SCL-90-R) Measures psychological symptoms across many areas Derogatis LR. SCL-90-R Administration, Scoring and Procedures Manual–II for the Revised Version. Towson, Md: Clinical Psychometric Research; 1983.	NCS Assessments. Web page describing the SCL-90-R questionnaire and order forms. Available for purchase from NCS Assessments. http://assessments.ncspearson.com/assessments/tests/scl90r.htm
Center for Epidemiologic Studies—Depression (CES-D) Measures depression Radloff L.S. The CES-D scale: a self-report depression scale for research in the general population. Appl Psychol Measurement. 1977;1:385-401.	University of Pittsburgh. Provides a portable document file ("pdf") of the measure and scoring instructions available via free download: www.wpic.pitt.edu/research/City/OnlineScreeningFiles/CesdDescription.htm

to screen for depressive symptoms. Considerations for the use of formal screening questionnaires include availability of resources to provide screening measures for all patients for whom it would be appropriate, availability of diabetes educator's time to review forms for severity of presentation, availability of immediate referral resources for patients identifying significant symptoms of depression (eg, immediate self-harm).

In the absence of formal assessment procedures, diabetes educators can incorporate simple screening questions into routine interviews to assess the presence/absence of depressive symptoms. Table 4.3 provides routine screening questions for depression (as well as questions pertinent to anxiety disorders and diabetes-related stress).

Prior studies have noted that healthcare providers who ask patients about psychosocial issues are more likely to have individuals identify issues affecting their health.[33] Depression has been shown to have direct negative effects on overall diabetes self-care behaviors. Identifying and addressing this component may be important in working with persons with diabetes to facilitate adherence to self-care regimens.

Anxiety

This section discusses the following:

- What are the major anxiety disorders?
- How common is anxiety in people with diabetes?
- Who is most at risk for an anxiety disorder?
- What are the unique aspects of the combination of anxiety and diabetes?
- What treatment options are available?
- What is the role of the diabetes educator in detecting anxiety in people with diabetes?

TABLE 4.3 Diabetes-Related Stress, Depression, and Anxiety Disorders: Informal Screening Questions
Depression • In the past 2 weeks, have you been feeling consistently depressed or down? • Have you had difficulty with feeling sad or blue? • Has your mood interfered with taking care of your diabetes?
Anxiety Disorders *Anxiety* • What concerns do you have about your diabetes? • Tell me about the aspects of diabetes you fret about. *Avoidance* • What parts of your diabetes self-care are the hardest for you to do? • Are there situations or activities you avoid because of your diabetes? *Fear* • What is scary about diabetes for you? • Are there things about diabetes that frighten you? *Worry* • What do you worry about regarding your diabetes? • Tell me some of the thoughts that run through your head about diabetes?
Diabetes-Related Stress *Identification of Specific Stressors* • What drives you crazy about your diabetes? • Describe your typical day for me, starting when you wake up and ending when you go to sleep. What stressors do you face on a typical day? *Assessment of Stress Levels* • How high has your stress level been since our last appointment? • On a scale from 0 to 10, with 0 being no stress and 10 being the worst stress imaginable, what number would you give your stress level today? *Assessment of Diabetes Burnout* • Do you ever feel frustrated, fed up, overwhelmed, or burned out by diabetes? • I notice managing your diabetes has been hard for you lately. Do you think stress may play a role?

Most people experience a certain amount of anxiety in their lifetimes, and anxiety is a normal part of living. However, when anxiety becomes frequent, intense, or prolonged, it may interfere with normal functioning and impact diabetes care.

What are the major anxiety disorders?

In some cases, symptoms of anxiety may be elevated to the degree that they meet criteria for an anxiety disorder. According to the American Psychiatric Association,[1] there are 12 distinct anxiety disorders. The following disorders are covered in this chapter:

- Panic Disorder
- Specific Phobia
- Generalized Anxiety Disorder
- Posttraumatic Stress Disorder
- Adjustment Disorder with Anxiety
- Anxiety Disorder Not Otherwise Specified (NOS)

Panic Disorder

According to the American Psychiatric Association, the essential feature of Panic Disorder is recurrent and unexpected panic attacks about which there is persistent concern.[1] A panic attack is a discrete period in which there is sudden apprehension, fear, or terror, often associated with feelings of impending doom, fear of "going crazy," or losing control. Physical symptoms may include shortness of breath, palpitations, chest pain, or choking. Panic attacks are often mistaken for cardiac problems. Although most panic attacks last only a few minutes, they may be perceived as lasting much longer.

Specific Phobia

The essential feature of a Specific Phobia is anxiety provoked by a specific feared object or situation that often leads to avoidance of the object or situation.[1] Most adults recognize that their fear is excessive and out of proportion to any real danger posed by the object or situation, but children may not. Social phobia, for example, is the fear of social situations that involve interaction with other people. The anxiety in social phobia usually concerns being judged and evaluated by others.

Generalized Anxiety Disorder

Generalized Anxiety Disorder (GAD) is characterized by at least 6 months of excessive anxiety and worry in 2 or more domains (eg, money, safety of children).[1] Anxiety in this condition is usually "free floating"; that is, it is not necessarily limited to a specific object or situation, as is the case with Specific Phobia.

Posttraumatic Stress Disorder

The essential feature of Posttraumatic Stress Disorder is the reexperiencing of an extremely traumatic event through nightmares, obsessive thoughts, and flashbacks (feeling as if the trauma is occurring again).[1] There is an avoidance of situations, people, and/or objects that are reminders of the trauma. There is increased anxiety in general, possibly with a heightened startle response (eg, very jumpy, startle easily by noises).

Adjustment Disorder With Anxiety

The essential feature of Adjustment Disorder with Anxiety is anxiety in response to an identifiable psychosocial stressor in excess of what would be expected given the nature of the stressor.[1] Psychosocial stressors associated with the Adjustment Disorder such as loss of a job, divorce, or geographical relocation are not necessarily traumatic as is required for diagnosis of posttraumatic stress disorder. Symptoms may include nervousness, worry, or jitteriness.

Anxiety Disorder Not Otherwise Specified

The essential feature of Anxiety Disorder Not Otherwise Specified (NOS) is symptoms of anxiety that do not meet criteria for one of the other anxiety disorders.[1]

Additional anxiety disorders that are beyond the scope of this chapter include Acute Stress Disorder and Obsessive-Compulsive Disorder.

How common is anxiety in people with diabetes?

Anxiety in Adults

Among those without diabetes, 7% of the population meets criteria for an anxiety disorder in any given month, and 15% do at some point during their lifetime in the United States.[34] In fact, anxiety disorders are the most common of all the psychiatric disorders. Anxiety disorders are also common in persons with diabetes. The most reliable evidence is for GAD and Panic Disorder.[35] Current and lifetime rates were 13.5% and 20.5% for GAD and 1.3% and 1.9% for Panic Disorder, respectively. Rates of other anxiety disorders were also high: for simple phobia, 21.6% and 24.8% and for Anxiety Disorder NOS, 26.5% and 39%. Some studies have found that rates of anxiety among people with diabetes are higher than among nondiabetic controls. However, this is difficult to conclude with certainty because most studies lack nondiabetic comparison groups.

Among adults with diabetes, rates of subclinical anxiety symptoms are significantly higher than rates of overt anxiety disorders.[35] Rates of elevated symptoms averaged 39%. Rates of elevated symptoms were significantly higher in women (55%) compared to men (33%), but there was no difference by diabetes type.

Anxiety in Children and Adolescents

Among children with diabetes, GAD appears to be the most common anxiety disorder. Maternal psychiatric disorder has been shown to be a risk factor for pathology among children at diabetes diagnosis.[36]

Greatest risk is child's first year with diabetes:

The highest rates of any psychological disturbance among children with diabetes are during the year after diagnosis.

The overall high prevalence rates for anxiety disorders in adults and children highlight the need to assess for anxiety symptoms and anxiety disorders.

Who is most at risk for an anxiety disorder?

With the exception of risk conferred by female gender, evidence of risk factors for anxiety disorders among persons with diabetes is limited, because of the small number of studies. Epidemiological studies from the nondiabetic population have identified a number of risk factors for anxiety disorders. The following all have a higher rate of anxiety than individuals in other groups:[34]

- Women
- Individuals under age 45
- Family history of psychiatric disorder
- Separated or divorced
- Low socioeconomic groups

Also at increased risk for anxiety:

- Individuals with depression, especially the elderly

Older Adults. Although rates of anxiety disorders decrease with age, diabetes educators should be aware that they are still common among older adults. In community samples, the prevalence of any anxiety disorder among persons aged 65 years or older is 5.5%.[37]

Anxiety disorders are a mental health concern in older adults:

Anxiety disorders are the most prevalent mental disorders among community-dwelling older adults,[38] more common than even dementia. As with younger persons, rates are higher in older women compared with older men.

The prevalence of anxiety disorders among older adults in institutions also is a concern. A study of older adults in nursing homes found that 3.6% had 1 or more anxiety disorders.[39] Risk factors for anxiety among nursing home residents include the following:[40]

- Female
- Depression
- Lack of social support
- Poor physical health
- Functional impairment
- Cognitive impairments

Race, Ethnicity, Cultural Influences. Race and ethnicity may also play a role in risk for anxiety disorders. Early data suggested that African Americans had the same prevalence of anxiety disorders as the white population; however, recent data suggests that rates are actually higher among African Americans. The way in which African Americans experience and express their anxiety may not be detected by conventional mental health surveys, some have suggested. Furthermore, some racial and ethnic groups may be more at risk for certain types of anxiety disorders than other types. For example, Native Americans are at higher risk for Posttraumatic Stress Disorder than other anxiety disorders.[41] Certain immigrant populations who have experienced political or religious persecution may also be at risk for Posttraumatic Stress Disorder.[42]

What are the unique aspects of the combination of anxiety and diabetes?

Similarity in Symptoms of Anxiety and Hypoglycemia

The anxiety disorders have unique implications for diabetes and its treatment. First, clinicians must differentiate anxiety from symptoms of hypoglycemia. The adrenergic symptoms of anxiety and hypoglycemia can masquerade as each other, including sweating, tremulousness, weakness, dizziness, lack of concentration, and nervousness. Irritability, restlessness, poor memory, and indecisiveness may also occur in both conditions. Individuals who report these symptoms should be encouraged to self-monitor blood glucose while symptomatic. If symptoms occur during periods of euglycemia, anxiety disorders should be considered a possible cause and assessed.

Impact of Anxiety on Glycemic Control

Although the data are not entirely consistent, anxiety may impact glycemic control. The literature suggests that anxiety symptoms per se may not be associated with worsened glycemic control, but that overt anxiety has in fact been associated with worsened glycemic control.[43] Anxiety may directly impact glycemic control via counterregulatory hormones that are released during anxiety. Anxiety may also indirectly impact glycemic control by interfering with diabetes self-care behaviors.

Anxiety? Hypoglycemia?

Symptoms can be similar. Self-monitoring helps differentiate these two problems.

Specific Diabetes-Related Fears

Certain fears and anxieties are unique to diabetes. The following are discussed in this section:

- Fear of invasive procedures
- Fear of site rotation
- Fear of hypoglycemia
- Fear of long-term complications

Fear of Invasive Procedures. A Specific Phobia that is particularly problematic in diabetes management is fear of invasive procedures. This includes fear of injections and especially fear of procedures that involve blood, including self-monitoring of blood glucose (SMBG). People with extreme fear of injecting and fear of SMBG report higher levels of anxiety and depression, more fear of hypoglycemia and diabetes-related distress, lower levels of general well-being, and less frequent self-monitoring; as well, this fear is associated with higher A1C.[44] Research shows that rates of this type of Specific Phobia are relatively low among persons with diabetes.[45] However, subclinical symptoms of this sort are common and can compromise self-care behaviors.[46]

When this type of fear is present but self-care behaviors are performed nonetheless, the individual's quality of life is affected. People with this anxiety may be very resistant to initiating self-monitoring and insulin injections. Anxiety-reducing therapies can be helpful; also, these persons may benefit from newer insulin delivery technologies (insulin pens, inhaled insulin) and careful meter selection. A meter can be chosen that requires smaller amounts of blood and provides simplified blood sampling and alternate site blood sampling. Other patients may not fear the invasive procedure per se, but may be anxious about performing it in public due to a Social Phobia.

While there are numerous reasons people may avoid injections and SMBG, an individual who demonstrates any of the following should nonetheless be assessed for this type of phobia:

- Shows strong resistance to initiating or increasing the number of insulin injections
- Shows strong resistance to initiating or increasing the number of times SMBG is performed
- Does not change continuous subcutaneous insulin infusion sites as frequently as recommended
- Experiences significant distress when performing these tasks
- Requests that others (eg, family members) perform these tasks

Fear of Site Rotation. A related problem is fear of self-monitoring, injecting, or inserting a continuous subcutaneous insulin infusion site in a new location on the body. For example, a person may feel comfortable injecting in the arm, but be very resistant to injecting in the abdomen. This fear has been coined "site fright." The rates of "site fright" are not known; however, anecdotal accounts, particularly regarding children, suggest that it is not uncommon. Site fright can make site rotation a challenge, potentially resulting in lipohypertrophy and lipoatrophy at overused sites and subsequent problems with insulin absorption. Anxiety-reducing therapies can be used. These persons may also be good candidates for recent advances in technology such as novel injection devices, continuous subcutaneous insulin infusion set insertion devices, and inhaled insulin. An individual should be assessed for site fright in the following circumstances:

- Resists rotating sites
- Presents with hypertrophy or atrophy
- Shows evidence of otherwise unexplainable problems with insulin absorption

Fear of Hypoglycemia. People can also be fearful of experiencing hypoglycemia. Fear of hypoglycemia is common especially among type 1 diabetes, insulin users, those whose oral agents can induce hypoglycemia, those with hypoglycemia unawareness, and those who have experienced severe or embarrassing episodes of hypoglycemia in the past. Fear of hypoglycemia is related to greater blood glucose variability and lower mean daily blood glucose.[47] Parents of children with diabetes and spouses of those with diabetes may also experience fear of hypoglycemia for their loved one. Fear of hypoglycemia may develop in 2 ways.[48] First, hypoglycemic fear may result from recurrent hypoglycemia, leading to difficulty with symptom discrimination and the development of more pervasive and chronic anxiety and fear. Alternatively, chronically anxious individuals may be more likely either to fail to perceive the initial warning signs of hypoglycemia or to confuse these with anxiety. This may lead to increased anxiety and uncertainty concerning the onset of hypoglycemia.

Some people with fear of hypoglycemia may be hypervigilant about blood glucose levels, performing SMBG much more often than recommended. Others may deliberately undertreat their diabetes, allowing their blood glucose levels to run higher than the target range set by the healthcare provider in order to avoid hypoglycemic episodes. Someone who fears hypoglycemia may also avoid driving, public situations, being alone, or other situations in which a hypoglycemic episode could be dangerous or embarrassing.

Fear of hypoglycemia has also been documented as an important component of "psychological insulin resistance," a reluctance to transition from oral hypoglycemic agents to insulin therapy. [49] One study showed that 43% of insulin-naïve patients cited hypoglycemia as a reason for unwillingness to initiate insulin if prescribed by their healthcare provider.[50] An individual who demonstrates any of the following should be assessed for fear of hypoglycemia:

- Routinely performs SMBG far in excess of recommendation
- Shows chronically suboptimal glycemic control despite appropriate treatment recommendations
- Limits normal daily activities
- History of frequent or severe hypoglycemia
- History of dangerous or embarrassing hypoglycemic episodes

Fear of Complications. Worrying about the future and the possibility of serious long-term complications is often rated as the most distressing aspect of both type 1 and type 2 diabetes.[51] There is strong evidence that people with diabetes know more about complications that involve disability (eg, vision loss, amputation, dialysis) than life-threatening complications (eg, atherosclerotic disease and stroke)[52] and that those in ethnic minority groups may know less about their risk for some long-term complications than do people in the white population.[53] Because this fear is so ubiquitous, most persons with diabetes should be assessed for fear of long-term complications, especially if they are a caretaker for children or elders, live alone, have low social support, or express concern regarding complications.

What treatment options are available for people with diabetes and anxiety?

For people without diabetes, there are well-established, effective treatments for the various anxiety disorders. Effective treatments may include the following:

- Cognitive strategies to modify the person's worried thoughts
- Behavioral strategies to increase the person's successful exposure to the feared object or situation
- Relaxation training to decrease symptoms of arousal
- Medication to decrease symptoms of arousal

Pharmacotherapy

A few pharmacologic treatments for anxiety in diabetes have been tested in small studies, and, in general, they show benefit for anxiety and promising effects on A1C. One study compared 8 weeks of alprazolam up to 2 mg per day) to placebo among persons originally in poor glycemic control. At the end of treatment, both groups showed decreased anxiety, but only the alprazolam group showed improved A1C.[54] Another study compared 20 mg per day of fluoxetine to 20 mg per day of paroxetine for symptoms of depression and anxiety in type 2 diabetes. At the end of treatment, both groups showed decreased anxiety symptoms, and the fluoxetine group showed a promising benefit for reduced A1C.[55] A third study showed that 12 weeks of treatment with fludiazepam decreased anxiety and A1C in persons with type 2 diabetes.[56]

Behavioral Therapies

There is also some support for nonpharmacologic treatment of anxiety in diabetes. There is some evidence for cognitive-behavioral strategies for reduction of anxiety in diabetes.[57] A group program has shown benefits for coping with fears of long-term complications.[58] Behavioral methods have also been shown to be effective for treatment of injection phobias in children with diabetes.[59] Educational and psychological methods have also been described for decreasing psychological insulin resistance.[60]

Treatments designed for diabetes-related problems other than anxiety have also shown benefits for anxiety. For example, Blood Glucose Awareness Training-2 (BGAT-2), which was designed to help individuals better estimate their blood glucose levels as an adjunct to SMBG, resulted in a decrease in fear of hypoglycemia.[61] There is no evidence that behavioral treatments have a hyperglycemic effect, and none are contraindicated in diabetes. In general, diabetes educators should know that anxiety disorders are usually very responsive to treatment.

Opportunities in Diabetes Education

In addition to making referrals for psychological treatment delivered by a mental health professional, educators can directly help anxious patients in several ways, including the following.

- Distinguish symptoms of anxiety from hypoglycemia to help facilitate the appropriate treatment approach
- When appropriate and available, recommend less invasive diabetes care technologies
- As appropriate, practice glucose self-monitoring, insulin injections, or site rotation during office visits
- Clarify inaccurate information patients may have regarding risk for long-term complications
- Normalize the initiation of intensive treatment in a nonjudgmental manner, as appropriate

Educators should avoid using scare tactics to promote regimen adherence and should also avoid using initiation of insulin as a threat for those persons in suboptimal control on oral agents. These coercive strategies often have the undesirable and unintended effect of actually increasing anxiety and decreasing readiness to improve self-care.

What is the role of the diabetes educator in the detection of anxiety in people with diabetes?

People may not volunteer their anxieties to the educator. Therefore, educators must be vigilant for signs and symptoms of anxiety and assess for it. Table 4.3 includes routine screening questions for anxiety disorders (as well as questions on depression and diabetes-related stress). Table 4.4 lists tools for assessing anxiety in persons with diabetes.

Educators must also be aware that different groups may express their anxiety differently. For example, anxious children may regress, displaying behaviors typical of a younger child (eg, secondary nocturnal enuresis). Anxious children may have difficulty separating from caretakers, they may refuse to attend school, or they may somaticize (ie, experience and express their anxiety in physical complaints). Adults may also somaticize, reporting vague physical symptoms for which there are no underlying medical explanations. For example, higher prevalence of anxiety disorders is found in persons with medically unexplained gastrointestinal symptoms. Among persons with diabetes, gastrointestinal distress is also more prevalent among persons with anxiety.[62] There is also evidence that Asian Americans[63] and African Americans[64] may describe their anxiety in somatic terms. For example, African Americans associated the following symptoms with anxiety: talking fast, smelling strange smells, heart palpitations, fainting, sleeplessness, and gas/bloating.[64] Shenjing shuairuo is a Chinese illness concept characterized by physical and mental fatigue, dizziness, pain, concentration difficulty, sleep disturbance, and other signs that suggest disturbance of the branch of the nervous system involved in anxiety disorders. Because of these various presentations, educators should become familiar with culturally specific manifestations of anxiety in the patient populations they regularly serve.

Somatization must be differentiated from malingering (faking). Unlike malingering, somatization is not used for secondary gain (eg, attention, financial compensation). Persons who somaticize truly experience the physical symptoms they report. Reporting physical complaints may also reflect culturally appropriate help-seeking behaviors. In cases of suspected somatization, diabetes educators must first rule out any potential underlying medical problems, with referrals to medical specialists if necessary (eg, chest pains should be evaluated by a cardiologist). When findings are negative, assessment of anxiety should be initiated.

Diagnosis of anxiety disorders is beyond the scope of the diabetes educator's practice. When symptoms of anxiety exceed the limits of the educator's professional training, or when the educator's strategies to manage diabetes-related

TABLE 4.4 Anxiety in Persons With Diabetes: Assessment Tools

Assessment Tool	*Citation*
Fear of Hypoglycemia Survey (FHS) Self-report measure of fear and avoidance of hypoglycemia	Cox DJ, Irvine A, Gonder-Frederick L, Nowacek G, Butterfield J. Fear of hypoglycemia: quantification, validation, and utilization. Diabetes Care. 1987;10(5):617-21.
Fear of Hypoglycemia Self-report measure of fear of hypoglycemia designed specifically for children	Kamps JL, Roberts MC, Varela RE. Development of a new fear of hypoglycemia scale: preliminary results. J Pediatr Psychol. 2005;30(3):287-91. Epub 2005 Feb 23.
Diabetes Fear of Injecting and Self-Testing Questionnaire (D-FISQ) 30-item self-report questionnaire; has subscales that measure fear of self-injecting and fear of self-testing	Snoek FJ, Mollema ED, Heine RJ, Bouter LM, van der Ploeg HM. Development and validation of the diabetes fear of injecting and self-testing questionnaire (D-FISQ): first findings. Diabet Med. 1997;14(10):871-6.
Measure of Invasiveness as a Reason for Skipping SMBG (MISS) 7-item self-report questionnaire assessing the tendency to skip SMBG because of procedure's invasiveness	Wagner J, Malchoff C, Abbott G. Invasiveness as a barrier to self-monitoring of blood glucose in diabetes. Diabetes Technol Ther. 2005;7(4):612-9.
Fear of Progression of Chronic Disease 43-item self-report measure of fear of progression of chronic disease, including, but not exclusively designed for, diabetes	Herschback P, Berg P, Dankert A, Duran G, Engst-Hastreeiter U, Waadt S, Keller M, Ukat R, Henrich G. Fear of progression in chronic diseases: psychometric properties of the Fear of Progression Questionnaire. J Psychosom Res. 2005;58(6):505-11.
Diabetes-Related Fears Self-report measure of diabetes-related fears related to long-term complications, lifestyle changes, hypoglycemia, and weight gain	Taylor EP, Crawford JR, Gold AE. Design and development of a scale measuring fear of complications in type 1 diabetes. Diabetes Metab Res Rev. 2005;21(3):264-70.

fears are unsuccessful, referral to a mental health professional should be made. When in doubt, the educator should err on the side of making the referral. After the referral is made, the educator should work closely with the mental health professionals to coordinate care and track progress.

Eating Disorders

This section addresses the following:

- What are the major eating disorders?
- How common are eating disorders in people with diabetes?
- Who is most at risk for an eating disorder?
- What are the unique aspects of the combination of eating disorders and diabetes?
- What treatment options are available for eating disorders in people with diabetes?
- What is the role of the diabetes educator in detecting eating disorders?

Diabetes educators can play an important role in the identification and treatment of eating disorders. Although not as common as other psychological conditions described in this section, the combination of diabetes and an eating disorder can pose serious health consequences. Furthermore, individuals with eating disorders often do not seek help until the situation is serious. The American Diabetes Association recommends that the assessment of history and/or treatment of eating disorders be included as one of the core components of a comprehensive diabetes evaluation.[65] Ideally, all health professionals should be aware of the signs and symptoms of these conditions and help facilitate the identification and treatment of eating disorders in people with diabetes.

This section describes the major categories of eating disorders, along with their diagnostic criteria; prevalence rates for eating disorders; risk factors for eating disorders; and characteristics and consequences of eating disorders unique to people with diabetes. Current practice guidelines for treatment of eating disorders are summarized. Practice-based tips are offered to assist diabetes educators in identifying and working with individuals with eating disorders, along with information on screening and assessment.

What are the major eating disorders?

The American Psychiatric Association has 3 diagnostic categories for eating disorders:[1]

- Anorexia Nervosa
- Bulimia Nervosa
- Eating Disorders Not Otherwise Specified (EDNOS), which includes binge-eating disorder

The EDNOS category is used for eating-related disorders that do not fit clearly into the categories of anorexia and bulimia. Binge-eating disorder, an EDNOS, will be described in this section along with anorexia and bulimia.

Anorexia Nervosa

Table 4.5 lists diagnostic criteria for Anorexia Nervosa (and Bulimia Nervosa).[1] The primary clinical features are these:

- Refusal to maintain normal body weight
- Intense fear of becoming fat even though underweight
- Body image issues

In addition, people with anorexia may display strange eating habits, such as cutting their food into very small pieces or not eating in front of others, and they often obsess about food. Other associated features include self-esteem issues and general obsessive-compulsive features.

Bulimia Nervosa

Table 4.5 lists diagnostic criteria for Bulimia Nervosa (and Anorexia Nervosa).[1] The primary clinical signs include the following:

- Repeated episodes of binge eating involving a sense of loss of control
- Compensatory behaviors to prevent weight gain, such as self-induced vomiting, fasting, excessive exercise, and/or misuse of diuretics, laxatives, enemas, or other medications for weight-loss purposes
- Body image issues

Binge-Eating Disorder

Table 4.6 lists proposed diagnostic criteria for Binge-Eating Disorder. The primary clinical signs are repeated episodes of binge eating as in bulimia, but in the absence of compensatory behaviors to prevent weight gain and accompanied by marked distress about the binge eating.

As noted earlier, eating disorders do not always totally conform to these diagnostic symptoms, and other types will receive a diagnosis of EDNOS. Therefore, even though an individual may not have all of the symptoms of a particular eating disorder or may have some symptoms of both, that person may still receive an eating disorder diagnosis (ie, EDNOS) and still need intervention. Another factor to consider is that there are even more individuals with subclinical eating disorders or eating-disordered behaviors who can benefit from assistance with their unhealthy behaviors. Although the diagnostic criteria for the major eating disorders have been provided here, the reader is referred to the APA's Diagnostic and Statistical Manual of Mental Disorders, Fourth Edition, Text Revision[1] (DSM-IV-TR) and the suggested readings at the end of this chapter for more information on eating disorders.

TABLE 4.5 Anorexia Nervosa and Bulimia Nervosa: Diagnostic Criteria

Anorexia Nervosa	**Bulimia Nervosa**
A Refusal to maintain body weight at or above a minimally normal weight for age and height (eg, weight loss leading to maintenance of body weight less than 85% of that expected; or failure to make expected weight gain during period of growth, leading to body weight less than 85% of that expected). B Intense fear of gaining weight or becoming fat, even though underweight. C Disturbance in the way in which one's body weight or shape is experienced, undue influence of body weight or shape on self-evaluation, or denial of the seriousness of the current low body weight. D In postmenarcheal females, amenorrhea, ie, the absence of at least three consecutive menstrual cycles. (A woman is considered to have amenorrhea if her periods occur only following hormone, eg, estrogen administration.)	A Recurrent episodes of binge eating. An episode of binge eating is characterized by both of the following: 1. Eating, in a discrete period of time (eg, within any 2-hour period), an amount of food that is definitely larger than most people would eat during a similar period of time and under similar circumstances. 2. A sense of lack of control over eating during the episode (eg, a feeling that one cannot stop eating or control what or how much one is eating). B Recurrent inappropriate compensatory behavior in order to prevent weight gain, such as self-induced vomiting; misuse of laxatives, diuretics, enemas, or other medications; fasting; or excessive exercise. C The binge eating and inappropriate compensatory behaviors both occur, on average, at least twice a week for 3 months. D Self-evaluation is unduly influenced by body shape and weight. E The disturbance does not occur exclusively during episodes of Anorexia Nervosa.
Specify Type: *Restricting Type:* During the current episode of anorexia nervosa, the person has not regularly engaged in binge-eating or purging behavior (ie, self-induced vomiting or the misuse of laxatives, diuretics, or enemas). *Binge-Eating/Purging Type:* During the current episode of anorexia nervosa, the person has regularly engaged in binge-eating or purging behavior (ie, self-induced vomiting or misuse of laxatives, diuretics, or enemas).	*Specify Type:* *Purging Type:* During the current episode of Bulimia Nervosa, the person has regularly engaged in self-induced vomiting or the misuse of laxatives, diuretics, or enemas. *Nonpurging Type:* During the current episode of Bulimia Nervosa, the person has used other inappropriate compensatory behaviors, such as fasting or excessive exercise, but has not regularly engaged in self-induced vomiting or the misuse of laxatives, diuretics, or enemas.

Source: Reprinted with permission from the Diagnostic and Statistical Manual of Mental Disorders, 4th ed., text revision. Copyright 2000. American Psychiatric Association.

How common are eating disorders in people with diabetes?

In a review of the general literature on the prevalence of eating disorders, average prevalence rates (in the general population, not just those with diabetes) were as follows:[66]

- *Anorexia Nervosa:* 0.3% in young females (few studies included males)
- *Bulimia Nervosa:* 1% in young females and 0.1% in males
- *Binge-Eating Disorder:* Estimated to be at least 1%

Among the Diabetic Population. Many studies have also examined the prevalence of these disorders in people with diabetes. One recent meta-analysis of controlled studies examined differences in the prevalence of eating disorders in females with type 1 diabetes compared with those without diabetes.[67] This meta-analysis included only controlled studies from 1987 to 2003 that used interview-based diagnoses using the DSM (III or IV) criteria. In the 8 identified controlled studies, including a total of 748 females with type 1 diabetes and 1587 without diabetes, the average prevalence was this:

TABLE 4.6 Binge-Eating Disorder: Proposed Diagnostic Criteria

A Recurrent episodes of binge eating. An episode of binge eating is characterized by both of the following:
1. Eating, in a discrete period of time (eg, within any 2-hour period), an amount of food that is definitely larger than most people would eat in a similar period of time under similar circumstances
2. A sense of lack of control over eating during the episode (eg, a feeling that one cannot stop eating or control what or how much one is eating)

B The binge-eating episodes are associated with 3 (or more) of the following:
1. Eating much more rapidly than normal
2. Eating until feeling uncomfortably full
3. Eating large amounts of food when not feeling physically hungry
4. Eating alone because of being embarrassed by how much one is eating
5. Feeling disgusted with oneself, depressed, or very guilty after overeating

C Marked distress regarding binge eating is present.

D The binge eating occurs, on average, at least 2 days a week for 6 months.

E The binge eating is not associated with the regular use of inappropriate compensatory behaviors (eg, purging, fasting, excessive exercise) and does not occur exclusively during the course of Anorexia Nervosa or Bulimia Nervosa.

Source: Reprinted with permission from the Diagnostic and Statistical Manual of Mental Disorders, 4th ed., text revision. Copyright 2000. American Psychiatric Association.

- Anorexia Nervosa: 0.27%
- Bulimia Nervosa: 1.71%

The prevalence of anorexia was not significantly higher in females with diabetes compared with those without diabetes (0.27% vs. 0.06%), but bulimia was significantly higher in this group (1.73% vs. 0.69%, respectively). Males and those with binge-eating disorders were, notably, not included in this meta-analysis.[67] In the largest study in the meta-analysis, including 356 females (12 to 19 years old) with type 1 diabetes and 1098 age-matched controls, the presence of both clinical and subclinical eating disorders was approximately twice as common in females with diabetes.[68]

In a multicenter study that included a total of 340 men and women with insulin-dependent diabetes mellitus (IDDM) and 322 with non–insulin-dependent diabetes mellitus (NIDDM), prevalence rates for 4 eating disorders (anorexia, bulimia, binge-eating disorder, and EDNOS excluding binge-eating disorder) were identified using a 2-step process. The process involved completing self-report screening measures followed by clinical interviews based on the DSM-IV criteria.[69] The study found the following:

- Overall point prevalence rate (current state) across the 4 types of eating disorders: 5.9% (lifetime prevalence, 10%)
- Overall prevalence rate for people with IDDM: 5.3% (lifetime prevalence, 10%)
- Prevalence rate for those with NIDDM: 6.5% (lifetime prevalence, 9.5%)
- For women (N = 355), prevalence rate was 8.2% (lifetime prevalence, 14.7%), compared with 3.3% (lifetime prevalence of 4.6%) for men

Anorexia was found only in women with IDDM, and both bulimia and EDNOS were infrequently found in males. Binge-eating disorder was found in all groups, but was more common in those with NIDDM and overweight or obese individuals.

Screen for eating disorders across all groups

The prevalence rates cited above underscore the importance of screening for eating disorders across all groups. Diabetes educators can use these prevalence rates as a guide to become aware of groups at greatest risk for each disorder type.

In another study, 3000 primary care patients were assessed for binge-eating disorders (ie, bulimia and binge-eating disorder) using self-report measures.[70] This study found a current prevalence of eating disorders of 7% overall and 7.8% in people with diabetes. This indicates a significantly higher rate compared with other chronic medical conditions, which further supports the importance of screening for eating disorders in people with diabetes.

Who is most at risk for an eating disorder?

Several possible risk factors have been identified for eating disorders (ie, anorexia and bulimia), especially these:[71]

- Age: adolescence and early adulthood
- Gender: female
- Race/ethnicity: white populations
- Occupation/athletics that focus on weight
- Higher socioeconomic status (only anorexia)
- Family history of obesity, eating, and other mental health disorders (eg, depression)
- Premorbid experiences (eg, sexual abuse) and characteristics (eg, low self-esteem)

Little is known about risk factors for EDNOS, including binge-eating disorder. Awareness of risk factors can help the diabetes educator detect these disorders.

Age. Age is a risk factor for eating disorders and tends to display a bimodal distribution:[66]

- The peak age for anorexia occurs during the adolescent years (15 to 19 years of age)
- The peak age for bulimia occurs later (20 to 24 years of age)

Gender. Females have a much higher risk of developing eating disorders than males. Men are rarely diagnosed with anorexia. Overweight and obese men, however, are most likely to have a binge-eating disorder,[72] which points to the need to also screen for problem eating behaviors in men. Being overweight or obese, notably, was found to be associated with binge-eating disorder in both genders.[72]

Anorexia is more common in women of higher socioeconomic status and in Western societies.[71] In the United States, anorexia is more common in women of white populations than in African American females.[73] The risks for bulimia are similar except that there is a more even distribution across socioeconomic status.[71] Some have suggested that African American girls are more accepting of being overweight, more satisfied with their body image, and feel less social pressure to be thin.[74] Although much of the research has focused on women of white populations in developed countries, research has also found clinical eating disorders and disordered eating behaviors in developing countries as well as in black populations and those of Asian descent.[66,75] One study included women from black and white populations with binge-eating disorder who sought treatment compared with each other and with black and white community samples.[76] In this study, women with binge-eating disorder from black and white populations who sought treatment were not different in terms of age; education; dietary restraint; binge-eating frequency; or eating, shape, and weight concerns. They were only different on body mass index (BMI): black women who sought treatment had significantly higher BMIs than white women. When compared with community samples, more differences were found between groups that suggested that, in comparison to white women, black women may endure greater distress about their bodies or eating behavior before seeking treatment. In both groups, older women and heavier women were more likely to seek treatment.

In addition, family history of obesity (especially in bulimia) and certain mental health disorders (eg, eating disorders, depression, substance misuse—especially alcoholism in bulimia, premorbid experiences (eg, adverse parenting; sexual abuse; family dieting; and criticism around eating, shape, or weight), and individual characteristics (eg, low self-esteem; perfectionism—especially in anorexia; anxiety; obesity—especially in bulimia; and early menarche—especially in bulimia) may put the person at increased risk of developing an eating disorder.[71]

What are the unique aspects of the combination of eating disorders and diabetes?

There are several aspects of diabetes and its treatment that may make people with diabetes more vulnerable to eating disorders.[77] A number of situations related to diabetes may increase an individual's vulnerability to an eating disorder. For example, the initial weight loss associated with the onset of type 1 diabetes followed by weight gain with the initiation of insulin may increase the risk of an eating disorder in adolescent females, especially those who may have other characteristics (eg, body image issues, weight concerns). In addition, routine dietary recommendations may challenge the vulnerabilities of those prone to eating disorders. Such individuals may interpret recommendations in an extreme manner. For example, a recommendation to monitor intake of simple carbohydrates may be interpreted as "never eat sweets" and a recommendation to get regular physical activity may be interpreted as "exercise every day for 2 hours." Restrained eating in response to weight concerns or perceived dietary restrictions might make people with diabetes more vulnerable to binge eating. One study found, notably, that about 90% of people with type 2 diabetes reportedly developed their eating disorders prior to the diagnosis of diabetes;[72] this suggests that these factors are associated with binge-related eating disorders even in the absence of diabetes.

Intentional Insulin Omission

People with diabetes have been known to intentionally omit insulin shots for weight-control purposes. Misuse of medication for weight control is included as a type of compensatory behavior in the diagnostic criteria for bulimia.

Across all groups in the multicenter study, 4.1% of people with diabetes reported intentional insulin omission (5.6% of females, 2.6% of males).[69] Other studies have reported much higher rates,[68,78,79] suggesting that this is an important problem behavior that needs to be regularly assessed in individuals at risk. One study examined psychological predictors (eg, anxiety, depression, eating attitudes) and behavioral predictors (eg, "severe insulin omission," self-induced vomiting, binge characteristics) of A1C in females with type 1 diabetes with binge-eating problems.[80] This study found that "severe insulin omission" was the best predictor of elevated A1C levels. This study underscores the importance of considering insulin omission as a possible explanation for elevated A1C levels in young women with weight concerns and/or known eating disorder symptoms.

Negative Health Consequences of the Eating Disorders in People With Diabetes

The negative health consequences of the combination of diabetes and eating disorders has been recognized for many years and has even been described as a "deadly combination."[81] The combination puts the person at greater health risk than either alone and creates a serious situation. Although there are inconsistencies in the literature,[72] most studies found that individuals with diabetes and eating disorders or subclinical disordered eating behaviors experience increased risk of short-term (eg, elevated A1C levels) and long-term diabetes-related complications (eg, retinopathy, neuropathy) compared with those without such problems.[68,80,82-86] Furthermore, in a recent study, mortality rates for females with concurrent diabetes and anorexia were much greater than for those with either alone.[87]

Ideally, diabetes educators should be aware of these potential vulnerabilities to eating disorders and be especially careful about dietary, physical activity, and weight-related recommendations.

What are the treatment options available for eating disorders in people with diabetes?

The APA evidence-based practice guidelines for treatment of eating disorder support a combination of nutritional rehabilitation/counseling, psychosocial intervention, and medication.[88] The decision to treat as inpatient or outpatient is an important consideration, especially for anorexia. The decision to hospitalize a person should be based on psychiatric, behavioral, and general medical factors, especially including weight, cardiac, and metabolic status.

Anorexia Nervosa

In those with anorexia, the first goal is to restore a healthy weight through nutritional rehabilitation and counseling approaches.[88] Once weight gain is underway, individual psychotherapy should be initiated and may need to be supported with family, couples, and/or group therapy approaches. Psychotropic medications are not recommended as the primary or sole treatment approach with anorexia, but may be helpful (eg, antidepressants) once a healthy weight has been restored to prevent relapse and to help manage other problems, such as depression.

Bulimia Nervosa

For most people with bulimia, the combination of psychotherapy and psychotropic medication, particularly SSRIs, is the treatment of choice, along with adjunctive nutritional counseling.[88] Cognitive behavioral therapy has received the strongest research support, but interpersonal therapy, behavioral therapy, psychodynamic or psychoanalytic therapies, and family therapy have all been found to be useful.

Binge-Eating Disorder

For people with binge-eating disorder, cognitive behavioral therapy appears most promising.[88] Medication alone or in combination with cognitive behavioral therapy has also shown positive results.

The few controlled studies of the treatment of eating disorders in people with diabetes have been consistent with the general literature supporting the use of a variety of psychosocial interventions in treating eating disorders. For example, one randomized, controlled trial found that 2 different types of psychotherapy were effective in improving binge eating and A1C levels in people with type 2 diabetes.[89]

Special care needs to be taken in treating individuals with eating disorders and diabetes. Inpatient treatment needs to carefully monitor glycemic control and adjust insulin levels as the person's eating, physical activity, and weight change. Diabetes educators and dietitians need to work closely with mental health members of the treatment team to carefully coordinate care and give consistent messages about eating, weight, and physical activity.

What is the role of the diabetes educator in detecting eating disorders in people with diabetes?

This section summarizes the material presented above on eating disorders and offers the diabetes educator practice tips to help facilitate identification and treatment of individuals with diabetes who have eating disorders. Although it is not the role of the diabetes educator to diagnose and treat eating disorders, the educator should be familiar with the clinical features of each of these disorders based on the APA diagnostic criteria; also, the educator should recognize the numerous physical symptoms or lab abnormalities associated with eating disorders. The most common physical symptoms and lab abnormalities related to anorexia are presented in Table 4.7. In addition, in the presence of other signs and/or risk factors for eating disorders, unexplained elevations in A1C levels suggest the need for further evaluation of an eating disorder.

Ask directly about eating-related problems:

Healthcare professionals have generally believed that people with eating disorders deny their eating problems; however, recent research indicated otherwise:[90]

- 57% of individuals with disordered eating behaviors spontaneously disclosed their problem to a health professional
- Of those who did not volunteer information, the majority (91%) disclosed their problem when asked directly about it

This suggests that diabetes educators can increase the likelihood of identifying people with eating disorders simply by asking about eating-related problems. This is best done using a direct, nonjudgmental, supportive approach (chapter 25, on assessment, can be of help). The educator can introduce the topic by noting that having diabetes can make people more vulnerable to eating-related problems so questions about eating behaviors are asked of everyone. Some examples of questions to ask appear in Table 4.8. In addition, suggested

TABLE 4.7 Anorexia Nervosa: Common Medical Problems

Skin • Lanugo *Cardiovascular System* • Hypotension • Bradycardia • Arrhythmias *Hematopoietic System* • Normochromic, normocytic anemia • Leukopenia • Diminished polymorphonuclear leukocytes	*Fluid and Electrolyte Balance* • Elevated blood urea nitrogen and creatinine concentrations • Hypokalemia • Hyponatremia • Hypochloremia • Alkalosis *Gastrointestinal System* • Elevated serum concentration of liver enzymes • Delayed gastric emptying • Constipation	*Endocrine System* • Diminished thyroxine level with normal thyroid-stimulating hormone level • Elevated plasma cortisol level • Diminished secretion of luteinizing hormone, follicle-stimulating hormone, estrogen, or testosterone *Bone* • Osteoporosis

Source: Reprinted with permission from First M, Tasman A, eds. DSM-IV-TR Mental Disorders: Diagnosis, Etiology, and Treatment. Hoboken, NJ: John Wiley & Sons Limited; 2005.

TABLE 4.8 Eating Disorders: Informal Screening Questions

Weight Concerns
- How do you feel about your weight?
- Do you think you are overweight or worry about becoming overweight?
- Do you avoid getting on the scale?
- Would you weigh yourself in front of others?

Body Image Issues
- How do you feel about your appearance? Weight? Shape? Body size?
- What is your ideal body weight?

Binge Eating
- Are there certain foods you try to totally avoid eating? (Ask for details.)
- How often do you binge eat? (May need to define.)
- Describe your last binge episode.
- Do you ever feel like you cannot control your eating?

Compensatory Behaviors
- Have you ever induced vomiting or taken laxatives, diuretics, or enemas to lose weight?
- Have you ever reduced or skipped an insulin dose for weight purposes?
- Do you exercise regularly? (Ask for details)

Weight History
- What was your lowest and highest adult weight (Ask about adolescent weights where appropriate.)
- At what weight are you happiest?
- Have you experienced any rapid weight changes? (Ask for details.)

Unusual Eating Behaviors
- Are you uncomfortable eating in front of others?
- Do you have any eating habits your friends or family have told you were unusual?

self-report screening tools for eating disorders are listed in Table 4.9.

When the educator thinks that an individual may have an eating disorder, referral to a mental health professional with expertise in diabetes is critical. The mental health professional can conduct a full evaluation and provide treatment as needed. The educator must nevertheless work closely with the mental health professional to carefully coordinate care and give consistent messages about eating, weight, and physical activity.

Carefully construct dietary and physical activity recommendations:

When providing diabetes care and education to people with a suspected or known eating disorder, be careful with dietary and physical activity recommendations. These individuals tend to go to extreme with these behaviors. Minimize food restrictions and encourage eating healthy, including eating a variety of foods and getting regular (but not excessive) physical activity.

TABLE 4.9 Eating Disorders: Screening Tools

Assessment Tool	*Citation*
Eating Attitudes (EAT) 26-item survey assessing dieting and food restriction	Garner DM, Olmsted MP, Bohr Y, Garfinkel P. The Eating Attitudes Test: psychometric features and clinical correlates. Psychol Med. 1982;12:871-8.
Eating Disorders Inventory (EDI; EDI-2) 64-item survey assessing eating disorders symptoms	Garner DM, Olmsted MP, Polivy J. Development and validation of a multidimensional eating disorder inventory for anorexia nervosa and bulimia. Int J Eat Disord.1983;2:15-34.
Diabetes Eating Problems Survey (DEPS) Survey to assess eating-related problems, including manipulation of insulin for weight-control purposes, in people with diabetes	Antisdel JE, Laffel L, Anderson G. Improved detection of eating problems in women with type 1 diabetes using a newly developed survey. Diabetes. 2001;50 Suppl: A47.

Special Topics And Populations

What other psychiatric problems are related to diabetes?

Persons with diabetes are at increased risk for any dementia—and Alzheimer's dementia specifically.[91] People with schizophrenia[92] and bipolar disorder[93] have disproportionately high rates of diabetes, in part because some drugs used to treat these disorders increase risk for type 2 diabetes.[94] Despite this risk, these drugs are often prescribed because they are more efficacious and better tolerated than similar drugs that do not increase risk for type 2 diabetes. Persons with these psychiatric problems tend to have lower diabetes knowledge[95] and are less likely to receive diabetes care than their counterparts without mental illness.[96]

Diabetes education for this population needs to account for a range of cognitive abilities in attention, memory, problem solving, and judgment. Persons with cognitive deficits may have difficulty understanding medical information. Diabetes education should be delivered in a simple, organized, structured fashion with a limited amount of information delivered per session.

Persons with cognitive deficits may have poor functioning in activities of daily living and performance of complex behaviors, such as those required to maintain glycemic control. Environmental adaptation can compensate for some cognitive deficits. The educator should saturate the person's environment with cues, instructions, and memory aids to support diabetes self-care. For example, place important prompts (eg, reminders to perform SMBG, lists of healthy snack options, instructions for sick days) written in large, colorful letters in prominent places. The educator should also assist the person in rearranging the physical environment to be more conducive to self-care (eg, using a weekly pill organizer for oral agents and using automatic refill options for prescriptions). Whenever possible, educators should include significant others or support persons (eg, family members, neighbors, case workers, mental health professionals) in diabetes education since these individuals can help support the person in diabetes care.

These disorders have a variable course, and therefore educators should be alert to signs of decompensation (symptom exacerbation), including changes in hygiene, sensory perception, thought content, mood, memory, and attention. Changes should be promptly reported to the individual's mental health professional. During periods of decompensation, support persons (eg, family, caseworkers) may be required to assume responsibility for diabetes management at home. If psychiatric hospitalization becomes necessary, educators should collaborate closely with psychiatry hospital staff to ensure diabetes care plans are followed.

What do we know about psychological adjustment in women with diabetes during pregnancy?

Women with diabetes during pregnancy represent a special group. Included in this special category are 3 subgroups:

- Those with preexisting type 1 diabetes who become pregnant
- Those with preexisting type 2 diabetes who become pregnant
- Those newly diagnosed with gestational diabetes mellitus (GDM)

Diabetes during pregnancy puts both the mother and baby at risk of negative health outcomes. In addition, self-management is complex and behaviorally demanding. For those with preexisting diabetes, the management of diabetes may be intensified with additional glucose self-tests and insulin shots.[97] For those who are newly diagnosed, there is the need to learn all about diabetes and its management as well as adhere to the complex daily self-care regimen. The regimen, either intensified or new, may be accompanied by emotional and behavioral challenges. To date, however, few controlled studies have focused on psychosocial aspects of diabetes during pregnancy.

The few controlled studies that have been conducted have indicated that pregnant women with diabetes, especially those newly diagnosed with gestational diabetes, may experience an initial increase in negative emotions, such as anxiety and hostility.[98] These symptoms often do not reach clinical levels and usually improve and return to baseline levels over time during the pregnancy and the early postpartum period.[98-102] A few studies have examined stress in pregnant women with diabetes. Findings suggest that women with higher levels of stress have associated elevations in glucose levels.[103]

Concerns have also been raised about the potential negative impact of screening for diabetes in pregnancy[104] and about the intensified treatment of diabetes in pregnancy. One study found that women in both groups (GDM and controls) felt positively about being tested for gestational diabetes in the current pregnancy and preferred to be tested in future pregnancies. This finding suggests that the negative emotional impact of screening is minimal.[99] Studies examining the impact of intensified treatment of gestational diabetes, including self-monitoring and liberal insulin use, found that these approaches do not increase anxiety or depression in these women.[99-100] Although the research suggests that women may quickly adapt to the diagnosis of gestational diabetes and intensified treatment, pregnancy for both those with preexisting and those with newly diagnosed diabetes still may put women at higher risk for emotional challenges. Thus, pregnant women with diabetes should be assessed over the course of their pregnancy for problems with adjustment. In addition, more controlled studies are needed to better understand the emotional response patterns of pregnant women with diabetes.

More information on pregnancy complicated by diabetes can be found in chapter 11, on pregnancies with preexisting diabetes, and chapter 12, on GDM.

What do we know about stress in people with diabetes?

Living with diabetes is stressful. The unrelenting demands of diabetes self-care, feeling deprived of food, and failure to achieve treatment goals can be chronic stressors.[105] Interactions with healthcare providers, coworkers, family, and friends around diabetes can be difficult and unpleasant. Everyday diabetes experiences can also be burdensome, including carrying diabetes supplies and interrupting normal daily activities for self-care behaviors. Major diabetes transitions, such as the conversion from oral medication to insulin or the onset of long-term complications, are also stressful. Moreover, diabetes-related stressors are superimposed on other life stressors not related to diabetes.

Diabetes-related stress is very common,[106] and it can negatively impact diabetes self-care, glycemic control, and overall quality of life. Among adults, individuals' serious concerns regarding diabetes are related to poorer self-care, worsened glycemic control, and higher rates of long-term complications.[107] Children and adolescents also report high rates of diabetes-related concerns,[108] especially regarding family, peers, school, and transition from parental supervision to independence.

Risk factors for high levels of diabetes-related stress include the following:[109,110]

- Diagnosis of type 1 diabetes
- Insulin use
- Younger age
- Female gender
- Significant psychiatric history
- Recent hypoglycemia or DKA
- Poor general health
- Economic disadvantage
- Limited access to health care
- Social isolation

Stress is a subjective experience. That is, individuals differ in the situations they perceive to be stressful as well as in the way they cope with these stressful situations. Diabetes educators have an important role in helping people with diabetes deal with stress—by helping individuals modify their appraisals of common diabetes-related stressors and helping individuals develop more effective coping strategies.

A coping mechanism works to the degree that it is a good fit for the demands of the particular stressor. Successful coping strategies can buffer the effect of stress on diabetes.[111]

Appreciating that stress is experienced both physically and psychologically is important. Stress can have a direct effect on diabetes outcomes by affecting metabolic and cardiovascular functioning via the "fight or flight" response. Fight or flight is an involuntary mobilization of physical and psychological resources for fighting or fleeing from dangerous situations. This response is generally adaptive in individuals without diabetes who are facing an acute physical stressor. However, this response can be maladaptive and put the individual at health risk if stress becomes chronic, the stressor is psychological rather than physical, or if the person has diabetes and is therefore more vulnerable to metabolic or cardiovascular perturbations. If this stress response continues over a long period of time, an individual can reach a stage of physical and psychological exhaustion. In diabetes, psychological exhaustion has been called "burnout."[112] Burnout can hinder routine diabetes self-care behaviors (eg, skipped SMBG, less physical activity) and medical care (eg, missed appointments), and it can also increase unhealthy behaviors (eg, smoking, overeating, and alcohol or substance use). Stress also increases the likelihood of mental health problems such as depression and anxiety.

Psychosocial Interventions

Psychosocial interventions can decrease diabetes-related stress.[113] Coping skills training in adults results in improvements in stress and coping[114,115] as well as glycemic control.[116,117] Coping skills training has also been shown to be effective with adolescents.[117] Cognitive-behavioral group training has been shown to improve confidence in self-management, diabetes-related stress, and mood.[118] The evidence is mixed as to whether stress management and relaxation training produce glycemic benefits in adults or children, although several studies show benefits; there is no evidence to suggest that these interventions worsen glycemic control.[119-121] More frequent interactions with healthcare providers may be beneficial. Intensive diabetes education and nurse case-management have both shown positive effects.[122,123] Considered all together, the literature suggests that a variety of psychosocial treatments may help individuals with diabetes manage their stress more effectively, some of which may also improve glycemic control.

Opportunities in Diabetes Education

In addition to referring patients for formal psychosocial interventions, diabetes educators play an important role in helping those with diabetes manage diabetes-related stress. Educators can assess stress (see Table 4.3 for informal questions and Table 4.10 for formal assessment tools)

TABLE 4.10 Diabetes-Related Stress: Screening Tools

Assessment Tool	*Citation*
Problem Areas in Diabetes (PAID) 20-item questionnaire on patient's subjective feelings about difficulties with diabetes	Polonsky WH, Anderson BJ, Lohrer PA, Welch G, Jacobson AM, Aponte JE, Schwartz CE. Assessment of diabetes-related distress. Diabetes Care. 1995;18(6):754-60.
Diabetes Distress Scale (DDS) 17-item measure of distress associated with various aspects of living with diabetes	Polonsky WH, Fisher L, Earles J, Dudl RJ, Lees J, Mullan J, Jackson RA. Assessing psychosocial distress in diabetes: development of the diabetes distress scale. Diabetes Care. 2005;28(3):626-31.
Diabetes Hassles Scale to assess extent to which everyday demands of diabetes represent "hassles" or annoyances	Cox DJ, Taylor AG, Nowacek G, Holley-Wilcox P, Pohl SL, Guthrow E. The relationship between psychological stress and insulin dependent diabetic blood glucose control: preliminary investigations. Health Psychol. 1984;3:63-75.
World Health Organization–Wellbeing Questionnaire (WHO W-BQ) 22-item questionnaire designed to be sensitive to positive psychological benefits of treatment programs as well as more commonly measured symptoms of distress	Bradley C. The Wellbeing Questionnaire. In: Handbook of Psychology and Diabetes: A Guide to Psychological Measurement in Diabetes Research and Practice. Bradley C, ed. Chur, Switzerland: Harwood Academic Publishers; 1994.
Questionnaire on Stress in Diabetes (QSD-R)	Herschbach P, Duran G, Waadt S, Zettler A, Amm C, Marten-Mittag B. Psychometric properties of the Questionnaire on Stress in Patients with Diabetes–Revised (QSD-R). Health Psychol. 1997;16:171–4.

and implement stress management strategies. In particular, educators can help patients minimize the effect of stress on glycemic control. Because the effect of stress on glycemia is dependent upon numerous factors, it is difficult for patients to predict what effect stress will have on glucose levels. The educator can help by collaborating on a plan for managing high-stress days, including preparing meals and snacks ahead of time, performing more frequent SMBG, scheduling relaxation breaks throughout the day, and enlisting the help of support persons for diabetes care (chapter 5, on social support, can be of value). Patients with busy schedules or many life stressors may benefit from additional efforts to ensure continuity in the clinical relationship, such as regularly coordinated contact via telephone, email, or fax. Useful interpersonal strategies include focusing on diabetes successes, supporting problem-solving skills, involving the family in care, and building the person's emotional strength by creating an atmosphere of hope, optimism, and even humor regarding diabetes.[124] Overall, the literature shows that behavioral interventions delivered by diabetes educators can improve glycemic control.[125]

In cases when diabetes burnout is suspected, the diabetes educator might also give individuals permission to take a brief "vacation" from their diabetes self-care, during which they would follow a modified and less intensive self-management regimen within clearly outlined safe parameters for a limited period of time. The support and positive experiences that are available from joining diabetes support groups, participating in diabetes fundraising events, or volunteering for their local chapter of the American Diabetes Association or Juvenile Diabetes Research Foundation can also be of value. Children and adolescents may benefit from attending diabetes summer camp. See chapter 5 for more information on social support.

Practice-Based Strategies for Diabetes Educators

Screening

Although diagnosis and treatment of psychological disorders is outside the scope of practice for diabetes educators, educators should be aware of the signs and symptoms of these conditions so they can identify when referrals are needed. Screening for emotional and psychological problems is an important role of the educator. Signs and symptoms of depression, anxiety, and eating disorders have been presented in this chapter to help the educator identify these problem areas. Once the diabetes educator has determined that a patient has signs or symptoms of a disorder, a referral to a mental health professional or primary care physician, where appropriate, is warranted to pursue thorough assessment and treatment where needed.

Referrals

Within Care Team. Ideally, the diabetes care team should include a mental health professional (eg, psychiatrist, psychologist, social worker). This streamlines the referral process and coordination of care.

To Community Resources. If a mental health professional is not available within the practice setting, the diabetes education team should identify one in the community, preferably an individual who has experience working with people with diabetes. Psychologists, social workers, psychiatric nurses, and psychiatrists may be appropriate referrals, depending on their type of clinical practice. Although many private practitioners list their practices in the phone directory, contacting professional associations (eg, psychology, social work, psychiatrists) through state or national registries, such as the National Register of Health Service Providers in Psychology, can help locate referral sources.

Collaboration. When the referral is made, the mental health professional benefits from receiving as much information as possible from the educator, especially observed or reported signs and symptoms of the suspected disorder, beginning and duration of the symptoms, severity of the symptoms, and level of interference with diabetes and other life areas. To help facilitate communication and collaboration, the patient can sign a reciprocal release of information to avoid any concerns regarding breach of confidentiality when interacting with the multidisciplinary team. Educators are encouraged to seek advice from their institutions and its Health Insurance Portability and Accessibility Act (HIPAA) advisor on this topic.

The diabetes educators should communicate closely with the mental health professional throughout the treatment process to best coordinate the patient's care and give consistent messages, especially with eating disorders. As noted earlier, when working with people with a suspected or known eating disorder, dietary and physical activity recommendations must be carefully given because these individuals tend to go to extreme with these behaviors. In particular, be careful about recommendations regarding food restrictions and be sure to encourage healthy eating and regular (but not excessive) physical activity. Be sensitive to body image issues and weight concerns when discussing weight recommendations.

Coordination of Care. As noted, the diabetes educator is in an important position to facilitate care for mental health disorders by working closely with the patient, the mental health professional, and other members of the diabetes care team. Table 4.11 highlights a number of steps that diabetes educators can take to facilitate mental health treatment and coordinate care for their patients.

TABLE 4.11 Strategies to Facilitate Mental Health Assessment and Treatment

- Educate patients and the diabetes care team about common emotional responses to being diagnosed and living with diabetes; cover also the conditions or circumstances under which these emotional responses become problematic.
- Provide information to patients about depression, anxiety, and eating disorders and their impact on diabetes.
- Provide information to diabetes care team about signs and symptoms of common psychological disorders.
- Screen at-risk patients for common psychological disorders.
- Discuss the assessment process and treatment options with patients identified to have symptoms of psychological disorders. Explore with patients any stigma or concerns they may have about the assessment and treatment of mental health disorders.
- When symptoms of a disorder are identified and patient expresses interest, make a referral to a mental health professional. Be aware of local mental health resources.
- Be aware of appropriate options when symptoms of a disorder are identified and the situation is urgent (eg, suicidal intent) or the patient is not willing to pursue further assessment and treatment (eg, Anorexia Nervosa). Know the local emergency mental health services. Network with a mental health professional in your practice setting or community who can provide advice in these cases.
- Provide information to patients about local mental health resources. Encourage patients to ask about their mental health insurance benefits before contacting the mental health professional.
- Maintain ongoing communication with the mental health professional regarding treatment and agree on consistent messages to give the patient. Promote adherence with mental health treatment approaches in educational sessions.
- Educate the mental health professional about diabetes, its complications, and the patient's treatment regimen. Ask the mental health professional to promote adherence to the diabetes regimen.
- Assess the impact of emotional and psychological problems on routine personal and diabetes self-care. Reinforce and support patients in maintaining optimal routine and diabetes self-care, including healthful eating, regular physical activity, proper sleep habits, adherence with medication regimens, and regular glucose self-monitoring.
- Regularly reassess emotional and psychological symptoms during educational visits.
- Follow up with patients about mental health referrals at subsequent visits. Review barriers to care. Reinforce strategies for good mental health self-care.

Recent studies have demonstrated that coordinated care by primary care providers, nursing staff, and mental health professionals has the capacity to effectively treat depression in persons with type 1 and type 2 diabetes.[27,28] By sharing their assessment of the patient's presentation to all allied providers, diabetes educators can increase coordination and continuity of care for the whole person.

Role for Diabetes Education

Although diabetes education is not an effective treatment for clinical presentations of depression, anxiety, or eating disorders, studies have shown that diabetes education *is* effective in assisting patients with the diabetes self-management difficulties associated with these psychological disorders.[82] In some cases, lack of information or misinformation on diabetes, its treatment, and consequences may contribute to the negative emotions experienced by persons with diabetes. In these cases, providing general diabetes education on these topics will give such individuals a more thorough and accurate understanding of their situation and may help relieve their anxiety or sadness.

Diabetes educators can also play a key role in providing patients with information about specific conditions, such as depression, and their treatment. A person with diabetes may not be aware of the role these conditions may play in influencing glycemic control and interfering in self-care behaviors, such as eating healthy and getting physical activity. Diabetes educators can help validate that these conditions are treatable and facilitate communication and coordinate care with primary care and other allied health providers.

Resources for Patient Education

Educators are encouraged to contact organizations that publish educational brochures and information for patients. For example:

- National Institute for Mental Health
- National Association of Mental Illness
- American Psychological Association
- American Psychiatric Association

In addition, educators may guide patients to Internet resources, advising patients to obtain information from reputable Web sites. The educator is encouraged to identify and carefully review available Web sites and make specific recommendations to patients.

Finally, diabetes educators play a crucial role in providing patients with information about diabetes self-management that contributes to good mental health. Good nutrition, exercise, effective glycemic management, and adherence to medication regimens contribute to quality of life and positively reinforce mental health treatment. Chapter 34 on healthy coping contains more information that can be of value. Educators can inquire about psychotherapy and/or medication use for mental health treatment. Educators can also reinforce and support patients' behavioral strategies in caring for their psychological disorders in addition to diabetes self-management goals. Such discussion validates the value of both sets of interventions and supports persons with diabetes as they work to care for themselves in body and mind.

Focus on Education: Pearls for Practice

Teaching Strategies

- **Support the individual's mental health.** At each contact, promote good nutrition, regular physical activity, and proper sleep habits and offer problem solving to assist with adherence to medication regimens.
- **Seek team collaboration.** Maintaining ongoing communication with all members of the diabetes care team and mental health professionals is crucial for the appropriate care of individuals with these problems.
- **Regularly incorporate screening.** Be familiar with screening tools and comfortable in initiating screening for symptoms of mental health problems during the education and care process. Increase comfort with the referral process and establish communication lines with mental health professionals.

Messages for Patients

- **Discuss openly.** Individuals with diabetes may experience mental health problems, including depression, anxiety, and eating disorders. Talking about the possibility of this and creating awareness may offer quicker recognition and allow treatment opportunities to be scheduled sooner.
- **Consider mental health part of good diabetes control.** Mental health problems may interfere with diabetes self-management and diabetes control. Periodically monitoring mental health and feelings is an important part of routine diabetes care.
- **Help is available.** Persons dealing with both diabetes and matters of mental health need to know they are not alone; help and support are available. Offer handouts or Web site addresses with information on where to find additional support or information. Make an appointment with a mental health professional as the need arises.

Suggested Readings

Depression

Anderson BJ, Rubin RR, eds. Practical Psychology for Diabetes Clinicians: Effective Techniques for Key Behavioral Issues, 2nd ed. Washington, DC: American Diabetes Association; 2002.

Rubin RR, Ciechanowski P, Egede L, Lin E, Lustman PJ. Recognizing and treating depression in patients with diabetes. Curr Diab Rep. 2004(2):119-25.

Anxiety

Kelly MN. Recognizing and treating anxiety disorders in children. Pediatr Ann. 2005;34(2):147-50.

Lauderdale SA, Sheikh JI. Anxiety disorders in older adults. Clin Geriatr Med. 2003;19(4):721-41.

Rubin RR, Peyrot M. Psychological issues and treatments for people with diabetes. J Clin Psychol. 2001 Apr;57(4):457-78.

Snoek FJ, TC Skinner, eds. Psychology in Diabetes Care. West Sussex, England: Wiley & Sons Limited; 2005.

See also Anderson, under category of Depression

Eating Disorders

American Psychiatric Association. Practice Guidelines for the Treatment of Patients With Eating Disorders, 2nd ed. Arlington, Va: American Psychiatric Association; 2000.

Fairburn CG. Eating disorders. Lancet 2003;361:407-16.

Kelly SD, Howe CJ, Hendler JP, Lipman TH. Disordered eating behaviors in youth with type 1 diabetes. Diabetes Educator. 2005;34(4):572-83.

Working With Mental Health Professionals

Gelfand K, Geffken G, Lewin A, et al. An initial evaluation of the design of pediatric psychology consultation service with children with diabetes. J Child Health Care. 2004;8(2):113-23.

Working With Children With Diabetes

Silverstein J, Klingensmith G, Copeland K, et al. Care of children and adolescents with type 1 diabetes: a statement of the American Diabetes Association, Diabetes Care 2005;28:186-212.

References

1. American Psychiatric Association. Diagnostic and Statistical Manual of Mental Disorders, 4th ed., text revision. Washington, DC: American Psychiatric Association; 2000.
2. Landrine H, Klonoff EA. Cultural diversity and health psychology. In: Handbook of Health Psychology. Baum A, Revenson TA, and Singer JE, eds. New Jersey: Lawrence Erlbaum Associates; 2001:851-91.
3. Anderson RJ, Freedland KE, Clouse RE, Lustman PJ. The prevalence of comorbid depression in adults with diabetes. Diabetes Care. 2001;24(6):1069-78.
4. Gary TL, Crum RM, Cooper-Patrick L, Ford D, Brancati FL. Depressive symptoms and metabolic control in African-Americans with type 2 diabetes. Diabetes Care. 2000;23(1):23-9.
5. Gross R, Olfson M, Gameroff M, et al. Depression and glycemic control in Hispanic primary care patients with diabetes. J Gen Intern Med. 2004;20:460-6.
6. Grandinetti A, Kaholokula J, Crabbe K, Kenui C, Chen R, Chang H. Relationship between depressive symptoms and diabetes among native Hawaiians. Psychoneuroendocrinol. 2000;25:239-46.
7. de Groot M, Hockman E, Wagner J. Depression in a multicultural sample of diabetes expo attenders. Diabetes. 2003;52 Suppl 1:A411.
8. Peyrot M, Rubin RR. Persistence of depressive symptoms in diabetic adults. Diabetes Care. 1999;22:448-52.
9. Grey M, Whittemore R, Tamborlane W. Depression in type 1 diabetes children: natural history and correlates. J Psychosom Res. 2002;53:907-11.
10. Jacobson AM, Hauser ST, Willett JB, et al. Psychological adjustment to IDDM: 10-year follow-up of an onset cohort of child and adolescent patients. Diabetes Care. 1997;20:811-8.
11. Katz L, Swami S, Abraham M, et al. Neuropsychiatric disorders at the presentation of type 2 diabetes mellitus in children. Pediatric Diabetes. 2005;6:84-9.
12. Katon W, Von Korff M, Ciechanowski P, et al. Behavioral and clinical factors associated with depression among individuals with diabetes. Diabetes Care. 2004;27:914-20.
13. Lustman PJ, Griffith LS, Clouse RE. Depression in adults with diabetes: results of 5-year follow-up study. Diabetes Care. 1988;11:605-12.

14. Carnethon M, Kinder L, Fair J, Stafford R, Fortmann S. Symptoms of depression as a risk factor for incident diabetes: findings from the National Health and Nutrition Examination Epidemiologic Follow-Up Study, 1971-1992. Am J Epidemiol. 2003;158:416-23.

15. Jacobson AM, Weinger K, Hill TC, Parker JA, Suojanen J, Jimerson D, Soroko D. Brain functioning, cognition and psychiatric disorders in patients with type 1 diabetes. Diabetes. 2000;49 Suppl 1:A132.

16. McEwen BS, Magarinos AM, and Reagan L P. Studies of hormone action in the hippocampal formation: possible relevance to depression and diabetes. J Psychosom Res. 2002;53:883-90.

17. Lustman PJ, Anderson RJ, Freedland KE, de Groot M, Carney RM, Clouse RE. Depression and poor glycemic control: a meta-analytic review of the literature. Diabetes Care. 2000;23:934-42.

18. de Groot M, Anderson RJ, Freedland KE, Clouse RE, Lustman PJ. Association of depression and diabetes complications: a meta-analysis. Psychosom Med. 2001;63:619-30.

19. Ciechanowski PS, Katon WJ, Russo JE. Depression and diabetes: impact of depressive symptoms on adherence, function, and costs. Arch Intern Med. 2000;160:3278-85.

20. Egede LE, Zheng D, Simpson K. Comorbid depression is associated with increased health care use and expenditures in individuals with diabetes. Diabetes Care. 2002;25:464-70.

21. Egede LE. Diabetes, major depression and functional disability among U.S. adults. Diabetes Care. 2004;27:421-8.

22. Zhang X, Norris SL, Gregg EW, Cheng YJ, Beckles G, Kahn HS. Depressive symptoms and mortality among persons with and without diabetes. Am. J Epidemiol. 2005;161:652-60.

23. Jacobson AM, de Groot M, Samson, JA. The effects of psychiatric disorders and symptoms on quality of life in patients with type I and type II diabetes mellitus. Qual Life Res. 1997;6:11-20.

24. Gaynes BN, Burns B, Tweed D, Erickson P. Depression and health-related quality of life. J Nerv Ment Dis. 2002;190:799-806.

25. Garrison M, Katon W, Richardson L. The impact of psychiatric comorbidities on readmissions for diabetes in youth. Diabetes Care. 2005;28:2150-4.

26. Lustman PJ, Griffith LS, Freedland KE, Kissel SS, Clouse RE. Cognitive behavior therapy for depression in type 2 diabetes mellitus: a randomized, controlled trial. Ann Intern Med. 1998;129:613-21.

27. Katon WJ, Von Korff M, Lin EH, et al. The Pathways Study: a randomized trial of collaborative care in patients with diabetes and depression. Arch Gen Psychiatry. 2004;61:1042-9.

28. Williams JW, Katon W, Lin EHB, et al. The effectiveness of depression care management on diabetes-related outcomes in older patients. Ann Intern Med. 2004;140:1015-24.

29. Goodnick PJ. Use of antidepressants in treatment of comorbid diabetes mellitus and depression as well as in diabetic neuropathy. Ann Clin Psych. 2001;13:31-41.

30. Lustman PJ, Griffith LS, Clouse RE, et al. Effects of nortriptyline on depression and glycemic control in diabetes: results of a double-blind, placebo-controlled trial. Psychosom Med. 1997;59:241-50.

31. Lustman PJ, Freedland KE, Griggith LS, Clouse RE. Fluoxetine for depression in diabetes: a randomized double-blind placebo-controlled trial. Diabetes Care. 2000;23:618-23.

32. Goodnick PJ, Kumar A, Henry JH, Buki VM, Goldberg RB. Sertraline in coexisting major depression and diabetes mellitus. Psychopharmacol Bull. 1997;33:261-4.

33. Robinson JW, Roter DL. Psychosocial problem disclosure by primary care patients. Soc Sci Med. 1999;48:1353-62.

34. Regier DA, Narrow WE, Rae DS. The epidemiology of anxiety disorders: the Epidemiologic Catchment Area (ECA) experience. J Psychiatr Res. 1990;24 Suppl 2:3-14.

35. Grigsby AB, Anderson RJ, Freedland KE, Clouse RE, Lustman PJ. Prevalence of anxiety in adults with diabetes: a systematic review. J Psychosom Res. 2002;53:1053-60.

36. Kovac M, Goldsone D, Obrosky DS, Bonar LK. Psychiatric disorders in youths with IDDM: rates and risk factors. Diabetes Care. 1997;20:36-44.

37. Regier DA, Boyd JH, Burke JD Jr, Rae DS, Myers JK, Kramer M, et al. One-month prevalence of mental disorders in the United States: based on five Epidemiologic Catchment Area sites. Arch Gen Psychiatry. 1988;45:977-86.

38. Hybels CR, Blazer DG. Epidemiology of late-life mental disorders. Clin Geriatr Med. 2003;19:663-96.

39. Burns BJ, Larson DB, Goldstrom ID, et al. Mental disorder among nursing home patients: preliminary findings from the National Nursing Home Survey Pretest. Int J Geriatr Psych. 1988;3:27-35.

40. Smalbrugge M, Pot AM, Jongenelis K, Beekman AT, Eefsting JA. Anxiety disorders in nursing homes: a literature review of prevalence, course and risk indicators. Tijdschr Gerontol Geriatr. 2003;34:215-21.

41. Beals J, Novins DK, Whitesell NR, Spicer P, Mitchell CM, Manson SM. Prevalence of mental disorders and utilization of mental health services in two American Indian reservation populations: mental health disparities in a national context. Am J Psychiatry. 2005;162:1723-32.

42. Eissenman DP, Gelberg L, Liu H, Shapiro MF. Mental health and health-related quality of life among adult Latino primary care patients living in the United States with previous exposure to political violence. JAMA. 2003;290:627-34.

43. Anderson RJ, Grigsby AB, Freedland KE, et al. Anxiety and poor glycemic control: a meta-analytic review of the literature. Int J Psychiatry Med. 2002;32:235-47.

44. Berlin I, Bisserbe JC, Eiger R, et al. Phobic symptoms, particularly the fear of blood and injury, are associated with poor glycemic control in type I diabetic adults. Diabetes Care. 1997;20:176-8.

45. Mollema ED, Snoek FJ, Heine RJ, Van der Ploeg HM. Phobia of self-injecting and self-testing in insulin-treated diabetes patients: opportunities for screening. Diabet Med. 2001;18:671-4.

46. Wagner J, Malchoff C, Abbott G. Invasiveness as a barrier to self-monitoring of blood glucose in diabetes. Diabetes Technol Ther. 2005;7:612-9.

47. Irvine AA, Cox D, Gonder-Frederick L. Fear of hypoglycemia: relationship to physical and psychological symptoms in patients with insulin-dependent diabetes mellitus. Health Psychol. 1992;11:135-8.

48. Polonsky WH, Davis CL, Jacobson AM, Anderson BJ. Correlates of hypoglycemic fear in type I and type II diabetes mellitus. Health Psychol. 1992;11:199-202.

49. Snoek, FJ. Breaking the barriers to optimal glycaemic control—what physicians need to know from patients' perspectives. Int J Clin Pract Suppl. 2002;129:80-4.

50. Polonsky WH, Fisher L, Guzman S, Villa-Caballero L, Edelman SV. Psychological insulin resistance in patients with type 2 diabetes: the scope of the problem. Diabetes Care. 2005;28:2543-5.

51. Snoek FJ, Pouwer F, Welch GW, Polonsky WH. Diabetes-related emotional distress in Dutch and U.S. diabetic patients: cross-cultural validity of the problem areas in diabetes scale. Diabetes Care. 2000;23:1305-9.

52. The Diabetes-Heart Disease Link. A report on the attitudes toward and knowledge of heart disease risk among people with diabetes in the U.S. American Diabetes Association and the American College of Cardiology; 2002.

53. Wagner J, Lacey K, Abbott G, de Groot M, Chyun D. Knowledge of heart disease risk in a multicultural community sample of people with diabetes. Ann Behav Med. In press 2006.

54. Lustman PJ, Griffith LS, Clouse RE, et al. Effects of alprazolam on glucose regulation in diabetes: results of double-blind, placebo-controlled trial. Diabetes Care. 1995;18:1133-9.

55. Gulseren L, Gulseren S, Hekimsoy Z, Mete L. Comparison of fluoxetine and paroxetine in type II diabetes mellitus patients. Arch Med Res. 2005;36:159-65.

56. Okada S, Ichiki K, Tanokuchi S, Ishii K, Hamada H, Ota Z. Improvement of stress reduces glycosylated haemoglobin levels in patients with type 2 diabetes. J Int Med Res. 1995;23:119-22.

57. Snoek FJ, van der Ven NC, Lubach CH, chatrou M, Ader HJ, Heine RJ, Jacobson AM. Effects of cognitive behavioural group training (CBGT) in adult patients with poorly controlled insulin-dependent (type 1) diabetes: a pilot study. Patient Educ Couns. 2001;45:143-8.

58. Zettler A, Duran G, Waadt S, Herschbach P, Strian F. Coping with fear of long-term complications in diabetes mellitus: a model clinical program. Psychother Psychosom. 1995;64(3-4):178-84.

59. Rainwater N, Sweet A, Lynne E. Systematic desensitization in the treatment of needle phobias for children with diabetes. Child Fam Beh. Ther. 2001;45:143-8.

60. Funnel MM, Kruger DF, Spencer M. Self-management support for insulin therapy in type 2 diabetes. Diabetes Educ. 2004;30:274-80.

61. Cox DJ, Gonder-Frederick L, Polonsky W, Schlundt D, Kovatchev B, Clarke W. Blood glucose awareness training (BGAT-2): long-term benefits. Diabetes Care. 2001;24:637-42.

62. Talley SJ, Bytzer P, Hammer J, Young L, Jones M, Horowitz M. Psychological distress is linked to gastrointestinal symptoms in diabetes mellitus. Am J Gastroenterol. 2001;96:1033-8.

63. Hsu SI. Somatisation among Asian refugees and immigrants as a culturally-shaped illness behaviour. Ann Acad Med Singapore. 1999;28:841-5.

64. Heurtin-Roberts S, Snowden L, Miller L. Expressions of anxiety in African Americans: ethnography and the epidemiological catchment area studies. Cult Med Psychiatry. 1997;21:337-63.

65. American Diabetes Association. Standards of medical care in diabetes. Diabetes Care. 2005;38 Suppl 1: S24-31.

66. Hoek HW, van Hoeken, D. Review of the prevalence and incidence of eating disorders. Int J Eat Disord. 2003;34:383-96.

67. Mannucci E, Rotella F, Ricca V, Moretti S, Placid GF, Rotella CM. Eating disorders in patient with type 1 diabetes: a meta-analysis. J Endocrinol Invest. 2005;28:417-9.

68. Jones JM, Lawson ML, Daneman D, Olmsted MP, Rodin G. Eating disorders in adolescent females with and without type 1 diabetes: cross-sectional study. BMJ. 2000;320:1563-6.

69. Herpertz S, Wagener R, Albus C, et al. Diabetes mellitus and eating disorders: a multicenter study on the comorbidity of the two diseases. J Psychosom Res. 1998;44:503-515.

70. Goodwin RD, Hoven CW, Spitzer RL. Diabetes and eating disorders in primary care. Int J Eat Disord. 2003;33:85-91.

71. Fairburn CG. Eating disorders. Lancet. 2003;361:407-16.

72. Herpertz S, Albus C, Wagener R, et al. Comorbidity of diabetes and eating disorders: does diabetes control reflect disturbed eating behavior? Diabetes Care. 1998;21:1110-6.

73. Zhang AY, Snowden LR. Ethnic characteristics of mental disorders in five U.S. communities. Cultur Divers Ethnic Minor Psychol. 1999;5:134-46.

74. Striegel-Moore RH, Fairbun CG, Wilfley DE, Pike KM, Dohm FA, Kraemer HC. Toward an understanding of risk factors for binge-eating disorder in black and white women: a community-based case-control study. Psychol Med. 2005;35:907-17.

75. Hoek HW, van Harten PN, Hermans KM, Katzman MA, Matroos GE, Susser ES. The incidence of anorexia nervosa on Curacao. Am J Psychiatry. 162;4:748-52.

76. Grilo CM, Lozano C, Masheb RM. Ethnicity and sampling bias in binge eating disorder: black women who seek treatment have different characteristics than those who do not. Int J Eat Disord. 2005;38:257-62.

77. Daneman D, Olmsted M, Rydall A, Maharaj S, Rodin G. Eating disorders in young women with type 1 diabetes: prevalence, problems and prevention. Horm Res. 1998;50 Suppl 1:79-86.

78. Bryden KS, Neil A, Mayou RA, Peveler RC, Fairburn CG, Dunger DB. Eating habits, body weight, and insulin misuse: a longitudinal study of teenagers and young adults with type 1 diabetes. Diabetes Care. 1999;22:1956-60.

79. Polonsky WH, Anderson BJ, Lohrer PA, Aponte JE, Jacobson AM, Cole CF. Insulin omission in women with IDDM. Diabetes Care. 1994;17:1178-85.

80. Takil M, Komaki G, Uchigata Y, Maeda M, Omori Y, Kubo C. Differences between bulimia nervosa and binge-eating disorder in females with type 1 diabetes: the important role of insulin omission. J Psychosom Res. 1999;47:221-31.

81. Hillard JR, Hillard PJ. Bulimia, anorexia nervosa, and diabetes: deadly combinations. Psychiatry Clin North Am. 1984;7:367-79.

82. Affenito SG, Backstrand JR, Welch GW, Lammi-Keefe CJ, Rodriguez NR, Adams CH. Subclinical and clinical eating disorders in IDDM negatively affect metabolic control. Diabetes Care. 1997;20:182-4.

83. Cantwell R, Steel JM. Screening for eating disorders in diabetes mellitus. J Psychosom Res. 1995;40:15-20.

84. Marcus MD, Wing RR, Jawad A, Orchard TJ. Eating disorders symptomology in a registry-based sample of women with insulin-dependent diabetes mellitus. Int J Eat Disord. 1992;12:425-30.

85. Rydall AC, Rodin GM, Olmsted MP, Devenyi RG, Daneman D. Disordered eating behavior and microvascular complications in young women with insulin-dependent diabetes mellitus. N Engl J Med. 1997;336:1849-54.

86. Steel JM, Young RJ, Lloyd GG, Clarke BF. Clinically apparent eating disorders in young diabetic women: associations with painful neuropathy and other complications. BMJ. 1987;294:859–62.

87. Nielsen S, Emborg C, Molbak AG. Mortality in concurrent type 1 diabetes and anorexia nervosa. Diabetes Care. 2002;25:309-12.

88. American Psychiatric Association. Practice Guidelines for the Treatment of Patients With Eating Disorders, 2nd ed. Arlington, Va: American Psychiatric Association; 2000.

89. Kenardy J, Mensch M, Bowen K, Green B, Walton J. Group therapy for binge eating in Type 2 diabetes: a randomized trial. Diabet Med. 2002;19:234-9.

90. Becker AE, Thomas JJ, Franko Dr, Herzog DB. Disclosure patterns of eating and weight concerns to clinicians, educational professionals, family, and peers. Int J Eat Disord. 2005;38:18-23.

91. Leibson CL, Rocca WA, et al. Risk of dementia among persons with diabetes mellitus: a population-based cohort study. Am J Epidemiol. 1997;145:301-8.

92. Sokal J, Messias E, Dickerson FB, et al. Comorbidity of medical illnesses among adults with serious mental illness who are receiving community psychiatric services. J Nerv Ment Dis. 2004;192:421-7.

93. McIntyre RS, Konarsky JZ, Misener VL, Kennedy SH. Bipolar disorder and diabetes mellitus: epidemiology, etiology, and treatment implications. Ann Clin Psychiatry. 2005;17:83-93.

94. American Diabetes Association; American Psychiatric Association; American Association of Clinical Endocrinologists; North American Association for the Study of Obesity. Consensus development conference on antipsychotic drugs and diabetes. Diabetes Care. 2004;27:596-601.

95. Dickerson FB, Goldberg RW, Brown CH, et al. Diabetes knowledge among persons with serious mental illness and type 2 diabetes. Psychosomatics. 2005;46:418-24.

96. Cradock-O'Leary J, Young AS, Yano EM, Wang M, Lee ML. Use of general medical services by VA patients with psychiatric disorders. Psychiatric Services. 2002;53:874-8.

97. Tuffnell DJ, West J, Walkinshaw SA. Treatments for gestational diabetes and impaired glucose tolerance in pregnancy (review). Cochrane Database Syst Rev. 2003;(3):CD003395.

98. Langer N, Langer O. Emotional adjustment to diagnosis and intensified treatment of gestational diabetes. Obstet Gynecol. 1994;84:329-34.

99. Daniells S, Grenyer BF, Davis WS, Coleman KJ, Burgess JA, Moses RG. Gestational diabetes mellitus: is a diagnosis associated with an increase in maternal anxiety and stress in the short and intermediate term? Diabetes Care. 2003;26:385-9.

100. Langer N, Langer O. Pre-existing diabetics: relationship between glycemic control and emotional status in pregnancy. J Matern Fetal Med. 1998;7:257-63.

101. Spirito A, Williams C, Ruggiero L, Bond A, McGarvey ST, Coustan D. Psychological impact of the diagnosis of gestational diabetes. Obstet Gynecol. 1989;73:562-6.

102. York R, Brown LP, Persily CA, Jacobsen BS. Affect in diabetic women during pregnancy and postpartum. Nurs Res. 1996;45:54-6.

103. Barglow P, Hatch R, Berndt D, Phelps R. Psychosocial childbearing stress and metabolic control in pregnant diabetes. J Nerv Ment Dis. 1985;173:615-20.

104. US Preventive Services Task Force. Screening for gestational diabetes mellitus: recommendations and rationale. Obstet Gynecol. 2003;101:393-5.

105. Rubin RR, Peyrot M. Psychological issues and treatments for people with diabetes. J Clin Psychol. 2001;57:457-78.

106. Welch GW, Jacobson AM, Polonsky WH. The problem areas in diabetes scale: an evaluation of its clinical utility. Diabetes Care. 1997 May;20(5):760-6.

107. Polonsky WH, Anderson BJ, Lohrer PA, et al. Assessment of diabetes-related distress. Diabetes Care. 1995;18:754-60.

108. Davidson M, Penney Ed, Muller B, Grey M. Stressors and self-care challenges faced by adolescents living with type 1 diabetes. Appl Nurs Res. 2004;17:72-80.

109. Snoek FJ, Pouwer F, Welch GW, Polonsky WH. Diabetes-related emotional distress in Dutch and U.S. diabetic patients: cross-cultural validity of the problem areas in diabetes scale. Diabetes Care. 2000 Sep;23:1305-9

110. Centers for Disease Control and Prevention (CDC). Serious psychological distress among persons with diabetes—New York City, 2003. MMWR Morb Mortal Wkly Rep. 2004;53:1089-92.

111. Peyrot MF, McMurry JF. Stress buffering and glycemic control: the role of coping styles. Diabetes Care. 1992;15:842-6.

112. Polonsky WH. Diabetes Burnout: Preventing It, Surviving It, Finding Inner Peace. Alexandria, Va: American Diabetes Association; 1999.

113. Snoek FJ, Skinner TC. Psychological counselling in problematic diabetes: does it help? Diabet Med. 2002;19:265-73.

114. Grey M, Berry D. Coping skills training and problem solving in diabetes. Curr Diab Rep. 2004;4(2):126-31.

115. Rubin RR, Peyrot M, Saudek CD. The effect of a diabetes education program incorporating coping skills training on emotional well-being and diabetes self efficacy. Diabetes Educator. 1993;19:210-4.

116. Karlsen B, Idsoe T, Dirdal I, Rokne Hanestad B, Bru E. Effects of a group-based counselling programme on diabetes-related stress, coping, psychological well-being and metabolic control in adults with type 1 or type 2 diabetes. Patient Educ Couns. 2004;53(3):299-308.

117. Grey M, Boland EA, Davidson M, Tamborlane WV. Coping skills training for youth with diabetes mellitus has long-lasting effects on metabolic control and quality of life. J Pediatr. 2000;137:107-13.

118. van der Ven NC, Hogenelst MH, Trom-Wever AM, et al. Short-term effects of cognitive behavioral group training (CBGT) in adult type 1 diabetes patients in prolonged poor glycaemic control: a randomized controlled trial. Diabet Med. 2005;22:1619-23.

119. Surwit RS, van Tilburg MA, Zucker N, McCaskill CC, Parekh P, Feinglos MN, et al. Stress management improves long-term glycemic control in type 2 diabetes. Diabetes Care. 2002:25;30-4.

120. McGinnis RA, McGrady A, Cox SA, Grower-Dowling KA. Biofeedback-assisted relaxation in type 2 diabetes. Diabetes Care. 2005;28:2145-9.

121. Aikens JE, Kiolbasa TA, Sobel R. Psychological predictors of glycemic change with relaxation training in non-insulin-dependent diabetes mellitus. Psychother Psychosom. 1997;66:302-6.

122. Keers JC, Groen H, Sluiter WJ, Biouma J, Links TP. Cost and benefits of a multidisciplinary intensive diabetes education programme. J Eval Clin Pract 2005;11:293-303.

123. Gabbay RA, Lendel I, Saleem TM, et al. Nurse case management improves blood pressure, emotional distress and diabetes complication screening. Diabetes Res Clin Pract. 2006;71(1):28-35. Epub 2005 Jul 12.

124. Rubin RR. Counseling and psychotherapy in diabetes mellitus. In: Psychology in Diabetes Care. Snoek FJ, Skinner TC, eds. England: Wiley & Sons Limited; 2005.

125. Ismail K, Winkley K, Rabe-Hesketh S. Systematic review and meta-analysis of randomized controlled trials of psychological interventions to improve glycemic control in patients with type 2 diabetes. Lancet. 2004;363:1589-97.

CHAPTER

5

Social Support: Conceptualization, Issues, and Complexities

Authors

Anne H. Skelly, PhD, RN, CS, ANP
Dorothy Burns, PhD, RN

Key Concepts

Despite the limitations of research to date, members of the diabetes care team need a clear understanding of the concept of social support. To effectively evaluate and employ social support in clinical situations and be able to predict outcomes, healthcare professionals must understand how social support works and under what circumstances. To aid the diabetes care team in evaluating and activating an individual's social support resources, this chapter addresses the following key concepts:

- The concept of social support and its forms (types) and sources, including ways in which social support may exert a positive influence on health
- Variables affecting support, including influences of culture and ethnicity
- Measurement (informal and formal) of social support, including issues and limitations
- The state of the science of social support in diabetes care: studies looking at social support in children and adolescents, adults, families, and members of different ethnic and cultural groups
- Considerations for the use of support in the clinical care of diabetes, including resources and clinical pearls for educators and other healthcare professionals

Introduction

Healthcare providers and professional organizations have long recognized the important role social support plays in helping individuals manage their diabetes and cope with the daily burden of a chronic illness. One example is support groups (both formal and informal), which are frequently used in diabetes care. Such groups can help individuals develop coping skills, manage frustration and diabetes "burnout," and learn new strategies for dealing with the daily burden of diabetes care.[1] Use of diabetes support groups is consistent with the recognition of the positive efficacy of support. Other sources of social support include family, friends, community resources, support groups, lay advisors, and others. In 2 reviews of stress and coping in the nursing literature, social support was the most frequent coping resource mentioned.[2]

Social support can contribute to positive health states and behaviors and is widely accepted as an important strategy to decrease stress and promote healthy coping. Inadequate and ineffective social support can also have negative effects. This chapter reviews evidence from the literature on the value and effect of social support and guides those on the diabetes care team to carefully evaluate and employ effective social support strategies.

Influence on Self-Care Behaviors. Social support, as a function of psychosocial adaptation or healthy coping for living with diabetes, affects the individual's ability to perform important self-care behaviors. Each of the AADE 7 Self-Care Behaviors™—Healthy Eating, Being Active, Taking Medication, Monitoring, Problem Solving, Healthy Coping, Reducing Risks—can be positively and/or negatively affected by social support.

Evidence Base. Researchers have reported, since the early 1980s, on the positive effects that social support has on morbidity, mortality, and a variety of disease outcomes.[3] Diabetes, arthritis, heart disease, and asthma self-management are among the chronic illnesses that have been examined.[4-6] Early studies showed that greater levels of social support correlated with improved diabetes self-management,[7-9] possibly by influencing the performance of self-care behaviors.[10-11]

Early research into the concept of social support was characterized by methodological problems and often produced equivocal findings on the benefits of social support. Methodological problems included the use of different conceptual and operational definitions of support and a diversity of measurement tools, many of which lacked psychometric support.[12-13] Some of these same methodological concerns and lack of clarity in the conceptualization of support persist to this day. In addition, despite the abundance of research in this area, the mechanisms by which support influences health are still not well understood.[14] Current self-management discussions mention social support as a potentially important positive influence, but often little attention is paid to the specifics of the relationship, such as an examination of the roles of significant others.

Social Support: The Concept

When asked about their coping, individuals with diabetes most frequently report social support as a strategy. Despite its importance, social support has suffered from a lack of consistency and clarity in both definition and conceptualization. This lack of clarity has affected its generalizability across different situations and groups of people. Broadly defined, social support refers to the assistance and protection given by one individual or group to another.[15-17] Conceptualizations of social support typically consider the type and source of support, the relationship between social support and health outcomes, and variations across diverse individuals and populations.

Types of Support

Researchers studying social support most frequently measure it in terms of an individual's *perception* rather than as an objective measure of actual support. In part, this is because individual perception of support is a more powerful determination of satisfaction than the objective level of support. Research into social support has attempted to describe types, or attributes, of support. Although specific labels vary depending upon the conceptual model used, commonly identified types of support include the following: emotional, informational, instrumental, and affirmational. The list below summarizes the attributes of each.

Each of the 4 types of support described in this list is hypothesized to play a role in improving health and wellbeing.[17,24] Further research is needed to better understand the types of support that are most useful for individuals in specific situations and under certain environmental conditions.[24-26]

Sources of Support

To increase the consistency of findings across studies, research has stressed the importance of differentiating "sources" of support from "types" of support. Sources of support can be categorized as follows:

- Individual, group, or network of providers
- Individuals with similar experiences
- Lay versus professional support

Perception vs. Reality

Perceived support is more important to satisfaction than objectively measured support

Types of Social Support

Emotional Support

- Involves caring, empathy, love, and trust
- Ranks as most important category through which the perception of support is conveyed to others, according to House[18]
- When instances of support are described, emotional support far outnumbers all other types[17,19]

Informational Support

- Information provided to another during a time of stress[18,20]
- Found to assist in problem-solving[21]

Instrumental Support

- Providing tangible goods and services;[18,22] concrete assistance
- The type of support most individuals are referring to when they talk about "help"

Affirmational Support

- Expressed by statements that affirm the appropriateness of acts or statements made by another; thus, its role is greater in self-evaluation than problem-solving[23]

Social Networks. Research has explored the comprehensiveness of an individual's social network and its relationship to perceived levels of support.[27] However, studies to date have not demonstrated that the size of a social network is related to either satisfaction with social support or enhanced outcomes.[28-29]

Suitable and Preferred Sources. Sources of support differ in the types of support they are best suited to provide. For example, a health professional may be better suited than a friend in providing an individual newly diagnosed with diabetes with the informational support needed for successful coping. Culture also influences the acceptability of different sources of support and the degree to which professional support is valued and sought.[30] For example, Latinas may prefer family and lay sources of support during childbearing, while middle-class white women more frequently consult professional sources of support.[31] Additional research is needed to identify the cultural and socioeconomic influences on preferred sources of support.

Relationship to Outcomes

Support is thought to exert its effect through main, mediating, and moderating roles. The terms "mediator," "moderator," and "buffer" have been used inconsistently, and statistical tests of these relationships have contributed to confusion in the literature regarding the efficacy of social support. In addition, a particular aspect of social support may be more relevant to the model than another.[26] When evaluating findings (or results), healthcare professionals need to understand clearly what specific aspects of support a conceptual model is testing and be assured that the statistical tests used are appropriate. The summary below clarifies the roles of social support, showing how it can function as the main effect and in moderating and mediating roles.

Outcomes. Positive health states or behaviors are the most frequently studied outcomes or effects of support. Some researchers consider psychological well-being to be the most important outcome of social support, with other outcomes comprising components of psychological well-being.[17] The following positive health states and behaviors have been mentioned:

- Life satisfaction and psychological well being[28]
- Increased personal competence
- Decreased anxiety and depression[37]
- Coping abilities[38]
- Increased competence in times of stress[39]
- Positive affect and increased sense of self-worth[33]
- Improved diabetes self-management skills[40]

Two additional considerations in the evaluation of social support are the cost to the recipient of obtaining support and matters of reciprocity. In the social science and nursing literature, the reciprocal nature of support and the cost of obtaining support have received attention in studies dealing with the burden of caregiving.[26]

Cost. Generally, social support is conceptualized as cost-free; however, clinicians should assume that any support, even in a professional relationship, may carry emotional, economic, and/or physical costs.[13,26]

Reciprocity. Reciprocity addresses whether outcomes are enhanced when persons are able to give as well as receive support. It implies a burden of obligation when support is received but not returned. Stevens identified a positive relationship between life satisfaction and the receiving of social support as well as the giving of social support. [41] Riegel and Gocka, in a study of myocardial infarction patients, found that reciprocity in providing support was only an issue for women, suggesting that it may be gender-specific.[42]

Relationship to Diabetes Self-Management

Psychosocial adaptation, or healthy coping in learning to live with diabetes, is 1 of the 7 AADE Self-Care Behaviors™. Healthcare providers and professional organizations have long recognized the important role social support plays in helping individuals manage their diabetes and cope with the daily burden of a chronic illness. They also recognize

Various Roles of Social Support

Main Effect

Models that propose a main effect for social support describe a direct relationship between support and an outcome variable such as improved glycemic control or quality of life. This main effect has been supported in several studies. For example, using the Norbeck Social Support Questionnaire (NSSQ), Frey found that perceived availability of social support has a significant effect on family health among parents of children with diabetes, but not on children's health.[32]

Moderating, or Buffering, Role

Moderators are antecedent conditions that interact with a stressor to affect an outcome. In a moderating role, social support is thought to protect an individual from a stressor. This may occur through social support's influence on an individual's appraisal of a stressor (eg, as less harmful) or its role as a shield that protects an individual from exposure to stress. Several studies have demonstrated the moderating or buffering effect of social support.[25,33] For example, using the NSSQ in a study of 133 teens with asthma, Kang et al found that social support buffered stress. [34]

Mediating Role

Social support has also been proposed as a mediator of the relationship between stress and an outcome variable. A mediator is defined as a variable that significantly accounts for the relationship between 2 other variables such that, when it is not present, that relationship is no longer significant. In a study of caregiver burden, social support and coping were evaluated as mediators of the relationship between the burden of caregiving for individuals with multiple sclerosis and the caregiver's health and life satisfaction.[35] Similarly, a study of the relationship between maltreatment as a child and adult adjustment confirmed the role of social support as a mediator.[36]

the importance of understanding variations in the way social support influences diabetes self-management across different types and sources of support and individual self-care regimens. This type of information is essential to the design of effective self-management interventions.

Positive Support. Family members and others in the social network may facilitate diabetes management in a number of ways. For example, they may provide emotional support and affirmations or hands-on help with self-care activities. Churches can have various types of groups that function as social support. Family members and significant others may also provide instrumental assistance by paying bills, completing insurance forms, or doing housekeeping.

Regimen-Specific Support. It has been hypothesized that in chronic illness, regimen-specific support may be more effective than the more global type of support.[43] For example, in a study of disease-related and psychosocial correlates of quality of life in persons with diabetes, Aalto and Uutela found that support related to illness management was more predictive of health outcomes than general support.[44]

Negative Support. Social interactions can also negatively influence self-management, such as when family members or friends offer inappropriate advice that conflicts with self-management recommendations or directly or indirectly promote unhealthy behaviors.[43] See the section “Issues and Directions” toward the end of the chapter for more information.

Mediating Effects. The effect of social support on diabetes self-management may be mediated by self-efficacy as well as other psychological mechanisms, such as motivation, coping, and psychological well-being.[3,45] These effects may vary according to the type of self-management required. For example, with the stress of more demanding and complex regimens, support may become more important. Support may also be more important during periods of crisis and uncertainty. Self-care activities that are more observable, such as diet, are more open to influences by family members and friends than activities usually done alone.

Antecedents of Support

For social supportive behaviors to occur, a social network with a quality of connectedness that is known as embeddedness must be in place to generate an atmosphere of helpfulness and protection. Three characteristics—social network, social embeddedness, and social climate—are considered antecedents of support:[17]

- *Social Network.* Vehicle through which social support is provided.[23] It may consist of a single individual or a group of individuals. A social network can be thought of as the structure of an interaction, while social support is the function.
- *Social Embeddedness.* The connectedness people have to significant others in their social network.[46] To obtain support from an environment, some degree of social connectedness or embeddedness must exist.
- *Social Climate.* The personality of an environment.[47] Qualities of the social climate that foster support are helpfulness and protection.

Age, gender, and ethnicity are 3 variables contributing to social support that have received increased attention in recent years. The findings listed above suggest that support needs to be evaluated on an individual basis—one that considers the individual’s perceptions of what meets his or her needs as well as the meaning and value the individual ascribes to social support.

Measurement of Social Support

While research has documented the beneficial effects of social support on a variety of positive disease outcomes, many of these studies contain a variety of methodological flaws and different conceptualizations or definitions of the construct social support.[3,43] One of the major distinctions among these studies is whether the support measured was general or specific to a self-care regimen. In general, the majority of studies focused on the functional, as opposed to the structural, aspects of support. The most common dimension of social support assessed was perceived instrumental and emotional support, followed by satisfaction with the support provided and desired support. With few exceptions, most samples were convenience samples, typically of outpatient groups using cross-sectional, descriptive, or correlational designs.

Social support can be measured formally using instruments designed to capture attributes of support or informally as part of the clinical encounter.

Informal Assessment. Informally, the healthcare practitioner can approach the issue of support as part of the review of the diabetes self-management regimen, by placing it in the context of how individuals are managing their diabetes. With the person’s permission, family members and significant others may be invited to participate in the visit and share their perspectives. This type of shared problem-solving strengthens the management plan. If family members are not available, the healthcare professional can inquire about what family members do to facilitate (or hinder) self-care and what the person with diabetes may need from family members to make their self-care easier.[55] The healthcare professional must remember that people are often protective of their families and may not reveal that they are receiving little support; the practitioner needs

Variables Across Individuals and Populations

Age

There are fewer studies specifically focused on children apart from family than those with adults. This may be partially due to the need to develop appropriate measures of support sensitive to developmental levels. Also, social support as it relates to families has been studied less frequently than at the individual level. This is especially important since people most frequently call on family members in times of stress. In a study of family members caring for elderly parents, Fink found that social support together with hardiness and socioeconomic status explained 65% of the variance in well-being for family members.[48] More on age-related social support can be found in the "State of the Science" section later in this chapter.

Gender

There is also evidence that social support is affected by gender, although these findings are not uniformly consistent.[26] Allen and Stoltenberg found that college freshmen women felt more supported and satisfied with support than male students.[49] In contrast, in a study of individuals with multiple sclerosis, Gulick[50] found greater perceptions of social support in men compared to women, while studies by McColl and Friedland[51] and Willey and Silliman[52] found no relationship between gender and support. More on gender-specific aspects of social support can be found in the "State of the Science" section later in this chapter.

Ethnicity

In examining the role of social support in an African American sample, Picot found a positive, but weak correlation between social support and confrontive coping in women caring for relatives with Alzheimer's disease.[53] Studying Korean families, Choi found that differing philosophical outlooks may influence the appraisal of support.[54] More on ethnic and cultural influences can be found in the "State of the Science" section later in this chapter.

TABLE 5.1 Assessing Social Support Available to People With Diabetes

1. Who helps you in your effort to manage your diabetes? What does each of these persons do that you find helpful?
2. Does anyone provide you with practical or emotional support for managing your diabetes?
3. Does anyone important to you make it harder to manage your diabetes? What does this person do that makes it harder for you to manage your diabetes?
4. What would you like in the way of support for day-to-day diabetes management that you are not getting now?
5. What one thing could you do to make it more likely you will get the support you want? Anything else?
6. What can I do to help you get the support you want? (Suggest options such as joint meeting with family, materials for family to read, educational or support group programs to attend.)

Source: Adapted with permission from A Core Curriculum for Diabetes Education: Diabetes Education and Program Management, 4th ed. Franz MJ, ed. Rubin R, Napora, J. Psychosocial Assessment. Chicago, Il: American Association of Diabetes Educators; 2001:46.

to remain sensitive and aware of clues that may indicate this is the case. Often, gentle probing and support by the healthcare professional is sufficient to identify the problem. Table 5.1 presents questions to elicit available support.[56]

Formal Instruments. Instruments to measure various aspects or attributes of support have been developed and can be used in the clinical setting or as part of a research design using quantitative methods. However, few of these quantitative measures have been adequately tested for reliability and validity or tested with minority populations.[13] Qualitative studies have been instrumental in helping explicate the conceptual basis and mechanism of support and provide new directions for exploration of the concept.[57-59]

Three instruments—the NSSQ,[60] Personal Resources Questionnaire (PRQ),[61,62] and Tilden Interpersonal Relationship Inventory (IPR)[63]—have been adequately tested for reliability and validity and extensively used to measure social support with diverse community and clinical populations. Because they are theory-based, these 3 instruments have contributed to professional understanding of the concept of support.[13] They are summarized below along with a few other instruments. The list is by no means exhaustive; readers may wish to review these references for sources presenting more information.

Measuring Social Support With Formal Instruments

Norbeck Social Support Questionnaire (NSSQ)

Based on attachment theory, the NSSQ measures affect, affirmation, aid, network properties, and recent losses.[60,64] Sources of support are rated on a 5-point scale in relation to the amount of aid, affect, or affirmational support provided. Total scores are obtained for 1) functional support and 2) network properties. Internal consistency is reported as .89 and .78 to .84.[32] Test-retest reliability for the subscales ranges from .85 to .92.[26] The NSSQ has been used in a study of children with diabetes and their parents[32] and families.[64]

Personal Resources Questionnaire (PRQ)

Based on Weiss' conceptualization of social relationships, the PRQ measures 5 dimensions of social support: intimacy, social integration, nurturance, worth, and assistance.[61,62] The PRQ has 2 parts: part 1 measures support needs for the past 6 months, with satisfaction rated on a 6-point scale from very satisfied to very dissatisfied, and part 2 rates the 5 dimensions of social support on a 7-point scale from strongly disagree to strongly agree. Internal consistency ranges from .87 to .91.[65] Intimacy/assistance, integration/affirmation, and reciprocity are 3 factors revealed by factor analysis.[26,64] The PRQ has been used in a study of persons with diabetes.[66]

Tilden Interpersonal Relationship Inventory (IPR)

Measures costs and benefits of support and relationships and is based on social-exchange theory and equity theory. The IPR consists of 39 items measuring perceived states and enacted behaviors using a 5-point scale. The social support, reciprocity, and conflict subscales are scored separately.[63] Internal consistency is reported as .83 to .92 and test-retest reliability as .81 to .91.[63] Construct validity of the scales has been supported through quantitative and qualitative studies.[65]

Interpersonal Support Evaluation List (ISEL)

A 40-item questionnaire assessing perceived availability of general support. Measures 4 functions of support: appraisal, tangible support, self-esteem, and belonging. Internal consistency is reported as .90 for the entire scale with test-retest reliability at .70 over a 6-week interval.[67]

Family Environment Scale[68]

Composed of 3 subscales assessing the degree of commitment, help, and support family members provide for one another. Used in research with African American families and children 10 years of age and older. Internal consistency ranges from .61 to .78. Test-retest reliabilities range from .68 to .86 at 2 months.[68] Other instruments that have been used to measure support in children are the *People in My Life* scale[69] and *Perceived Social Support from Family (PSS-FA)*.[70]

Other Instruments

Other instruments used to measure social support include the *Duke-UNC Functional Social Support Questionnaire*,[71] *Medical Outcomes Study Social Support Survey*,[72] *Duke Social Support and Stress Scale*,[73] and *Perceived Social Support from Family* scale.[70]

Instruments Specific to Diabetes

When examining the relationship between social support and chronic illness outcomes, diabetes is the most commonly studied disease. In particular, the focus has been on the relationship between support and aspects of the diabetes self-care regimen. Most studies measure diabetes self-management by self-report, with dietary compliance the most common self-management behavior examined.[43] This involves measurement of the concept of support (or the attribute of interest), the self-care behavior, and outcome variables.

In studies of persons with diabetes, social support has been measured using a variety of instruments. Many investigators have developed measures of support for their individual studies or adapted existing instruments. Unfortunately, this often occurs without reporting the psychometric data to support the new (or adapted) instrument. Four instruments that have been developed to measure support in diabetes are listed below as examples. Each differs in how support is conceptualized and measured and is briefly summarized.

This list of studies on diabetes-specific tools is by no means exhaustive; see also the references themselves and the texts by Bradley[81] and McDowell and Newell.[82]

In summary, problems remain in the measurement of social support. The theory underlying the measurement tool should be explained, and specifics on how social support is being conceptualized should be provided, even if only studying an attribute of social support rather than the full construct. This knowledge is necessary if we are

Diabetes-Specific Instruments for Measuring Social Support

Diabetes Family Behavior Checklist II

Measures support from family members for the performance of diabetes self-care activities, specifically for those with type 2 diabetes.[76] It has 2 parts: part 1 rates the frequency of supportive-nonsupportive actions related to the individual's diabetes self-care regimen, and part 2 asks respondents to rate these same actions in terms of their perceived helpfulness or unhelpfulness.[76] Internal consistency has been reported at .71 for the positive summary score and .64 for the negative summary score, and test-retest reliability at .97 at 2 weeks.[40]

Diabetes Care Profile (DCP)

Measures social and psychological factors related to diabetes and its treatment.[77] Subscales assess a person's attitude toward diabetes (including support), diabetes beliefs, adherence to the diabetes self-care regimen, and difficulties with self-care. Reliability and validity have been established in 2 separate populations with a reported internal consistency of .60 to .95 in one population and .66 to .94 in the other population.

Diabetes Social Support Questionnaire—Family Version

A 52-item instrument measuring perceived family support for 5 areas of diabetes care: insulin, blood testing, diet, exercise, and emotions.[78] It has been validated with adolescent populations and demonstrated an internal consistency of .95 for the total scale.

Diabetes Self-Management Assessment Tool (DSMART)—Support and Confidence Subscale

A 3-item scale measuring family/friend support, professional support, and confidence in diabetes self-management on a 4-point Likert scale.[79] Higher scores indicate greater support and confidence in living with diabetes. Internal consistency is reported as .94 with good reliability.[79-80] (Currently being revised.)

to better understand how social support affects health outcomes. Healthcare professionals are urged to seek out well-established instruments to help build the evidence for support. In evaluating instruments, Ducharme, Stevens, and Rowat suggest that healthcare professionals clearly identify the following 3 aspects.[83] This degree of rigor is necessary to build a body of evidence for the relationship between social support and diabetes.[26]

- Components of support being measured
- Unit of measurement
- Validity and reliability of the instrument

State of the Science

Studies focusing on diabetes self-management and support may assess general support, a specific aspect of support (eg, support for diet or physical activity), or both. Studies also may focus on the characteristics of families and their effect on support. In recent years, interest in looking at the influences of ethnicity and gender on support has increased. Below is a brief review of select studies highlighting some of the key findings pertinent to the "state of the science." These research summaries are organized by category, as follows:

- Support for children and adolescents with type 1 diabetes
- Support for adults with type 2 diabetes
- Characteristics of supportive families
- Influences of gender and ethnicity

Support in Children and Adolescents With Type 1 Diabetes

Management of type 1 diabetes is especially burdensome for children and adolescents as they learn to integrate what is often a complex regimen into their daily lives. Adolescence, in particular, is often a period when self-management routines may be disrupted, and this is a concern in preventing and delaying later complications.[84] Bearman and La Greca have stressed the importance of better understanding the match between what children and families with diabetes

> ***What's Important to Teens***
>
> For adolescents, consider peer support especially important, but reinforce family involvement in care

need, the type of treatments available to them, and the role of the family in providing support.[78] Glasgow and Anderson have recommended increased attention to the social context of adolescents, including explanatory models of how the family influences the child's adaptation to diabetes.[85]

Roles of Family and Peers. Researchers studying social support and diabetes in children and adolescents have responded to the call for increased attention to this subject by focusing on the roles of family and peers, with the role of peers gaining increasing importance as children age.[86,87] Peers are especially important sources of emotional and affirmational support for adolescents with diabetes; this support is associated with metabolic control and, perhaps, well-being.[88,89] Highlights of 3 studies are given below.

- *Pendley et al.* Studied social support and peer and family involvement in 68 youths between the ages of 8 and 17 diagnosed with type 1 diabetes.[90] They found that adolescents perceived greater support from peers than do school-age children. Although, in this study, perceived peer and family support were not correlated with metabolic control, peer participation in a later intervention was correlated with metabolic control. The researchers concluded there is a developmental shift in perceptions of peer support that underscores the importance of developing appropriate measures of support that are sensitive to developmental level.[26]
- *La Greca and colleagues.* Studied the support provided by family members and friends for the diabetes care of 74 adolescents with type 1 diabetes.[88] Using a structured interview, respondents were asked to describe how family members and friends provided support for insulin shots, blood glucose monitoring, eating proper meals, exercising, and helping them "feel good about their diabetes." The researchers found that families provided more instrumental support than did friends for insulin injections, blood glucose monitoring, and meals, and this was related to younger age, shorter duration of disease, and better treatment adherence. Friends provided more emotional support. The researchers stressed the importance of encouraging parents to remain active in their adolescents' diabetes management.
- *Skinner, John, and Hampson.* Studied 52 adolescents with type 1 diabetes to examine whether peer support and illness representation mediate the link between family support, diabetes self-management, and well-being.[91] They found that beliefs about the effectiveness of the diabetes treatment regimen were predictive of improved dietary self-care. Support from family and friends also predicted better dietary self-care. Perceptions of supportive family and friends were predictive of participants' well-being.

Common themes in the body of research on children's social support:

- Importance of addressing social context of children's lives (particularly for adolescents)
- Personal models of well-being
- The unique contributions of family to the management of type 1 diabetes
- The influence of peers

Support for Adults

Adults with diabetes receive social support from a variety of sources that may vary during their lifetime and differentially affect diabetes self-management. Among these, family members are the most common source of support. Highlights of 11 studies are given below.

- *Wilson et al.* In a study of 208 men and women with type 2 diabetes, measured the perceived availability of tangible, appraisal, self-esteem, and belonging support using the *Interpersonal Support Evaluation List* (*ISEL*).[67] They found that diabetes-specific support predicted all self-care behaviors.
- *Sherbourne.* In a study of 1198 adults between the ages of 19 and 97 years, using a composite measure of 4 types of support, emotional ties, and interpersonal functioning, found that perceptions of the availability of support increased adherence for diabetes.[92]
- *Lloyd et al.* Using the *ISEL* in a study of 592 persons with type 1 diabetes, found greater support predicted better self-care.[93]
- *Glasgow and Toobert.* Studying 127 persons with type 2 diabetes, measured the frequency of supportive and nonsupportive behaviors related to medications, glucose-testing, exercise, and diet using the *Diabetes Behavior Checklist II*.[76] They found a relationship between the relevant regimen-specific score and adherence.
- *Ruggiero et al.* Using the *Diabetes Social Support Questionnaire* in a study of 98 pregnant females with gestational diabetes, found greater support was related to improved diet and insulin adherence.[94] In a later study, Ruggiero et al found that perceptions of greater support were related to better self-care.[96]

- *Garay-Sevilla et al.* Using an adapted version of the *Diabetes Social Support Questionnaire*, in a study of 200 individuals between the ages of 19 and 85 with type 2 diabetes, found that support predicted better adherence to diet and medication.[97]
- *Pham et al.* In a study of 76 individuals with type 2 diabetes who were amputees, looked at perceived support using the *Diabetes Health Belief Scale*.[98] While they found no relationship between support and other self-care, they did find that greater support predicted better adherence to diet and exercise.
- *Tillotson and Smith.* In a study of 465 individuals with type 2 diabetes, looked at self-reported adherence to a weight-control regimen and found that greater support predicted greater adherence.[99] When perceptions of support were low, they found a negative relationship between locus of control and weight management.
- *Whittemore, D'Eramo-Melkus, and Grey.* In a study of metabolic control, self-management, and psychological adjustment in 53 women with type 2 diabetes, found that enhanced social support and self-confidence in diabetes self-management may improve metabolic control and psychosocial adjustment to diabetes.[80]
- *Kawakami et al.* In a study of job strain, social support in the workplace, and glycemic control in a sample of Japanese men, found a relationship among higher concentrations of A1C, the highest quartile of job strain and the lowest quartile of social support at the workplace, indicating a need to consider the social context of support.[100]

Common theme from the body of research on adults' social support:

- Support is important to improved self-care activities and thereby health outcomes for adults with diabetes. This is particularly true for regimen-specific support.

Despite different conceptualizations and measures, the body of research on adults' social support suggests supports' importance to self-care and health outcomes. Adults with diabetes face different developmental issues than younger people face (eg, childbearing, child-rearing, retirement, aging). Their situations may be confounded by possible discrimination in the workplace and financial and insurance concerns. Support needs need to be evaluated on an individual basis, based on the individuals' requirements and their perceptions of what meets their needs. What types of support would be most effective, when, from whom, and under what circumstances—these are important considerations when looking at social support for adults with diabetes. Also important are variations due to gender, ethnicity, and changes over time.

Characteristics of Supportive Families

While some researchers have studied the types of support provided by families, others have concentrated on the characteristics of supportive and nonsupportive families. The characteristics of supportive families have been studied more in families of individuals with type 1 diabetes than those with type 2 diabetes.

- *Fisher et al.* Defined the social network/context of diabetes as residing in the family and proposed a family-centered approach to diabetes care that they explored in later studies.[101]
- *MacLean and Lo.*[74] In a study of 95 individuals with type 2 diabetes, measured intention to succeed with exercise, glucose testing, and diet and failure to comply, using the *Perceived Social Support from Family* scale.[87] Although they found that family support was related to intended success but unrelated to failure to comply, a later study, using the same tool, found that family support positively predicts success.[75]
- *Trief et al.* Investigated whether family system variables were related to metabolic control or psychosocial adaptation in 150 insulin-requiring adults. Using 2 family system measures (the *Family Environment Scale* and *Diabetes Family Behavior Checklist*), found that family system variables were not related to metabolic control, but were related to better psychosocial adaptation to diabetes. When family members were perceived to be supportive of the diabetes care regimen, those with diabetes were more satisfied with their adaptation to the illness and reported less interference with their ability to take care of their diabetes due to emotional problems.[102]
- *Gerstle, Varenne, and Contento.* In an ethnographic study of 5 families of women with diabetes over a 2.5-year period, looking at family adaptation after nutrition education, found that home and family routines had changed in the women with improved glycemic control. They concluded that nutrition education should be directed towards existing family social support.[103]
- *Herpetz et al.* In a multicenter study of the association of psychosocial stress and the use of psychosocial support in 253 patients with diabetes, found that family members were the main source of support.[104]

Common themes in the body of research on characteristics of family support:

- More work needs to be done with families to describe characteristics that contribute to a helpful environment for diabetes management
- More work needs to be done to identify geographical, ethnic, and socioeconomic barriers to support

Healthcare professionals need strategies to work with families to enhance support.[80] Additional research is needed on how families can be supported in their care of individuals with diabetes, including how best to use resources such as support groups, lay health advisors, and other community resources. Chapter 6 on community and society may also be of help.

Gender Differences

The social support literature provides growing evidence that support may differ between genders, indicating a need for gender-specific approaches. Highlights of 6 studies are given below:

- *Murphy, Williamson, and Nease.* Found that men were more likely to have a family member to help with their diabetes self-care, and while men's helpers were usually their wives, women's helpers were more likely their adult daughters.[105]
- *Riegal and Gocka* and *Conn, Taylor, and Abel.* In a study of men and women, 1 month following myocardial infarction, Riegal and Gocka found that women received significantly more emotional support than men, although there were no differences in the need for support.[42] In a similar study of patients 1 to 2 years postinfarct, Conn, Taylor, and Abel reported a negative correlation between age and social support for men but not for women.[106]
- *Rubin and Peyrot.* Found that men with diabetes report more general social support than women.[107]
- *Mercado & Vargas.* Report more support for diet in men.[108]
- *Lloyd et al.* In a study of 592 individuals with type 1 diabetes over the age of 18, found that gender was associated with diabetes self-care activities; women reported more self-care than men.[93]

Factoring in gender:

While the research findings are not consistent (Willey and Silliman, for example, found gender unrelated to social support[52]), a growing body of evidence suggests this:

- Gender differences in social support exist and need to be taken into consideration, particularly for culturally defined gender roles

Noting gender differences may be especially relevant for culturally defined gender roles and how they may influence perceptions of need for support and the acceptability of support.[57-59] For example, the traditional multicaregiving role of older African American women, as caretakers of their family, may interfere or conflict with their ability to comfortably receive support from family members for their diabetes care.[109]

Ethnic and Cultural Differences

Culture determines the conduct and content of social relationships, including the provision and receipt of social support. In the past, research into social support has focused more on white, middle-class adults.[1] However, more recent research has begun to identify cultural or ethnic differences in social support that can be of value in tailoring self-management interventions to specific populations.

Most of the research into ethnic and cultural differences has been done with African Americans with diabetes in the United States. However, an increasing number of studies with participants from other diverse populations are further enhancing professional understanding of cultural differences and, thereby, improving health outcomes for underserved minorities. The African American population in the United States is heterogeneous in socioeconomic status, religion, and geographic origin. However, given the strong role of the extended family in African American culture and the influence of the African American family on its members—especially its elders—ethnic and cultural differences in perceptions of social support are important to consider.[43,110] Highlighted in the paragraphs that follow are specific studies pertinent to ethnicity and social support:

- 10 studies among African American populations and 1 of black South Africans
- 4 more studies examining age and gender influences among African Americans
- Studies specific to Latino and Native American populations—2 individual studies and a review looking at 12 studies

African American and Black Populations

- *Neighbors and Jackson.* Considered *types* and *sources* of social support in African Americans.[111] Using data from the *National Survey of Black Families and Households*, they found that informal help was used more often than formal help by African Americans. Eighty-seven percent of respondents reported they had talked with an informal helper (spouse, children, parents, siblings, friend, or neighbor), compared with 48% who had consulted a formal source of support (healthcare provider, social services, minister, lawyer, police, employment agency). In this survey, individuals with a chronic illness were more likely to seek informal help than those without a physical problem.

- *Taylor.* Examined the impact of familial and demographic factors on the receipt of social support from family members in a sample of 2107African Americans, as part of the *1979-1980 National Survey of Black Americans.*[112] Taylor found that the majority of respondents received support from their family members. Particularly important in the informal social network of elders were adult children. Factors that influenced receipt of support included age, income, contact with the family, subjective closeness, and proximity of relatives.
- *Silverstein and Waite.* Found no differences between African Americans and whites in providing and receiving instrumental and emotional support.[113]
- *Luckey.* Found that informal social support was vital in maintaining the elderly in African American communities.[114]
- *Walls.* In looking at the role of church and family support in the lives of older African Americans, stressed the importance of considering the church when studying support networks of African American elders.[115] Participants reported receiving instrumental support from church members that contributed to feelings of well-being. Perceptions of the church as supportive generated the feelings of well-being, not the ideology (spiritual aspects) or involvement in organizational aspects of the church.
- *Belgrave and Lewis.* In considering social support in African Americans with diabetes, in a study of 78 African Americans with diabetes, found that social support was significantly associated with appointment-keeping behavior and adherence to health activities.[116]
- *Fitzgerald et al.* In a study of 178 men and women with type 2 diabetes, 41% of whom were black and 59% white, found a beneficial effect of support for whites but not blacks.[77]
- *Ford, Tilley, and McDonald.* Examined the role of social support in promoting diabetes management and improving glycemic control in African American adults with type 2 diabetes.[117] Their findings indicate that African Americans tend to rely more heavily than whites on their informal social networks to meet disease management needs; also, that social support is significantly associated with improved diabetes management. In an earlier paper discussing a theoretical framework for examining the relationship between social support and glycemic control,[118] the authors suggested that informal support may be particularly relevant for members of this population, who may be isolated from formal support services by economic or cultural barriers.
- *Westaway et al.* In a study of effects of social support on health, well-being, and management of diabetes in a sample of 263 black South Africans, identified socioemotional and tangible support as the underlying dimensions of social support.[119] Emotional support was found to be the most important determinant of health and well-being. In this study, social support was only beneficial for 1 aspect of diabetes management: blood pressure control.
- *Gavin and Landrum.* Suggest that denial could impact the degree to which African Americans and other individuals seek support from family, friends, or others.[120] They further suggest that family members can help by letting the individual with diabetes express their emotions, asking what is hardest for them and what seems to work for them in regard to their diabetes care. Additional approaches include asking ways family members might be of help without being the "diabetes police," reminding individuals of their strengths, and assisting with problem-solving.

Among African Americans, studies have also found some influences dependent on gender and age:

- *Bryant and Rakowski.* Found that social contacts provide a greater health benefit for African American men than for African American women.[121]
- In a qualitative study of the relationship between perceived social support and diabetes self-management with 12 African American women, participants expressed that members of their social network lack an understanding of their needs.[58] The women felt that although those who provided informational support seemed to care, they often misunderstood the type of support needed or how best to deliver it. Positive support was seen as more of a motivator than negative support.
- Participants in a descriptive study of 9 African American women with type 2 diabetes stated that being reminded by a family member about what they should eat was helpful at times, but at other times made them angry.[57] Other strategies for dealing with their diabetes were talking with others who had diabetes and trust in God.

- *Mutran.* In a study of socioeconomic and cultural influences on intergenerational family support among blacks and whites, found that black elders gave and received more help than white elders after controlling for age and sex. Mutran saw this as related to socioeconomic, rather than cultural, factors. The increased amount of help provided by black elders to the middle and younger generations reflected a combination of both cultural and socioeconomic factors. Mutran concluded that attitudes of respect for each generation among black families play a part in determining family support.[122]

Latinos and Native Americans

- *Gleeson-Krieg, Bernal, and Woolley.* In a study of the self-management of diabetes among 95 Latino participants, found that social support was not strongly related to diabetes self-management.[123] Participants had large networks composed mostly of family members to turn to for assistance. Professional support was provided mainly by community health nurses. Participants were least satisfied with the help they received for their diabetes self-care, personal care, and financial assistance. The authors concluded that education and resources need to be provided for support persons and the support network of persons with diabetes should be evaluated not only for the availability of support, but also for satisfaction with support.
- *Sarkisian et al.* In a review of 12 studies of diabetes self-care interventions for older African American or Latino adults, found that characteristics of successful interventions included cultural or age-tailoring the intervention, use of group counseling or support, and involvement of spouses and adult children.[124]
- *Epple et al.* Investigated the relationship between active family nutritional support and improved metabolic outcomes for Diné (Navajo) individuals with type 2 diabetes. Found active nutritional support significantly associated with improved triglyceride, cholesterol, and A1C levels, suggesting that the family (rather than the individual alone) is a useful unit for interventions to improve diabetes self-care.[125]

Common theme in the body of research on ethnicity:

- The heterogeneity of an ethnic or cultural group must always be considered

Although the types and sources of support may vary, the role of social support as a strategy for coping with the burden of diabetes is almost universally seen across all ethnic groups. Where differences exist, socioeconomic as well as cultural factors need to be considered. Further research is needed to help explicate factors influencing diabetes self-management in various cultures. This includes development and testing of culturally sensitive instruments to capture the multidimensional concept of support in diverse populations. It also calls for longitudinal research designs to assess changes in the support network with aging and in response to changes in the healthcare delivery system. See Table 5.2 for considerations for addressing social support in diverse groups.

TABLE 5.2 Key Points in Looking at Social Support in Diverse Groups

- Provide time to listen to clients and family members or support persons about their concerns
- Be sensitive to and aware of who the support persons are; discuss with them (with the client's permission) the management of the family member's diabetes
- Teach family members or other support persons how to help the individual with diabetes self-manage their diabetes
- Assist the client and support persons to locate and use available culturally sensitive resources in the community
- Remain aware that ethnic groups are often heterogeneous; do not assume you know all about a group based on interactions with a few members

Adapted from the following sources: Burns D, Skelly AH. African American women with type 2 diabetes meeting the daily challenges of self-care. J Multicultural Nurs & Health. 2005;11(3):63-7.

Gleeson-Kreig, Bernal, Woolley. The role of social support in the self-management of diabetes mellitus among a Hispanic population. Public Health Nurs. 2002 May-Jun;19(3):215-22.

Ford, Tilley, McDonald. Social support among African-American adults with diabetes. Part 1: Theoretical framework (review). J Natl Med Assoc. 1998 Jun;90(6):361-5.

Ford, Tilley, McDonald. Social support among African-American adults with diabetes, Part 2: A review (review). J Natl Med Assoc. 1998 Jul;90(7):425-32.

Case in Point: An Older, African American Woman Identifies Social Supports

MH was a 53-year-old African American with type 2 diabetes of 7 years' duration. She was a widow and worked part-time as a school bus assistant, which she felt gave her a "little extra money" to make ends meet. This also got her home in time to provide after-school care for her 3 grandchildren, which was an important part of her life. MH felt defeated and hopeless about her ability to "stay on track" with her diabetes. On previous visits, the nurse practitioner offered some ideas to help MH improve her diabetes self-management routine, such as walking in the mall and delegating some household duties (grocery shopping, laundry) to her daughters who live nearby. MH had not followed through with these suggestions. While this perplexed the nurse practitioner, she was aware that the need for support varies among individuals including what is considered acceptable and under what circumstances it is acceptable.

- Besides diabetes, MH was being treated for hypertension and hypercholesterolemia, both of which had been under good control
- Too young for Medicare and with income over that required by Medicaid, her medication costs were a major burden on an already stretched income
- Over the 7 years she has had diabetes, MH's A1C ranged from 8.2% to 9.5%. This she attributed to difficulty obtaining and cooking the "right" foods, lack of physical activity ("too tired," "have to watch the kids"), and a weight gain of 15 lb
- MH had developed some protein in her urine and intermittent numbness and tingling in her toes, which concerned her

The Patient's Perspective

At the next visit, circumstances had not changed. The nurse practitioner began the visit with a review of MH's self-management goals and engaged MH in a discussion of her progress towards these goals and what MH *felt* might be beneficial to her diabetes self-management:

- MH discussed her family, her pride in them and the importance of her role as head, or caregiver, of the family. She did not want to place any additional burdens on her daughters who were working outside of the home and required her support in the form of child care.
- However, she felt that having someone to talk things over with, someone not in the family (who would worry), who would listen and provide support might be helpful.
- She did not feel, at this time, that she would benefit from professional help, saying "I'm not crazy yet!"

The nurse practitioner and MH then began to brainstorm what resources were available in the community to provide that support.

- MH was a member of a local community church and attended services on a weekly basis, but did not participate in any of the church groups. She was aware that the church had a Women's Health group that met monthly and discussed African American women's health issues, including diabetes. She had been meaning to contact the leader for a list of topics being discussed, but hadn't had the chance.
- She also felt she might ask her daughters to attend with her so they might learn more about diabetes.
- MH volunteered that she was interested in the church's *Prayer Circle* and felt that she might call and add her name to the prayer list. She had done this before, during her husband's last illness, and felt a spiritual benefit.

Aligning Comfortable Support

The nurse practitioner encouraged MH to follow through. At the next visit, MH reported that she had contacted the *Prayer Circle.* She felt her spirits were improving and that she seemed to have more energy. In addition, she had made an appointment for later in the week to speak with her pastor, on the suggestion of the *Prayer Circle* coordinator. While she had not contacted the women's health group, she had begun to walk every other day in the morning before work with a neighbor who also had diabetes.

Case Wrap-Up

The interest demonstrated by the nurse practitioner in helping MH gain better control of her diabetes provided MH with the incentive to reach out to sources of support that were meaningful and acceptable to her. This example illustrates the importance of *starting with the patient* and avoiding a cookbook approach in recommending types and sources of support. In the African American and Latino communities in particular, churches may provide a variety of types of support, including affective/emotional, affirmative, informational, and instrumental support to church members. However, for support to be effective, the patient's preferred type and sources of support are the most important considerations. This is why questions like, "What would help you get better control of your diabetes?" and "What kinds of help would work for you?" are important approaches to helping patients succeed.

Issues and Directions

Although there is continuing debate about the nature of social support and which attributes best predict health outcomes, the importance of social support as a coping strategy in diabetes self-management cannot be overlooked. Current issues and directions in research on social support involve the following. Each of these topics is discussed briefly below.

- Negative aspects of social support
- Further investigations into the role and quality of social networks, including self-help groups and lay advisors
- Technology-aided approaches to delivering social support
- Better understanding of the role of support in different ethnic and cultural groups

Negative Aspects of Social Support

Questions have been raised over whether the concept of social support has overemphasized positive exchanges and given less attention to the more negative aspects of support.[13] In several studies, the following have been found to correlate more strongly with decreased perceived support and increased psychological symptoms than positive interactions:[43,65,126-127]

- Conflict
- Poor communication
- Negative interactions
- Lack of stability

> ***Support Strategies***
>
> When employing and evaluating social support, consider both supportive and nonsupportive aspects of relationships

Therefore, since the effects seen may depend more on the absence of conflict than the presence of positive support, both the supportive and nonsupportive aspects of a relationship should be considered.

Quality of Networks

Continuing inquiry into the role and quality of networks may be beneficial in understanding the role of support as a buffer of stress.[26] This includes the relationship of the family context to outcomes in diabetes as well as the use of self-help groups and lay, or peer, advisors. Consumer and self-help movements, in which members exchange information, exist for most chronic illnesses. Such groups have the potential to extend networks and supply emotional, informational, affirmational, and occasionally tangible support.[128]

One mode of applied research relevant to support-focused interventions is participatory research, which is defined as cooperative inquiry by both the researcher and the members of a community who are the subjects of the study.[129] The participatory paradigm can be used to further study the role of self-help groups and use of lay advisors in improving diabetes self-management and health outcomes.

Technology-Aided Social Support

Innovative methods of delivering social support include use of the following:

- Telephone assurance programs
- Computer-based interactive programs
- Internet-based support groups
- Other telecommunication technology

Highlights of 2 studies that used technology to aid social support are given below.

- *Smith and Weinert.* Tested the use of telecommunication technology to deliver diabetes education and social support to 30 rural women as part of the Women to Women Diabetes Project and found that improving health and higher educational levels positively influenced social support and quality of life.[130]

- *Barrera et al.* Tested an Internet-based support group in a randomized trial of 160 adults with type 2 diabetes.[131] They reported significant increases in support on a diabetes-specific support measure and a general support scale in individuals in the 2 support conditions.

Cultural Congruence

To be effective, diabetes self-management and diabetes self-management education must be culturally congruent. Both approaches (management and education) must be sensitive to how support is viewed by members of a particular group and what is acceptable. Although, more studies are being conducted with members of minority groups, most of the present knowledge of social support pertains to the white, middle-class in Western civilization. There are also no measures of social support for members of ethnic or cultural groups with diabetes, although some existing measures have been adapted to non-white cultures. This places the responsibility on the healthcare provider to provide culturally sensitive care, and the provider may be challenged to withhold judgment about how members of a network should provide support.

A Broader View

In summary, social support's effects on diabetes self-management are only one aspect of its potential to influence health and well-being. To better appreciate the social influences that may be operating, healthcare professionals need to take a broader view of social conditions. This may entail considering the following:[3,52]

- Impact of shared norms about health practices and behaviors
- Access to material resources
- Economic, social, and political influences
- Social and cultural role obligations on diabetes self-management

Acknowledgments

The authors wish to acknowledge Dr. Jennifer Leeman, Ms. Amanda Hill, and Ms. April Soward for their invaluable contributions to this chapter.

Focus on Education: Pearls for Practice

Teaching Strategies

- **Identify the individual's sources of support.** Remember that support is in the eye of the beholder, meaning each person has his or her own belief about and unique needs regarding desired and acceptable forms of support. Assist in identifying who currently provides support, how, what type, when, and where.

- **Personalize the education plan.** Teaching and discussions need to start where the patient is. Consider age, gender, and ethnicity/culture. Then begin to add information. Consider also person, place, and time (social context, social influences, social/cultural role).

- **Solicit feedback to confirm a plan's feasibility.** Ask the person with diabetes "Will this work" and "Is this plan acceptable?"

Messages for Patients

- **Use your support system wisely.** Know the strengths and weaknesses of your support system—who to go to for what kind of support, when other supports need to be found. Recognize when relationships and social influences may have negative effects on diabetes management, health, and well-being—devise alternatives and solutions.

- **Recognize areas of conflict.** Identify when expectations of your familiar role or cultural background conflict with your diabetes care regimen, health, and well-being.

Suggested Readings

To learn more about social support:

Gallant MP. The influence of social support on chronic illness self-management: a review and directions for research. Health Educa Behav. 2003;30(2):170-95.

Stewart MJ. Integrating social support in nursing. Newbury Park, Calif: Sage Publications, Inc; 1993.

Underwood PW. Social support: the promise and the reality. In: Handbook of Stress, Coping and Health: Implications for Nursing Research, Theory and Practice. Rice VH, ed. Thousand Oaks, Ca: Sage Publications; 2000;367-92.

To learn more about measuring social support specific to diabetes:

Bradley C, ed. Handbook of Pyschology and Diabetes. Chur, Switzerland: Harwood Academic Publishers; 1994.

To learn more about social support in general:

McDowell I, Newell C. Measuring Health: A Guide to Rating Scales and Questionnaires, 2nd ed. New York: Oxford University Press; 1996.

References

1. Rubin R, Peyrot M. Helping patients develop diabetes coping skills. In: Practical Psychology for Diabetes Clinicians: Effective Techniques for Key Behavioral Issues, 2nd ed. Anderson BJ, Rubin RR, eds. Alexandria, Va: American Diabetes Association; 2002:63-71.
2. Ruiz-Bueno J, Underwood P. Resources as Moderators/Mediators of the Stress-Health Outcome Linkage. Chicago, Ill: Midwest Nurs Res Soc; 2000.
3. Berkman L, Glass T. Social integration, social networks, and health. In: Berkman LF, Kawachi I, eds. Social Epidemiology. New York: Oxford University Press; 2000:137-73.
4. Lorig K, Holman H. Arthritis self-management studies: a twelve-year review. Health Educ Q. 1993;20:17-28.
5. Holroyd KA, Creer TL, eds. Self-Management of Chronic Disease. New York: Academic Press; 1986.
6. Goodall TA, Halford WK. Self-management of diabetes mellitus: a critical review. Health Psychol. 1991;10:1-8.
7. Levy RL. Social support and compliance: a selective review and critique of treatment integrity and outcome measurement. Soc Sci Med. 1983;17:1329-88.
8. Kaplan RM, Hartwell SL. Differential effects of social support and social network on physiological and social outcomes in men and women with type II diabetes mellitus. Health Psychol. 1987;6:387-98.
9. Schafer LC, McCaul KD, Glasgow RE. Supportive and nonsupportive family behaviors: relationships to adherence and metabolic control in persons with Type I diabetes. Health Psychol. 1986;9:179-85.
10. Uchino BN, Cacioppo JT, Kiecolt-Glaser JK. The relationship between social support and physiological processes: a review with emphasis on underlying mechanisms and implications for health. Psychol Bull. 1996;119:488-531.
11. Gottlieb NH, Green L. Life events, social network, lifestyle and health: an analysis of the 1979 National Survey of Personal Health Practices and Consequences. Health Educ Q. 1984;11:91-105.
12. Artinian NT. Resources: factors that mediate the stress-health-outcome relationship. In: Barnfather JS, Lyon BL, eds. Stress and coping: State of the Science and Implications for Nursing Theory, Research and Practice. Indianapolis, Ind: Sigma Theta Tau International; 1993b.
13. Stewart M, Tilden V. The contributions of nursing science to social support. Int J Nurs Stud. 1995;32(6):535-44.
14. Bloom JR. The relationship of social support and health. Soc Sci Med. 1990;30:635-7.
15. Shumaker SA, Bronwell A. Toward a theory of social support: closing conceptual gaps. J Soc Issues. 1984;40(4):11-33.
16. Wortman CB, Dunkel-Schetter C. Conceptual and methodological issues in the study of social support. In: Baum A, Singer JE, eds. Handbook of Psychology and Health. Hillsdale, NJ: Lawrence Erlbaum Associates; 1987:63-108.
17. Langford CPH, Bowsher J, Maloney JP, Lillis PP. Social support: a conceptual analysis. J Adv Nurs. 1997;25:95-100.

18. House J. Work stress and social support. Englewood Cliffs, NJ: Prentice Hall; 1981.

19. Gottlieb B. The development and application of a classification scheme of informal helping behaviors. Can J Behav Sci. 1978;10:105-15.

20. Krause N. Social support, stress, and well-being. J Gerontol. 1986;41(4):512-9.

21. Cronenwett LR. Network structure, social support, and psychological outcomes of pregnancy. Nurs Res. 1985a;34(2):93-9.

22. Cutrona CE, Russell DW. Type of social support and specific stress: toward a theory of optimal matching. In: Sarason BR, Sarason IG, Pierce GR, eds. Social Support: An Interactional View. New York: John Wiley & Sons; 1990:319-66.

23. Kahn R, Antonucci TC. Convoys over the life course: attachment, roles and social support. In: Baltes PB and Brim O, eds. Life Span Development and Behavior, vol. 3. New York: Academic Press; 1980:253-86.

24. Nyamathi A. The coping responses of female spouses of patients with myocardial infarction. Heart Lung. 1987;16:86-92.

25. Cobb S. Social support as a moderator of life stress. Psychosom Med. 1976;38:300-14.

26. Underwood PW. Social support: the promise and the reality. In: Rice VH, ed. Handbook of Stress, Coping, and Health: Implications for Nursing Research, Theory, and Practice. Thousand Oaks, Calif: Sage Publications Ltd; 2000:367-92.

27. Berkman L, Syme L. Social networks, host resistance, and morality: a nine year follow-up study of Alameda County residents. Am J Epidemiol. 1979;109:186-204.

28. Lambert VA, Lambert CE, Klipple GL, Meshaw EA. Social support, hardiness and psychological well-being in women with arthritis. Image: J Nurs Sci. 1989;21:128-31.

29. Powers BA. The meaning of nursing home friendships. Adv Nurs Sci. 1991;14(2):42-58.

30. Vaux A, Harrison D. Support network characteristics associated with support satisfaction and perceived support. Am J Commun Psychol. 1985;13(3):245-67.

31. Underwood PW. Psychosocial variables: their prediction of birth complications and relationship to perception of childbirth. Ann Arbor, Mich: University Microfilms, International; 1986.

32. Frey M. Social support and health: a theoretical formulation derived from King's conceptual framework. Nurs Sci Q. 1989;2:138-48.

33. Cohen S. Psychosocial models of the role of social support in the etiology of physical disease. Health Psychol. 1988;7(3):269-97.

34. Kang D, Coe C, Karaszewski J, McCarthy D. Relationship of social support to stress responses and immune function in healthy and asthmatic adolescents. Res Nurs Health. 1998;21:117-28.

35. O'Brien R, Wineman N, Nealon N. Correlates of the caregiving process in multiple sclerosis. Scholarly Inquiry for Nurs Pract. 1995;9:323-42.

36. Runtz M, Schallow J. Structural characteristics of social networks and their relationship with social support in the elderly: who provides support. Soc Sci Med. 1988;26:737-49.

37. Buschmann MB, Hollinger LM. Influence of social support measure. Clin Gerontologist. 1994;14(4):13-28.

38. Stewart MJ. Integrating social support in nursing. Newbury Park, Calif: Sage Publications Ltd; 1993.

39. Krause N. Understanding the stress process: linking social support with locus of control beliefs. J Gerontol. 1987;42(6):589-93.

40. Skelly AH, Marshall J, Haughey B, Davis P. Self-efficacy and confidence in outcomes as determinants of self-care practices in inner-city Afro-American women with NIDDM. Diabetes Care. 1995;21:38-46.

41. Stevens ES. Reciprocity in social support: an advantage for the aging family. J Contemp Human Services. 1992:533-41.

42. Riegel BJ, Gocka I. Gender differences in adjustment to acute myocardial infarction. Heart Lung. 1995;24:457-66.

43. Gallant MP. The influence of social support on chronic illness self-management: a review and directions for research. Health Educ Behav. 2003;30(2): 170-95.

44. Aalto AM, Uutela A, Aro AR. Health related quality of life among insulin-dependent diabetics: disease-related and psychosocial correlates. Patient Edu Couns. 1997;30:215-25.

45. Wortman CB, Conway TL. The role of social support in adaptation and recovery from physical illness. In: Cohen S, Syme L, eds. Social Support and Health. Orlando, Fla: Academic Press; 1985:281-302.

46. Barrera M. Distinctions between social support concepts, measures, and models. Pub Med. 1986;14(4):413-45.

47. Moos R, Lemke S. Sheltered care environment scale manual. Palo Alto, Calif: Department of Veterans Affairs and Stanford University Medical Centers; 1992.

48. Fink S. The influence of family demands on the strains and well-being of caregiving families. Nurs Res. 1995;44:139-46.

49. Allen S, Stoltenberg C. Psychological separation of older adolescents and young adults from their parents: an investigation of gender differences. J Psychosoc Oncol. 1995;73:542-6.

50. Gulick EE. Model for predicting work performance among persons with multiple sclerosis. Nurs Res. 1992;41:266-72.

51. McColl M, Friedland J. Social support, aging, and disability. Topics in Geriatr Rehabil. 1994;9:54-71.

52. Willey C, Silliman R. The impact of disease on the social support experiences of cancer patients. J Psychosoc Oncol. 1990;8:79-95.

53. Picot S. Rewards, costs, and coping of African American caregivers. Nurs Res. 1995;44:147-52.

54. Choi EC. Nursing research in Korea. Annu Rev Nurs Res. 1994;12:215-29.

55. Franz MJ, ed. A Core Curriculum for Diabetes Education: Diabetes Education and Program Management, 4th ed. Chicago, Ill: American Association of Diabetes Educators; 2001.

56. Rubin RR, Napora JP. Psychosocial assessment. In: Franz MJ, ed. A Core Curriculum for Diabetes Education: Diabetes Education and Program Management, 4th ed. Chicago, Ill: American Association of Diabetes Educators; 2001:25-46.

57. Burns D, Skelly AH. Type 2 diabetes: meeting the daily challenges of self-care. J Multicult Nurs Health. 2005; 11(3):63-7.

58. Carter-Edwards L, Skelly AH, Cagle C, Appel S. "They care but they don't understand": social support of African American women with type 2 diabetes. Diabetes Educ. 2004;30(4):1-21.

59. Cagle C, Appel S, Skelly AH, Carter-Edwards L. Mid-life African American women with type 2 diabetes: influence on work and the multicaregiver role. Ethn Dis. 2002;12(4):555-66.

60. Norbeck J. The Norbeck Social Support Questionnaire. Birth Defects: Original Article Series. 1984;20(5):45-55.

61. Brandt P, Weinert C. The PRQ—a social support measure. Nurs Res. 1981;35:4-9.

62. Weinert C, Brandt P. Measuring social support with the Personal Resources Questionnaire. West J Nurs Res. 1987;9:589-602.

63. Tilden VP, Nelson C, May B. The IPR inventory: development and psychometric characteristics. Nurs Res. 1990b;39:337-43.

64. Norbeck J. Social support: a model for clinical research and application. Adv Nurs Sci. 1981;3(4):43-59.

65. Tilden VP, Nelson C, May B. Use of qualitative methods to enhance content validity. Nurs Res. 1990a;39:172-5.

66. White N, Richter J, Fry C. Coping, social support, and adaptation to chronic illness. West J Nurs Res. 1992;14:211-24.

67. Wilson W, Ary DV, Bigland A, Glasgow RE, Toobert DJ, Campbell DR. Psychosocial predictors of self-care behaviors and glycemic control in NIDDM. Diabetes Care. 1986;9:614-22.

68. Moos R, Moos B. A typology of family social environments. Fam Process. 1981;15:357-71.

69. Harter S. "People in My Life" Social Support Scale for Children. Denver, Colo: University of Denver; 1985.

70. Procidiano ME, Heller K. Measures of perceived social support from friends and from family: three validation studies. Am J Community Psychol.1983;11:1-24.

71. Broadhead WE, Gehlbach SH, De Gruy FV, Kaplan BH. The Duke-UNC Functional Social Support Questionnaire: measurement of social support in family medicine patients. Med Care. 1988;26(7):709-723.

72. Sherbourne CD, Stewart AL. The MOS Social Support Survey. Soc Sci Med. 1991;32:705-14.

73. Parkerson GR Jr, Michener JL, Wu LR, et al. Associations among family support, family stress, and personal functional health status. J Clin Epidemiol. 1989;42:217-29.

74. MacLean D, Lo R. The non-insulin-dependent diabetic: success and failure in compliance. Aust J Adv Nurs. 1998;15:33-42.

75. Lo R. Correlates of expected success at adherence to health regimen of people with IDDM. J Adv Nurs. 1999;30:418-24.

76. Glasgow RE, Toobert DJ. Social environment and regimen adherence among Type II diabetic patients. Diabetes Care. 1988;11:377-86.

77. Fitzgerald JT, Davis WK, Connell CM, Hess GE, Funnell MM. Development and validation of the Diabetes Care Profile. Eval Health Professions. 1996;19(2):208-30.

78. Bearman KJ, La Greca AM. Assessing friend support of adolescents' diabetes care: The Diabetes Social Support Questionnaire—Friends Version. J Pediatr Psychol. 2002;27(5):417-28.

79. Mulcahy K, Peeples M, Tomky D, Weaver T. National Diabetes Education Outcomes System: application to practice. Diabetes Educator. 2000;26:957–64.

80. Whittemore R, D'Eramo-Melkus G, Grey M. Metabolic control, self-management and psychosocial adjustment in women with type 2 diabetes. J Clin Nurs. 2005;14:195-203.

81. Bradley C, ed. Handbook of Psychology and Diabetes. Chur, Switzerland: Harwood Academic Publishers; 1994.

82. McDowell I, Newell C. Measuring Health: A Guide to Rating Scales and Questionnaires, 2nd ed. New York: Oxford University Press; 1996.

83. Ducharme F, Stevens B, Rowat K. Social support: conceptual and methodological issues for research in mental health nursing. Issues Ment Health Nurs. 1994;15:373-92.

84. Johnson SB, Kelly M, Henretta JC, et al. A longitudinal analysis of adherence and health status in childhood diabetes. J Pediatr Psych. 1992;17:537-53.

85. Glasgow RE, Anderson BJ. Future directions for research on pediatric chronic disease management: lessons from diabetes. J Pediatr Psychol. 1995;20(4):389-402.

86. Wysocki T, Greco P, Harris MA, Bubb J, White NH. Behavior therapy for families of adolescents with diabetes: maintenance of treatment effects. Diabetes Care. 2001;24(3):441-6.

87. Anderson BJ, Vangsness L, Connell A, Butler D, Goebel-Fabbri A, Laffel LMB. Family conflict, adherence, and glycemic control in youth with short duration Type 1 diabetes. Diabet Med. 2002;19:635-42.

88. La Greca AM, Auslander WF, Greco P, Spetter D, Fisher EB Jr, Santiago JV. I get by with a little help from my family and friends: adolescents' support for diabetes care. J Pediatr Psychol. 1995;20(4):449-76.

89. Skinner TC, White J, Johnston C, Hixenbaugh P. Interaction between social support and injection regimen in predicting teenagers' concurrent glycosylated haemoglobin assays. J Diabetes Nurs. 1999;3:140-4.

90. Pendley JS, Kasmen L, Miller D, Donze J, Swenson C, Reeves G. Peer and family support in children and adolescents with type 1 diabetes. J Pediatr Psychol. 2002;27:429-38.

91. Skinner TC, John M, Hampson SE. Social support and personal models of diabetes as predictors of self-care and well-being: a longitudinal study of adolescents with diabetes. J Pediatr Psychol. 2000;25(4):257-67.

92. Sherbourne CD, Hays RD, Ordway L, DiMatteo MR, Kravitz RL. Antecedents of adherence to medical recommendations: results from the Medical Outcomes Study. J Behav Med. 1992;32:S5-20.

93. Lloyd CE, Wing RR, Orchard TJ, Becker DJ. Psychosocial correlates of glycemic control: The Pittsburgh Epidemiology of Diabetes Complications (EDC) Study. Diabetes Res Clin Pract. 1993;21:187-95.

94. Ruggiero L, Spirito A, Coustan D, McGarvey ST, Low KG. Self-reported compliance with diabetes self-management during pregnancy. Int J Psychiatry Med. 1993;23:195-207.

95. Schlenk EA, Hart LK. Relationship between health focus of control, health value, and social support and compliance of persons with diabetes mellitus. Diabetes Care. 1984;7:566-74.

96. Ruggiero L, Spirito A, Bond A, Coustan D, McGarvey S. Impact of social support and stress on compliance in women with gestational diabetes. Diabetes Care. 1990;13:441-3.

97. Garay-Sevilla ME, Nava LE, Malacara JM, et al. Adherence to treatment and social support in patients with non-insulin dependent diabetes mellitus. J Diabetes Complications. 1995;9:81-6.

98. Pham DT, Fortin F, Thibaudeau MF. The role of the health belief model in amputees' self-evaluation of adherence to diabetes self-care behaviors. Diabetes Educ. 1995;22:133-9.

99. Tillotson LM, Smith MS. Locus of control, social support, and adherence to the diabetes regimen. Diabetes Educ. 1996;22:133-9.

100. Kawakami N, Akachi K, Shimizu H, Haratani T, Koyayashi F, Ishizaki M, et al. Job strain, social support

in the workplace, and hemoglobin A1c in Japanese men. Occup Environ Med. 2000;57:805-9.

101. Fisher L, Chesla CA, Bartz RJ, et al. The family and type 2 diabetes: a framework for intervention. Diabetes Educ. 1998;24:599-607.

102. Trief PM, Grant W, Elbert K, Weinstock RS. Family environment, glycemic control, and the psychosocial adaptation of adults with diabetes. Diabetes Care. 1998;21(2):241-5.

103. Gerstle JF, Varenne H, Contento I. Post-diagnosis family adaptation influences glycemic control in women with type 2 diabetes mellitus. J Amer Diet Assoc. 2001;101(8):918-22.

104. Herpertz S, Johann B, Lichtblau K, Stadtbaumer M, Kocnar M, Kramer-Paust R, Paust R, Heinemann H, Senf W. Patients with diabetes mellitus: psychosocial stress and use of psychosocial support: a multicenter study. Med Klin (Munich). 2000;95(7):369-77.

105. Murphy DJ, Williamson PS, Nease DE Jr. Supportive family members of diabetic adults. Fam Pract Res J. 1994;14:323-31.

106. Conn VS, Taylor SG, Abel PB. Myocardial infarction survivors: age and gender differences in physical health, psychosocial state and regime adherence. J Adv Nurs. 1991;16:1026-34.

107. Rubin RR, Peyrot M. Psychological issues and treatments for people with diabetes. J Clin Psychol. 2001;57(4):457-78.

108. Mercado F, Vargas PN. Disease and the family: differences in metabolic control of diabetes mellitus between men and women. Women Health. 1989;15:111–21.

109. Samuel-Hodge C, Headon S, Skelly AH, Elasy T, Ammerman A, Keyserlying T. Spirituality, stress, multicaregiving role and other contextual factors in Type 2 diabetes. Diabetes Care. 2000;23:928-33.

110. Davis L, Wykle ML. Self-care in minority and ethnic populations: the experience of older Black Americans. In: Ory MG, DeFriese GH, eds. Self-Care in Later Life. New York: Springer; 1998:170-9.

111. Neighbors HW, Jackson JS. Four patterns of illness behavior in the Black community. Amer J Community Psychol. 1984;12(6):629-44.

112. Taylor JR. Receipt of support among Black Americans: demographic and familial differences. J Marriage Fam. 1986;48:67-77.

113. Silverstein M, Waite L. Are blacks more likely than whites to receive and provide social support in the middle and old age? yes, no and maybe so. J Gerontol. 1993;48 Suppl 4:S212-S222.

114. Luckey I. African American Elders: the support network of generational kin. Families in Society: J Contemp Human Sci. 1994:82-89.

115. Walls CT. The role of church and family support in the lives of older African Americans. Generations. 1992 summer:33-36.

116. Belgrave FZ, Lewis DM. The role of social support in compliance and other health behaviors for African Americans with chronic illnesses. J Health Soc Policy. 1994;5(3/4):55-68.

117. Ford ME, Tilley BC, McDonald PE. Social support among African American adults with diabetes, Part 2: a review. J Natl Med Assoc. 1998;90(7):425-32.

118. Ford ME, Tilley BC, McDonald PE. Social support among African American adults with diabetes, Part 1: a review. J Natl Med Assoc. 1998;90(6):361-5.

119. Westaway MS, Seager JR, Rheeder P, Van Zyl DG. The effects of social support on health, well-being and management of diabetes mellitus: a black South African perspective. Ethn Health. 2005;10(1):73-89.

120. Gavin JR III, Landrum S. Dr. Gavin's health guide for African Americans. Canada: Small Steps Press; 2004.

121. Bryant S, Rakowski W. Predictors of mortality among elderly African Americans. Res on Aging. 1992;14(5):50-67.

122. Mutran E. Intergenerational family support among blacks and whites: response to culture or to socioeconomic differences. J Geront. 1985;40(3):382-89.

123. Gleeson-Kreig J, Bernal H, Woolley S. The role of social support in the self-management of diabetes among a Hispanic population. Public Health Nurs. 2002;19(3):215-22.

124. Sarkisian CA, Brown KC, Wintz RL, Mangione CM. A systematic review of diabetes self-care interventions for older, African American, or Latino adults. Diabetes Educ. 2003;29(3):467-79.

125. Epple C, Wright AL, Joish VN, Bauer M. The role of active family nutritional support in Navajos' type 2 diabetes metabolic control. Diabetes Care. 2003;26:2829-34.

126. Coyne JC, Downey G. Social factors and psychopathology: stress, social support and coping processes. Annu Rev Psychol. 1991;42:401-25.

127. Schuster T, Kessler R, Aseltin R. Supportive interactions, negative interactions and depressed mood. Am J Community Psychol. 1990;18(3):423-38.

128. Katz AH. Self-help in America: A Social Movement Perspective. New York: Twayne; 1993.

129. Ramphele M. Participatory research: the myths and realities. Social Dynamics. 1990;16(2):1-15.

130. Smith L, Weinert C. Telecommunication support for rural women with diabetes. Diabetes Educ. 2000;26(4):645-55.

131. Barrera M, Glasgow RE, McKay HG, Boles SM, Feil EG. Do internet-based support interventions change perceptions of social support? an experimental trial of approaches for supporting diabetes self-management. Am J Community Psychol. 2002;30(5):637-54.

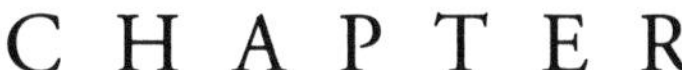

CHAPTER

6

Community and Society Support for Diabetes Self-Management

Authors

Carol A. Brownson, MSPH
Sarah L. Lovegreen, MPH
Edwin B. Fisher, PhD

Key Concepts

- An ecological approach asserts that self-management behavior is influenced by—and in turn influences—the environment.
- A model of "Resources and Supports for Self-Management" delineates what individuals need to manage their diabetes successfully.
- Influences at the levels of communities, organizations, and society are too often unrecognized but very important in diabetes prevention and control.
- The AADE 7 Self-Care Behaviors™ can be supported through community and organizational health promotion campaigns.

Introduction

Diabetes requires management for the rest of an individual's life. Individuals with diabetes cannot achieve disease management through *isolated medical interventions*, such as surgery or even periodic injections. Nor can they achieve sustained management through *periodic participation* in intensive treatments or regimens, such as residential weight-loss programs or periodic hospitalizations. Rather, persons with diabetes must carry out their plans for use of medicines, healthy eating, and physical activity throughout their daily lives and in the places where they live, work, and play. Diabetes management, thus, must be considered squarely within the settings of those daily lives—in the family and community—and recognized to be substantially influenced by them.

The importance of interventions that will support diabetes management in daily life is reflected in research. For example, research has shown that the best predictor of change in metabolic control is the duration of self-management programs.[1,2] "Interventions with regular reinforcement are more effective than one-time or short-term education."[1] Recognizing that the importance of ongoing support in the settings of daily life is not limited to diabetes is also helpful; the importance of sustained support is reflected in other reviews and meta-analyses in health promotion[3] and, for example, in key reviews of interventions for smoking cessation.[4,5]

An Ecological Approach to Self-Management

The importance of sustained support and resources in individuals' daily lives poses a challenge for self-management programs. How can those who plan and implement such programs—programs that conventionally focus on teaching skills for buying and preparing food, managing medications, and so on—address worksites, communities, families, friends, or coworkers? This challenge was evident in the work to develop plans for the Diabetes Initiative of the Robert Wood Johnson Foundation. The Diabetes Initiative was intended to demonstrate real-world, sustainable programs for self-management. Ecological models guided plans for the Initiative. Ecological perspectives were of value in considering how influences at the levels of family, group, neighborhood, community, and government might complement individual patient education and care and lead to sustained self-management.[6] Thus, in addition to self-management classes or collaborative goal setting within the clinical encounter, Diabetes Initiative projects address family and peer support; community-based programs and activities; and community resources that can reinforce, facilitate, and sustain individuals' self-management efforts.

Ecological perspectives recognize that individuals and communities interact with their physical and sociocultural environments.[7,8] "Conceptualizing health as a product, in part, of social conditions facilitates the identification of relationships between social determinants and health outcomes that may be amenable to change."[9(114)]

Recognizing Societal Levels that Affect Behavior and Influence Each Other

The simplest ecological model includes 3 societal levels:[8]

- Individual
- Interpersonal
- Community

Although numerous ecological models exist[8,10] with varying numbers of levels and different taxonomies, the underlying premise is the same: behavior influences and is influenced by multiple levels of the environment.

> ### *What Influences Behavior?*
>
> Behavior influences and is influenced by the environment. Issues at individual, interpersonal, and community levels influence each other, ultimately affecting individual self-care behavior.

Influences Among Influences. In addition to the broad assertion that behavior is influenced by and influences the environment, ecological models emphasize another important point: that the different levels influence each other. Thus, worksite or health system programs and policies may influence family practices, which, in turn, influence the management and behaviors of individuals within those families.

Yoo has described this kind of "influence among influences" by positing that at each level in the ecological model, one can identify an issue, an intervention, and a desired outcome. Further, the success of the intervention is directly influenced by the issue at the next higher level.[11] For example:

- *Influence at Individual Level.* If the issue at the individual level is poor diet and the intervention is a meal plan, the success of that intervention is directly influenced by issues in the individual's immediate social circle—friends, family, and coworkers.
- *Influence at Family Level.* If the corresponding issue at the family level is that the individual has no role in food purchase and preparation in a family whose eating patterns include no fruits and vegetables, the likelihood of that individual's success in changing her or his meal plan (the desired outcome) is greatly diminished. If, on the other hand, the family embraces healthy eating, the person's chances of success skyrocket.
- *Influence at Community Level.* Taking that to the community level, the family's success will be greatly influenced by the availability of affordable healthy foods from which to choose and so on.

This approach makes it possible to model complex problems and see points of intervention and connections among intervention approaches. Figure 6.1 portrays such

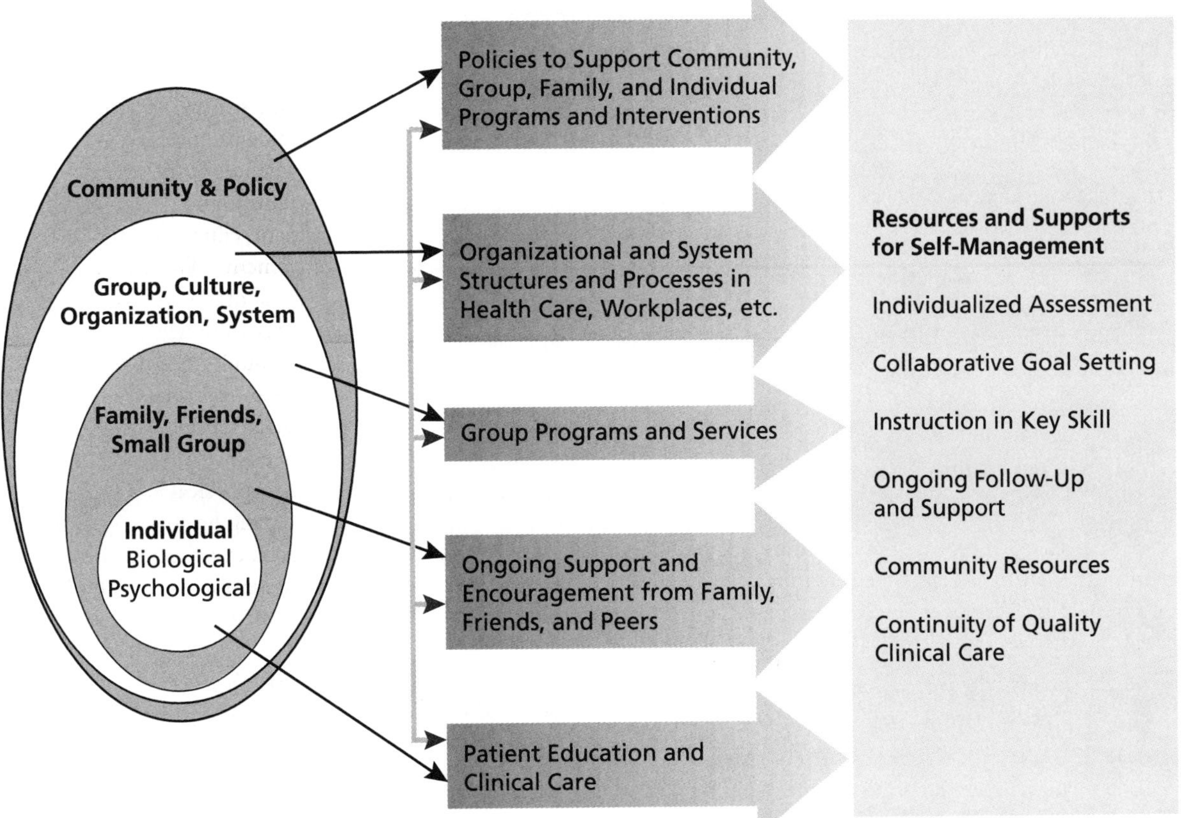

FIGURE 6.1 Relationships Among Ecological Levels, Policies and Organizational/System Factors, Programs and Services, and Resources and Supports for Self-Management as Available to Individuals With Diabetes

Note: Indicated paths are exemplary, not inclusive. That there are multiple connections among ecological levels, programs and services, and Resources and Supports available to individuals is an emphasis of ecological perspectives.

relationships among ecological levels, policy influences, programs and services, and aspects of the Resources and Supports for Self-Management, which will be described more fully below.

Historical Perspective:
Moving from the Individual to the Community

Ecological perspectives can be seen to have emerged through an evolution of views of health and illness and the contributions of interventions in various channels and areas. See the sidebar summarizing the evolution from the 1920s to the present.

The Evolving Focus of Health Care

Medical Phase: 1920 to 1960

The years from 1920 to 1960 have been characterized as the "medical phase," which saw growth in the numbers of hospitals, development of health specialties, and support for biomedical research.[12] Despite this growth and investment, by the middle of the 20th century, the major accomplishments of medicine—through control of infectious disease, for example—were not leading to improvements in population health proportionate to the resources being invested. Leading causes of death in the United Sates were transitioning from acute and infectious diseases to chronic conditions.

Health Promotion Phase: 1960 to 1990s

By the late 1970s, recognition that a significant percentage of the causes of morbidity and mortality were attributable to lifestyle and behavior[13] led to a "health promotion phase."[12] Documents like Healthy People 2000[14] and, subsequently, Healthy People 2010[15] set a national agenda for disease prevention and health promotion. Concurrently, developments in behavioral medicine[16] and understanding of diabetes[17] increased the awareness of the importance of the individual's behavior in prevention and management of chronic disease and of interventions to help individuals live healthy lives.

Community Health Phase: From mid-1990s

Beginning in the mid-1990s and aided by the pioneering work of *Amick et al*,[18] social epidemiology made an important contribution to society's understanding of and approach to diseases in populations. We might call this the "community health" phase.

Social epidemiology focuses on social groups versus individuals and the social characteristics of communities that shape them. Social determinants of health are factors that positively or negatively affect a wide array of health conditions.[19]

- Supportive community environments and policies make good health and healthy choices possible.
- Conversely, poverty, inequalities, stress, social isolation, and lack of access to health care negatively affect health.

Negative factors such as poverty and inequalities affect health directly and indirectly by limiting access to resources and opportunities for maintaining health. The social meaning of poverty or being disenfranchised is also known to have a negative influence on health.[20] Consistent with ecological perspectives, the societal factors that affect health operate at both the individual and community levels. At the community level, these social determinants tend to be concentrated among the same people and to exacerbate each other's effects, thereby furthering disparities in disease burden.

Much has been learned about the pathways by which social conditions affect health.[18,20-23] Table 6.1 provides examples of how such social conditions and determinants directly or indirectly affect health in general and diabetes specifically.

Resources and Supports for Self-Management

The ecological perspective highlights the importance of social and community influences on each other and on the behavior of those subject to them. When what is needed to live with diabetes is considered from the point of view of the individual, the ecological model highlights the importance of a range of services, resources, types of assistance, opportunities, and other resources and supports for diabetes management. These resources and supports come from the individual's care providers as well as families, friends, workplaces, neighborhoods, governments, and so on. They have been articulated in the Diabetes Initiative as a set, entitled Resources and Supports for Self-Management.[6] Using this model, individuals are seen to have need for the following types of support:

- Individualized assessment
- Collaborative goal setting
- Instruction in key skills
- Ongoing follow-up and support
- Community resources
- Continuity of quality clinical care

Table 6.2 provides descriptions of each category. Figure 6.1 relates elements of the Resources and Supports for Self-Management model to ecological influences.

Resources and Supports for Self-Management constitutes a model of *what individuals need* from varied sources in order to manage their disease. Very likely, no single agency or source could provide them all, and no

TABLE 6.1 Examples of Social Determinants of Health and Their Impacts on Health and Diabetes

Social Determinant	*Impacts on Health and Diabetes*
Social gradient	Within and across social strata, people at lower ends of the social ladder experience disease and premature death at much higher rates. Low socioeconomic status is associated with a heightened prevalence of diabetes.[1, 2]
Stress	Inability to cope and feelings of worry and anxiety are damaging to health and may lead to premature death. People on lower ends of the social gradient experience relatively more stress. Depression occurs at much higher rates among people with diabetes than those without it.[3] Depression and stress exacerbate diabetes and impair diabetes management.[4]
Social exclusion	"Life is short where its quality is poor."[5] Deprivation, discrimination, and social exclusion result in premature death.
Work	While having a job is generally better for health than not, health suffers when people have little control over their work or are unable to use their skills. Diabetes is a predictor of lower productivity at work, increasing with length of diagnosis and consequent complications.[6] Impacts on diabetes of work conditions providing flexibility for employees to manage diabetes.[7]
Unemployment	Both the psychological and financial effects of unemployment lead to illness and premature death; conversely, job security improves health and well-being. Income loss due to diabetes results from early retirement, increased sick days, disability, and premature mortality.[8]
Social support	Poverty increases social isolation and poorer health. Strong, supportive social networks have a protective effect on health. Social support has been shown to buffer the physical and emotional consequences of stressors among people with diabetes.[9,10]
Access to food	Having access to affordable nutritious foods influences diet more than education. People with low incomes are less able to afford healthy food; there are more fast-food and convenience stores in low-income neighborhoods.
Transportation	Mechanization and urban sprawl have engineered a great deal of physical activity out of our daily lives. "Healthy transportation" promotes physical activity through biking, walking, and use of public transportation. Studies are underway to reduce diabetes risk and burden through increased access to and promotion of walking trails.[11]
Heath care	Access to quality, affordable, culturally competent health care affects health. Disparities exist in health care of patients by race and ethnicity and by insurance status.[12]

References

1. Everson SA, Maty SC, Lynch JW, Kaplan GA. Epidemiologic evidence for the relation between socioeconomic status and depression, obesity, and diabetes. J Psychosom Res. 2002;53(4):891-5.
2. Robbins JM, Vaccarino V, Zhang H, Kasl SV. Socioeconomic status and diagnosed diabetes incidence. Diabetes Res Clin Pract. 2005;68(3):230-6.
3. Anderson RJ, Freedland KE, Clouse RE, Lustman PJ. The prevalence of comorbid depression in adults with diabetes: a meta-analysis. Diabetes Care. 2001;24(6):1069-78.
4. Lin EHB, Katon W, Von Korff M, et al. Relationship of depression and diabetes self-care, medication adherence, and preventive care. Diabetes Care. 2004;27(9):2154-60.
5. Wilkinson R, Marmot M. Social Determinants of Health: The Solid Facts, 2nd ed. Copenhagen, Denmark: World Health Organization; 2003.
6. Lavigne JE, Phelps CE, Mushlin A, Lednar WM. Reductions in individual work productivity associated with type 2 diabetes mellitus. PharmacoEconomics. 2003;21(15):1123-34.
7. Heins JM, Arfken CL, Padgett D, Nord W. Management of diabetes mellitus (DM) at work. Diabetes. 1990;39 Suppl.:167A.
8. Vijan S, Hayward RA, Langa KM. The impact of diabetes on workforce participation: results from a national household sample. Health Serv Res. 2004;39(6 Pt 1):1653-69.
9. Gallant MP. The influence of social support on chronic illness self-management: a review and directions for research. Health Educ Behav. 2003;30(2):170-95.
10. Griffith LS, Field BJ, Lustman PJ. Life stress and social support in diabetes: association with glycemic control. Int J Psych Med. 1990;20(4):365-74.
11. Brownson RC, Hagood L, Lovegreen SL, et al. A multilevel ecological approach to promoting walking in rural communities. Prev Med. 2005;41(5-6):837-42.
12. Smedley BD, Stith AY, Nelson AR, eds (Committee on Understanding and Eliminating Racial and Ethnic Disparities in Health Care). Unequal Treatment: Confronting Racial and Ethnic Disparities in Health Care. Washington, DC: National Academy Press; 2002.

TABLE 6.2 Resources and Supports for Self-Management	
Individualized Assessment	Assessment of individual status, experience with diabetes, history of self-management activities, areas of success and areas presenting challenges, personality, family, and cultural perspectives pertinent to diabetes management
Collaborative Goal-Setting	Discussion with individuals, families, or groups to set goals for self-management, including necessary steps to accomplishing them, likely barriers, needed skills
Instruction in Key Skills	Instruction, practice, feedback, revised instruction in key skills for self-management, including monitoring blood sugar, taking medications, healthy eating, physical activity, healthy coping and management of negative emotions, cultivation of supportive relationships, problem solving
Ongoing Follow-Up and Support	Monitoring success in self-management and achievement of self-management goals, encouragement, social support, assistance in adjusting self-management plans, arrangement for renewed individualized assessment, collaborative goal setting, etc, occasioned by change in status or circumstance
Community Resources	Access to key resources for self-management, including availability of healthy, affordable food that is congruent with cultural perspectives; availability of affordable medications and supplies for self-management; safe and attractive places for physical activity; accessible health information and care
Continuity of Quality Clinical Care	Regular clinical care as per American Diabetes Association recommendations, delivered through culturally competent clinicians who cultivate a proactive, individualized, collaborative relationship with patients

Definition of Key Terms

- Community resources
- Ongoing follow-up and support

Community influences on diabetes management are the focus of this chapter. In the framework of Resources and Supports for Self-Management, this clearly includes community resources such as access to healthy food and to attractive, safe places for physical activity. Another community-based influence on self-management is community-based ongoing follow-up and support, such as that received from peer groups, community health workers, local promotional campaigns to increase awareness of diabetes and understanding of the needs of those with the disease, and campaigns to promote healthy eating or physical activity. The category of ongoing follow-up and support also includes professionally based resources and services such as follow-up by clinic-based nursing staff. For the purposes of this chapter, however, the domain of community resources and supports is considered to include community resources and only those aspects of ongoing follow-up and support that are delivered through community-based channels or by peers, neighbors, community health workers, and the like, as opposed to healthcare professionals.

single policy could guarantee them all. However, planning of self-management programs may be enhanced by considering what access to these resources and supports a program's intended audience may have and how gaps may be addressed. As will be seen in considerations of the clinician's role, below, just recognizing unmet needs for community resources may enhance the effectiveness of individual advice and counseling.

From this model, 2 elements stand out as especially pertinent to persons with diabetes in their efforts to sustain self-management where it occurs, in the settings of their daily lives:

- Ongoing follow-up and support
- Community resources

These 2 elements are especially important in meeting the needs of those who must manage diabetes throughout the course of their lives. The remainder of this chapter focuses on ways in which programs and policies might enhance what a community provides in these 2 areas. The chapter draws from research on applications of the ecological perspective to prevention of other diseases and from the more limited research applying the ecological perspective to diabetes management. The chapter also draws lessons from projects of the Robert Wood Johnson Foundation Diabetes Initiative and other diabetes practice models. As the chapter concludes, it highlights policies that must provide a base for community resources and supports, controversies and areas requiring additional knowledge, and suggestions for clinicians and practitioners in addressing these issues.

Community Health Promotion Outside of Diabetes Management

A number of developments in public health, community, prevention, and disease management interventions, such as the Healthy Cities and Healthy Communities Movement,[24,25] pose models for community approaches to diabetes management. Early lessons came from major projects that began in the 1970s on community-based prevention of cardiovascular disease—programs that focused, for example, on weight management, physical activity, smoking cessation, and detection and control of hypertension.[26-32]

Lessons in Community-Based Prevention

Learning from the Cardiovascular Programs

Stanford, Pawtucket, and Minnesota Studies. The Stanford, Pawtucket, and Minnesota heart disease prevention studies addressed key cardiovascular risks, diet, weight, blood pressure, physical activity, and smoking in populations identified through the communities in which they lived. The Stanford 3- and 5-City Community Studies examined combinations of intensive instruction through individual and group programs and extensive media campaigns.[33] In the Minnesota and Pawtucket Heart Health Programs, there was extensive emphasis on planning and implementation of programs through community-based committees in order to enhance community support for the programs and their objectives.[34-36] In general, results of these programs have not been as compelling as expected, although positive findings have included improved diet and physical activity in some analyses, improved blood pressure control, and some improvements in rates of smoking cessation.[26,28,29,37-40]

That the results of these major community projects have been less strong than anticipated has been discussed in light of the clear evidence of secular trends suggesting substantial effects of broad campaigns to reduce risk factors such as smoking[41-43] and hypertension.[44] This has led to the assertion that aspects of the research design of these community programs have limited their impacts, especially by constraining the local initiative, flexibility in program development, and recruitment of informal and peer social influences to promote program objectives. For example, an editorial[45] discussing the similarly modest results of a large trial of community-based approaches to smoking cessation, COMMIT,[46,47] noted that interventions were planned by a national steering committee and only disseminated through community boards and governance structures. The program-to-be-implemented included 58 mandated activities and the possibility of proscribing locally chosen activities if they were viewed as deviating from the overall plan. In some cases, locally chosen plans were vetoed by the national coordinators.[48] Given such constraints posed by research methodologies, the problem may not be that research has found community health promotion to be weak in its effects—the epidemiologic trends make clear that the effects of broad community campaigns are substantial[42]—but that conventional designs have been found to be weak in capturing those effects and advancing understanding of them.[45]

North Karelia Project. The North Karelia project has been the most successful in changing a variety of risk factors and reducing cardiovascular mortality. This project used probably the broadest range of interventions, from mass media to cooperation with agricultural and food merchandising groups, to improve the availability of healthy foods.[30] Importantly, this project emanated from the Department of Epidemiology of the National Public Health Institute within North Karelia, with field offices at the level of county departments of health and local advisory boards. Community organization in North Karelia included collaboration with existing official agencies and voluntary health organizations so that "the new health service activities initiated by the Project became part of formal public health activities in the area."[30(166)] National and regional media campaigns were integrated with community-level campaigns and promotion in local newspapers and media. Training activities targeted physicians and nurses and also social workers, representatives of voluntary health organizations, and informal opinion leaders. Training was organized through county-level or other local organizations. Attention to the health system included reorganizing treatment for hypertension and care following myocardial infarction. This included training and development of treatment guidelines. Cooperation with other local organizations included not only the voluntary health agencies but also the critical food industry (eg, dairies and sausage factories) and grocery stores.[30] Results included impressive reductions in cardiovascular risk factors[31] and mortality[49] as well as reductions of cancer risk factors.[32] Two characteristics appear to have been critical in the North Karelia community organization: (1) the variety of activities included and (2) the attention in all areas to implementation through and in collaboration with local organizations.

Other Community Interventions. Additional community interventions have been demonstrated in promoting physical activity,[50] promoting weight management and healthy eating,[51-54] and smoking cessation.[55, 56] The Missouri Bootheel Heart Health Project,[57] focusing on risk reduction through use of community coalitions, showed a 6.8% increase in physical activity among those living in an area with an active community coalition. Increased cholesterol screening was another outcome. Other community-based programs to increase fruit and vegetable intake or decrease fat intake have used churches[58,59] and WIC clinics.[60]

Integrating programs across levels of influence strengthens interventions:

Successful approaches create connections—for example, building coalitions, using community organizations, and changing resources to better meet needs and then promoting these resources through communication campaigns.

As noted earlier in the chapter, a key characteristic of ecological perspectives is their emphasis on multiple levels of influence and connections among them. Community-level approaches exemplify this by combining (*1*) environmental strategies that change health behavior by changing community resources, such as places for physical activity, with (*2*) promotional and health education campaigns to encourage use of those community resources.[61] Success of community-based interventions has been documented in the use of already established community organizations and through development and use of community coalitions. These interventions have more sustaining power due to their integration into the fabric of the community and the involvement of multiple partners to achieve the health goal.

Learning from Smoking Prevention and Cessation Initiatives

The value of integrating a broad range of ecologic levels of influence (community, organization, policy, individual, and group) in health promotion is perhaps most clearly illustrated in the steady decline in smoking since the 1964 Surgeon General's Report,[62] from 42% among persons 18 years of age and older in 1965 to 23% in 2001. Considering that smoking is addictive, that it is relatively inexpensive and convenient, and that cigarettes are promoted by the culture's most heavily financed marketing campaign, the changes that have occurred constitute what C. Everett Koop called "a revolution in behavior. . .a major public health success" in his preface to the 1989, 25th anniversary Surgeon General's Report.[43] What brought about this unprecedented "revolution in behavior" has been a wide range of influences, including information about the impact of smoking on disease and death, dissemination of this information to the public, surveillance and evaluation of prevention and cessation programs, campaigns by advocates for nonsmokers' rights, restrictions on cigarette advertising, counter advertising, policy changes (ie, enforcement of minors' access laws, legislation restricting smoking in public places, and increased taxation), improvements in treatment and prevention programs, and an increased understanding of the economic costs of tobacco use.[43]

Statewide programs exemplifying this range of factors promoting nonsmoking—such as in California and Massachusetts—have not relied on "magic bullets," but have included broad campaigns of public education (including "hard hitting" counter marketing), increased taxes on cigarettes, support services for cessation, smoking prevention programs aimed at youth, and multicultural approaches, all coordinated through community-based coalitions.[63] Such broad, multilevel, comprehensive approaches have yielded impressive results. In California, such campaigns have reduced deaths from heart disease.[64]

In his summary of a major review of smoking cessation research,[4] Kottke articulated well the importance of broad, varied approaches to smoking cessation and the lessons they provide for how efforts to promote diabetes management need to consider community resources and supports:

> Success was not associated with novel or unusual interventions. It was the product of personalized . . . advice and assistance, repeated in different forms by several sources over the longest feasible period . . . given clearly, repeatedly, and consistently through every feasible delivery system; personalized advice; printed materials; the mass media; and . . . medical, work, school, and home environments.[4(2888-2889)]

Community Approaches to Diabetes Prevention

The major chronic conditions—cancer, heart disease, obesity, diabetes—share common risk factors. Poor diet, sedentary lifestyle, and tobacco use, for example, account for an estimated 33.5% of actual deaths in the United States.[65,66] Ecological approaches to diabetes prevention apply as well to prevention of other major and chronic illnesses. Diabetes prevention exemplifies the utility of ecological perspectives in tying together a wide variety of influences:[67]

- Individual risk perception and decision making
- Group behavior change programs
- Community norms and influences
- Social and ethnic disparities and policies

The results of the Diabetes Prevention Program point especially toward the importance of research on weight loss, dietary change, and physical activity. Major reviews in these areas have included review of interventions promoting physical activity as part of the Task Force on Community Preventive Services[68] organized by the Centers for Disease Control and Prevention (CDC) and review of interventions promoting healthy diet, such as in a report of the Agency for Healthcare Research and Quality.[69] Both these reports reflected the present emphases on community influences in concluding that effective program characteristics include these characteristics:

- Supporting behavior change through as many channels and levels (individual, group, community) as possible
- Sustaining interventions over as long a period as possible

Prevention Programs in Organizational Settings

The report of the Agency for Healthcare Research and Quality[69] and a review of weight-loss interventions in diabetes[70] both emphasized interventions at the organizational level, especially schools and worksites. Their reviews of such interventions are summarized below. Church-based interventions are also discussed. Tactics employed in successful studies are also summarized.

School-Based Interventions. Of course, schools are organizations that are especially pertinent to diabetes prevention. In general, school-based interventions that have been successful have focused on multiple levels of intervention, including the following:[71-73]

- Classroom instruction by teachers
- Environmental change, such as cafeteria food choices
- Family involvement, for example through dietary-related homework, activity packets, or group meetings

The CATCH trial demonstrated that altering school lunch and physical education environments can influence dietary behaviors of children.[54,74,75]

Workplace Interventions. Organizational settings have also included worksites. Successful programs most often employed multiple strategies across multiple levels, such as by opening interventions or activities to workers' families[76] or by initiating environmental changes such as increasing availability of healthy food choices.[77] Tactics in successful programs include the following:[76-78]

- Screenings
- Nutrition classes
- Goal setting
- Changes in food available in cafeterias and vending machines
- Individualized feedback on food intake
- Mailed self-help materials
- Family components
- Participatory approaches, such as employee advisory boards to help plan interventions

Focusing on naturally occurring groups, one successful worksite program was organized around informal cliques of blue-collar employees.[79]

Church-Based Interventions. In African American communities particularly, churches have had a long history of addressing the community's health and social needs and serving as a setting for intervention activities.[80,81] Classes, support groups, health messages from the pulpit, and peer advisor programs are among the approaches that have been used effectively. In a study by McNabb and colleagues,[82] a church-based weight-loss program run by trained community volunteers for urban African American women at risk for diabetes was effective in demonstrating clinically significant weight loss as compared to a control group. In another study, the addition of spiritual strategies resulted in clinically important cardiovascular improvements among African American women in a church-based program when compared to the standard nutrition and physical activity intervention.[83]

Tactics of Note

Tactics in successful diabetes prevention programs have included the following:

- Attention to self-management strategies
- Family components[84]
- Emphasis on peers or lay instructors[52,60,85,86]
- Combination of home visits and newsletters[87]
- Community-based classes[88]
- Altering supermarket environments[89]
- Combined channels, such as reaching adolescent females through Girl Scout troops and then using them to reach their parents[90]

Community Resources and Diabetes Prevention

Community Resources for Physical Activity

In addition to health education and health promotion interventions delivered through community and organizational settings, research over the past decade has examined how the "built environment" in communities influences behavior and health. In a study in North Carolina communities, availability of walking trails and places for physical activity were associated with engaging in recommended amounts of physical activity after control for demographic and other environmental factors.[91] More generally, "urban sprawl" and the corresponding absences of compact, walkable neighborhoods are associated with greater obesity and hypertension but less walking.[92]

Availability of Healthy Food

Research has also examined the impacts of policy and environmental factors on the availability of healthy food.[53] Brownell's 2004 book *Food Fight: The Inside Story of the Food Industry, America's Obesity Crisis, and What We Can Do About It*[93] describes an "obesigenic" environment and outlines policy initiatives to address it. This attention to environmental and policy influences on healthy eating, obesity, and diseases such as diabetes and cardiovascular disease has begun to emulate policy-level initiatives combating cigarette smoking.[41,63,64]

Task Force Recommendations

In 1996, the Task Force on Community Preventive Services was charged with "developing recommendations for interventions that promote health and prevent diseases in our nation's communities and healthcare systems."[9(ix)] The task force met over an 8-year period to conduct systematic reviews and evaluation of the scientific evidence for population-based interventions in high-priority health topics. The first results were published in *The Guide to Community Preventive Services* (*Community Guide*)[9] in 2005. These are also available on the Internet at http://thecommunityguide.org. The Web site posts new reviews as they become available. Pertinent to this chapter, the *Community Guide* covers diabetes and a number of its key risk factors (eg, physical activity, nutrition, and tobacco product use). In the *Community Guide*, the level of evidence for the effectiveness of an intervention is categorized as strong, sufficient, or insufficient, based on "the number of available studies, the suitability of their designs and quality of execution, and the consistency and size of reported effects" [9(444)]

What's working in community interventions:

For physical activity, the *Community Guide* reported *strong evidence* for the following:

- Community-wide campaigns
- School-based physical education
- Nonfamily social support
- Individually adapted health behavior change
- Creation of and/or enhanced access to places for physical activity combined with informational outreach activities

The task force found sufficient evidence for the effectiveness of "point-of-decision" prompts, such as signs placed by elevators or escalators to encourage use of nearby stairways. Other strategies were investigated, but could not be recommended based on the strength of the evidence currently available. While those interventions may, in fact, work, the findings indicate that additional research is needed.

Reflecting years of anti-tobacco work on many fronts, the *Community Guide* reported strong evidence for a number of strategies: smoking bans and restrictions, increasing the unit price for tobacco, integrating media campaigns with in-person interventions, combining provider education with provider reminder systems, and adding telephone support to cessation interventions. It reported sufficient evidence for programs that reduce costs to patients of smoking cessation services and of systems to remind providers which of their patients smoke, what progress they may have made toward quitting, or how they may approach those patients' smoking.

Rural Prevention Program to Increase Physical Activity

A community-based program, called Project WOW: Walk the Ozarks to Wellness, that is currently in use seeks to reduce incidence or delay onset of type 2 diabetes through increased physical activity. Through use of a regional steering committee, interventions at 3 levels of the ecological perspective (individual, interpersonal, and community) are implemented.

- *At the Individual Level:* The individual-level interventions included tailored newsletters, individual glucose screenings through health fairs, and physician counseling.
- *At the Interpersonal Level:* Regular walking groups were the focus of interpersonal interventions.
- *At the Community Level:* Community level interventions included events such as community contests, community walks, media campaigns, and walking trail enhancements (eg, lighting, water fountains).

Year 1 follow-up analyses showed that those community members with medium or high exposure to Project WOW interventions were 3 times more likely to meet moderate physical activity recommendations through walking than those with no exposure.[94]

Rural Prevention Program for an Ethnic Community

In Canada, a community-based diabetes prevention program was implemented among a rural Aboriginal population.[95] The program included weight management, aerobic classes, and walking clubs. A community advisory board and a tribal recreation coordinator provided direction and support. Changes were observed in body mass index, systolic blood pressure, and knowledge of diabetes, but these were not significantly greater than changes in comparison communities. The authors argue that insufficient time (2 years) and attention to community process resulted in insufficient activation of the community, an important consideration for community organization approaches. This also illustrates a challenge in evaluating community programs amid broader secular trends that may obscure program effects.[42,45]

Self-Management Behaviors: An Ecological Perspective

In diabetes management as well as in diabetes prevention programs, community resources and supports are a factor to consider. This section looks at community resources and supports as they apply to each of the AADE 7 Self-Care Behaviors™. All 7 of the behaviors—Healthy Eating, Being Active, Monitoring, Taking Medication, Problem Solving, Healthy Coping, and Reducing Risks—may be addressed through interactions at the individual level, such as through clinical settings. Additionally, family and group interventions may work in support of many of these behaviors. Organizational and community settings can also promote these self-care behaviors. Table 6.3 provides examples of how these behaviors might be promoted in organizational- and community-level interventions.

Most of the AADE 7 Self-Care Behaviors™ reduce health risks for all individuals:

Five of the 7 self-care behaviors outlined by the AADE reflect healthy lifestyle behaviors that are appropriate for

TABLE 6.3 Organizational and Community Level Interventions for Self-Care Behaviors

AADE 7 Self-Care Behaviors™	*Organizational-Level Interventions*	*Community-Level Interventions*
Healthy Eating	Healthy food choices in workplaces, schools, and places of social gathering; reduced pricing for healthy vending machine options	Availability of affordable healthy foods in local food stores and from providers of ready-to-eat foods; nutrition labeling at points of food purchase, including restaurants; development of food policy councils
Being Active	Worksite polices that allow exercise on company time (eg, walk breaks; point-of- decision prompts for taking the stairs); adding and lengthening PE classes in schools	Improved sidewalks and lighting; community walking trails; improved access to community exercise facilities; focus on recreational activity
Monitoring Health Status	Worksite policies that provide breaks and suitable settings for monitoring blood sugar	Public education to increase awareness, destigmatize diabetes, and change social norms regarding chronic disease management; insurance policies that provide access to care
Taking Medication	Electronic pharmacy records; patient education at point of medication purchase	Prescription drug benefits that ensure access to needed medications
Problem Solving	Critical thinking skills in school curricula; worksite policies that encourage supervisors to be flexible in working out arrangements for employees' needs for self-management	Policies and readily available resources that encourage individuals to do what they need to do to take care of their diabetes (eg, directing family food choices toward healthy eating)
Healthy Coping	Human resource policies that are family-friendly, encourage employee input in policies, and minimize unnecessary strain or stress in the work situation; classes or programs for stress management skills; support groups; employee assistance programs	Community resources and supports for healthy coping and supportive relationships. Resources for adequate food, housing, and transportation. Access to classes and services that promote healthy coping skills; availability of counseling services for individuals and families
Reducing Risks	Organization-based screenings (eg, worksite, church, school), health education and health promotion programs	Policies, resources, and services that encourage healthy lifestyles for all individuals, not just those with identified diseases

all people in maximizing health and reducing risk of preventable diseases:

- Healthy Eating
- Being Active
- Problem Solving
- Healthy Coping
- Reducing Risks

Recognizing the pertinence of these AADE 7 Self-Care Behaviors™ for all adults, not just those with diabetes, can have 2 desired effects:

- Reducing the stigma individuals with diabetes face in pursuing these behavioral goals
- Expanding the base of individuals and groups calling for community resources to support them

Research on Community Resources and Supports for Diabetes Management

Community Resources and Supports Influential in Diabetes Management

Community Resources

- Stores selling healthy, affordable food
- Safe and attractive locations for physical activity and recreation
- Safe walking areas
- Organizational and community practices providing flexibility for those with diabetes to manage their disease (eg, monitoring blood glucose)
- Accessible places to obtain affordable medications and supplies, information about self-management, and assistance in implementing self-management plans

Ongoing Follow-Up and Support

- Continued assistance in refining problem-solving plans and skills
- Encouragement in the face of less-than-perfect performance and success
- Assistance in responding to new problems that may emerge
- Assistance that may entail linking patients back to primary care providers or other parts of the disease management team

The sidebar on community resources and supports offers examples of measures that can influence diabetes management. The evidence in support of using community resources and supports for diabetes management is discussed below.

The literature related to community resources and supports for diabetes management is not extensive. A review of literature from the years 1996 through 2005 found few published pieces on interventions for diabetes management that addressed community resources.[6] The same review found appreciable literature on interventions to provide ongoing follow-up and support, but much of this examined interventions administered not by peers or community-based health workers, but by nurses or other clinic-based staff (eg, phone follow-up programs).[96-100]

Community Resources

The research that exists on community resources in diabetes management includes community approaches to identifying and developing resources for physical activity and healthy eating[101-103] using pharmacists to provide self-management resources in individuals' daily circumstances,[104,105] and an individualized, multilevel intervention to provide support for maintenance of improvements brought about through a self-management program.[106] Additional studies have found that information resources and discussion groups available through the Internet are well accepted and used by those with type 2 diabetes.[107,108]

A popular and effective approach to providing follow-up and support is through community-based peers such as community health workers, who are also known as lay health educators, outreach workers, health coaches, or, in Spanish, as *promotores de salud.* The AADE position statement on diabetes community health workers describes them as "community members who work as bridges between their ethnic, cultural, or geographical communities and health-care providers to help their neighbors prevent diabetes and its complications through self-care management and social support, including community engagement."[109] Consistent with roles outlined in the position statement, the literature offers numerous examples of community health worker involvement in care teams and in providing individualized assessment, goal setting, and teaching skills as well as providing follow-up and support.[110-112] The Diabetes Initiative projects demonstrate the widespread use of community health workers in individualized, peer-based patient education, problem-solving, and ongoing support and encouragement in both clinic and community settings.

Support from community health workers:

Research indicates several characteristics of community health workers that may be especially beneficial, including the following:

- Easy access to these community members
- Limited constraints on the extent or focus of their service[113]
- Support that is nondirective (cooperating without taking control, accepting recipient's perspectives rather than prescribing correct courses of action)[114, 115] or enhances autonomy[116]

Surmounting Individuals' Reluctance

Individuals are not always eager to engage in programs that are intended to provide them with follow-up and support. Interest in receiving support may vary among individuals with diabetes. For example, lower levels of interest in supportive interventions were found among adults with diabetes who also smoke cigarettes than among those who do not smoke.[117] Some efforts to provide support receive very modest response from those they seek to help. In one study, only 41% of participants attended even one meeting of monthly support groups over a 3- to 12-month period following a 4-hour education program.[118]

Phone-Based Intervention. Given the reluctance of people to participate in some interventions designed to provide follow-up and support, the success of phone-based interventions for follow-up and support in diabetes is interesting to note.[96-100,119] Two features of such interventions are noteworthy:

- Convenience to the recipient
- Ability of the provider to deliver phone interventions without active attendance by the recipient

These suggest again the strategic importance of community-based support that can be convenient to individuals and require little effort on their part.

Interventions for Follow-Up and Support

Grantees of the Diabetes Initiative of the Robert Wood Johnson Foundation have identified key aspects of interventions that provide ongoing follow-up and support for diabetes management. In reviewing these, one should consider that psychological research has long recognized that the factors that lead to ongoing performance and maintenance may be very different than those that encourage initial learning.[120] Similarly, Prochaska's model of "stages of change"[121] holds that "maintenance strategies" are different than those for individuals in "action" stages of behavioral change (see chapter 3). In the Diabetes Initiative, the key aspects of maintenance strategies or approaches to ongoing follow-up and support are these:

- Based in an ongoing relationship with the source or provider
- Available on demand and as needed by the recipient
- Proactive through low-demand contact initiated by provider on a regular basis (eg, every 2 to 3 months)
- Motivational
- Not limited to diabetes (eg, can address a variety of concerns or challenges the recipient faces)
- Includes (*1*) monitoring the need for and (*2*) promoting appropriate access to other components of the Resources and Supports for Self-Management model (ie, individualized assessment, collaborative goal setting, enhancing skills, community resources, and continuity of quality clinical care).

Practice Models

Within the diabetes field, several programs have demonstrated models for engaging community and social resources.

Diabetes Today

The CDC's Division of Diabetes Translation developed the Diabetes Today program in 1992 to train state and local health departments on community-based diabetes prevention and control programs. Using a "train the trainer" format, state and local level public health workers provided training to community health advocates on planning, implementation, and evaluation of programs. Currently, the Diabetes Today program is implemented in both English and Spanish and over 1000 public health professionals have been trained.[122]

REACH 2010

In 1999, the CDC launched REACH 2010—Racial and Ethnic Approaches to Community Health—as its key strategy to address racial and ethnic disparities in health. REACH projects focus on 6 priority areas: cardiovascular disease, immunizations, breast and cervical cancer screening and management, diabetes, HIV/AIDS, and infant mortality. Ethnic groups targeted include African Americans, American Indians, Alaska Natives, Asian Americans, Hispanics, and Pacific Islanders.

The CDC's Web site, at www.cdc.gov/nccdphp/publications/aag/reach.htm, emphasizes the attention to coalitions and partnerships in the REACH 2010 program that ". . .supports community coalitions in designing, implementing, and evaluating community-driven strategies to eliminate health disparities. Each coalition comprises a community-based organization and three other organizations, of which at least one is either a local or state health department or a university or research organization."

More than a dozen REACH 2010 projects around the country are focusing on diabetes. In Detroit, Michigan, a community steering committee is working to reduce risk factors for type 2 diabetes and its complications among African American and Latino residents. Community residents were trained as Family Health Advocates to provide five 2-hour courses to increase knowledge and skills related to healthy eating, physical activity, and stress reduction for diabetes prevention and self-management. From pretest to posttest, behavioral changes were seen in various diet behaviors including improved food preparation techniques and increased consumption of fruits and vegetables and whole grain bread. A mean decrease of 0.8% was seen in A1C values among those who participated in the intervention. The REACH 2010 Detroit diabetes program successfully used a community committee and community health workers (Family Health Advocates) to reduce risk behaviors associated with diabetes and its complications.[123]

HEED

In 1999, the East Side Village Health Worker Project in Detroit identified diabetes as a priority, which gave birth to HEED (Healthy Eating and Exercising to Reduce Diabetes). The HEED project sought to reduce risks or delay onset of type 2 diabetes through in-depth education, increasing community resources for physical activity and healthy eating, addressing social and physical environmental characteristics that impact diabetes, and strengthening partnerships within the community. The HEED project trained 18 community residents on detailed information on diabetes, how healthy eating and physical activity prevent and help manage diabetes, nutrition label reading, recipe modification, and strategies for working within communities. As a result, the trained HEED advocates began a walking club for seniors, hosted numerous diabetes education activities for all age groups, held culturally appropriate cooking demonstrations, and performed community audits. The audits showed a lack of availability of high-quality produce. Through education on individual and social factors that impact diabetes, community residents learned to identify connections among health, environment, and social factors and identified intervention points, such as addressing a lack of available produce. This led to weekly "minimarkets" that were held at a local community center to increase access to quality produce.[22]

Project DIRECT

In North Carolina, Project DIRECT (Diabetes Interventions Reaching and Educating Communities Together) was the first and largest comprehensive community-based diabetes project in an African American community in the United States.[124] Initiated as a pilot project in 1993, Project DIRECT aimed to demonstrate and document the effectiveness of a model diabetes program for state and local health departments to reduce the burden of diabetes and its complications among communities of African Americans through a high level of community involvement and with culturally appropriate interventions. The project was supported primarily by funds from the CDC. An important distinction between Project DIRECT and other large-scale community-based studies, such as the cardiovascular diseases trials, is that DIRECT included all 3 levels of preventions: primary, secondary, and tertiary. Interventions were targeted in health promotion to improve diet and physical activity, outreach to improve case finding and awareness, and diabetes care to improve access and quality.[125] In addition to improvement in some health outcomes, the project offered many important lessons about the development of community partnerships as an approach to diabetes interventions.[126]

Diabetes Initiative of the Robert Wood Johnson Foundation

As noted earlier, the Diabetes Initiative of the Robert Wood Johnson Foundation was designed to demonstrate diabetes self-management programs that are feasible in real-world settings. Through 14 demonstration projects around the country, the Initiative examines ways to advance diabetes self-management in primary care settings and to improve the network of community supports for self-management. Six projects were selected to demonstrate that comprehensive models of diabetes self-management can be delivered in primary care settings and can significantly improve patient outcomes. Eight projects were chosen to build supports for diabetes management in communities in recognition that diabetes management takes place primarily in settings of individuals' daily lives. All sites chosen for the Initiative serve patient populations that are predominantly indigent, medically underserved, and/or from varied cultural and linguistic backgrounds.

The Diabetes Initiative projects have been especially resourceful in developing ways to address community resources and supports in their programs. Even in the individually focused services of primary care, the ecological perspective can be useful. For example, a primary care site in the Initiative has included in individuals' charts information about patients' proximity to stores selling healthy food and to places for safe physical activity. This is to facilitate counseling by providers that at a minimum is cognizant of the challenges individuals may face in gaining access to key resources. The sidebar on community supports and community resources describes other approaches taken by members of the Initiative.

Policy

Policy and environmental approaches are key to initiating and sustaining changes at multiple ecological levels that will in turn lead to improved health.[127] Policy initiatives can be relatively low cost, affect large numbers of people, and

Community Supports

Used by the Diabetes Initiative

- Extensive use of community health workers, or *promotores*, from the communities to be served in 9 of the 14 projects
- Incorporation of "talking circles" in American Indian sites to influence norms around health behaviors and diabetes management and to stimulate ongoing support through peer channels
- Participation in networks of social service providers to facilitate patients' access to basic needs and support services
- Inclusion of patients and program participants in planning programs and services to ensure a fit with their needs
- Cultivation and support of employees at worksites to encourage physical activity among peers

Community Resources

Used by the Diabetes Initiative

- Development of community- and peer-based services to provide information and guidance on walking as regular physical activity
- Facilitating community residents' requests to food stores to carry attractive, healthy, culturally appropriate foods
- Placement and promotion of diabetes educational materials in public libraries
- Improved access to community fitness facilities through clinic-community partnership involving referrals and incentives for physical activity
- Recipe contests with local restaurants to engage chefs and increase availability and enhance awareness of foods appropriate for people with diabetes
- Drop-in community location for "diabetes watchers" to assist with diabetes monitoring and weight management

create an environment supportive of future, more targeted interventions. For example, school-based education on healthy eating may follow changes in policies regarding food available in vending machines within schools.

Community resources and supports raise important questions that extend beyond immediate issues of costs and benefits and lead to consideration of policies. But policies also reflect a society's fundamental values and models of the roles of individuals, communities, governments, and organizations. Consider the issues surrounding access to resources for safe and healthy physical activity. Evidence is emerging that the availability of resources for routine, moderate physical activity (eg, walking paths) enhances individual health. Substantial policy issues are then raised regarding the responsibility of governments to provide such opportunities or to assure equal access to them. As wealthy communities are able to provide more of such resources for themselves, what is the responsibility of government to assure comparable resources for those in less wealthy or impoverished communities? More and more, healthcare is coming to be viewed as a fundamental right, one to be assured or guaranteed by government. In this context, expanding healthcare to include features such as community resources and supports raises substantial and complex issues of values, ethics, and policy.

Issues of Access. The importance of access to healthy and affordable food raises additional policy issues. As noted earlier, it is well documented that considerable disparities exist in access to food among different neighborhoods. One problem is that for families that are financially challenged, calories associated with foods of poor nutritional value are considerably less expensive than calories in healthy foods. Thus, for parents to keep their children from feeling hungry, economic constraints may drive purchase patterns toward foods of poor nutritional quality.

Issues of Business Values. A larger question is raised about the role of business organizations in American culture. A reportedly common response of supermarket chains to questions about healthy food in poor neighborhoods is that efforts to sell more healthy food in low-income neighborhoods meet with poor consumer response and, consequently, poor profits. This tends to be accepted as reasonable justification for the failure of supermarkets to provide attractive, healthy, and affordable produce evenly across their locations in a region. This line of reasoning reflects a more fundamental and widely held assumption that the primary responsibility of business management is to return a profit to the company's shareholders. This is widely accepted in the United States as almost intrinsically justified. However, one could argue that it is the responsibility of management and corporations to balance (1) the needs of shareholders for return on investment with (2) the needs of employees for healthy working conditions and a reasonable standard of living and (3) the needs of the broader community for goods and services that enhance rather than detract from quality of life and community well-being. One could argue, for example, that supermarkets should be required (1) to maintain outlets within all neighborhoods within regions in which they choose to be active and (2) to provide comparable food offerings in all their stores. Aside from its merits, such a suggested policy illustrates the kinds of values that lie beneath policies and practices in these areas, values that should be considered and appraised rather than merely assumed.

Food Policy Councils. Among innovative approaches to addressing food inadequacies and inequities is the formation of food policy councils. These were begun in Knoxville, Tennessee in 1982 by a man who questioned the lack of a governmental department to address food as a basic need since there were departments of housing, transportation, water, and so on. Following Knoxville's example, food policy councils have been formed in cities, states, and other countries.[128] They are comprised of community stakeholders from various segments of the food system. Their goal is to assess the operation of the food system—its cost, availability, accessibility—and develop improvements in food supply, distribution, public awareness, and public health.

The relationship between society and health and health inequities is obviously complex.[21] Glasgow argues for embracing this complexity to create movement toward innovative solutions.[129] Ruger suggests "an integrated and multifaceted approach to health improvement that involves multiple institutions making simultaneous progress on various fronts."[19(364)] For example, she proposes integrating "horizontal" and "vertical" public policy initiatives. Horizontal approaches in diabetes would include simultaneous and integrated approaches to diabetes prevention and control across the ecological levels. As discussed earlier, efforts to control tobacco use model this approach well.[130] Vertical approaches use "reinvented" community partnerships to link health and social policies so they will be mutually reinforcing. For example, communities could respond to the unavailability of healthy foods in neighborhoods by improving access to sources of healthy foods through enhanced public transportation and explicitly linking their marketing of those services to healthy food access.

Challenge of Influencing Community-Level Resources and Supports

For professionals or organizations that provide services to individual patients or clients, addressing community and social influences on diabetes management presents numerous challenges. Within their clinical roles, professionals are well placed to reach government agencies, worksites, community organizations or groups, or the social structures that surround their patients' or clients' lives. Also, many professionals are not trained in community organization or organization development skills. These are complex skills to which extensive training is devoted in graduate programs in social work, public health, and related areas. It may seem as though it is "common sense" to "get all the stakeholders together," but good sense in this area is not common and getting groups together with diverse agendas, priorities, resources, and constraints is difficult.[131]

In addition to challenges in the area of professional skills and training, current approaches to financing of health and social services also limit the ability of professionals and organizations to address community influences. For those dependent on reimbursement for delivery of direct services, taking time to develop collaborations and address community influences may be very difficult to justify and sustain. This illustrates again the principle of the ecological model that influences at several levels are interrelated. Policies regarding financing of services directly affect the ability of organizations and professionals to address the distal and environmental influences on their patients' and clients' behavior.

What Healthcare Professionals Can Do

In spite of the barriers to influencing social influences, community resources, or policies from the clinic or consulting room, healthcare professionals and healthcare organizations are important within communities and cultures. Their influence regarding policy issues can often be great. Influence may be expressed by acting as concerned citizens, lending expertise and prestige to advocacy efforts. It may also be expressed through collaborations with similar organizations to address community, state, or even national policies regarding health and social services and support for expanding the increased breadth of such services. Even at the level of working with individual patients or clients, considering the extent to which the individual's behavior is influenced by such community and social factors may increase the professional's empathy and rapport with his or her patient or client and, so, increase the effectiveness of services delivered.

Five ways health professionals may consider and address community resources and supports are described in the paragraphs that follow. In brief, these are to (*1*) heighten awareness, (*2*) expand the agenda of problem solving, (*3*) expand the scope of programs, (*4*) expand programs through partnerships, and (*5*) advocate.

Heighten Awareness. Healthcare professionals need to gain understanding of the many ways in which the social and environmental factors over which they may have no control will nevertheless have great influence on the behavior of their patients or clients. As noted above, this can make individual counseling more effective at least by enhancing understanding and, consequently, rapport between provider and patient. It can also help professionals increase the pertinence of their counseling to the realities of their patients' circumstances.

Expand Agenda of Problem Solving. A second way that consideration of community resources and supports may enhance professional services is by identifying topics important to address in implementing self-management plans. In addition to considering clients' commitment to specific goals or plans and their skills for achieving them, professionals need to consider their patients' and clients' opportunities and resources for executing plans and the barriers to their success. An example of this is the Diabetes Initiative project noted above that included in patients' files their proximity to resources for buying healthy food and getting physical activity. This should prompt attention to such availability by professionals. If the problem, for example, is an unsafe neighborhood in which to walk, counseling may not be able to solve the problem of where to walk in the neighborhood, but it may assist in identifying alternatives, such as exercise that clients can complete within their homes or efforts to identify other safe, attractive locations for exercise, such as at a mall.

Expand Scope of Programs. A third approach to addressing community resources and supports may be to expand the scope of programs themselves. Individual clinicians and educators can take advantage of opportunities to maximize the effects of their programs and services by linking them to trends or events or by coordinating with other efforts occurring simultaneously. For example, an educator may offer a class in a new community center so that participants also become aware of and familiar with the exercise facilities at the center.

Provider agencies may create linkages by increasing their involvement in the community. A community health center might facilitate organizing groups of neighborhood residents to walk together. Similarly, a health center might work with groups of its patients to request improvements in food available at community supermarkets. Recognizing the importance of community norms in supporting self-management efforts, the provider agency might increase its activity in community events, health fairs, presentations at local churches, and so on to raise awareness among all community residents of (*1*) the needs of those with diabetes and other chronic diseases and (*2*) the overlap between healthy lifestyles for those with diabetes and healthy lifestyles for all persons who are interested in long and satisfying lives.

Expand Programs Through Partnerships. Provider agencies may be ready and have the capacity to build referral networks or partnerships among healthcare and community agencies. The AADE's position paper "Diabetes Education and Public Health"[132] discusses the need for clinicians to work with public health and nontraditional partners in a holistic approach to diabetes prevention and control. The National Diabetes Education Program: A Diabetes Community Partnership Guide offers tips on selecting partners and suggestions for community activities. Information can be found at their Web site: http://betterdiabetescare.nih.gov/WHATcommunityexamples.htm.

The mechanisms for working together are vast and require time, commitment, and leadership. A number of terms—sometimes used interchangeably—describe working across organizations (eg, networks, collaboratives, partnerships, consortia, coalitions). This chapter uses "partnership" broadly to encompass the range of structures under which agencies combine resources and work together to effect changes they are unable to bring about individually.

There are levels of partnerships that require progressively greater resources, commitment, and involvement of partners.[133]

- *Exchange networks* that involve sharing information for mutual benefit require the least investment. Referrals would fall into this category.
- *Partner agencies*, at the next level, contribute or pool resources for a mutual goal. This requires joint planning and division of roles, so the investment and risk are greater.
- *Systemic networks* are the highest level of partnership, in which partners collaborate fully and create something new together—sharing the potential risks and rewards.

While it is beyond the scope of this chapter to delve into the nuances of the various types of partnerships, a number of lessons can be learned from those who have worked together successfully. See the sidebar on lessons in partnerships.

Advocate. Healthcare professionals can play important roles in advocating for changes in policies that influence community resources and supports. This should begin "at home," with examination of organizations' own worksite policies regarding how they support healthy choices. Professionals and organizations need to educate policy makers about evidence-based and promising practices. With sharpened recognition of the importance of policies in shaping the ways in which communities influence individual health and through local chapters and national activities of the AADE, American Diabetes Association, American Dietetic Association, or other

Lessons in Partnerships

- The partnership must have a clear purpose, a structure that supports its work, and the ability to bring diverse groups together.
- Partnerships develop over time. Highly effective, mature partnerships or networks are seamless and comprehensive. They are based on shared leadership, shared vision, participatory decision making, constructive conflict resolution, shared resources, trust, open communication, and good management.[131,134,135]
- Outcomes of partnerships can be evaluated from the perspective of patients, partnering organizations, and/or the community.

professional, health advocacy, public health, or political organizations, professionals can work for supportive community resources and policies for people with diabetes.

While clinicians and educators are certainly not responsible for the whole of social change, taking these steps and an ecological view of diabetes can enhance community resources and supports for diabetes prevention and management. The significance of this cannot be overstated. In the absence of changes in community policies and supportive environments, communities will continue to have more individuals with the conditions we are trying to prevent or control, thus taxing resources.

Finally, the ecological perspective also may help providers and educators avoid a common strategic error of many health promotion programs. This is the mis-

Questions and Controversy

How to extend diabetes care to address community resources and support is a major question that is being considered. Also, viewing diabetes for so long from a medical treatment perspective has limited the field's development of perspective that emphasize influences and interventions outside the clinic. Thus, along with increased research and knowledge, there is a need to expand perspectives. One aspect of this entails the roles of professionals. Today's professionals have been trained to provide direct services of a quality for which they can take responsibility and be held responsible. Expanding their activities to include community and social characteristics and forces over which they have little control and for which they cannot be responsible entails a major shift in their views of their roles. Such an extension of professional role may be uncomfortable for many and unacceptable for some.

A second area of challenge is establishing a knowledge base for community interventions. As outlined in this chapter, such a base exists in prevention programs, especially those that have addressed heart disease prevention.[30,31,49-60] A base for future programs also exists in some programs evaluating community approaches to diabetes and chronic disease management and in projects, such as those of the Diabetes Initiative, that demonstrate program approaches in real-world settings. Still, the knowledge base is modest relative to the documented importance of community resources and community support in lifestyle behaviors, self-management, and chronic disease management.

In addition to study of interventions addressing diabetes and other chronic diseases, research should address improved understanding of how the ecological levels and influences interact in shaping and guiding behavior and health. Although there is widespread support for the importance of community-based interventions and coalitions and partnerships in promoting health, there is insufficient articulation of what specific approaches to community organization may be most effective for what problems, in what settings, with what populations, and with what organizational resources and barriers at hand. Similarly, great interest attends social capital, community and neighborhood resources, social support, social networks, and related concepts. How these interact with each other, how they influence health, and how they may be recruited to improve health promotion programs, however, is not well understood.

Closely related to the challenge of a modest knowledge base are several methodological issues. One concerns measures of outcomes. Current outcome evaluation relies heavily on individual-level measures and indices. These have their place, but from the perspectives of populations and community-level influences, community- and population-level indicators are also important.[136] For example, given the solid documentation of the broad contributions of modest physical activity to prevention and management of diabetes and other diseases, documentation of increased use of community-based resources for physical activity should be taken as evidence of the value of community programs to promote such use, without requiring documentation of individual-level changes. This same case can be made, for example, regarding use of supermarket sales data to document the utility of programs promoting healthy food purchases. This is not to say that individual-level change is not important, but that community-focused programs would be well evaluated by documentation of community-level changes.

A second methodological issue concerns the choice of research designs and evaluation methods for studying community and social influences. Along with emphases on community approaches, community organization,[137] and community-based participatory research,[131] state-of-the-art evaluation approaches have evolved that combine diverse methods such as from educational evaluation, qualitative and participatory research, and evaluation of process improvements and systems change.[138] Within education, community psychology, social work, and many areas of public health, these approaches have become the state of the art for evaluation. However, they have not been embraced by many areas of health scholarship, including prestigious and general readership journals and grant-review policies of the National Institutes of Health.

A central barrier to promoting research on community and social resources and supports is the special status ascribed to the randomized, controlled trial (RCT) in health research. The RCT is widely acknowledged to be an extremely strong design for evaluating (*1*) discreet interventions, (*2*) the key ingredients of which are not dependent on their contexts. Investigative medications meet these 2 criteria quite well, but community interventions do not. Indeed, the assumption of randomized trials that effective components of interventions can be isolated from their contexts runs counter to the overriding emphasis of the ecological model on the importance of relations among different levels of context and influence. One can try to control community influences, such as mass media or volunteer support, but this may constrain or hamstring areas of influence that community programs need to maximize and document. Alternatively, one can try to isolate community programs from such community and social influences, but this may lead to evaluation of community programs stripped of some of their most powerful components, a strategy likely to underestimate substantially the true impact of such programs.[42, 45] Health research in these areas needs liberation from the hegemony or domination of the RCT and to recognize and promote the legitimacy of alternative evaluation models such as those noted above.

placed effort of responding to superficial manifestations of problems or symptoms rather than to more fundamental causes. For example, if working conditions are unfavorable to self-management behaviors for people with diabetes, stress management classes may be of limited use in improving the health of people in that work environment. With or without stress management classes, effort might also be spent meeting with human resources or general management to educate them about ways they could support health for people with diabetes in the work environment. If implemented and successful, these could result in reduced stress among workers, while at the same time creating an environment in which stress management classes would be most appropriate and effective.

Focus on Education: Pearls for Practice

Teaching Strategies

- **Value community resources, then educate others.** Community agencies and other resources such as recreational facilities, senior centers, libraries, and support groups can assist in reinforcing and facilitating behavior change and helping sustain individuals' self-management efforts.

- **Promote the community.** Integrate the ecological perspective as a vital part of every teaching event by recognizing community resources. Compile and hand out a list of community agencies and other resources that are available in the area. Partner with an agency to expand available services and advertise how to apply for or access the service.

- **Successful teaching tactics.** Include resources as its own topic in the curriculum. Emphasize to all instructors the use of newsletters, printed media, CDs, and DVDs of prepared content for participants to take home. This provides reinforcement of community information classes. To reinforce information, repeat clear and consistent messages about community resources and use phone or electronic follow-up for convenience.

Messages for Patients

- **Expand network of resources.** Recognize the importance of expanding knowledge and building skill. Consider a variety of options in the community in which to participate to learn and reinforce new information. Examples are using the library and computer to look up information, attending an education event in the community on a specific topic, participating in grocery store "classes" on shopping. Become a member of the American Diabetes Association to obtain the monthly magazine. Participate in community diabetes expositions, trade shows, and other local health events.

- **Promote community resource awareness.** Volunteer in local diabetes advocacy groups, such as the American Diabetes Association, Juvenile Diabetes Research Foundation, and local diabetes education programs. Contact local and national legislatures to advocate and promote the passing of diabetes-related bills. Contact local diabetes education program staff to seek additional education and update information annually. Participate in satisfaction surveys.

References

1. Norris SL, Engelgau MM, Narayan KM. Effectiveness of self-management training in type 2 diabetes: a systematic review of randomized controlled trials. Diabetes Care. 2001;24:561-87.
2. Norris SL, Engelgau MM, Narayan KM. Effectiveness of self-management education for adults with type 2 diabetes: a meta-analysis of the effect on glycemic control. Diabetes Care. 2002;25:1159-71.
3. Mullen PD, Green LW, Persinger GS. Clinical trials of patient education for chronic conditions: a comparative meta-analysis of intervention types. Prev Med. 1985;14:753-81.
4. Kottke TE, Battista RN, DeFriese GH. Attributes of successful smoking cessation interventions in medical practice: a meta-analysis of 39 controlled trials. JAMA. 1988;259:2882-9.
5. Fiore MC, Bailey WC, Cohen SJ, et al. Treating Tobacco Use and Dependence: Clinical Practice Guideline. Rockville, Md: US Department of Health and Human Services, Public Health Service; 2000.
6. Fisher EB, Brownson CA, O'Toole ML, Shetty G, Anwuri VV, Glasgow RE. Ecologic approaches to self-management: the case of diabetes. Am J Public Health. 2005;95(9):1523-35.
7. Institute of Medicine: Committee on Health and Behavior: Research Practice and Policy. Health and

Behavior: the Interplay of Biological, Behavioral, and Societal Influences. Washington, DC: National Academy Press; 2001.

8. Sallis JF, Owen N. Ecological models of health behavior. In: Health Behavior and Health Education: Theory, Research, and Practice, 3rd ed. Glanz K, Lewis FM, Rimer BK, eds. San Francisco, Calif: Jossey-Bass; 2002:462-84.

9. Zaza S, Briss PA, Harris KW, eds. The Guide to Community Preventive Services: What Works to Promote Health? New York: Oxford University Press; 2005.

10. McLeroy K, Bibeau D, Steckler A. An ecological perspective on health promotion programs. Health Educ Q. 1988;15:351-77.

11. Yoo S, Weed NE, Lempa ML, Mbondo M, Shada RE, Goodman RM. Collaborative community empowerment: an illustration of a six-step process. Health Promot Pract. 2004;5(3):256-65.

12. Green LW, Anderson C. Community health. St. Louis, Mo: CV Mosby; 1982.

13. Lalonde M. A New Perspective on the Health of Canadians. Ottawa: Health and Welfare Canada; 1974.

14. US Department of Health and Human Services. Healthy People 2000: National Health Promotion and Disease Prevention Objectives. Washington, DC; 1990. Publication No. 017-001-00474-0.

15. US Department of Health and Human Services. Healthy People 2010, 2nd ed. With Understanding and Improving Health and Objectives for Improving Health. 2 vols. Washington, DC; Nov 2000.

16. Matarazzo JD, Weiss SM, Herd JA, Miller NE, Weiss SM, eds. Behavioral Health : A Handbook of Health Enhancement and Disease Prevention. New York: Wiley; 1984.

17. Etzwiler DD. Diabetes management: the importance of patient education and participation. Postgrad Medi. 1986;80:67-72.

18. Amick III BJ, Levine S, Tarlov AR, Chapman Walsh D. Society and Health. New York: Oxford University Press; 1995.

19. Ruger JP. Ethics of the social determinants of health. Lancet. 2004;18(364):1092-7.

20. Wilkinson R, Marmot M. Social Determinants of Health: The Solid Facts, 2nd ed. Copenhagen, Denmark: World Health Organization; 2003.

21. Jack Jr L. Beyond lifestyle interventions in diabetes: a rationale for public and economic policies to intervene on social determinants of health. J Public Health Manage Pract. 2005;11(4):357-60.

22. Schulz AJ, Zenk S, Odoms-Young A, et al. Healthy eating and exercising to reduce diabetes: exploring the potential of social determinants of health frameworks within the context of community-based participatory diabetes prevention. Am J Public Health. 2005;95(4):645-51.

23. Smedley BD, Stith AY, Nelson AR, eds (Committee on Understanding and Eliminating Racial and Ethnic Disparities in Health Care). Unequal Treatment: Confronting Racial and Ethnic Disparities in Health Care. Washington, DC: National Academy Press; 2002.

24. Ashton J, Seymour H. The New Public Health. Philadelphia, Pa: Open University Press; 1988.

25. Ashton J, Grey P, Barnard K. Healthy Cities—WHO's new public health initiative. Health Promot. 1986;1:319-23.

26. Fortmann SP, Winkleby MA, Flora JA, Haskell WL, Taylor CB. Effect of long-term community health education on blood pressure and hypertension control: The Stanford Five-City Project. Am J Epidemiol. 1990;132(4):629-46.

27. Fortmann SP, Taylor CB, Flora JA, Jatulis DE. Changes in adult cigarette smoking prevalence after 5 years of community health education: The Stanford Five-City Project. Am J Epidemiol. 1993;137(1):82-96.

28. Luepker RV, Murray DM, Jacobs DR Jr, et al. Community education for cardiovascular disease prevention: risk factor changes in the Minnesota Heart Health Program. Am J Public Health. 1994;84(9):1383-93.

29. Carleton RA, Lasater TM, Assaf AR, Feldman HA, McKinlay S, Pawtucket Heart Health Program Writing Group. The Pawtucket Heart Health Program: community changes in cardiovascular risk factors and projected disease risk. Am J Public Health. 1995;85:777-85.

30. Puska P, Nissinen A, Tuomilehto J, et al. The community-based strategy to prevent coronary heart disease: conclusions from the ten years of the North Karelia Project. Ann Rev Public Health. 1985;6:147-93.

31. Vartiainen E, Puska P, Jousilahti P, et al. Twenty-year trends in coronary risk factors in North Karelia and in other areas of Finland. Int J Epidemiol. 1994;23:495-504.

32. Luostarinen T, Hakulinen T, Pukkala E. Cancer risk following a community-based programme to prevent cardiovascular diseases. Int J Epidemiol. 1995;24:1094-9.

33. Farquhar JW, Fortmann SP, Maccoby N, et al. The Stanford Five City Project: an overview. In: Behavioral Health: A Handbook of Health Enhancement and Disease Prevention. Matarazzo JD, Weiss SM, Herd JA, Miller NE, Weiss SM, eds. New York: Wiley; 1984.

34. Blackburn H, Luepker RV, Kline FG, et al. The Minnesota Heart Health Program: a research and demonstration project in cardiovascular disease prevention. In: Behavioral health: A Handbook of Health Enhancement and Disease Prevention. Matarazzo JD, Weiss SM, Herd JA, Miller NE, Weiss SM, eds. New York: Wiley; 1984.

35. Elder JP, McGraw SA, Abrams DB, et al. Organizational and community approaches to community-wide prevention of heart disease: the first two years of the Pawtucket Heart Health Program. Prev Med. 1986;15:107-17.

36. Lasater T, Abrams D, Artz L, et al. Lay volunteer delivery of a community-based cardiovascular risk factor change program: The Pawtucket Experiment. In: Behavioral Health: A Handbook of Health Enhancement and Disease Prevention. Matarazzo JD, Weiss SM, Herd JA, Miller NE, Weiss SM, eds. New York: Wiley; 1984.

37. Farquhar JW, Fortmann SP, Flora JA, et al. Effects of community-wide education on cardiovascular disease risk factors: The Stanford Five-City Project. JAMA. 1990;264:359-65.

38. Lando HA, Pechacek TF, Pirie PL, et al. Changes in adult cigarette smoking in the Minnesota Heart Health Program. Am J Public Health. 1995;85(2):201-8.

39. Young D, Haskell W, Taylor C, Fortmann S. Effect of community health education on physical activity knowledge, attitudes, and behavior. Am J Epidemiol. 1996;144:264-74.

40. Eaton C, Lapane K, Garber C, Gans K, Lasater T, Carleton R. Effects of a community-based intervention on physical activity: The Pawtucket Heart Health Program. Am J Public Health. 1999;89(11):1741-4.

41. Fisher EB, Brownson RC, Luke DA, Sumner WI, Heath AC. Cigarette smoking. In: Health Behavior Handbook, vol II. Raczynski J, Bradley L, Leviton L, eds. Washington, DC: American Psychological Association; 2004.

42. Susser M. The tribulation of trials: intervention in communities. Am J Public Health. 1995;85(2):156-8.

43. US Department of Health and Human Services. Reducing the Health Consequences of Smoking: 25 Years of Progress. A Report of the Surgeon General. Public Health Service. 1989; DHHS Publication No. (CDC) 89-8411.

44. Lenfant C, Roccella E. Trends in hypertension control in the United States. Chest. 1992;2(3):296-305.

45. Fisher EB, Jr. Editorial: the results of the COMMIT trial. Am J Public Health. 1995;85(2):159-60.

46. The COMMIT Research Group. Community Intervention Trial for Smoking Cessation (COMMIT): I. Cohort results from a four-year community intervention. Am J Public Health. 1995;85(2):183-92.

47. The COMMIT Research Group. Community Intervention Trial for Smoking Cessation (COMMIT): II. Changes in adult cigarette smoking prevalence. Am J Public Health. 1995;85(2):193-200.

48. Lichtenstein E, Hymowitz N, Nettekoven L. Community Intervention Trial for Smoking Cessation (COMMIT): adapting a standardized protocol for diverse settings. In: Interventions for Smokers: An International Perspective. Richmond R, ed. Baltimore, Md: Williams & Wilkins; 1994:259-91.

49. Puska P, Vartiainen E, Tuomilehto J, Salomaa V, Nissinen A. Changes in premature deaths in Finland: successful long-term prevention of cardiovascular diseases. Bull World Health Organ. 1998;76:419-25.

50. Brownson RC, Housemann RA, Brown DR, et al. Promoting physical activity in rural communities: walking trail access, use, and effects. Am J Prev Med. 2000;18:235-41.

51. Auslander WF, Haire-Joshu D, Houston C, Dreitzer D, Williams JH. The eat well, live well nutrition program—dietary changes in African American women by activation. Paper presented at: NIH Conference on Psychosocial Treatments; 1996; Bethesda, Md.

52. Haire-Joshu D, Brownson R, Schechtman K, Nanney S, Houston C, Auslander W. A community research partnership to improve the diet of African Americans. Am J Health Behav. 2001;25:140-6.

53. Haire-Joshu D, Nanney MS. Prevention of overweight and obesity in children: influences on the food environment. Diabetes Educ. 2002;28(3):415-23.

54. Perry CL, Lytle LA, Feldman H, et al. Effects of the Child and Adolescent Trial for Cardiovascular Health (CATCH) on fruit and vegetable intake. J Nutr Educ. 1998;30:354-60.

55. Fisher EB, Jr, Auslander WF, Munro JF, Arfken CL, Brownson RC, Owens NW. Neighbors For a Smoke Free North Side: evaluation of a community organization approach to promoting smoking cessation among African Americans. Am J Public Health. 1998;88(11):1658-63.

56. Secker-Walker RH, Flynn BS, Solomon LJ, et al. Helping women quit smoking: results of a community intervention program. Am J Public Health. 2000;90:940-6.

57. Brownson RC, Smith C, Pratt M, et al. Preventing cardiovascular disease through community-based risk reduction: The Bootheel Heart Health Project. Am J Public Health. 1996;86(2):206-13.

58. Campbell MK, Demark-Wahnefried W, Symons M, et al. Fruit and vegetable consumption and prevention of cancer: the Black Churches United for Better Health project. Am J Public Health. 1999;89:1390-6.

59. Campbell MK, Honess-Morreale L, Farrell D, Carbone E, Brasure M. A tailored multimedia nutrition education pilot program for low-income women receiving food assistance. Health Educ Res. 1999;14:257-67.

60. Havas S, Anliker J, Damron D, Langenberg P, Ballesteros M, Feldman R. Final results of the Maryland WIC 5-A-Day Promotion Program. Am J Public Health. 1998;88:1161-7.

61. Glanz K, Lankenau B, Foerster S, Temple S, Mullis R, Schmid T. Environmental and policy approaches to cardiovascular disease prevention through nutrition: opportunities for state and local action. Health Educ Q. 1995;22:512-27.

62. US Public Health Service. Smoking and Health: Report of Advisory Committee to the Surgeon General of the Public Health Service. US Department of Health, Education, and Welfare, Public Health Service, Center for Disease Control; 1964. PHS Pub. No. 1103.

63. Siegel M. The effectiveness of state-level tobacco control interventions: a review of program implementation and behavioral outcomes. Annu Rev Public Health. 2002;23:45-71.

64. Fichtenberg CM, Glantz SA. Association of the California Tobacco Control Program with declines in cigarette consumption and mortality from heart disease. N Engl J Med. 2000;343(24):1772-7.

65. Mokdad AH, Marks JS, Stroup DF, Gerberding JL. Actual causes of death in the United States, 2000. JAMA. 2004;291(10):1238-45.

66. Mokdad AH, Marks JS, Stroup DF, Gerberding JL. Correction: actual causes of death in the United States, 2000. JAMA. 2005;293(3):293-4.

67. Fisher EB, Walker EA, Bostrom A, Fischhoff B, Haire-Joshu D, Johnson S. Behavioral science research in the prevention of diabetes: status and opportunities. Diabetes Care. 2002;25:599-606.

68. Task Force on Community Preventive Services. Increasing Physical Activity: A Report on Recommendations of the Task Force on Community Preventive Services. MMWR Recommendations and Reports, 2001;Volume 50, Number RR-18. Morbidity and Mortality Weekly Reports Recommendations and Reports. Vol 50: Centers for Disease Control; 2001.

69. Agency for Healthcare Research and Policy. The Efficacy of Interventions to Modify Dietary Behavior Related to Cancer Risk. 2001. Evidence Report/Technology Assessment Number 25.

70. Wing RR, Goldstein MG, Acton KJ, et al. Behavioral science research in diabetes: lifestyle changes related to obesity, eating behavior, and physical activity. Diabetes Care. 2001;24(1):117-23.

71. Domel SB, Baranowski T, Davis H, et al. Development and evaluation of a school intervention to increase fruit and vegetable consumption among 4th and 5th grade students. J Nutr Educ. 1993;25:345-9.

72. Luepker RV, Perry CL, McKinlay SM, et al. Outcomes of a field trial to improve children's dietary patterns and physical activity: the Child and Adolescent Trial for Cardiovascular Health (CATCH). JAMA. 1996;275(10):768-76.

73. Perry CL, Bishop DB, Taylor G, et al. Changing fruit and vegetable consumption among children: the 5-a-Day Power Plus program in St. Paul, Minnesota. Am J Public Health. 1998;88:603-9.

74. Nader PR, Stone EJ, Lytle LA, et al. Three-year maintenance of improved diet and physical activity: the CATCH cohort. Child and Adolescent Trial for Cardiovascular Health. Arch Pediatr Adolesc Med. 1999;153:695-704.

75. Stone EJ, Osganian SK, McKinlay SM, Wu WC, Webber LS. Operational design and quality control in the CATCH multicenter trial. Prev Med. 1996;25:384-99.

76 Tilley BC, Glanz K, Kristal AR, et al. Nutrition intervention for high-risk auto workers: results of the Next Step Trial. Prev Med. 1999;28(3):284-92.

77. Sorensen G, Thompson B, Glanz K, et al. Work site-based cancer prevention: primary results from the Working Well Trial. Am J Public Health. 1996;86:939-47.

78. Sorensen G, Morris DM, Hunt MK, et al. Worksite nutrition intervention and employees' dietary habits: the Treatwell program. Am J Public Health. 1992;82:877-80.

79. Buller DB, Morrill C, Taren D, et al. Randomized trial testing the effect of peer education at increasing fruit and vegetable intake. J Nat Cancer Institute. 1999;91(17):1491-1500.

80. Ammerman A, Washington C, Jackson B, et al. The PRAISE! Project: a Church-based nutrition intervention designed for cultural appropriateness, sustainability, and diffusion. J Health Promot Pract. April 2002;3:286-301.

81. Peterson J, Atwood JR, Yates B. Key elements for church-based health promotion programs: outcome-based literature review. Public Health Nurs. 2002;19(6):401-11.

82. McNabb W, Quinn M, Kerver J, Cook S, Karrison T. The Pathways church-based weight loss program for urban African-American women at risk for diabetes. Diabetes Care. 1997;20:1518-23.

83. Yanek LR, Becker DM, Moy TF, Gittelsohn J, Matson-Koffman D. Project Joy: faith-based cardiovascular health promotion for African American women. Public Health Report. 2001;116 Suppl 1:68-81.

84. Fitzgibbon ML, Stolley MR, Avellone ME, Sugerman S, Chavez N. Involving parents in cancer risk reduction: a program for Hispanic American families. Health Psychol. 1996;15:413-22.

85. Havas S, Treiman K, Langenberg P, et al. Factors associated with fruit and vegetable consumption among women participating in WIC. J Am Diet Assoc. 1998;98(10):1141-8.

86. Auslander W, Haire-Joshu D, Williams JH, Houston C, Krebill H. The short-term impact of a health promotion program for African-American women. Res Soc Work Pract. 2000;10:78-97.

87. Knutsen SF, Knutsen R. The Tromso Survey: the Family Intervention study—the effect of intervention on some coronary risk factors and dietary habits, a 6-year follow-up. Prev Med. 1991;20:197-212.

88. Hartman TJ, McCarthy PR, Park RJ, Schuster E, Kushi LH. Results of a community-based low-literacy nutrition education program. J Community Health. 1997;22:325-41.

89 Rodgers AB, Kessler LG, Portnoy B, et al. 'Eat for Health': a supermarket intervention for nutrition and cancer risk reduction. Am J Public Health. 1994;84:72-6.

90. Cullen KW, Bartholomew LL, Parcel GS. Girl scouting: an effective channel for nutrition education. J Nutr Educ. 1997;29:86-91.

91. Huston SL, Evenson KR, Bors P, Gizlice Z. Neighborhood environment, access to places for activity, and leisure-time physical activity in a diverse North Carolina population. Am J Health Promot. 2003;18:58-69.

92. Ewing R, Schmid T, Killingsworth R, Zlot A, Raudenbush S. Relationship between urban sprawl and physical activity, obesity, and morbidity. Am J Health Promot. 2003;18:47-57.

93. Brownell KD, Horgen KB. Food Fight: The Inside Story of the Food Industry, America's Obesity Crisis, and What We Can Do About It. New York: McGraw-Hill; 2004.

94. Brownson RC, Hagood L, Lovegreen SL, et al. A multilevel ecological approach to promoting walking in rural communities. Prev Med. 2005;41(5-6):837-42.

95. Daniel M, Green LW, Marion SA, et al. Effectiveness of community-directed diabetes prevention and control in a rural Aboriginal population in British Columbia, Canada. Soc Sci Med. 1999;48:815-32.

96. Piette JD, McPhee SJ, Weinberger M, Mah CA, Kraemer FB. Use of automated telephone disease management calls in an ethnically diverse sample of low-income patients with diabetes. Diabetes Care. 1999;22:1302-9.

97. Piette JD, Weinberger M, Kraemer FB, McPhee SJ. Impact of automated calls with nurse follow-up on diabetes treatment outcomes in a Department of Veterans Affairs Health Care System: a randomized controlled trial. Diabetes Care. 2001;24:202-8.

98. Piette JD, Weinberger M, McPhee SJ. The effect of automated calls with telephone nurse follow-up on patient-centered outcomes of diabetes care: a randomized, controlled trial. Med Care. 2000;38:218-30.

99. Piette JD, Weinberger M, McPhee SJ, Mah CA, Kraemer FB, Crapo LM. Do automated calls with nurse follow-up improve self-care and glycemic control among vulnerable patients with diabetes? Am J Med. 2000;108:20-7.

100. Weinberger M, Kirkman MS, Samsa GP, et al. A nurse-coordinated intervention for primary care patients with non-insulin-dependent diabetes mellitus: impact on glycemic control and health-related quality of life. J Gen Intern Med. 1995;10:59-66.

101. Reid L, Hatch J, Parrish T. Commentary: the role of a historically black university and the black church in community-based health initiatives: the Project DIRECT experience. J Public Health Manage Pract. 2003;Nov(Suppl):S70-73.

102. Nasmith L, Cote B, Cox J, et al. The challenge of promoting integration: conceptualization, implementation, and assessment of a pilot care delivery model for patients with type 2 diabetes. Family Med. 2004;36:40-50.

103. Dillinger TL, Jett SC, Macri MJ, Grivetti LE. Feast or famine? supplemental food programs and their impacts on two American Indian communities in California. International J Food Sci Nutr. 1999;50:173-87.

104. Cranor CW, Bunting BA, Christensen DB. The Asheville Project: long-term clinical and economic outcomes in a community pharmacy diabetes care program. J Am Pharm Assoc. 2003;43:173-84.

105. Cranor CW, Christensen DB. The Asheville Project: short-term outcomes of a community pharmacy diabetes care program. J Am Pharm Assoc. 2003;43:149-59.

106. Toobert DJ, Strycker LA, Glasgow RE, Barrera M, Bagdade JD. Enhancing support for health behavior change among women at risk for heart disease: the Mediterranean Lifestyle Trial. Health Educ Res. 2002;17:574-85.

107. Goldberg HI, Ralston JD, Hirsch IB, Hoath JI, Ahmed KI. Using an internet comanagement module to improve the quality of chronic disease care. Joint Commission J Qual Safety. 2003;29:443-51.

108. Zrebiec JF, Jacobson AM. What attracts patients with diabetes to an internet support group? a 21-month longitudinal website study. Diabetic Med. 2001;18:154-8.

109. American Association of Diabetes Educators. Diabetes Community Health Workers (position statement). Diabetes Educ. 2003;29(5):818-24.

110. Swider SM. Outcome effectiveness of community health workers: an integrative literature review. Public Health Nurs. 2002;19:11-20.

111. Corkery E, Palmer C, Foley ME, Schechter CB, Frisher L, Roman SH. Effect of a bicultural community health worker on completion of diabetes education in a Hispanic population. Diabetes Care. 1997;20:254-7.

112. Zuvekas A, Nolan L, Tumaylle C, Griffin L. Impact of community health workers on access, use of services, and patient knowledge and behavior. J Ambu Care Manage. 1999;22:33-44.

113. Fisher EB. A behavioral-economic perspective on the influence of social support on cigarette smoking. In: Advances in Behavioral Economics, vol 3. Green L, Kagel JH, eds. Norwood, NJ: Ablex; 1996:207-36.

114. Fisher EB Jr, La Greca AM, Greco P, Arfken C, Schneiderman N. Directive and nondirective support in diabetes management. Int J Behav Med. 1997;4:131-44.

115. Fisher EB, Todora H, Heins J. Social support in nutrition counseling. On the Cutting Edge: Diabetes Care and Education. 2003;24(4):18-20.

116. Williams GC, Rodin GC, Ryan RM, Grolnick WS, Deci EL. Autonomous regulation and long-term medication adherence in adult outpatients. Health Psychol. 1998;17:269-76.

117. Solberg LI, Desai JR, O'Connor PJ, Bishop DB, Devlin HM. Diabetic patients who smoke: are they different? Annals Fam Med. 2004;2:26-32.

118. Banister NA, Jastrow ST, Hodges V, Loop R, Gillham MB. Diabetes self-management training program in a community clinic improves patient outcomes at modest cost. J Am Diet Assoc. 2004;104:807-10.

119. Kim HS, Oh JA. Adherence to diabetes control recommendations: impact of nurse telephone calls. J Advanced Nurs. 2003;44:256-61.

120. Rachlin H. Introduction to Modern Behaviorism, vol 3. San Francisco, Calif: Freeman; 1991.

121. Prochaska JO, Redding CA, Evers KE. The Transtheoretical Model and Stages of Change. In: Health Behavior and Health Education: Theory, Research, and Practice, 3rd ed. Glanz K, Lewis FM, Rimer B, eds. San Francisco, Calif: Jossey-Bass/Pfeiffer; 2002:99-120.

122. Damond M, Winters A, Jack LJ, Cropper D, Londono M, Stoddard R. Mobilizing communities: local applications of the Diabetes Today National

Training Center Project. J Public Health Manage Pract. 2003;9(6S):S15-18.

123. Two Feathers J, Kieffer EC, Palmisano G, et al. Racial and Ethnic Approaches to Community Health (REACH) Detroit partnership: improving diabetes-related outcomes among African American and Latino adults. Am J Public Health. 2005;95(9):1552-60.

124. Project DIRECT Management Plan. Raleigh, NC: North Carolina Department of Health and Human Services; May 2001.

125. Engelgau MM, Narayan KMV, Geiss LS, et al. A project to reduce the burden of diabetes in the African-American community: Project DIRECT. J Nat Med Assoc. Mar 1998;90(10):605-13.

126. Goodman RM, Liburd LC, Green-Phillips A. The formation of a complex community program for diabetes control: lessons learned from a case study of Project DIRECT. J Public Health Manage Pract. May 2001;7(3):19-29.

127. Economos CD, Brownson RC, DeAngelis MA, et al. What lessons have been learned from other attempts to guide social change? Nutr Rev. Mar 2001;59(3 Pt 2):S40-56.

128. Webb K, Hawe P, Noort M. Collaborative intersectoral approaches to nutrition in a community on the urban fringe. Health Educ Behav. 2001;28(3):306-19.

129. Glasgow RE, Lichtenstein E, Marcus AC. Why don't we see more translation of health promotion research to practice? rethinking the efficacy-to-effectiveness transition. Am J Public Health. Aug 2003;93(8):1261-7.

130. Yach D, McKee M, Lopez AD, Novotny T. Improving diet and physical activity: 12 lessons from controlling tobacco smoking. BMJ. 2005;330(7496):898-900.

131. Israel BA, Eng E, Schulz AJ, Parker EA, eds. Methods in Community-Based Participatory Research for Health. San Francisco, Calif: Jossey-Bass; 2005.

132. American Association of Diabetes Educators. Diabetes education and public health. Diabetes Educ. 2000;26:607-9.

133. Alter C, Hage J. Organizations Working Together. Thousand Oaks, Calif: Sage Publishers; 1993.

134. Mizrahi T, Rosenthal BB. Complexities of coalition building: leaders' successes, strategies, struggles, and solutions. Soc Work. 2001;46(1):63-78.

135. Sofaer S. Working Together, Moving Ahead: A Manual for Effective Community Health Coalitions. New York: School of Public Affairs, Baruch College, City University of New York; 1999.

136. Leventhal H, Safer MA, Cleary PD, Gutmann M. Cardiovascular risk modification by community-based programs for life-style change: comments on the Stanford study. J Consult Clin Psychol. 1980;48(2):150-8.

137. Minkler M, ed. Community Organizing and Community Building for Health, 2nd ed. New Brunswick, NJ: Rutgers University Press; 2005.

138. Moen RD, Nolan TW, Provost LP, eds. Quality Improvement Through Planned Experimentation. New York: McGraw-Hill; 1999.

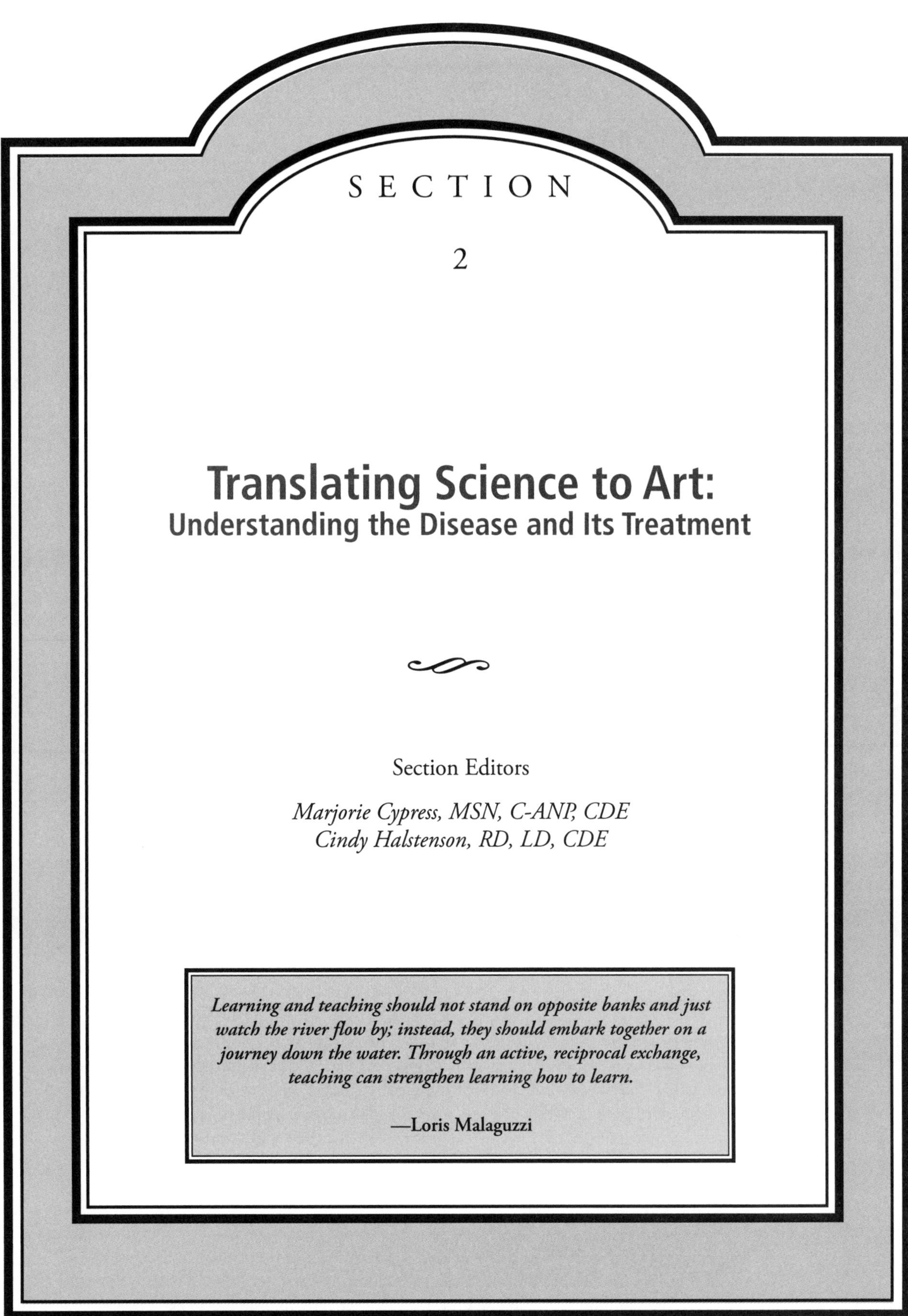

SECTION

2

Translating Science to Art:
Understanding the Disease and Its Treatment

Section Editors

Marjorie Cypress, MSN, C-ANP, CDE
Cindy Halstenson, RD, LD, CDE

> *Learning and teaching should not stand on opposite banks and just watch the river flow by; instead, they should embark together on a journey down the water. Through an active, reciprocal exchange, teaching can strengthen learning how to learn.*
>
> —Loris Malaguzzi

SECTION 2 OVERVIEW

Marjorie Cypress, MSN, C-ANP, CDE
Cindy Halstenson, RD, LD, CDE

Learning and teaching should not stand on opposite banks and just watch the river flow by; instead, they should embark together on a journey down the water. Through an active, reciprocal exchange, teaching can strengthen learning how to learn.

—Loris Malaguzzi[1]

Like other health professionals on the diabetes care team, diabetes educators are expected to have a foundation of medical knowledge. This core of knowledge encompasses a current understanding of the science of diabetes, its treatment options, and diabetes-related complications. There is a notable difference in the way educators use this information, in comparison to others on the team: the educator must not only understand the science and apply it in decision making, but also must translate medical concepts and information into messages that can contribute to effective diabetes self-management education (DSME).

Levels of learning

As healthcare professionals, we develop our expertise in stages, moving from concrete facts to abstract thinking. Competency requires both knowledge and experience and takes time to acquire. Bloom[2] defines levels of abstraction that include knowledge, comprehension, application, analysis, synthesis, and evaluation. Learning skills progress from knowledge based on simple recall to comprehension, when knowledge is interpreted and translated into a new situation or context, to the application of information, concepts, and theories. Analysis involves the ability to organize and recognize patterns, and synthesis is the ability to relate a body of knowledge into predictions and conclusions. Finally, evaluation is demonstrated by the ability to assess, discriminate between ideas, and verify the value of theories and evidence.

The chapters in this section show how learning progresses, how information is organized and integrated into problem-solving strategies. While we may recognize this progression in ourselves, we need to appreciate our patients' need to apply new and sometimes intricate knowledge in new situations and the challenge they face in applying information as they strive to become competent in self-management. Bloom's taxonomy provides us with direction in DSME, but also reminds us how complex this new knowledge can be—both to us and to our patients.

From medicine to messages

For the diabetes educator, the focus in this information-rich section of the *Desk Reference* is on understanding and using medical information to promote behavior change and self-management. Thus, rather than follow the framework of the medical model in presenting this information, these chapters emphasize how this body of scientific and medical knowledge is integrated into the educator's practice setting. The chapters are approached as one may approach a patient: taking an initial history, drawing on knowledge to probe for more information, making a diagnosis, developing a plan of care, and evaluating.

In dealing with the constant changes of a chronic progressive disease, the diabetes educator is further challenged to continually modify and adapt self-management education. Case studies are used in many of the chapters. These help elucidate the experience of the individual living with the disease and draw out important points for diabetes education. The cases follow a patient through descriptions of the symptoms, physiology, and treatment options and, finally, to explore how the healthcare team member can use his or her own experience and knowledge to help the individual affected by the disease.

As healthcare professionals, we learn about disease by studying the basic science and medical concepts and reading the published literature. As knowledge advances, we must stay current with the literature and evolution of the practice. Using evidence-based practice, we synthesize the scientific evidence to improve the quality and effectiveness of health care[3] and DSME. The science of medicine is transformed into the art of diabetes education when the educator is able to appropriately incorporate and translate medical concepts into assessments, plans, interventions, and interactions.

Diabetes care is a multidisciplinary and interdisciplinary challenge. Physicians, nurses, dietitians, pharmacists, behaviorists, and exercise physiologists contribute their expertise, working in teams to provide comprehensive care. The interdisciplinary approach is clearly evident in this section of the book; chapter authors incorporate knowledge from the various health specialties, but frame it in the context of diabetes education. Material is organized into 3 content areas: the disease itself, its therapies and management, and chronic complications. Chapters within each topic area review and summarize current knowledge and relate to points relevant for diabetes education.

First, we review the pathophysiology of diabetes. True to the book's focus, the authors of chapters 7 through 12 detail how the disease presents in individuals. Diabetes and hyperglycemia are described as they present in youths, teenagers, young adults, pregnancy, adulthood, and later adulthood. Patients often ask why certain things are happening to their bodies, and these chapters provide a lot of answers. Understanding the pathophysiology enables the educator to not only interpret the signs and symptoms being experienced, but also to be proactive in the approach to self-management education.

The next 7 chapters focus on therapies and disease management. The heart of diabetes self-management is integrating food, activity, frequent monitoring, and medications into a daily regimen. Chapters 13 through 19 summarize important technical knowledge pertinent to these self-management issues: medical nutrition therapy, physical activity, pharmacologic therapies for glucose management, pattern management, intensifying insulin therapy, pharmacologic therapies for hypertension and dyslipidemia, and complementary therapies. In each chapter, the science is presented, the research is discussed, and implications for diabetes education are highlighted. Chapters elucidate why certain treatments are used, how this translates to the individual with diabetes, and how individuals choose to manage their disease. Since comorbid conditions often affect the individual with diabetes, other chronic illnesses, specifically hypertension and dyslipidemia, are included. Finally, with the current interest and research into alternatives to Western medicine, and efforts to blend it with other approaches, the chapter on complementary therapies provides information important to the healthcare professional working in DSME. Whether health professionals use or recommend these therapies is not as relevant in diabetes education as being aware of the alternative remedies people may be using and how those therapies interact with recommended or prescribed treatments.

Diabetes-related complications are addressed at length in chapters 20 through 24. We begin with a chapter of overview on the various physical and psychological systems affecting the individual with diabetes. Issues of macrovascular disease, eye disease, diabetic kidney disease, and neuropathy are then dealt with in individual chapters. Current information on the etiology of chronic complications is presented, and strategies for primary, secondary, and tertiary prevention are highlighted. The case study approach helps show how specific conditions can affect an individual and progress in an individual; the cases consider current treatments and what is recommended.

The challenge to change

As the profession of diabetes education continues to move from a content-driven method of teaching to an approach that is individualized and outcome centered, practitioners are urged to recognize that their own methods of learning must change as well. Personal philosophies and experiences, moral and ethical positions, understanding and knowledge about science and behavior change—all of these color and enrich the patient-provider interaction. The unique work of diabetes education, and its ultimate goal of positively affecting the person with diabetes, involves taking evolving diabetes knowledge and applying it to individuals and populations.

Competence in the science, theory, and research is an underpinning of diabetes education. With this grounding, those responsible for DSME begin the art of their work: using their talents, personalities, and gifts in a therapeutic manner and integrating personal meanings and values into meaningful interactions with patients and clients.[4,5] Readers are challenged to recognize how they and their patients learn so they can best apply the complex medical information in the delivery of DSME. The diabetes educator's success in translating, explaining, and interpreting difficult information enables those with diabetes to become experts in their own care.

References

1. Loris Malaguzzi (1920–1994), Italian early childhood education specialist. Quoted in The Hundred Languages of Children: the Reggio Emilia approach to early childhood education, chapter 3, by Edwards CP, Gandini L, Forman GE. Norwood, NJ: Ablex Publishing Corp;1993.
2. Bloom BS. Taxonomy of Educational Objectives. Boston, Mass: Allyn and Bacon; 1984.
3. Evidence-based practice center overview. Agency for Healthcare Research and Quality. Rockville, Md; Feb 2005. Available on the Internet at: www.ahrq.gov/clinic/epc. Accessed 16 Mar 2006.
4. Carper BA. Fundamental patterns of knowing in nursing. In: Perspectives on Philosophy of Science in Nursing: An Historical and Contemporary Anthology. Polifroni EC, Welch M, eds. Philadelphia, Pa: Lippincott; 1999:12-19
5. Chinn PL, Kramer ML. Integrated Knowledge Development in Nursing. St. Louis, Mo: Mosby; 2004.

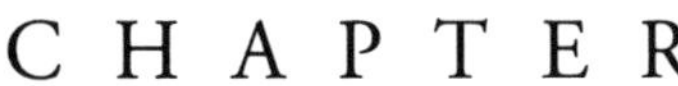

CHAPTER

7

Pathophysiology of the Metabolic Disorder

Authors

Joan K. Bardsley, RN, MBA, CDE
Robert E. Ratner, MD, FACP, FACE

Key Concepts

- Diabetes is a disease characterized by abnormal metabolism of carbohydrates, proteins, and fats. Understanding normal fuel metabolism and its hormonal control is important in appreciating the abnormalities that occur in diabetes.
- Newly discovered hormones and systems that regulate energy balance have increased understanding of normal physiology and the pathophysiology of diabetes. This has resulted in improved treatment modalities for diabetes.
- An estimated 7% of the US population has diabetes. The disease is more prevalent among Hispanics, Native Americans, African Americans, and Pacific Islanders.
- Arbitrary glycemic limits are used to diagnose prediabetes and diabetes. Frequently, diabetes is suspected on the basis of acute symptoms, including frequent urination and excessive thirst and hunger. Many practitioners prefer the fasting plasma glucose (FPG) for diagnosing diabetes, while others prefer the oral glucose tolerance test (OGTT). The 2006 ADA Standards of Medical Care indicate that either the 1-step OGTT or the 2-step FPG method can be used.
- Type 1 diabetes results from autoimmune beta-cell destruction, leading to absolute insulin deficiency. Type 1 diabetes is characterized by the abrupt onset of clinical signs and symptoms associated with marked hyperglycemia and a strong propensity for ketoacidosis.
- Type 2 diabetes is a multihormonal pathophysiology involving a progressive insulin secretory defect along with insulin resistance. This disease progresses from an early asymptomatic state with insulin resistance, to mild postprandial hyperglycemia, to clinical diabetes requiring pharmacologic intervention. Obesity, weight gain in adulthood, and physical inactivity are environmental factors affecting the progression at all points along the continuum.
- Diabetes includes 4 clinical classes: type 1 diabetes, type 2 diabetes, gestational diabetes, and other specific types of diabetes (eg, caused by genetic defects in beta-cell function or insulin action, diseases of the exocrine pancreas, or drugs).

State of the Problem

Diabetes is a chronic, progressive metabolic disorder characterized by abnormalities in the ability to metabolize carbohydrate, fat, and protein, leading to a hyperglycemic state. This chronic metabolic dysregulation is associated with long-term damage to various organs, including the eyes, kidneys, nerves, heart, and blood vessels.

Diabetes has become an epidemic in the United States, with 21 million people (7% of the population) affected by the disorder.[1] Nearly one-third are unaware they have the disease.[2] Although plasma glucose levels are controlled within a narrow range in individuals without diabetes, slow decompensation of the system results in a progressive increase in fasting and postchallenge glucose levels. International bodies have determined categorical cutoffs in glucose levels to define diabetes. These cutoffs correlate with the epidemiologic risk of developing microvascular complications, particularly retinopathy specific to diabetes. However, vascular problems may pose a threat to individuals even at glycemic levels that do not approach the diagnostic definition of diabetes; these levels are termed prediabetes. **Prediabetes** can be defined in terms of impaired glucose tolerance (IGT) or impaired fasting glucose (IFG), depending on which diagnostic test is used.

Although hyperglycemia plays a role in the complications of diabetes (which are caused by abnormalities in the structure and function of blood vessels and nerves), other pathological processes and additional risk factors are major, and sometimes independent, factors. The diabetes educator is encouraged to consider the pathophysiology of diabetes not only as a problem of carbohydrate metabolism, but also as abnormalities in fat metabolism, feeding behavior, and vascular biology.

Although improvements in technology and scientific knowledge are providing more tools to help people with diabetes, the diabetes educator must nonetheless recognize that diabetes is primarily a self-managed disease. The person with diabetes owns the responsibility of making the daily decisions that may affect the disease consequences. Healthcare professionals are challenged to understand the impact self-management has on the outcome of disease management. The AADE focuses on self-care as an outcome of diabetes self-management education (DSME). Seven core, evidence-based self-care behaviors— known as the AADE 7 Self-Care Behaviors™—are described as having an impact on diabetes management.[3] As understanding of the disease entity increases, health professionals must use this information to support clients in making their self-care behavior decisions.

A glossary of key terms related to pathophysiology appears at the end of this chapter

Normal Fuel Metabolism

To understand the abnormalities in fuel metabolism characterized by diabetes, a basic understanding of normal fuel metabolism is needed. The sidebar describes the 5 phases of fuel homeostasis described by Chipkin et al.[4]

The concentration of plasma glucose depends on the rate at which the glucose enters and the rate at which it is removed from the circulation. In adults without diabetes, the fasting plasma glucose concentration remains within a narrow range (70 to 100 mg/dL). This occurs because glucose appearance, which under fasting conditions is largely the rate of glucose output from the liver (endogenous glucose), and glucose disposal, which reflects the rate at which

Fuel Homeostasis: 5 Phases

Phase I is the fed state (0 to 3.9 hours after eating), in which circulating glucose predominantly comes from an exogenous source. Plasma insulin levels are high, **glucagon** levels are low, and triglycerides are synthesized in liver and adipose tissue. Insulin inhibits breakdown of **glycogen** and triglyceride reservoirs. The brain and other organs use some of the glucose that has been absorbed from the gastrointestinal tract, with the remaining excess glucose stored in hepatic, muscle, adipose, and other tissue reservoirs.

Phase II is the postabsorptive state (4 to 15.9 hours after food consumption), in which blood glucose originates from glycogen breakdown and hepatic **gluconeogenesis**. Plasma insulin levels decrease and glucagon levels begin to increase. Energy storage (anabolism) ends in this phase and energy production (catabolism) begins. Carbohydrate and lipid stores are mobilized. Hepatic glycogen breakdown provides maintenance of plasma glucose and ensures an adequate supply of glucose to the brain and other tissues. **Adipocyte** triglyceride begins to break down and free fatty acids (FFA) are released into the circulation and used by the liver and skeletal muscle as a primary energy source and as a **substrate** for gluconeogenesis. The brain continues to use glucose, provided mainly by gluconeogenesis (35% to 60%), because of its inability to use FFA as fuel.

Phase III is the early starvation state (16 to 47.9 hours after food consumption), in which blood glucose originates from hepatic gluconeogenesis and **glycogenolysis**. Gluconeogenesis continues to produce most of the hepatic glucose. In this phase of starvation, **lactate** makes up half of the gluconeogenic substrate. Amino acids, specifically alanine, and glycerol are other major substrates. Insulin secretion is markedly suppressed, and counterregulatory hormone (eg, glucagon, cortisol, growth hormone, and epinephrine) secretion is stimulated.

Phase IV is the preliminary prolonged starvation state (48 hours to 23.9 days after food consumption), in which blood glucose originates from hepatic and renal gluconeogenesis. By 60 hours of starvation, gluconeogenesis provides more than 97% of hepatic glucose output. Insulin secretion is markedly suppressed, and counterregulatory hormone (eg, glucagon, cortisol, growth hormone, and epinephrine) secretion is stimulated.

Phase V is the secondary prolonged starvation state (24 to 40 days after food consumption), in which blood glucose originates from hepatic and renal gluconeogenesis, the same source as in Phase IV. In Phase V, the rate of glucose being used by the brain diminishes, as does the rate of hepatic gluconeogenesis.

glucose is taken up by peripheral tissues, are well matched. Ingestion of a meal containing carbohydrates (exogenous glucose) increases circulating glucose dramatically because the gastrointestinal tract becomes a second source of glucose entering the circulation.[5]

The Role of Hormones

Pancreatic (glucoregulatory) hormones:

- Insulin
- Amylin

In adults without diabetes, the sudden increase in exogenous glucose stimulates the pancreatic beta cells, which respond by exocytosis of secretary granules.[5] These granules contain 2 glucoregulatory peptide hormones, insulin and the recently discovered **amylin**, which are released into the portal vein and then appear in the systemic circulation; their release into the bloodstream limits an abnormal rise in glucose concentration.[6] The hormones insulin and amylin act together to coordinate the rate of glucose appearance and disappearance in the circulation.[5]

Insulin

Insulin controls postprandial glucose via 2 mechanisms:

- Insulin stimulates the uptake of glucose into insulin-sensitive peripheral tissues.
- Insulin inhibits hepatic glucose output and inhibits glucagon secretion from the pancreatic beta cells.[5]

Amylin

The discovery of amylin has contributed to the understanding of postprandial glucose homeostasis.[7,8] Amylin, a 37–amino acid polypeptide hormone, is secreted from the pancreatic beta cells, along with insulin, in response to nutrient stimuli.[9] Amylin may complement the effects of insulin in postprandial glucose control via 3 mechanisms.[5]

- Amylin suppresses postprandial glucagon secretion;[10] thus, glucagon-stimulated hepatic glucose output is reduced during the postprandial period.
- Amylin regulates the rate of gastric emptying from the stomach to the small intestine.[11]
- Amylin also may suppress appetite.[5,12]

Incretin (intestinal) hormones:

- Glucose-dependent insulin-releasing polypeptide (GIP)
- Glucagon-like peptide-1 (GLP-1)

In addition to a better understanding of pancreatic hormones, recent advances have furthered understanding of the role of incretin hormones in normal physiology. Incretin hormones are intestinal hormones, which are released in response to food intake, and potentiate the glucose-induced insulin response.[13] The 2 peptide hormones primarily responsible for this incretin effect are GIP and GLP-1.

Glucose-Dependent Insulin-Releasing Polypeptide

GIP is secreted by K cells from the upper small intestine.[13] GIP, along with GLP-1, is released following a meal; together, these hormones act on the beta cells to increase their sensitivity to glucose, although they do not stimulate insulin secretion by themselves.[14]

Glucagon-Like Peptide-1

GLP-1 is predominantly produced in the enteroendocrine L cells located in the distal intestine.[13] As noted above, it is released after a meal and works with GIP to increase the beta cells' sensitivity to glucose. GLP-1 appears to be the major mediator of the incretin effect in humans. GLP-1 potentiates the glucose-stimulated insulin secretion following a carbohydrate meal. The incretin effect is seen in comparisons of insulin secretion after an oral glucose tolerance test versus an intravenous glucose tolerance test in nondiabetic volunteers. A significantly greater insulin response occurs after the oral test, despite identical glucose stimuli (see Figure 7.1).[15] GLP-1 accounts for 70% to 80% of the endogenous incretin effect.[15]

In addition to its effects on insulin secretion, GLP-1 exerts other significant actions to modulate intermediary metabolism, including stimulation of insulin biosynthesis, inhibition of glucagon secretion and gastric emptying, reduced food intake, and trophic effects on the pancreatic islet cells.[15]

GIP and GLP-1 both are rapidly degraded into inactive metabolites by the enzyme dipeptidyl-peptidase-IV (DPP-IV),[13] which is produced by endothelial cells and circulates in the plasma.[16] DPP-IV is a key regulator of incretin hormones.[17,18]

Other Hormones and Factors Affecting Fuel Metabolism

- Peptide-YY
- Endocannabinoid system

Peptide-YY. The hormone peptide-YY (PYY) is a 36–amino acid peptide secreted from the L cells of the gastrointestinal tract postprandially in proportion to the calorie content of the meal. The gut hormone peptide $YY_{3\text{-}36}$ (PYY) reduces food intake via hypothalamic Y2 receptors in the brain. Preliminary data show that infusion of postprandial concentrations of $PYY_{3\text{-}36}$ significantly decreases food intake at a buffet meal.[19,20] Its site of action is the

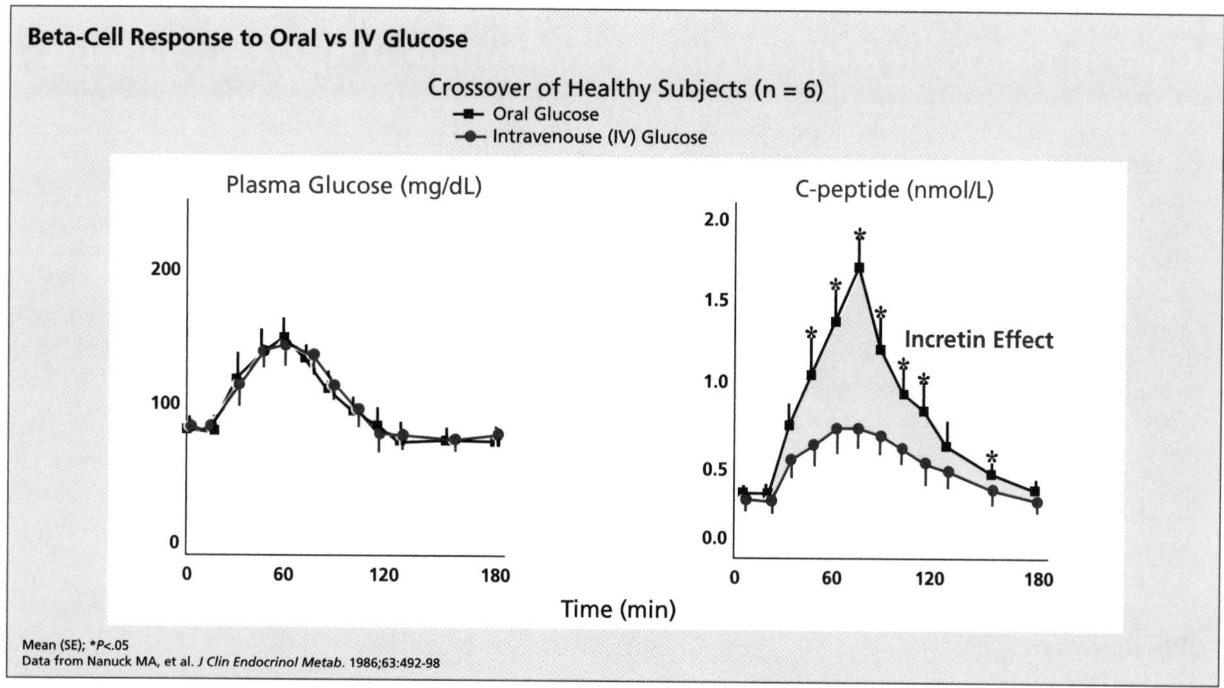

FIGURE 7.1 The Incretin Effect

arcuate nucleus of the hypothalamus, an area known to be involved in regulating food intake.[19]

Endocannabinoid System. The newly discovered endocannabinoid system further contributes to the physiological regulation of energy balance, food intake, and lipid and glucose metabolism through both central and peripheral effects.[21-24] This system consists of endogenous ligands and 2 types of G-protein-coupled cannabinoid receptors: CB_1 (which is located in several brain areas and in various peripheral tissues including adipose tissue, the gastrointestinal tract, the pituitary and adrenal glands, sympathetic ganglia, heart, lung, liver, and urinary bladder)[21, 25,26] and CB_2 (in the immune system).[27]

Activation of the central endocannabinoid system increases food intake and promotes weight gain.[28] The observation that endocannabinoid activation is not reversible with a 5% weight loss may suggest that this activation is a cause rather than a consequence of obesity. The endocannabinoid system is overactivated in response to exogenous stimuli, such as excessive food intake,[29] leading experts to believe that overeating promotes more overeating.

Insights into the endocannabinoid system have been derived from studies in animals with genetic deletion of CB_1. These animals have a lean phenotype and are resistant to diet-induced obesity and associated insulin resistance.[21,30] Further information comes from investigation of pharmacologic blockade of CB_1 receptors with the selective CB_1 blocker rimonabant, which produces weight loss and ameliorates metabolic abnormalities in obese animals.[29]

Exogenous cannabinoids and endocannabinoids increase food intake and promote weight gain by activating central endocannabinoid receptors.[28,31-34] These normal endocrine processes provide the framework for research that may further our understanding of the pathophysiology leading to diabetes as well as insight into potential sites of pharmacologic intervention.

Diagnosis

Diabetes consists of a group of metabolic diseases characterized by inappropriate hyperglycemia that results from defects in insulin secretion, insulin action, or both. The arbitrary glycemic limits used to diagnose diabetes have been modified many times over the years based on current understanding of the epidemiological relationship between glucose levels and diabetes-specific microvascular complications (see Table 7.1). As will be described subsequently in this chapter, the processes by which diabetes occurs take place over a prolonged period of time, with a wide variety of compensating mechanisms. The disease is continuous, even though the glucose definitions are fixed. Frequently, the diagnosis of diabetes is made on the basis of acute symptoms, including frequent urination, excessive thirst and hunger, weight loss, blurred vision, fatigue, headache, occasional muscle cramps, and poor wound healing. Signs and symptoms of chronic hyperglycemia include growth impairment; susceptibility to certain infections; and renal, retinal, peripheral vascular, connective tissue, and neuropathic syndromes. Acute life-threatening consequences of diabetes include hyperglycemia with

Case in Point: An African American Woman at Risk for Diabetes

CS, a 29-year-old African American female, was noted to have a random glucose of 125 mg/dL on a "blood test" obtained as part of a visit to the local health clinic. She had no symptoms of diabetes and thought her blood sugar was okay during her last pregnancy. She had been told to "watch her sugars" and to exercise. She had been healthy, but recently had complained of frequent yeast infections. Her family history included a mother and 2 older sisters with type 2 diabetes. Her grandmother died from diabetes after she started on the "the shot." CS smoked cigarettes, at a rate of a pack per day since age 18. She tried stopping because of the cost, but had been unsuccessful. She worked evenings and her husband worked days to cover childcare. They had 2 children, ages 3 and 5 years old.

Physical Exam

- Height: 63 in
- Weight: 203 lb
- Blood pressure: 138/94 mm Hg
- Waist circumference: 40 in
- Skin: Acanthosis nigricans on neck, trace edema; otherwise normal
- A1C: 6.4% (normal, 4% to 6%)
- 1-hour postprandial glucose: 132 mg/dL

Diagnosis and Classification

- Prediabetes
- Type 1 diabetes
- Type 2 diabetes
- Other types of diabetes
- Gestational diabetes mellitus

TABLE 7.1 Prediabetes and Diabetes: Diagnostic Tests

Diagnosing Prediabetes—2 Testing Options	
Fasting plasma glucose:	100 mg/dL to 125 mg/dL (5.6 to 6.9 mmol/L)
or	
2-hour plasma glucose:	140 mg/dL to 199 mg/dL (7.8 to 11.0 mmol/L) during oral glucose tolerance test (75-g glucose)
Diagnosing Diabetes—3 Testing Options	
Acute symptoms plus casual plasma glucose:*†	≥200 mg/dL (11.1 mmol/L)
or	
Fasting plasma glucose:‡	≥126 mg/dL (7.0 mmol/L)
or	
2-hour plasma glucose:	≥200 mg/dL (11.1 mmol/L) during oral glucose tolerance test (75-g glucose)

Note: Unless unequivocal symptoms of hyperglycemia are present, these criteria must be confirmed by repeat testing on a subsequent day

*Classic symptoms of diabetes: polyuria, polydipsia, polyphagia, and unexplained weight loss

†Casual implies any time of day without regard to time since last meal

‡Fasting is defined as no caloric intake for at least 8 hours

ketoacidosis (DKA), hyperosmolar hyperglycemic state (HHS), and therapy-induced hypoglycemia (these are the subject of chapter 8).

Distinctions among the various conditions that encompass diabetes are described below.

Prediabetes: Diagnosis

Hyperglycemia not sufficient to meet the diagnostic criteria for diabetes is categorized as prediabetes. This condition is identified through a fasting plasma glucose (FPG) or an oral glucose tolerance test (OGTT).[35] Prediabetes has been shown to be a risk factor for diabetes and cardiovascular disease (CVD).[35]

Type 1 Diabetes: Diagnosis

People with type 1 diabetes generally present with acute symptoms associated with markedly elevated blood glucose levels. Because of the acute onset of symptoms, type 1 diabetes usually is detected soon after symptoms develop, although the autoimmune process causing the disease may precede the clinical presentation by many years.[36] Approximately three-quarters of all cases of type 1 diabetes are diagnosed in individuals younger than age 18.[35]

Type 2 Diabetes: Diagnosis

Type 2 diabetes frequently is not diagnosed until complications appear. This is because many of the symptoms are absent or attributed to other causes.[35]

Notes on Diagnostic Testing for Diabetes

Diagnosis in Children. Distinction between type 1 and type 2 diabetes in children can be difficult because ketosis may be present in those with otherwise straightforward type 2 diabetes (including obesity and acanthosis nigricans). Such a distinction at diagnosis is critical because the natural history, treatment regimens, educational approaches, and dietary counsel differ markedly between the 2 diagnoses.[35] Chapters 9 and 10, on type 1 and type 2 diabetes, respectively, discuss this further.

Confirmation. There are 3 acceptable ways to diagnose diabetes (see Table 7.1), and each must be confirmed on a subsequent day unless unequivocal symptoms of hyperglycemia are present.

Test Selection. Although the 75-g OGTT is more sensitive and modestly more specific than FPG to diagnose diabetes, the OGTT is used less commonly. Ease of use, acceptability to patients, and lower cost have made the FPG the preferred diagnostic test, despite its significantly lower sensitivity to identify true disease.

Case—Part 2: Screening and Diagnostic Testing

With a random blood glucose of 125 mg/dL, CS did not meet the criteria for diabetes. However, she had several risk factors, physical evidence of insulin resistance, and an indication of hyperglycemia:

- High-risk racial group
- Family history of type 2 diabetes
- Obesity
- Acanthosis nigricans
- Recurrent yeast infections

Her family physician ordered a fasting blood glucose level:

- FPG: 112 mg/dL (when repeated, 108 mg/dL)

CS was diagnosed with prediabetes and advised to lose weight and exercise.

Classification

This section describes characteristics of type 1 and type 2 diabetes and the other types of diabetes. Diabetes includes 4 clinical classes:

- *Type 1 Diabetes:* the result of autoimmune beta-cell destruction, leading to absolute insulin deficiency
- *Type 2 Diabetes:* a multihormonal pathophysiology involving a progressive insulin secretory defect along with insulin resistance; usually associated with obesity
- *Other Specific Types of Diabetes:* diabetes due to other causes (for example, genetic defects in beta-cell function, genetic defects in insulin action, diseases of the exocrine pancreas, and disease induced by drugs or chemicals)
- *Gestational Diabetes:* diabetes diagnosed during pregnancy[35]

Type 1 Diabetes: Classification

- Develops at any age, but in most cases is diagnosed before age 30
- Characterized by autoimmune destruction of the beta cells of the islets of Langerhans with resulting absolute insulin deficiency

- Undiagnosed or untreated individuals experience significant weight loss, polyuria, and polydipsia characterized by the abrupt signs and symptoms associated with marked hyperglycemia and the strong propensity for the development of ketoacidosis
- Subjects are dependent on exogenous insulin to prevent ketoacidosis and sustain life
- Coma and death can result from delayed diagnosis and/or treatment

Type 2 Diabetes: Classification

- Approximately 90% of people in the United States with diabetes have type 2 diabetes, with disproportionate representation among the elderly and certain ethnic groups.
- Usually diagnosed after age 30, but its onset can occur at any age. Onset in adolescence is becoming more common among individuals in American Indian, Hispanic, and African American communities. Type 2 diabetes now accounts for 30% to 50% of childhood-onset diabetes.
- Frequently asymptomatic at the time of diagnosis, but as many as 20% may present with end-organ complications (eg, retinopathy, neuropathy, and nephropathy).
- Endogenous insulin levels may be normal, increased, or decreased, with a variable need for exogenous insulin.
- Insulin resistance occurs early and persists through prediabetes and subsequent clinical diabetes.
- Not prone to ketosis except in rare cases of severe physiologic stress.
- Approximately 50% of men and 70% of women are obese at the time of diagnosis.[37]

Other Forms of Diabetes: Classification

Other forms of diabetes are diagnosed when diabetes occurs as a result of another disorder or treatment. Treatment of these underlying disorders or discontinuation of diabetogenic agents may result in amelioration of the diabetes. Frequently, however, reversing the underlying disorder or stopping the offending agent is not possible. Therapy, then, is similar to diabetes therapy in general—using the modalities of medical nutrition therapy, physical activity, and medications. The following disorders are classified as other kinds of diabetes:

- Known genetic defects associated with Maturity Onset Diabetes of the Young (MODY), glycogen synthase deficiency, and mitochondrial DNA markers
- Pancreatic disorders, such as hemochromatosis, chronic pancreatitis, and pancreatectomy
- Hormonal disorders, such as Cushing syndrome (excess amounts of corticosteroids), pheochromocytoma (excess catecholamines), and acromegaly (excess growth hormone)
- Other disorders, such as cystic fibrosis, congenital rubella syndrome, and Down syndrome
- Concomitant diabetogenic drug therapy (eg, glucocorticoids, protease inhibitors, and pentamidine)

Gestational Diabetes: Classification

Gestational diabetes mellitus (GDM) is a diagnosis that applies only to women in whom glucose intolerance develops or is first discovered during pregnancy. GDM affects about 4% of all pregnant women—about 135,000 cases in the United States each year.[2] Risk assessment for gestational diabetes should be undertaken at the first prenatal visit. Women with clinical characteristics consistent with a high risk for gestational diabetes (those with marked obesity, personal history of gestational diabetes, glycosuria, or a strong family history of diabetes) should undergo glucose testing as soon as possible.[38] High-risk women not found to have the disorder at the initial screening and average-risk women should be tested between 24 and 28 weeks of gestation. Some authors have suggested that a substantial percentage of gestational diabetes is in fact only the identification of preexisting carbohydrate intolerance because of increased surveillance.[39] Although this may be true in a large percentage of individuals, the subsequent normalization of carbohydrate tolerance postpartum suggests that impaired glucose handling is an acquired defect inherent in the pregnant state.[37]

After pregnancy, the diagnostic classification may be changed to previous abnormality of glucose tolerance, type 1 or type 2 diabetes, or prediabetes. After pregnancy, 5% to 10% of women with gestational diabetes are found to have type 2 diabetes. Women who have had gestational diabetes have a 20% to 50% chance of developing diabetes in the next 5 to 10 years.[2] Women whose diabetes predates the pregnancy are not included in the gestational diabetes classification.

Gestational diabetes is associated with insulin resistance due to pregnancy and perhaps obesity and genetic predisposition.[40] Failure to augment beta-cell insulin response to the insulin resistance is the hallmark of the disorder.[41] The condition is usually asymptomatic, but is dangerous for the developing fetus. Maternal risks include hypertension, polyhydramnios, and cesarean delivery. See chapter 12 for a complete discussion of GDM.

Epidemiology

The increasing incidence of diabetes mellitus can be further appreciated when broken down into its effect on various age ranges:

- About 176,500 people age 20 or younger have diabetes
- Approximately 1 in every 400 to 600 children and adolescents has type 1 diabetes
- Of those age 20 or older, 20.6 million people (9.6% of all people in this age group) have diabetes
- Of those age 60 or older, 10.3 million (20.9% of all people in this age group) have diabetes (see Figure 7.2)[2]

Type 1 diabetes may account for 5% to 10% of all diagnosed cases of diabetes. Risk factors for type 1 diabetes include genetic, autoimmune, and environmental factors.[2]

Physical and behavioral characteristics used to identify people at risk for type 2 diabetes and prediabetes include the following:

- Obesity
- Sedentary lifestyle
- History of hypertension
- Dyslipidemia
- Family history of diabetes
- Gestational history
- Ethnicity

These risk factors may be assessed by various means, including community health screening, media campaigns, annual health maintenance exams, and self-administered risk assessment tools.[42]

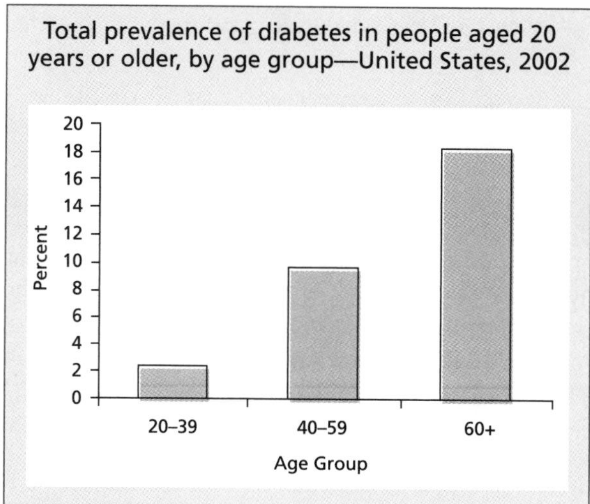

FIGURE 7.2 Diabetes Prevalence in the United States

Source: 1999-2001 National Health Interview Survey and 1999-2000 National Health and Nutrition Examination Survey estimates projected to year 2002.

The prevalence of diabetes in the United States continues to rise in epidemic proportions. This increase parallels the rising rates of obesity and overweight.[43-45] As body mass index (BMI) increases, the risk of developing type 2 diabetes increases in a dose-dependent manner.[46,47] The prevalence of type 2 diabetes is 3 to 7 times higher in obese than in normal-weight adults, and those with a BMI >35 kg/m^2 are 20 times more likely to develop diabetes than those with a BMI between 18.5 and 24.9 kg/m^2.[48,49] Weight gain during adulthood is directly correlated with an increased risk of type 2 diabetes.[50-52] Clinic-based reports and regional studies indicate that type 2 diabetes is becoming more common among Native American/American Indian, African American, and Hispanic and Latino children and adolescents.[2]

The actual rate of diagnosis of type 2 diabetes remains extremely poor, with almost 30% of those affected not aware they have diabetes. Microvascular complications are found in approximately 20% of newly diagnosed individuals with type 2 diabetes. Type 2 diabetes may be present, on average, for about 6 to 12 years prior to identification and treatment. The prevalence of coronary artery disease in those with type 2 diabetes is twice that of the nondiabetic population, and cardiovascular and total mortality are 2- to 3-fold greater than in nondiabetic individuals.[53]

Heredity plays a major role in the expression of type 2 diabetes. Although there is no recognized HLA linkage, offspring of individuals with type 2 diabetes have a 15% chance of developing the disease and a 30% risk of developing impaired glucose tolerance.[54] A greater than 90% concordance rate exists between monozygotic twins if one has type 2 diabetes, suggesting the primacy of the genetic defect in this form of the disease.

Identification of specific gene defects in certain groups with exceptionally high prevalence of type 2 diabetes has resulted in their designation as other specific types of diabetes. MODY is a series of 6 familial disorders characterized by early onset and mild hyperglycemia. MODY is associated with distinct genetic defects of beta-cell function and minimal or no defects in insulin action.[14,55] Six genes on different chromosomes have been identified that cause MODY. Each abnormality leads to impaired insulin secretion. Numerous other specific mutations have also been identified in insulin, the insulin receptor, and mitochondrial DNA that result in the development of diabetes.[14,47]

Type 1 Diabetes: Pathogenesis and Physiology

Type 1 diabetes develops when the body's immune system destroys **pancreatic beta cells**, the only cells in the body that make the hormones insulin and amylin. This form of diabetes usually occurs in children and young adults, although disease onset can occur at any age.

Type 1 diabetes is characterized by the abrupt onset of clinical signs and symptoms associated with marked hyperglycemia and a strong propensity for ketoacidosis. The disease begins to develop long before the clinical signs become evident. Pathologic and biochemical changes may occur as long as 9 years before clinical identification of type 1 diabetes. The 5 stages of development are shown in Table 7.2.

Genetic Propensity. There is a genetic propensity for type 1 diabetes. The risk of type 1 diabetes in the general population ranges from 1 in 400 to 1 in 1000.[56] That risk is substantially increased (from approximately 1 in 50 to 1 in 20) in the offspring of people with diabetes. The genetic predisposition to type 1 diabetes is the result of the combination of HLA-DQ coded genes for disease susceptibility offset by genes that are related to disease resistance. Genes that produce resistance are frequently dominant over those that produce disease susceptibility. HLA-DR3 and/or HLA-DR4 appear to be present in greater than 90% of Caucasians with type 1 diabetes. However, 95% of these individuals are found to have HLA-DQA1*0301, HLA-DQA1*0302. This HLA **genotype** is strongly associated with the occurrence of type 1 diabetes among African American, Caucasian, and Japanese populations. Dominant protection from developing diabetes results from the presence of the genotype HLA-DQB-1*0602 or HLA-DQW1.2.

Not all individuals at genetic risk for type 1 diabetes develop the disease. Although 40% of Caucasian individuals express the DR-3 or DR-4 haplotype, fewer than 1% develop diabetes.[57] A 50% discordance rate of type 1 diabetes exists between identical twins, suggesting that specific genes are necessary but not sufficient conditions for disease development.

Trigger for Expression. A trigger is necessary for the expression of the genetic propensity for type 1 diabetes; environmental triggers have long been suspected.

TABLE 7.2 Pathophysiologic Stages in the Development of Type 1 Diabetes

Stage 1	Genetic predisposition
Stage 2	Environmental trigger
Stage 3	Active autoimmunity
Stage 4	Progressive beta-cell dysfunction
Stage 5	Overt diabetes mellitus

- *Viral triggers* are suggested by the association of type 1 diabetes with congenital rubella syndrome and Coxsackie B4 infection.
- *Bovine serum albumin* (BSA) has been thought to be an environmental trigger by some investigators. BSA-specific antibodies are found in the majority of children with newly diagnosed diabetes. Thus, early exposure to cow's milk may be a potential determinant of type 1 diabetes, increasing disease risk by as much as 1.5 times.[58] Structural similarities exist between BSA and an islet cell surface antigen referred to as ICA-69. The cross-reactivity of circulating anti-BSA antibodies with ICA-69 would provide a link between the environmental trigger and the subsequent development of autoimmunity, causing type 1 diabetes. Long breastfeeding, exclusive breastfeeding in particular, and supplementation with vitamin D in infancy have been reported to confer partial protection against beta-cell autoimmunity and type 1 diabetes.[59] Other researchers, however, have not supported the hypothesis that infant diet is related to the occurrence of type 1 diabetes.[60] Some researchers suggest that type 1 diabetes is most likely the result of oxidative stress, due to high local levels of nitric oxide (NO) and oxygen radicals (O_2), on the beta cells of the pancreas, which eventually leads to their destruction.[61]
- *Additional environmental factors* that have been suggested as triggers for type 1 diabetes include sex steroids as seen in puberty and during pregnancy, environmental toxins (including N-nitroso derivatives and the rodenticide vacor), or possibly insulin itself.[62]

Epidemiologic studies have suggested that the incidence of type 1 diabetes is increased in both the spring and fall and is coincidental with various viral disorders.[37] Older studies relating apparent epidemic outbreaks of type 1 diabetes in populations previously affected by outbreaks of mumps provide strong circumstantial evidence. The finding of activated T cells and active autoimmunity in as many as one-third of individuals suffering from congenital rubella syndrome further supports a viral contribution.[37] The finding of a beta-cell cytotropic Coxsackie B virus in a young child dying of ketoacidosis when presenting with type 1 diabetes was the first apparent demonstration of direct viral attack on the beta cells.[37] Although this direct viral hypothesis remains controversial, it is evident that several viruses have the potential to either directly destroy islets or induce changes leading to a slow autoimmune destruction of the beta cells.[37]

The dilemma in identifying specific triggers involves the apparent long latency period between the triggering of active autoimmunity and the subsequent clinical development of diabetes. Thus, identifying which insult over the past 7 to 10 years may have been the actual trigger of the disease process is difficult. More likely is the possibility that a wide variety of viral or environmental agents may trigger expression of the genetic predisposition to the disease.

Autoimmunity. Regardless of the trigger, early type 1 diabetes is first identified by the appearance of active autoimmunity directed against pancreatic beta cells and their products. Fifty percent of relatives with high-titer islet cell antibodies (ICAs) have diabetes within 5 years of follow-up. ICA negativity has a 99.9% probability of freedom from the development of type 1 diabetes. Glutamic acid decarboxylase (GAD), a 64,000 Mr protein appears to be the best immunologic predictor for the future development of type 1 diabetes.[63] Additional islet cell autoantibodies that may play a permissive or pathologic role in the causation of type 1 diabetes are shown in Table 7.3.

There is also an immunologic attack on insulin, the product of the beta cells. In the early stages of the disease, markers of immune destruction of the beta cells are found, including ICAs, insulin autoantibodies (IAAs), and autoantibodies to GAD. Beta-cell destruction occurs at varying rates and is usually faster among younger patients, accounting for the classic abrupt clinical manifestation. Beta-cell destruction is slower in adults, which sometimes leads to an incorrect diagnosis of type 2 diabetes.[14] Seventy-eight percent of future cases of type 1 diabetes found in ICA-positive individuals arose from the subset with multiple autoantibodies; thus, the combination of positive antibody titers provides both increased sensitivity and specificity for disease progression.[64]

The combination of autoimmune attack on beta cells and on insulin by IAAs progressively diminishes the effective circulating insulin level. Before the clinical onset of diabetes, intravenous (IV) glucose tolerance testing demonstrates a progressive decline in first-phase insulin secretion (the insulin released within the first 5 minutes following an IV glucose stimulus) in individuals with positive immunologic markers. More than 50% of individuals with positive ICAs, but normal glucose tolerance tests have first-phase insulin secretion that falls within the 10th percentile of the normal population.[65] Hyperglycemia and symptoms consistent with diabetes develop only after >90% of the secretory capacity of the beta cells have been destroyed.

TABLE 7.3 Islet Cell Antibodies (ICAs) Observed in Type 1 Diabetes
Glutamic acid decarboxylase (GAD)
Insulin and proinsulin
Glycolipids, ganglioside GT3
Carboxypeptidase H, PM-1 polar antigen
Islet cell proteins of varying size and unknown function—37 or 40 kd, 38 kd, 52 kd, 69 kd
Peripherin
Heat shock protein 65
Insulin receptor
Endocrine cell antigens
Cytoskeletal proteins—tubulin actin, reticulin
Nuclear antigens—single-stranded DNA and RNA
Autoantibodies against islet tyrosine phosphatase (Islet Antigen A2 and A2 beta)

Adapted from: Boitard C. The differentiation of the immune system towards anti-islet autoimmunity: clinical prospects. Diabetologia. 1992;35(12):1101; Atkinson MA, Maclaren NK, The pathogenesis of insulin-dependent diabetes mellitus. N Engl J Med 1994;331(21):1428.

Clinical Onset. The clinical onset of diabetes may be abrupt, but the pathophysiologic insult is a slow, progressive phenomenon. At any time during the progressive decline in beta-cell function, overt diabetes may be precipitated by either acute illness or stress, thus increasing the insulin demand beyond the reserve of the damaged islet cells. Hyperglycemia will ensue until such time as the acute illness or stress is resolved; then, the individual may revert to a compensated state for a variable time period in which the beta cells are able to maintain normal glycemia. This "honeymoon period" is a variable period of noninsulin dependency following acute decompensation. Continued beta-cell destruction occurs, and the individual will require insulin within 3 to 12 months.

Latent Autoimmune Diabetes of Aging (LADA) may account for as many as 10% of cases of insulin-requiring diabetes in older individuals and represents a slow, progressive form of type 1 diabetes that is frequently confused with type 2 diabetes. People with LADA may remain insulin-independent for many years, even though they experience the autoimmune beta-cell deterioration associated with the traditional type 1 diabetes.[66]

Slow and Silent Progression

Although the clinical onset of diabetes may be abrupt, the pathophysiologic insult occurs slowly and progressively.

Implications for Prevention and Cure. Identifying these multiple stages in the development of type 1 diabetes provides a framework for potential interventions that focus on prevention and cure. For example:

- Identifying HLA markers may allow recognition of populations at risk at the time of birth.
- Developing specific vaccines against identified environmental triggers, or the simple avoidance of suspected environmental toxins such as bovine serum albumin, may prevent triggering of autoimmunity.
- Identifying active autoimmunity by measuring ICAs may serve as a marker for individuals who are destined to develop type 1 diabetes.

Three large randomized, controlled trials designed to delay or prevent type 1 diabetes—two DPT-1 trials[67] (one using subcutaneous insulin therapy in high-risk individuals and the other using oral insulin in a lower risk population) and the European Nicotinamide Diabetes Intervention Trial (ENDIT)[68]—failed to demonstrate a treatment effect. Notably, of the myriad of interventions that showed preclinical efficacy, both DPT-1 and the ENDIT Trial used interventions with low toxicity in their attempts to interdict the type 1 diabetes disease process. Thus, one should not conclude that it is impossible to delay or prevent type 1 diabetes; rather, testing of more potent interventions or combinations of therapies may be required. This work may be guided by better understanding of the immunopathogenesis of the disease to attenuate or ameliorate the destructive immune process that leads to type 1 diabetes.

Case—Part 3: Inattention to Modifiable Risk Factors

For 2 years, CS felt fine and despite being advised to try to exercise and lose weight, she had been unable to incorporate this into her busy life. That summer, however, she experienced progressive fatigue and found she was very thirsty. She assumed this was from the heat of summer. She noticed a red, shiny patch of skin under her breasts and went to her local health clinic. A random blood glucose at that time was 203 mg/dL.

Type 2 Diabetes: Pathogenesis and Physiology

Current research characterizes type 2 diabetes' pathophysiology as progressive and multihormonal. Insulin resistance in the liver and muscle and impaired function of the beta cells play a major role in the pathogenesis of type 2 diabetes. First, in the basal state, the liver overproduces glucose despite high fasting insulin levels, causing fasting hyperglycemia. Because this overproduction reflects enhanced gluconeogenesis rather than breakdown of glycogen, drugs that inhibit gluconeogenesis could aid in diabetes therapy. Second, in the insulin-stimulated state after glucose ingestion, muscle glucose uptake is reduced by more than 50%.[18]

The third component is the pancreas. In response to the insulin resistance and hyperglycemia, the beta cells increase their secretion of insulin. However, with fasting hyperglycemia >140 mg/dL, the compensatory insulin response cannot be maintained, insulin secretion declines progressively, and diabetes emerges. About 70% of beta-cell function has been lost when the 2-hour glucose value during the OGTT reaches 120 to 140 mg/dL.[69]

Acquired defects in beta-cell activity have been noted in response to hyperglycemia and referred to as glucose toxicity. Beta cells chronically exposed to hyperglycemia and to increased free fatty acids (lipotoxicity) become progressively less efficient in responding to subsequent glucose challenges. Thus, beta-cell dysfunction may be either primary or acquired in the pathogenesis of type 2 diabetes; in any event, it remains a necessary component of carbohydrate intolerance. Further progression of the disease is marked by an absolute insulin deficiency.

The islet in type 2 diabetes is characterized by a deficit in beta-cell mass, increased beta-cell apoptosis, and impaired insulin secretion. Some but not all studies suggest that a decrease in beta-cell mass contributes to the impaired insulin secretion of type 2 diabetes.[70] In sum, relative beta-cell volume, and therefore the presumptive beta-cell mass, is decreased in both obese and lean individuals with type 2 diabetes compared with their nondiabetic age- and weight-matched counterparts. People with prediabetes have a decreased relative beta-cell volume, suggesting that this is an early process and mechanistically important in the development of type 2 diabetes. Finally, the decrease in beta-cell mass may be caused by an increase in the frequency of beta-cell apoptosis with the rate of new islet formation being unaffected. Thus, in striving to prevent type 2 diabetes, strategies to avoid the increased frequency of beta-cell apoptosis may be useful. Also, in people with established type 2 diabetes, inhibition of this 3- to 10-fold increased rate of apoptosis may lead to restoration of beta-cell mass, because islet neogenesis appears intact.[71]

In type 2 diabetes, adipocytes (fat cells) are resistant to the antilipolytic effect of insulin and pour fat into the bloodstream, resulting in elevated plasma free fatty acid (FFA) levels. In this fourth component, the elevated FFA levels exacerbate liver and muscle insulin resistance, drive gluconeogenesis in the liver, and impair beta-cell insulin secretion.[72] The dysfunctional adipocytes produce multiple cytokines that contribute to inflammation and atherosclerosis as well as insulin resistance.[73]

Recently, gastrointestinal incretin hormones have been implicated as a fifth factor in the pathogenesis of type 2 diabetes. GLP-1 is deficient in people with type 2 diabetes and prediabetes, contributing to the excessive hepatic glucose production, failure to suppress postprandial glucagons, and unrestrained eating.

DPP-IV activity is increased in the fasting state in subjects who have type 2 diabetes. This may be one reason type 2 diabetes is associated with impaired postprandial GLP-1 secretion. One therapeutic strategy in type 2 diabetes has been to develop DPP-IV antagonists to enhance the natural incretin effects of these hormones.[15]

The insulinotropic effects of GLP-1 and GIP are enhanced by use of DPP-IV inhibitors.[74,75] The potential advantage of DPP-IV inhibitors over GLP-1 agonists is that DPP-IV inhibitors can be given orally. GLP-1 agonists, by causing greater serum GLP-1 levels, may be associated with more gastrointestinal side effects and more weight loss than DPP-IV inhibitors.[15]

Obesity, aging, weight gain in adulthood, and physical inactivity are environmental factors affecting the progression of diabetes at all points along the continuum. Type 2 diabetes progresses from an early asymptomatic state with insulin resistance, to mild postprandial hyperglycemia, to clinical diabetes requiring pharmacologic intervention.

Early suggestions of impaired insulin receptor function have not been demonstrated. Rare individuals have been identified as having altered insulin receptor structure or function. However, in the vast majority of individuals with type 2 diabetes, insulin binding to its receptor, insulin receptor number, and insulin receptor activity appear to be normal.[76]

Prevention and Intervention

These premises, along with the public health demands of recognizing an insidious disorder associated with substantial morbidity and mortality, led the National Institutes of Health to propose a prevention trial for type 2 diabetes.[77] The Diabetes Prevention Program (DPP) screened over 14,000 high-risk individuals for the presence of prediabetes. Subsequent interventions with intensive lifestyle modifications (eating habits, exercise, and subsequent weight loss) versus a pharmacologic intervention using metformin to improve endogenous insulin action were aimed at ameliorating the specific defects prior to decompensation to a hyperglycemic state. The results for the DPP study showed that lifestyle intervention reduced the incidence by 58% (95% confidence interval, 48% to 66%) and metformin by 31 percent (95% confidence interval, 17% to 43%), as compared with placebo; the lifestyle intervention was significantly more effective than metformin. To prevent one case of diabetes during a period of 3 years, 6.9 persons would have to participate in the lifestyle-intervention program, and 13.9 would have to receive metformin.[78]

Additional clinical trials examining the impact of lifestyle intervention in the area of diabetes and obesity are underway. These include The Diabetes Prevention Program Outcomes Study (DPP-OS) and Look AHEAD (Action for Health in Diabetes) and STOPP-T2D (Stop Pediatric Type 2 Diabetes).[35]

Identifying people at risk for diabetes is the first step in preventing the disease. The term prediabetes was adopted in 2002 to describe IGT or IFG, to promote awareness of the importance of prediabetes screening and to spread the news that diabetes may be preventable.[35] See chapters 1 and 2 for more information on prevention and related interventions.

In summary, knowledge of the pathophysiology of diabetes is increasing, and diabetes educators can use this new knowledge to guide their clients in managing their diabetes to ameliorate complications.

Case Wrap-Up

There were numerous clues that if dealt with earlier may have prevented or delayed the onset of type 2 diabetes for CS. Diabetes education could have played a vital role in primary prevention in this case. Care should have included early recognition and intervention to counsel CS about her risk factors (and her children's risk), treating her prediabetes, and emphasizing the need for follow-up. The fact that this did not occur caused continued and progressive metabolic abnormalities that may have resulted in decreased beta-cell function.

Questions and Controversies

Metabolic Syndrome

Discussions are taking place regarding the implications of the cluster of clinical entities that comprise what is known as the metabolic syndrome. Clinicians have been advised to avoid labeling patients with the term metabolic syndrome, yet to aggressively treat the risk factors associated with the cluster.[79] Randomized trials need to be completed to find appropriate pharmacologic treatment for this syndrome.

Hormones as Targets of Therapy

We are beginning to understand the defects in hormones other than insulin in those with diabetes. These include GLP-1, amylin, and DPP-IV. Medications targeted toward these defects have been or are in development for use in people with diabetes. We need to increase our understanding of these defects in those with IGT or IFG.

Some of the questions regarding hormone and other therapies are these:

- Is there a role for such medications for uses other than those currently indicated, perhaps to prevent diabetes and aid in weight loss?
- Although knowledge of defects has increased, patients still must work with existing treatments. How do those with diabetes accept the treatments that are available?
- What is the effect of multiple injections on quality of life over time?

Focus on Education: Pearls for Practice

Teaching Strategies

- **Stay abreast of evolving concepts.** Stay current. Know all specific signs, symptoms, and classification of the different types of diabetes. These are important in intervening with appropriate treatment. Stay informed about the changing knowledge of pathophysiology and the implications for treatment; for example, attend local and national meetings and retain membership in organizations that provide frequent updates and latest research. Bring this information back to the practice setting and inform peers and patients when teaching.

- **Heed diagnosing information.** The diagnosis of diabetes may have life-altering, major lifestyle implications. Thus, the following steps are essential: diagnostic criteria must be followed, testing must be completed, and test results with future implications (such as the need for follow-up or annual retesting) must be discussed.

Messages for Patients

- **Prediabetes is a time to act.** Lifestyle changes can prevent diabetes. Recognize also that having diabetes or even having risk factors for diabetes increases the chance that relatives may also have the same problem. Healthy lifestyles can improve the future health of a family.

- **The person with diabetes is part of the care team.** Be an active participant on the healthcare team. Being involved right from the beginning is the first step toward implementing preventive medicine and is revolutionizing the concept of health management through lifestyle modification.

- **Staying up to date can help your health.** Keep current with the new ideas about diabetes management, new treatment options, and other new and pertinent information. Attend educational sessions annually. Use Web sites, the educator on the team, and diabetes publications.

Acknowledgments

We gratefully acknowledge Rachel Schaperow, Writer-Editor, MedStar Research Institute, for her assistance in the research and preparation of this chapter.

Suggested Reading

Flier JS. Diabetes: the missing link with obesity? Nature. 2001;409:292-3.

Fujimoto WY, Bergstrom RW, Boyko EJ, et al. Preventing diabetes: applying pathophysiological and epidemiological evidence. Br J Nutr. 2000;84(suppl 2):173-6.

Ong KK, Dunger DB. Thrifty genotypes and phenotypes in the pathogenesis of type 2 diabetes. J Pediatr Endocrinol Metab. 2000;13(suppl 6):1419-24.

Enriori PJ, Harz K, Woelfle J, Cowley MA, Reinehr T. Peptide YY is a regulator of energy homeostasis in obese children before and after weight loss. J Clin Endocrinol Metab. 200;90(12):6386-91.

le Roux CW, Batterham RL, Aylwin SJ, et al. Attenuated peptide YY release in obese subjects is associated with reduced satiety. Endocrinology. 2006 Jan;147(1):3-8. Epub 2005 Sep 15.

Suggested Internet Resources

Centers for Disease Control and Prevention: National Diabetes Fact Sheet

www.cdc.gov/diabetes/pubs/factsheet05.htm

General information and national estimates on diabetes in the United States, 2003, rev ed. Atlanta, Ga: US Department of Health and Human Services, Centers for Disease Control and Prevention; 2004.

Diabetes Roundtable

www.diabetesroundtable.com

For healthcare professionals. Features a slide library, literature update, online continuing medical education courses, physician tools and patient education resources, recent news, and a semiannual newsletter of case studies. Sponsored by Washington Hospital Center, of Washington, DC, with its affiliates MedStar Diabetes Institute, MedStar Research Institute, and Union Memorial Hospital.

American Diabetes Association

www.diabetes.org/about-diabetes.jsp

Has a well-developed section for healthcare professionals. Clinical practice guidelines are posted online, including, for example, diabetes diagnostic and classification information. The diabetes research database is useful for information on the latest in research on the pathophysiology of diabetes, genetics, islet cell biology, and immunology. Several journals published by the ADA can be searched and viewed online.

Glossary of Key Terms

Adipocyte. A fat cell that serves as the primary storage for excess calories. Now known to be the source of many hormones and cytokines important in controlling appetite, weight, inflammation, and intermediary metabolism.

Amylin. A 37–amino acid polypeptide hormone, co-secreted from the pancreatic beta cells in conjunction with insulin in response to nutrient stimuli. Amylin, in the immediate postprandial period, may mediate part of its effect by the slowing of gastric emptying and by suppressing glucagon secretion, resulting in the suppression of hepatic glucose production.

Genotype. The specific description of a defined region of a chromosome.

GLP-1. Glucagon-like peptide-1, which is secreted by the small intestine in response to meals, promotes glucose-mediated insulin secretion, inhibits glucagon secretion, has a satiety effect on the brain, and delays gastric emptying.

Glucagon. A hormone produced by the alpha cells of the pancreatic islets of Langerhans and a counterregulatory hormone to insulin. Glucagon release results in an increase in the circulating glucose level by stimulating gluconeogenesis.

Gluconeogenesis. The process of glucose production in the liver from precursors, such as lactate and amino acids.

Glycogen. A complex carbohydrate that serves as the primary storage form of glucose in the liver and muscle.

Glycogenolysis. The metabolic conversion of glycogen into glucose.

Lactate. An incomplete breakdown product in the anaerobic metabolism of glucose; can serve as a precursor for subsequent glucose synthesis in the process of gluconeogenesis.

Pancreatic beta cells. The only cells in the body that make the hormone insulin.

Prediabetes. A term used to distinguish people who are at increased risk of developing diabetes. People are considered to have prediabetes if they have impaired fasting glucose (IFG) and/or impaired glucose tolerance (IGT). IFG is a condition in which the fasting blood sugar level is elevated (between 100 and 125 mg/dL after an overnight fast). IGT is a condition in which the blood sugar level is elevated (between 140 and 199 mg/dL after a 2-hour oral glucose tolerance test).

Substrate. A material that may be acted upon by enzymes in a metabolic process (ie, lactate is a substrate for gluconeogenesis).

References

1. Centers for Disease Control, US Department of Health and Human Services. National Diabetes Fact Sheet. 2005. On the Internet: http://www.cdc.gov/diabetes/pubs/factsheet05.htm. Accessed 2 Nov 2005.
2. American Diabetes Association. National Diabetes Fact Sheet. 2002. On the Internet: http://www.diabetes.org/diabetes-statistics/national-diabetes-fact-sheet.jsp. Accessed 22 Sep 2005.
3. Mulcahy K, Maryniuk M, Peeples M, et al. Diabetes self-management education core outcomes measures. Diabetes Educ. 2003;5:768-803.
4. Chipkin SR, Kelly KL, Ruderman NB. Hormone-fuel interrelationships: fed state, starvation, and diabetes mellitus. In: Joslin's Diabetes Mellitus, 13th ed. Kahn CR, Weir GS, eds. Philadelphia, Pa: Lea & Febiger; 1994:97-115.
5. Amylin Pharmaceuticals. The Role of the Hormone Amylin in Glucose Homeostatsis: A Scientific Monograph. Amylin Pharmaceuticals; 2003.
6. Kruger DF, Gatcomb PM, Owen SK. Clinical implication of amylin and amylin deficiency. Diabetes Educ. 1999;25:389-98.
7. Heptulla RA, Rodriguez LM, Bomgaars L, Haymond MW. The role of amylin and glucagon in the dampening of glycemic excursions in children with type 1 diabetes. Diabetes. 2005;54:1100-7.
8. Nyholm B, Orskov L, Hove KY, et al. The amylin analog pramlintide improves glycemic control and reduces postprandial glucagon concentrations in patients with type 1 diabetes mellitus. Metabolism. 1999;48:935-41.
9. Young A, Denaro M. Roles of amylin in diabetes and in regulation of nutrient load. Nutrition. 1998;14:524-7.
10. Gedulin BR, Rink TJ, Young AA. Dose-response for glucagonostatic effect of amylin in rats. Metabolism. 1997;46:67-70.
11. Samsom M, Szarka LA, Camilleri M, Vella A, Zinsmeister AR, Rizza RA. Pramlintide, an amylin analog, selectively delays gastric emptying: potential role of vagal inhibition. Am J Physiol. 2000;278: G946-51.
12. Bhavsar S, Watkins J, Young A. Synergy between amylin and cholecystokinin for inhibition of food intake in mice. Physiol Behav. 1998;64:557-61.
13. Gautier JF, Fetita S, Sobngwi E, Salaun-Martin C. Biological actions of the incretins GIP and GLP-1 and therapeutic perspectives in patients with type 2 diabetes. Diabetes Metab. 2005 Jun;31(3 pt 1):233-42.
14. Burant CF. Medical Management of Type 2 Diabetes, 5th ed. Arlington, Va: American Diabetes Association; 2004.
15. Uwaifo GI, Ratner, RE. Novel pharmacologic agents for type 2 diabetes. In: Type 2 Diabetes and Cardiovascular Disease: Endocrinology and Metabolism Clinics of North America (series). Einhorn D, Rosenstock J, eds. Philadelphia, Pa: Saunders; 2005;34:155-97.
16. Rotella CM, Pala L, Mannucci E. Glucagon-like peptide 1 (GLP-1) and metabolic diseases. J Endocrinol Invest. 2005;28:746-58.
17. Lankas GR, Leiting B, Roy RS, et al. Dipeptidyl peptidase IV inhibition for the treatment of type 2 diabetes: potential importance of selectivity over dipeptidyl peptidases 8 and 9. Diabetes. 2005;54:2988-94.
18. DeFronzo RA. New concepts in pathophysiology: incretins in type 2 diabetes. In: Clinical Highlights Newsletter: The Role of Incretin Mimetics and Potentiating Agents in the Prevention and Treatment of Type 2 Diabetes. 2004;1:3-4.
19. Hung CC, Pirie F, Luan J, et al. Studies of the peptide YY and neuropeptide Y2 receptor genes in relation to human obesity and obesity-related traits. Diabetes. 2004;53:2461-6.
20. Batterham RL, Cowley MA, Small CJ, et al. Gut hormone PYY(3-36) physiologically inhibits food intake. Nature. 2002;418:650-4.
21. Van Gaal LF, Rissanen AM, Scheen AJ, Ziegler O, Rössner S, and the RIO-Europe Study Group. Effects of the cannabinoid-1 receptor blocker rimonabant on weight reduction and cardiovascular risk factors in overweight patients: 1-year experience from the RIO-Europe study. Lancet. 2005;365:1389-97.

22. Di Marzo V, Bifulco M, De Petrocellis L. The endocannabinoid system and its therapeutic exploitation, Nat Rev Drug Discov. 2004;3:771-84.

23. Cota D, Marsicano G, Tschop M, et al. The endogenous cannabinoid system affects energy balance via central orexigenic drive and peripheral lipogenesis. J Clin Invest. 2003;112:423-31.

24. Di Marzo V, Goparaju SK, Wang L, et al. Leptin-regulated endocannabinoids are involved in maintaining food intake. Nature. 2001;410:822-5.

25. Croci T, Manara L, Aureggi G, et al. In vitro functional evidence of neuronal cannabinoid CB1 receptors in human ileum. Br J Pharmacol. 1998;125:1393-5.

26. Bensaid M, Gary-Bobo M, Esclangon A, et al. The cannabinoid CB1 receptor antagonist SR141716 increases Acrp30 mRNA expression in adipose tissue of obese fa/fa rats and in cultured adipocyte cells. Mol Pharmacol. 2003;63:908-14.

27. Howlett AC, Breivogel CS, Childers SR, Deadwyler SA, Hampson RE, Porrino LJ. Cannabinoid physiology and pharmacology: 30 years of progress. Neuropharmacology. 2004;47(suppl 1):345-58.

28. Engeli S, Bohnke J, Feldpausch M, et al. Activation of the peripheral endocannabinoid system in human obesity. Diabetes. 2005;54:2838-43.

29. Ravinet Trillou C, Arnone M, Delgorge C, et al. Anti-obesity effect of SR141716, a CB1 receptor antagonist, in diet-induced obese mice, Am J Physiol Regul Integr Comp Physiol. 2003;284:R345-53.

30. Kunos G, Batkai S. Novel physiologic functions of endocannabinoids as revealed through the use of mutant mice. Neurochem Res. 2001;26:1015-21.

31. Jamshidi N, Taylor DA. Anandamide administration into the ventromedial hypothalamus stimulates appetite in rats. Br J Pharmacol. 2001;134:1141-54.

32. Williams CM, Kirkham TC. Observational analysis of feeding induced by Delta9-THC and anandamide. Physiol Behav. 2002;76(2):241-50.

33. Williams CM, Kirkham TC. Anandamide induces overeating: mediation by central cannabinoid (CB1) receptors. Psychopharmacology (Berl). 1999;143:315-7.

34. Cota D, Marsicano G, Lutz B, et al. Endogenous cannabinoid system as a modulator of food intake. Int J Obes Relat Metab Disord. 2003;27:289-301.

35. American Diabetes Association. Standards of medical care in diabetes. Diabetes Care. 2006(Suppl 1): S4-36.

36. Babaya N, Nakayama M, Eisenbarth GS. The stages of type 1A diabetes. Ann N Y Acad Sci. 2005;1051:194-204.

37. Ratner RE. Type 2 diabetes mellitus: the grand overview. Diabetes Med. 1998;15(Suppl 4):S4-7.

38. American Diabetes Association: gestational diabetes mellitus (position statement). Diabetes Care. 2004;27 (Suppl 1):S88-90.

39. Harris MI. Gestational diabetes may represent discovery of preexisting glucose intolerance. Diabetes Care. 1988;11:402-11.

40. Mulcahy K, Lumber T. The Diabetes Ready Reference for Health Professionals, 2nd ed. Arlington, Va: American Diabetes Association; 2004.

41. Weisz B, Cohen O, Homko CJ, Schiff E, Sivan E. Elevated serum uric acid levels in gestational hypertension are correlated with insulin resistance. Am J Perinatol. 2005;22(3):139-44.

42. American Association of Diabetes Educators. The scope of practice, standards of practice, and standards of professional performance for diabetes educators. Diabetes Educ. 2005;31:487-512.

43. Klein S, Sheard NF, Pi-Sunyer X, et al. Weight management through lifestyle modification for the prevention and management of type 2 diabetes: rationale and strategies. Diabetes Care. 2004; 27:2067-73.

44. Harris MI, Flegal KM, Cowie CC, et al. Prevalence of diabetes, impaired fasting glucose, and impaired glucose tolerance in U.S. adults: the Third National Health and Nutrition Examination Survey, 1988-1994. Diabetes Care. 1998;21:518-24.

45. Mokdad AH, Ford ES, Bowman BA, et al. The continuing increase of diabetes in the U.S. Diabetes Care. 2001;24:412.

46. Colditz GA, Willett WC, Stampfer MJ, et al. Weight as a risk factor for clinical diabetes in women. Am J Epidemiol. 1990;132:501-13.

47. Must A, Spadano J, Coakley EH, Field AE, Colditz G, Dietz WH. The disease burden associated with overweight and obesity. JAMA. 1999;282:1523-9.

48. Mokdad AH, Ford ES, Bowman BA, et al. Prevalence of obesity, diabetes, and obesity-related health risk factors, 2001. JAMA. 2003;289:76-9.

49. Field AE, Coakley EH, Must A, et al. Impact of overweight on the risk of developing common chronic diseases during a 10-year period. Arch Intern Med. 2001;161:1581-6.

50. Hu FB, Manson JE, Stampfer MJ, et al. Diet, lifestyle, and the risk of type 2 diabetes mellitus in women. N Engl J Med. 2001;345:790-7.

51. Carey VJ, Walters EE, Colditz GA, et al. Body fat distribution and risk of non-insulin-dependent diabetes mellitus in women: the Nurses' Health Study. Am J Epidemiol. 1997;145:614-9.

52. Chan JM, Rimm EB, Colditz GA, Stampfer MJ, Willett WC. Obesity, fat distribution, and weight gain as risk factors for clinical diabetes in men. Diabetes Care. 1994;17:961-9.

53. Ratner RE. Pathophysiology of the diabetes disease state. In: A Core Curriculum for Diabetes Education: Diabetes and Complications, 5th ed. Franz, MJ, ed. Chicago, Ill: American Association of Diabetes Educators; 2003:3-18.

54. Redondo MJ, Fain PR, Eisenbarth GS. Genetics of type 1A diabetes. Recent Prog Horm Res. 2001;56:69-89.

55. Florez JC, Hirschhorn J, Altshuler D. The inherited basis of diabetes mellitus: implications for the genetic analysis of complex traits. Annu Rev Genomics Hum Genet. 2003;4:257-91.

56. Redondo MJ, Fain PR, Eisenbarth GS. Genetics of type 1A diabetes. Recent Prog Horm Res. 2001;56:69-89.

57. Thai A-C, Eisenbarth GS. Natural history of IDDM. Diabetes Rev. 1993;1:1-14.

58. Wasnuth HE, Kolb H. Cow's milk and immune-mediated diabetes. Proc Nutr Soc. 2000;59:573-9.

59. Knip M, Akerblom HK. Early nutrition and later diabetes risk. Adv Exp Med Biol. 2005;569:142-50.

60. Sipetic S, Vlajinac H, Kocev N, Bjekic M, Sajic S. Early infant diet and risk of type 1 diabetes mellitus in Belgrade children. Nutrition. 2005;21(4):474-9.

61. Persaud DR, Barranco-Mendoza A. Bovine serum albumin and insulin-dependent diabetes mellitus; is cow's milk still a possible toxicological causative agent of diabetes? Food Chem Toxicol. 2004;42(5):707-14.

62. Vaarala O, Hyoty H, Akerblom HK. Environmental factors in the aetiology of childhood diabetes. Diabetes Nutr Metab. 1999;12(2):75-85.

63. Atkinson MA, MacLaren NK, Scharp DW, Lacy PE, Riley WJ. 64,000 Mr autoantibodies as predictors of insulin-dependent diabetes. Lancet. 1990;35:1357-60.

64. Bingley PJ, Christie MR, Bonifacio E, et al. Combined analysis of autoantibodies improves prediction of IDDM in islet anti-body positive relatives. Diabetes. 1994;43:1304-10.

65. Maclaren NK. How, when and why to predict IDDM. Diabetes. 1988;37:1591-94.

66. Pozzilli P, Di Mario U. Autoimmune diabetes not requiring insulin at diagnosis (latent autoimmune diabetes of the adult): definition, characterization, and potential prevention. Diabetes Care. 2001;24:1460-7.

67. Diabetes Prevention Trial-Type 1 Diabetes Study Group, effects of insulin in relatives of patients with type 1 diabetes. N Engl J Med. 2002;346:1658-91.

68. European Nicotinamide Diabetes Intervention Trial (ENDIT) Group. European Nicotinamide Diabetes Intervention Trial (ENDIT): a randomized controlled trial of intervention before the onset of type 1 diabetes. Lancet. 2004;363:925-31.

69. Gastaldelli A, Ferrannini E, Miyazaki Y, et al. Beta-cell dysfunction and glucose intolerance: results from the San Antonio metabolism (SAM) study. Diabetologia. 2004;47:31-9.

70. Butler AE, Jang J, Gurlo T, Carty MD, Soeller WC, Butler PC. Diabetes due to a progressive defect in beta-cell mass in rats transgenic for human islet amyloid polypeptide (HIP Rat): a new model for type 2 diabetes. Diabetes. 2004 Jun;53(6):1509-16.

71. Butler AE, Janson J, Bonner-Weir S, Ritzel R, Rizza RA, Butler PC. Beta-cell deficit and increased beta-cell apoptosis in humans with type 2 diabetes. Diabetes. 2003 Jan;52(1):102-10.

72. Kashyap S, Belfort R, Gastaldelli A, et al. A sustained increase in plasma free fatty acids impairs insulin secretion in nondiabetic subjects genetically predisposed to develop type 2 diabetes. Diabetes. 2003;52:2461-74.

73. Bays H, Mandarino L, DeFronzo RA. Role of the adipocyte, free fatty acids, and ectopic fat in pathogenesis of type 2 diabetes mellitus: per oxisomal proliferators-activated receptor agonists provide a rational therapeutic approach. J Clin Endocrinol Metab. 2004;28:463-78.

74. Deacon CF, Danielsen P, Klarskov L, Olesen M, Holst JJ. Dipeptidyl peptidase IV inhibition reduces the degradation and clearance of GIP and potentiates its insulinotropic and antihyperglycemic effects in anesthetized pigs. Diabetes. 2001;50:1588-97.

75. Deacon CF, Hughes TE, Holst JJ. Dipeptidyl peptidase IV inhibition potentiates the insulinotropic

effect of glucagon-like peptide 1 in the anesthetized pig. Diabetes. 1998;47(5):764-9.

76. Gerich JE. Is insulin resistance the principal cause of type 2 diabetes. Diabetes Obes Metab. 1999;1:257-63.

77. The Diabetes Prevention Program Research Group. The Diabetes Prevention Program: baseline characteristics of the randomized cohort. Diabetes Care. 2000;23:1619-29.

78. Diabetes Prevention Program Research Group. Reduction in the incidence of type 2 diabetes with lifestyle intervention or metformin. New Engl J Med. 2002;346:393-403.

79. Kahn R, Buse J, Ferrannini E, Stern M. The metabolic syndrome: time for a critical appraisal. Diabetes Care. 2005;28:2289-2304.

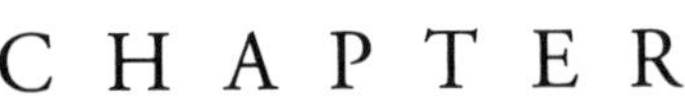

CHAPTER

8

Hyperglycemia

Authors

Marilynn S. Arnold, MS, RD, LD, CDE
Dace L. Trence, MD, FACE

Key Concepts

This chapter helps the reader recognize symptoms of acute hyperglycemia, understand principles of evaluation and treatment, and prevent recurrent episodes in individuals with diabetes.

- **Diabetic ketoacidosis** (DKA) occurs when there is so little insulin available to transport glucose into cells that glucose accumulates in the blood, raising levels to 250 mg/dL or greater (mean 475 mg/dL).[1] DKA can evolve quickly (within 24 hours), causing dehydration and ketosis and electrolyte imbalance and acidosis. This condition requires immediate treatment.
- **Hyperosmolar hyperglycemic state** (HHS) occurs when hyperglycemia and dehydration slowly exacerbate each other until both are extreme. Blood glucose levels rise greater than 600 mg/dL but with few, if any, ketones. HHS occurs primarily in undiagnosed or elderly individuals with type 2 diabetes and is especially common in residents of long-term care facilities. HHS is even more life-threatening than is DKA.
- **Chronic hyperglycemia** is glucose that is persistently elevated. With a few exceptions, everyone with diabetes experiences chronic hyperglycemia to some extent. How high and how often glucose levels rise over the reference range varies greatly. People with high blood glucose may not feel well, but typically continue with their usual activities and responsibilities. Very high glucose levels are acute and serious and can evolve from chronic hyperglycemia. The ramifications of ongoing hyperglycemia are well known and are addressed in full in other chapters.

State of the Condition

Hyperglycemia is defined as blood glucose above normal. In persons with diabetes, significant hyperglycemia is the objective finding of diabetes out of control. A gradual or abrupt decline of insulin production or availability, typically in conjunction with insulin resistance, contributes to elevated blood glucose levels. Stress, whether psychologic or metabolic, can exacerbate insulin resistance, which in turn stimulates hepatic glucose production to further elevate blood glucose. People with diabetes may suffer long-term complications from chronic hyperglycemia as well as acute episodes of life-threatening complications with severely high glucose levels. This chapter addresses acute states of elevated blood glucose; for information on ongoing hyperglycemia, see chapters 7, on pathophysiology, and 21, on macrovascular disease.

Diabetic Ketoacidosis

Pathology

Diabetic ketoacidosis (DKA) occurs more often in people with type 1 diabetes, but can also be seen in individuals with type 2 diabetes during acute illness and/or after they have become insulin deficient.[1] DKA also appears as an acute presentation of unrecognized diabetes as a new diagnosis, particularly in certain ethnicities.[2-5] Type 1 diabetes, by definition, is characterized by insulin deficiency. Treatment provides insulin in an amount designed to match the amount required for glucose uptake into the cells. Available insulin and insulin delivery systems have improved tremendously, but remain imperfect. Even with usually effective and stable food, medication, and activity regimens, some

Case in Point: DKA in a Busy Woman With Type 1 Diabetes

GT was a 24-year-old female with type 1 diabetes since age 12. She had been using an insulin pump for 8 years and checked her blood glucose 4 to 6 times per day. She did not understand why others she had met did not take their diabetes more seriously. GT was 5 ft 8 in and 160 lb. Her latest A1C was 6.2 %, and her daily glucose readings ranged from 50 to 200 mg/dL. She had no evidence of complications and other than diabetes was a healthy young adult. She was a full-time student working toward an MBA and also worked part-time as an accountant for a gift shop.

Precipitating Events

GT usually ate regularly, matched insulin to carbohydrate, exercised, and slept 7 to 8 hours a night. Since mid-November, though, life was chaotic as extra hours at work, end-of-semester exams, and personal holiday preparations converged. Some days she skipped meals, grabbed a sandwich, or snacked from the vending machine. She had missed most of her scheduled times at the gym. She was tired and began drinking more coffee and diet soda to keep going. Increased commitments had disrupted her routine.

GT was anxiously awaiting her next 3-month shipment of diabetes supplies, which seemed to be delayed in the mass of holiday packages. She began spacing out her blood glucose monitoring to conserve strips and hoped the new shipment arrived before her holiday trip to visit with family. As soon as the semester was finished, she was flying to Maine for a quick visit with her grandparents before heading home for Christmas.

situations (often illness) can quickly and substantially elevate blood glucose.[6] Other conditions, such as persistent untreated hyperglycemia, newly prescribed medications, or missed insulin can disrupt the perfect match. Anything that increases blood glucose and decreases insulin action can contribute to the development of DKA.

Ingested Glucose

Eating more food or more carbohydrate than usual, without changing insulin dosing, elevates blood glucose. This happens frequently to people who take fixed doses of insulin but not fixed quantities of food. Hyperglycemia itself can stimulate hunger, leading to further food intake. Food intake alone is not sufficient to cause DKA, but may cumulatively contribute to it. Two small, but recent studies of pediatric patients reported consumption of large volumes of high-calorie beverages before admission for DKA,[7,8] and in type 2 diabetes, alcohol has been associated with DKA development.

Inadequate Insulin

Glucose levels rise directly from deficient insulin production and/or an inability to effectively use the insulin produced. People with type 1 diabetes—or, to a lesser extent, people with type 2 diabetes requiring insulin—can be receiving inadequate insulin from poorly designed or poorly followed treatment plans. Inadequate insulin impacts other physiological functions that elevate glucose levels indirectly.

Glucose stored in the liver as glycogen is available to provide fuel between meals and during sleep. Ideally, hepatic glucose offers stored energy as needed to maintain blood glucose levels, support exercise, and provide extra fuel for extraordinary events such as surgery or fighting a grizzly bear. When adequately available, insulin turns off this hepatic feeding function as soon as there is sufficient glucose available to hungry cells.

When there is inadequate insulin, the liver keeps producing glucose, as there is no ability to sense that the problem is inadequate insulin availability to promote glucose entry into cells. This process of glycogenolysis and even gluconeogenesis (the production of glucose from amino acids obtained from protein breakdown) floods the bloodstream with unwelcome sugar molecules. Multiple forms of stress (illness, trauma, menses, pregnancy, fear, worry, excitement, and other physical or emotional stressors) and some medications stimulate the counterregulatory and stress hormones. These hormones stimulate hepatic glucose production and, at the same time, interfere with insulin effectiveness and glucose uptake in the peripheral tissues. Glucagon, secreted in response to meal ingestion, is another hormone that stimulates hepatic glucose production and exacerbates an already disruptive situation.

Ketones

A homeostatic mechanism to feed cells when glucose cannot enter cells is to break down fat (lipolysis) into glucose and ketone bodies. As the concentration of ketones increase, the kidneys via osmotic diuresis excrete both glucose and ketones. The increasing amount of water lost in the process causes dehydration. Dehydration concentrates serum glucose and further increases hyperglycemia. Increased hyperglycemia drives further dehydration.

With dehydration and the increasing accumulation of ketones in the serum, sodium and potassium (key electrolytes that impact muscle and other organ function) are affected. Potassium is involved with the regulation of heart rhythm, and loss of potassium may be life threatening. Further, as potassium is imperative to facilitate insulin action, hypokalemia can inhibit the ability of provided insulin to be therapeutic.

When ketone accumulation is excessive, blood becomes too acidic to support life. DKA can be termed mild, moderate, or severe, depending on parameters of blood glucose levels, acidity, and ketone formation.[6] Prompt treatment is essential.

Precipitating Situations

Inadequate Insulin

There are numerous factors that contribute to inadequate insulin. The onset or acute decompensation of subclinical type 1 diabetes accounts for 30% of DKA cases.[9] Increases in insulin resistance or suboptimal treatment plans are other reasons for inadequate insulin being available. However, in many instances insulin injections may be skipped for psychosocial reasons, lack of adequate planning, or a patient's lack of knowledge about adequate self-management. Some examples:

- *Insulin Omitted to Control Weight:* Insulin omission can be a form of bulimia. In a study of subjects age 11 to 25 years, 36% reported insulin misuse to control weight.[10] The Ahead survey show 10.3% of females reported skipping insulin and 7.4% reported taking less insulin to control their weight.[11] Omission of or undertreatment with insulin may be the most important contributor to DKA in urban African Americans with type 2 diabetes.[9]
- *Psychological Problems Complicated by Eating Disorders:* May be a factor in 20% of recurrent ketoacidosis.[6]
- *Insulin Omitted to Avoid Hypoglycemia, Especially When Home Alone or During Active Work Days:*[6] May be seen as a patient self-initiated safety measure.
- *Insulin Omitted to Avoid the Inconvenience or Embarrassment of Injecting in a Public Situation:* Many feel uncomfortable injecting insulin in a restaurant or asking permission to leave their work site.
- *Inadequate or Poorly Timed Insulin Due to Inadequate Organization:* Some people never seem to have all the supplies they need in the right place at the right time.
- *Insulin Dose Reduced to Save Money*
- *Insulin Dose Reduced or Omitted When Ill:* Some believe they need less insulin if they eat less. Because nausea, vomiting, and stomach pain are symptoms of DKA, omitting insulin for gastrointestinal symptoms may only push glucose levels higher and make symptoms worse.
- *Using Insulin That Is Outdated, Improperly Stored, Inaccurately Measured, or Incorrectly Injected:* Can provide a lower dose than planned.

Excess Hepatic Glucose

Stress, whether physical, emotional, or psychological, can dramatically elevate hepatic glucose and acutely increase blood glucose levels. All forms of stress increase adrenal glucocorticoid production and catecholamine levels, both of which raise glucose levels through increased hepatic glucose production. This can increase the risk of DKA if there is no intervention to either decrease the instigating stress or provide compensatory insulin adjustment. The following are examples of situations that increase hepatic glucose:

- Infection—the most common precipitating factor
- Pneumonia and urinary tract infections—account for 30% to 50% of DKA
- Gastrointestinal bleeding
- Cerebrovascular accident (CVA)
- Alcohol abuse
- Pancreatitis
- Myocardial infarction
- Trauma
- Pregnancy
- Drugs that affect carbohydrate metabolism (corticosteroids, thiazides, dobutamine, terbutaline, cocaine)[9]

Prevention

Preventing or at least greatly limiting the severity of DKA due to causes other than acute decompensation or development of type 1 diabetes mellitus is possible. Early recognition of hyperglycemia and appropriate treatment can prevent acute complications and reduce fatalities. When hyperglycemia is ignored or occurs unexpectedly, coma and even death are possible.

Some people with diabetes purposely avoid insulin during work hours or as a weight-loss tool, and disadvantaged children are more vulnerable to episodes of DKA.[12]

> ***Inadequate Insulin***
>
> If an individual intentionally omits or is deprived of insulin for any reason, discussing DKA prevention may be ineffective unless underlying problems are also addressed.

Intentionally omitting insulin for any reason suggests there are other problems that need to be addressed before further discussing DKA prevention.

Education regarding glucose self-management during illness and stress management are essential to prevent DKA. Patients benefit from having sick day management information reinforced over and over again during routine appointments. See sidebar below.

Also provide information about possible causes and how to recognize symptoms of DKA. Identifying the cause or risks for DKA in the individual's specific situation may help prevent the problem. Common contributors to acute hyperglycemia include the following:

- Relying on "how you feel" to assess glucose levels
- Skipping insulin when not eating
- Inadequate monitoring during illness

Other possible causes for acute hyperglycemia include the following:

- Use of expired insulin
- Increased insulin needs during growth or hormonal spurts
- Preoccupation with other priorities and missing (or not learning to recognize) symptoms of escalating glucose levels

The more patients understand how their medications work, the more able they are to use them to their advantage. Learning to supplement with extra insulin for high glucose levels and for ketones prepares them to handle acute situations.

Remaining attentive to the symptoms of hyperglycemia and monitoring glucose in the midst of other priorities could prevent many incidents of DKA. Finding and using resources, including knowing when to contact the physician, can ease the burden of living with diabetes.

Ultimately, information is essential, but to prevent DKA, patients and their families require more than information. The individual must be prepared to effectively employ self-management strategies to prevent severe hyperglycemia and intervene early when at risk.

Assessing Hyperglycemia

Diabetic Ketoacidosis: Signs, Symptoms, and Laboratory Indicators

The symptoms of hyperglycemia may mimic other diseases or conditions. Assessment of the following helps accurately diagnose the problem:

Sick Day Management

	Type 1	*Type 2*
Hydration	• 8 oz fluid per hour • Every third hour, consume this 8 oz as a sodium-rich choice such as bouillon	Same
SMBG	• Every 2-4 hours while BG is elevated or until symptoms subside	Same
Ketones	• Every 4 hours or until negative	Determine for the individual
Medications adjustments	• Continue as able • Adjust insulin doses to correct hyperglycemia • Hold metformin during serious illness • Instruct patients to call their healthcare provider for specific instructions if they have not previously received them	Same
Food and beverage selections	• Guide patients to consume 150-200 g carbohydrates daily, in divided doses • Switch to soft foods or liquids as tolerated • Provide patients lists of foods and beverages with 15 g carbohydrates	Same
Contact healthcare professionals	Provide guidelines on conditions that require the patient to call: • Vomiting more than once • Diarrhea more than 5 times or for longer than 6 hours • BG levels >300 on 2 consecutive measurements that are not responsive to increased insulin and fluids • Moderate or large urine ketones or blood ketones >0.6 mmol/L	Same

- Hyperglycemia
- Dehydration
- Electrolyte status
- Ketosis
- Acidosis
- Osmolality

The physical signs and symptoms and the laboratory findings consistent with DKA relate physiologically to one of these markers: hyperglycemia, dehydration, electrolyte imbalance, ketosis, or acidosis. Patients can present with a spectrum of low energy to confusion, lethargy to coma, abdominal pain, polyuria, and polydipsia. Table 8.1 summarizes these markers.

Initial Evaluation Findings

- *Blood Glucose:* Fingerstick blood glucose of >250 mg/dL if outpatient; serum glucose will be obtained in urgent or acute care settings
- *Urine Ketones:* Positive

Confirmation of Diagnosis (either of the following)

- *Arterial pH:* <7.3
- *Serum Bicarbonate:* <16 mEq/L

Identification of Precipitating Factors

- *History and Full Clinical Exam:* To identify precipitating etiologies; includes looking for potential sources of infection such as perirectal abscess or cellulitis
- *Vital Signs:* Such as weight, blood pressure in the supine and upright positions, and pulse rate to assess hydration status
- *Laboratory Evaluation:*[1] Serum electrolyte values (with calculated anion gap), blood urea nitrogen (BUN)/creatinine levels, beta-hydroxybutyric acid (or serum ketones, if not available), calcium and phosphorus concentrations, serum osmolality, complete blood cell count with differential, electrocardiogram (EKG)

TABLE 8.1 Markers of Diabetic Ketoacidosis

	Hyperglycemia	*Dehydration*	*Electrolyte Imbalance*	*Ketosis*	*Acidosis*
Physical Signs	Polyuria Polydipsia Blurred vision Polyphagia Weight loss if insulin deficiency is present long enough (days to weeks)	Decreased intravascular volume Decreased neck vein filling from below while person is lying absolutely flat Orthostatic hypotension (systolic blood pressure drop of 20 mm Hg after 1 min of standing) Poor skin turgor: seen earlier in children "Soft eyeballs": late sign of profound dehydration in adults		'Fruity' or acetone breath Nausea Vomiting Abdominal pain	Kussmaul respirations (hyperpnea)
Laboratory Tests	Glucose >250 mg/dL	Hemoglobin Hematocrit Total protein values are often mildly elevated Creatinine Blood urea nitrogen (BUN)	Sodium: low, medium, or high Potassium: low, medium, or high Phosphorus: medium, or high	Positive ketones	Low pH (<7.2) Low HCO_3 (<15 mEq/L) Low PCO (<35 mm Hg)

- *Additional Tests, as Needed:*[9] Bacterial blood cultures if infection suspected, urine analysis for urinary tract infection, chest X-ray, EKG, A1C (to identify whether DKA was an isolated event or the cumulative result of undiagnosed or poorly controlled diabetes), pregnancy (if of childbearing age)

Additional Notes on Markers of DKA

Hyperglycemia

Elevated glucose is a marker of DKA, but not a good index of the severity. DKA does occur with lower glucose levels, especially in children, pregnant women, and persons who have been vomiting frequently.

Dehydration

Due to dehydration, the labs values listed are likely to be mildly elevated before treatment of DKA but to correct themselves after treatment. Elevated creatinine or BUN after rehydration suggests further assessment for renal problems.

Electrolyte Imbalance

- *Sodium.* Dehydration causes a profound loss of total body sodium (Na^+) that serum levels can not accurately measure. The results of testing serum sodium may appear low, normal, or high, depending on whether the sodium lost was greater, equal to, or less than the relative amount of water lost.
- *Potassium.* Similarly, total body depletion of potassium always occurs with DKA, but lab values of serum potassium (K^+) can test low, normal, or high. As with sodium, serum potassium reflects the relative amounts of water lost compared with potassium lost. Potassium may be low before treatment or fall as it enters the cells, with glucose and fluids reducing the serum concentration. Status of renal function should be ascertained before any potassium is replaced.
- *Phosphate.* Phosphate concentrations are usually high or high-normal initially and decrease with insulin therapy, sometimes markedly, to very low levels over the next day or two. Phosphate replacement remains controversial at this time, as it is felt that with rapid access to oral normal food intake, phosphate can be replaced without need for parenteral phosphate.[6]

Ketosis

One ketone produced during DKA, acetoacetate, converts to acetone and is excreted by the lungs. Acetone has a fruity odor that may be detectable on the breath of someone in ketosis. Beta-hydroxybutyric acid is the most prevalent ketone in DKA, and measurement of this acid is the most reliable way to measure treatment progress. Beta-hydroxybutyric acid is measured by serum assessment using the nitroprusside method.

Acidosis

Very deep and sometimes rapid breathing unrelated to exertion or the inability to "catch one's breath" is a symptom of acidosis called Kussmaul respiration or hyperpnea. This form of hyperventilation is an effort to correct the metabolic acidosis by blowing off carbon dioxide.

Increased Osmolarity

Mental status changes seem to correlate best with serum osmolality and less so with glucose levels. People with DKA may be alert, obtunded, stuporous, or in frank coma. The changes in mentation, rather than the status itself, offer clues to diagnosis.

Others Significant Symptoms of DKA

- *Nonspecific Symptoms.* Include weakness, lethargy, malaise, and headache.
- *Acute Abdomen.* A common condition; marked by tenderness to palpation, diminished bowel sounds, and some muscle guarding, especially in children. A few patients may have more severe signs (absent bowel sounds, rebound tenderness, board-like abdomen) that suggest a surgical emergency. These signs can be due to profound DKA and disappear after treatment, but can present a challenge to diagnose, as appendicitis or cholecystitis can be a precipitating cause of DKA.
- *Hypotonia.* Signs that do not appear until late in the progression of DKA and suggest a poor prognosis are uncoordinated ocular movements and fixed, dilated pupils.
- *Hypothermia.* Common during DKA, making the presence of a fever a strong indicator of infection.

Symptoms of DKA that Are Probably Insignificant

- Increased amylase alone does not suggest pancreatitis. In DKA, salivary glands, not the pancreas, release most of the amylase.
- Increased white blood cells (WBC) with DKA do not indicate infection. The differential count may be helpful with increased immature WBCs (>10% band forms), but clinical exam findings, such as fever, can supersede laboratory findings.[10]

- Mildly elevated liver function tests (LFTs) usually do not suggest liver damage and return to normal in several weeks.
- Serum creatinine can be elevated at initial evaluation. This needs to be followed, as often the creatinine will fall as fluid replacement is initiated, but the issue as to when potassium replacement is safe requires that the creatinine be followed closely.

Although the symptoms of poorly controlled diabetes may be present for several days, the metabolic alterations typical of ketoacidosis usually occur within a short time frame (typically less than 24 hours). Occasionally, DKA may develop more acutely with no prior signs or symptoms.[2]

Treatment of Diabetic Ketoacidosis

The first part of this section describes treatment of moderate-to-severe DKA. Mild DKA is covered at the end of this section. Goals of DKA treatment,[1] listed in Table 8.2, are discussed individually below.

Mortality for moderate-to-severe DKA is high:

Hospitalization may be required for appropriate treatment of DKA that is moderate to severe. Mortality remains high, even in teaching institutions. Treatment always requires supplemental fluids (first), followed by additional insulin.

Although hyperglycemia is the cause of osmotic diuresis that leads to dehydration, the dehydration must be treated first, then the hyperglycemia—particularly when hypotension indicates potential impending circulatory collapse. Eventually, providing additional glucose is necessary to stop cellular starvation and intracerebral swelling. Treatment of DKA would not be complete without providing information and coaching to help prevent future episodes.

TABLE 8.2 Treatment Goals for Diabetic Ketoacidosis
1. Provide adequate fluids to rehydrate
2. Provide adequate insulin to restore and maintain normal glucose metabolism
3. Correct electrolyte deficits and acidosis if needed
4. Prevent complications
5. Provide source of glucose when needed
6. Provide patient and family education and follow-up

Source: Davidson MB, Schwartz S. Hyperglycemia. In: A Core Curriculum for Diabetes Education: Diabetes and Complications, 5th ed. Franz MJ, ed. Chicago, Ill: American Association of Diabetes Educators; 2003:27-8.

DKA Case—Part 2: Diagnosis and Identification of Precipitating Factors

The holiday commitments GT tried to meet that fall were additional stressors, known to stimulate counterregulatory hormones and hepatic glucose release. With less sleep and poor eating habits, compounded by hyperglycemia from increasingly poorer glycemic control, GT was at risk for an infection.

She began to feel nauseous and noted decreasing energy. While studying for finals with her roommates, GT started to vomit and complained of stomach cramps. Her friends escorted her to the emergency room. The hospital staff suspected DKA when they learned GT had type 1 diabetes and heard about the nausea, vomiting, and abdominal pain, which were signs of ketones in her blood. The result of a fingerstick glucose reading was 350 mg/dL. Urinary ketones were large.

Diagnosis

GT's laboratory work was compatible with DKA diagnosis (see chart listing DKA, HHS, and reference range values):

- Serum glucose was 395 mg/dL
- The test for beta-hydroxybutyric acid confirmed ketosis
- Low serum bicarbonate and arterial pH confirmed acidosis
- Previous lab work had suggested slight anemia, but hemoglobin and hematocrit were now both elevated, as were BUN and creatinine—signs of dehydration

- Increased serum osmolality conveyed the extent to which glucose was elevated and fluids lost
- Sodium was slightly low, potassium slightly high—dehydration caused the potassium number to look higher than it was. Excess loss lowered the actual amount of sodium in the blood. In addition, high glucoses caused factitious lowering in the sodium level

Identification of Precipitating Cause

To look for the precipitating cause of DKA, cultures were obtained of GT's blood and urine, as was a pregnancy test. GT's blood glucose had probably been running higher than usual for several weeks as she became increasingly less focused on her diabetes self-management. The diet soda was less hydrating than the water she usually chose to drink, and with decreasing fluid intake accompanying diuresis from hyperglycemia, GT's fluid deficit was increasingly larger over time. The hormonal changes of increasing estrogen (accompanying menses) and the stress of incident infection quickly elevated blood glucose and precipitated ketone production.

GT's Lab Values: Comparing Diabetic Ketoacidosis and Hyperosmolar Hyperglycemic State With Reference Range

Test	*Reference Range**	*DKA*†	*HHS*†
Serum glucose (mg/dL)	70–40	>250	>600
Serum osmolality (mOsm/kg)	275–295	>320	>320
Sodium bicarbonate (mEq/L)	22–26	<15	>15
Arterial pH	7.36–7.44	<7.2	>7.3
Serum beta-hydroxybutyrate (mmol/L)	0.02–0.27	>1.1 mmol/L	
Ketones	absent	moderate to high	absent to small
Increases Due to Dehydration			
BUN (mg/dL)	5–20	32	61
Serum creatinine (mg/dL)	0.17–.093	1.1	1.4
Losses Often Masked by Dehydration			
Serum potassium (mmol/L)	3.5–5.0	4.5	3.9
Serum sodium (mmol/L)	135–145	134	149
Serum phosphorus (mg/dL)	2.3–4.3		

*Reference ranges from Bakerman S. Bakerman's ABC's of Interpretive Laboratory Data. Scottsdale, Ariz: Interpretive Laboratory Data, Inc.: 2002.

†Nugent BW. Hyperosmolar hyperglycemic state. Emerg Med Clin North Am. 2005:Aug 23(3):629-48.

Goal 1: Provide Adequate Fluids to Rehydrate

Begin fluid replacement. In all cases, adequate fluid replacement is critical to maintain circulation, expand volume, and restore renal perfusion.[1]

Initial Fluid Replacement

Initiate rapid administration of saline and reduce rate after first hour. Initial fluid replacement uses one-half normal (0.45%) or normal (0.9%) saline, depending on serum sodium and state of hydration. Avoid changes in osmolality by more than 3 mOsm per kilogram per hour.

- *For adults.* The average adult requires 1 to 2 L in the first hour, after which the patient's status is reassessed.[1,8,11]
- *For children.* Deliver 10 to 20 mL per kilogram of body weight in the first hour. If no urination occurs, continue giving 20 mL per kilogram of body weight of fluid during the second and third hours.

Subsequent Fluid Replacement

The level of fluid replacement is monitored and adjusted based on maintenance needs, replacement requirements, and ongoing losses. The rate is adjusted to avoid fluid overload for renal and cardiac patients.

- Hyperglycemia will persist (even with appropriate insulin therapy) if fluid replacement is inadequate.
- Hydration status should typically correct within 48 hours. Several hours of hydration may be necessary before some patients will be able produce urine. If there is no urine flow after 4 hours of appropriate hydration, bladder catheterization may be warranted.

Goal 2: Provide Adequate Insulin to Restore and Maintain Normal Glucose Metabolism

All patients with DKA need insulin. Regular insulin by continuous intravenous infusion is the treatment of choice.[2]

- *Insulin Type:* Regular or rapid-acting insulin offers relatively fast results in reducing glucose levels.
- *Delivery Method:* Insulin delivery via intravenous rather than injections offers these advantages: (1) more predictable decreases in glucose and (2) reduced risk of cerebral edema.
- *Pediatrics:* Rapid-acting insulin delivered via subcutaneous injections may be a cost-effective way to treat DKA in a pediatric population without admission to the hospital.[13] Target decreases in plasma glucose of 50 to 75 mg/dL per hour.

Goal 3: Correct Electrolyte Deficits and Acidosis If Needed

Potassium

Total body potassium depletion is associated with DKA. All patients with urine flow eventually need potassium repletion to avoid hypokalemia. Hypokalemia, if not treated properly, can lead to death. Prolonged hyperglycemia will be blunted in the setting of hypokalemia.

- The patient is observed closely for clinically significant signs of potential hypokalemia such as cardiac arrhythmias; serum potassium is checked periodically (ie, every 2 to 4 hours until level stable or glucose stable).
- Once urine output is documented, depending on the serum potassium level, 20 to 30 mEq of potassium per liter of fluid to be infused is added.[3]

Serum potassium concentration is frequently monitored, as it is essential to guide therapy. Serum potassium concentrations can drop rapidly from the initial results obtained before therapy. With increased hydration, the intravascular volume expands and renal perfusion increases renal excretion of potassium. With insulin administration, more potassium enters the cells contributing to a drop in serum potassium while restoring total body potassium.

Phosphate

Serum phosphate (PO_4) levels are monitored. Research does not support routine supplementation with phosphate, as oral intake of food can promptly replace deficits.

Acidosis

Adequate insulin is continued to resolve acidosis. Acidosis takes longer to reverse than does hyperglycemia treated with insulin. The time required to resolve acidosis has not been well studied because the serial pH measurements necessary to measure acidosis have not been done.

Sodium Bicarbonate

Treating acidosis with sodium bicarbonate ($NaHCO_3$) is controversial. It may be appropriate in special circumstances (as with acute cardiorespiratory arrest or hyperkalemia-induced cardiac arrhythmias). Caution is warranted for the following reasons:

- No clinical benefit has been documented
- Sodium bicarbonate increases risk for hypokalemic-induced arrhythmias because it causes potassium levels to drop so quickly
- There is some evidence that bicarbonate increases risk for cerebral edema[11]

Hyperchloremic Acidosis

Expect hyperchloremic acidosis following DKA to be transient and require no treatment.[1] In hyperchloremic acidosis, bicarbonate levels plateau at approximately 15 to 20 mEq/L (15 to 20 mmol/L), usually between 12 to 24 hours after treatment began. At this time, chloride levels remain elevated, pH has returned to normal, and serum ketone bodies have dropped to low or absent.

Goal 4: Provide Source of Glucose When Needed

- When glucose reaches 250 mg/dL, 5% to 10% dextrose is added to the intravenous solution.[9] Starvation perpetuates ketosis. In addition, sudden drops in glucose can be associated with cerebral edema.

- Ketones are monitored. Ketosis is usually reversed in 12 to 24 hours, although occasionally urinary ketone bodies may be present for several days. If ketones persist, adequacy of dietary intake is evaluated.

Goal 5: Prevent Complications

Hypoglycemia, hypokalemia, and hyperglycemia are frequent complications of overzealous treatment with insulin, use of bicarbonate, or inadequate insulin delivery during the transition from intravenous to subcutaneous administration. A 2-hour overlap between infused insulin and initiation of subcutaneous insulin helps avoid gaps in insulin delivery.

Delay in diagnosis and misdiagnosis adds to severity:

Identification and treatment of the initial cause of hyperglycemia as well as early intervention substantially improve clinical outcomes following DKA.

Two common errors—delay in diagnosis and misdiagnosis—delay treatment and make the consequences of DKA worse than they need to be. The longer treatment is delayed, the more severe the DKA episode and the more complex the treatment. DKA is often misdiagnosed as gastroenteritis or appendicitis. Hypokalemia and cerebral edema may also go unrecognized, causing critical delays in beginning appropriate therapy for these conditions.

Most deaths occur in older patients with medical complications other than DKA.[11] Older age and depth of coma predict mortality risk. Death is usually due to infection, arterial thrombosis, shock, or an unrecognized precipitating event that is not treated adequately. Complications such as aspiration and pulmonary edema may occur even in the most rigorously controlled treatment environment.

Cerebral Edema. Cerebral edema occurs rarely and is more common in children with DKA. It occurs early in the course of treatment, typically in the first 24 hours and usually in the first 12 hours of treatment. The following help minimize the risks for this complication:

- Assess mental status frequently (every 1 to 2 hours), especially in children, who are more susceptible to cerebral edema than adults.
- Monitor for headache, lethargy, and mental status changes, all are symptoms of cerebral edema.
- Suspect cerebral edema if improvement in lethargy and mental function is followed by deterioration, while metabolic status continues to improve and normalize.
- Avoid rapid drops in blood glucose, which may be a factor in the development of cerebral edema. To moderate the rate of glucose drop, add intravenous glucose to the regimen as the serum glucose level reaches about 250 mg/dL.
- If cerebral edema does occur, include IV osmotic diuretics (mannitol) and possibly high-dose glucocorticoids (dexamethasone) in the treatment.

The earlier the treatment, the better the prognosis. Treatment of cerebral edema at early stages may be beneficial, but is usually ineffective at later stages. Once clinical symptoms (seizures, incontinence, bradycardia, respiratory arrest) appear, mortality rate is >70% with only 7% to 14% recovering completely.[6]

Goal 6: Provide Patient and Family Education and Follow-up

After an episode of DKA, patients and their families may be more receptive to learning how they might avoid a repeat hospitalization. A multidisciplinary team approach, including psychosocial intervention, may be needed to address concerns of patients with recurrent episodes of DKA. See the earlier section on prevention of DKA and also the section on questions and controversies at the end of this chapter.

Self-Care Behaviors in the Prevention of Severe Hyperglycemia

The AADE 7 Self-Care Behaviors™ provide a framework for prevention of severe hyperglycemia. Table 8.3 demonstrates how the AADE 7 Self-Care Behaviors™ can be used in the prevention of DKA. More detail on fostering specific self-care behaviors is provided in the chapters in section 3 of this book.

Treating Mild DKA

Some milder cases of DKA can be treated at home without hospitalization or an emergency room visit.[14] The following are parameters:

- The patient can still drink and retain oral fluids without difficulty, and
- The patient or patient's family can provide accurate blood glucose values and results of urine ketone tests, and
- A knowledgeable healthcare professional is available to guide therapy over the phone.

DKA Case—Part 3: Treatment, Including Education Components

Before the laboratory results were back, the medical staff started an IV of normal saline to replace GT's fluids. Then, they added regular insulin at the recommended dose (0.1 units per kilogram per hour) to slowly lower blood glucose. Glucose and insulin doses were routinely entered into a flow sheet in her medical record.

- After 1 hour, glucose was 260 mg/dL. Because this drop exceeded the target rate for lowering glucose, the physician reduced the insulin drip to 0.08 units per kilogram per hour. GT provided blood for another set of labs: glucose, sodium, potassium, and phosphorus.
- When the second set of lab results came back, glucose was down to 248 mg/dL. Other results were potassium 3.9 mEq/L, sodium 135 mEq/L, and phosphate 2.5 mg/dL. The rate of IV insulin was maintained. Potassium was already being supplemented, and the lab finding was in the reference range. However, potassium would drop further as her glucose level fell and took potassium with it back into cells. Additional potassium was added as potassium phosphate.
- After another hour, glucose was 214 mg/dL and urine ketones were moderate. Glucose was added to GT's IV.
- The next day, GT's labs were much improved. Electrolytes were within the reference range, glucose ranged from 150 to 220 mg/dL, and ketones were small.

As GT chatted with her nurse, she began to see what had happened in the days leading to this DKA episode. In retrospect, she could see how little by little, meals had became erratic, replaced with caffeine to help keep her going, and insulin doses had been missed. GT had not realized her growing fatigue probably reflected her climbing glucose levels—something she would have known if she had continued to test regularly. The two reviewed sick day guidelines and reviewed why GT's body required insulin even when she was not eating as much as usual. The office provided sample strips to support her blood glucose testing at home until the mail-order strips arrived and a new prescription for ketone test strips was filled.

The review of sick day management principles helped GT. If GT checked and found her blood glucose over 250 mg/dL, she would do a urine test for ketones. If ketones were positive, she could take her usual supplemental insulin dose to lower glucose. Because ketones increase insulin resistance, to effectively lower blood glucose GT would need to take more supplemental insulin than usual. That information made more sense now. The first time she had heard it, GT had believed DKA would never happen to her; she now knew better.

TABLE 8.3 Applying Self-Care Behaviors to Prevention of Diabetic Ketoacidosis

AADE 7 Self-Care Behaviors™	*Concept*	*Application*
Being Active	Being safely active: • Exercising without adequate insulin can dangerously elevate blood glucose (BG). • Maintaining hydration is also important.	• If glucose before exercise is high (>250 mg/dL), check for ketones. Presence of ketones indicates glucose is high due to inadequate insulin. Do not exercise until ketones are gone. • To compensate for fluids lost during physical activity, drink adequately before, during, and after, especially on hot days.
Healthy Eating	• Matching premeal insulin and carbohydrate to manage glucose levels. • Having sick day plan and supplies (food and fluids).	Identify acceptable, easy-to-digest foods for sick days. Avoid an extreme carbohydrate load with a large volume of sweetened beverages.

TABLE 8.3 Applying Self-Care Behaviors to Prevention of Diabetic Ketoacidosis

AADE 7 Self-Care Behaviors™	*Concept*	*Application*
Taking Medication	Exogenous insulin is essential to life for people with type 1 diabetes. Taking the right insulin in the right amount at the right time helps prevent very high BG. Other drugs may help improve/stabilize glucose.	• Inadequate insulin dosing or poor timing of insulin action increases the risk for DKA. Omitting insulin almost guarantees it. To reduce risks for acute hyperglycemia, understand how insulin works and maintain the skills needed to take it appropriately. Everyone with type 1 diabetes needs this understanding.
Monitoring	Monitoring BG and ketone levels provides feedback about the treatment plan and early warning of impending DKA.	• Monitor regularly to help identify hyperglycemia before it becomes life threatening and enable early intervention and progress assessment. • Increase monitoring frequency when not eating or ill. • Do not rely strictly on "how you feel"—this has been shown to be an inaccurate measure of BG values. Monitor to obtain accurate BG levels. • Access to monitoring supplies may be a barrier to self-monitoring of BG. Address issues of concern. • Assess problems with monitoring. Resistance to monitoring may have multiple causes.
Problem Solving	Applying information to individual situations so information already learned helps solve problems—avoiding initial events as well as recurrence.	• Review the circumstances preceding a DKA episode. Identify precipitating factors to obtain clues to prevent another episode. Questions to reduce risk may relate to delaying exercise, limiting carbohydrate intake, monitoring blood glucose, or adjusting medication. • Review factors contributing to DKA and learn to recognize signs and symptoms to prevent recurrence.
Reducing Risks	Reducing the risk as well as the impact of DKA is possible. Unlike most diabetes management decisions, reducing complications from DKA treatment is primarily a provider responsibility.	• Delayed treatment, excessive insulin, and inadequate insulin are common complications of treating DKA. Reduce complications with prompt diagnosis, adjusting insulin to glucose response, and beginning injected insulin before stopping IV. • Discuss sick days—interventions for nausea, fever, loss of appetite; correction factors for hyperglycemia and further corrections for ketones; when to seek medical care and after-hours procedures.
Healthy Coping	Eating well, taking medications, testing BG, and using results to problem-solve are difficult, never-ending aspects of self-management.	• Use information, support, and encouragement to help lower the barriers that interfere with optimal prevention of DKA. Acknowledge the inevitable struggle that is part of living with diabetes to lighten the load. • Discuss growth and hormonal spurts. • Discuss inattention to signs and distractions of life. • Identify resources and situations in which to seek medical attention.

Note: See also the chapters on each behavior in section 3 of this book.

Attention to physical symptoms, timely monitoring, and ability to adjust insulin all contribute to reducing the incidence and severity of DKA. Treatment at this stage can focus on oral hydration and supplemental insulin.

Oral Hydration

Provide 3 to 5 oz sugar-containing fluids per hour. The amount may be better tolerated if offered in smaller doses every 20 to 30 minutes (or at every television commercial). Broths containing sodium may be more efficacious if there are no contraindications (congestive heart failure, hypertension).

Adequate Insulin to Restore and Maintain Normal Glucose Metabolism

Provide supplemental insulin to compensate for hyperglycemia and for ketosis in addition to usual insulin. The amount needed depends on the patient's known sensitivity to insulin and current level of ketosis.

- *For Children.* 0.25 to 0.5 units per kilogram of regular insulin every 4 to 6 hours, or rapid-acting insulin every 3 to 4 hours as needed.[1]
- *For Adults.* 4 to 10 units or 10% to 20% of the usual total daily dose. Monitor frequently and adjust insulin for slow drop in glucose and resolution of ketosis.

Treatment of DKA depends on the severity of the episode, the abilities of the person with diabetes, and access to competent support. When someone with diabetes successfully treats mild DKA at home, clinical follow-up is still appropriate to reinforce information and support efforts to prevent DKA.

Hyperosmolar Hyperglycemic Nonketotic Syndrome

A blood glucose level greater than 600 mg/dL without significant ketones characterizes hyperosmolar hyperglycemic state (HHS).[13] HHS can occur whether or not diabetes medications are part of usual treatment.[13] Elevated blood glucose can escalate for days before it becomes a serious, acute threat.

In HHS, extreme dehydration is the primary precipitating factor:

Extreme dehydration, more than profound insulin deficiency, is the primary precipitating factor. Profound dehydration, with subsequent hyperosmolarity and electrolyte losses, compounds the seriousness of this acute complication. HHS occurs most frequently in undiagnosed or older adults with type 2 diabetes, but also occurs in children and in people with type 1 diabetes. In 30% to 40% of HHS cases, HHS is the initial presentation of type 2 diabetes. While about 25% of new pediatric cases present with DKA, an estimated 4% of newly diagnosed children present with symptoms of HHS.[12]

Because HHS develops slowly (average 12 days) and does not cause the gastrointestinal pain associated with DKA, it is often overlooked or misdiagnosed.[15] Lack of treatment prolongs the osmotic diuresis secondary to hyperglycemia and worsens the clinical outlook. Due to delayed treatment as well as other medical conditions common in an older population, the mortality rate is about 15%, higher than the rate for DKA.

Pathophysiology of HHS

HHS is similar to DKA except that insulin deficiency is less profound and dehydration plays a much more significant role. When blood glucose levels exceed 180 mg/dL, the kidneys are no longer able to reabsorb glucose. The concomitant renal water loss reduces renal perfusion and further dehydration. The water loss and concomitant inability to make up this water loss with oral intake causes the more extreme levels of hyperglycemia and osmolarity in HHS than those found with DKA. The alterations in consciousness seen with HHS and the risk for morbidity are related to the degree of osmolarity.

Without significant ketone formation, related symptoms typical of DKA like ketosis, acidosis, gastrointestinal discomfort, and Kussmaul respirations do not occur. Without the physical discomfort of ketosis, patients and their caregivers do not recognize a problem and the need for medical care. The mutual exacerbation of hyperglycemia and dehydration can begin with either problem (elevated glucose or inadequate fluids) and steadily escalate.

Precipitating Situations

Elevated Blood Glucose

Anything that elevates blood glucose or reduces hydration can contribute to development of HHS. For example:

- New onset type 2 diabetes
- Infection—a precipitating factor in 60% of cases[16]
- Surgery
- Myocardial infarction
- Gastrointestinal hemorrhage
- Uremia
- Arterial thrombosis
- Pancreatitis
- CVA
- Pulmonary embolism
- Medications that impact carbohydrate metabolism such as glucocorticoids, thiazides, phenytoin, and β-blockers

Decreased Water Intake and Access to Fluids

- Osmotic diuresis due to hyperglycemia—this is primary
- Fever
- Severe burns
- Diarrhea
- Peritoneal and hemodialysis
- Diuretic medications
- Hypertonic feeding
- Impaired thirst mechanism
- Inability to replace fluids may initiate dehydration

Particularly vulnerable are elderly people who must depend on others for their daily care (as in a hospital or nursing facility) and have difficulty communicating. Older people with impaired thirst who live alone may drink little unless prompted in some way. There are many opportunities to disrupt the development of HHS with regular monitoring and attention to those at risk.

Maintaining Adequate Fluids

Emphasize avoiding becoming dehydrated. Situations that warrant extra care include physical activity, illness, institutionalized care settings (hospital, long-term care), forgetfulness, and aversion to drinking water or other hydrating fluids.

Assessing Hyperglycemia

Hyperosmolar Hyperglycemic State: Signs, Symptoms, and Laboratory Indicators

The signs and symptoms of HHS are similar to DKA, with some important exceptions.

Case in Point: HHS in an Elderly Man With Type 2 Diabetes

Early in October, GT's Grandpa Joe had fallen and broken his hip while shopping. GT understood that the surgery had gone smoothly and that Grandpa was making reasonable progress with physical therapy, but Grandma said he seemed a bit confused and slept more and more during the day. Before the fall, Grandpa had been active despite a little arthritis. He had managed his type 2 diabetes with a careful eye on what he ate and had kept his A1C less than 6%. After his fall, Joe needed the help of a long-term care setting. His doctor saw no reason for Grandpa to check his own blood glucose at home, like his granddaughter with "the serious kind" of diabetes needed to do.

GT delayed her trip to visit her grandparents in Maine until after Christmas. Grandpa Joe was still in the nursing home so she took a cab straight there after her flight. Both grandparents welcomed her warmly and wanted to hear more about her DKA episode. As she talked, she noticed Grandpa nodding off or jumping into the conversation with comments about his "54 Chevy." Grandma was cheery but her face signaled her worry about Grandpa's slow recovery. GT was now setting a timer on her watch to let her know when it was time to check an after-meal blood glucose. She went ahead and did the test, explaining what she was doing and learning to her grandparents, who had not previously seen a home glucose monitor.

Grandma thought it would be a wonderful idea if GT checked Grandpa's blood glucose. After some minor protests and without a thought to nursing home protocol, GT got Grandpa's cooperation to poke his finger and test a drop of blood. They were all flabbergasted when the result read "high," meaning the glucose level was too high for the meter to read it. They called the nurse to double-check that number.

Precipitating Events

It is not unusual for the stress of surgery to elevate glucose levels. As is typical, Grandpa had little appetite after surgery so his losing a little weight did not alarm anyone. In fact, he had begun to eat a little more with Grandma there with him for most meals. What no one noticed was that Grandpa was not drinking. He ate rather than drank his calories at meals and left the containers of water on his bedside table untouched as he slept most of the day.

Slowly, Grandpa became more and more dehydrated, concentrating glucose and further increasing hyperglycemia. Without pain, Grandma and the nursing home staff did not perceive a problem to address.

The primary markers of HHS are these:

- Severe hyperglycemia
- Profound dehydration
- Neurologic changes
- Absence of significant ketosis

Severe Hyperglycemia. Blood glucose levels in HHS are greater than 600 mg/dL. The reported mean glucose is greater than 1000 mg/dL, with elevations as high as 1500 mg/dL due to the extreme concentration of intravascular fluids.[16]

Profound Dehydration. Profound dehydration is marked by plasma osmolality greater than 320 mOsm per kilogram. Deficits of 20% to 25% of total body water or 12% to 15% of body weight may be observed. Physical symptoms include dry mucous membranes, poor skin turgor, and sunken eyes. Weakness, anorexia, leg cramps, dizziness, lethargy, and confusion may be signs of worsening hydration status. Coma affects about 20% of cases.[16]

Electrolyte losses of sodium, potassium, phosphorus, and magnesium accompany fluid losses. Sodium and potassium losses usually require supplementation but due to their concentration from dehydration, laboratory results may initially appear high and do not represent actual status. BUN, serum creatinine, hematocrit, and many other routine blood chemistry levels may appear high, but will resolve without treatment following hydration. Persistent elevations in BUN signal follow-up evaluation of renal function, and normal hematocrit when dehydrated is likely to indicate anemia. Access to medical history and information regarding usual lab results helps the provider focus on the most relevant parameters.

Neurologic Changes. The neurologic changes of decreased mentation (eg, lethargy and mild confusion) are more common in HHS than in DKA and the result of extreme dehydration. Patients with HHS may have focal neurological signs (hemisensory deficits, hemiparesis, aphasia, and seizures) that mimic a CVA. These signs will reverse completely as biochemical status returns to normal. As in DKA, decreases in mentation best correlate with serum osmolality.

Absence of Significant Ketosis. Ketone bodies are not present in significant quantities. Starvation and dehydration may elevate serum ketones slightly. If present, gastrointestinal symptoms are usually milder than those found in DKA, and Kussmaul respirations are rare. Arterial pH greater than 7.3 mm Hg and bicarbonate level greater than 15 mEq/L are typical of HHS.

Other Tests

Other tests are necessary to determine the precipitating cause of HHS:

- Cultures of blood, urine, and sputum
- Chest X-ray
- EKG

An EKG is used to assess cardiac status in a population at risk for cardiac complications as well as to quickly evaluate potassium status. Serial EKGs can monitor and guide potassium replacement therapy.

Treatment of Hyperosmolar Hyperglycemic State

HHS requires hospitalization for appropriate and effective treatment. Treatment goals for HHS are similar to those for DKA. Table 8.4 lists treatment goals for HHS. Each is discussed separately below.

Goal 1: Provide Adequate Fluids to Rehydrate

The cornerstone of treatment of HHS is to expand intravascular volume and restore renal perfusion. A guideline for fluid replacement is to infuse half of the fluid deficit over the first 12 hours and the remainder during the following 12 to 24 hours. Glucose levels may drop as much as 80 to 200 mg/dL per hour from rehydration alone.[16]

- *Elderly.* Particularly with an elderly person, care must be taken to adjust the hydration rate to the patient's individual needs and consider the person's current hydration, cardiovascular, and renal status.

TABLE 8.4 Treatment Goals for Hyperosmolar Hyperglycemic State
1. Provide adequate fluids to rehydrate
2. Correct electrolyte deficits
3. Provide adequate insulin to restore and maintain normal glucose metabolism
4. Prevent complications
5. Treat underlying medical condition
6. Provide patient and family education and follow-up

Source: Davidson MB, Schwartz S. Hyperglycemia. In: A Core Curriculum for Diabetes Education: Diabetes and Complications, 5th ed. Franz MJ, ed. Chicago, Ill: American Association of Diabetes Educators; 2003:33-6.

- *Renal Insufficiency.* For people with renal insufficiency, restoring blood flow is critical, but especially for older patients with compromised cardiovascular status, fluid loss must be replaced with saline slowly and cautiously to avoid fluid overload and congestive heart failure.
- *Cardiovascular Disease.* Patients with a previous history of cardiovascular disease must be monitored by central venous pressure or Swan-Ganz catheter.

Goal 2: Correct Electrolyte Deficits

Laboratory tests provide critical information to guide replacement decisions for electrolytes.

Potassium

The EKG provides immediate feedback regarding potassium status. Potassium replacement is similar to that required for DKA even though losses tend to be greater. However, insulin therapy needs to be withheld if initial laboratory results are less than 3.3 mEq/L, indicating profound deficiency. Potassium supplementation begins once renal function is known to be normal.

Sodium

Sodium levels can be falsely low in HHS from extreme glucose concentration. The following correction provides a more accurate assessment of hydration status. Note that if the corrected sodium is high, dehydration is extreme.

$$\text{Correct (Na)} = 1.6 \times (\text{glucose} - 100)/100$$

Phosphorus and Magnesium

Phosphorus and magnesium laboratory readings may come back high or normal, indicating some losses with dehydration, but the levels tend to normalize without replacement therapy.

Routine Blood Work

Routine blood work is similarly elevated with dehydration. Monitor and reassess metabolic status after hydration.

Goal 3: Provide Adequate Insulin to Restore and Maintain Normal Glucose Metabolism

Hydration is essential to lower glucose levels. Following hydration, insulin administration is usually but not always required to restore normal glycemia.

- *Insulin.* Treatment of acidosis is not a part of HHS, so insulin requirements are typically not as high as for DKA. Infuse insulin separately. Once insulin is started, do not interrupt delivery until hyperglycemia is adequately resolved.
- *Serum Glucose.* Expect serum glucose to fall 50 to 75 but less than 100 mg/dL per hour. If serum glucose falls less than 50 mg/dL, consider whether to add or increase insulin and increase hydration. When glucose values reach acceptable levels (~300 mg/dL), reduce insulin and add 5% dextrose to infusion.[13] Monitor glucose hourly.

Goal 4: Prevent Complications

- Monitor frequently for blood pressure, fluid, electrolyte, and glucose levels.
- Watch for complications of underlying atherosclerosis and consider low-dose heparin for at-risk individuals.
- Once insulin is started, do not interrupt delivery until euglycemia is assured.
- Hypoglycemia is unlikely.
- Pay attention to goal 5.

Goal 5: Treat Any Underlying Medical Condition

Treatment of the underlying medical condition(s) is critical to resolving HHS. In an elderly population, potential contributors to HHS are multiple and require thorough exploration and follow-up. It is difficult to prevent excessive fluid losses or control hyperglycemia without identifying the source of the problem.

Goal 6: Provide Patient and Family Education and Follow-Up

The risks for HHS include inadequate fluid intake, excessive fluid losses, and prolonged hyperglycemia. The tools to prevent or at least moderate the devastating impact of HHS are not complicated, but they require understanding and attention to daily habits. Regularly monitoring blood glucose and promptly treating mild hyperglycemia can interrupt the cycle leading to HHS before it is much of a problem.

Self-Care Behaviors in the Prevention of HHS

The AADE 7 Self-Care Behaviors™ provide a framework for prevention of HHS. Table 8.5 demonstrates how the

TABLE 8.5 Applying Self-Care Behaviors for Prevention of Hyperosmolar Hypoglycemic State

AADE 7 Self-Care Behaviors™	*Concept*	*Application*
Being Active	Activity continues to lower insulin resistance and improve blood glucose (BG) levels. • Be safely active at all ages. • Maintain adequate hydration.	To compensate for fluids lost during physical activity, drink adequately before, during, and after, especially on hot days.
Healthy Eating	• Matching timing of food with medication activity. • Having sick day plan and supplies (food and fluids).	To avoid high BG, do not consume extra carbohydrate without taking extra insulin. It is easy to consume extra carbohydrate with liquids. A large soft drink at a fast-food restaurant offers as much carbohydrate as 5 slices of bread.
Taking Medications	If glucose goals are not met with activity and meal planning, medication is necessary.	Inadequate levels of diabetes medication, especially reluctance to initiate insulin when needed, significantly contributes to high glucose levels.
Monitoring - Blood Glucose	Monitoring provides feedback about the treatment plan and warning of impending hyperosmolar hyperglycemic state.	• Monitor regularly to help identify hyperglycemia before it becomes life threatening; this is true even for those not treated with medication, especially during illness or other stress. Monitoring allows early intervention and progress assessment. • Discuss usual monitoring routine and what to do when not eating or ill. • Do not rely strictly on "how you feel"—this has been shown to be an inaccurate measure of BG values. Monitor to obtain an accurate BG level. • Access to monitoring supplies may present a barrier to self-monitoring of BG. Address issues of concern. • Assess problems with monitoring. Resistance to monitoring may have multiple causes.
Problem Solving	Applying information already learned to individual situations helps solve problems.	• Review the circumstances preceding the HHS episode to look for clues to prevent another. Would a system for drinking fluids, monitoring blood glucose, or a change in medication have reduced the risk? • To prevent recurrence, review signs, symptoms, and treatment.
Reducing Risks	Reducing the risk as well as the impact of HHS is possible. HHS also increases risks for many concomitant conditions.	• As HHS usually occurs in an older, more vulnerable population, individualize and carefully monitor therapy for these persons to help prevent complications. • Discuss sick days—interventions for nausea, fever, loss of appetite; correction factors for hyperglycemia; when to seek medical care and after-hours procedures.
Healthy Coping	Eating well, taking medications, testing blood glucose, and using the results to problem solve are difficult, never-ending aspects of self-management.	• Use information, support, and encouragement for caregivers as well as patients to help prevent HHS. • Identify resources and situations in which to seek medical attention.

Note: See also the chapters on each behavior in section 3 of this book.

AADE 7 Self-Care Behaviors™ can be used in the prevention of HHS. For more detail on fostering specific self-care behaviors, see appropriate chapters in section 3 of this book. Most essentially, educators can assist individuals in avoiding HHS by encouraging hydration and identifying individuals at high risk.

Encourage Hydration

Encourage adequate hydration for everyone with diabetes. Many will need frequent reminders and suggestions for specific ways to include more fluids before they will be able to do so.

- *Living Alone.* Individuals who live alone may require help devising a system for remembering to drink fluids, such as keeping fluids within reach or offering them every 2 hours.
- *Dependent on Others.* Intake of adequate fluids can be a special challenge when the individual is dependent on others (for example, older adults in a hospital or nursing home and those who cannot communicate a request for water). These individuals depend on the institution to monitor fluid intake, evaluate fluid status, and establish a plan that keeps residents adequately hydrated.

Identify High Risk

Identify high-risk individuals and when dealing with them, put special emphasis on the basics. Examples are the elderly in nursing homes, hospitals, or other settings where dehydration may not be noticed and persons being treated with glucocorticoids or other medications that may precipitate hyperglycemia. Offer information to both the person with diabetes and the person's family and caregivers. Be sure they have the opportunity to understand the rationale for and have the supplies necessary to accomplish the following:

- Obtain adequate fluids
- Monitor blood glucose regularly
- Manage sick days that may include fever and vomiting
- Keep sick day supplies on hand and accessible (eg, thermometer, acceptable and easy-to-eat food and drink, contact numbers for physician and urgent care services)
- Know the signs and symptoms of HHS and the critical need for medical attention should they appear
- Know how and when to contact their healthcare provider

Identify Vulnerabilities

Help individuals, especially those at high risk, understand the problems that may occur, signs and symptoms, precipitating factors, and appropriate actions. Provide education to help prevent DKA and HHS.

HS Case—Part 2: Diagnosis and Treatment

Soon after the nurse took another fingerstick blood glucose that was "high," the physician arrived to examine Grandpa. The physician could tell from looking at Grandpa's skin that he was dehydrated. The physician quickly ordered lab work and had the staff start an IV of normal saline, just as someone had done for GT a few weeks ago; however, for Grandpa, the rate was slower. The physician explained that in a person her Grandpa's age, the lab results needed to be examined to be sure Grandpa's heart and kidneys could tolerate a higher infusion rate. The physician also did not start insulin, but told GT and Grandma that because Grandpa Joe's blood was so concentrated, just adding fluids could lower his blood glucose.

- Initial lab results were glucose 699 mg/dL, potassium 3.9 mEq/L, phosphorus 3.3 mmol/L, and serum osmolality 340 mOsm/kg.
- An hour later, glucose was 652 mg/dL, potassium 3.8 mEq/L, and serum osmolality 337 mOsm/kg. Serum osmolality had fallen the maximum 3 mOsm/kg, so the normal saline remained at the slower rate. However, as glucose was still quite elevated, insulin infusion was started.
- It was the better part of a week before Grandpa Joe began acting like his old self again. Because the A1C in Grandpa's chart was in the normal range, the hospital staff unfortunately had not monitored his glucose in the hospital.

(continued)

HS Case—Part 2: Diagnosis and Treatment (continued)

With a little persuading from his granddaughter, it was clear Grandpa, too, was going to self-monitor his blood glucose from now on. A dietitian came in to brainstorm options to increase Grandpa's fluid intake. Knowing he did not like the taste of water, the dietitian brought a list of several calorie-free products with a few samples for him to try. The staff at the nursing home also met to discuss ways to improve how they monitor the fluid intake of their patients. Slowly but surely, Grandpa became more alert and eager to complete therapy so he could return home to his own bed and Grandma's cooking.

Case Wrap-Up: DKA and HHS

- Overall, to treat their respective conditions, Grandpa (experiencing HHS) required more fluids and GT (experiencing DKA) required more insulin
- GT needed to test ketones when her blood glucose was high; Grandpa did not
- Both agreed they would put more effort into drinking fluids, regular monitoring, and responding to monitoring results
- Grandma joined them for a class on sick day management and learned how to treat a fever, what to eat when they did not feel like eating, and when to call the doctor

They all left feeling a little more confident they could prevent a repeat of recent experiences.

Case in Point: Preventing Hyperglycemia in an Institutional Care Setting

A skilled-care facility supervisor called for advice regarding a patient with type 2 diabetes of known 16-year duration. JM was an 85-year-old man who had been in the skilled nursing facility after a cerebrovascular accident (CVA) that resulted in some difficulty ambulating unassisted. He appeared fatigued and somewhat lethargic, and the symptoms seemed to have been slowly more perceptible over the past 3 days. There had been no acute change in overall well-being, but the patient just seemed to appear somewhat different than usual. The CVA also left JM with mild dysarthria, which was exacerbated when he was fatigued, making him more difficult to understand. He was seen in his primary care clinic within the last week, and a thiazide was started to target better control of hypertension. The family members who typically visited JM once a week and were very involved with his care had been out of town, so the supervisor was relying on staff reports of patient change. Staff had not been able to speak with family about their observations. That day, there was concern regarding JM's increasing lethargy, and a fingerstick blood glucose of 390 mg/dL was obtained.

Case Wrap-Up

Applying the principles presented in the text of this chapter, hydration would be imperative and then a discussion on the effects of a thiazide, a medication that can potentiate hyperglycemia.[17,18] Many commonly prescribed pharmacologic agents for treatment of diabetes comorbidities such as hypertension and dyslipidemia can potentiate hyperglycemia.[19]

Inadequate access to water or hydrating fluids is a major confounder of hyperglycemia,[20] and neurologic deficits can be a barrier to appropriate fluid intake.[21,22] The recognition of inadequate water intake can be challenging in a skilled care facility.

Additionally, many metabolic disease states common in the older population can be associated with hyperglycemia; in particular, hyperthyroidism,[23] Cushing syndrome,[23] and even hyperparathyroidism[24] can potentiate hyperglycemia that responds to treatment of the specific instigating metabolic problem.[19] Identification of the hyperosmolar nonketotic state early and prompt initiation of treatment is directly associated with survival.[25]

Key Aspects of Treatment, Prevention, and Education

Treatment

- *Why infuse dextrose when blood glucose is 250 mg/dL?*
  To prevent cerebral edema
- *Why not give insulin when blood glucose is 1000 mg/dL?*
  Insulin increases the risk of further lowering potassium, and the potassium is already low at <3.3 mmol/L
- *How to adjust sodium for elevated glucose:*
  To correct for dilution from glucose when concentration is very high:[16]

  Correct (Na) = 1.6 × (glucose -100)/100

- *Testing for ketones:*
  Measure beta-hydroxybutyrate to evaluate DKA and monitor progress[26]
- *When to consider phosphorus supplementation:*
  To avoid skeletal and cardiac muscle weakness and respiratory depression in patients with cardiac dysfunction, anemia, or respiratory depression if PO_4 <1.0 mg/dL[26]
- *When to consider bicarbonate supplementation:*
  If pH is <6.9, although no research substantiates benefit[26]
- *Ketoacidosis without DKA:*
  Starvation and alcoholic ketoacidosis (AKA)

Educational Topics

For patient:

- Sick day management
- When to call physician
- Medication adjustments during illness
- Need for no-calorie fluids

For family, caregivers, school personnel:

- Recognizing symptoms of hyperglycemia
- Knowing what to do about hyperglycemia

For primary care providers:

- Patient instruction for supplemental insulin during illness
- Who benefits from home blood glucose monitoring

For nursing home/hospital staff, caregivers:

- How to monitor glucose, hydration, and mentation
- How to identify at-risk patients

Prevention

Monitoring supplies:

- How to time monitoring when strips are limited

Hydration:

- Getting fluids when not thirsty and do not like

Questions and Controversy

Intensive Management

New approaches to intensive case management aimed at identifying severe hyperglycemia and managing it earlier are emerging. Telephone care was one aspect of a study examining intensive case management for individuals experiencing recurrent DKA (see chapter 6's discussion of phone-based intervention). Individual institutional procedures, guidelines, and protocols must be in place to prevent mishap and protect the healthcare team providing this service before such an approach can be fully implemented and embraced by the community.

As mentioned earlier in this chapter, when severe hyperglycemia is a recurrent problem, attention needs to be paid to underlying factors, and interventions need to be tailored to the problem. Intensive case management, disease management interventions, and follow-up by phone guided by written protocols may be one solution.[27]

There will continue to be interest in proving the effectiveness (both in terms of cost and quality of life) of case and disease management strategies for recurrent hyperglycemia, as this becomes more costly and time-intensive for the patient and the care provider. "Case management is effective . . . in conjunction with disease management when delivered. . . . With one or more educational, reminder, or support interventions."[28] Patient care and management may be intensified with a number of innovative electronics under study.

Focus on Education: Pearls for Practice

Teaching Strategies

- **Know signs and symptoms.** Diabetes educators should be very familiar with signs and symptoms of impending hyperglycemia so they can recognize it and intervene early.
- **Relate monitoring to prevention.** Teaching the benefits of blood glucose monitoring can often prevent severe hyperglycemia. Monitoring recognizes low as well as high blood glucose. Teach the concept of testing. Teach also that carrying (eating) carbohydrate can often prevent severe hypoglycemia, especially before driving and exercise.
- **Show how planning leads to prevention.** Planning ahead is an important part of preventing hyperglycemia. This includes having proper supplies (blood glucose kit and ketone testing equipment) (and not running out of them), testing and treating with insulin, and calling the healthcare provider.
- **Be alert for issues among adolescents and elderly adults.** Teenagers or young adults with type 1 diabetes who have recurrent DKA may be purposely omitting insulin for weight loss or attention. In elderly adults, underlying illness, the cause of high blood glucose, dehydration, and medication compliance can be a concern. Assess the patient and family for referral for counseling.
- **Identify high-risk situations.** Identify potential high-risk situations, such as the following: young adults going off to college, teenagers beginning to drive, elderly in nursing homes who may become dehydrated, and persons being treated with glucocorticoids or other medications that may precipitate hyperglycemia.
- **Provide a "when to call" list.** Give patients a prepared list of situations on when to call the physician. Include contact information for days, nights, and weekends. This reassures patients' that it is necessary to call if they have concerns and calling is not a bother.
- **Prepare family members.** Educate family members to recognize high-risk situations and intervene early enough to prevent development of severe, life-threatening hyperglycemia.
- **Educate emergency personnel.** Offer a hyperglycemia refresher course to local emergency rooms, hospital floor nurses, paramedics, school nurses, and others. Bring equipment for hands-on blood testing and ketone testing. Reinforce the need for ketone testing equipment in the home for early detection and intervention. For HHS, urge earlier identification by recognizing dehydration status, underlying illness, and potential causes.
- **Offer telephone care for mild DKA.** In some cases in which DKA is mild and recognized early, it can be treated with insulin and oral fluids via telephone consults. Know also when this is not appropriate.
- **Evaluate and reeducate.** Always carefully assess the reasons for a DKA or HHS occurrence so that preventive strategies can be taught and instituted.

Messages for Patients

- **Ensure others understand what puts you at high risk.** Family members and friends need to recognize high-risk situations and be able to respond with early interventions to prevent the development of severe, life-threatening hyperglycemia. Recognizing the underlying cause of high blood glucose, such as illness, bad insulin, or an inadequate insulin amount, is important.
- **Distribute handouts so others can help you.** Provide family, friends, roommates, work, school, and leaders of groups you participate in with information handouts and contact information for emergency medical care. Invite family and close friends to attend education and clinic visits. Teach appropriate people in your life how to test your blood glucose and ketones. Remind these people, especially if you are an older adult, about the importance of getting adequate fluids.

References

1. Davidson MB. Diabetic ketoacidosis and hyperosmolar nonketotic coma. In: Diabetes Mellitus: Diagnosis and Treatment, 4th ed. Davidson MB, ed. New York, NY: WB Saunders Company; 1998:159-94.
2. Tan KC, Mackay IR, Zimmet PZ, et al. Metabolic and immunologic features of Chinese patients with atypical diabetes mellitus. Diabetes Care. 2000;23(3):335-8.
3. Westphal SA. The occurrence of diabetic ketoacidosis in non-insulin-dependent diabetes and newly diagnosed diabetic adult. Am J Med. 1996;101:19-24.
4. Wilson C, Krakoff J, Gohdes D. Ketoacidosis in Apache Indians with non-insulin-dependent diabetes mellitus. Arch Intern Med. 1997;157(18):2098-100.
5. Balasubramanyam A, Zern JW, HYman DJ, et al. New profiles of diabetic ketoacidosis: type 1 vs type 2 diabetes and the effect of ethnicity. Arch Intern Med. 1999;159(19):2317-22.
6. American Diabetes Association. Hyperglycemic crises in patients with diabetes mellitus (position statement). Diabetes Care. 2004;24 Suppl 1:S94-102.
7. McDonnell CM, Pedreira CC, Vadamalayan B, et al. Diabetic ketoacidosis, hyperosmolarity and hypernatremia: are high-carbohydrate drinks worsening initial presentation? Pediatr Diabetes. 2005 Jun;6:90-4.
8. Kershaw MJ, Newton T, Barrett TG, et al. Childhood diabetes presenting with hyperosmolar dehydration but without ketoacidosis: a report of three cases. Diabet Med. 2005;22:645-7.
9. Charfen MA, Fernandez-Frackelton M. Diabetic ketoacidosis. Emerg Med Clin N Am. 2005;23:609-28.
10. Peveler RC, Bryden KS, Neil HA, et al. The relationship of disordered eating habits and attitudes to clinical outcomes in young adult females with type 1 diabetes. Diabetes Care. 2005;28:84-8.
11. Neumark-Sztainer D, Patterson J, Mellin A, et al. Weight control practices and disordered eating behaviors among adolescent females and males with type 1 diabetes. Diabetes Care. 2002;25:1289-96.
12. Agus MS, Wolfsdorf JI. Diabetic ketoacidosis in children. Pediatr Clin North Am. 2005;52:1147-63.
13. Kitabchi AE, Umpierrez GE, Murphy MB, et al. Management of hyperglycemic crises in patients with diabetes mellitus (technical review). Diabetes Care. 2001;224:131-53.
14. Trachtenbarg DE. Diabetic ketoacidosis. Am Fam Physician. 2005;71(9):1705-14.
15. Della MT, Steinmetz L, Campos PR, et al. Subcutaneous use of a fast-acting insulin analog: an alternative treatment for pediatric patients with diabetic ketoacidosis. Diabetes Care. 2005;28:1856-61.
16. Nugent BW. Hyperosmolar hyperglycemic state. Emerg Med Clin N Am. 2005;23:629-48.
17. Bressler P, DeFronzo RA. Drugs and diabetes. Diabetes Rev. 1994;2(1):53-84.
18. Fonseca V, Phear DN. Hyperosmolar non-ketotic diabetic syndrome precipitated by treatment with diuretics. BMJ. 1982;284:36-7.
19. Trence DL, Hirsch IB. Hyperglycemic crises in type 2 diabetes mellitus. Endocrinol and Metab Clin. 2001;30(4):817-31.
20. Ennis ED, Stahl E JVB, Kreisberg RA. The hyperosmolar hyperglycemic syndrome. Diabetes Rev. 1994;2(1):115-26.
21. Lorber D. Non-ketotic hypertonicity in diabetes mellitus. Med Clin North Am. 1995;79:39-52.
22. Maccario M. Neurologic dysfunction associated with nonketotic hyperglycemia. Arch Neurol. 1968;19:525-34.
23. Berelowitz M, Go EH. Non-insulin-dependent diabetes mellitus secondary to other endocrine disorders. In: Diabetes Mellitus. LeRoith D, Taylor SI, Olefsky JM, eds. Philadelphia, Pa: Lippincott-Raven Publishers: 1996:496-502.
24. Akgun S, Ertel NH. Hyperparathyroidism and coexisting diabetes mellitus: altered carbohydrate metabolism. Arch Intern Med. 1978;138(10):1500-2.
25. Wachtel TJ, Silliman Ra, Lamberton P. Predisposing factors for the diabetic hyperosmolar state. Arch Int Med. 1987;147:499-501.
26. American Diabetes Association. Hyperglycemic crises in patients with diabetes mellitus (position statement). Diabetes Care. 2004;24 Suppl 1:S94-102.
27. Weinberger M, Kirkman MS, Samsa GP, et al. A nurse-coordinated intervention for primary care patients with non-insulin-dependent diabetes mellitus: impact on glycemic control and health-related quality of life. J Gen Intern Med. 1995;10:59-66.
28. Norris SL, Nichols, PJ, Caspersen CJ, et al. The effectiveness of disease and case management for people with diabetes: a systematic review. Am J Prev Med. 2002;22(4):15-38.

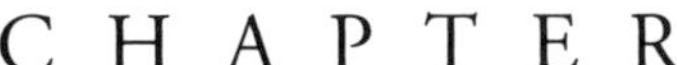

CHAPTER

9

Type 1 Diabetes Throughout the Life Span

Authors

Carolyn Banion, RN, MN, CPNP, CDE
Virginia Valentine, CNS, BC-ADM, CDE

Key Concepts

- Clinical management of diabetes relies on patient and family self-management.
- Diabetes education is an essential and crucial component of the care and management of individuals with type 1 diabetes. Education must be ongoing through the course of the disease.
- There are important differences in the diabetes education and management of children and adolescents versus adults. Learning materials, content, demonstration of skills, and expectations must be appropriate for the age, abilities, and attention span of each child, adult, and family member.
- The primary goals of treatment are achievement of optimal glycemic goals, avoidance of acute and chronic complications, positive psychosocial adjustment to diabetes, and normal growth and development in children.
- To achieve the desired goals of diabetes management, the person with diabetes and the person's family must integrate a comprehensive and rigorous diabetes regimen into their daily lives.
- In caring for children and adolescents with diabetes, healthcare providers need to understand the importance of involving adults in diabetes management for these youths.

Introduction

Type 1 diabetes affects all ages, and management and education is an ongoing process throughout an individual's life span. There are a variety of issues, new situations, and physical and emotional differences that present at distinct ages and life stages. The diabetes educator must appreciate that diabetes self-management education (DSME) in children, adolescents, and adults presents challenges. The goals for treatment are twofold: to promote normal physical and psychological growth and development and to avoid both acute and chronic complications of diabetes. This chapter focuses on DSME in type 1 diabetes throughout the life span. Issues in providing care to children and teens are given primary attention. As appropriate though, throughout the chapter, information pertinent to adults with type 1 diabetes is provided. Transition to adult care and development of type 1 diabetes in adults are addressed at the end of the chapter.

State of the Disease

Type 1 diabetes is an autoimmune disease in which hyperglycemia is secondary to insulin deficiency, which is caused by destruction of pancreatic beta cells. Type 1 diabetes accounts for 5% to 10% of all diagnosed cases of diabetes.[1] Age at diagnosis was the initial classification criteria used to describe what was clearly a distinct form of diabetes. Recent classification systems abandoned both age and treatment as criterion and now attempt to identify etiology of disease to classify different types of diabetes.

Seventy percent of cases of type 1 diabetes are diagnosed before the person reaches 30 years of age, but onset can occur at any age. Type 1 diabetes is one of the most common childhood illnesses and in the United States approximately 1 in every 400 to 500 children and adolescents under 20 years of age has type 1 diabetes.[1] The worldwide prevalence and incidence of type 1 diabetes varies from one geographic location to another, with the highest incidence being in the Scandinavian countries of Sweden, Finland, and Norway and lowest incidence in Japan. Evidence suggests that the incidence of type 1 diabetes is increasing globally at a rate of about 3% per year. In some regions, this increase is reported to be greater in children under the age of 5 years.[2] This trend, it has been speculated, is more likely related to environmental changes, such as exposure to viral infections, than to differences in genetic susceptibility.[3]

The current standards for diabetes management reflect the need to maintain glucose control as near to normal as safely possible in both children and adults. The Diabetes Control and Complications Trial (DCCT) and the follow-up study Epidemiology of Diabetes Interventions and Complications (EDIC) have shown that intensive treatment and the maintenance of glucose concentrations close to the normal range clearly decrease the frequency and severity of the macrovascular and microvascular complications of diabetes.[4,5] These trials have involved adults and only a small cohort of adolescent patients. Since special consideration must be given to the unique differences of children with diabetes, the American Diabetes Association (ADA) has published a statement on standards of care pertaining to children and adolescents with type 1 diabetes.[6] The ideal goal of near-normalization of blood glucose levels may be more difficult to attain in children and adolescents after the honeymoon period, the consequences of hypoglycemic events are distinctly different between adults and children, and the risk for diabetic complications are likely influenced by puberty.[6] The plasma blood glucose and A1C goals for type 1 diabetes in children are shown in Table 9.1 See also the section on type 1 in adults, at the end of this chapter.

TABLE 9.1 Plasma Blood Glucose and A1C Goals for Type 1 Diabetes in Children

	Plasma Blood Glucose Goal Range (mg/dL)			
Values by Age	*Before Meals*	*Bedtime/ Overnight*	*A1C*	*Rationale*
Toddlers and preschoolers (<6 years)	100–180	110–200	<8.5% (but >7.5%)	High risk and vulnerability to hypoglycemia
School age (6–12 years)	90–180	100–180	<8%	Risks of hypoglycemia and relatively low risk of complications prior to puberty
Adolescents and young adults (13–19 years)	90–130	90–150	<7.5%*	Risk of hypoglycemia Developmental and psychological issues
Key Concepts in Setting Glycemic Goals:				
Goals should be individualized and lower goals may be reasonable based on benefit–risk assessment				
Blood glucose goals should be higher than those listed above in children with frequent hypoglycemia or hypoglycemia unawareness				
Postprandial blood glucose values should be measured when there is a disparity between preprandial blood glucose values and A1C levels				

*A lower goal (<7.0%) is reasonable if it can be achieved without excessive hypoglycemia

Source: Copyright © 2005 American Diabetes Association. Modified with permission from the American Diabetes Association. Silverstein J, Klingensmith G, Copeland K, et al. Care of children and adolescents with type 1 diabetes. Diabetes Care. 2005;28:193.

Case in Point: Type 1 Diabetes—Infancy to Young Adulthood

JJ is now a 22-year-old college student who was diagnosed with type 1 diabetes at 9 months of age.

- His diabetes was diagnosed when his parents took him to his primary care physician because he was waking frequently and soaking through many diapers during the night and would drink anything given to him.
- He was hospitalized at a children's hospital in moderate diabetic ketoacidosis (DKA) for metabolic stabilization, initiation of insulin therapy, and education of his family.
- Family history included a maternal aunt with type 1 diabetes, who incidentally had been a subject in the Diabetes Control and Complications Ttrial (DCCT) before JJ's diagnosis.

The case study in this chapter follows a young male from diagnosis at infancy through young adulthood. Issues the boy and his family faced at different stages are highlighted.

Diagnosis

The onset of type 1 diabetes is usually acute, with symptoms ranging from incidental glycosuria to life-threatening DKA. The diagnosis of diabetes in infants is rare, and children less than 4 years of age more often present in DKA than do older children or adults. About 30% of children with new-onset type 1 diabetes present in DKA, requiring intravenous rehydration and insulin.[7] Many require treatment in an intensive care unit. At the time of diagnosis, 80% to 90% of the beta cells have been destroyed. Most children present with complaints of nocturia and enuresis and a several-week history of polyuria, polydipsia, and weight loss. Adults with type 1 diabetes often present with polyphagia, but this is rarely seen in children. Other common symptoms include blurred vision, drowsiness, poor stamina, nausea and vomiting, frequent skin and bladder infections, and vaginitis in females. Laboratory values indicate hyperglycemia, glycosuria, ketonemia, and ketonuria.

Diagnosis of type 1 diabetes in children is usually clear-cut and requires little or no specialized testing. An elevated blood glucose concentration must be documented to diagnose diabetes. The incidental discovery of hyperglycemia in the absence of classic symptoms does not necessarily indicate new-onset diabetes, especially in young children with acute illness.[6]

The criteria for the diagnosis of diabetes are presented in Table 9.2. In the absence of unequivocal hyperglycemia, these criteria should be confirmed by repeat testing on

TABLE 9.2 Diagnosing Type 1 Diabetes

3 Options		
Acute Symptoms[*] Plus Casual[†] Plasma Glucose ≥200 mg/dL (11.1 mmol/L)	**Fasting Plasma Glucose[‡]** ≥126 mg/dL (7.0 mmol/L)	**2-Hour Plasma Glucose** ≥200 mg/dL (11.1 mmol/L) during oral glucose tolerance test (75-g glucose)[§]

Note: Unless unequivocal symptoms of hyperglycemia are present, these criteria must be confirmed by repeat testing on a subsequent day.

[*]Classic symptoms of diabetes include polyuria, polydipsia, and unexplained weight loss.

[†]Casual is defined as any time of day without regard to time since last meal.

[‡]Fasting is defined as no caloric intake for at least 8 hours.

[§]See text for discussion of when the oral glucose tolerance test is appropriate.

Source: Silverstein J, Klingensmith G, Copeland K, et al. Care of children and adolescents with type 1 diabetes: a statement of the American Diabetes Association. Diabetes Care. 2005;28:187.

a different day. The oral glucose tolerance test (OGTT) is not recommended for routine clinical use, but may be required in the evaluation of patients when diabetes is still suspected despite a normal fasting plasma glucose.[8] Glucose tolerance testing is rarely required to diagnose type 1 diabetes, except in atypical cases or very early disease. Because of the risk of rapid clinical deterioration, especially in untreated children with type 1 diabetes, unnecessary delays in the diagnosis must be avoided and a definitive diagnosis should be made promptly.[6]

As the incidence of type 2 diabetes in children and adolescents increases, differentiating newly diagnosed type 1 from type 2 diabetes has become more important. In the slender prepubertal child, type 2 diabetes would be very unlikely. In the overweight adolescent, measurement of islet autoantibodies may be necessary to differentiate the diagnosis. Between 85% to 95% of individuals with type 1 diabetes have circulating antibodies directed against one or more islet cell components. Regardless of the type of diabetes, insulin will be required for the child who presents with significant fasting hyperglycemia, metabolic derangement, and ketonemia.[6]

The diagnosis of diabetes, as in other chronic illnesses, often causes individuals to grieve the loss of their health or parents to grieve the loss of their healthy child. Frequently, parents feel guilty about the diagnosis of diabetes in their child because of the genetic component of the disease. Parents may have numerous unexpressed questions, and they may fear they did something to cause the diabetes.

The diabetes educator can be instrumental in initiating discussion of and normalizing these feelings. Parents and family must be reassured that there is nothing they could have done to prevent the disease and that the combination of genes from both parents increases the risk for type 1 diabetes in their offspring. New technology, medications, and treatment strategies have changed diabetes management dramatically in recent years; explaining this to families is usually reassuring. The parents and family need to understand the difference in pathophysiology and treatment of type 1 and type 2 diabetes. DSME is essential for all individuals with newly diagnosed diabetes. Planning and provision of diabetes education should recognize the following:

- *Infants and Preschoolers.* Education is directed toward the parents and primary caregivers (babysitters, grandparents, older siblings). The tremendous responsibility of care and fear of hypoglycemia are extremely stressful for these families. [9]
- *School-Age Child.* Parents need to assume most of the responsibility, but the child will be able to learn some of the skills needed for self-management.
- *Adolescents.* For most (depending on their cognitive and emotional development), education should be directed primarily toward the adolescent, with parents included.
- *Adults.* Spouses or significant others should also receive self-management education.

Case—Part 2: Provision of Family Education and Support

Once JJ's DKA was treated, the educational process with his family was initiated by a team of healthcare professionals, including a pediatric endocrinologist, diabetes nurse educator, dietitian, and medical social worker. JJ's parents experienced the usual shock, grief, anger, sadness, and denial that most parents do when their child is diagnosed. JJ's mother grew up with a sibling with type 1 diabetes so she had some preconceived ideas about diabetes management. Due to the high prevalence of type 2 diabetes, other friends and family members who had experience with type 2 diabetes offered conflicting advice about the management of JJ's diabetes. This heightened JJ's parents' fears. Both parents had a real fear of hypoglycemia because of the increase in frequency of hypoglycemia the mother's sister had experienced with intensive insulin therapy during the DCCT. The diagnosis can be particularly devastating for families who have had experience with the complications of diabetes.

Education needed to be individualized and communicated in a way that addressed the age and developmental stage of the child, family dynamics, past experiences with diabetes, and issues facing the entire family. In JJ's case, his family needed to understand that there are different types of diabetes and that everyone's experience with diabetes may be different. The family needed to be reassured that they could not have prevented the diagnosis of diabetes. Diabetes education regarding survival skills was foremost, and this education included JJ's siblings and other caretakers, such as grandparents. The pace of teaching followed the progress the family was making in learning the necessary skills. The diabetes educator, by learning more about the cultural preferences and beliefs in the family, was able to integrate this into the teaching and treatment regimen.

Survival skills: the focus of the first week

The initial teaching focuses on survival skills:

- Testing blood glucose and urine or blood ketones
- Measuring and administering insulin
- Insulin actions
- Meal planning
- Prevention, recognition, and treatment of hypoglycemia

Because of the strong emotions (shock, anger, grief) felt at this time, most patients and their families do not comprehend much more than survival skills in the first week. Others may seem to adapt more quickly and move forward at a quicker pace; sometimes, however, these same families may experience the grief and anger at a later time.

The education provided must be culturally appropriate, personalized to the needs of its recipients (child, individual, family), sensitive to family resources, paced to accommodate individual needs, and provided for all caregivers. Siblings should not be overlooked, as they sometimes feel left out because of the attention being given to the child with diabetes.

The educational process needs to be an open-ended, ongoing experience between the individual with diabetes, family, friends, and the diabetes team.[10] Developing effective stress management/coping skills and problem-solving skills is considered as important to successful therapy as insulin administration, nutrition therapy, monitoring, and exercise.[11]

The content provided will be the same whether the individual with new-onset diabetes is in the inpatient or outpatient setting. About 70% of children with new onset diabetes are not acutely ill and do not require hospitalization for medical management. However, hospitalization is not inappropriate for these children for initiation of insulin therapy and education. If there is an outpatient facility equipped to do outpatient education and management for individuals and their families, these children will not require hospitalization. To do this successfully, a multidisciplinary team must teach the patient and family how to safely use insulin at home and be available to troubleshoot by phone if problems arise. Initial care and education costs are substantially lower than those associated with inpatient care.[12,13] Families may be directed to additional educational support through the ADA and AADE, who can refer them to a diabetes educator or diabetes education team.

> Near-continuous blood glucose monitoring may dramatically alter diabetes management.

To achieve the desired goals for glycemic control, patients and families must integrate a comprehensive and rigorous diabetes management plan into their daily lives.

Key components of type 1 diabetes management: Monitoring, Taking Medication, Healthy Eating, Being Active

Management of type 1 diabetes includes the following key components:

- *Monitoring:* Measurement of blood glucose 4 or more times daily
- *Taking Medication:* Insulin infusion therapy or 2 or more injections of insulin per day
- *Healthy Eating:* Attention to food intake
- *Being Active:* Regular exercise

Monitoring

Blood Glucose Monitoring

Frequent monitoring of blood glucose levels is necessary for optimal glycemic control. In a number of studies, the frequency of blood glucose monitoring has been strongly associated with glycemic control.[14,15] In a study of 7- to 16-year-olds, frequency of testing was the most important predictor of A1C levels.[16]

Blood glucose: tested at least 4 times a day

A minimum of 4 blood glucose measurements should be performed each day to determine patterns of hypoglycemia and hyperglycemia and to enable individuals to make adjustments in food, exercise, scheduling, and/or insulin.

- *Preprandial Blood Glucose*
- *Postprandial Blood Glucoses:* Also important in determining if premeal insulin dose was correct
- *Overnight Blood Glucose:* Valuable in determining doses and detecting nocturnal hypoglycemia, especially after unusual exercise, hypoglycemia, illness, or poor food intake
- *Frequent Testing:* Essential in young children or anyone who has hypoglycemic unawareness

Meters. Many good blood glucose meters are available. Often, third party payors dictate which meter the individual uses. Several of the newer meters allow alternate-site testing (eg, arm or leg), which some people find more comfortable than finger-sticks. There is some concern that alternate-site testing may not reflect arterial glucose values as quickly as finger-stick capillary blood glucose measurements, thus creating a delay in evaluating hypoglycemia when the glucose level is changing rapidly.[17,18]

Data Log. Blood glucose test results are important to document in a logbook or by downloading from the meters. Almost all meters contain a memory chip that allows individuals and care providers to download blood glucose test results. Interpretation of results and use of this information for calculating dose is essential in achieving good metabolic control. Individuals/families should be taught to review this data frequently to look for blood glucose patterns and make appropriate dose adjustments or call their healthcare provider for assistance.

Near-Continuous Monitoring. New technology is now offering near-continuous blood glucose monitoring. These devices hold promise for improved assessment of metabolic control and the avoidance of hypoglycemia, which is often the most significant barrier to optimal control. Continuous glucose monitoring devices may dramatically alter the management of diabetes; such devices may be particularly beneficial in the following situations:[19]

- Young child
- Hypoglycemic unawareness
- Nocturnal hypoglycemia

Healthy Coping

When a family has a child with type 1 diabetes, developing effective stress management/coping skills and problem-solving skills is as important as insulin administration, nutrition therapy, monitoring, and exercise.

Case—Part 3: Tools of Therapy

During baby JJ's hospitalization, his parents were taught survival skills for diabetes management.

Monitoring

- Blood glucose
- Blood or urine ketones

JJ's parents were instructed on the use of a blood glucose meter that used a small sample of blood. They were instructed on record keeping and the importance of using this data for pattern management.

Insulin Therapy

JJ was started on BID regular and NPH insulins. JJ's parents were instructed on the measurement of insulin and the administration and rotation of insulin injections. When JJ's mother expressed reluctance because she did not want to hurt her baby, the educator had the parents practice giving each other saline injections.

Meal Planning

Ensuring adequate nutrition and calories was a primary consideration, as it is essential in the growing child. At the time JJ was diagnosed, JJ's parents met with a pediatric registered dietitian. Food was one of their biggest concerns, as is often the case for parents of infants and toddlers. The educator explained that because infants require a frequent feeding schedule, getting glucose values with even a 2-hour fast is often difficult and 'feeds' often do not match the peaks of insulin.

Physical Activity

The activity level of a 9-month old, such as JJ at the time of his diagnosis, is unpredictable and in general cannot be planned for or controlled. That is one of the many challenges of managing diabetes in an infant. It was important for JJ's parents to understand how his activity level, sleep, and nap patterns affected his blood glucose levels so they could make appropriate adjustments in food and insulin.

Hypoglycemia

The fear of hypoglycemia is one of the major barriers to achieving optimal glycemic control for all individuals with diabetes and is one of the biggest fears for parents of children with diabetes. Severe hypoglycemia can affect the growing brain of the child, and recognizing the early warning signs of hypoglycemia in a very young child may be difficult. However due to the seriousness of hypoglycemia, the importance of prevention and early adequate treatment must be stressed. JJ's parents were instructed on the signs, symptoms, and treatment of hypoglycemia, including use of glucose gel and glucagon. They were encouraged to do frequent monitoring of blood glucose to validate hypoglycemic episodes.

When baby JJ was discharged from the hospital his parents had learned an entire new set of skills and had the challenge of raising a child with diabetes.

- Frequent DKA
- Unexplained glucose excursions
- Gastroparesis

Current testing provides incomplete data, giving a snapshot of the blood glucose at that moment. Further improvements of continuous sensors are in development. The challenge for healthcare providers will be to learn how to interpret this data in an efficient way and to teach patients how to respond to and use the data to achieve the best possible metabolic control. Chapter 17, on intensifying insulin therapy, and chapter 32, on monitoring, also discuss this new technology.

Ketone Testing

The general recommendation for ketone testing is to test when blood glucose levels exceed 300 mg/dL (16.6 mmol/L) and during illness.

Some centers advise routine ketone testing before breakfast as an indicator of overnight or antecedent insulin deficiency. Overnight (antecedent) insulin deficiency—referred to as the "dawn phenomenon"—is fasting hyperglycemia related to the normal rise in growth hormone, cortisol, and other hormones that can raise blood glucose levels in the absence of insulin.[20]

Ketones can be tested in either urine or blood. Blood ketone testing gives more current results, but the blood testing strips are much more expensive than the urine testing strips. Testing the urine for ketones is a commonly taught skill; however, more recent meters are available that test both blood glucose and blood ketones.[1] Some families may find this meter more convenient for those times when obtaining a urine sample is difficult.

The presence of persistent moderate or large amounts of ketones in the urine or concentrations of greater then 0.6 mmol/L in the blood suggests the possibility of impending DKA and should prompt individuals to adjust insulin or seek assistance from their healthcare provider. Additional fluids and/or insulin are often required to clear ketosis.

Taking Medication

Insulin Injection Therapy

Insulin is the mainstay of treatment for type 1 diabetes. Subcutaneous insulin injections are begun at the time of diagnosis, or once ketoacidosis is resolved in those in whom it was present. There are many different insulin preparations available. The various preparations are genetically engineered to have different onsets, peaks, and duration of activity (see chapter 15). These insulins are used in combination or individually and can be delivered by syringe, or in some cases, a pen, pump, or, as recently approved for adults only, an inhaler.

Regimen and Dose Determinations

Infants and Toddlers. The small insulin needs of infants and toddlers may require diluted insulin to allow for more precise dosing and measurement of insulin in less than 1-unit increments. Diluents are available for specific types of insulins from the insulin manufacturers. Insulin

Considerations for Insulin Injections in Children and Teens[22]

- Usual injection sites for young children are the legs, arms, and the buttocks. Abdominal injections may not be advisable in young children with little subcutaneous abdominal fat. Injections can be given in the abdomen of school-age children and adolescents if they have adequate subcutaneous tissue.
- Rotating sites in a consistent manner (eg legs in the morning, arms in the evening, buttocks at bedtime) may provide a more consistent rate of absorption. It may also prevent lipohypertrophy of sites.
- Avoid giving injections into hypertrophied areas to achieve the best absorption possible.
- Use 31-gauge, short- or mini-needles for more comfortable injections and to avoid intramuscular injection.
- Use the smallest barrel possible (eg, 30-unit syringe for doses less than 30 units, 50-unit syringe for doses between 30 and 50 units) for the most accurate dosing.
- Half-unit increments can now be measured on certain insulin syringes.
- An automatic injector (Inject-Ease or similar device) may be useful for some.
- Needle phobias are common in children and adults (parents or patients). *Always* assess.
- Having parents give each other practice saline injections reassures parents that giving insulin injections to their child is not the trauma they envision.
- For older children, seeing family members giving themselves a practice saline injection may be supportive, making it less frightening for the child.

can be diluted either at a pharmacy or at home, once parents are trained. BID lispro and NPH insulins are one option for infants; a basal/bolus regimen using a long-acting insulin analog plus a rapid-acting insulin with food intake may also be a good insulin regimen for children this age.

Children. Most children are started on 2 to 4 injections per day, using either of the following:

- A combination of a rapid-acting insulin/intermediate-acting insulin BID, *or*
- A basal/bolus regimen of a long-acting insulin with rapid-acting insulin before meals

Children's insulin requirements are based on body weight, age, and pubertal status. Children with newly diagnosed type 1 diabetes usually require an initial total daily dose of 0.5 to 1.0 units per kilogram. Younger and prepubertal children usually require lower doses, while the presence of ketoacidosis, use of steroids, and puberty all dictate the need for higher doses.

Adults. For adults newly diagnosed with diabetes, a basal/bolus regimen is common: that is, use of a long-acting insulin plus rapid-acting insulin before meals. Adults, on average, require between 0.4 to 1.0 units per kilogram per day.[1]

Decreased Insulin Needs During Honeymoon Period. Once blood glucose levels are normalized, and endogenous insulin production increases during the first month after diagnosis, most individuals with type 1 diabetes enter a honeymoon, or remission, period. During this phase of diabetes, insulin requirements decrease significantly, to as little as 0.1 to 0.3 units per kilogram per day.[1] Many children can maintain acceptable metabolic control with a BID rapid-acting and intermediate-acting insulin regimen during this period. However, some healthcare providers prefer to use a basal/bolus insulin regimen from the start of insulin therapy.

The duration of the honeymoon period varies, but typically lasts between 3 and 12 months. Parents and patients need to be prepared for this period of decreasing insulin needs and minimal fluctuation in blood glucose values so they do not question the diagnosis of diabetes. Beta-cell destruction continues during the honeymoon period. The end of this remission period is characterized by the following:

- Increased variability of blood glucose levels
- Increased insulin requirements
- Greater need to attend to diabetes management

Some patients who have had a prolonged and significant honeymoon period have described the end of the honeymoon period as "getting diabetes all over again."

Increased Insulin Needs With Growth and Puberty. Insulin requirements increase with growth and particularly during puberty. Insulin requirements during puberty may increase to as much as 1.5 units per kilogram per day due to the hormonal influences of increased growth hormone and sex hormone secretion. Insulin therapy regimens must be based on the individual needs of the child, adolescent, adult, and family, including meal, school and work schedules, supervisory issues, and glycemic patterns.

Metabolic Control. The DCCT demonstrated that individuals on basal/bolus insulin therapy with multiple daily injections (MDI) or a continuous subcutaneous insulin infusion (pump therapy) achieved better metabolic control compared to those on twice-daily insulin dosing.[4]

Regimen Flexibility. A basal/bolus insulin regimen uses a long-acting insulin analog (most often given at bedtime, although it can be given at other times) combined with a rapid-acting insulin analog given before meals and snacks. Using an insulin-to-carbohydrate ratio in determining the rapid-acting insulin dose before meals and snacks allows flexibility for the timing and amount of food consumed (see chapter 17 for more information on carbohydrate counting). Other factors involved in determining the dose are the current blood glucose and the anticipated level of physical activity in the coming hours.

For children, whose intake is unpredictable, giving the insulin immediately following the meal,[21] so that actual food intake and insulin are matched more closely, may be efficacious in minimizing the potential for hypoglycemia. However, postprandial glucose control may not be as good when insulin is given after the meal.

One of the most difficult times to control postprandial glucose is after the morning meal. In some instances, such as a high blood glucose premeal, giving the rapid-acting insulin analog 10 to 20 minutes before the meal may help so that the insulin begins to lower the blood glucose before the meal is ingested.

The multiple snacks consumed by some children and adolescents may translate into multiple injections if the basal/bolus plan is strictly followed. An alternative may be to use small amounts of intermediate-acting insulin for coverage of some snacking and for lunch if a child is in a situation where insulin cannot be administered with lunch. For example, some regimens use NPH insulin in the morning to cover either the lunch meal or the after-lunch snack so the child does not have to take an additional injection of rapid-acting insulin during the day.

The number of insulin injections may be a barrier to good control using an MDI regimen with carbohydrate (CHO) counting, even though it allows flexibility of eating times and amounts. Some patients and families may consider insulin infusion therapy when injections are required too frequently. Omission of injections may increase when regimens become too difficult.

Premixed Insulins. Commercially prepared premixed insulins do not allow for the flexibility of daily dosage adjustment based on blood glucose values and exercise levels, which are especially variable in children, and therefore may not be appropriate for people with type 1 diabetes. However, these insulins may be useful for those who are unable or unwilling to regularly adjust insulin doses.

Continuous Subcutaneous Insulin Infusion

Continuous subcutaneous insulin infusion (CSII) has been demonstrated to improve control, decrease fluctuations in blood glucoses, decrease the risk of severe hypoglycemia, and allow more flexibility in food intake. These advantages make CSII an appealing option for pediatric patients with diabetes, and results from several studies indicate that CSII is safe and effective in the pediatric population.[23-28] (See chapter 17.) There are some pump issues that are unique to children, including use at school or camp and adjustments for sports.

Use at School, Day Care, and Camp. One issue is management of the pump in the school setting, day care, or camp. The child may need help counting carbohydrates and bolusing correctly. The child may also need help troubleshooting the pump (eg, what to do for air bubbles, alarms, dislodgment of insulin infusion sets). Either the school nurse or other school or camp staff will require training to perform these tasks for or with the child. Camp counselors, camp nurses, and day care staff should be familiar with the mechanics of the insulin pump and know how to problem solve and who to contact if there is a problem with the pump.

Adjusting for Sports. Managing insulin infusion therapy during sports requires some special adjustments. For sports that require the pump to be disconnected (swimming, soccer, football, basketball, hockey, and tennis), the individual and his or her parents usually learn by trial and error how to adjust for the missed basal. If the blood glucose is above target after the activity, a starting place is to give one-half of the missed basal prior to disconnecting. It is best if the pump is disconnected for no longer than 2 hours. Frequent blood glucose monitoring is essential so the individual can learn what adjustments work. For sports that do not require the pump to be disconnected, temporary basal rates and decreasing boluses usually work well.

Glycemic Control. Unfortunately, even with CSII, approximately 30% of subjects remain in suboptimal glycemic control.[27]

Nearly 1 in 3 pump users falls short of glycemic goals

The primary reasons for suboptimal glycemic control in children using CSII are missed meal boluses and inadequate testing so that blood glucose levels are not corrected.

Studies show that for every 4 to 5 missed meal boluses per week, the A1C increases by 1%.[4,29] The use of meal bolus alarms may be helpful, and an effective partnership between the child and parent is essential. Adult supervision is often required while the child is away from parents.

Case—Part 4: Insulin Infusion Therapy to Improve Glycemic Control

When JJ was 14 years old, he was taking multiple daily injections, and his A1C was in the 8% to 9% range. He had one severe nocturnal hypoglycemic episode and was experiencing fairly frequent mild to moderate hypoglycemic episodes, often related to his competitive ski racing. JJ and his parents decided they wanted to pursue insulin infusion therapy.

Insulin pump therapy should be a joint decision by the patient, family, and diabetes management team. It requires more in-depth self-management education and performance of self-care behaviors. JJ and his family received extensive diabetes self-management education including adequate nutrition for his activity, the need for more frequent blood glucose monitoring, problem solving, calculating insulin dosages, and mechanics of the insulin pump. JJ had to demonstrate his ability to operate the pump and manage his diabetes safely and appropriately. With help from the diabetes management team, JJ learned to adjust his pump for his skiing and reduce the number of hypoglycemic episodes. JJ and his parents also discussed the use of pump therapy with JJ's coach.

Children in preschool or day care need an adult to supervise pump programming; school-age children and in some instances adolescents may require supervision as well.

Healthy Eating

Eating is usually one of the biggest concerns for all individuals with new-onset diabetes. Because of "old wives tales," people may fear they will never again eat sweets or other foods they like. An important role of the educator is to help the patient and the patient's family understand how to incorporate the foods the patient likes into a healthful food plan. The clinical goals of medical nutrition therapy (MNT) for children and adolescents with diabetes are the same as for all individuals with type 1 diabetes, with the addition of maintenance of normal growth and development.[30,31]

Nutrition Assessment. Nutritional recommendations for children and adolescents are based on a nutrition assessment. This assessment involves evaluating parameters such as age, weight, height, growth percentiles on a growth chart, body mass index, gender, recommended daily allowances (RDAs) for caloric range, schedules, treatment modalities, and blood glucose patterns for each child.

Calorie Consumption and Normal Growth. In general, children need sufficient calories for growth and pubertal development without excessive hypoglycemic episodes. The child's height and weight should be plotted on a growth chart at each visit to determine trends. If growth patterns are appropriate for age, the child's meal plan includes calories adequate for growth and development. Children and teens who are of normal weight do not need to focus on weight-control issues, other than to follow prudent recommendations important for the general population. For children who are above an ideal weight range, encouraging alterations in food selection and physical activity levels can decrease possible insulin resistance and increase metabolic status.[30]

Meal Plans and Insulin Regimen. Meal plans must be individualized to match food preferences, cultural influences, family eating patterns and schedules, age, weight, activity level, and insulin action peaks. Insulin therapy can be integrated into usual eating and exercise habits. Therefore, it is important to determine the meal plan before determining an insulin regimen. The child's appetite should be considered when determining the total caloric level provided in the meal plan.[22] Young children require smaller portions of food and need to eat more frequently than adults. Infants and toddlers have changing and unpredictable eating patterns.

Most children newly diagnosed with type 1 diabetes have experienced some weight loss that must be restored with insulin initiation, hydration, and adequate energy intake. Once their weight is restored to normalcy, their appetite and caloric intake will decrease significantly.

Appetite changes require dose adjustments

When the person recovers from the acute onset of diabetes and his or her appetite decreases, the insulin dose must be decreased to avoid hypoglycemia. The patient should be forewarned this may occur, and the family must be alerted to watch for this.

Adolescents, especially girls, are often pleased with the weight loss they incurred as diabetes developed and do not want to regain the weight. When and as appropriate, these teens should be given guidance to help them minimize their weight gain.

Using an insulin-to-carbohydrate ratio (chapter 17) for determining premeal insulin dose allows for more flexibility in food intake, whereas food intake will need to be more consistent for individuals on fixed insulin regimens. The diabetes educator should discourage parents from withholding food or having the child overeat consistently without an appetite for food in an effort to control blood glucose. Withholding food can feel punitive to a child and eventually promote reluctance to honestly report extra food or high glucose values. Forcing children to eat when they are not hungry or when they are no longer hungry should also be avoided.[22]

Children under the age of 6 years typically desire 3 meals per day plus 3 snacks. Most children over the age of 6 want 3 meals per day plus snacks in midafternoon and at bedtime.[22] Carbohydrate counting principles are the same for children as they are for adults. Carbohydrate counting can allow greater flexibility and alternatives in a child's meal plan if an insulin pump or MDI therapy is used (see chapter 13, on medical nutrition therapy, for more detail). Children and their caregivers need to be carefully instructed to not withhold carbohydrates in an effort to control blood glucoses; doing so can result in inadequate caloric intake for growth. Additional carbohydrate intake is often needed before physical activity to decrease the risk of a hypoglycemic episode during or after exercise.

Chapters 13 and 29, on medical nutrition therapy and self-management behaviors related to healthy eating, provide further information.

Being Active

Physical activity has many benefits, but in type 1 diabetes increased attention must be given to age, consistency, insulin dosing, and changes in blood glucose levels.

Increased frequency in blood glucose testing is a requirement, as is education on how to respond before, during, and after the period of physical activity.

Adjusting for Activity Levels. The activity level of a 9-month-old child is unpredictable and in general cannot be planned for or controlled. That is one of the many challenges of managing diabetes in an infant. Individuals of all ages with diabetes need to make adjustments in their diabetes regimen for changes in activity levels.

Benefits of Physical Activity. Intervention strategies that promote lifelong physical activity should be encouraged for all individuals with diabetes because of the health-promoting benefits of a regular exercise program. Benefits of exercise in type 1 diabetes are detailed in an ADA Technical Review [32] and include the following:[32,33]

- Lower plasma glucose levels
- Greater sense of well-being
- Weight management
- Improved physical fitness
- Improved cardiovascular fitness with lower pulse and blood pressure
- Improved lipid profile

These advantages apply to children as well as adults. All individuals with type 1 diabetes should adhere to the recommendations of the Centers for Disease Control and Prevention and the American Academy of Sports Medicine:[6]

- *Recommendation:* At least 30 to 60 minutes of moderate physical activity daily

Hypoglycemia Prevention. More frequent blood glucose monitoring (before, during, and after exercise) may be necessary to avoid hypoglycemia during or after exercise. The decision of whether to adjust food or insulin is determined by the individual's diabetes management goals and is further affected by whether the exercise was planned. When exercise is planned sufficiently in advance, the preference is to adjust the insulin acting during the period of physical activity to minimize hypoglycemia risk.[34] If exercise is not planned far enough ahead to modify the relevant insulin dose, a carbohydrate snack should be taken. Planning or predicting physical activity in very young children is especially difficult. For school-age children and adolescents, the intensity and duration of a sports practice, physical education period, and sports game may vary greatly from day to day so adjusting insulin may be difficult for them as well. With the increasing prevalence of obesity in all age groups, exercise is often important for weight management and if additional food is consumed to cover increases in activity, the benefits of exercise for weight management are lost.

Depending on the glucose value at the start of exercise and the intensity and duration of the activity, carbohydrate intake may be necessary before, during, and/or after exercise.[34] Recommendations must be individualized but a general guideline is to consume 10 to 20 g of carbohydrate for every 30 minutes of moderate activity (chapter 14 provides more information on physical activity).

In the pediatric population, 10% to 20% of hypoglycemic episodes are associated with exercise that is of greater-than-usual intensity, duration, or frequency. Increased hepatic glucose output in association with vigorous exercise secondary to both β- and α-adrenergic stimulation may cause hyperglycemia during and immediately after exercise. Hypoglycemia may follow within 1 to 16 hours of completion of exercise due to glucose transport into skeletal muscle tissue and hepatic glycogen depletion.[35] School-age children and adolescents are frequently involved in different sports at various times of the year, all requiring different adjustments in their diabetes regimen. Their activities are often during the late afternoon and evening, and the delayed hypoglycemia that can occur is likely to occur during the night if appropriate adjustments are not made in insulin or carbohydrate intake.

Blood glucose monitoring at bedtime is crucial

In 1 study, examining the effect of exercise on overnight hypoglycemia in children with diabetes, 36% of the 50 study participants experienced nocturnal hypoglycemia even when the blood glucose was greater than 130 mg/dL at bedtime.[36]

Use of an electrolyte-containing sports drink or other source of a readily absorbable carbohydrate may be helpful in preventing hypoglycemia both during and after exercise. Chapter 14 offers more information on encouraging fluid intake.

See chapters 14 and 30 for more information on physical activity and self-management behaviors related to being active.

Healthy Coping

Many parents equate having a newly diagnosed child with diabetes with leaving the hospital with their first-born child. The parents can be overwhelmed with fears and the stress of learning new skills and having new responsibilities associated with having a child with newly diagnosed diabetes. The stressful, changed situation may create tension among family members. Mothers and fathers may argue and siblings may feel frightened and can become resentful as all the attention is directed towards the family member with diabetes. The potential for family dysfunction is great. The diabetes educator can be instrumental in assisting families dealing with these issues by initiating discussion about these feelings and suggesting referral for family counseling. Including the entire family in the diabetes education process helps support all family members and provides everyone the opportunity to participate in the care of the person with diabetes.

Psychosocial issues for the patient and the entire family change throughout the child's lifetime. The diabetes educator needs to understand normal developmental tasks at different developmental stages in order to identify and circumvent potential problems. Major developmental issues and their effect on diabetes in children and adolescents are summarized in Table 9.3.

Psychosocial Issues: Infants and Toddlers

Normal characteristics in the development of young children must be taken into account when diabetes management regimens are determined. Normal growth and development for infants and toddlers (from birth to age 3) progresses rapidly and predictably. An understanding of normal developmental tasks of children is essential when developing the diabetes management plan.

One of the developmental tasks of infancy is to develop a trusting relationship with caregivers. Parents often worry that "hurting" their child (finger pokes and injections) will hamper this "bonding" process. Parents should be encouraged to develop a matter-of-fact attitude for the management tasks with the provision of incentives, like hugs, positive verbal reinforcement, or reading a book immediately after the poke or injection. In normal development, differentiation begins at around 4 to 5 months of age, and tentative experimentation with separation-individuation begins at around 6 months. Infants become much more mobile when they begin crawling, at around 9 months of age and walking at about 10 to 15 months of age. Their energy expenditure increases greatly once they become mobile; insulin dose adjustments or extra snacks may thus be necessary to prevent hypoglycemia.[22]

In infancy, feedings not only provide nutrition to maintain life and physiologic well-being, but also build a relationship. A positive feeding interaction between the infant and caregiver fosters the ingestion of an appropriate amount of food. Infants usually nurse or eat predictably, but for breastfed infants it is difficult to know how much breast milk they are getting. A feeding pattern that imitates family meal times should evolve by the end of the first year of life to incorporate the infant into the family's normal meal schedule.[22]

Toddlers develop a sense of mastery and autonomy, and they begin to separate and individuate, testing their separateness by saying "no" and behaving in an oppositional manner. Most parents know this as the "terrible two's." Providing choices at this age can give the toddler with diabetes some control, but the choices need to be framed in such a way that the child is not allowed to make important decisions.[22] For example, asking, "which finger shall we do?" works better than asking "Do you want to do your blood test now?" Some families have "cute" names for finger pokes and injections. Naming the meter and decorating it with stickers can take some of the fear out of the testing procedure. Injections should not be called "shots" because children may confuse this with the shot of a gun.

Appetite may become erratic in toddlers when rapid growth begins to subside. Food can become problematic for parents and caretakers. If a toddler will not eat, favorite foods or alternatives can be offered, but parents should avoid becoming short-order cooks for a demanding toddler.[22] A basal/bolus regimen, adjusting insulin for food intake, and giving insulin immediately after consumption of food may work best. Insulin infusion therapy is also an option in this age group (see chapter 17 on insulin pump therapy). Normal activity in toddlers is sporadic and spontaneous, interspersed with sudden bursts of whole body movement. To prevent hypoglycemia, activity needs to be balanced with extra food or beverages such as milk or juice.[22]

Hypoglycemia is often a constant fear for parents of infants and toddlers

Parents must rely on frequent blood glucose monitoring to distinguish normal infant and toddler behaviors from symptoms of hypoglycemia. Infants and toddlers are often defiant, demanding, sleepy, or cranky as part of their normal development.[22] Temper tantrums cannot be ignored until hypoglycemia has been ruled out with a blood test.

Psychosocial Issues: Preschool Years

The preschool years are from age 3 to 5. Physical growth slows after the toddler stage, but is still relatively rapid. Development of fine motor skills continues, and cognitive language is rapid. Children engage in magical thinking; they believe that if they think or wish something, they can cause it to happen.[37] Separation-individuation continues as children learn to distinguish themselves as being separate from their parents. Body integrity and confidence in their ability to accomplish tasks is important. Fear of intrusive procedures is characteristic of this age, and children may act out their anxieties at the times when insulin injections and blood testing are done. The use of adhesive bandages is helpful to the preschool child, as they help address concerns about body integrity.[22] Even though they often lack the fine motor skills, cognitive development, and impulse

TABLE 9.3 Major Developmental Issues and Their Effect on Diabetes in Children and Adolescents

Developmental Stage (Approximate Ages)	*Normal Developmental Tasks*	*Type 1 Diabetes Management Priorities*	*Family Issues in Type 1 Diabetes Management*
Infancy 0–12 months	• Developing a trusting relationship/ "bonding" with primary caregiver(s)	• Preventing and treating hypoglycemia • Avoiding extreme fluctuations in blood glucose levels	• Coping with stress • Sharing the "burden of care" to avoid parent burnout
Toddler 13–36 months	• Developing a sense of mastery and autonomy	• Preventing and treating hypoglycemia • Avoiding extreme fluctuations in blood glucose levels due to irregular food intake	• Establishing a schedule • Managing the "picky eater" • Setting limits and coping with toddler's lack of cooperation with regimen • Sharing the burden of care
Preschooler and Early Elementary School Age 3–7 years	• Developing initiative in activities and confidence in self	• Preventing and treating hypoglycemia • Unpredictable appetite and activity • Positive reinforcement for cooperation with regimen • Trusting other caregivers with diabetes management	• Reassuring child that diabetes is no one's fault • Educating other caregivers about diabetes management
Older Elementary School Age 8–11 years	• Developing skills in athletic, cognitive, artistic, social areas • Consolidating self-esteem with respect to the peer group	• Making diabetes regimen flexible to allow for participation in school/peer activities • Child learning short- and long-term benefits of optimal control	• Maintaining parental involvement in insulin and blood glucose monitoring tasks while allowing for independent self-care for "special occasions" • Continue to educate school and other caregivers
Early Adolescence 12–15 years	• Managing body changes • Developing a strong sense of self-identity	• Managing increased insulin requirements during puberty • Diabetes management and blood glucose control become more difficult • Weight and body image concerns	• Renegotiating parents and teen's roles in diabetes management to be acceptable to both • Learning coping skills to enhance ability to self-manage • Preventing and intervening with diabetes-related family conflict • Monitoring for signs of depression, eating disorders, risky behaviors
Later Adolescence 16–19 years	• Establishing a sense of identity after high school (decision about location, social issues, work, education)	• Begin discussion of transition to a new diabetes team • Integrating diabetes into new lifestyle	• Supporting the transition to independence • Learning coping skills to enhance ability to self-manage • Preventing and intervening with diabetes-related family conflict • Monitoring for signs of depression, eating disorders, risky behaviors

Source: Copyright © 2005 American Diabetes Association. Modified with permission from the American Diabetes Association. Silverstein J, Klingensmith G, Copeland K, et al. Care of children and adolescents with type 1 diabetes: a statement of the American Diabetes Association. Diabetes Care. 2005(28):186-212.

control to do diabetes management tasks independently, allowing preschoolers to do "bits and pieces" of procedures is important (such as placing the meter and lancing device on the table or getting the syringe out of the box).

Preschoolers have difficulty understanding the need for insulin injections and blood tests, particularly if they are feeling well. Describing the need in terms of "keeping you healthy" fosters a positive outlook. Allowing the child to have some control by providing limited choices can be helpful;[22] for example, asking "Do you want mashed potatoes or macaroni for dinner?" Preschoolers need positive reinforcement (verbal praise, sticker charts) for their cooperation with the regimen. Diabetes management tasks should not be used as rewards or punishment.

Children establish a balance between their inner life and reality by continually exploring and testing through their play. Guided play, or play therapy, provides a forum and vehicle for children to express their concerns. Play therapy provides a mechanism for emotional release, by helping the child learn to deal with these issues through creative expression. Giving a child a "safe" syringe, family and health professional dolls, a meter, and other diabetes supplies provides an opportunity for the child to play out their personal life issues and concerns about having diabetes. Bears with colored patches for injections and finger pokes are useful for this and are available from the Juvenile Diabetes Research Foundation (JDRF). Forms of artwork also help young children express themselves.[22]

Appetites may be very erratic and are often unpredictable in the preschool child. Variability in eating is not considered harmful but, rather, normal from a developmental point of view. Children may eat only a few foods or may want the same item meal after meal. (For example, children may want to eat only bananas and peanut butter for days at a time, and then they will switch to grilled cheese sandwiches and apples.) These eating patterns typically last a few days or weeks. When treated casually, the behaviors are forgotten after a brief period. Increased appetites tend to precede growth spurts, and food intake is usually balanced over a period of weeks. This erratic eating makes glucose control difficult for this age group and parents worry about hypoglycemia when their child will not eat. Parents can allow the child some control over eating by providing reasonable choices without allowing the child to control eating situations. By giving young children limited choices, parents may avoid a battle of wills.[22]

Many preschool-age children are able to identify symptoms of hypoglycemia and can at least alert adults that they do not feel well. This is especially important since many children are in preschool or day care settings at this age. Undetected hypoglycemia is still a risk in the preschool years and is especially worrisome to parents when their child is in the care of others.

The responsibility of caring for a young child with diabetes and fear of hypoglycemia are extremely stressful for families[9]

In two-parent families, both parents should be involved in the day-to-day management of the child's diabetes. In single-parent families, the single parent needs to identify others who can provide support and respite care. Healthcare providers can often assist parents in identifying support systems that can be helpful in easing the burden of care and avoiding parental burnout. Support groups, involvement in professional organizations such as the American Diabetes Association, the Juvenile Diabetes Research Foundation, or other local organizations may be a source of support for families, not only for families with young children but for children of all ages.

Psychosocial Issues: School-Age Children

A school-age child (6 to 11 years old) is physically well-coordinated, has a vivid fantasy life, speaks fluently, has a conscience, and is able to share and cooperate. The child has concrete reasoning and likes repetition, which is played out in sports, games, and skills. Although the school-age child has increasing need for independence, the power and protection of the parent are very important to the child's feeling of well-being. One of the greatest drives of school-age children is to avoid failure. They acquire strategies to keep from feeling different from peers.[22]

One study shows that immediately following the diagnosis of diabetes in the school-age child, mild depression and anxiety are common.[38] This usually resolves by 6 months after diagnosis.

Anxiety and depression are a concern for school-age children with diabetes

After the first 1 to 2 years, depressive symptoms increase, and anxiety decreases for boys but increases for girls over the first 6 years after diagnosis.[38] The increase in depression may be associated with the end of the "honeymoon" period, when children come to realize that the disease will not go away and that it is more difficult to manage.[37] Support groups, individual counseling, or diabetes camps can be useful in assisting the child in resolving these feelings. Determining the child's individual coping skills, supporting adaptive strategies, and providing interventions should be initiated early and should be a part of follow-up care.[22] Chapter 4 provides more information on depression and anxiety in the child with diabetes.

Parent and Child Roles in Diabetes Management. In terms of diabetes management, the parent's role is to perform diabetes care tasks while moving the child toward independence through supervision, encouragement, and support. At times, the child may be willing and able to perform blood glucose monitoring, prepare his or her own snacks, and administer insulin (and may do so with supervision). At other times, a parent will need to perform the test or administer insulin. Parent-child sharing of these responsibilities is essential during the school-age years and beyond.[22] Several studies have shown that a child's early and independent participation in the diabetes regimen was significantly associated with poorer control.[39,40] Parents of the school-age child with diabetes may be more understandably protective than other parents. This attitude can make it difficult for the child with diabetes to attain the same level of independence as a child of the same age without diabetes. Diabetes management planning for special events and activities is important to promote independence and minimize differences. By planning ahead, most children can safely participate in all childhood activities.[22]

Monitoring, eating special snacks, taking injections, and fear of peers witnessing symptoms of hypoglycemia can alter diabetes self-care routines and ultimately affect self-esteem. Helping the child fit diabetes management into normal routines both at home and at school can minimize feelings of being different. For example, a snack break can be implemented for all children in the classroom. If children desire, they should be able to check glucose in the classroom. However, school policies vary, and not all schools allow blood glucose testing in the classroom. Some are concerned about other children coming in contact with another student's blood and the school's liability if the blood test result is not reported correctly. Children should carry a source of carbohydrate with them at all times and need to be able to treat hypoglycemia in the classroom. An adult or other student should accompany the student with diabetes to the clinic if the student is not feeling well.

Blood glucose values are often seen as "good" or "bad," and a child's level of control can also affect self-esteem. Because of school-age children's desire to please adults and their fear of failure, children in this age group sometimes falsify blood glucose results or report results when tests were omitted. When a child's A1C result is incompatible with the day-to-day glucose testing results, there is a high level of suspicion that this is occurring.

School-age children usually accept a greater variety of foods and develop increased autonomy regarding eating behaviors. As children spend their time in school and other organized activities, meal times and snacks are less frequent than with preschoolers.

Care in School Settings. Because school-age children spend a large portion of their day in school, expecting school personnel to become informed about diabetes care is reasonable. The school can present significant challenges or be a source of support to the child with diabetes.[6] This topic is well covered in the ADA's position statement on diabetes care in the school and day care setting[41] and another publication, Helping the Student with Diabetes Succeed: A Guide for School Personnel, by the National Diabetes Education Program, which is available on the Internet (http://ndep.nih.gov/diabetes/pubs/catalog.htm). School districts and personnel are obligated to provide an individualized plan to accommodate a child's special healthcare needs. Certain federal laws address these issues. The Education for All Handicapped Act of 1975,

Key Points on Arranging Diabetes Care in School Settings

Information from Parent. Parents need to provide the school with basic information about diabetes, the causes of hypoglycemia, the specific requirements of their child's daily management plan, and their child's usual signs and symptoms of hypoglycemia and hyperglycemia.

Plan of Care. The information provided by the parent is used to develop a plan of care that satisfies the needs of the child, parents, and school policies.[22] This written plan includes who will administer the care, the location of the supplies, and where the treatment will take place in the school setting.

Glucagon Administration. The administration of glucagon in schools must be provided if recommended by the student's healthcare provider.[41] When an order is provided by the healthcare provider, the school must designate a person to administer glucagon in the written plan of care.

Scheduling Changes. When scheduling changes occur in the daily school routine (eg, field trips or parties), the school needs to notify parents prior to the event so appropriate care can be administered or arranged. However, parents cannot be required to attend all field trips.

Meal Plan. A review of the food/meal plan basics provides school personnel with a general awareness of what the child eats. Providing a plan to enable the child to manage parties and snacks in school is also beneficial.[38] Some instruction on carbohydrate counting will be necessary if the student is using an insulin-to-carbohydrate ratio for calculating insulin dose for lunch and snacks.

commonly referred to as Public Law No. 94-142, is a federal mandate that entitles all physically, developmentally, emotionally, and other health-impaired children to free, appropriate public education.[42] Any school that receives federal funding or facility considered open to the public must reasonably accommodate the special needs of children with diabetes.[41] The other law, Section 504, is a more general civil rights law that makes it illegal for any agency or organization that receives federal funds to discriminate in any way against qualified people with disabilities.[43] See the sidebar summarizing key points on facilitating appropriate diabetes care in school settings.

The current standards for diabetes management reflect the need to maintain glucose control as near to normal as safely possible. To achieve this level of control, many children will be on intensified management. Intensified therapy requires not only blood glucose testing, but also insulin administration by injection or insulin infusion pump and some attention to food intake and the increased risk for hypoglycemia during the school day. This requires flexibility and close communication between the child, parents, school personnel, and healthcare team.[41]

Each school year should begin with a conference involving the child with diabetes, parents, and school personnel to establish a plan of care, communication, and a means of addressing important issues and concerns.

Psychosocial Issues: Adolescence

There are many differences in behavior and development between early, middle, and late adolescence, the time between 12 and 21 years of age. Characteristics of each of these 3 stages are outlined in Table 9.4.

Adolescence is a period of rapid biological change and increasing physical, cognitive, and emotional maturity. These changes may occur slowly or rapidly and are determined by genetic familial factors, economy, nutrition, health, and habitat.

Diabetes affects normal adolescent development. Identity and self-image concerns can revolve around diabetes concerns such as the appearance of the injection site or self-identification as "a diabetic." Normal independence issues may be thwarted as a result of parental protectiveness or the teen's failure to assume responsibility for self-care. Adolescents with diabetes can become particularly concerned about their growth and sexual maturation even though they usually display normal growth patterns and normal onset and progression of pubertal development.

Metabolic control tends to deteriorate in adolescence[38]

Attitudes of experimentation and rebellion and risk-taking behaviors normally associated with adolescence can affect diabetes issues such as taking insulin regularly, monitoring, and the quality and quantity of food consumption.

TABLE 9.4 Developmental Characteristics at Each Stage of Adolescence

Early Adolescence, 12 years old:

- The child becomes acutely aware of body image
- Dependent versus independent struggles begin between parent and child
- There may be great vacillation between childlike and adult behaviors
- There is less social involvement with family and more with peers
- Parental criticism becomes difficult to accept
- Turmoil and conflict within the parent-child relationship may begin

Middle Adolescence, 13 to 15 years old:

- Peer group allegiance develops
- Greater experimentation and risk taking occurs
- Physical and social activity increases
- Opposite sex relationships emerge and are important
- Formal operational thinking begins along with abstract reasoning

Late Adolescence, 16 to 21 years old:

- Teens and parents experience conflict in their relationship
- Cognitive abilities and abstract morals develop
- The peer group loses its primary importance
- There is increasing separation from the family unit
- Teens become future oriented
- Conscience can stand without support or validity from others

Source: Grey M, Cameron ME, Lipman TH, et al. Psychosocial status of children with diabetes in the first 2 years after diagnosis. Diabetes Care. 1995:18:1330-6.

Risky Behaviors. Healthcare providers must be aware of and address issues of substance abuse (tobacco, alcohol, and drug use), use of steroids or other supplements to enhance muscle growth, and sexual practices and attitudes in their assessment of adolescent diabetes management. Risk taking and lack of health-promoting behaviors is widespread, especially among adolescents.[38] Alcohol use can result in severe hypoglycemia several hours after drinking if adequate food is not ingested. Some individuals may need to lower their basal insulin through the night. Alcohol also can affect judgment and impair an individual's ability to recognize and adequately treat the symptoms of hypoglycemia.

Eating Habits. Food intake becomes less consistent due to issues such as participation in athletics, busier schedules, preoccupation with body weight and/or appearance, and the search for self-identity. Proper eating habits are still important to ensure continued growth and development and to develop good patterns to be used for a lifetime. Adolescents give low priority to their nutritional needs regarding recommended amounts and type of food. Typical food-related behaviors include skipping meals, eating away from home, experimenting with fad diets, and attempting to change their weight.[38] Educating adolescents, especially boys, about the effect of poor metabolic control on growth, can sometimes be a motivating factor for improving control.

Issues Involving Reproductive Health. Issues of sexuality, sexual functioning, and reproductive health should be addressed with teens and young adults, as well as adults, in a relaxed, comfortable manner. Reproductive health must be discussed in those of childrearing age. Comfort in discussing sexual topics comes with practice and a sense of control over the subject matter. The comfort level of the healthcare provider is communicated to the patient and sets the tone for discussions. Sex education should begin in the preteen years so that it becomes a routine part of diabetes assessment and education. Use of unbiased, gender-neutral language is important when assessing sexual orientation, practice, frequency, use of contraceptives, and consistency of contraceptive practices.[38]

Adolescent females with diabetes must be taught the importance of planning pregnancy and meticulously using contraception to avoid an unwanted pregnancy. Their instruction should include a frank dialogue about the potential fetal/maternal health risks of an unplanned pregnancy in a woman with diabetes.[22] (See the section on teens in chapter 11, on pregnancy with preexisting diabetes.)

Conditions Associated With Poor Glycemic Control and/or Health Outcomes[22]

- Biologically, the adolescent's heightened insulin resistance combined with earlier and greater epinephrine responses to drops in blood glucose concentrations may contribute to some of the lability in metabolic control.
- Adolescent rebellion/experimentation, a chaotic home environment, chronic family stress, parent-child conflicts, or parental over- or under-involvement can contribute to poor metabolic control for children and adolescents. While adolescents can perform the tasks necessary for diabetes management, they may not always follow the treatment regimen, and they still need help making decisions about insulin dose adjustments. Adolescents whose parents maintain some guidance and supervision in the management of diabetes have better metabolic control.[40,44]
- Developmental delays or learning disabilities, in either the adolescent child or a parent, may hamper understanding of diabetes care and thus self-management.
- Emotional disturbance can cause disequilibrium and precipitate frequent episodes of ketoacidosis. Insulin insufficiency may occur by insulin omission or in response to physical or emotional stress, resulting in overproduction of counter-regulatory hormones.[44] Repeated episodes of DKA warrant investigation, as DKA can be deliberately induced to displace family tensions. Family patterns of interaction may reveal family enmeshment, rigidity, poor communication, and overprotectiveness.[42] Treatment may include family counseling and aggressive insulin therapy when illness, stress, or ketones appear. Adolescents sometimes develop DKA because they fail to take their insulin. Insulin doses can be missed when parents are not involved in an adolescent's diabetes management.[42,45]
- Adolescents may decide to skip injections for the purpose of weight control, which is a variant of an eating disorder (see chapter 4). This most often occurs in females but can also occur in males. Diabetes and the regimen may provide the right conditions for those who are at risk of developing an eating disorder because of the focus on food and discipline required. Healthcare providers need to be aware of the possibility of pathologic eating behaviors, particularly among adolescent and young adult females.
- Needle anxiety occurs in almost everyone to some degree. If severe or persistent and left unresolved, diabetes control may suffer because of missed injections, inadequate testing, and avoidance of health care follow-up visits. When a parent has needle fears, the child will most likely have the same fears. Any patient who has a persistently high A1C should be evaluated for needle phobias. Desensitization therapy, biofeedback, assistance with relaxation, distraction, and use of an automatic injector (Inject-Ease or similar device) have proven helpful.[46]

Females may experience more vaginal candidiasis, especially if metabolic control is less than optimal. Adolescent males may have concerns about sexual dysfunction, since this is a fairly common complication in adults with diabetes. Discussing this with them can sometimes be a motivating factor to strive for good control. Teens should be reminded that abstinence is the only 100% effective contraceptive method for preventing pregnancy, sexually transmitted diseases (STDs), and acquired immune deficiency syndrome (AIDS). They need to be taught that use of a condom during sexual activity will help prevent STDs and AIDS, but is not the most effective method of preventing pregnancy.[22] Table 11.9, in chapter 11, summarizes the efficacy and safety of female contraceptive methods for those with diabetes.

Driver Safety. Driving is a serious adult responsibility that can be given as a privilege to teens. The use of appropriate self-care skills and safety precautions must be taught and reinforced in teens and adults who drive themselves to school or work or otherwise operate a motorized vehicle. Healthcare professionals and parents of teens who are approaching legal driving age should begin discussions with the teen about the responsibility of safety when driving. Students heading off to college with a car should be frequently reminded to drive responsibly and take the self-care steps necessary to ensure safety of the driver, passengers, and those on the road. Guidelines for safety while driving[22] are summarized in Table 9.5.

TABLE 9.5 Driving Safely With Diabetes

Issues to Discuss:

- Responsible diabetes self-care
- Desire or motivation to consider the safety of self and others
- Monitoring before driving
- Testing blood glucose at 2-hour intervals while driving
- Carrying appropriate supplies, including carbohydrates
- Wearing a medical ID
- Never driving with signs of hypoglycemia

Case—Part 5: Acute Complications: Hypoglycemia and DKA

JJ was never hospitalized again in DKA. He did, however, experience one nocturnal hypoglycemic seizure, at the age of 13 years, after a very active day of skiing.

Hypoglycemia

The fear of hypoglycemia is one of the major barriers to achieving optimal glycemic control for all individuals with diabetes, and it is one of the biggest fears for parents of children with diabetes. The definition of hypoglycemia is controversial, but studies have shown cognitive impairment at blood glucose concentrations <60 mg/dL (3.3 mmol/L).[47] There is some reduction in mental function during the acute phase of hypoglycemia, and sometimes this persists beyond the acute phase. Hypoglycemia that interferes with normal thinking can make schoolwork difficult. It also makes riding a bicycle, driving a car, or operating machinery dangerous. While diabetes itself is not associated with cognitive deficits, some investigations have found an increase in cognitive dysfunction in individuals who have experienced repeated or prolonged episodes or severe hypoglycemia before the age of 5 years.[48-50] Glycemic goals are higher for children under 5 years of age because of the deleterious effects of hypoglycemia in this age group.

Hypoglycemia is more frequent in individuals with lower A1C levels, a prior history of severe hypoglycemia, or higher insulin doses and in younger children.[51] Frequent hypoglycemia, even if it is mild, can cause hunger and overeating, thus contributing to excessive weight gain and subsequent hyperglycemia. Repeated episodes of hypoglycemia or long diabetes duration may result in abnormality of the counterregulatory system and loss of adrenergic symptoms, leading to hypoglycemia unawareness. Frequent blood glucose monitoring is necessary to avoid recurrent episodes.

Hypoglycemia can be categorized according to severity. The precise blood glucose level at which patients develop symptoms or the level they will experience a mild, moderate, or severe hypoglycemic episode is difficult to define. Symptoms generally occur when the blood glucose is less than 60 mg/dL (3.3 mmol/L).

Mild Hypoglycemia

Mild hypoglycemia is associated with mild adrenergic symptoms (sweating, pallor, palpitations, and tremors) and occasionally mild neuroglycopenic symptoms (headache and behavior change). Except in infants and toddlers, these can usually be self-treated with 10 to 15 g of easily absorbed carbohydrate, such as 3 to 4 glucose tablets or 4 oz of juice or regular soda. Additional intake of a more complex carbohydrate may be necessary, depending on timing for the next meal or snack. Treatment is individualized and most individuals learn what and how much works best for them. Excessive intake should be avoided.

Moderate Hypoglycemia

Moderate hypoglycemia requires that someone else help with treatment, but the treatment can be administered orally. Typical symptoms are aggressiveness, drowsiness, and confusion. Usually, at least 15 to 30 g of an easily absorbed glucose in a gel form is required, with an additional snack to follow.

Severe Hypoglycemia

Severe hypoglycemia is associated with altered states of consciousness, including coma or seizure, and requires treatment with glucagon or intravenous glucose. Glucagon may be required for the treatment of severe hypoglycemia, such as when the patient cannot safely swallow, is combatant to efforts to intervene, or is unable to cooperate with treatment. Doses for infants and children are significantly different than for adults. Table 9.6 lists recommended doses.[52] Glucagon can be given intramuscularly or subcutaneously in the deltoid or anterior thigh region. Parents, roommates, spouses, and significant others should be taught how to mix, draw up, and administer glucagon.

Following a hypoglycemic episode, the plasma glucose threshold for autonomic activation is lowered, thus increasing the potential for further hypoglycemic events. Any severe episode of hypoglycemia should be reported to the healthcare provider so that changes in therapy can be made when indicated.

Also see the section on hypoglycemia in chapter 15, on pharmacologic therapies for glucose management.

Diabetic Ketoacidosis

DKA is a result of insulin deficiency leading to hyperglycemia, an accumulation of ketone bodies in the blood, dehydration, and subsequent metabolic acidosis. DKA is potentially a life-threatening emergency and occurs in a variety of circumstances. Approximately 30% of children with new-onset diabetes present in ketoacidosis.[7] In the patient with known diabetes, the most common cause is omitted insulin injections or mismanagement of insulin infusion therapy. DKA also results when inadequate dose adjustments are made for intercurrent illnesses, trauma, surgery, or other physiological stress. In the child or adolescent with recurrent episodes of DKA, it is almost always due to insulin omission. These children have a higher incidence of psychiatric illness, especially depression, and are more likely to omit insulin, come from single-parent homes, and be underinsured than their peers.[45]

Because of the significant morbidity and mortality associated with DKA, prevention is of paramount importance. Prevention can be achieved by:

- Public awareness of the signs and symptoms of untreated diabetes
- Education of friends, roommates, and other caregivers about the signs and symptoms of early DKA
- Increased recognition that insulin omission due to psychological problems and lack of financial resources is the most common cause of DKA in patients with established diabetes
- Improved detection of families at risk
- Education about ketone monitoring
- 24-hour telephone availability and encouragement to contact the healthcare team when blood glucose levels are high, when there is ketonuria or ketonemia, and especially during intercurrent illnesses [6]

Chapter 8 provides detailed information on hyperglycemia.

TABLE 9.6 Recommended Doses for Glucagon

Adults and children >20 kg: 1 mg subcut or IM*
Children <20 kg: 0.5 mg subcut or IM or 20 to 30 mcg per kilogram (9.1 to 13.6 mcg per pound) of body weight*

*If necessary, the dose may be repeated after 15 minutes.

Source: Banion C, Chase HP. Hypoglycemia. In: Understanding Diabetes, 11th ed. Chase HP, ed. SFI: Denver, Colo; 2006.

Associated Autoimmune Disorders

Thyroid Disorders

Thyroid disorders are the most common autoimmune disorder associated with type 1 diabetes, with an incidence of about 17%. Patients with thyroid autoimmunity may be euthyroid, hypothyroid (most common), or hyperthyroid.[53]

Individuals with type 1 diabetes should be screened for autoimmune thyroid disease shortly after diabetes diagnosis, when metabolic control has been established. Thyroid antibodies are measured to identify thyroid autoimmunity and identify patients at risk for developing thyroid disease. Measurement of thyroid-stimulating hormone (TSH) may be the most sensitive way to identify persons with thyroid dysfunction. Subclinical hypothyroidism has been associated with an increased risk of symptomatic hypoglycemia and with reduced linear growth. Patients with elevated TSH levels should be treated with thyroid replacement therapy. Patients with a normal TSH who have no thyromegaly or growth abnormality should be screened every 1 to 2 years.[6]

Case—Part 6: Associated Autoimmune Disorders

At the age of 11 years, JJ was diagnosed with hypothyroidism on a routine screening test. He denied symptoms (fatigue, dry skin, constipation), his physical exam did not reveal thyromegaly, and his linear growth was normal. He was started on thyroid replacement therapy. At age 13, he was diagnosed with celiac disease, after 2 positive TG antibodies, which was confirmed, by a gastroenterologist, via a small-bowel biopsy. JJ also had no symptoms of celiac disease.

The dietitian instructed JJ and his parents on a gluten-free diet. The diagnosis of another chronic illness can be difficult for patients and their families. The affected individual often feels that his or her entire body is failing. This may be especially difficult for adolescents, who are working to develop a strong sense of identity.

Celiac Disease

Celiac disease is an immune-mediated disorder that is also more common in individuals with type 1 diabetes, with a prevalence of 1% to 16%.[54] Immune-mediated damage to the mucosa of the small intestine occurs after exposure to gluten, leading to destruction of the villi of the small intestine. Symptoms of celiac disease include diarrhea, weight loss or poor weight gain, growth failure, abdominal pain, chronic fatigue, irritability, an inability to concentrate, malnutrition due to malabsorption, and other gastrointestinal problems. Symptoms of celiac disease in persons who also have diabetes may include unpredictable blood glucose levels, unexplained hypoglycemia, and deterioration in glycemic control. Individuals with confirmed celiac disease should be provided guidance so they are able to follow a gluten-free diet to prevent unexpected hypoglycemia due to absorptive abnormalities and to prevent the other nutritional, metabolic, and oncologic consequences of celiac disease.[6]

There are no controlled trials to guide recommendations for asymptomatic individuals with elevated autoantibody levels and normal small-bowel biopsies. Likewise, there is little literature to guide the optimal frequency of repeat antibody testing of those with negative antibody levels.

Ongoing Care

Individuals with type 1 diabetes should see their diabetes healthcare provider every 3 months for evaluation of

Case—Part 7: Ongoing Care

JJ's most recent A1C was 6.9%. Over the years, he had regular quarterly visits, and his parents had always been involved in his care. His most recent eye exam was normal as were his urine microalbumin excretion tests. He was successful using continuous insulin infusion therapy and experienced infrequent hypoglycemia. He followed a gluten-free diet. Since starting college, he had experienced some depression and had been taking an antidepressant.

therapy and ongoing education. Studies suggest that delivery of intensive diabetes case management, telephone availability of the healthcare team, and regular in-person care improves A1C and decreases hospitalizations.[55-59] Knowledge and skills should be evaluated regularly by a diabetes educator. Frequency of hypoglycemia and the presence of hypoglycemia unawareness should be assessed at every visit. If hypoglycemia unawareness is present, blood glucose targets should be reassessed. For children, height and weight measurements are essential and should be plotted on growth charts at each visit. Poor diabetes control can lead to poor linear growth and poor weight gain, as well as a delay in pubertal and skeletal maturation. Poor growth with adequate metabolic control should raise suspicion of hypothyroidism or celiac disease.

Quarterly Follow-Up With Healthcare Provider

Each quarterly follow-up visit with the healthcare provider should include the following:

- Height, weight, and BMI calculation (and comparison to age- and sex-specific norms)
- Blood pressure determination (and comparison to age-, sex-, and height-related norms)
- A1C determination
- Evaluation of results of blood glucose monitoring, ketone testing, and patient's use of data
- Physical examination with specific emphasis on injection or pump sites (lipoatrophy or lipohypertrophy) and finger or alternative sites for blood glucose testing. Physical examination should also include funduscopic, oral, cardiac, abdominal (hepatosplenomegaly), hand/finger, foot, skin (acanthosis nigricans, necrobiosis lipoidica diabeticorum), and neurological examinations
- Interval history should include recent or current infections or illnesses; current or recent use of medications; frequency and treatment of hypoglycemia; presence of hypoglycemia unawareness; physical activity and exercise habits; meal plan;

psychosocial factors that may influence diabetes management; use of tobacco, alcohol, and/or recreational drugs; and contraception and sexual activity (if applicable)

- Review of systems should include gastrointestinal function (including symptoms of gluten intolerance) and symptoms of other endocrine disorders, especially thyroid and Addison disease
- Assessment of knowledge, skills, and coping level with referral to appropriate diabetes healthcare provider (diabetes nurse educator, dietitian, behavioral specialist) for intervention
- Assessment of emergency preparedness, including availability of glucagon to parents, roommates, and significant others knowledgeable about administering it, wearing of diabetes identification (wallet cards are not adequate), testing before driving, and the availability of a source of glucose in the car; for those living alone, identification of someone to check in if they fail to show for work or school

Yearly Assessments and Screenings

- *Ophthalmologic Evaluation:* Starting at 10 years of age with diabetes duration of 3 to 5 years[6]
- *Microalbuminuria:* Starting at 10 years of age with diabetes duration of 5 years[6]
- *Lipid Profile:* Starting at 2 years of age if positive or unknown family history for CVD; starting at puberty if family history is negative
- *Celiac and Adrenal Antibodies, TSH:* Every 1 to 2 years (more frequently if symptomatic or poor growth)
- *Depression Screening:* Starting at 10 years of age
- *Diabetes Nurse Educator and Dietitian:* Yearly visit is the minimum; many individuals may benefit from this quarterly or even more frequently, especially during the first year of diagnosis
- *Behavioral Specialist:* To enhance support and empowerment, to identify and discuss ways to overcome barriers in successful diabetes management, and, in pediatrics, to maintain family involvement in diabetes care tasks[6]

Vaccinations

Children with diabetes and children who have family members with type 1 diabetes should receive all immunizations in accordance with the recommendations of the American Academy of Pediatrics. Large studies have shown no causal relationship between childhood vaccination and type 1 diabetes.[6]

Transition to Adult Care

The individual with diabetes, the family, the pediatric diabetes team and the adult care providers should determine the appropriate time to transition young adults to adult care providers. Issues for adults with diabetes usually include college, marriage, family, employment and establishment of a career, and finances. Adult care providers may be more knowledgeable about dealing with these issues.

Type 1 Diabetes in Adults

Although type 1 diabetes is most frequently diagnosed in children, the diagnosis can occur at any age. When diabetes is diagnosed in adults, differentiating type 1 from type 2 diabetes is sometimes more difficult. One way to identify the person with the autoimmune type of diabetes (type 1) versus the insulin-resistant form (type 2) is to look for the presence or absence of islet autoantibodies. Laboratory markers of immune destruction of the beta cell include islet cell autoantibodies, autoantibodies to insulin, and autoantibodies to glutamic acid decarboxylase (GAD_{65}). One and usually more of these autoantibodies are present in 85% to 90% of individuals when fasting hyperglycemia is initially detected.[60] See chapter 8, on pathophysiology, for a more in-depth discussion on latent autoimmune diabetes in adults (LADA).

The rate of β-cell destruction can be rapid in some adults (as it almost always is in infants and children) and slow in others. While some authors differentiate rapid-onset type 1 diabetes in adults from LADA,[61] most clinicians now recognize the term LADA to describe the adult form of type 1 diabetes. Adults with LADA have similar HLA genetic susceptibility as well as autoantibodies to islet antigens. However, they may retain sufficient residual ß-cell function so that treatment of their diabetes does not require insulin initially, and they appear clinically to be affected by type 2 diabetes. Adults with LADA usually require insulin for survival after about 6 years, and they are at risk for ketoacidosis at that time. At this latter stage of the disease, there is little or no insulin secretion, as manifested by low or undetectable levels of plasma C-peptide.[60]

Associated Autoimmune Disorders

Adults with type 1 diabetes are also prone to other autoimmune disorders, such as Graves disease, Hashimoto thyroiditis, Addison disease, vitiligo, celiac sprue, autoimmune hepatitis, myasthenia gravis, and pernicious anemia.[60] The proportion of male patients is significantly higher (70%) than those diagnosed as children (57.5%).[62]

Clinical Presentation

The clinical presentation of adults with rapid-onset type 1 diabetes and the initial management of their diabetes and treatment with insulin is similar to children with new-onset diabetes as discussed earlier in this chapter. The clinical presentation of the adult with LADA may include the following:

- Lean body mass,
- Family history of type 1 diabetes or autoimmune disease, and/or
- Age 35 to 60 years

Diagnosis

In addition to the usual glucose diagnostic tests, the clinician may want to measure anti-GAD antibodies; if positive, this confirms the diagnosis of LADA. Subsequent measurement of C-peptide can delineate progression to insulin dependency. Attention should be paid to diagnose such individuals because therapy may influence the speed of progression toward insulin dependency, and in this respect, efforts should be made to protect residual C-peptide secretion.[63]

Treatment

No specific guidelines for management of LADA currently exist, but treatment to achieve normoglycemia to prevent complications is warranted. Most individuals with LADA will become insulin dependent within 6 to 8 years, and many clinicians progress to insulin sooner rather than later, although in the initial stages, LADA can be managed with therapies used for type 2 diabetes.

As stated earlier, adults newly diagnosed with diabetes often employ a basal/bolus regimen, using a long-acting insulin plus rapid-acting insulin before meals. Adults, on average, require between 0.4 to 1.0 units per kilogram per day.[1]

Primary Treatment Goals for All Individuals With Type 1 Diabetes

- To achieve optimal glycemic goals with a flexible, individualized diabetes management plan
- To avoid severe hypoglycemia, symptomatic hyperglycemia, and ketoacidosis
- To promote and maintain day-to-day clinical and psychological well-being[1]

Summary

Type 1 diabetes is not only a disease of the very young. It affects people throughout the life span and presents many challenges to both the person with diabetes and the friends and families of that person. The self-management behaviors and skill sets required to be successful and effective are very demanding, and this is in addition to the issues and stages that an individual goes through as they age. It is important that not only normal physical growth and development be a goal for this population, but that emotional growth and development be addressed. In addition, self-management depends on socioeconomic support as well as emotional and physical support. Wishing to participate in intensive management, but not being able to afford the supplies needed may be one of many barriers the individual with type 1 diabetes and the family will face. Focusing only on blood glucose values and judging blood glucose numbers as "good" or "bad" will only lead to resentment and can affect self esteem. The diabetes educator is a very important part of the diabetes care team and plays a crucial role in helping families cope with the many anticipated and unanticipated events and changes that occur.

Questions and Controversy

Despite many advances in pharmacologic therapy, monitoring blood glucose levels, and data management systems, many individuals with type 1 diabetes are still unable to achieve and maintain optimal glycemic control. There are known clinical barriers to achieving glycemic goals: fear of hypoglycemia, weight gain, postprandial hyperglycemia, and fluctuations in blood glucoses.

One aspect of the DCCT that is not often discussed is the frequency of contact with healthcare providers for the intensively managed cohort. Is that another major factor missing in the traditional care of individuals with diabetes? Do individuals need more frequent contact for motivation and education? Do we need to spend more time empowering patients to achieve optimal control? Diabetes management has gotten more and more complex—with more technology, carbohydrate counting, and use of insulin-to-carbohydrate ratios for dosing insulin—which seems to indicate that more, rather than less, education is required. Who will pay for more intensive management? Is the cost worth the benefit?

Focus on Education: Pearls for Practice

Teaching Strategies

- **Teaching plans.** There is no *one* right way to provide diabetes self-management education in type 1 diabetes, whether working with children or adults. All have different desires, needs, and expectations. Flexibility, creativity, and options for different learning styles and ages are needed—for example, use of games and puppets for small children; demonstrations and media-based materials (videos, handheld and electronic games) for teens and young adults; and models, problem-solving discussions, and demonstrations for adults.

- **After this new diagnosis, life changes.** Assist in anticipating common problems and feelings. Use role playing and discussion to openly validate feelings, and think about examples of how to handle some of the day-to-day occurrences (eg, relationships, overnight travel, party food choices).

- **The person becomes the "expert."** Coach children or adults that they are the "expert" in their diabetes. Assist them to plan a topic-specific presentation in their school or support group (in a safe environment). Include family and friends. This reinforces information and may help self-esteem.

Messages for Patients

- **Knowledge is power.** Learn as much as you can about taking care of diabetes. Attend classes offered through a local clinic or diabetes-affiliated organization at every reasonable opportunity.

- **Change is inevitable.** Expect that at different stages of life and in different situations glucose control will change and require adjustments in how it is managed. The diabetes educator and care team will help with these unexpected or unanticipated events. Include the child with diabetes in care issues, teaching school personnel, and involving the whole family.

- **Diabetes is unpredictable.** Everything can be done "right" and still perfection is not achieved. Generally speaking, life is not perfect. The focus should not be on making life perfect; rather, it needs to be more about how to cope with change. Everyone needs support—use friends, family, and your medical team for support. Ask for help; ask for what you need to achieve your goals. Use the diabetes educator and health team as consultants. Diabetes care needs to be flexible, dynamic, and individualized. There are many different ways to achieve optimal control. If one method or plan does not work, try a different approach.

Additional Readings

American Diabetes Association. Clinical Practice Recommendations 2005. Diabetes Care. 2006;29 suppl.

Betschart J. Diabetes Care for Babies, Toddlers and Preschoolers. New York, NY: John Wiley and Sons; 1999.

Betschart J, Thom S. In-Control: A Guide for Teens With Diabetes. New York, NY: John Wiley and Sons: 1995.

Brackenridge B, Rubin R. Sweet Kids: How to Balance Diabetes Control and Good Decision Making With Family Peace. Alexandria, Va: American Diabetes Association; 1996.

Chase HP. Understanding Diabetes, 10th ed. SFI, Denver, Colo; 2006. (Available for purchase at www.childrensdiabetesfdn.org or free online at www.uchsc.edu/misc/diabetes/ud10.html).

Loy VN. Real Life Parenting of Kids With Diabetes. Alexandria, Va: American Diabetes Association; 2001.

Satter E. How to Get Your Child to Eat . . . But Not Too Much. Palo Alto, Calif: Bull Publishing; 1987.

Satter E. Child of Mine—Feeding with Love and Good Sense. Palo Alto, Calif: Bull Publishing; 1987.

Siminerio L, Betschart J. Raising a Child With Diabetes, 2nd ed. Alexandria, Va: American Diabetes Association; 2000.

Wysocki T. The Ten Keys to Helping Your Child Grow Up With Diabetes. Alexandria, Va: American Diabetes Association; 1997.

References

1. American Diabetes Association. Medical Management of Type 1 Diabetes. Alexandria, Va: American Diabetes Association; 2004.
2. Onkamo P, Vaananen S, Karvonen M, et al. Worldwide increase in incidence of type 1 diabetes—the analysis of the data on published incidence trends. Diabetologia. 1999;42:1395-403.
3. Libman IM, LaPorte RE. Changing trends in epidemiology of type 1 diabetes mellitus throughout the world: how far have we come and where do we go from here. Pediatr Diabetes. 2005;6:119-20.
4. Diabetes Control and Complications Trial Research Group. The effect of intensive treatment of diabetes on the development and progression of long-term complications in insulin-dependent diabetes mellitus: the Diabetes Control and Complications Trial Research Group. N Engl J Med. 1993;329:977-86.
5. The Epidemiology of Diabetes Interventions and Complications (EDIC) Study. Sustained effect of intensive treatment of type 1 diabetes mellitus on development and progression of diabetic nephropathy. JAMA. 2003;290:2159-67.
6. Silverstein J, Klingensmith G, Copeland K, et al. Care of children and adolescents with type 1 diabetes. Diabetes Care. 2005;28:186-212.
7. Scibilia J, Finegold D, Dorman J, et al. Why do children with diabetes die. Acta Endocrinol Suppl. 1986;279:326-33.
8. American Diabetes Association. Diagnosis and classification of diabetes mellitus (position statement). Diabetes Care. 2004:27 suppl 1;S5-10.
9. Banion C, Miles M, Carter M. Problems of mothers in management of children with diabetes. Diabetes Care. 1983:6:548-51.
10. Boland E, Grey M. Coping strategies of school-age children with diabetes mellitus. Diabetes Educ. 1996; 22:592-7.
11. Drash, A, Becker D. Behavioral issues in patients with diabetes mellitus with special emphasis on the child and adolescent. In: Ellenberg and Rifkin's Diabetes Mellitus Theory and Practice, 4th ed. Rifkin H, Porte D Jr, eds. New York, NY: Elsevier Publishing; 1990:922-33.
12. Escobar O, Becker D, Drash A. Management of the child with diabetes. In: Pediatric Endocrinology, 4th ed. Lifshitz F, ed. New York, NY: Maarcel Dekker, 2004:653-67.
13. Kostraba JN, Gay EC, Rewers M, et al. Increasing trend of outpatient management of children with newly diagnosed IDDM. Colorado IDDM Registry, 1978-1988. 1992;15:95-100.
14. Mortensen HB, Hougaard P. Comparison of metabolic control in a cross-sectional study of 1,873 children and adolescents with IDDM from 18 countries. Diabetes Care. 1997;20:714-20.
15. Anderson B, Ho J, Brackett J, et al. Parental involvement in diabetes management tasks: relationships to blood glucose monitoring adherence and metabolic control in young adolescents with insulin-dependent diabetes mellitus. J Pediatr. 1997;130:257-65.
16. Levine BS, Anderson BJ, Butler DA. Predictors of glycemic control and short-term adverse outcomes in youth with type 1 diabetes. J Pediatr. 2001;139:197-203.
17. Greenhalgh S, Bradshaw S, Hall CM, et al. Forearm blood glucose testing in diabetes mellitus. Arch Dis Child. 2004;89:516-8.
18. Fedele D, Corsi A, Noacco D, et al. Alternative site blood glucose testing: a multicenter study. Diabetes Technol Ther. 2003;5:983-9.
19. Valentine V. Continuous glucose monitoring has left the station: are you on board? Diabetes Educ. 2005;31:649-62.
20. International Society for Pediatric and Adolescent Diabetes. Consensus Guidelines 2000. ISPAD Consensus Guidelines for the Management of Type 1 Diabetes Mellitus in Children and Adolescents. Medical Forum International; 2000.
21. Rutledge KS, Chase HP, Klingensmith GJ, et al. Effectiveness of postprandial Humalog in toddlers with diabetes. Pediatrics. 1997;100:968-72.
22. Roemer JB, McGee T. Type 1 diabetes in youth. In: A Core Curriculum for Diabetes Education: Diabetes Management Therapies, 5th ed. Franz MJ, ed. Chicago, Ill: American Association of Diabetes Educators; 2003.
23. Mack-Fogg JE, Orlowski CC, Jospe N. Continuous subcutaneous insulin infusion in toddlers and children with type 1 diabetes mellitus is safe and effective. Pediatr Diabetes. 2005;6:17-21.
24. Ahern JAH, Boland EA, Doane R, et al. Insulin pump therapy in pediatrics: a therapeutic alternative to safely lower HbA1c levels across all age groups. Pediatr Diabetes. 2002;3:10-5.

25. Fox LA, Buckloh LM, Smith SD, et al. A randomized controlled trial of insulin pump therapy in young children with type 1 diabetes. Diabetes Care. 2005;28:1277-81.

26. Wilson DM, Buckingham BA, Kunselman EL, et al. A two-center randomized controlled feasibility trial of insulin pump therapy in young children with diabetes. Diabetes Care. 2005;28:15-9.

27. Plotnick LP, Clark LM, Brancati FL, et al. Safety and effectiveness of insulin pump therapy in children and adolescents with type 1 diabetes. Diabetes Care. 2003; 26:1142-6.

28. Maniatis AK, Klingensmith FJ, Slover RH, et al. Continuous subcutaneous insulin infusion therapy for children and adolescents: an option for routine diabetes care. Pediatrics. 2001;107:351-6.

29. Burdick, JC, Chase HP, Slover RH, et al. Missed insulin meal boluses and elevated hemoglobin A1C levels in children receiving insulin pump therapy. Pediatrics. 2004;113:221-4.

30. American Diabetes Association. Evidence-based nutrition principles and recommendations for the treatment and prevention of diabetes and related complications. Diabetes Care. 2003;26 suppl 1:S51-61.

31. Holzmeister LA. Medical nutrition therapy for children and adolescents with diabetes. Diabetes Spectrum. 1997;10:268-74.

32. Wasserman DH, Zinman B. Exercise in individuals with IDDM. Diabetes Care. 1994;17:924-37.

33. Austin A, Warty V, Janosky J, et al. The relationship of physical fitness to lipid and lipoprotein levels in adolescents with IDDM. Diabetes Care. 1993;16:421-5.

34. American Diabetes Association. Intensive Diabetes Management. Alexandria, Va: American Diabetes Association; 2003.

35. MacDonald MJ. Postexercise late-onset hypoglycemia in insulin-dependent diabetic patients. Diabetes Care. 1987;10:584-8.

36. The Diabetes Research in Children Network (DirectNet) Study Group. Impact of exercise on overnight glycemic control in children with type 1 diabetes mellitus. J Pediatr. 2005;147:528-34.

37. Kovacs M, Iyengar S, Goldston D, et al. Psychological functioning of children with insulin-dependent diabetes: a longitudinal study. J Pediatr Psychol. 1990;15:619-32.

38. Grey M, Cameron ME, Lipman TH, et al. Psychosocial status of children with diabetes in the first 2 years after diagnosis. Diabetes Care. 1995:18:1330-6.

39. Fonagy P, Moran GS, Lindsay MK, et al. Psychological adjustment and diabetic control. Arch Dis Child. 1987; 62:1009-13.

40. Follansbee DS. Assuming responsibility for diabetes management: what age? what price? Diabetes Educ. 1989;15:347-53.

41. American Diabetes Association. Diabetes care in the school and day care setting (position statement). Diabetes Care. 2005;28 suppl 1:S43-9.

42. Numbers that Add Up to Educational Rights for Children With Disabilities. Washington, DC: Children's Defense Fund; 1989.

43. Grey M, Boland EA, Yu C, et al. Personal and family factors associated with quality of life in adolescents with diabetes. Diabetes Care. 1998;21:909-14.

44. Anderson BJ, Auslander WC. Research on diabetes management and the family: a critique. Diabetes Care. 1980; 3:696-702.

45. Rewers A, Chase HP, Mackenzie T, et al. Predictors of acute complications in children with type 1 diabetes. JAMA. 2002; 287:2511-6.

46. Temple-Trujillo R, Chase HP. Psychosocial Adjustment. In: Understanding Diabetes, 11th ed. Chase HP, ed. Denver, Colo: SFI (in print).

47. Ryan CM, Atchison J, Puczynski S, et al. Mild hypoglycemia associated with deterioration of mental efficiency in children with insulin-dependent diabetes mellitus. J Pediatr. 1990;117:32-8.

48. Northam EA, Anderson PJ, Werther FA, et al. Neuropsychological complications of IDDM in children 2 years after disease onset. Diabetes Care. 1998;21:379-84.

49. Rovet J, Alvarez M. Attentional functioning in children and adolescents with IDDM. Diabetes Care. 1997;20:803-10.

50. Bjorgaas M, Gimse R, Vik T, et al. Cognitive function in type 1 diabetic children with and without episodes of severe hypoglycemia. Acta Paediatr. 1997;86:148-53.

51. Davis EA, Keating B, Byrne GC, et al. Impact of improved glycaemic control on rates of hypoglycaemia in insulin dependent diabetes mellitus. Arch Dis Child. 1998;78:111-5.

52. Banion C, Chase HP. Hypoglycemia. In: Understanding Diabetes, 11th ed. Chase HP, ed. Denver, Colo: SFI; 2006.

53. Roldan MB, Alonso M Barrio R. Thyroid autoimmunity in children and adolescents with type 1 diabetes mellitus. Diabetes Nutr Metab. 1999;12:27-31.

54. Holmes GK. Screening for celiac disease in type 1 diabetes. Arch Dis Child. 2002; 87:495-8.

55. Beck JK, Logan KJ, Hamm RM, et al. Reimbursement for pediatric diabetes intensive case management: a model for chronic diseases? Pediatrics. 2004;113: e47-50.

56. Svoren BM, Butler D, Levine BS, et al. Reducing acute adverse outcomes in youths with type 1 diabetes: a randomized, controlled trial. Pediatrics. 2003;112:914-22.

57. Howells L, Wilson AC, Skinner TC, et al. A randomized control trial of the effect of negotiated telephone support on glycaemic control in young people with type 1 diabetes. Diab Med. 2002;19:643-8.

58. Couper JJ, Taylor J, Fotheringham MJ, et al Failure to maintain the benefits of home-based intervention in adolescents with poorly controlled type 1 diabetes. Diabetes Care. 1999; 22:1933-7.

59. Mortensen HB, Tobertson KJ, Aanstoot HJ, et al. Insulin management and metabolic control of type 1 diabetes mellitus in childhood and adolescence in 18 countries. Hvidore Study Group on Childhood Diabetes. Diabet Med. 1987;15:752-9.

60. American Diabetes Association. Diagnosis and classification of diabetes mellitus. Diabetes Care. 2005;28: S37-42.

61. Rosario PWS, Reis JS, Amim R, et al. Comparison of clinical and laboratory characteristics between adult-onset type 1 diabetes and latent autoimmune diabetes in adults. Diabetes Care. 2005;28:1803-4.

62. Sabbah E, Savola K, Ebeling T, et al. Genetic, autoimmune and clinical characteristics of childhood- and adult-onset type 1 diabetes. Diabetes Care. 2000;23:1326-32.

63. Pozzilli P, DiMario U. Autoimmune diabetes not requiring insulin at diagnosis (latent autoimmune diabetes of the adult). Diabetes Care. 2001;24:1460-7.

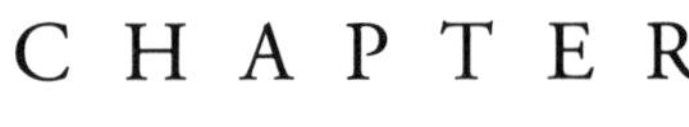

CHAPTER

10

Type 2 Diabetes Across the Life Span

Author

Geralyn R. Spollett, MSN, ANP, CDE

Key Concepts

- Type 2 diabetes, while historically a disease affecting older individuals, is affecting children, teenagers, young and older adults at alarming rates. Each age group has specific problems requiring specific strategies.
- Risk factors for developing type 2 diabetes include ethnic background, family history, obesity, and a sedentary life style.
- Type 2 diabetes is also associated with hypertension, hyperlipidemia, and cardiovascular disease.
- Treatment primarily consists of physical activity, healthy eating, and multiple medications, which present challenges to the diabetes educator, individual with diabetes, and family.

Introduction

This chapter examines type 2 diabetes across the life span. Discussion begins with the concept of diabetes as a progressive disease. A case study is used to provide a brief overview of the pathophysiologic deficits and diagnostic criteria for type 2 diabetes. Next, treatment is discussed, using the clinical practice recommendations of the American Diabetes Association (ADA). The basic principles of care are then outlined for 2 age groups with numerous special considerations: elderly adults and children and adolescents. Similarities and differences in approaches to care for each of these age-specific populations are explored. Questions and controversies are highlighted at the end of the chapter.

State of the Problem

Clinical Presentation

Type 2 diabetes is a disease characterized by hyperglycemia. The dual defects of insulin resistance, primarily at the cell receptor sites of muscle tissue, and a progressive decrease in insulin secretory capacity, result in hyperglycemia.[1]

The deficiency of pancreatic beta-cell function, which progresses over time, limits insulin production. Without adequate insulin amounts to compensate for insulin resistance, the transportation of glucose from the bloodstream into the cell cannot occur. Insulin resistance and a reduction in insulin production and secretion are present in varying degrees, depending upon the duration of the disease.

- *Phase 1:* The natural progression of type 2 diabetes appears to start with insulin resistance and impaired insulin sensitivity, followed by compensatory insulin hypersecretion.
- *Phase 2:* In the second phase, now referred to as prediabetes, impairment of pancreatic beta-cell secretion of insulin produces an abnormal rise in postmeal and fasting glucose levels.
- *Phase 3:* In the third phase, overt diabetes appears due to progressive impairment of beta-cell insulin secretion and lack of insulin sensitivity accompanied by increased hepatic glucose production.[2]

In the third phase, fasting glucose levels are greater than or equal to 126 mg/dL; however, many people with type 2 diabetes are unaware they have the disease since the mild elevations in glucose levels do not produce physical signs and symptoms prompting medical evaluation. Based on the number of persons who have long-term complications at initial presentation, scientists have estimated that diabetes may have been present for 4 to 7 years prior to the clinical diagnosis.[3]

Unlike the abrupt onset of type 1 diabetes, which presents with the classic symptoms of polyuria, polydipsia, and polyphagia, type 2 diabetes is usually insidious and progresses gradually. The first symptoms may be fatigue, poor wound healing, dry mouth, or other poorly differentiated symptoms. Alternately, type 2 diabetes that has gone undetected for a period of time can present with many of the overt symptoms usually attributed to type 1 diabetes. This wide range of presenting symptoms reflects the level of insulin resistance and the degree of beta-cell dysfunction at diagnosis.

Incidence and Prevalence

In 2005, the Centers for Disease Control and Prevention (CDC) announced that 20.8 million people, or 7% of the US population, have diabetes. Nearly a third of these Americans are undiagnosed. Of those diagnosed, 85% to 90% have type 2 diabetes.

Generally Increases With Age. In looking at how type 2 diabetes affects the demographic groups, the fastest-growing segment of the population diagnosed with this disease are those aged 65 years and older. Prevalence of diabetes increases with age. The incidence may vary between the sexes from one population to another, but in general men and women are afflicted equally.[4]

Children and Adolescents Now Also a Concern. The National Diabetes Fact Sheet 2005 notes that type 2 in children is still rare but of growing concern.[5] Although type 2 diabetes typically presents in adults over 30 years old, diagnosis of children with type 2 diabetes, particularly among the high-risk ethnic groups (eg, Hispanics, African American, and Native American) has increased over the past 5 years.

Genetics and Environment are Factors. Genetics and environmental/behavioral factors also play an important role in the development of type 2 diabetes. Chapter 2 on diabetes prevention discusses these aspects more fully.

Diabetes is reaching epidemic proportions throughout the world. The CDC and World Health Organization estimate that by the year 2025, 330 million people will have diabetes, predominantly type 2. The greatest areas of growth are in Asia and Africa, where the shift to more industrialized economies, sedentary lifestyles, and Westernized diets has increased the incidence of type 2 diabetes dramatically.[4]

As this explosion in the number of persons with diabetes reaches epidemic proportions, healthcare economics will be seriously affected. The healthcare system will be straining its capacity to effectively and efficiently diagnose, treat, and educate those affected. Prevention and early detection of diabetes play a significant role in controlling this epidemic (see chapter 2).

Risk Factors for Type 2 Diabetes

Most important risk factors for type 2 diabetes:

- Heredity, which is nonmodifiable
- Obesity, which is modifiable
- Physical inactivity, which is also modifiable

Obesity is the most powerful predictor for the development of type 2 diabetes. In high-risk populations, such as the Pima Indians, members of the at-risk group who are not obese have a lower incidence of diabetes. The interplay of other risk factors, however, such as family history with obesity, can increase incidence.

Summary of risk factors for type 2 diabetes:

The following list summarizes risk factors.[6] In addition, some public health experts and planners have noted that the economically disadvantaged have increased risk and some groups are targeting public health programs to this group—for example, Healthy People 2010.[7]

- Age of at least 45 years: The elderly especially have increased risk
- Overweight (body mass index [BMI] ≥25 kg/m^2): May not be correct for all ethnic groups; see chapter 2 for more information regarding Asian populations
- First-degree relative with diabetes
- Habitual physical inactivity
- Member of a high-risk ethnic population: African American, Hispanic, Native American, Asian American, Pacific Islander
- Previously identified prediabetes: impaired glucose tolerance (IGT) or impaired fasting glucose (IFG)
- History of gestational diabetes mellitus or the delivery of a baby that weighed more than 4.1 kg (9 lb)
- Hypertension ≥140/90 mm Hg
- High-density lipoprotein level of up to 35 mg/dL or a triglyceride level of at least 250 mg/dL
- Polycystic ovarian syndrome
- History of vascular disease

Diagnosis of Type 2 Diabetes

The American Diabetes Association has outlined 3 options for diagnosing type 2 diabetes.[8] See Table 10.1 for a summary. Findings should be confirmed by repeat testing on a different day.

TABLE 10.1 Diagnosing Type 2 Diabetes in Adults

3 Options		
Acute Symptoms* Plus Casual† Plasma Glucose ≥200 mg/dL (11.1 mmol/L)	**Fasting Plasma Glucose‡** ≥126 mg/dL (7.0 mmol/L)	**2-Hour Postload Glucose** ≥200 mg/dL (11.1 mmol/L) during oral glucose tolerance test (75-g glucose)§

Note: These results should be confirmed by repeat testing on a different day

*Classic symptoms of diabetes include polyuria, polydipsia, and unexplained weight loss

†Casual is defined as any time of day without regard to time since last meal

‡Fasting is defined as no caloric intake for at least 8 hours

§The oral glucose tolerance test is not recommended for routine clinical use

Source: Data from the American Diabetes Association. Diagnosis and classification of diabetes mellitus. Diabetes Care. 2004;27 Suppl 1:S9.

Treatment of Type 2 Diabetes

At diagnosis of type 2 diabetes, the person with diabetes and the healthcare professional work together to create an individually tailored management plan that will focus on the treatment of hyperglycemia present as well as the underlying physiologic deficits. The plan addresses the following:

- Medical nutrition therapy
- Physical activity and exercise plan
- Blood glucose control
- Reduction of risks for chronic complications
- Medication as the disease progresses

This multifaceted approach requires that the patient and provider consider a significant range of options. Much of the initial treatment aims to reduce troublesome symptoms such as polyuria and dry mouth and restore physiologic balance.

Lifestyle Interventions

For newly diagnosed patients with diabetes, medical nutrition therapy (MNT) is an essential first step in controlling glucose levels. Increasing physical activity is also important. The case in this chapter exemplifies this; more information on these topics can be found in chapters 13 and 29 (on nutrition) and 14 and 30 (on physical activity).

Reducing Complications

The major cause of death in persons with type 2 diabetes is related to cardiovascular disease. In 2001, an estimated 19% of all deaths for which cardiovascular disease was listed as the primary cause of death were attributed to diabetes. This accounted for 108,000 (58%) of all deaths attributable to diabetes.[10] Both nutrition plans and exercise plans for individuals with type 2 diabetes must incorporate prevention of cardiovascular disease. Reducing saturated fat, limiting sodium use, encouraging physical fitness and weight reduction when appropriate are all components of a healthy-heart strategy. After the diagnosis of diabetes, screening for hypertension and hypercholesterolemia is appropriate; if these comorbidities are present, aggressive treatment is initiated.

Blood Glucose Control

The following target goals have been established by the ADA to minimize the effects of the disease and its chronic complications:[11]

- *Before-meal glucose*: 90 to 130 mg/dL
- *Bedtime glucose:* 110 to 180 mg/dL
- *A1C:* below 7%

Studies such as the Diabetes Control and Complications Trial (DCCT)[12] and the UK Prospective Diabetes Study (UKPDS)[13] demonstrated that maintaining glycemic control with an A1C of <7% significantly reduced the microvascular complications associated with diabetes.

Self-Monitoring. Self-monitoring of glucose is an essential component to self-care. Self-monitoring empowers those with diabetes to make needed adjustments in their daily care and gives them the necessary data to evaluate those changes.

Glucose meters for home use are simple to use, requiring only 2 to 3 steps in the procedure. A small sample of capillary blood, which can be taken from a variety of sites, is applied to a testing strip; results are reported in 5 to 45 seconds. Small and portable, meters can use either language

> ***Heart Disease is the Leading Threat***
>
> More than half of all deaths attributable to diabetes are due to cardiovascular disease.

Case in Point: An Adult Develops Type 2 Diabetes

EB, a widowed Hispanic woman age 46, noted that in the past year she had had a 15-lb weight gain, recurrent vaginitis, and a tendency to become fatigued after her main meal. She attributed these problems to her stressful life, which included caring for both her ill mother and a new grandchild in her home. Her past medical history was significant for hypertension and dyslipidemia, notably an elevated triglyceride and decreased HDL level. Her social history revealed that she had never smoked and drank red wine approximately 1 to 2 times per month. She had not been sexually active since the death of her husband 3 years prior. During the medical evaluation for urinary tract infection and the subsequent follow-up laboratory testing, the following data were gathered:

- Urine analysis: glycosuria
- BMI: 35
- BP: 130/85 mm Hg
- Skin: marked acanthosis nigricans in folds of neck and axillae
- Fasting glucose: 199 mg/dL and 233 mg/dL

The lab data confirmed the diagnosis of diabetes. EB was upset but not surprised by the diagnosis. Her mother, two sisters and a brother all had type 2 diabetes; she had wondered in the past if she, too, had diabetes. During the course of the visit, EB stated she knew very little about managing diabetes and could not see herself incorporating changes in diet or exercise into her already busy life. She expressed fear at the possible development of blindness and kidney disease and worry that her children will be burdened with her care.

Since coming to the United States from Puerto Rico 4 years ago, EB was learning to speak English, but still preferred to read in Spanish. Her children, particularly her daughter who lived with her, usually assisted in language interpretation at EB's medical appointments.

Discussion

The diagnosis of type 2 diabetes in EB signifies the increased incidence of the disease among certain ethnic groups, in this case among Hispanic Americans. With a significant family history, EB had a genetic predisposition: 4 first-degree relatives already diagnosed with diabetes. A history of obesity with further weight gain, diminished exercise, and significant life stressors may have been the environmental and behavioral triggers that led to the manifestation of type 2 diabetes. The presence of acanthosis nigricans, a thickening of the stratum corneum that becomes pigmented, was a marker for the presence of insulin resistance. Insulin and IGF-1 receptors were present and respond to high levels of insulin. This hyperinsulinemia promotes keratinocyte proliferation resulting in acanthosis nigricans and/or skin tags.[9]

EB had a significant number of risk factors for diabetes. She was obese with a BMI of 35, and although active, had limited exercise. Her family history was strongly positive for diabetes and her ethnicity further increased risk. EB also had a past medical history of hypertension and elevated lipid values.

In those with underlying pathophysiologic changes indicative of prediabetes, the overt presentation of type 2 diabetes often occurs after an illness or other stressor. In EB's case, she had the physical stress and exhaustion of being a multigenerational caregiver. Determining whether the underlying and as-yet untreated diabetes exacerbated the urinary tract symptoms, which brought her to the clinic, or if the UTI was an initial symptom of the diabetes is difficult. Often, UTI or vaginitis are the presenting symptom in a woman with abnormal glucose levels.

The presence of glucose in the urine indicated that the level of serum glucose had exceeded approximately 180 mg/dL, the level considered the usual adult renal threshold. Urine results are not diagnostic, but heighten the suspicion for the diagnosis of diabetes. Renal threshold is reduced in children and pregnant women and elevated in the aged. Applying the diagnostic criteria (Table 10.1) to EB's lab results shows that her glucose values are indicative of diabetes.

or symbols to prompt the person to perform the next step of the procedure. Most meters now have a memory to store the time, date, and testing results of multiple glucose tests. The person with diabetes tests blood at certain times of the day to assess a response to food intake, medication, and/or exercise. Recording these results creates a diary of diabetes care that can act as a reference to assist in future therapeutic decisions.

A point to consider for the diabetes educator is the psychomotor and cognitive ability of the individual performing the skill of blood glucose monitoring. Even for patients who have experience with a glucose-testing device, these skills must be demonstrated at least once to the diabetes educator. During the evaluation, the diabetes educator assesses the individual's ability to properly calibrate or code the meter, insert strips, obtain the sample, replace the battery, and troubleshoot meter errors.

Pharmacologic Interventions

The pathways to controlling blood glucose levels and achieving the target goals vary for each person with diabetes. Initially, lifestyle modifications may be sufficient, but as the disease progresses, the pathophysiologic changes diminish insulin sensitivity and beta-cell production, requiring medications to reach target goals.

Individualized Plan

The provider must tailor the medication regimen to the individual and adjust it as necessary to maintain glycemic control. During the first few years of type 2 diabetes, the use of oral medications, usually in a multiple drug regimen, are effective in reaching target goals.

Oral medications (discussed in depth in chapter 15) used for the treatment of diabetes address the various pathophysiologic deficits:

Biguanides (metformin):	Reduce hepatic glucose output
Sulfonylureas (glyburide, glipizide):	Improve insulin secretion
Thiazolidinediones (rosiglitiazone, pioglitazone):	Increase insulin sensitivity
Meglitinides (repaglinide, nateglinide):	Increase circulating insulin levels but have a shorter duration than the sulfonylureas
Alpha-glucosidase inhibitors (miglitol, acarbose):	Act within the intestinal wall to prevent/delay the breakdown of certain carbohydrates

As diabetes progresses, oral agents may need to be supplemented with additional medications. Injectable exenatide may be added to the regimen, or insulin therapy may be initiated. In addition to the traditional injectable formulation, an inhaled form of insulin was approved by the US Food and Drug Administration in January 2006. (See chapter 15 for more information on medications.) With increasing duration of disease, many people with type 2 diabetes require insulin therapy to remain in a healthy glycemic range. Both the person with diabetes and the healthcare professional need to determine when to add or convert to insulin therapy.

The decision to start an injectable therapy, particularly insulin, can be a difficult one. Fear of needles or injections, myths and fallacies about insulin therapy, concerns about hypoglycemia when using insulin, and alterations in lifestyle due to the use of injectable therapies all can present barriers to initiation of this therapy. (See chapter 4 for more information on anxieties and diabetes-specific fears.) Those who did not adhere to their diabetes regimen may have been threatened with the prospect of insulin therapy, further compounding their reluctance to switch to this therapy when the time is appropriate. Coercion of this type increases fear and resistance to using this safe and effective drug.

There are many different types of insulin and various delivery devices. Patient education is a critical component of management of type 2 diabetes with insulin therapy. Not only must the individual with diabetes and ancillary caregivers understand how to administer the insulin; they must also learn about the type, timing, and action of insulin. Chapters 15 and 31 provide detailed information.

Type 2 Diabetes in Older Adults

Undiagnosed and untreated diabetes is more common in older adults than in any other age group. Approximately 20.9% of all people age 60 or older have diabetes.[5] Those age 65 and older account for almost 50% of the population with diabetes.[5] In 2004, the prevalence of diagnosed diabetes among people aged 65 to 74 years (16.7%) was approximately 12 times that of people less than 45 years of age (1.4%).[14] The risk of developing diabetes increases with age, but diminishes after the age of 80.

Screening and Diagnosis of Older Adults

Diagnostic criteria for diabetes do not alter or become less stringent for older adults. The same set of criteria is applied to the nonpregnant adult regardless of age (only in the case of pregnancy do guidelines for screening and diagnosing

Case—Part 2: Implementing the Adult's Treatment Plan

Although EB had stated her reservations about attempting lifestyle changes, the individualized approach to nutrition, presented in a step-wise manner, addressed these concerns and endeavors so that the necessary adjustment could be made.

Nutrition Plan

MNT involves a thorough assessment of the person's current lifestyle, eating patterns, ethnic, and cultural or traditional food preferences as well as nutritional requirements for stages of growth and development. MNT also incorporates nutritional changes necessary to prevent or treat other health conditions, such as dyslipidemia or osteoporosis. For EB, her nutrition plan would incorporate the following key elements:

- She could eat the Hispanic foods she loved, but was encouraged to limit portion sizes where appropriate to enhance weight loss
- During early phases of treatment, reduction of carbohydrates such as juices and concentrated sweets would be emphasized to lower the glycemic load, which would help reduce insulin resistance from glucose toxicity

Physical Activity Plan

EB's life was very active, but she was doing little to improve her cardiovascular system or to increase her metabolism to burn calories and contribute to weight loss. An increase in aerobic exercise would address both of these concerns. In addition, weight loss and exercise might improve her lipid values—raising HDL and lowering triglycerides. Exercise would also provide a healthy outlet for the stress EB experienced in her role as caregiver. Although beginning an exercise program can be daunting, most patients find a walking program an easy and effective way to increase aerobic activity. Planning brief 10- to 15-minute periods of time to walk throughout the day helps improve insulin sensitivity, reduce weight, and improve cardiovascular fitness.

Blood Glucose Control

A significant part of EB's treatment plan focused on obtaining and maintaining blood glucose ranges in accordance with target goals established by the ADA. The role of maintaining glycemic control in reducing microvascular complications was an important and empowering message for EB, who feared blindness and renal disease.

Monitoring. To monitor changes in blood glucose levels and the response to treatment, EB needed to learn to check her glucose at home. Self-monitoring of glucose is an essential component to self-care. It empowers the patient to make needed adjustments in their daily care and gives them the necessary data to evaluate those changes. EB had been checking her mother's glucose level at home sporadically. She had never self-tested. She told the diabetes educator she felt confident using the brand of meter she had used for her mother and did not feel the need for further instructions. EB demonstrated proper techniques in the use of her glucose meter and agreed to test before breakfast and again before supper. She was given an instruction sheet written in Spanish that delineated the steps needed to periodically check the accuracy of the meter, including the help-line number for the meter manufacturer.

Medication

EB needed not only MNT, but also medication because she was symptomatic. She was started on metformin (Glucophage). She received all written instructions and material in both Spanish and English. During the appointment, her daughter had been helpful in translating certain difficult English words to Spanish for EB; however, once EB was at home, she would need to be able to read and formulate her own questions regarding her therapy.

After receiving a prescription to treat the UTI, a sample of metformin, and instructions to increase her fluid intake while on the antibiotics, EB was scheduled for an appointment for follow-up care in 1 week, at which time she would bring her glucose test results diary for discussion and participate in further dietary instruction.

gestational diabetes change, relying on an oral glucose tolerance test to determine the diabetes state).

Older adults should be screened annually for diabetes. Although measuring fasting plasma glucose increases detection of diabetes in the young, this test may actually miss 31% of cases in older adults.[15]

Recommended screening method for older adults:

For older adults, a 2-hour oral glucose tolerance test may better reveal the presence of diabetes than measuring plasma glucose increases.

Clinical Presentation

As in the younger adult population, type 2 is the most common type of diabetes in older adults. Older adults with diabetes rarely present with the typical symptoms of hyperglycemia.[16] Physiologic changes associated with aging may diminish thirst and increase dehydration. Glycosuria at the usual levels may not be seen because of the advance in renal threshold associated with aging.

Older, Lean Patients. Lean older adults may exhibit signs of autoimmune changes like that usually seen in type 1. Latent autoimmune diabetes of adults (LADA) does occur, presenting in older adults who are not obese. Often, this presentation creates a confusing clinical picture of acute hyperglycemia because this population normally is diagnosed with type 2 diabetes. To be well controlled, LADA requires insulin treatment to preserve beta-cell function and promote euglycemia. Although the rates of occurrence are small, the healthcare professional must be aware of the possibility of this diagnosis in older lean patients. A laboratory blood test to measure antiglutamic acid decarboxylase (anti-GAD) or islet cell antibodies (ICAs) can confirm the autoimmune state and improve treatment of the person with LADA.[17]

Other Presentations. Others may present with glucose elevations due to an acute illness, a transient medical condition, or the introduction of a certain medication (steroids, antihypertensives, cardiac medications). This increase in plasma glucose levels may be a clue to previously undiagnosed diabetes, IGT, or IFG and present an opportunity for further assessment and treatment.

Care With Older Adults

Interventions must carefully consider nutrition and exercise limitations and medication side effects pertinent to the older adult's situation.

Considerations Regarding Older Adults

Older adults are a heterogeneous group; some may be active and functional, providing their own self-care, while others may suffer from multiple comorbidities and require assistance or total care. The following factors must be carefully considered in planning education and care for the unique needs of individuals in this age group:

- Medical complications
- Physical limitations
- Other prescribed medications
- Effects of aging
- Greater risk of hypoglycemia

Complications

Older persons with type 2 may have a long duration of diabetes with an increase in complications, both macrovascular and microvascular. The UKPDS showed that macrovascular complications of diabetes are 1.5 to 2 times more prevalent in the older diabetic populations than in the nondiabetic population.[18] Based on diabetes mortality and morbidity rates collected from Medicare claims data on the elderly population in the United States, the following conclusions have been drawn:[19]

- Leading causes of morbidity are ischemic heart disease and stroke
- Gangrene, amputation, and lower extremity infection make up the next cohort of diseases associated with morbidity
- Acute complications (hypoglycemia, ketoacidosis, hyperosmolar syndrome) comprise the last group

Physical Limitations

Older adults with diabetes are about 1.5 times more likely to have physical limitations and alterations in the activities of daily living than those without diabetes.[20] Disabilities may be directly linked to eye disease, strokes, cardiovascular disease, neuropathies, and peripheral vascular disease. Older persons with diabetes may also respond more symptomatically to both hyperglycemia and hypoglycemia. Coupled with additional comorbidities, the long tenure of diabetes may contribute to frailty. Physical limitations necessitate adjustment in management goals and interventions.

Polypharmacy

Older adults with diabetes may also be on multiple medications for a variety of ailments. This can lead not only to dosing and timing errors, but also the heightened possibility of drug interactions. The healthcare professional must use caution when prescribing certain diabetes medications for older adults.

Cautions with diabetes medication in older adults:[21]

- *Metformin.* In patients >80 years of age, evaluate renal function with creatinine clearance; if <60 mg/dL, do not administer drug. Serum creatinine is a poor correlate of renal health because of the low muscle mass characteristic of the elderly person.
- *Thiazolidinediones.* Contraindicated in Class 3 and 4 congestive heart failure (CHF); avoid if CHF is present, determine benefit versus risk.
- *Sulfonylureas.* Beware of long half-life and propensity for hypoglycemia; caution in liver and renal dysfunction.
- *Insulin.* Risk of severe hypoglycemia increases with age.

Aging

Physiologic changes in aging affect signs and symptoms associated with diabetes and its complications. Below are facets of normal aging that can significantly impact diabetes care:

- Diminished taste and olfactory sense
- Reduced metabolic rate that alters digestion
- Decreased renal clearance
- Altered pain perception

Higher Risk for Hypoglycemia

Slowed counterregulation of hormones, erratic food intake, certain medications (beta-blockers), and slowed intestinal absorption place the older adult at higher risk for hypoglycemia. The adrenergic response to low blood glucose levels may be diminished or absent. Instead, the initial symptoms, such as lack of motor skills or confusion, represent a neuroglycopenia that may be misdiagnosed or pose a safety risk to the individual.

In light of all of the changes in the older adult's health, close attention must be paid to nutrition and exercise interventions and medication side effects. The healthcare professional must keep in mind the individual's preferences and physiologic alterations.

Factors Influencing Education Strategies

For those with diabetes who are still hardy, diabetes self-care and management goals must reflect their capabilities. Despite the fact that age can affect the processing of information, the capacity to learn and integrate new information remains intact throughout the life cycle. In the educational process, accommodations should especially be made for the following:

- Hearing changes
- Visual changes
- Cognitive status

Paced Learning and Feedback. As with all adult learners, older persons with diabetes benefit from a step-wise approach to education that recognizes their past experience and builds upon it. In addition, several studies have demonstrated that some older adults with type 2 diabetes may experience some mental slowing that affects the ability to perform diabetes self-care behaviors.[22,23] The diabetes educator must assess older patients for comprehension and memory through both verbal and skill feedback.

Equipment Difficulties. Self-care devices that require technical skill and manipulation, such as those for self-monitoring of glucose and insulin administration, have become much easier for the older adult with diabetes to use.

- Glucose meters have larger display screens, audible beeping prompts, reduced sample size, and ergonomically designed easy-to-grip bodies to facilitate ease of use. Some meters have test strips in drums or cartridges that are easier for arthritic hands to maneuver.
- *Insulin administration.* Insulin pens have made self-administration of insulin safer for the older person with diabetes. Since it is easier to read dosage marks on insulin pens than on syringes, accuracy of dosing is increased. These devices reduce dosage errors and do not require the manual dexterity of the vial and syringe method. The advantages and disadvantages of inhaled insulin delivery may also be considered as products in this category become available.

Since some third party payors do not routinely reimburse for some of these devices, the diabetes educator must endeavor to educate third party payors regarding the need for these devices and to advocate on behalf of the patient.

Other Barriers. In an older, retired population, financial concerns, insurance issues, and transportation difficulties can become staggering problems, confounding the delivery of health care and health maintenance. For the person with type 2 diabetes, expenses can be a concern—both the expense of medication for diabetes and its comorbidities and the cost of coverage for multiple medical visits plus podiatric, dental, and eye care. The healthcare provider must be aware of these issues and seek to ameliorate them whenever possible. For example, prescribing medications that are preferred and offer maximal reimbursement or coverage whenever possible reduces the financial burden of the person with diabetes.

Institutional Settings. Many older adults live in long-term care facilities; a large proportion of them have diabetes. In addition to all of the usual therapeutic considerations for type 2 diabetes, in this population, skin care takes on heightened importance—so that infections, ulcerations, and amputations can be avoided. Reduced circulation, neurological impairment, diminished range of motion, and compromised nutritional status contribute to the fragility of the skin. People with diabetes who are no longer capable of self-care depend on healthcare providers to develop effective care strategies to maintain glycemic control and prevent or reduce health-altering consequences. The diabetes educator can help establish strategies to ensure the following:

- Glucose levels are appropriately monitored and acted upon
- Acute complications of hypoglycemia and hyperglycemia are avoided when possible and treated if present
- Insulin and other diabetes medications are given accurately and in a timely manner; other medications are checked for potential negative interactions
- Nutrition intervention supplies sufficient calories and is delivered in a manner that best suits the patient's needs and preferences
- Skin and foot care become an integral part of the daily care regimen to promote circulation and avoid breakdown

Type 2 Diabetes in Children and Adolescents

Type 2 represents 8% to 45% of all diabetes reported among children and adolescents.[24] Of this group, 94% belonged to minority groups.

Diagnosis of Type 2 Diabetes in Children and Teens

Risk Factors

Type 2 diabetes in children and adolescents has increased as the frequency of obesity has risen in the United States. At diagnosis, 85% of children with type 2 diabetes are overweight or obese.[25] Nearly all children diagnosed have a positive family history of type 2 diabetes, with 74% to 100% having a first- or second-degree relative with type 2 diabetes and 45% to 80% having a parent with diabetes. Many of these children are of non-European descent (eg, African American, Hispanic, and Native American).

Clinical Presentation

In general, children and adolescents diagnosed with type 2 diabetes have glycosuria without ketonuria, mild thirst, some increase in urination, and little-to-no weight loss; however, up to 33% will have ketonuria at diagnosis, with 5% to 25% having ketoacidosis unrelated to stress, illness, or infection.[25] Polycystic ovarian syndrome (PCOS) and acanthosis nigricans, disorders associated with insulin resistance, are commonly seen[24] as well as lipid disorders and hypertension. There are ethnic differences in lipids, lipoproteins, and blood pressure with further indications of the metabolic syndrome in this high-risk population.

At times, the clinical picture of the child with diabetes can be confusing, making it difficult to differentiate type 1 from type 2 without laboratory studies. A variation on the presentation of type 2 diabetes occurs in children with a positive family history of early-onset diabetes. Although the child presents in diabetic ketoacidosis, which is usually seen in type 1 diabetes, the antibody tests are negative (both anti-GAD and ICA), and insulin is not required once the acute episode is resolved. These children have elevated C-peptide levels, which indicates a hyperinsulinemia as opposed to reduced insulin levels found in type 1 diabetes. Many of these children are of African American descent.

Due to the difficulty in establishing the type of diabetes in children by presentation alone, in an ideal situation type 1 diabetes would be confirmed by a test for autoantibodies, while type 2 diabetes would use a test for insulin resistance such as the fasting C-peptide.[26]

Insulin Resistance. The pattern for development of type 2 diabetes in children appears to follow the insidious pathway seen in adult type 2. Insulin levels may be normal or elevated, but first-phase insulin release is not sufficient to compensate for insulin resistance, which leads to hyperglycemia. Just as in adults with type 2 diabetes, obesity and a lack of physical activity promote overt diabetes. Both of these lifestyle factors promote insulin resistance. The onset of type 2 frequently occurs around the time of puberty, a time when insulin sensitivity declines. This evidence further supports the importance of insulin resistance in the pathogenesis of the disease.

Intrauterine Environment. The intrauterine environment, specifically birth weight and maternal hyperglycemia, may have possible links to type 2 diabetes in children. Low birth weight predicts type 2 diabetes in middle age.[27] Low birth weight has also been associated with the development of diabetes in teens and adolescents. Higher levels of amniotic fluid insulin at 33 to 38 weeks' gestation were a strong predictor of later IGT.[28] Children born to mothers with gestational diabetes also appear to have a higher risk of developing type 2 diabetes.[29]

Diagnostic Criteria

With the current explosion in the number of new cases of diabetes and the importance of screening, controversies concerning the criteria and the most effective testing method for screening for diabetes, particularly type 2 in children, abound. At present, the same diagnostic criteria are applied to children; however, whether these established cut-points are valid in a younger population is not known.

Public Health Interventions. The advent of type 2 diabetes in children and adolescents carries with it a significant public health problem. The onset of the disease in younger populations leads to earlier onset of complications, both macrovascular and microvascular. The estimated financial costs and loss of productivity resulting from these health problems represent a significant economic burden. Earlier diagnosis and aggressive treatment may help in preventing or delaying these costly complications, making a strong case for screening. In 2000, the ADA outlined recommendations for testing children at substantial risk for type 2 diabetes. See Table 10.2.

TABLE 10.2 Diagnosing Type 2 Diabetes in Children

*Criteria for Considering Screening for Diabetes**
Overweight (BMI 85th percentile for age and sex, weight for height 85th percentile, or weight 120% of ideal for height)
Plus any 2 of the following risk factors: • Family history of type 2 diabetes in first- or second-degree relative • Race/ethnicity (American Indian, African American, Hispanic, Asian/Pacific Islander) • Signs of insulin resistance or conditions associated with insulin resistance (acanthosis nigricans, hypertension, dyslipidemia, PCOS)
Age of Initiation:
Age 10, or at onset of puberty if puberty occurs at a younger age
Frequency:
Every 2 years
Test:
Fasting plasma glucose preferred

*Clinical judgment should be used to test for diabetes in high-risk subjects who do not meet these criteria.

Source: Data from the American Diabetes Association. Type 2 diabetes in children and adolescents (consensus statement). Diabetes Care. 2000;23(3):381-9.

Considerations Regarding Children and Teens

Once a child or adolescent learns he or she has type 2 diabetes, the approach to care must incorporate the youth's developmental needs and psychosocial concerns. Since many of the children and teens diagnosed with type 2 diabetes are overweight or obese, they have already faced issues that may separate them from their peers. Personal appearance (issues of both style and size), participating in competitive athletics, and congregating at fast-food restaurants or malls are often integral aspects of growing up in the United States. Adjustments in lifestyle that help reduce weight and control diabetes can seem to run counter to the norm and become problematic. Striving for independence and developing a sense of self are important developmental tasks that are made more difficult in the presence of diabetes. While parental support and guidance are a necessary part of dealing with a medical condition such as diabetes, at this time of life, the adolescent desires less parental involvement.

For adolescents and children with type 2 diabetes, the goals of therapy are the same as for any person with diabetes:

- To achieve physical and psychological well-being while maintaining long-term glycemic control and to avoid microvascular and macrovascular complications

Lifestyle Interventions

Medical nutrition therapy and increased physical activity are the cornerstone of therapy for all age groups; however, weight management in children and adolescents must take into consideration health growth and development needs. Thus, aggressive weight-loss programs are not recommended for these age groups. The approach must be one of substitution and reduction, rather than elimination. The following are important dietary adjustments that still leave room for the adolescent lifestyle:

- Learning to make healthy choices at fast-food restaurants
- Reducing fatty, calorie-dense foods
- Drinking less sugary beverages
- Choosing healthy snacks

Obese youths may lack the stamina and athletic prowess to compete in sports. Therefore, physical activities can be a source of self-degradation and ridicule by peers and can contribute to low self-esteem. In the treatment of type 2 diabetes, physical activity lowers insulin resistance and helps maintain weight loss. The challenge is to make this important therapy agreeable to an audience that usually eschews it.

Rather than focusing on competitive activities, the child needs encouragement to improve fitness through individual activities such as roller-blading, biking, or dancing.[30] Reducing television and computer time and substituting any type of physical movement has benefits. See the list of Web sites with information to help counter childhood obesity at the end of chapter 30.

Pharmacologic Interventions

Many children with type 2 diabetes will require medication in addition to lifestyle modification to achieve glucose goals. Some will need medication at diagnosis. Currently, the US Food and Drug Administration (FDA) approves 2 pharmacologic agents for use in children and adolescents:

- Metformin (an oral agent)
- Insulin (injectable formulations)

A third class of medications, the thiazolidinediones, is being investigated for safety and efficacy in this population.

Metformin. The oral agent metformin (Glucophage), a biguanide, has been approved for use in children 10 to 16 years of age with type 2 diabetes. In controlled trials in subjects ages 8 to 16 years with type 2 diabetes, metformin significantly decreased fasting plasma glucose and A1C levels when compared to placebo.[31] The drug has 2 common adverse effects:

- Diarrhea
- Nausea

To minimize adverse effects, metformin should be taken with food and the dosage titrated slowly, starting with one 500-mg tablet per day until the effective dosage is achieved. The extended-release preparation of metformin may lessen or minimize the adverse effects. For children, the maximum dosage of metformin is 2000 mg (in adults it is 2550 mg).

In girls with type 2 diabetes and PCOS, use of metformin may normalize ovulatory abnormalities and increase the risk of unplanned pregnancy; therefore, girls of childbearing age using this therapy should be counseled regarding this risk.[24] See also the section on teens in chapter 11, on pregnancy with preexisting diabetes.

Insulin. Insulin therapy has a long history of usage in the pediatric population. Healthcare professionals prescribe insulin for children, whether type 1 or type 2, who present with diabetic ketoacidosis, hyperosmolar hyperglycemic state, moderate ketosis, or symptomatic glycemic levels. The need for insulin in the hyperglycemic state complicated by insulin resistance may persist for weeks after diagnosis. However, once glycemic levels decrease and lifestyle measures are in place, some children are able to maintain euglycemic levels with metformin.

Insulin therapy should be used if oral agents are not effective or when the disease worsens and clinical goals are no longer met with oral agents alone. Insulin can be used as monotherapy or in combination with metformin.

Some children have been able to meet target goals with 1 injection of a long-acting insulin per day, such as insulin glargine, while others have needed multiple daily injections (MDI) using a basal-bolus regimen. Insulin therapy must be tailored to the physical as well as psychosocial needs of the person with diabetes. Despite the flexibility of an MDI regimen, adolescents may at times feel encumbered by it and switch to prefilled mixed insulin pens to maximize convenience and have a respite from the demands of self-care.[30] In the presence of insulin resistance in type 2 diabetes, larger amounts of insulin are necessary to adequately control glycemic levels. This is also true in children and particularly adolescents who have type 2 diabetes. During puberty and growth spurts, insulin resistance increases, necessitating compensatory dosing of insulin. Irrespective of ethnicity, insulin sensitivity is reduced while fasting levels are increased in both obese and nonobese children during Tanner stages II through IV of pubertal development.[32]

Other Medications. Sulfonylureas, glucosidase inhibitors, and meglitinides may be effective in treating type 2 diabetes in children, but more research must be conducted to determine the risks of using these drugs in this population. In particular, researchers must explore whether insulin secretagogues such as sulfonylureas, accelerate beta-cell demise in this group, especially in the presence of autoimmunity.[33] Inhaled insulin has been approved for adults in some instances (see chapter 15), but has not been approved for children.

Social Support

No matter the therapy selected, patient education and family support are vital components of diabetes management in children and teens. Ideally, a diabetes care team will be able to assess, treat, evaluate, and support the youth and family during the initial stages of the disease. Not all communities have access to such services. In many cases, school counselors and nurses, coaches, teachers, family friends, and peers can assist in providing information, supporting dietary changes, encouraging physical activity, and becoming a sounding board for the frustrations and concerns of the young person with diabetes.

Self-Care Behaviors

The self-care behaviors described in the AADE 7 Self Care Behaviors™ are applicable throughout the life span for those with type 2 diabetes. Each behavior is critical in attaining self-sufficiency in the management of diabetes. However, each behavior must be modified to incorporate the particular developmental needs of the person with diabetes to reflect the individual's physical capabilities and self-care responsibilities. Strategies pertinent to each behavior are covered more fully in the chapters in section 3 of this book.

Being Active

All persons with type 2 diabetes need to maintain a program of physical fitness, the definition of which will vary according to age and ability. Motivation for exercise, creating a program that is sustainable, and integrating it into daily routine may be quite different for a child compared to a nursing home resident, yet for both exercise is an integral factor in reducing insulin resistance and improving cardiovascular health.

Healthy Eating

Nutritional management skills such as knowing how, when, and how much to eat are the basis of self-care in diabetes. Modifications for age, caloric requirements, and activity level individualize this therapy.

Adults and Older Adults. Adults with diabetes must learn to replace harmful dietary habits with healthy ones. Selecting nutritious foods that are easier to chew and digest that are also appetizing and healthy may pose a problem for some older adults. The elderly adult may also experience social isolation and a reduction in appetite. Financial limitations can also affect healthy eating behaviors.

Teens. Learning how to cope with the typical diet of their peers while maintaining glycemic control is a daunting task for teens. Alcohol consumption and eating disorders, particularly overeating, may also prove a threat (see chapter 4).

Taking Medication

Polypharmacy in adults and older persons with diabetes can create problems in accuracy and adherence. Issues of vision and manual dexterity complicate this task. For children, medications can be dispensed by a responsible adult or taken under supervision. Despite this, the child needs an age-appropriate understanding of the importance of the medication regimen and the ability to recognize and treat possible side effects such as hypoglycemia.

Monitoring

Learning to accurately monitor glucose levels is a basic skill that is integral to self-managing diabetes, regardless of age. The young and the old both experience lifestyle changes that can radically alter glucose levels. In such cases, self-monitoring of blood glucose is an important safety tool for avoiding critical low or high levels.

Problem Solving

Understanding glucose data or interpreting signs and symptoms of acute complications and being able to make appropriate therapeutic adjustments are complex skills that require education and mentoring. Caregivers for those who are home-bound or in nursing facilities may assume this task when the person with diabetes is unable to make these decisions alone. In these situations, diabetes healthcare professionals need to educate and support ancillary care providers to ensure that standards of diabetes care are upheld.

Reducing Risks

For the young, much of self-care education focuses on improving glycemic control to prevent future complications. Risk reduction for cardiovascular disease is of paramount importance in obese, type 2 children. Smoking abstinence or cessation and control of lipids and blood pressure are also important in reducing risk. Diabetes educators have the task of informing communities of the lifestyle modifications necessary to prevent and treat diabetes in youth. For older persons with diabetes, vigilance and screening for complications is also important to delay or prevent complications. Eye exams, prophylactic foot care, flu and pneumonia vaccines, and dental care all help to maintain functional status among elderly adults.

Healthy Coping

Psychosocial adaptations are required. Living with a chronic disease requires support, creative coping skills, and a certain hardiness. Remaining motivated in the face of a somewhat capricious disease such as diabetes can be very difficult.

The life stressors present for young and old add considerable burden, and it is not uncommon for persons with diabetes to become depressed. Healthcare providers must help patients learn a variety of coping skills to meet the challenges of life with diabetes and be ready to appropriately screen and treat depression. Chapters 4 and 34 provide more information on depression.

Questions and Controversies

Limited Experience With Children and Teens

The increased incidence of type 2 diabetes in children and adolescents has sparked a number of questions with regard to the following:

- Criteria for screening and diagnosis
- Best screening methods
- Best treatment options

The lessons learned in type 2 diabetes and best-practice scenarios may not be applicable to the younger populations. Many questions remain to be answered through research.

Safe Blood Glucose Targets

The American College of Endocrinologists has recommended lower target levels for diabetes control, specifically these: A1C levels ≤6.5%, fasting and premeal glucose values of <110 mg/dL, and postprandial glucose values of <140 mg/dL.[34] The important issue is, however, safety; these targets must be individualized. In the older adult with a long duration of diabetes and comorbidities, setting less-intensive glycemic goals is reasonable.[35] There is no research that A1C values <7% are beneficial in the very elderly over 80 years of age.

In children with type 2 diabetes, who face increased risks of vascular complications related to the potentially long duration of diabetes, goals for control are normal fasting blood glucose values, which are defined as <126 mg/dL and A1C <7%.[36]

Obesity Prevention

Obesity is the most prevalent risk factor for type 2 diabetes and yet no long-term effective strategies are in place to prevent or reduce the incidence of obesity in children or adults.

Older Adults: Frail vs. Functional

Although there is a decline in function with age that can be more severe in people with diabetes, too often diabetes therapy in this population fails to meet target goals. While important to acknowledge that the frail elderly may need more relaxed glucose goals, the functional elderly must be treated to the standard of care.

Summary

Type 2 diabetes is a major problem affecting all ages. With the incidence and prevalence of this disease rising to epidemic proportions, the healthcare professional must address the factors that contribute to development of diabetes as well as those that contribute to the development of diabetic complications. Obesity, genes, and family history are the prime risk factors; however, attention to interpersonal, intrapersonal, community, and societal issues can help promote healthy lifestyles for those with diabetes.

- To prevent type 2 diabetes, interventions at the individual, family, and community levels are crucial to reduce the levels of obesity in Western society.
- Important steps to improve diabetes care include these: community awareness of lifestyle modifications necessary to reduce risk, appropriate screening for diabetes among those at highest risk, and promotion and adherence to diabetes standards of care.
- To be effective, education and medical management must be tailored to the individual, taking into consideration age, socioeconomic status, and cultural and religious affiliations.

By recognizing the needs of individuals with type 2 diabetes throughout the life span, the health professional is better prepared to offer appropriate treatment and guidance.

Focus on Education: Pearls for Practice

Teaching Strategies

- **Be sensitive to issues of age and culture.** Type 2 and LADA affect a wide range of age groups. Give simple, clear information and messages, in a step-wise approach. Tailor content to the age group. Seek out questions that need to be answered first. Establish rapport, then begin to offer information and handouts.

- **Create a milieu.** Think about a wide range of ages, previous experience with diabetes in the family or with friends, and how to deliver content with more than a single approach. For example, teens and adults who drink soft drinks benefit from actually measuring teaspoons of sugar found in a "real" soft drink. This gives a visual of calorie and glycemic value of a commonly used beverage. Adults and teens also respond to seeing test tubes filled with fat that equal the fat in food products such as hamburger, steak, and chicken.

- **Identify polypharmacy problems.** Polypharmacy may be a problem, particularly in older adults. Routinely review all medications the person is taking, including over-the-counter products and dietary supplements. Discuss use and misuse (for example, use in combination with other medicines and street drugs).

- **Recognize psychological concerns.** Changes in self-esteem, for example, are a concern to all age groups. Accepting diabetes as a chronic disease may be especially difficult for younger individuals, but belief in the chronicity and care needed is of concern to all age groups. As an elderly person's medical and mental status changes, the person may be placed at risk for adverse events. Family involvement is advised for support.

Messages for Patients

- **Screening visits protect health longer.** Schedule health visits for screening and then schedule follow-up appointments without delay. Doing so helps individuals with diabetes know what they are most at risk for, helps avoid and delay complications related to having diabetes, and improves the chances for effective treatment.

- **Physical activity helps at every age.** All age groups engage in fitness. Although competitive sports may be culturally encouraged, fitness and endurance are true primary focus. Walking and workout programs are examples.

- **Involve family.** Involving family and/or significant others at all levels of education from basic information to participation in exercise is encouraged.

References

1. American Diabetes Association. Standards of medical care in diabetes (position statement). Diabetes Care. 2006;29 Suppl 1: S4-42.
2. Kahn SE. The relative contributions of insulin resistance and beta cell dysfunction to the pathophysiology of type 2 diabetes. Diabetologia. 2003; 46:3-19.
3. Nathan DM. Insulin treatment of type 2 diabetes mellitus. In: The Diabetes Mellitus Manual: A Primary Care Companion to Ellenberg and Rifkin's, 6th ed. Inzucchi S, ed. New York: McGraw-Hill; 2005:138-49.
4. American Diabetes Association. Diabetes population statistics. In: Diabetes 4-1-1: Facts, Figures and Statistics at a Glance. Alexandria, Va: American Diabetes Association; 2005:34-46.
5. Centers for Disease Control and Prevention. National diabetes fact sheet: general information and national estimates on diabetes in the United States, 2005. Atlanta, Ga: US Department of Health and Human Services, Centers for Disease Control and Prevention, 2005. On the Internet: www.diabetes.org/diabetes-statistics.jsp. Accessed 1 Feb 2006.
6. Inzucchi SE, Sherwin RS. The prevention of type 2 diabetes mellitus. Endocrin Metab Clin North Am. 2005;34(1):199-219.
7. Healthy People 2010 Consortium. Diabetes. In: Healthy People 2010 (vol 1), 2nd ed: Objectives for Improving Health. US Department of Health and Human Services, Office of Disease Prevention and Health Promotion. Nov 2000.
8. American Diabetes Association. Classification and diagnosis of diabetes mellitus. Diabetes Care. 2004;27 Suppl 1: S9.
9. Danish RK, West BB. Rapid progression from prediabetes to severely ill diabetes while under "expert care": suggestions for improving screening for disease progression. Diabetes Spectrum. 2005;18(4):229-39.
10. American Diabetes Association. Diabetes mortality rates. In: Diabetes 4-1-1: Facts, Figures and Statistics at a Glance. Alexandria, Va: American Diabetes Association; 2005:75-7.
11. American Diabetes Association. Clinical practice recommendations. Diabetes Care. 2006;29 Suppl 1:
12. The DCCT Research Group. The effect of intensive treatment of diabetes on the development and progression of long-term complications in insulin-dependent diabetes mellitus. N Engl J Med. 1993;329:977-86.
13. UK Prospective Diabetes Study Group. Intensive blood glucose control with sulphonylureas or insulin compared with conventional treatment and risk complications in patients with type 2 diabetes (UKPD 33). Lancet. 1998;352:837-53.
14. Centers for Disease Control and Prevention, National Center for Health Statistics, Division of Health Interview Statistics, data from the National Health Interview Survey. Centers for Disease Control and Prevention, Atlanta, Ga. On the Internet: Prevalence of Diagnosed Diabetes by Age, US, 1980-2004; from the National Diabetes Surveillance System of the National Center for Chronic Disease Prevention and Health Promotion. Accessed 6 Feb 2006.
15. Harris MI, Flegal KM, Cowie CC, et al. Prevalence of diabetes, impaired fasting glucose, and impaired glucose tolerance in US adults: the Third National Health and Nutrition Examination Survey 1988-1994. Diabetes Care. 1998;21:518-25.
16. The DECODE Study Group. Is fasting glucose sufficient to define diabetes? epidemiological data from 20 European studies. Diabetologia, 1999;42:647-54.
17. Meneilly GS, Tessier D. Diabetes in elderly adults. J Gerontol Med Sci. 2001;56A:M5-13.
18. Ahmann AJ, Riddle MC. Oral pharmacological agents. In: Medical Management of Diabetes Mellitus. Leahy JL, Clark NG, Cefalu WT, eds. New York: Marcel Dekker, Inc; 2000:267-83.
19. Stratton IM, Adler AI, Neil HA, et al. Association of glycaemia with macrovascular and microvascular complications of type 2 diabetes (UKPDS 35): prospective observational study. BMJ. 2000;321(7258):405-12.
20. Bertoni AG, Krop JS, Anderson GF, Brancati FL. Diabetes-related morbidity and mortality in a national sample of US elders. Diabetes Care. 2002;25(3): 471-5.
21. Songer TJ. Disability in diabetes. In: Diabetes in America, 2nd ed. Harris MI, Cowie CC, Stern MP, Boyko EJ, Bennet PH, eds. Bethesda, Md: National Institute of Diabetes and Digestive and Kidney Diseases; 1995:259-83.
22. Chau D, Edelman SV. Clinical management of diabetes in the elderly. Clin Diabetes. 2001; 19(4):172-5.
23. Sommerfield AJ, Deary IF, Grier BM. Acute hyperglycemia alters mood and impairs cognitive performance

in people with type 2 diabetes. Diabetes Care. 2004;27:2335-40.

24. Sinclair AJ, Girling AJ, Bayer A. Cognitive dysfunction in older subjects with diabetes mellitus: impact on diabetes self-management and use of care services. Diabetes Res Linc Pract. 2000;50:203-12.

25. American Diabetes Association. Type 2 diabetes in children and adolescents (consensus statement). Diabetes Care. 2000;23(3):381-9.

26. Sinha R, Fisch G, Teague B, et al. Prevalence of glucose tolerance among children and adolescents with marked obesity. N Engl J Med. 2002;346:802-10.

27. Alberti G, Zimmet P, Shaw J, Bloomgarden Z, Kaufman F, Silink M. Type 2 diabetes in the young: the evolving epidemic. Diabetes Care. 2004;27:1798-1811.

28. Phillips DI. Birthweight and the future development of diabetes: a review of the evidence. Diabetes Care.1998;21 Suppl 2:B150-55.

29. Silverman BL, Metzger BE, Cho NH, Loeb CA. Impaired glucose tolerance in adolescent offspring of diabetic mothers: relationship of fetal hyperinsulinism. Diabetes Care. 1995;18:611-17.

30. Pettit DJ, Nelson RG, Saad MF, Bennett PH, Knowler WC. Diabetes and obesity in the offspring of Pima Indian women with diabetes during pregnancy. Diabetes Care. 1993;16:310-4.

31. Schreiner B. Promoting lifestyle and behavior change in overweight children and adolescents with type 2 diabetes. Diabetes Spectrum. 2005;18(1):9-12.

32. Copeland KC, Becker D, Gottschalk M, Hale D. Type 2 diabetes in children and adolescents: risk factors, diagnosis and treatment. Clin Diabetes. 2005;23(4):181-5.

33. Jones KL, Arslanian S, Peterokova VA, et al. Effect of metformin in pediatric patients with type 2 diabetes: a randomized controlled trial. Diabetes Care. 2002;25:89-94.

34. Amiel SA, Sherwin RS, Simonson DC, Lauritano AA, Tamborlane WV. Impaired insulin action in puberty, a contributing factor to poor glycemic control in adolescents with diabetes. N Engl J Med. 1986;315:215-9.

35. American College of Endocrinologists. ACE consensus development conference on guidelines for glycemic control. Endocrine Practice Supplement. 2001.

36. American Diabetes Association. Standards of medical care in diabetes, 2006. Diabetes Care. 2006;29 Suppl 1:S4-S42.

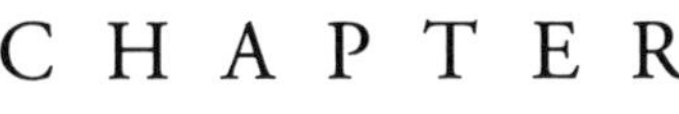

CHAPTER

11

Pregnancy with Preexisting Diabetes

Author

Alyce Thomas, RD

Key Concepts

- Higher incidences of maternal and fetal complications are associated with poor glycemic control in preexisting diabetes
- Optimal blood glucose levels are associated with lower perinatal mortality rates
- Preconception counseling should be available to all women with preexisting diabetes to decrease the risk of congenital anomalies and spontaneous abortions
- Strategies to improve outcomes include maternal and fetal testing and self-management skills
- Weight-gain goals based on current recommendations from the Institute of Medicine are established at the initial prenatal visit
- Health professionals involved in the care of pregnant women with preexisting diabetes should develop an understanding of the pathophysiology that occurs with the mother and fetus
- Unless contraindicated, breastfeeding is recommended for all women with preexisting diabetes

Introduction

The most prevalent medical complication in pregnancy is diabetes mellitus. Preconceptional diabetes is estimated to affect 1% of all pregnancies in the United States.[1] Approximately 34% of pregnant women with preexisting diabetes have type 1 diabetes. In recent years, intensive insulin therapy and greater attention to diabetes self-management have resulted in better maternal glycemic control. The current perinatal mortality rate in women with preexisting diabetes is 2%, which is comparable to women without diabetes.[2]

While the survival rates for infants of women with preexisting diabetes have risen, maternal and fetal complications continue to be higher than in the normal pregnant population. Congenital anomalies account for 40% to 50% of fetal deaths and occur in 6% to 12% of all infants born to women with diabetes.[3]

The two main strategies to improve outcomes for pregnant women and their offspring are these:

- *Preconception Counseling.* The American College of Obstetricians and Gynecologists (ACOG) recommends preconception counseling for women with preexisting diabetes as a beneficial and cost-effective service.[4] Counseling that focuses on achieving euglycemia prior to and during the critical period of organogenesis may help prevent anomalies.
- *Euglycemia Throughout Pregnancy.* Focusing on glycemic control is another important way to decrease fetal risks and infant morbidity associated with maternal hyperglycemia. The woman will have the greatest success in maintaining optimal glycemic control throughout her pregnancy when working with a multidisciplinary team and receiving targeted self-management education. Key components of care include medical tests, of both the mother and fetus, and effective use of self-management skills.

Definition and Classification for Pregnancy Complicated by Diabetes

Diabetes in pregnancy is divided into 2 groups:

- Women with *preexisting diabetes,* which includes type 1 and type 2 diabetes
- Women with *gestational diabetes mellitus* (GDM), which is defined as any degree of glucose intolerance with onset or first recognition during pregnancy[5]

Type 1 diabetes is characterized by a cellular-mediated autoimmune destruction of the beta cells of the pancreas, this form of diabetes accounts for 5% to 10% of all cases of diabetes. Type 2 diabetes encompasses individuals with insulin resistance with either absolute or relative insulin deficiency.

Classification systems have been developed to identify risk factors in pregnant women with diabetes.

White's Classification. The White classification system was, for many years, the most widely applied system for assessing the risk factors of pregnancy complicated by diabetes.[6] White observed that the age of onset of maternal diabetes, duration, and the presence of vascular complications were factors affecting the outcome of pregnancy. This classification of diabetes in pregnancy does not include any underlying fetal risks or guidelines for insulin treatment for gestational diabetes. However, the White system continues to be used by some healthcare providers.

Buchanan and Coustan's Classification. In their classification, Buchanan and Coustan[7] divided pregnant women with diabetes into 2 groups: pregestational and gestational diabetes. Maternal risks are based on the type of diabetes, the degree of metabolic control, and the presence of vascular complications. These factors appear to be more important predictors of perinatal outcome than either the age at onset or the duration of maternal diabetes.

This chapter addresses pregnancy with preexisting diabetes; information on gestational diabetes appears in chapter 12.

Complications

Because of the diabetes, both the mother and fetus are at risk for complications. Specific complications are described in the paragraphs that follow.

Maternal Complications

Complications can predate the pregnancy (retinopathy, nephropathy, neuropathy, hypertension, and diabetic ketoacidosis) or occur during pregnancy (hypertensive disorders, pyelonephritis, polyhydramnios, and oligohydramnios).

Diabetic Retinopathy. Hormones, such as growth hormone and insulin-like growth factor (IGF-1), and the rise in estrogen, progesterone, and cortisol levels may accelerate retinopathy.[8,9] Rosenn et al[10] found that pregnancy-induced or preexisting chronic hypertension was the most important risk factor associated with progression of retinopathy in pregnancy. Rapid normalization of blood glucose can cause acute progression of retinopathy.[11] Pregnant women with diabetes who have no background of mild retinopathy are less likely to have progression than those with advanced retinopathy. In most situations, background retinopathy that occurs during pregnancy regresses after delivery. If the woman has untreated proliferative retinopathy, pregnancy should be delayed until after laser photocoagulation.

Diabetic Nephropathy. Hypertension, increased glomerular filtration rate, increased protein intake and excretion, and glycemic control are factors that contribute to the development of diabetic nephropathy. Diabetic nephropathy is associated with poor pregnancy outcome. Optimal maternal hypertensive and glycemic control may improve renal function and slow the progression of nephropathy during and after pregnancy. ACE inhibitors are contraindicated during pregnancy because of potential fetal risks; methyldopa is used for hypertension control.

Hypertension. Hypertension in pregnancy is classified into 4 categories based on the guidelines by the National Institutes of Health Working Group Report on High Blood Pressure in Pregnancy (Table 11.1).[12] As a result of poor glycemic control, the incidence of hypertensive disorders in pregnancy is higher in women with diabetes.[13]

Diabetic Ketoacidosis (DKA). DKA is more common in women with type 1 diabetes than in women with type 2 diabetes. Increased insulin resistance and accelerated starvation ketosis play a role in the higher incidence of DKA in pregnant women with type 1 diabetes than in nonpregnant women with type 1 diabetes. In pregnancy, DKA increases the risk of fetal demise. Other factors associated with diabetic ketoacidosis include hyperemesis; gastroparesis; and treatment with corticosteroids or betamimetic, tocolytic medications, such as terbutaline or ritodrine.[4]

Complications Associated With Obesity. Obesity is a risk factor in the higher perinatal mortality and morbidity rate found in type 2 diabetes, including congenital malformation and macrosomia.[14-16] Complications associated with obesity in pregnancy include chronic hypertension, obstructive sleep apnea, preeclampsia, increased urinary tract infections, and higher rates of cesarean and difficult deliveries in the mother.[17]

Fetal Complications

Fetal complications associated with maternal hyperglycemia include congenital malformations, neonatal hypoglycemia, macrosomia, stillbirth, respiratory distress syndrome (RDS), hyperbilirubinemia, hypocalcemia, and polycythemia.

Congenital Malformations. Congenital anomalies occur during organogenesis, the first 8 weeks of gestation.[18] In a large Danish study that compared pregnancy outcomes in type 1 diabetic pregnancies with a nonpregnant population, the perinatal complications in the former group were higher in women with increasing A1C levels

TABLE 11.1 Hypertensive Disorders in Pregnancy

Preeclampsia	Diagnosed after the 20th week of gestation: systolic BP >140 mm Hg or a diastolic BP ≥90 mm Hg and proteinuria
Eclampsia	Preeclampsia with unexplained seizures
Chronic hypertension	Hypertension diagnosed before the 20th week of gestation: systolic BP >140 mm Hg or a diastolic BP ≥90 mm Hg
Preeclampsia superimposed on chronic hypertension	Preeclampsia that occurs in women with hypertension. Suspected if: • Hypertension and proteinuria occur before 20 weeks' gestation • Sudden increase in proteinuria • Sudden increase in BP in a woman with previously well-controlled BP • Thrombocytopenia: platelet count <100 000 cells/mm^3
Gestational hypertension.	Elevated BP detected for the first time after midpregnancy; no proteinuria present

Source: Report of the National High Blood Pressure Education Program Working Group on High Blood Pressure in Pregnancy. Am J Obstet Gynecol. 2000;183:S1-S22.

and poor self-care.[19] Wren et al found a fivefold increase in the risk of cardiovascular malformations in the infants born to women with preexisting diabetes than in nondiabetic women.[20] Birth defects associated with preexisting diabetes in pregnancy are listed in Table 11.2.

Macrosomia. ACOG defines macrosomia as a birth weight greater than 4000 g.[21] Macrosomic infants have trunks and shoulders that are disproportionally larger than the head, which increases the risk for shoulder dystocia, Erb palsy, and brachial plexus palsy. A cesarean section is often indicated if infant birth weight exceeds 4500 g.[22]

Neonatal Hypoglycemia. Neonatal hypoglycemia may result if the infant continues to produce excessive insulin after delivery once the maternal glucose supply has ended. In term infants, neonatal hypoglycemia is defined as a plasma glucose value less than 35 mg/dL (1.92 mmol/L); in preterm infants, the number is less than 25 mg/dL (1.37 mmol/L). The most efficient and safest treatment to prevent neonatal hypoglycemia is initiation of early oral feeding.

Organogenesis—A Critical Period

Women with diabetes must be extremely careful the first 8 weeks after conception—to protect the fetus during organogenesis and avoid perinatal complications and birth defects.

TABLE 11.2 Congenital Malformations in Infants Born to Women With Preexisting Diabetes

Cardiovascular • Transposition of great vessels • Ventricular septal defect • Atrial septal defect
Central nervous and skeletal • Sacral agenesis • Anencephalus • Hydrocephalus • Neural tube defects
Genitourinary • Renal agenesis • Hydronephrosis • Ureteral duplication • Anal/rectal atresia
Gastrointestinal • Duodenal atresia • Anorectal atresia

Sources:

1. Wren C, Birrell G, Hawthorne G. Cardiovascular malformations in infants of diabetic mothers. Heart. 2003;89:1217-1220.
2. Farrell T, Neale L, Cundy T. Congenital anomalies in the offspring of women with type 1, type 2 and gestational diabetes mellitus. Diabetes Med. 2002;19:322-326.
3. Landon MB, Gabbe SG. Diabetes Mellitus. In: Barron WM, Lindheimer MD, Davison JM, eds. Medical Disorders in Pregnancy. St. Louis, Mo: Mosby; 2000.

> ***Preventing Neonatal Hypoglycemia***
>
> Early oral feeding is the safest, most efficient way to prevent neonatal hypoglycemia.

Respiratory Distress Syndrome (RDS). If a preterm infant's lungs are not fully mature at delivery, RDS can result. When maternal glycemic levels are in good control, delivery can be delayed until term and the need for RDS testing can be eliminated.

Other Fetal Complications. Incidences of *hypocalcemia*, *hyperbilirubinemia*, and *polycythemia* are reduced when the mother maintains good glycemic control during the third trimester.

Preconception Care and Education

Both the ADA and ACOG recommend that diabetes care and education begin prior to conception.[1,4] However, in a study that examined preconception counseling rates in managed care, only 52% of the women recalled any discussion with their healthcare provider on glucose control and 37% received advice on family planning.[23] Ideally, preconception care should begin when the female with diabetes reaches childbearing age. Sufficient time must be allowed to evaluate the mother's health status and to normalize or maximize glycemic control, thereby offering the best chance for the fetus. Receiving preconception counseling at least 3 to 4 months before becoming pregnant can give the woman sufficient time to achieve glycemic control and see a change in the glycated hemoglobin level. See also the section on "Teens—A Special Population" later in this chapter.

With the increased incidence of women with type 2 diabetes during their childbearing years, the potential for new cases of pregnancy among women with type 2 diabetes exceeds that of type 1 diabetes. Yet, studies have indicated that women with type 2 diabetes are not referred for preconception care as often as their type 1 counterparts.[24] A 12-year outcome analysis of pregnant women with type 2 diabetes showed a twofold greater risk of stillbirth, a 2.5-fold greater risk of perinatal mortality, and a 3.5-fold of neonatal death than in the general population.[25] In an Australian study, 27.8% of women with type 1 diabetes received preconception counseling, but only 12% of those with type 2 diabetes received it.[26] Dunne suggested that the higher rate of perinatal mortality and congenital anomalies in type 2 women results from the perception that type 2 diabetes is a benign condition and not as serious as type 1 diabetes.[24]

> ***Importance of Euglycemia***
>
> Maintaining normal maternal blood glucose levels is extremely important in preventing perinatal complications. Euglycemia is the ultimate goal in management of diabetes and pregnancy.

Care and Education During Pregnancy

Pathophysiology of Type 1 Diabetes

The fetus depends upon an adequate but not excessive supply of fuel from maternal sources. Glucose, which is transported across the placenta via facilitated diffusion, is the fuel source preferred by the fetus over any other energy-producing nutrient.[27] The first trimester is often characterized by lower maternal glucose levels than those of nonpregnant women. As hormonal levels (estrogen, progesterone, human placental lactogen) progressively increase in the second and third trimesters, higher fasting and postprandial levels are observed. This results in increased insulin resistance and decreased insulin sensitivity. Fetal growth accelerates in the third trimester as free fatty acids are mobilized for maternal energy needs. This allows for more placental transfer of glucose to the developing fetus. Maternal insulin does not cross the placenta.

In the first trimester, women with type 1 diabetes may actually experience a drop in their insulin requirements as their glycemic levels fall and insulin sensitivity increases.[28,29] As the pregnancy progresses, the absence of maternal pancreatic beta cell function increases the concentration of glucose, fatty acids, ketones, and amino acids transported across the placenta to the fetus. Exogenous insulin requirements may increase twofold to threefold over prepregnant amounts to maintain euglycemia and reduce the risk of fetal complications. Pedersen hypothesized that maternal hyperglycemia is the primary reason for fetal hyperinsulinemia resulting from an overstimulation of the fetal pancreatic beta cell.[30] Other factors, such as insulin growth factors, leptin, and tumor necrosis factor, have been identified that affect fetal growth.[31]

Pathophysiology of Type 2 Diabetes

Type 2 diabetes is characterized by insufficient insulin receptors in response to a given degree of glycemia. As insulin resistance increases, beta cell function declines and glucose levels rise. Insulin resistance can be substantially greater in women with type 2 diabetes than in women with type 1 because women with type 2 are more likely to be obese. If glycemic levels are elevated around conception and the organogenesis period, the risk of congenital malformations and spontaneous abortions increases. Hyperglycemia is a particular problem in the second and third trimesters, when the levels of maternal hormones increase. Throughout the pregnancy, insulin requirements increase; self-management education should prepare the woman for this expected occurrence.

Complications in Pregnancy With Type 2 Diabetes

- *Fetal Complications:* Similar to those of type 1 diabetes.
- *Diabetic Ketoacidosis:* Not usually associated with type 2 diabetes.
- *Complications Associated With Obesity:* See earlier discussion at the end of the section on maternal complications.

Diabetes Care During Labor and Delivery

The key to successful intrapartum management is to monitor blood glucose levels frequently and administer insulin and glucose as necessary. One regimen used to manage blood glucose levels during labor and delivery is this:

1. Administer the usual dose of intermediate-acting insulin at bedtime.
2. Withhold the morning dose of insulin and begin an intravenous infusion of normal saline.
3. Once active labor begins or glucose levels decrease to less than 70 mg/dL, change the infusion to dextrose to keep blood glucose levels below 110 mg/dL.[4] The rate of dextrose administered is 2.0 to 2.5 mg per kilogram per minute.
4. Measure maternal blood glucose values every hour.
5. Administer short-acting insulin by multiple subcutaneous doses or by continuous intravenous infusion as necessary to maintain euglycemia and help prevent neonatal hypoglycemia.[32]

Postpartum Care and Education

Postpartum diabetes care and education begin while the woman is still in the hospital, caring for the infant and recovering from the delivery. About 2 weeks after the woman has been home with her infant, a follow-up phone call by a diabetes nurse educator is appropriate. By 6 weeks after delivery, the woman should have a scheduled office visit with both the diabetes educator and registered dietitian. Topics for education include the following:

- Planning for lactation, including possible delays in lactation
- Glycemic control with decreasing insulin requirements
- More frequent self-monitoring of blood glucose
- Balancing infant care with self-care for the new mother
- Depression and stress
- Readjusting the insulin regimen
- Readjusting the food plan, if breastfeeding or not
- Weight loss or weight management
- Contraception (see Table 11.3)

Self-Care Behaviors

Evidence shows that intensive diabetes management can improve perinatal outcome. The AADE 7 Self-Care Behaviors™, summarized in Table 11.4, provide a framework to assess and evaluate outcomes from preconception to postpartum. Points pertinent to self-care throughout a pregnancy are discussed individually below.

Healthy Eating

During a pregnancy with diabetes, medical nutrition therapy (MNT) has 3 important goals:

- Provide adequate nutrients for maternal and fetal health
- Assist in appropriate gestational weight gain that is neither subnormal nor excessive and avoid maternal ketosis
- Minimize blood glucose excursions

Nutritional recommendations similar for pregnant women without diabetes can be followed by women with preexisting diabetes. An individualized food plan is important to optimize blood glucose control.

Weight Gain. Healthcare providers use the Institute of Medicine's recommendations for weight gain during pregnancy, which are based on prepregnancy body mass index (BMI) (Table 11.5).[33] Weight loss is contraindicated in all BMI categories. Strauss and Dietz found higher rates of intrauterine growth retardation with low maternal weight gain (<0.3 kg per week) in the second and third trimesters independent of the prepregnancy BMI.[34] Weight loss in the first trimester was not a significant factor.

TABLE 11.3 Contraceptive Use in Women With Preexisting Diabetes

Contraceptive Type	*Efficacy*	*Safety*
Barrier methods: diaphragm, condoms, spermicides, cervical caps	70% to 97% depending on method and if used alone or in combination with another method	No contraindications
Intrauterine devices (IUD)	98% to 99%	Not recommended if high-risk exposure to sexually transmitted diseases
Oral contraceptives	97% to 99.5%	Low-dose progestin or combination lowest progestin/estrogen dose preferred for women without vascular complications or strong family history of myocardial disease
Non-oral hormonal contraceptives (eg, implants, injections, transdermal patches)	99%	May have effect on glucose and lipid levels

Sources:

1. Kim C, Seidel KW, Begier EA, et al. Diabetes and depot medroyprogesterone contraception in Navajo womem. Arch Inter Med. 2001;161.
2. Chuang CH, Chase GA, Bensyl DM, Weisman CS. Contraceptive use by diabetic and obese women. Women's Health Issues. 2005;15(4):167-173.
3. Kjos SL, Buchanan TA. Postpartum management, lactation, and contraception. In: Reece EA, Coustan DR, Gabbe SG, eds. Diabetes in Women: Adolescence, Pregnancy and Menopause. Philadelphia, Pa. Lippincott Williams & Wilkins; 2004:441-449.
4. Kjos SL. Postpartum care of women with diabetes. Clin Obstet Gynecol. 2000;43:46-55.

TABLE 11.4 AADE 7 Self-Care Behaviors™ for Pregnancy With Preexisting Diabetes

Healthy Eating	• Consume adequate calories to avoid weight loss and ketone production • Consume adequate nutrient intake for maternal stores and fetal growth and development • Avoid alcohol and other substances • Avoid foods that can lead to foodborne illnesses
Being Active	• Participate in daily physical activity, if no contraindications • Carry extra carbohydrate for hypoglycemia prevention
Monitoring	• Test blood glucose levels daily; frequency determined by healthcare provider • Test ketones as instructed by healthcare provider • Keep food records as instructed by registered dietitian • Increase frequency of monitoring during lactation
Taking Medications	• Understand the increased insulin requirements as pregnancy progresses • Understand that oral agents may be discontinued until after delivery
Problem Solving	• Identify symptoms and treatment of hyperglycemia • Identify criteria for when to contact healthcare provider • Schedule follow-up visits for review of self-management skills
Reducing Risks	• Understand risk of maternal hyperglycemia on fetal outcome • Manage weight to decrease long-term health risks
Healthy Coping	• Understand the necessity of a higher degree of intensive care, including more frequent healthcare visits • Obtain support and referral, as necessary

TABLE 11.5 Recommended Ranges of Total Weight Gain for Pregnant Women

Weight-for-Height Category	*Recommended Total Weight Gain*
Underweight (BMI* <19.8)	28–40 lb (12.7–18.2 kg)
Normal weight (BMI 19.8–26.0)	25–35 lb (11.2–15.9 kg)
Overweight (BMI 26.0–29.0)	15–25 lb (6.8–11.3 kg)
Obese (BMI >29)	~15 lb (6.8 kg)
Twin gestation	35–45 lb (15.9–20.5 kg)
Triplet gestation	45–55 lb (20.5–25.0 kg)

*BMI=weight/height^2

Source: National Academy of Sciences. Nutrition During Pregnancy. Washington, DC: National Academy Press, 1990.

Energy Requirements. Adequate calories are necessary to provide for fetal growth and to avoid ketonemia either from ketoacidosis or accelerated starvation ketosis in all pregnant women.[35,36] Adjustments to the food plan may be necessary to compensate for erratic blood glucose levels caused by fluctuating hormonal levels.

The Dietary Reference Intakes (DRIs)[37] are used to determine the estimated energy requirements (EER) in pregnancy, which are based on age, height, weight, and physical activity level. The EERs for pregnancy are as follows:

- *1st trimester:* Adult EER + 0
- *2nd trimester:* Adult EER + 160 kcal (8 kcal/wk × 20 wk) + 180 kcal
- *3rd trimester:* Adult EER + 272 kcal (8 kcal/wk × 34 wk) + 180 kcal

The 8 kcal per week represents the change in total energy expenditure due to pregnancy; the 180 kcal is the mean energy deposition during pregnancy.

Protein. The Recommended Dietary Allowance (RDA) for protein in the nonpregnant woman is 0.80 g per kilogram per day or 46 g per day. Protein requirements increase to 1.1 g per kilogram per day or 25 g extra per day for a singleton gestation and 50 g extra for twin pregnancies.[37]

Carbohydrate. The DRI for carbohydrate in pregnant women ages 19 to 50 is a minimum of 175 g per day to provide an adequate source of glucose for fetal growth (approximately 33 g per day) and to supply glucose for the maternal brain.[37] The amount and distribution of energy intake and carbohydrates are individualized and based on the woman's food preferences, blood glucose records, and physical activity level.

Vitamins and Minerals. Adequate calcium, iron and folate, vitamin D, and magnesium intakes are especially important in pregnancy. DRIs in pregnancy are listed in Table 11.6.

Other nutrition-related issues during pregnancy are morning sickness and the safety of what is consumed. Guidelines on nonnutritive sweeteners, alcoholic beverages, mercury-contaminated fish, and foods that can lead to listeriosis infection are highlighted below.

Safe eating during pregnancy:

Morning Sickness. Can present a challenge to pregnant women. If vomiting occurs after taking a premeal rapid-acting or short-acting insulin dose, glucagon can be administered to help prevent hypoglycemia until the vomiting subsides. The woman is advised to contact her healthcare provider if vomiting becomes severe.[38]

Nonnutritive Sweeteners. The Food and Drug Administration (FDA) has approved 5 nonnutritive sweeteners: saccharin, aspartame, acesulfame K, sucralose, and neotame. All were shown to be safe for use during pregnancy.[39]

Alcohol. Use of all alcoholic beverages during pregnancy is discouraged because of the risks of fetal alcohol spectrum disorders.[40]

Mercury-Contaminated Fish. The FDA has recommended that pregnant women and women of childbearing age avoid eating shark, swordfish, jack mackerel, and tilefish. These fish often contain high levels of methylmercury, a potent human neurotoxin, which readily crosses

TABLE 11.6 Dietary Reference Intakes (DRIs) for Pregnant and Lactating Women

Nutrient	*Pregnant Woman*	*Lactating Woman*
Protein (g)	+25	+25
Vitamin A (mcg)		
14–18 years	750	1200
19–50 years	770	770
Vitamin D (mcg)	5	5
Vitamin K (mcg)		
14–18 years	75	75
19–50 years	90	90
Vitamin C (mg)		
14–18 years	80	115
19–50 years	85	120
Thiamin (mg)	1.4	1.4
Riboflavin (mg)	1.4	1.6
Niacin (mg NE)	18	17
Vitamin B_6 (mg)	1.9	2.0
Folate (mcg FE)	600	500
Vitamin B_{12} (mcg)	2.6	2.8
Calcium (mg)		
14–18 years	1300	1300
19–50 years	1000	1000
Phosphorus (mg)		
14–18 years	1250	1250
19–50 years	700	700
Magnesium (mg)		
14–18 years	400	360
19–50 years	360	320
Iron (mg)		
14–18 years	27	10
19–50 years	27	9
Zinc (mg)		
14–18 years	12	13
19–50 years	11	12
Iodine (mcg)	220	290
Selenium (mcg)	60	70

Source: Trumbo P, Schlicker S, Yates AA, Poos M. Dietary reference intakes for energy, carbohydrate, fiber, fat, fatty acids, cholesterol, protein and amino acids. J Am Diet Assoc. 2002;102:1621-1630.

the placenta and has the potential to damage the fetal nervous system.[41] Women should consult their local health department for further fish advisories in their area.

Listeriosis. Food safety is of primary concern in pregnancy. The Centers for Disease Control and Prevention estimates a fivefold risk of contracting listeriosis during pregnancy. Approximately 1/3 of all listeriosis cases involve pregnant women. Listeriosis can be transmitted to the fetus via the placenta. The risks of listeriosis are preterm delivery, spontaneous abortions, and other complications. Pregnant women are advised to avoid the following:

- Deli meats, hot dogs, or luncheon meats, unless reheated until steaming hot
- Soft cheeses (such as feta, Brie, Camembert, blue-veined) and quesos blanco fresco (but hard cheeses and pasteurized cheese are recommended)
- Refrigerated patés or meat spreads (but canned or shelf-stable paté and meat spreads can be consumed)
- Refrigerated smoked seafood, unless cooked
- Raw or unpasteurized milk

Lactation. As challenging as it may be to achieve desired metabolic control while establishing lactation, breastfeeding is recommended for women with preexisting diabetes.[42] Early separation of the mother and infant, for example, may delay lactogenesis.[43]

Key education points regarding lactation:

- *Insulin:* Breastfeeding mothers may require less insulin because of the calories expended during nursing
- *Snack:* Breastfeeding mothers may need a carbohydrate-containing snack either before or during breastfeeding or require an evening or late-night snack to avoid hypoglycemia[42]
- *Monitoring:* Breastfeeding mothers may need more frequent self-monitoring of blood glucose

The EER for lactation is estimated from total energy expenditure, milk energy output, and energy mobilization from tissue stores.[37] In the first 6 months postpartum, lactating women experience an average weight loss of 0.8 kg per month, which is equivalent to 170 kcal per day. The milk energy output is approximately 500 kcal per day. As the infant is introduced to solid foods, usually at 6 months, the amount of milk produced is reduced and the milk energy output decreases to 400 kcal per day. The EER for lactation is as follows:

- *1st 6 months:* EER + 500 – 170 (milk energy output – weight loss)
- *2nd 6 months:* EER + 400 – 0 (milk energy output – weight loss)
- *RDA for protein:* 1.1 g per kilogram per day or an additional 25 g per day (same as in pregnancy)[37]
- *RDA for carbohydrate:* 210 g per day[37]
- *Lactation:* Table 11.7 lists DRIs of other nutrients for lactating women

Being Active

Physical activity can have a beneficial effect on blood glucose levels as well as overall well-being during pregnancy. See chapter 30, Being Active, for more information.

Frequency and duration of exercise:

- *Goal of 30 minutes daily.* In the absence of medical or obstetric complications, pregnant women should accumulate 30 minutes or more of moderate-intensity physical activity on most, if not all, days of the week, state the Dietary Guidelines of America (DGA).[44] Active women can continue similar activities during pregnancy.
- *Intervals as short as 10 minutes can be effective.* The physical activity can be short bouts of 10 minutes each, accumulated over the course of the day
- *Sedentary lifestyle.* Pregnancy generally is not a time for a woman who was previously sedentary to initiate strenuous activity; however, walking is possible for most women, and a 15- to 20-minute walk can lower blood glucose by 20 to 40 mg/dL

Precautions on exercise and physical activity:

Diabetes education should include the following:

- Explain to the woman that, as with physical activity for any person with diabetes, planning, adjustments, and education for safety are needed
- Instruct her to always carry additional carbohydrate in case of hypoglycemia; advise those taking insulin of the risk for hypoglycemia and the need to test blood glucose before and after exercise
- Teach the woman to palpate her uterus during physical activity and to stop if she detects contractions
- Caution the woman against becoming dehydrated, overheated, tachycardic (heart rate >140 bpm), or dyspneic
- Advise those taking insulin of the risk for hypoglycemia and the need to test blood glucose before and after exercise
- Advise the woman of contraindications for exercise in pregnancy, which include preterm labor, premature rupture of the membranes, and abnormally high or low blood glucose levels (see Table 11.7)[45]

Monitoring

Although there is a lack of agreement regarding precise glucose thresholds and timings, maintaining normal blood glucose levels remains the ultimate goal in management of diabetes and pregnancy. Table 11.8 summarizes the range of plasma glucose targets recommended by the ADA, ACOG, and other experts. Until consensus is reached, glycemic profiles should be individualized in women with preexisting diabetes. Target glucose goals are not always attainable.

TABLE 11.7 Exercise Guidelines for Pregnant Women With Preexisting Diabetes

- Discuss with healthcare provider to determine safety, type, and duration of exercise
- Get screened for proliferative retinopathy, neuropathy, and cardiovascular disease
- Monitor blood glucose levels before, during, and after exercise; avoid exercise if glycemic levels are <60 mg/dL or >200 mg/dL
- Be aware of immediate and prolonged hypoglycemia after exercising
- Carry readily available form of glucose at all times to treat hypoglycemia
- Avoid injecting insulin into an extremity to be used during exercising
- Avoid exercising during peak insulin action times
- Learn to palpate uterus to detect contractions

Sources:

1. Thomas AM, Gutierrez YM. American Dietetic Association Guide to Gestational Diabetes Mellitus. Chicago, Ill: American Dietetic Association; 2005.
2. American College of Obstetricians and Gynecologists: Committee on Obstetric Practice. ACOG Committee Opinion No. 267. Exercise during pregnancy and the postpartum period. Obstet Gynecol. 2002;99(1):171-173.
3. Carpenter MW. The role of exercise in pregnant women with diabetes mellitus. Clin Obstet Gynecol. 2000;43:56-64.

Adapted from: Thomas AM, Gutierrez YM. American Dietetic Association Guide to Gestational Diabetes Mellitus. Chicago, Ill: © American Dietetic Association; 2005. Adapted with permission.

TABLE 11.8 Blood Glucose Goals in Diabetic Pregnancy

	During Pregnancy	*Preconception*
Fasting	60 to 100 mg/dL (3.3 to 5.6 mmol/L)	
Premeal	60 to 115 mg/dL (3.3 to 6.4 mmol/L)	80 to 110 mg/dL (4.4 to 6.1 mmol/L)
1-h postprandial	<145 mg/dL (<8.1 mmol/L)	
2-h postprandial	<135 mg/dL (<7.5 mmol/L)	<155 mg/dL (<8.8 mmol/L)
2 h to 6 h	>60 to 135 mg/dL (3.3 to 7.5 mmol/L)	

Sources: Adapted from the following:

1. Jovanovic L, ed. Medical Management of Pregnancy Complicated by Diabetes, 3rd ed. Alexandria, Va: American Diabetes Association; 2000:7.
2. Kitzmiller JL. Antepartum and intrapartum obstetric care. In: Lebovitz HE. Therapy for Diabetes Mellitus and Related Disorders, 3rd ed. Alexandria, Va: American Diabetes Association; 1998: 36-43.
3. American Diabetes Association. Preconception care of women with diabetes. Diabetes Care. 2003;26 Suppl 1:S91-93.
4. Klingensmith GJ, ed. Intensive Diabetes Management, 3rd ed. Alexandria, Va: American Diabetes Association; 2000:68.
5. Landon MB, Gabbe SG. Insulin treatment of the pregnant patient with diabetes mellitus. In: Reece EA, Coustan DR, Gabbe SG, eds. Diabetes in Women: Adolescence, Pregnancy and Menopause. Philadelphia, Pa: Lippincott Williams & Wilkins; 2004:257.

In a study by Kitzmiller et al, 90% of the patients achieved mean blood glucose levels of 104 to 160 mg/dL (5.8 to 8.9 mmol/L) during organogenesis, with no excess of congenital anomalies.[46] Diabetes control is monitored through measurements of glycemic levels, ketones, and A1C—each discussed separately below.

Blood Glucose. Self-monitoring of blood glucose is needed pre- and postprandially in women with type 1 diabetes to evaluate the effectiveness of rapid-acting or short-acting insulin. No studies have specifically compared preprandial versus postprandial blood glucose monitoring in type 2 diabetes. Studies in women with type 1 diabetes and GDM have shown that postprandial testing is more closely associated with a lower incidence of maternal and fetal complications.[47] Blood glucose records are verified by the use of memory meters to help identify glucose patterns.

Ketones. Ketones cross the placenta, and ketone testing is necessary during illness, weight loss, or a reduction in calorie intake caused by nausea and/or vomiting. The presence of ketones with normal or low blood glucose levels is suggestive of starvation ketosis and usually indicates inadequate food intake. A registered dietitian will need to evaluate the food plan to determine the appropriate calorie level. Studies have demonstrated an association between elevated plasma ketone levels and lower IQ scores in offspring.[48,49]

A1C. Measurements of A1C may be obtained every 4 to 6 weeks. A1C should be within 1% of the normal range.[1] Relatively mild elevations of A1C have been associated with increased fetal morbidity.[1]

Premature labor:
Caution with tocolytic agents

Tocolytic agents such as ritodrine or terbutaline used to treat premature labor have been reported to cause deterioration of blood glucose control and ketosis in pregnant women with diabetes.[50] These agents should not be the first line of therapy for women with diabetes; if they are used, blood glucose levels must be carefully monitored.

Medication

Insulin is often required during pregnancy, and certain medications are not appropriate for the pregnant woman. Throughout a pregnancy, medication regimens are frequently modified to achieve optimal glycemic control. Use of insulin and insulin analogs, incretin mimetic hormones, pump therapy, and oral agents during pregnancy is discussed in this section. See also the questions and controversy section near the end of the chapter and chapter 15 on pharmacological therapies for glucose management.

Insulin and Insulin Analogs. Human-based insulin is recommended in pregnancy over animal-based insulin because of human insulin's faster absorption and less allergenic profile. Use of rapid-acting insulin analogs (lispro, aspart) in pregnancy has yielded results comparable to short-acting insulin.[50-55] In pregnancy, intensive insulin therapy requiring 3 or 4 injections is used to achieve the best glycemic control. The usual insulin regimen is this:

- *Morning:* Intermediate- and rapid-acting or short-acting insulin
- *Lunch:* Rapid-acting insulin
- *Dinner:* Rapid-acting or short-acting insulin
- *Bedtime:* Intermediate-acting insulin

Brief information on the insulin analogs glargine (Lantus) and insulin detemir (UK brand name Levemir) is given below. See also the discussion at the end of this chapter on questions and controversy in using insulin analogs and chapter 15 on pharmacological therapies for glucose management.

- *Glargine (Lantus)* is a long-acting insulin analog that provides a 24-hour peakless basal pattern. It is listed by the FDA as a Category C drug, which means the medication is only used in pregnancy if the potential benefits justify the potential risks to the fetus.
- *Insulin Detemir (Levemir, UK brand name)* is another long-acting insulin analog. It is used in combination with short- or rapid-acting insulin. No clinical studies have been conducted on use of detemir in pregnancy, although animal studies have shown no embryotoxicity or teratogenicity; thus, it is not recommended for use in pregnancy at this time.

Incretin Mimetic Hormones. Brief information is given below on pramlintide acetate (Symlin) and exenatide (Byetta). See also the questions and controversy section near the end of this chapter and chapter 15 on pharmacological therapies for glucose management.

- *Pramlintide (Symlin)* is a synthetic analog of amylin, a neuroendocrine hormone that is synthesized by the pancreatic beta cell. It is used in treatment of both type 1 diabetes and type 2 diabetes for postprandial glucose control.
- *Exenatide (Byetta)* is an incretin mimic used in type 2 diabetes. It works by suppressing inappropriate glucagon levels, promoting satiety and decreasing food intake, and slowing the absorption rate.

Insulin Requirements (Daily Dose). Insulin requirements in pregnancy are based on current weight, gestational age, blood glucose monitoring results, and caloric intake. The daily dose per kilogram per day generally ranges during trimesters; see Table 11.9.

Pump Therapy. Continuous subcutaneous insulin infusion therapy (CSII), use of the insulin pump, delivers insulin in a pattern similar to the normal physiologic secretion of insulin. Insulin pump therapy lowers

TABLE 11.9 Insulin Requirements During Pregnancy

	Insulin (units/kg)
First trimester	0.7 to 0.8
Second trimester	0.8 to 1.0
Third trimester	0.9 to 1.2
With obesity (>150% of desirable body weight)	1.5 to 2.0, secondary to insulin resistance

Source: American College of Obstetricians and Gynecologists. Pregestational diabetes mellitus. Practice bulletin No. 60. Obstet Gynecol. 2005;105:680.

the amount of circulating basal insulin, thereby decreasing the incidence of premeal hypoglycemia while efficiently controlling the more dramatic rise in postprandial glucose common during pregnancy.[56] Other advantages of insulin pump therapy during pregnancy include more rapid and predictable insulin absorption, decreased severe hypoglycemia, enhanced lifestyle flexibility, and simplified morning sickness management.[57] Women continuing on insulin pump therapy postpartum have been shown to have significantly lower A1C levels 1 year following delivery compared to women receiving multiple daily injections of insulin.[58]

Pregnant women using insulin pumps must be highly motivated and compliant. Complications can arise, such as frequent and severe hypoglycemia if there is an interruption in the delivery of insulin or an infection at the infusion site.[59]

Oral agents warning:

Women with type 2 diabetes who take oral agents for diabetes treatment are usually switched to insulin. The ACOG recommends limiting and individualizing the use of oral agents until more data is available regarding their safety and efficacy.[4]

Problem Solving

A pregnant woman with preexisting diabetes may or may not have received self-management instructions prior to conception. She may not, thus, be aware of the importance of glycemic control and how best to avoid perinatal complications, birth defects, or emergency situations requiring hospitalization during pregnancy. Without the preparation of preconceptual counseling, the women may not be well prepared to apply problem-solving and self-management skills to the critical situations that arise quickly in early pregnancy. As mentioned in the chapter introduction, preconception counseling goes a long way toward reducing risks. Plans for diabetes education during pregnancy must thus factor in whether or not the woman began with preconception care.

Preconception Counseling Occurred. Diabetes care and pregnancy care get off to a more reassuring start when the woman has had adequate preconception counseling. During pregnancy, particularly in the first trimester, topics for diabetes education are these:

- Assist in making minor adjustments to keep glycemic levels in optimal control during pregnancy
- Reiterate that more frequent visits with the diabetes team are necessary at the beginning of pregnancy during the critical organogenesis period
- Reinforce ongoing performance of successful self-management skills used prior to pregnancy

Women in Suboptimal Control and Those Not Counseled Before Conception. Women in suboptimal diabetes control, especially during the first trimester, and those who did not have preconception counseling will need to learn self-management skills quickly to achieve and maintain euglycemia through the rest of the pregnancy. Specifically, the woman must develop the flexibility to make adjustments to the care plan, including the following:

- Recognizing and treating hypoglycemic episodes
- Consistency in monitoring
- More frequent interactions with care team, including (1) discussing food plan adjustments with registered dietitian, (2) follow-up diabetes education visits to assess self-management skills, and (3) when to contact the appropriate healthcare provider to discuss her plan of care

Preconception Counseling Advisory

Hospitalizations, spontaneous abortions, birth defects, and congenital anomalies can be best prevented by reaching glycemic control before conception.

Reducing Risks of Diabetes Complications

Women with preexisting diabetes have a higher incidence of poor perinatal outcomes than women with GDM. As reiterated throughout this chapter, to decrease both maternal and fetal complications, all women with diabetes or at high risk for developing diabetes should be referred for preconception counseling. If no preconception care occurs, hospitalization may be necessary to begin intensive diabetes control and education. Indications for hospitalization include the following:

- To begin intensive diabetes control and education
- Hyperemesis
- Maternal hyperglycemia with ketones
- Noncompliance to previous instructions
- Obstetric complications, such as preeclampsia or preterm labor

Self-management skills reinforced or taught for the first time during pregnancy also have a long-term benefit for the mother, setting her up with good habits to continue beyond the postpartum period. As glycemic levels remain within the normal ranges, the woman's risk of developing long-term complications associated with diabetes is reduced.

Healthy Coping

Although women with preexisting diabetes can be experts at self-management, a pregnant woman may not be prepared for the degree of intensive care associated with pregnancy. With a growing fetus, interaction with a new healthcare provider or team (obstetrician and/or perinatal center), and more frequent healthcare visits and tests, she may sometimes feel overwhelmed. Diabetes education helps the woman prepare mentally for the more intensive care. Points to discuss:

- *Tests.* Ultrasonography, additional laboratory tests, and weekly or biweekly biophysical profiles are just some of the testing that will be performed during pregnancy. Nonstress tests or contraction stress tests, maternal serum alpha fetal protein, and amniocentesis may also be performed.
- *Changes to Insulin Regimen.* Women with type 1 diabetes will have their insulin regimens changed several times during the pregnancy.
- *Injections.* Women with type 2 diabetes may be resistant to switching from oral medications to insulin injections or more frequently monitoring.

The role of the diabetes educator is to assure the woman that adjustments are necessary to help reduce the risks associated with diabetes and pregnancy. Barriers to self-care may not always be mental or emotional; financial barriers can also be posed by the added costs of testing supplies and the loss of days off work because of hospitalization or office visits. The diabetes educator offers support by referring the woman to appropriate sources.

Case in Point: Type 1 Diabetes—A Pregnancy With Preconception Care

PB was a 33-year-old woman with type 1 diabetes of 18 years' duration who was referred by a diabetes treatment center to a tertiary level center for obstetrical care. At her first prenatal visit, she was confirmed at 7 weeks' gestation. This was her third pregnancy; her previous pregnancies ended in first-trimester spontaneous abortions 4 and 5 years ago (at 8 weeks' and 10 weeks' gestation, respectively). In planning this pregnancy, she was instructed by the diabetes center to delay conception again until her blood glucose levels were at optimal control.

- PB used oral contraceptives for 6 months prior to conception
- Pertinent family history included her father with type 2 diabetes who is on metformin (Glucophage) and a 25-year-old brother with type 1 diabetes (diagnosed 9 years ago)
- She had proliferative retinopathy, for which she received laser photocoagulation therapy 7 years ago; a history of DKA, with the last episode 3 years ago; and began experiencing neuropathy in her feet at age 24
- Her appetite had decreased in the past 2 weeks because of early morning nausea and occasional vomiting; no other gastrointestinal discomforts were noted

Preconception Care and Education

PB received preconception care and counseling, which according to the American Diabetes Association (ADA) helps decrease the risk of spontaneous abortions and congenital anomalies in infants of women with diabetes. She delayed conception, for 6 months using contraception, until her A1C was within 1% above the upper limit of normal. Regarding diabetes education, the following protocol was established so that PB would achieve optimal diabetes control before attempting conception.

- Discuss safe and realistic goals (include her partner, if applicable)
- Assess any vascular complications, including a dilated retinal examination; thyroid function tests; kidney function testing to determine creatinine, creatinine clearance, and microalbumin; and an EKG
- Refer for genetic counseling because of the family history of diabetes
- Refer to a registered dietitian for adjustments to her food plan
- Begin folic acid supplementation of 400 mcg per day[44]
- Assess her self-management skills, including insulin administration, glucose monitoring, and treatment of hypoglycemic episodes
- Continue contraception until glucose goals are attained

Care and Education During Pregnancy

Pathophysiology in Type 1 Diabetes

PB started her pregnancy with planning and implementation of efforts to optimize her glycemic control and improve the outcomes of her pregnancy.

Diabetes Management During Pregnancy

Early in the pregnancy, PB received confirmation of her pregnancy and benefited from care planning. At her first prenatal visit, PB brought her last laboratory tests, which were performed 10 weeks ago, and her blood glucose records. Her A1C was 6.3% and hemoglobin and hematocrit were 13.8 mg/dL and 40.6%, respectively. Her recent assessment of kidney function (24-h urine for protein and creatinine) were within normal limits. Her body mass index was 22.4. Her fasting blood glucose ranged from 75 to 115 mg/dL (4.2 to 6.4 mmol); premeal 58 to 132 mg/dL (3.2 to 7.4 mmol); and postprandial 115 to 145 mg/dL (7.1 to 8.1 mmol). PB was testing her blood glucose 7 times a day (fasting, premeal, postmeal, and bedtime), and her insulin regimen was 3 injections per day with short- and intermediate-acting insulin in the morning, short-acting before dinner, and intermediate at night.

Complications. Care and education were important to achieve and maintain optimal glycemic control and improve perinatal outcome. PB had background diabetic retinopathy and was at higher risk for progression of the condition during pregnancy. She also experienced DKA in the past. Since conception was delayed until her glycemic levels were at optimal control, the risk for fetal complications was decreased.

Healthy Coping. Facing a lot of stressful and fearful situations, PB needed support from the diabetes care team and her family. The diabetes center recommended CSII, which PB had avoided in the past but was now considering because of the pregnancy. She indicated she would comply with all instructions to ensure that this pregnancy was carried to term. Also at her initial visit, PB expressed cautious optimism because of her past obstetrical history.

Healthy Eating. PB denied use of alcohol and drugs. With early morning nausea and occasional vomiting, her appetite had decreased in the past 2 weeks.

Care Plan. As a result of preparations made early in the pregnancy and even before conception, the following elements of care were planned as optimal management during pregnancy.

- Maternal and fetal surveillance and testing (eg, ultrasound, nonstress test, biophysical profile, contraction stress test, maternal serum alpha fetal protein, amniocentesis)
- Referral to an ophthalmologist for a baseline eye exam to detect changes during pregnancy
- Referral to dietitian for medical nutrition therapy in pregnancy
- Referrals to other specialists, as necessary

Diabetes Education. The following were identified as topics for which PB required education and/or intervention.

- *Diabetic Ketoacidosis Prevention:* Teach PB how to prevent diabetic ketoacidosis
- *Risks:* Discuss with PB and her husband the risks associated with type 1 diabetes and pregnancy

(continued)

Case in Point: Type 1 Diabetes—A Pregnancy With Preconception Care (continued)

- *Intensity of Care:* Explain how prenatal care is more intensive than preconception care (during pregnancy, more frequent obstetrical visits and more tests are needed)
- *Hypoglycemia:* Assess the husband's knowledge of signs and symptoms of hypoglycemia and how to administer glucagon
- *Assessment of Social-Emotional Well-Being:* Assess PB's response to feelings about this pregnancy, since the two earlier pregnancies ended in miscarriage; as needed, refer the couple to a social worker or behavioral health specialist to discuss their feelings about this pregnancy

Medical Nutrition Therapy. Medical nutrition therapy was necessary to evaluate PB's eating habits. Referral to a registered dietitian was made, who provided PB with information on the following:

- Recommended weight gain and rate of gain according to her prepregnancy body mass index
- Managing nausea and vomiting to avoid hypoglycemia
- Managing other gastrointestinal discomforts that may occur (eg, heartburn, constipation, ptyalism)
- Use of nonnutritive artificial sweeteners during pregnancy
- Food safety issues
- Exercise and physical activity program, if there are no contraindications
- Infant feeding plans
- Keeping food records

To avoid hypoglycemia, PB had to try to maintain consistency in her meal and snack times and portion sizes. She was told that insulin-to-carbohydrate ratios may be different depending on the meal. For example, the insulin-to-carbohydrate ratio at breakfast may be larger than at other meals because of increased cortisol and growth hormone levels that appear to contribute to morning glucose intolerance. Monitoring of blood glucose levels, blood or urine ketones, appetite, and weight gain guided the registered dietitian in developing an appropriate individualized meal plan and in making adjustments to the meal plan throughout the pregnancy.[24]

Insulin Therapy. Aspects of insulin therapy that needed to be addressed through diabetes education included glucose targets during pregnancy and the need to adjust the insulin regimen as the pregnancy advances.

- *Glucose Targets.* Optimal blood glucose control was necessary to decrease the risk of complications in pregnancy. Treatment of hypoglycemia was necessary if blood glucose levels were below 60 mg/dL. Changes in blood glucose recommendations for pregnancy were discussed (these are lower than prepregnancy values). PB's last episode of diabetic ketoacidosis was 3 years ago. The signs, symptoms, and management of DKA were discussed. More frequent self-monitoring of her blood glucose levels was appropriate, especially if she experienced nocturnal hypoglycemia.
- *Changing Insulin Requirements.* PB was told that her insulin regimen would change throughout the pregnancy. Her requirements might decrease during the first trimester, but increase in the second and even triple her prepregnancy dosage by the third trimester. The benefits of CSII were discussed since this was suggested by the diabetes treatment center.

PB decided to delay switching to the insulin pump until after delivery. She was compliant with her diabetes and pregnancy regimen. She did not miss any appointments with her healthcare provider, diabetes educator, or registered dietitian. Blood glucose records were consistently kept and verified by her memory meter, as were food records, which she e-mailed to the dietitian. The results of both maternal and fetal surveillance were normal, and PB discovered during an ultrasound appointment that she was having a girl!

Diabetes Care During Labor and Delivery. PB's blood glucose levels were frequently monitored, and insulin and glucose were administered as necessary. After 6 hours of labor, she vaginally delivered baby Brianna, a 3540-g girl.

Postpartum Care and Education

Lactation. Soon after conceiving, PB decided she would breastfeed. Brianna spent a day in the neonatal intensive care unit to be assessed for any anomalies or complications. With no complications, she was reunited with her mother. Because PB knew her milk production might be delayed, she had begun pumping her breasts soon after delivery. She noticed a drop in her glucose level whenever Brianna nursed.

Assessment Phone Call. Two weeks after PB delivered her baby, the diabetes nurse educator phoned her to assess how she was adjusting to motherhood. PB told her that breastfeeding was going well and Brianna was gaining weight. PB's insulin requirements had decreased, and she had to monitor her glycemic levels more often. To assess for postpartum depression, the diabetes educator asked PB how she felt emotionally; PB denied any emotional changes.

Office Visit. PB made an appointment with the diabetes educator to discuss changes to her regimen during the postpartum period. Diabetes education stressed the need to maintain optimal glycemic control for the duration of the breastfeeding period and when she weans her daughter. Hypoglycemic awareness while she was breastfeeding was also emphasized, which may increase the frequency of self-monitoring of her glycemic level. During the appointment, PB told the diabetes educator that although she was happy being a new mother, she wanted to wait at least 2 years before attempting to conceive again. The educator reviewed contraceptives that were safe while breastfeeding and those for use after weaning. After her 6-week postpartum checkup, PB was scheduled to return to the diabetes center for care and to make an appointment with the registered dietitian to discuss weight loss and adjustments to her food plan.

Preconception care, as demonstrated with PB's case, is key to improving outcomes in pregnancies complicated by diabetes. Both the ADA and ACOG recommend that diabetes care and education begin before conception.[1,4] Sufficient time must be allowed to evaluate the mother's health status and to normalize or maximize glycemic control, thereby offering the best chance for the fetus.

Another Case in Point: Type 2 Diabetes—A Pregnancy Requiring Hospitalization

LR was a 27-year-old Hispanic woman referred for her first pregnancy at 13 weeks' gestation, which was confirmed while at an emergency room after fainting at home. She was admitted from the emergency room for glucose control when her random blood glucose level was 210 mg/dL (11.7 mmol). At her initial prenatal visit, LR weighed 248 lb. Her body mass index (BMI) was 42.5; height 64 in.

- Four years ago, LR was diagnosed with type 2 diabetes and prescribed glyburide and metformin (Glucovance), 500 mg twice a day, but she stopped taking it a year ago. When asked why, she replied that she forgot to take the drug on most days.
- LR received MNT when first diagnosed, but only followed the food plan for about 6 months.
- Her family history included diabetes in both maternal and paternal grandfathers.
- LR lived alone, having recently separated from her husband, and worked part time as a school bus aide.
- She denied use of alcohol, tobacco, and drugs.

Preconception Care and Education

LR did not receive preconception counseling.

Care and Education During Pregnancy

Pathophysiology of Type 2 Diabetes

LR presented for her first visit with many of the challenges of poorly controlled type 2 diabetes; her situation was further complicated by an unstable home situation. To help her deliver a healthy baby, the care

(continued)

Another Case in Point: Type 2 Diabetes—A Pregnancy Requiring Hospitalization (continued)

team needed many questions answered. LR needed the help of a comprehensive diabetes care team.

Diabetes Management During Pregnancy

LR was unsure of her prepregnancy weight, but weighed 248 lb at her initial prenatal visit (height 64 in, BMI 42.5). Her A1C was 11.0 %, and her hemoglobin was 12.5 mg/dL. She had complained of recurrent urinary tract infections (UTIs) and was currently on antibiotics.

Assessment. It was important to assess why LR discontinued her diabetes treatment plan, including her oral antidiabetic medications. There had been recent changes in LR's life, including an unplanned pregnancy and a recent separation: more information was needed about her current living conditions. Referral to a social worker or mental health professional was helpful in establishing baseline information on her willingness and ability to follow a care plan and then to develop and implement a care plan.

- What was her current relationship with her husband? Was there anyone who could assist her during the pregnancy?
- What was her financial situation? Did she have health insurance, and if not, would she be able to purchase the diabetes supplies, including insulin and syringes, test strips, and lancets?
- Was she willing to follow an intensive insulin regimen requiring her to self-inject insulin and monitor her blood glucose levels multiple times daily?

Complications. LR had experienced UTIs and might have been vulnerable to other complications associated with obesity—such as chronic hypertension, obstructive sleep apnea, preeclampsia, higher rates of cesarean, and difficult deliveries. Careful and comprehensive assessment for complications was required, and appropriate interventions were initiated. At each subsequent visit, LR was screened for UTI.

Insulin Therapy. LR was started on an insulin regimen of 3 injections daily: rapid-acting before meals; intermediate-acting before breakfast and at night. She monitored her blood glucose levels 4 times daily (fasting and 2-hour postprandial). LR was started on insulin immediately to quickly bring her glycemic levels to normal. Because of her BMI, the initial insulin initiation was calculated at 1.5 units/kg of actual body weight. She was told that as insulin resistance increases in the third trimester, the insulin dose may increase to 2.0 units per kilogram.

Medical Nutrition Therapy. LR received MNT during admission, but found the food plan difficult to follow at home. Before providing appropriate MNT, the registered dietitian needed to understand LR's lifestyle, eating preferences, and barriers to using a food plan for diabetes management. The original food plan was modified to include LR's food preferences. LR was income-eligible for WIC and Food Stamps and referred to these programs. By the third visit with the dietitian, LR was compliant with the food plan. She had decided to formula-feed the baby.

Diabetes Education. LR needed information about the risks she and her child face, healthy and reasonable expectations regarding weight gain, mental preparation for the increase in medical testing, and support regarding her use of the food plan.

Risks. LR needed assistance in understanding that obese pregnant women with type 2 diabetes are at higher risk for adverse pregnancy outcomes, including macrosomia.

- *Weight.* She received information on weight gain recommendations and the importance of avoiding weight loss to decrease the risk for starvation ketosis and intrauterine growth retardation. She was told that calorie restriction is not recommended during pregnancy because of the possible effect of ketonuria or ketonemia on the fetus.
- *Food Plan.* She was given information on how women with type 2 diabetes may benefit from a lower calorie food plan of no less than 1800 calories. Effective implementation of medical nutrition therapy could help LR avoid ketosis and excessive weight gain and provide adequate nutrients.
- *Medical Care.* She was informed about and prepared for her medical tests. Maternal and fetal testing would begin according to the gestational

week. Because of the elevated A1C at conception, in addition to the usual laboratory testing in diabetes and pregnancy, LR would be offered an amniocentesis to assess chromosomal abnormalities. She learned that frequent scanning was necessary to assess fetal well-being.

- *Glycemic Control.* She was informed about the value of good glycemic control in the short and long term, for the health of both her unborn child and herself.

Because LR worked split shifts, she was able to meet with the diabetes educator between bus runs. She expressed gratitude for the assistance she received. She met with the social worker and was referred for financial assistance to help with insulin and monitoring supplies. An amniocentesis was performed, and the test results were negative for Down syndrome and neural tube defects. Having learned from the diabetes educator that maternal glycemic levels can affect the fetus, LR complied with the insulin and monitoring schedule.

Postpartum Care and Education

LR delivered a 4630-g baby boy at 38 weeks via cesarean section. During pregnancy, the diabetes educator emphasized the importance of maintaining postpartum glycemia to levels as near to normal as possible to decrease the risk of complications. Four weeks after delivery, LR went back to her prescription of glyburide and metformin (Glucovance), taking it as prescribed. She scheduled an appointment with the registered dietitian to discuss weight loss and a new eating plan.

For most women with type 2 diabetes, referral for preconception counseling is rare. As in LR's case, pregnancy is the first introduction to diabetes self-care management. Ongoing diabetes care and medical care are important so the woman can continue using the skills learned during pregnancy and decrease the risk of microvascular complications. Self-care steps for women with type 1 diabetes can be followed by women with type 2 diabetes. Women with type 2 diabetes who are not breastfeeding can be switched back to oral medications soon after delivery; the breastfeeding woman with type 2 diabetes, however, needs to continue insulin for the duration of the lactation period.

Teens—A Special Population

The pregnant adolescent with preexisting diabetes poses additional challenges to the healthcare team. Meeting the needs of a pregnant teen involves more than the already-intense diabetes and pregnancy care required for adult women. Topics of diabetes education for adolescent girls span the following:

- Pregnancy prevention
- Preconception counseling
- Pregnancy management

Although studies have found delayed menarche in adolescent girls with type 1 diabetes,[60,61] research has not indicated any difference in the fertility rates compared to teenagers without diabetes. One study found that pregnant adolescent girls with diabetes had an unusually high frequency of pregnancy.[62] The following are unique aspects of providing diabetes education to this special population.

Teen pregnancy and education:

Preconception counseling should begin at puberty (childbearing age) for females with diabetes. Because the majority of teen pregnancies are unplanned, the higher risk of elevated A1C and poor glycemic control further increases the risk of fetal congenital malformations.

Higher Energy and Nutrient Requirements. Pregnant teenagers have higher energy and generally higher nutrient requirements than pregnant adults with diabetes because their bodies may not have reached full maturation.

Additional Stresses. The physiological stress of pregnancy is only one of the challenges facing the adolescent; emotional turmoil may also play a role. The situation becomes even more complicated if the teen does not inform her parents or guardians or waits to inform them about her pregnancy.

Legal Emancipation. In certain states, and depending on the person's age, a teenager may be considered emancipated. The emancipation of a minor generally refers to a teen given the rights to live on her own. This legal status allows the minor to obtain and make decisions about medical care without parental consent. Diabetes educators must be aware of the emancipation laws in states where they practice.

Questions and Controversy

Controversies about the use of certain medications in pregnancy are important to stay abreast of. Issues regarding use of insulin analogs, incretin mimetic hormones, and oral hypoglycemic agents in pregnancy are detailed below. Questions are also being asked about how diabetes is affected by menopause; see below.

Medications

Insulin Analogs. Recent studies have shown the safety and efficacy of rapid-acting insulin analogs in pregnancy,[50-55] and although acknowledged by the ACOG and ADA, neither association has recommended their use in pregnancy.[1,4] In a review article by Hirsch, randomized, controlled clinical trials are lacking on the use of insulin analogs in pregnancy; however, retrospective studies have not shown any significant difference between insulin lispro and short-acting insulin.[63] Glargine (Lantus) is considered a Category C drug (meaning the medication is only used in pregnancy if the potential benefits justify the potential risks to the fetus); however, no randomized trials have been conducted using glargine. Case reports found no teratogenic or embryotoxic effects.

New Injection Medications. Exenatide (Byetta), pramlintide acetate (Symlin), and insulin detemir (Levemir, UK brand name) (expected to be available in the United States in 2006) are relatively new injection medications for use in diabetes. Each is classified as Category C.

Use of Oral Agents. Use of oral hypoglycemic agents in pregnancy is controversial. The following can be said for specific drugs:

- *Glyburide:* Glyburide (Diabeta, Glynase, Micronase, Pres Tab) has been shown not to cross the placenta, and its use in GDM is increasing; however, women with type 2 diabetes will probably be switched from this oral agent to insulin
- *Metformin:* Women taking metformin (Glucophage), which is used in the treatment of infertility and polycystic ovary syndrome prior to pregnancy, may continue during their pregnancy; the ADA and ACOG have not recommended use of this oral agent in pregnancy until more data on the safety and efficacy of oral hypoglycemics become available

Menopause

Few studies have considered what happens with women with diabetes when they enter the menopausal stage of life, after the childbearing years have ended. Studies have found earlier[64] or no difference[65] in menopause in women with diabetes. Use of hormone-replacement therapy (HRT) is controversial, and although HRT is known to improve glycemic control and improve lipid levels, information is conflicting on the effect of these therapies on coronary heart disease in women with diabetes.[66,67] Discussion of menopause with a woman with diabetes must include the following:

- *Hormone Replacement Therapy:* Benefits and risks
- *Lifestyle Changes:* To decrease any age-related health risks, such as cardiovascular disease and osteoporosis

Curriculum Topics

Pregnancy is an excellent time to plan a variety of interesting and resourceful teaching strategies for the woman with preexisting diabetes. Information on how diabetes affects maternal and fetal outcomes will help the woman adhere to the diabetes regimen. The following material should be covered:

- *Pathophysiology.* Explain pathophysiology of diabetes and pregnancy, including an explanation of how glucose and ketones cross the placenta.
- *Euglycemia.* Communicate importance of maintaining euglycemia through entire pregnancy to decrease the risk of maternal and fetal complications.
- *Intensity of Care.* Explain the frequency of obstetric visits and antenatal testing appointments.
- *Insulin Use.* Explain role of insulin in pregnancy and need for higher insulin requirements as pregnancy progresses (the increase in placental hormones is antagonistic to insulin action). Explain that insulin does not cross the placenta.
- *Registered Dietitian.* Refer to registered dietitian for medical nutrition therapy.
- *Hypoglycemia.* Review signs, symptoms, causes, treatment, and prevention of hypoglycemia with the woman, her partner, and other appropriate family members or co-workers. Affirm the woman understands sick day rules and how to treat nausea and vomiting. Instruct family members on glucagon administration. Explain that to avoid excessively high glycemic levels, treatment recommendations may change from concentrated sources of carbohydrates (such as orange juice) to milk. Advise her to carry glucose tablets or gel or another source of carbohydrate at all times.
- *Blood Glucose.* Assess her blood glucose monitoring technique periodically. Occasionally verify her meter's accuracy with a laboratory plasma glucose test.
- *Injections.* Review injection sites and absorption times for different sites. Reassure her that the abdomen can be used as an injection site.
- *Physical Activity.* Review guidelines on physical activity and exercise.
- *Urgent Situations.* Provide instructions on when to contact the healthcare team, such as continual or severe vomiting, persistent presence of ketones, vaginal bleeding or discharge, uterine contractions, blurred vision, decreased fetal movement, edema, or severe headaches.
- *Continued Self-Management.* Explain that self-care management must continue following birth. Mothers tend to turn their attention to the baby while neglecting their own health. Careful diabetes management will help ensure future successful pregnancies and reduce the risk for long-term diabetes complications such as retinopathy and/or nephropathy.
- *Breastfeeding.* Assure the mother that breastfeeding is recommended for women with diabetes, unless contraindicated.

Focus on Education: Pearls for Practice

Preconception counseling has become the key for good perinatal outcomes. An increasing number of women are developing type 2 diabetes during their childbearing years. Growing, too, is the number of women with type 1 diabetes desiring to have children.

- **Encourage the woman to see herself as a vital part of the multidisciplinary team.** In both her preconception and antepartum care, the pregnant woman's willingness to work together with the other members of the healthcare team can result in an improved outcome.

Teaching Strategies

The diabetes educator has many opportunities to make important contributions during a woman's pregnancy and planning for motherhood. From preconception through to postpartum care, both the mother and her infant benefit from the diabetes educator's involvement.

- **Relieve the stress.** Diabetes educators are pivotal in helping coordinate the woman's care to decrease the anxiety and stress the mother-to-be feels. These women are concerned about not carrying a pregnancy to term and delivering an infant with major malformations.

- **Pace the pregnancy with attainable goals.** Attending to the immediate issues of glycemic control, pregnancy care, and diabetes self-management, the educator assists the woman in establishing achievable goals for the pregnancy. As pregnancy progresses, the two review these frequently (family also, if needed) and make changes necessary.

- **Develop the opportunity to improve woman's long-term health.** The educator helps the woman establish goals and habits that can last beyond pregnancy and childbearing—the woman gains knowledge that can be of value in subsequent pregnancies and has the opportunity to lower her risk of long-term complications.

Messages for Patient Education

Motivation is a key to the success of a good outcome in pregnancy.

- **Expect more intense care and monitoring requirements.** In pregnancy complicated by diabetes, additional testing and monitoring are performed, both in the preconception period and during the pregnancy. Glycemic control within the optimal range is necessary to decrease the risk of congenital malformations and spontaneous abortions. More frequent self-monitoring of blood glucose levels may be required; this is necessary so the need for any adjustments in insulin and or food intake can be evaluated.

- **Pay attention to plans for food and weight.** Weight gain goals will be established based on prepregnancy weight. Medical nutrition therapy will be based on current eating habits and the Dietary Reference Intakes for pregnant women.

- **Expect changes in medication.** Medication therapy changes frequently during pregnancy as the hormones of pregnancy impact insulin needs. Therapies also change at delivery and in the postpartum phase.

- **Breastfeeding is good.** Breastfeeding is encouraged because of the immunological benefits to the mother and infant. Lactation may be delayed because of early separation of the infant, but pumping the breasts soon after delivery can establish a steady milk supply.

Suggested Readings

American College of Obstetricians and Gynecologists. Pregestational diabetes mellitus. Practice bulletin No. 60. Obstet Gynecol. 2005;105:675-685.

American Diabetes Association. Diagnosis and classification of diabetes mellitus (position statement). Diabetes Care. 2005;28:S37-S42.

Bailey BK, Cardwell MS. A team approach to managing preexisting diabetes complicated by pregnancy. Diabetes Educator. 1996;22:111-115.

Berkus MD, Conway D, Langer O. The large fetus. Clin Obstet Gynecol. 1999;42:766-784.

Bernasko J. Contemporary management of type 1 diabetes mellitus in pregnancy. Obstet Gynecol Surv. 2004;59:628-636.

California Diabetes and Pregnancy Program. Sweet Success: Guidelines for Care. Campbell, Calif: Education Program Associates; 1998.

Evers IM, DeValk HW, Mol BE, et al. Macrosomia despite good glycemic control in type 1 diabetic pregnancy: results of a nationwide study in the Netherlands. Diabetologia. 2002;45:1484-1489.

Gamson K, Chia S, Jovanovic L. The safety and efficacy of insulin analogs in pregnancy. J Materna Fetal Neonat Med. 2004;15:26-34.

Homko CJ, Reece EA. Ambulatory management of the pregnant woman with diabetes. Obstet Gynecol Clin North Am. 1998;41:584-596.

Homko C J and Sargrad KR. Pregnancy With Preexisting Diabetes. In: Franz MJ, ed. A Core Curriculum for Diabetes Education: Diabetes in the Life Cycle and Research, 5th ed. (Franz MJ, ed.). Chicago, Ill: American Association of Diabetes Educators; 2003.

Jovanovic L, ed. Medical Management of Pregnancy Complicated by Diabetes, 3rd ed. Alexandria, Va: American Diabetes Association; 2000.

Reece EA, Coustan DR, Gabbe SG. Diabetes in Women: Adolescence, Pregnancy, and Menopause, 3rd ed. Philadelphia: Lippincott Williams & Wilkins; 2004.

Rosenn BM, Miodovnik M. Medical complications of diabetes mellitus in pregnancy. Clin Obstet Gynecol. 2000;43:17-31.

Shils ME, Olson JA, Shike M, et al. Modern Nutrition in Health and Disease. Philadelphia: JB Lippincott; 1999.

Worthington-Roberts BS, Rodwell Williams S. Nutrition in Pregnancy and Lactation. New York: McGraw Hill; 1996.

References

1. Martin JA, Hamilton BE, Sutton PD, et al. Births: final data for 2002. Natl Vital Stat Rep. 2003;52(10):1-113.
2. Engelgau MM, Herman WH, Smith PJ, et al. The epidemiology of diabetes and pregnancy in the US, 1988. Diabetes Care. 1995;18:1029-1033.
3. Kitzmiller JL, Buchanan TA, Kjos S, et al. Preconception care of diabetes, congenital malformation, and spontaneous abortions. Diabetes Care. 1996;19:514-541.
4. American College of Obstetricians and Gynecologists. Pregestational diabetes mellitus. Practice bulletin No. 60. Obstet Gynecol. 2005;105:675-685.
5. American Diabetes Association. Position statement. Gestational diabetes mellitus. Diabetes Care. 2004;27 Suppl 1:S88-S90.
6. White P. Pregnancy complicating diabetes. Am J Med. 1949;7:609-616.
7. Buchanan TA, Coustan DR. Diabetes mellitus. In: Burrows GN, Ferris TF, eds. Medical Complications During Pregnancy, 4th ed. Philadelphia: WB Saunders; 1994:29-61.
8. Jovanovic L. Diabetic retinopathy. In: Reece EA, Coustan DR, Gabbe SG, eds. Diabetes in Women: Adolescence, Pregnancy, and Menopause, 3rd ed. Philadelphia: Lippincott Williams & Wilkins; 2004:371-382.
9. Lauszus FF, Klebe JG, Bek T, et al. Increased serum IGF-I during pregnancy is associated with progression of diabetic retinopathy. Diabetes. 2003;52:852-856.
10. Rosenn B, Miodovnik M, Kranias G, et al. Progression of diabetic retinopathy in pregnancy: association with hypertension in pregnancy. Am J Obstet Gynecol. 1992;166:1214-1218.
11. Brinchmann-Hansen O, Dahl-Jorgensen K, Hanssen KF, et al. Effects of intensified insulin treatment on various lesions of diabetic retinopathy. Am J Ophthalmol. 1985;100:644-653.
12. Report of the National High Blood Pressure Education Program Working Group on High Blood Pressure in Pregnancy. Am J Obstet Gynecol. 2000;183:S1-S22.
13. Hinton AC, Sibai BM. Hyertensive disorders in pregnancy. In: Reece EA, Coustan DR, Gabbe SG, eds. Diabetes in Women: Adolescence, Pregnancy and Menopause, 3rd ed. Philadelphia: Lippincott Williams & Wilkins; 2004:363-370.
14. Cundy T, Gamble G, Townend K, et al. Perinatal mortality in type 2 diabetes mellitus. Diabet Med. 2000;17:33.

15. Ehrenberg HM, Mercer BM, Catalano PM. The influence of obesity and diabetes on the prevalence of macrosomia. Am J Obstet Gynecol. 2004;191:964-968.

16. Clausen TD, Mathiesen E, Ekbom P, et al. Poor pregnancy outcome in women with type 2 diabetes. Diabetes Care. 2005;28:323-328.

17. Weiss JL, Malone FD. Caring for the obese obstetric patient. Contemporary Ob/Gyn. 2001;6:13-23.

18. Mills JL, Baker L, Goldman AS. Malformations in infants of diabetic mothers occur before the seventh gestational week: implications for treatment. Diabetes. 1979;28:292-293.

19. Jensen DM, Damm P, Moelsted-Pedersen L, et al. Outcomes in type 1 diabetic pregnancies. Diabetes Care. 2004;27:2819-2823.

20. Wren C, Birrell G, Hawthorne G. Cardiovascular malformations in infants of diabetic mothers. Heart. 2003;89:1217-1220.

21. American College of Obstetricians and Gynecologists. Fetal Macrosomia. Washington, DC: ACOG; 2000. ACOG Bulletin No. 22.

22. Coustan DR. Delivery: Timing, mode, and management. In: Reece EA, Coustan DR, Gabbe SG, eds. Diabetes in Women: Adolescence, Pregnancy, and Menopause, 3rd ed. Philadelphia: Lippincott Williams & Wilkins; 2004:433-439.

23. Kim C, Ferrara A, McEwen LN, et al. Preconception care in managed care: the translating research into action for diabetes study. Am J Obstet Gynecol. 2005;192:227-232.

24. Dunne F. Type 2 diabetes and pregnancy. Sem Fetal Neonatal Med. 2005;10:333-339.

25. Dunne F, Brydin P, Smith K, et al. Pregnancy in women with type 2 diabetes: 12 years outcome data 1990-2002. Diabet Med. 2003;20:734-738.

26. McElduff A, Ross GP, Lagström JA, et al. Pregestational diabetes and pregnancy: an Australian experience. Diabetes Care. 2005;28:1260.

27. Koos BJ, Moore PJ. Maternal physiology during pregnancy. In: DeCherney AH, Nathan L, eds. Current Obstetric and Gynecologic Diagnosis and Treatment. New York: Lange Medical Books/McGraw-Hill; 2003:154-162.

28. Landon MB, Gabbe SG. Diabetes mellitus. In: Barron WM, Lindheimer MD, Davison JM, eds. Medical Disorders in Pregnancy. St. Louis: Mosby; 2000:71-100.

29. Catalano PM, Buchanan TA. Metabolic changes during normal and diabetic pregnancies. In: Reece EA, Coustan DR, Gabbe SG, eds. Diabetes in Women: Adolescence, Pregnancy and Menopause. Philadelphia: Lippincott Williams & Wilkins; 2004:129-145.

30. Pedersen J. The Pregnant Diabetic and Her Newborn, 2nd ed. Baltimore: Williams & Wilkins; 1977.

31. Eidelman AI, Samueloff A. The pathophysiology of the fetus of the diabetic mother. Sem in Perinatol. 2002;26:232-236.

32. Landon MB. Diabetes mellitus and other endocrine disorders. In: Gabble SG, Niebyl JR, Simpson JL, eds. Obstetrics: Normal and Problem Pregnancies. New York: Churchill-Livingston; 1991:1097-1136.

33. National Academy of Sciences. Nutrition During Pregnancy. Washington, DC: National Academy Press, 1990.

34. Strauss RS, Dietz WH. Low maternal weight gain in the second or third trimester increases the risk for intrauterine growth retardation. J Nutr. 1999;19:988-993.

35. Abrahms BF, Laros RK Jr. Prepregnancy weight, weight gain and birth weight. Am J Obstet Gynecol. 1986;154:503-509.

36. Rizzo TA, Dooley SL, Metzger BE, et al. Prenatal and perinatal influences on long-term psychomotor development in offspring of diabetic mothers. Am J Obstet Gynecol. 1995; 173:1753-1758.

37. Institute of Medicine of the National Academies. Dietary Reference Intakes: Energy, Carbohydrate, Fiber, Fat, Fatty Acids, Cholesterol, Protein, and Amino Acids. Washington, DC: The National Academies Press; 2002.

38. Jovanovic-Peterson L, ed. Medical Management of Pregnancy Complicated by Diabetes, 3rd ed. Alexandria, Va: American Diabetes Association; 2000:7.

39. American Diabetes Association. Evidence-based nutrition principles and recommendations for the treatment and prevention of diabetes and related complications (position statement). Diabetes Care. 2003;26 Suppl 1:S51-S61.

40. Centers for Disease Control and Prevention. Notice to readers: Surgeon General's advisory on alcohol use in pregnancy. MMWR. 2005;54(9):229.

41. Evans EC. The FDA recommendations on fish intake during pregnancy. J Obstet Gynecol Neonatal Nurs. 2002; 31:715-720.

42. Murtaugh MA, Ferris AM, Capacchione CM, et al. Energy intake and glycemia in lactating women with type 1 diabetes. J Am Diet Assoc. 1998;98:642-648.

43. Ferris AM, Dalidowitz CK, Ingardia CM, et al. Lactation outcome in insulin-dependent diabetic women. J Amer Diet Assoc. 1988;88:317-322.

44. US Department of Health and Human Services, Department of Agriculture. Dietary Guidelines for Americans. Washington: National Academies Press; 2005.

45. Thomas AM, Gutierrez YM. American Dietetic Association Guide to Gestational Diabetes Mellitus. Chicago: American Dietetic Association; 2005.

46. Kitzmiller JL, Gavin LA, Gin GD, et al. Preconception care of diabetes: Glycemic control prevents congenital anomalies. JAMA. 1991;265:731-736.

47. Manderson JG, Patterson CC, Hadden DR, et al. Preprandial versus postprandial blood glucose monitoring in type 1 diabetic pregnancy: a randomized controlled clinical trial. Am J Obstet Gynecol. 2003;189:507-512.

48. Churchill JA, Berendes HW. Intelligence of children whose mothers had acetonuria during pregnancy. In: Perinatal Factors Affecting Human Development. Pan American Health Organization Scientific Publication. Washington, DC: Pan American Health Organization; 1969;185:300.

49. Rizzo T, Metzger BE, Burns WJ, et al. Correlations between antepartum maternal metabolism and child intelligence. N Engl J Med. 1991;325:911-916.

50. Mordes D, Kreutner K, Metzger W, et al. Dangers of intravenous ritodrine in diabetic patients. JAMA. 1982;248:973-975.

51. Pettit DP, Kolaczynski JW, Ospina P, et al. Comparison of an insulin analog, insulin aspart and regular human insulin with no insulin in gestational diabetes mellitus. Diabetes Care. 2003;26:183-186.

52. Lapolla A, Dalfrà MG, Fedele D. Insulin therapy in pregnancy complicated by diabetes: are insulin analogs a new tool? Diabetes Metal Res Rev. 2005;21:241-252.

53. Gamson K, Chia S, Jovanovic L. The safety and efficacy of insulin analogs in pregnancy. J Materna Fetal Neonat Med. 2004;15:26-34.

54. Garg SK, Frias JP, Anil S, Gottlieb PA, MacKenzie T, Jackson WE. Insulin lispro therapy in pregnancies complicated by type 1 diabetes: glycemic control and maternal and fetal outcomes. Endocr Pract. 2003;9:187-193.

55. Cypryk K, Sobczak M, Pertyńska-Marczewska M, Zawodniak-Szalapska M, Szyczak W, Wilczyński J, Lewiński A. Pregnancy complications and perinatal outcome in diabetic women treated with Humalog (insulin lispro) or regular human insulin during pregnancy. Med Sci Monit. 2004;10:129-132.

56. Rudolf MC, Coustan DR, Sherwin RS, et al. Efficacy of the insulin pump in the home treatment of pregnant diabetics. Diabetes. 1981;30:891-895.

57. Kitzmiller J, Younger D, Hare J, et al. Continuous subcutaneous insulin therapy during early pregnancy. Obstetrics and Gynecology. 1985:66:606-611.

58. Gabbe SG. New concepts and applications in the use of insulin pump during pregnancy. J Matern Fetal Med. 2000;9:42-45.

59. Radermecker RP, Scheen AJ. Continuous subcutaneous insulin infusion with short-acting insulin analogues or human regular insulin: efficacy, safety, quality of life, and cost-effectiveness. Diabetes Metab Res Rev. 2004;20:178-188.

60. Danielson KK, Palta M, Allen C, et al. The association of increased total glycosylated hemoglobin levels with delayed age at menarche in young women with type 1 diabetes. J Clin Endocrinol Metab. 2005;90(12):6466-6471.

61. Codner E, Barrera A, Mook-Kanamori D, et al. Ponderal gain, waist-to-hip ratio, and pubertal development in girls with type 1 diabetes mellitus. Pediatric Diabetes. 2004;5:182-189.

62. Fennoy I. Contraception and the adolescent diabetic. Health Educ. 1989;20(6):21-23.

63. Hirsch IB. Insulin analogues. New Engl J Med. 2005;352:174-183.

64. Dorman JS, Steenkiste A, Foley T, et al. Menopause in type 1 diabetic women: is it premature? Diabetes. 2001;50:1857-1862.

65. Lopez-Lopez R, Huerta R, Malacare JM. Age at menopause in women with type 2 diabetes mellitus. Menopause. 1999;6(2):174-178.

66. Khoo CL, Perera M. Diabetes and the menopause. J Br Menopause Soc. 2005;11(1):6-11.

67. Lim SC, Caballero E, Arora S, et al. The effect of hormonal replacement therapy on the vascular reactivity and endothelial function of healthy individuals and individuals with type 2 diabetes. J Clin Endocrinol Metab. 1999;84:4159-4164.

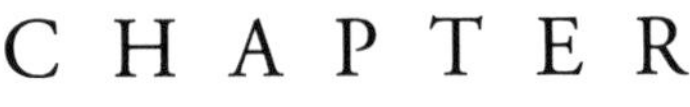

CHAPTER

12

Gestational Diabetes Mellitus

Author

Diane M. Reader, RD, CDE

Key Concepts

- Gestational Diabetes Mellitus (GDM) is a carbohydrate intolerance first recognized during pregnancy, and pregnancy is a progressive disorder that includes insulin resistance and relative insulin deficiency.
- Managing GDM requires balancing glucose control with the nutrient needs of a healthy pregnancy (ie, appropriate weight gain and adequate nutrient intake). Achieving glucose control should not compromise the outcomes of a healthy pregnancy; if unable to use nutrition therapy as monotherapy, oral or insulin therapy can be added concurrently.
- GDM signals the potential to develop type 2 diabetes; therefore, steps should be taken to prevent diabetes through weight control, food choices, and physical activity.
- Women with GDM have to learn and implement diabetes self-management in a very short period of time. Behavior change goals are important as changes must be accomplished quickly, and changes in glucose levels and, hence, therapy occur as the pregnancy progresses. From diagnosis to delivery can be only a matter of weeks.

State of the Disease

In the last 150 years, elevated glucose levels have been identified in older, more obese pregnant women who produced large babies and tended to develop diabetes later in life. In 1949, Priscilla White of the Joslin Clinic described diabetes first diagnosed during pregnancy as "Class A diabetes." The term gestational diabetes was first suggested by O'Sullivan in 1961. In 1979, at the First International Workshop-Conference on Gestational Diabetes, the current definition of gestational diabetes mellitus (GDM) as "carbohydrate intolerance of variable severity with onset or first recognition during pregnancy" was first suggested.[1] Today, both the American Diabetes Association (ADA) and American College of Obstetrics and Gynecology (ACOG) use this definition.[2,3]

Like type 2 diabetes, GDM is characterized by insulin resistance and relative insulin deficiency. This usually does not occur until the second trimester.

- *Insulin Resistance in the First Trimester:* Insulin resistance is diminished, resulting in a decrease in both fasting and postprandial glucose levels
- *Insulin Resistance in Second and Third Trimesters:* Insulin resistance increases dramatically due to increased levels of human placental lactogen, prolactin, estrogen, and free and bound cortisol

Insulin resistance leads to an increased demand on the pancreas to produce more insulin. As shown in Figure 12.1, in a normal pregnancy, insulin requirements are doubled or tripled by the time of delivery. Insulin resistance is a normal state of pregnancy, and most women can make the additional insulin required to maintain normal glycemia. However, some women are not able to produce the additional insulin required and thus show a relative insulin deficiency. These are the women who develop gestational diabetes.

Incidence, Risk Factors, and Ethnic Variables

About 1 in 15 pregnant women sitting in the waiting room of an obstetrician-gynecologist will be diagnosed with GDM.[2] Some may have undiagnosed type 2 diabetes.

Categories of Increased Risk. In addition to certain ethnicities (summarized separately below), any of the following factors signal the woman is at high risk for GDM:

- Women who are older
- Women who are heavier
- Women who have delivered a large-for-gestational age infant
- Women who have more children
- Women with a history of glucose intolerance
- Women with a family history of diabetes
- Women with a history of polycystic ovary disease may also have an increased risk for GDM

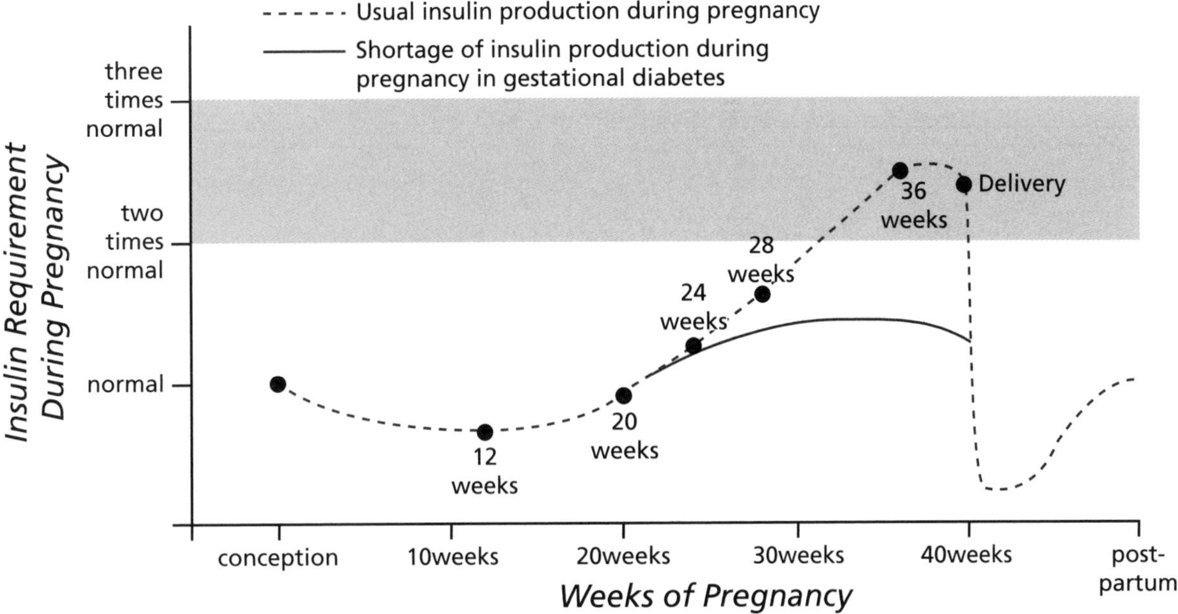

FIGURE 12.1 Insulin Requirements of Pregnancy

From *Gestational Diabetes BASICS* © 2005, International Diabetes Center, Minneapolis. U.S.A. Reprinted with permission.

Risk Associated With Ethnicity. GDM is more common in certain ethnic groups;[4] the rate parallels the rate of type 2 diabetes.

- *Highest Risk:* Native Americans and those of Hispanic, Asian, or Chinese descent
- *Lower Risk:* African women
- *Lowest Risk:* Non-Hispanic white women

Adolescence. The incidence of GDM in adolescence is unknown, but may be significant in populations with a high rate of type 2 diabetes and obesity in teenagers. For more information specific to pregnancy complicated by preexisting diabetes, see chapter 11.

Determining Risk, Screening, and Diagnosis

GDM is defined as glucose intolerance *first* recognized during pregnancy, even though these women may actually have had undiagnosed type 1 or type 2 diabetes prior to their pregnancy; this is one of the reasons for increased surveillance after the pregnancy ends. Unfortunately, defining glucose intolerance in pregnancy has been a challenge, and at this time there is no consensus.

Recommendations on Screening and Diagnosis

The American Diabetes Association and the World Health Organization use different criteria to diagnose GDM. The ADA recommends either the 1-step or 2-step approach to screen and diagnose GDM.[2]

1-Step Approach: The woman is given a 75-g Oral Glucose Tolerance Test (OGTT) between 24 to 28 weeks' gestation.

2-Step Approach: The first step is a 50-g Glucose Challenge Test (GCT) given at any time of the day. This screening test identifies 80% of women with GDM.[5] If the result 1 hour later is ≥140 mg/dL (7.8 mmol/L), then the second step, a 100-g OGTT, is scheduled. The woman reports to the lab, having fasted for at least 8 hours and consumed a normal carbohydrate load of at least 150 g for 3 days. Blood is drawn fasting and at 1, 2, and 3 hours. The woman cannot smoke or drink caffeine and is required to stay seated, resting. The diagnosis of GDM is made when 2 or more of the 4 tests are equal to or greater than the criteria in Figure 12.2.

Although no study has defined the relationship between OGTT and the need for insulin therapy, higher fasting glucose levels often indicate need for insulin therapy.[5,6] It is also important to note how many weeks of

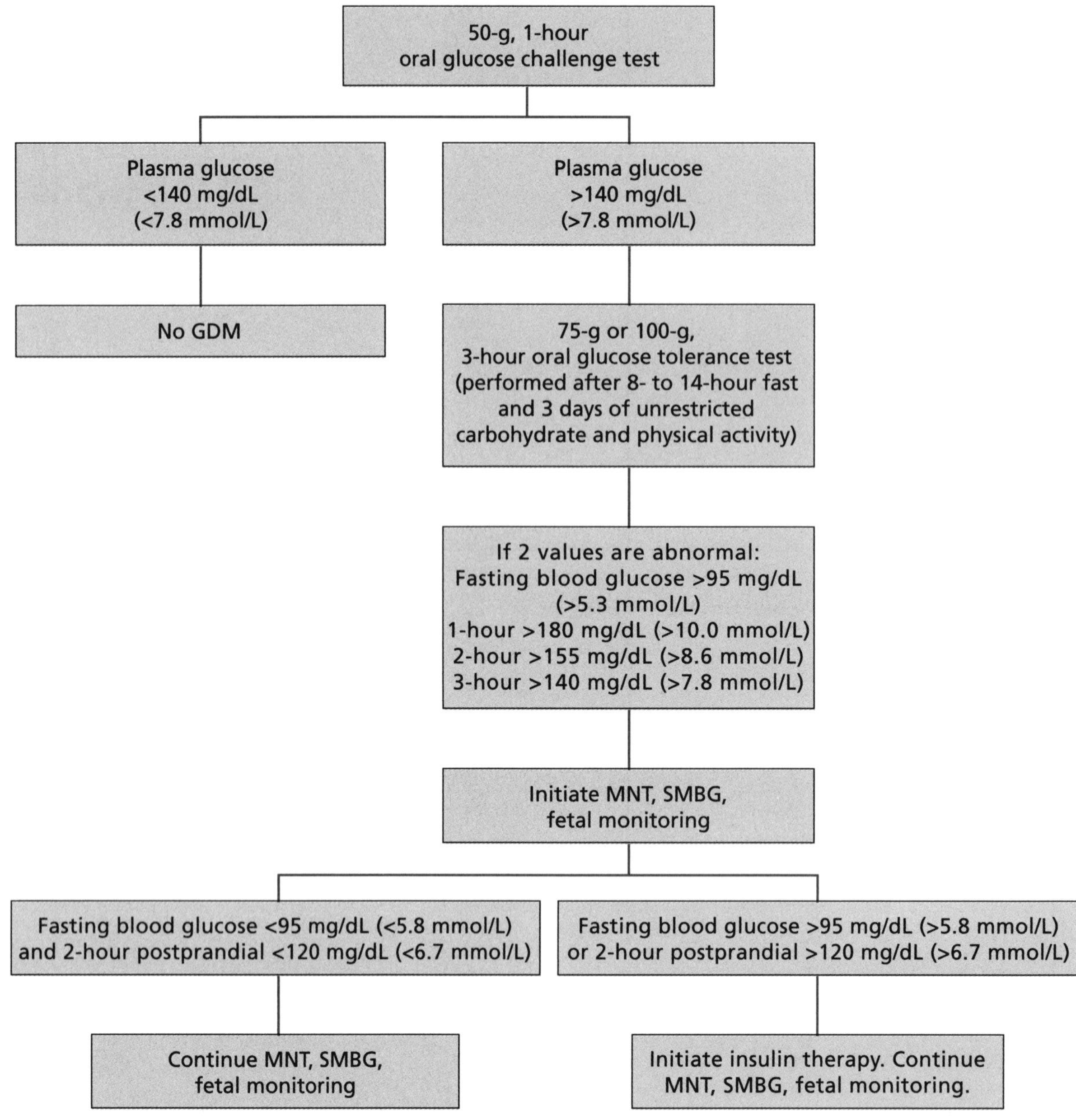

FIGURE 12.2 Screening and Diagnosis of Gestational Diabetes

Source: Copyright © 2000 American Diabetes Association. From Jovanovic L. Medical Management of Pregnancy Complicated by Diabetes (Clinical Education Series). Alexandria, Va: Reprinted with permission from *The American Diabetes Association.*

gestation the woman is, as insulin resistance of pregnancy continues to increase weekly until about 36 to 37 weeks.

Who to Screen. There is debate regarding who should be screened: all women or only those with risk factors. The recommendation from the Second and Third International Workshop-Conferences on Gestational Diabetes was that all pregnant women be screened for GDM between weeks 24 and 28 of pregnancy.[1]

When to Screen. The concept of risk assessment at the first prenatal visit was proposed in 1997 at the Fourth International Workshop-Conference on Gestational Diabetes.[5] The risk assessment would determine who would be screened for GDM and at what time during the pregnancy. Table 12.1 shows the risk categories, characteristics, and screening guidelines to be considered at the first prenatal visit.

TABLE 12.1 Risk Assessment at First Prenatal Visit

Risk Categories	*Characteristics*	*Screen*
High risk	History of large infant History of glucose intolerance or GDM Obese BMI >30 Strong family history of type 2 diabetes High-risk ethnic group	Glucose test at 1st prenatal visit If normal at 1st prenatal visit, then GCT between 24–28 weeks
Normal risk	Does not fit other categories	GCT between 24–28 weeks
Low risk	Young; < 25 years old No history of poor obstetrical outcome No first-degree family history of diabetes Normal or underweight Low-risk ethnic group	Not routinely screened Screened based on clinician assessment

Case in Point: A Pregnancy With GDM

MA had a number of risk factors for GDM:

- She was a member of a high-risk ethnic group
- She was both older and overweight
- She had a history of a large-for-gestational age infant
- Her mother and grandmother were living with type 2 diabetes

At MA's first prenatal appointment, her healthcare provider determined MA was at high risk for GDM and might have undiagnosed diabetes. After her appointment, MA went to the lab, drank a 50-g glucose solution, waited 1 hour and then a blood glucose level was drawn, which was reported as 123 mg/dL. With a blood glucose value of less than 140 mg/dL, MA passed the screening test, but needed to be screened again between weeks 24 and 28 of the pregnancy. MA was concerned and wanted to control her weight gain better during this pregnancy.

At 26 weeks, MA returned and took the 50-g glucose challenge test a second time. This time her result, of 155 mg/dL, was not normal. She returned within a week for the diagnostic OGTT. After an 8-hour fast, she consumed a 100-g glucose solution. Glucose levels were drawn fasting and at 1, 2, and 3 hours. Her results from the OGTT are shown below:

Blood Glucose After 100 g of Glucose	*Criteria: 2 or More Results Equal to or Greater Than:*	*MA's Test Results*
Fasting	≤95 mg/dL	93 mg/dL
1 hour	≤180 mg/dL	210 mg/dL
2 hour	≤165 mg/dL	176 mg/dL
3 hour	≤140 mg/dL	132 mg/dL

MA was diagnosed with GDM because at least 2 of the 4 tests were equal to or greater than the diagnostic criteria. The OGTT determines the diagnosis; however, it is interesting to ask if the OGTT also predicts her course with GDM. There appears to be a continuous relationship between increasing maternal glycemia and morbidities of pregnancy, so the higher the number the greater the likelihood MA will need insulin therapy.

Fetal and Maternal Risks With GDM

Fetal Complications

Macrosomia. The primary fetal risk is excessive growth. Macrosomia is often defined as an infant greater than 4000 g,[3] but this definition is not universal among researchers and clinicians. Macrosomia is significantly more common in infants of women with GDM than in the general population.[7] And it is the most common fetal complication in GDM, with a prevalence of 15% to 45%.[8]

The Pedersen hypothesis provides the best explanation for the link between macrosomia and gestational diabetes.[9] As the mother's blood circulates nutrients to her fetus, a high maternal level of glucose results in a high level of glucose in the fetus. Sensing elevated glucose levels, the fetal pancreas begins producing insulin to normalize this high level of glucose. As a growth hormone, insulin stimulates fetal growth. An increase in adipose tissue in the organs, chest, and abdomen means the trunk and shoulders become disproportionately larger than the head. A larger infant may lead the obstetrician to deliver via cesarean section to prevent birth trauma. Birth trauma may include items in the first bullet below;[8] the infants are also at increased risk for the other conditions listed:

- Shoulder dystocia, brachial plexus injury, Erb palsy, and asphyxia
- Having a higher body mass index (BMI)
- Developing glucose intolerance in their lifetime

Neonatal Hypoglycemia. Another fetal risk is neonatal hypoglycemia. The normal glucose level in the newborn is 40 to 120 mg/dL (2.2 to 6.7 mmol/L); therefore hypoglycemia is blood glucose less than 40 mg/dL (2.2 mmol/L). If the fetal pancreas has been overproducing insulin due to elevated circulating levels of glucose, low blood glucose will occur when the umbilical cord is clamped. This occurs within the first 12 hours of life and will require oral or intravenous glucose to return glucose levels to normal. Risks associated with neonatal hypoglycemia are seizures, cerebral damage, and death.[8]

Other Fetal Complications. Other problems associated with uncontrolled glucose levels in the infant include respiratory distress syndrome (RDS), hypocalcemia, polycythemia, and hyperbilirubinemia. Because GDM is a condition that begins in the second half of pregnancy, it is not associated with congenital malformations that may result from poor glucose control during organogenesis in the first trimester.

Maternal Complications

The maternal risks with GDM are *hypertension, polyhydramnios,* and *cesarean delivery.* In 1 study, the rate of cesarean section in women with GDM was 33% compared to 20.2% in the normal pregnant population, independent of the presence of macrosomia.[9]

Glucose control benefits mother and child:

- Excellent glucose control to prevent macrosomia helps women avoid assisted deliveries
- Macrosomia can result in immediate birth trauma for the infant and problems that become a factor later in life, such as high BMI and glucose intolerance
- The ADA, ACOG, and American Dietetics Association reflect the consensus that glucose control is critical to prevent the complications of GDM

Clinical Outcomes for GDM

Clinical studies in GDM and guidelines for nutrition, weight gain, and nutritional counseling are briefly summarized in this section. See also the questions and controversy section at the end of the chapter.

Clinical Studies

There are no landmark clinical trials, such as the Diabetes Control and Complications Trial (DCCT) or the UK Prospective Diabetes Study (UKPDS), that provide clear guidelines on management of GDM. Two studies are, however, of interest.

- The multinational Hyperglycemia and Adverse Outcome Study (HAPO) is underway. Its purpose is to clarify the associations between various levels of glucose intolerance during pregnancy and macrosomia, cesarean section rate, and hypertension among women of different cultures and ethnic groups.[10] For more detail, see the questions and controversy section at the end of this chapter.
- In June 2005, a randomized clinical trial was reported in the *New England Journal of Medicine* titled "Effect of treatment of gestational diabetes mellitus on pregnancy outcomes."[11] One thousand women with GDM were randomized to routine care or to intervention care that provided nutrition advice, blood glucose monitoring, and insulin as needed. The rate of serious perinatal complications was 1% in intervention care and 4% in routine care ($P = .01$). Ninety-two percent of the women in the intervention group saw a dietitian and 94% saw a nurse educator, compared to 10% and 11% respectively in the

routine care group. Four blood glucose tests per day were recommended, and target glucose was <95mg/dL (5.5 mmol/L) fasting and <126 mg/dL (7.0 mmol/L) at 2 hours.

Glucose Control

Clinical outcomes for GDM have been defined by the ADA and ACOG as well as by the American Dietetic Association in its publication *Nutrition Practice Guidelines for Gestational Diabetes Mellitus*.[2,3,12] Although there is some disagreement on specifics, there is agreement on overall goals. Glucose targets differ among organizations (see Table 12.2), but there is consensus that glucose control is critical to prevent the complications of GDM.

The summary and recommendations report of the Fourth International Conference-Workshop on GDM states this: "Prevention of adverse perinatal outcomes remains the primary focus of antepartum management of GDM. Information presented at the conference suggested a continuous relationship between increasing maternal glycemia and risk of perinatal morbidities, predominantly morbidities related to excessive fetal growth."[5] In short, blood glucose close to normal is the goal.

Nutrient and Weight Recommendations

- *Weight Gain:* All these organizations recommend following the Institute of Medicine guideline for weight gain during pregnancy, which is based on prepregnant body mass index (see Table 12.3)
- *Nutrients:* All agree that the woman with GDM should follow the same nutrient recommendations for a normal pregnancy: adequate calories and nutrients to support a health pregnancy and baby
- *Nutritional Counseling:* All these organizations recommend that the woman with GDM receive nutritional counseling by a registered dietitian when possible or by a qualified individual with experience in the management of GDM[2,3,5,12]

Nutrition practice guidelines of the American Dietetic Association are summarized in Figure 12.3. The

TABLE 12.2 Target Plasma Glucose in Pregnancy

Testing Times	*4th and 5th International Conference on GDM*[1]	*American Diabetes Association*[2]	*American College of Obstetric and Gyn.*[3]
Fasting	≤95 mg/dL (5.3 mmol/L)	≤105 mg/dL (5.8 mmol/L)	≤95 mg/dL (5.3 mmol/L)
1 hour	≤140 mg/dL (7.8 mmol/L)	≤155 mg/dL (8.6 mmol/L)	≤130 mg/dL (7.2 mmol/L)
2 hour	≤120 mg/dL (6.7 mmol/L)	≤130 mg/dL (7.8 mmol/L)	≤120 mg/dL (6.7 mmol/L)

Sources:

1. Metzger BE, Coustan DR, eds. Proceedings of the Fourth International Workshop-Conference on Gestational Diabetes Mellitus. Diabetes Care. 1998;21 Suppl 2:B164.
2. American Diabetes Association. Gestational diabetes mellitus (position statement). Diabetes Care. 2004;27 Suppl 1:S88-90.
3. American College of Obstetrics and Gynecology Committee on Practice Bulletins—Obstetrics. ACOG Practice Bulletin. Clinical management guidelines for obstetricians-gynecologists. Number 30, Sep 2001. Gestational Diabetes. Obstet Gynecol. 2001; 98:525-38.

Case—Part 2: Clinical Outcomes and Initial Therapy

What clinical outcomes needed to be set for MA? Glucose control was primary, as blood glucose levels within the normal range help prevent macrosomia and a large-for-gestational age infant, as MA had in her last pregnancy.

- *Self-Monitoring.* MA was taught self-monitoring of blood glucose and asked to test fasting and after her 3 largest meals of the day.
- *Weight Gain.* MA needed to control weight gain. With a BMI of 27, her weight gain target for the pregnancy was 15 to 25 lb.
- *Ketone Testing.* She was asked to test urine for ketones. She would be eating fewer carbohydrates in an attempt to control glucose and fewer calories to control weight gain, yet not so few as to develop starvation ketosis.
- *Records.* She also needed to eat a healthy diet, so she was asked to record her food intake as well as blood glucose values; these records would be assessed at a follow-up visit in 1 or 2 weeks.

Because MA's fasting result on the OGTT was less than 95 mg/dL, initial therapy for GDM was medical nutrition therapy.

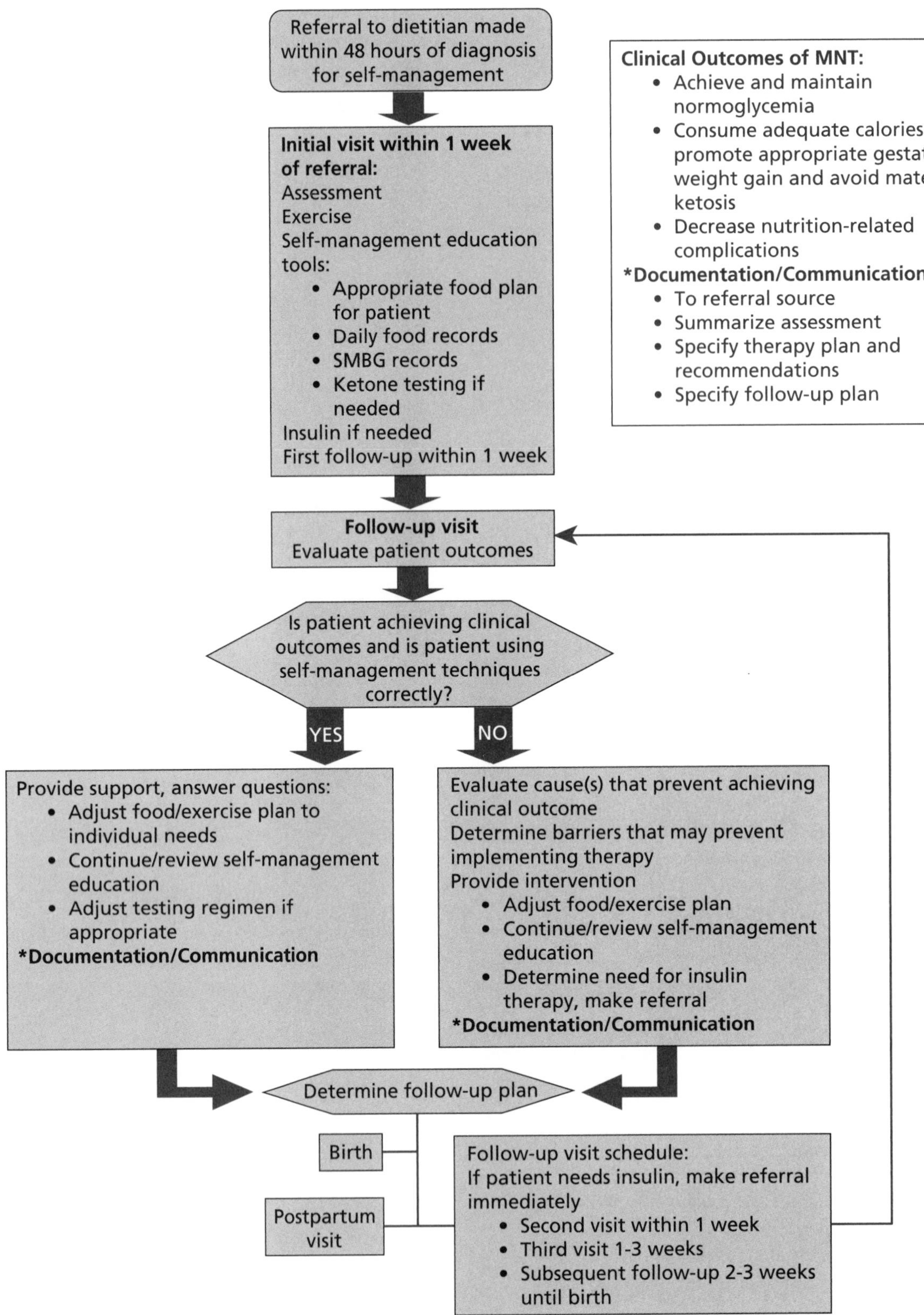

FIGURE 12.3 Nutrition Practice Guidelines for Gestational Diabetes

The process of providing medical nutrition therapy for women with gestational diabetes mellitus. Reprinted with permission from American Dietetic Association. Medical Nutrition Therapy Evidence-Based Guides for Practice: Nutrition Practice Guidelines for Gestational Diabetes Mellitus (CD-ROM). Chicago, Il: American Dietetic Association; 2001.

TABLE 12.3 Recommended Weight Gain for Pregnant Women

Prepregnant BMI	*Total Weight Gain*
Underweight <19.8	28–40 lb (12–18 kg)
Normal weight 19.8–26.0	25–35 lb (11–16 kg)
Overweight >26.0–29.0	15–25 lb (7–11 kg)
Obese >29.0	15 lb (7 kg)

Source: Institute of Medicine. Nutrition during pregnancy. Washington, DC: National Academy of Sciences; 1990.

nutrition prescription should be individualized and take into account the woman's weight status, activity level, lifestyle, and culture.

Achieving Clinical Outcomes Through Self-Management Education

Referral for self-management education varies from institution to institution. The education may occur in the diabetes education, endocrinology, health education, or obstetrics-gynecology department. Regardless of where the education happens, the woman diagnosed with GDM needs to learn all the self-monitoring practices everyone with diabetes should learn. The real challenge is that the pregnant woman must implement self-management tools immediately, as the outcome of the current pregnancy is affected.

Topics of Diabetes Education in GDM

The curriculum for diabetes self-management training for GDM contains the following important teaching objectives:[13]

- Define gestational diabetes and identify the risks of high blood glucose in pregnancy
- Describe normal glucose metabolism and pregnancy-related changes
- Explain diagnostic criteria
- Discuss treatment goals and strategies
- Explain rationale for blood glucose self-testing
- Identify testing times and targets
- Demonstrate and teach self-testing technique
- Discuss sharps disposal
- Teach ketone testing and identify targets and guidelines for action

The curriculum also needs to focus on the following nutrition therapy objectives:[13]

- Define food planning and identify goals, including weight-gain goals (see Table 12.3)
- Identify carbohydrate foods and how they affect blood glucose levels
- Instruct on carbohydrate counting or the plate method
- Demonstrate how to read food labels

Case—Part 3: Self-Management Education Begins

MA's healthcare provider referred her to the diabetes education center. She had her first appointment within a week of diagnosis, at 29 weeks' gestation.

The diabetes educator discovered that MA was very motivated to follow through with the protocol. Because her mother and grandmother had diabetes, she was familiar with blood glucose monitoring as well as how to give insulin. MA was surprised that her blood glucose targets were so much lower than the blood glucose values she saw her family members obtain. She was instructed to record her blood glucose tests 4 times per day on her food record form and test urine for ketones every other morning.

Healthy Eating. MA was very motivated to change her diet. She quit drinking regular soda pop when she was diagnosed with GDM. She readily admitted that she likes to eat, overeats, and could cut back on the fat in her diet.

Being Active. MA was physically active at work. She was busy at home with her family, but did not intentionally walk or exercise. MA started to consider whether a daily walk after dinner would be beneficial to her glucose control and desire to control weight gain.

Behavior Change Goals. MA and her diabetes team set up 3 behavior change goals at the first visit:

1. Test blood glucose every morning before breakfast and 1 hour after the start of each meal
2. Follow your food plan; count carbohydrates and record food intake
3. Test urine ketones every other morning

- Discuss use of food with added sugar
- Present a personal food plan
- Discuss timing of meals and snacks and the need for consistency
- Discuss weight gain
- Instruct on hyperglycemia
- Discuss the impact of physical activity of blood glucose levels
- Instruct on recording food and activity on record form
- Discuss gestational diabetes goals

Self-Management Behaviors in GDM

In GDM, as in other types of diabetes, appropriate self-care behaviors enhance health outcomes. In this section, points pertinent to improving and supporting the pregnant woman's performance of self-care behaviors are described. Table 12.4 describes, within the context of GDM, key facets of each behavior in the AADE 7 Self-Care Behaviors™. Because women with GDM have to learn and implement diabetes self-management in a very short period of time (and only for a short period of time), behavior change goals are important.

Healthy Eating

The American Dietetic Association's *Nutrition Practice Guidelines* for GDM state that "nutrition therapy for GDM is primarily a carbohydrate-controlled meal plan that promotes adequate nutrition with appropriate weight gain, normoglycemia, and the absence of ketonuria."[12] There is no single food plan or macronutrient combination that will achieve glucose control in the management of type 1 and type 2 diabetes.[14,15,16] Carbohydrate is the main nutrient that affects postprandial glucose levels.[17,18]

Achieving glucose control:

To achieve postmeal glucose targets, most women need to reduce mealtime carbohydrate and redistribute carbohydrate throughout the day into more meals and snacks.

Carbohydrates. The Nutrition Practice Guidelines suggest spreading carbohydrate intake into 3 small-

TABLE 12.4 AADE 7 Self-Care Behaviors™ in Gestational Diabetes

Self-Management Behaviors	*For Gestational Diabetes Mellitus*
Healthy Eating	Control total and per-meal carbohydrate; minimum of 175 g Eat 3 smaller meals and 2–4 snacks Avoid high-carbohydrate, low-nutrient foods, such as soda pop May need to reduce/restrict foods high in glycemic index Consume adequate intake of fruit, vegetables, milk, and protein
Being Active	Walk, or other physical activity, daily if no contraindications
Monitoring	Test blood glucose daily fasting and after breakfast, lunch, and dinner Test urine ketones fasting if recommended by healthcare provider Record food and beverage intake daily
Taking Medication	Use concurrent with nutrition therapy when needed: glyburide (Diabeta, Glynase, Micronase, Pres Tab) or insulin Understand risk and treatment for hypoglycemia
Problem Solving	Identify criteria for when to call with food, blood glucose, ketone, or medication questions or concerns Schedule follow-up visits with healthcare providers and diabetes educators
Healthy Coping	Acknowledge common emotional reaction to the diagnosis of GDM: fear, anger, guilt Offer support and referral if needed Guide development of a positive and cooperative response to lifestyle changes; emphasize benefits to the baby
Reducing Risks	Understand risk and treatment for hypoglycemia if on medication Describe risk of developing type 2 diabetes postpartum Encourage lifestyle changes that lead to diabetes prevention

to-moderate meals with 2 to 4 snacks.[12] This eating pattern accommodates the pregnant woman well because her stomach capacity shrinks as the pregnancy progresses. A starting food plan would suggest the following carbohydrate ranges for each meal and snack:

- *Breakfast:* 15 to 45 g
- *Lunch and Dinner:* 45 to 75 g each
- *Snacks:* 15 to 45 g

The most difficult blood glucose level to manage is the postbreakfast value, due to higher hormone levels in the morning. Consensus is to restrict carbohydrate at breakfast time to 15 to 45 g.[12] Breakfast cereals are often discouraged as the total amount of carbohydrate is higher than 45 g and postmeal blood glucose levels are higher than with other food choices. The glycemic index may help explain why some foods produce higher postmeal glucose levels. Highly processed breakfast cereals, sweet drinks, fast foods, and pizza are frequently found to raise postmeal levels higher than less-processed, higher fiber foods with the same amount of total carbohydrate. However, the total amount of carbohydrate is more significant than the type of carbohydrate, and controlling the amount of rice, pasta, potato, and other starches is the most important and initial message to the patient.[14]

Carbohydrate is a critical nutrient for fetal brain development. The 2002 Dietary Reference Intake for carbohydrate is 130 g per day for nonpregnant women and 175 g per day for pregnant women.[21] In an 1800-calorie food plan, if 40% of calories are from carbohydrate, 180 g of carbohydrate are provided, which is above the minimum amount of carbohydrate needed to produce enough glucose for the brain to function.

As women with GDM learn about controlling carbohydrate to manage GDM, they may inadvertently cut back on nutrient-rich carbohydrates such as fruit, milk, and starches. The diabetes educators and healthcare providers should review the food record and analyze the number of servings of fruit, milk or dairy, and grains to assure adequate intake. It is common to shift milk and fruit to snack time so that a more normal portion of starch can be consumed during meals.

Calories. Over the past 30 years, reducing total calorie intake has been studied for management of GDM. Severe restriction of calories has produced lower blood

Case—Part 4: Focus on the Food Plan

To help MA understand and quickly begin to use the food plan, the dietitian worked with her to create a sample 1-day intake that incorporated the changes suggested in this chapter. The dietitian assessed that MA would be capable of learning carbohydrate counting. The food plan gave a suggested starting range of carbohydrate choices based on the sample food plan they developed together. MA was instructed to record all of the food and beverage she consumed during the next week and return in 1 week. The chart below shows a typical day's intake for MA on the right and the new food plan and sample menu on the left. Also shown below is a table summarizing the dietitian's recommendations for modifying MA's food intake.

Typical Day	*Typical Day's Intake*	*New Food Plan*	*Sample Menu*
Breakfast, 9 AM	Cornflakes, whole milk, fruit, coffee	*Breakfast, 9 AM* *2 carb choices*	Slice of toast with peanut butter, 1 cup 1% milk
		Snack, 11 AM *1 carb choice*	Small piece of fruit
Lunch, 1 PM	Hamburger or sandwich, fries or chips, and 20-oz regular soda from a fast-food restaurant near work	*Lunch, 1 PM* *4 carb choices*	Sandwich, fruit, 1 carton light yogurt
		Snack, 4 PM *1–2 carb choices*	Carrots, 1/4 cup peanuts
Dinner, 8 PM	Traditional Mexican dinner of 4 tortillas made with rice, beans, chicken	*Dinner, 8 PM* *4–5 carb choices*	2 Rice-and-bean tortillas, salad, 1 cup 1% milk
		Bedtime snack, 11 PM *1–2 carb choices*	1 Tortilla with cheese, 1/2 cup juice

(continued)

Case—Part 4: Focus on the Food Plan (continued)

Summary of Dietitian's Recommendations for Modifying MA's Food Intake

Topic	*MA's Typical Intake*	*Recommendations*
Number of meals and snacks	3 meals, no snacks More than 12 hours between breakfast and dinner	Add afternoon snack Add bedtime snack to avoid so many hours without food
Intake of high-carbohydrate foods	Drinks regular soda Does not eat desserts: cookies, ice cream, pastries, candy	Discontinue regular soda May have 1–2 diet soda Good she does not have a sweet tooth
Total amount of carbohydrate at each meal and snack	Breakfast about 4 carbs Lunch about 8 carbs Dinner about 8 carbs	Reduce total carbs per meal; try 3–4 carbs per meal and test postmeal; add snacks
Estimate of calorie intake and weight-gain goal	Has gained 10 lb BMI category: overweight	Weight gain seems on track Gain 1/2 lb per week Weight gain goal 15–25 lb
Fat content of diet	Uses whole milk Prepares tortillas and beans with lard	Reduce fat content of milk to 2%, 1%, or skim Cook using monounsaturated oil; use less oil/fat
Anticipation of potential problems	Cornflakes at breakfast Fast foods	Avoid processed cereal at breakfast Avoid fast foods if postmeal reading is too high
Adequate nutrition in all food groups	Fruit: 1 serving per day Milk: on cereal only Protein: 2 servings per day Vegetables: at dinner	Increase fruit intake; add between meals or at lunch Increase milk to 3–4 servings per day; use milk instead of soda Protein intake adequate Add another serving vegetables with lunch or between meals

glucose levels, but has not provided adequate nutrients and has produced ketonemia.[19,20] Current thinking is that a modest calorie restriction, a minimum of 1800 calories, may help blood glucose control and still provide for adequate nutrients.[12] The Institute of Medicine report in 2002 provided a new formula to determine calories during pregnancy.[21] Calorie formulas are useful when problems arise. The more frequently used method to determine energy intake is to conduct a detailed assessment; develop an individualized food plan; and monitor appetite, food intake, blood glucose and ketone levels, and weight changes.

Ketone alert:

Ketonuria and ketonemia occur when a women does not eat enough calories or goes too long without eating. One study found a positive correlation between ketonemia and decreased intelligence test scores.[22] Avoiding ketone formation seems wise until further studies are done. To help the woman with GDM avoid going long hours without food, recommend eating smaller, more frequent meals and a bedtime snack.[12]

Protein. Protein intake for pregnancy is 1.1 g per kilogram per day or approximately 25 g per day above nonpregnant needs.[21] Protein does not raise blood glucose levels postprandially. Adding 1 or 2 oz of protein with breakfast or snacks is a method to add calories without affecting glucose levels.

Being Active

Physical activity has been shown to be an effective therapy to lower blood glucose levels and improve insulin resistance in people with type 2 diabetes and in GDM.[2,23] The ADA Clinical Practice Recommendation for Gestational Diabetes states, "Although the impact of exercise on neonatal complications awaits rigorous clinical trials, the beneficial glucose lowering effects warrants a recommendation that women without medical or obstetrical contraindication be encouraged to start or continue a program of moderate exercise as part of treatment."[2] The ACOG practice bulletin makes a similar recommendation.[24]

Physical activity recommendations should be individualized:

- Consider the physical activity of the woman before she became pregnant, current fitness level, and weeks of gestation.
- Low-impact activities, such as walking, swimming, or using a stationary bike, are preferred. Strenuous activities and contact sports are generally not recommended.
- Exercise may induce hypoglycemia if on insulin or oral hypoglycemic agents; therefore, monitoring blood glucose before and after exercise is recommended. To prevent hypoglycemia, the woman may need to add 15 to 30 g of carbohydrate.
- Exercising after a meal may improve postprandial glucose levels.
- Duration of exercise should not exceed 60 minutes; the woman should not exercise to exhaustion.

Monitoring

National organizations and committees agree that blood glucose monitoring is recommended for women with GDM to understand both the level of insulin resistance and insulin deficiency; however, there is no agreement regarding frequency and testing times.

A1C. The A1C test is the standard for overall glucose control in type 1and type 2; however, its role in gestational diabetes is not clear. The A1C may be used in women diagnosed with GDM in the first trimester.

Self-Monitoring. For most women, self-monitoring of blood glucose (SMBG) is the primary tool to determine if glucose control is adequate or inadequate and additional oral or insulin therapy is needed. If fasting blood glucose values are elevated, the woman will usually need to add exogenous insulin, as MNT does not impact fasting blood glucose very much. Postprandial testing guides food plan adjustments and confirms the need to add oral or insulin therapy. The results of 2 clinical research studies are highlighted below.

- *Premeal vs. Postmeal.* Postprandial testing has been shown in 1 study to provide better perinatal outcomes. DeVecianna randomized women with GDM who required insulin therapy to either premeal testing or postmeal testing.[25] Those who tested postmeal had fewer perinatal complications, smaller babies, and lower A1Cs. Total insulin doses were higher in the group testing postmeal compared to the premeal testers.
- *Conventional vs. Intensified.* In another study, 2500 women with GDM were randomized to conventional versus intensified management.[26] Conventional therapy, at the time of the study, was defined as 4 visually-read home blood glucose monitoring tests with weekly meter results from a clinic visit. Women in the intensified group received a reflectance meter and tested 7 times a day at home. Demographic characteristics and other potentially confounding variables were comparable in both treatment groups. The rate of insulin initiation was 63% versus 23% in intensified and conventional groups, respectively. The women in the conventional group had higher rates of cesarean section, shoulder dystocia, and large-for-gestational age infants. The women in the intensified group had maternal and infant outcomes similar to a matched control group. The study concluded that glycemic control clearly related to pregnancy outcomes.

Taking Medication

Not all women with GDM are able to manage with MNT and exercise therapy alone. The percentage of women who require concurrent medication is difficult to determine because the criteria for advancing therapy is inconsistent. A review of the literature regarding the approach to insulin management showed a wide range of insulin use from 7% to 66%.[27] Many recommend that if 2 or more blood glucose levels are outside the target range—within a short period of time and without dietary explanation—advancing therapy is recommended.[2,3,12]

Glyburide and Insulin. Historically, adding insulin was the only option for the woman with GDM. In 2000, the *New England Journal of Medicine* published "A comparison of glyburide and insulin in women with gestational diabetes."[28] Langer demonstrated that the oral hypoglycemic agent glyburide is a clinically effective alternative to insulin. Sulfonylurea drugs have not been used in pregnancy because of concern about teratogenicity and neonatal hypoglycemia. Glyburide was not detected in the cord serum of any infants in the glyburide group, eliminating worries that the drug would cause fetal problems. Since then, other studies have reported successful management of GDM using glyburide therapy. Glyburide (Diabeta, Glynase, Micronase, Pres Tab) is a second-generation sulfonylurea that stimulates the pancreas to produce more insulin. Starting doses are 2.5 mg once or twice a day; maximum dose is 20 mg. See also the discussion in the questions and controversy section at the end of this chapter.

Case—Part 5: Therapy Evolves as Pregnancy Progresses

Medical Nutrition Therapy

At 30 weeks' gestation, MA had her follow-up visit with the diabetes educators, 1 week after her initial visit. The diabetes educators assessed how she was progressing. Points discussed:[13]

- What her glucose levels were and how often she met her target levels
- How often she was able to follow her meal plan
- Whether she felt confident in her ability to calculate carbohydrates
- How often she found her hunger satisfied
- How happy she was with her weight gain
- What her urine ketone results had been

About half of MA's blood glucose readings were out of target. She demonstrated an ability to count carbohydrates and follow the food plan, but was frustrated because her postmeal readings were too high. She had cut back on her food intake more than she wanted to and now was very hungry. She lost 1 lb and spilled ketones the last 3 mornings.

From food records and her discussion with MA, the dietitian determined that MA understood and followed the food plan well. Her elevated postmeal blood glucose readings were not due to poor understanding or adherence to the food plan, but because she needed additional therapy beyond medical nutrition therapy. At 30 weeks' gestation, MA had lost 1 lb, was spilling ketones, and had a history of a large-for-gestational age infant. Although MA was willing to modify the diet further and add a daily walk, the diabetes educators agreed MA needed additional therapy.

Exercise Prescription

The diabetes care team provided MA guidance on implementing a safe physical activity plan that could help her manage her blood glucose level after meals. MA agreed to start with a daily walk after dinner.

Pharmacological Therapy

MA's healthcare provider recommended she try glyburide 2.5 mg (Diabeta, Glynase, Micronase, Pres Tab) at breakfast and dinner. MA was instructed to return to her initial food plan and continue to record food and blood glucose values. The diabetes educators worked with her on the following:[13]

- Explaining the purpose of the medication and how it works
- Defining hypoglycemia, its causes, and symptoms
- Explaining the rationale for eating a consistent amount of carbohydrate
- Describing how to treat hypoglycemia

Insulin Therapy

At 31 weeks' gestation, MA returned to see her healthcare provider. At 166 lb, she had gained 1 lb since diagnosis and was following the food plan well. Although postmeal blood glucose levels were lower, her fasting blood glucose values were over 100 mg/dL. Increasing the dose of glyburide (Diabeta, Glynase, Micronase, Pres Tab) was a possibility, but with 8 to 9 weeks remaining, insulin therapy was going to be needed. MA returned to the diabetes education center and learned insulin therapy. The educators worked with her on the following:[13]

- The 2 main kinds of injected insulin and how they work
- How to measure and inject insulin
- How to store insulin and dispose of sharps
- Relationship between carbohydrate and insulin
- Rationale for following the food plan and eating consistent amount of carbohydrate
- Reviewing hypoglycemia management

They calculated a starting dose of insulin using 0.5 units per kilogram as a guide. MA ate 6 times per day, so a regular/NPH insulin regimen twice a day was started. Two-thirds of the dose was given in the morning and 1/3 at dinner time. MA's starting insulin dose was calculated as follows:

166 lb/2.2 = 75 kg
75×0.5 = 38 units total units
38×0.66 = 26 units
given as 8 regular and 18 NPH
38×0.33 = 12 units
given as 6 regular and 6 NPH

Behavior Change

As with other women with gestational diabetes, MA had to learn and implement diabetes self-management in a very short period of time.

Many healthcare providers do not use glyburide therapy (Diabeta, Glynase, Micronase, Pres Tab) for women with GDM. Insulin therapy is still the preferred treatment when endogenous insulin production is inadequate. There is no one insulin regimen that has been shown to be the most effective in managing women with GDM. Human insulin is recommended for pregnancy compared to animal insulin. Insulin analogs are not approved for use in pregnancy; however, one study demonstrated improved postprandial blood glucose levels in women with GDM using NPH/lispro.[29] Regular and NPH insulin are the most commonly used insulins in pregnancy.

There is no protocol for starting insulin therapy in GDM; the ADA position statement recommends SMBG should guide the doses and timing of the insulin regimen.[2] Many women who need insulin during pregnancy will require basal insulin coverage with NPH insulin twice daily. Insulin resistance continues to increase dramatically during the third trimester, which means insulin doses need to be adjusted weekly until about 36 to 37 weeks of pregnancy. The dose of insulin at delivery is about 1.0 units per kilogram.[25]

Problem Solving

After initial instruction, follow-up visits are necessary to reinforce and review monitoring, food plan, and medications. The *Nutrition Practice Guidelines* suggest this:[11]

- 3 visits as a minimum for self-management for GDM
- A phone visit supplemented with food and blood glucose records obtained via fax or mail may be an option

Women who had GDM in a previous pregnancy may have a very thorough understanding of management goals, but most women need to be instructed on when to call their healthcare provider or diabetes educator. Coordination of care with the woman's obstetrician or endocrinologist is critical to assure that glucose control is achieved.

Healthy Coping

Pregnancy is an exciting time for most women, and those with GDM are generally motivated to follow the self-monitoring guidelines their providers and educators recommend. The desire to provide a healthy intrauterine environment is primary for most pregnant women. The fact that GDM is short-lived, usually only 10 to 12 weeks long, makes it more tolerable to do the many tasks that are required.

Despite the short duration of GDM, making lifestyle changes during pregnancy can be stressful and emotional. A number of issues related to diabetes self-management occur quite often, and the diabetes educator should look for and address these. Some common feelings and issues are listed below:

- *Guilt:* Many women feel guilty or embarrassed because they are overweight and know their food habits are not what they could be
- *Anger:* Some women may be angry they have to change their lifestyle through diet, monitoring, and giving injections
- *Fear:* Many women are fearful of insulin injections and may withhold or manipulate data about elevated blood glucose levels and food intake

See chapters 3, 4, and 5 for more information on addressing barriers to self-management. If a woman is not able to cope, referral to a psychologist or social worker who understands diabetes is recommended.

Reducing Risks

An important part of self-management education is teaching the woman using insulin or glyburide therapy (Diabeta, Glynase, Micronase, Pres Tab) how to recognize and treat hypoglycemic episodes. As the pregnancy progresses, the educator can assist the woman who has applicable risk factors in preparing for and understanding the various fetal monitoring procedures that may be appropriate in her situation. Another important task is helping the woman understand

Case—Part 6: Achieving Glucose Control

At 33 weeks

MA returned to her healthcare provider with food, blood glucose, and ketone records. Weight was 167, up 1 lb. She was comfortable with her food plan, and most blood glucose values were in target range. Knowing that insulin resistance would continue to increase, her insulin doses were increased slightly. She learned pattern control and how to increase each type of insulin dose by 1 or 2 units. She was instructed to call in her blood glucose values each week so insulin doses could be adjusted.

At 36 weeks

MA had her final visit for GDM management. She had done well and was happy with her blood glucose values. She had made many changes in her eating and activity habits that she planned to continue after delivery. She saw GDM as an opportunity to make changes that improved the health of her whole family. Now she was looking forward to delivery. During this visit, the guidelines for labor and delivery were discussed, including that when MA went into labor, she should stop taking insulin and discontinue eating.

that she is at increased risk for developing type 2 diabetes after the pregnancy and recognize factors that increase her risk and steps she can take that may help prevent it.

Hypoglycemia. The ADA and ACOG have not identified the lower limit of blood glucose in pregnancy; studies have shown that normal blood glucose levels are about 10 mg/dL lower in pregnant women.[8]

Hypoglycemia: the most common complication

The most common complication in GDM is hypoglycemia when a woman is on insulin or glyburide therapy (Diabeta, Glynase, Micronase, Pres Tab). Teaching the woman with GDM how to treat hypoglycemia is essential and the same as for someone who is not pregnant:

- Eat 15 g of carbohydrate
- After 15 minutes, test blood glucose to confirm level is back in normal range

Otherwise, long-term complications of diabetes are not an issue with GDM as it lasts only a few months or weeks.

Fetal Monitoring. Does GDM require additional fetal monitoring? Although pregnant women with type 1 diabetes undergo additional fetal testing near delivery, because of a lack of well-designed studies that question has not been answered for GDM.[2,3,5,9] In GDM, women with additional risk factors, such as hypertension, are often referred for additional testing, such as an ultrasound, non-stress tests, stress tests, and a biophysical profile. The educator can help the pregnant woman understand the need for and value of any increased fetal monitoring the healthcare provider may order.

Developing Type 2 Diabetes. Women who have had GDM are at higher risk for developing type 2 diabetes.[2,3,5,8] A systematic review of factors associated with the development of type 2 diabetes after GDM found that the cumulative incidence of diabetes varied widely, ranging from 2.6% to over 70% in studies that examined women 6 weeks to 28 years postpartum.[30] The incidence increased rapidly in the first 5 years postpartum and then appeared to plateau after 10 years. The most common predictor of future diabetes was an elevated fasting glucose level during the pregnancy. Other factors that impact the development of diabetes include ethnicity, postpartum BMI, and history of previous GDM. Noting a few studies, the rate of development of GDM at 5 years was 8% to 10% in whites, 30% in Zunis, 37% in a mixed population, and 62% in a mixed group of East Indians and blacks.[30] Factors that do not seem to impact the development of diabetes include weight gain during pregnancy, maternal age of GDM, and family history of diabetes.

Factors that increase the risk of developing GDM in a subsequent pregnancy, listed below, are appropriate to discuss during postpartum education:

- Amount of weight gained between pregnancies
- Hip-to-waist ratio
- Diet composition

Strategies for preventing type 2 diabetes are also appropriate to discuss. See chapter 1, on prevention, for topics. Also, lifestyle changes begun as a result of GDM can lead to a reduction in obesity, cardiovascular disease, and cancer. Changes can be reinforced and further promoted in postpartum education.

Case Wrap-Up

At 39 1/2 weeks, MA delivered an 8 lb 2 oz baby boy. Baby M's blood glucose was tested at 1 hour, and it was 70 mg/dL. He started breastfeeding and could stay with mom in her room. During her hospital stay, MA's blood glucose level was tested fasting the day after delivery. It was elevated, but she had not had insulin for 24 hours. When she left the hospital, she was instructed to continue to test her blood glucose levels once a week—fasting and 2 hours after eating—and to return in 6 weeks for an evaluation of glucose control.

At her 6-week postpartum visit, all blood glucose values were within the normal (nonpregnant) range: fasting <100 and 2 hour <140 mg/dL. To confirm that she did not have diabetes, her healthcare provider ordered a fasting glucose test. MA's was normal at less than 100 mg/dL. She continued with her food plan, walked every evening with her husband, and remained pleased to have lost 6 lb; she was feeling great. Her healthcare provider discussed her risk for getting type 2 diabetes and supported the excellent changes she had already made to her lifestyle. MA was instructed to return annually for a blood glucose test.

MA was told that if she becomes pregnant again, her risk for developing GDM again is 30% to 65%.[8] She was also made aware of factors that increase her risk: the amount of weight gained between pregnancies, hip-to-waist ratio, and diet composition.

Questions and Controversies

Randomized trials are, and always will be, difficult to do in pregnancy; thus, many research questions will never be answered definitively. At the Fifth International Workshop-Conference on GDM in November 2005, many controversial issues were discussed and debated.

Oral Agents. The most controversial issue at the conference was the use of oral hypoglycemic agents for glucose management in pregnancy. Langer's study has shown that glyburide does not cross the placenta and compared to insulin, maternal and infant outcomes were comparable.[26] Even though other trials have shown glyburide (Diabeta, Glynase, Micronase, Pres Tab) to be effective and safe, there is still hesitation to use it in pregnancy. Metformin (Glucophage) has not been indicated for use in the management of GDM, but it has successfully and safely been used in the first trimester for women with polycystic ovarian syndrome. It does cross the placenta and currently is being studied in gestational diabetes because it improves insulin resistance.

Insulin Analogs. Insulin analogs are not approved for use in pregnancy. Jovanovic-Peterson's study showed improved glucose control using insulin lispro in gestational diabetes and no adverse maternal or fetal outcomes.[29] Insulin analogs, both rapid-acting and long-acting, are becoming standard therapy for people with type 1 and type 2 diabetes because they have a more physiologic action compared to regular and NPH insulin. The major concern with insulin analogs is the unknown. More research is needed in this area.

HAPO Study. The results of the Hyperglycemia and Adverse Pregnancy Outcome (HAPO) study, due in 2007, are eagerly anticipated.[10] This multinational study will evaluate the outcomes of 25,000 women with GDM. The study hopes to identify the relationship between glucose and maternal and infant morbidities. The goal is for glucose levels for diagnosis and treatment to become universal around the world.

Focus on Education: Pearls for Practice

Teaching Strategies

- **Enable timely initial visits.** See new patients as soon as possible, within 1 week of referral
- **Involve team in glucose goals.** Achieve target glucose control as quickly as possible, within the context of a healthy pregnancy; get to know team members in obstetrics-gynecology, endocrinology, and family medicine and involve them in agreeing on targets, curriculum handouts, and content
- **Take action and offer support.** Women with GDM need more support than the person with type 1 or type 2 as there is so much to learn and implement in just a few weeks
- **Offer hope for a healthy future.** Present the information that implementing lifestyle changes now may lead to diabetes prevention as well as reduce their chances of becoming obese or developing cardiovascular disease or cancer
- **Model the lifestyle.** Consider how you and your team can best model positive approaches to lifestyle changes intended to lead to diabetes prevention and a reduction in obesity, cardiovascular disease, and cancer

Messages for Patients With GDM

- **Use your diabetes team.** Educators, clinicians, and specialty services are available to help you in any way to understand and manage GDM

- **Manage GDM.** Good control balances glucose control with the goals of a healthy pregnancy
- **Insulin is good medicine.** Do not be afraid of adding insulin as it is a hormone your body makes, not a drug; during the pregnancy, you may need extra insulin, via injection, to keep blood sugar under control
- **Guard your own health after delivery.** Knowing you had GDM is a clear signal you are at risk for developing diabetes; take steps to prevent diabetes by improving your eating and exercise habits and maintaining an appropriate weight after your baby is born; these healthy habits will not only help you, they will help your whole family

References

1. Gabbe S. The gestational diabetes mellitus conferences. Diabetes Care. 1998;21 Suppl 2:B1-2.
2. American Diabetes Association. Gestational diabetes mellitus (position statement). Diabetes Care. 2004;27 Suppl 1:S88-90.
3. American College of Obstetrics and Gynecology Committee on Practice Bulletins–Obstetrics. ACOG Practice Bulletin: clinical management guidelines for obstetricians-gynecologists. Number 30, September 2001. Gestational Diabetes. Obstet Gynecol. 2001;98:525-38.
4. King H. Epidemiology of glucose intolerance and gestational diabetes in women of childbearing age. Diabetes Care. 1998;21 Suppl 2:B9-13.
5. Metzger BE, Coustan DR, eds. Proceedings of the Fourth International Workshop-Conference on Gestational Diabetes Mellitus. Diabetes Care. 1998;21 Suppl 2:B1-167.
6. Sermer M, Naylor CD, Farine D, et al. The Toronto tri-hospital gestational diabetes project. Diabetes Care. 1998;21 Suppl 2:B33-42.
7. Sepe SJ. Gestational diabetes: incidence, maternal characteristics and perinatal outcome. Diabetes. 1985; 34 Suppl 2:13-6.
8. Thomas A, Gutierrez YM. American Dietetic Association Guide to Gestational Diabetes Mellitus. Chicago, Ill: American Dietetic Association; 2005.
9. Reece A, Coustan D. Diabetes Mellitus in Pregnancy. New York: Churchill Livingstone; 1995:79-92.
10. Metzger, B. The Hyperglycemia and Adverse Pregnancy Outcome (HAPO) Study: The end is in sight (abstract). Presented at 5th International Workshop-conference on Gestational Diabetes. 12 Nov 2005.
11. Crowther CA, Hiller JE, Moss JR, et al. Effect of treatment of gestational diabetes mellitus on pregnancy outcomes. N Engl J Med. 2005;352:2477-86.
12. Medical Nutrition Therapy Evidence-Based Guides for Practice: Nutrition Practice Guidelines for Gestational Diabetes Mellitus [CD-ROM]. Chicago, Ill: American Dietetic Association; 2001.
13. Reader D, Davidson J, Larson S. Gestational Diabetes BASICS Curriculum Guide. Minneapolis, Minn: International Diabetes Center, Park Nicollet Institute; 2005.
14. Franz MJ, Bantle JP, Beebe CA, et al. Evidence-based nutrition principles and recommendations for the treatment and prevention of diabetes and related complications (technical review). Diabetes Care. 2004;25:148-98.
15. Franz MJ, Monk A, Barry B, et al. Effectiveness of medical nutrition therapy provided by dietitians in the management of non-insulin-dependent diabetes mellitus: a randomized, controlled clinical trial. J Am Diet Assoc. 1995;95:1009-17.
16. Kulkarni K, Castle G, Gregory R, et al, for the Diabetes Care and Education Dietetic Practice Group. Nutrition practice guidelines for type 1 diabetes mellitus positively affect dietitian practices and patient outcomes. J Am Diet Assoc. 1998;98:62-70.
17. Major CA, Henry MJ, de Vecianna M, Morgan MA. The effects of carbohydrate restriction in patients with diet controlled gestational diabetes. Obstet Gynecol. 1998;7:456-70.
18. Peterson CM, Jovanovic-Peterson L. Percentages of carbohydrate and glycemic response to breakfast, lunch and dinner in women with gestational diabetes. Diabetes. 1990;39:234-40.
19. Magee MS, Knopp RH, Benedetti TJ. Metabolic effects of 1200 kcal diet in obese pregnant women with gestational diabetes. Diabetes. 1990;39:234-40.

20. Dornhorst A, Nicholls JS, Probst F, et al. Calorie restriction for treatment of gestational diabetes. Diabetes. 1991;40 Suppl 2:161-4.

21. Institute of Medicine. Dietary Reference Intakes for Energy, Carbohydrate, Fiber, Fat, Fatty Acids, Cholesterol, Protein, and Amino Acids (Macronutrients). Washington, DC: National Academy Press; 2002.

22. Rizzo T, Metzger BE, Burns WJ, Bursn K. Correlations between antepartum maternal metabolism and child intelligence. N Engl J Med. 1991;325:911-6.

23. American Diabetes Association. Standards of medical care in diabetes (position statement). Diabetes Care. 2004;27 Suppl 1:S15-35.

24. American College of Obstetrics and Gynecology Committee Obstetrics Practice. ACOG Committee Opinion. Number 267, January 2002: exercise during pregnancy and the postpartum period. Obstet Gyncol. 2002;99:171-3.

25. DeVencianna M, Major CA, Morgan MA, et al. Postprandial versus preprandial blood glucose monitoring in women with gestational diabetes mellitus requiring insulin therapy. N Engl J Med. 1995;333:1237-41.

26. Langer O, Rodriques D, Xenankis EMJ, McFarland MB, Berkus MD, Arredondo F. Intensified versus conventional management of gestational diabetes. Am J Obstet Gynecol 1994;170:1036-47.

27. Langer O. Maternal glycemic criteria for insulin therapy in gestational diabetes mellitus. Diabetes Care. 1998;21 Suppl 2:B91-8.

28. Langer O, Conway D, Berkus M, et al. A comparison of glyburide and insulin in women with gestational diabetes mellitus. N Engl J Med. 2000;343:1134-8.

29. Jovanovic-Peterson L, Ilic S, Pettitt D, et al. The metabolic and immunology effects of insulin lispro. Diabetes Care. 1999;22:1422-7.

30. Kim C, Newton KM, Knopp RH. Gestational diabetes and the incidence of type 2 diabetes. Diabetes Care. 2002;25:1862-8.

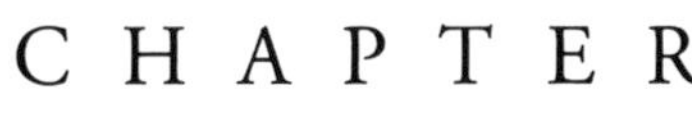

CHAPTER

13

Medical Nutrition Therapy

Authors

Janine Freeman, RD, LD, CDE
Marion J. Franz, MS, RD, LD, CDE

Key Concepts

- Medical nutrition therapy for persons with diabetes should be individualized, based on the person's metabolic needs, preferences, and willingness to make lifestyle changes.
- Weight loss through a reduction in food intake and an increase in physical activity is an important strategy in overweight or obese persons with insulin resistance or at risk for type 2 diabetes.
- Monitoring the amount of carbohydrate is a key strategy in achieving glycemic control in persons with type 1 and type 2 diabetes.
- Optimal nutrition through healthy eating remains an important goal for all persons with diabetes and should not be compromised to improve glycemia, lipids, or blood pressure control.
- Lifestyle modification to reduce intake of saturated fat, trans fat, and dietary cholesterol; increase physical activity; and promote weight loss (if needed) can improve lipids and reduce cardiovascular disease risk.
- Physical activity should be encouraged in all persons with diabetes to improve glycemic control, assist with maintenance of weight, and reduce the risk of cardiovascular disease.

Introduction

Nutrition therapy has been employed in the treatment of diabetes since diabetes was first discovered to be the "sweet urine" disease centuries ago. Nutrition recommendations have changed through the years based on the opinions of the era. Today, nutrition guidelines are based on available scientific evidence, which has dispelled many of the nutrition myths and misinformation of earlier times. Nutrition, like medicine, remains an ever-changing field as researchers and scientists learn more about the human body and how various components and combinations of foods and nutrients affect disease risk and management. The American Diabetes Association (ADA) now annually updates evidence-based nutrition recommendations to provide healthcare providers and persons with diabetes with the latest information on beneficial nutrition therapies and outcomes.[1]

Once thought of as a complex set of rigid calculations, today medical nutrition therapy (MNT) focuses on the individual needs and preferences of the person with diabetes. This focus sets the stage for the adoption of small, incremental lifestyle changes that include food/nutrition and physical activity to improve overall health and to reduce the risk of diabetes complications. MNT for diabetes should be delivered by registered dietitians (RDs) using the Nutrition Care Process, which includes nutrition assessment, nutrition diagnosis, nutrition intervention, and nutrition monitoring and evaluation.[2]

Evidence from clinical trials and observational studies supports the effectiveness of MNT in the primary, secondary, and tertiary prevention of diabetes (ie, preventing or delaying the development of diabetes and preventing and controlling the complications of diabetes).[3,4,5]

This chapter discusses the role of MNT in diabetes management and prevention; describes the role of MNT in glycemic control, weight control, and prevention and treatment of cardiovascular disease, including hypertension, dyslipidemia, and nephropathy; and discusses intervention strategies to achieve nutrition-related goals for youth and adults with diabetes.

Goals of Diabetes Medical Nutrition Therapy

Persons with diabetes and those at risk for diabetes should receive individualized MNT as needed to achieve treatment goals, preferably provided by a registered dietitian familiar with the components of diabetes MNT.[6] The person with diabetes should be involved in the decision-making process.

Goal of MNT for persons at risk for diabetes:[6]

- Reduce the risk for type 2 diabetes and cardiovascular disease by encouraging regular physical activity and weight loss for overweight or obese individuals.

Goals of MNT for all persons with diabetes:[6]

- Prevent and treat the chronic complications of diabetes by attaining and maintaining optimal metabolic outcomes, including blood glucose and A1C level, low-density lipoprotein cholesterol (LDL-C) and high-density lipoprotein cholesterol (HDL-C) and triglycerides levels, blood pressure, and body weight.
- Improve health through healthy food choices and physical activity.
- Address individual nutritional needs, taking into consideration personal and cultural preferences and lifestyle while respecting the individual's wishes and willingness to change.
- For individuals treated with insulin and/or insulin secretagogues, provide self-management education for treatment (and prevention) of hypoglycemia, acute illnesses, and exercise-related blood glucose problems.

A Healthy Eating Plan

With the emphasis on glycemic control and the immediate feedback provided through self-monitoring of blood glucose, healthcare providers and individuals with diabetes may tend to focus on normalizing glycemia with little regard to nutritional needs. Optimal nutrition through

Case in Point: Type 2 Diabetes Treated With Oral Agents

LW, an obese, 51-year-old African American female with type 2 diabetes of 5 years' duration, hypertension, and dyslipidemia was referred for diabetes education.

Clinical Data

Height: 64 in
Weight: 175 lb
Body mass index (BMI): 31 kg/m^2
A1C: 8.1%
HDL-C: 43 mg/dL
LDL-C: 160 mg/dL
TG: 234 mg/dL
BP: 148/88 mm Hg

Medications

Glimepiride (Amaryl) 4 mg daily
Metformin (Glucophage) 1000 mg bid
Simvastatin (Zocor) 20 mg daily, for dyslipidemia
Quinapril (Accupril) 20 mg daily, for hypertension

Nutrition Assessment

Assessment of LW's metabolic status revealed that she exhibited characteristics common in type 2 diabetes and metabolic syndrome. Markers of her increased cardiovascular risk were a pattern of dyslipidemia that included elevated LDL-C, low HDL-C, and hypertriglyceridemia along with hypertension and obesity (BMI $\geq$30 kg/m^2).

LW stated that she either skips breakfast or eats a light breakfast in her car, with lunch primarily at fast-food restaurants, and eats dinners out about 50% of the time. She occasionally snacked on chips or pork rinds in the afternoon and usually ate a bowl of sugar-free ice cream in the evening. She did not drink alcoholic beverages. A brief evaluation of LW's usual diet history revealed that her diet was high in total fat and saturated fat and appeared low in fiber and calcium with few fruits and vegetables. LW asked if a low-carbohydrate, high-protein diet would help her lose weight and improve her glucose control.

Physical Activity

LW's job was sedentary. She said she did not have the time or energy to go to the gym after work.

As the chapter progresses, readers gain insight into the following regarding LW's case: What initial lifestyle changes could be suggested to improve her glycemic control? What aspects of MNT could reduce her cardiovascular risk? What are the risks and benefits of using a low-carbohydrate diet to achieve her goals?

healthy food choices remains the underlying principle of the ADA nutrition recommendations.[1]

A healthy diet consists of the following:

- Multiple servings of fruits and vegetables, whole grains, low-fat dairy foods, fish, lean meats, poultry, and healthy fats

These recommendations are similar to evidence-based nutrition recommendations from the American Heart Association.[7]

For individuals with diabetes, macronutrient distribution should be individualized based on a nutrition assessment including clinical data, food preferences, and metabolic goals. There is no optimal percentage of carbohydrate, protein, and fat for everyone with diabetes. The Dietary Reference Intakes (DRIs) from the Food and Nutrition Board of the Institute of Medicine recommend that adults, in general, should consume 45% to 65% of calories from carbohydrate, 10% to 35% from protein, and 20% to 35% from fat.[8] Individuals with comorbidities such as metabolic syndrome, dyslipidemia/cardiovascular disease, or nephropathy may need more specific recommendations.

Vitamin and Mineral Supplementation

MNT should include education on how to acquire adequate amounts of vitamins and minerals from food sources. There is no clear evidence of benefit from vitamin and mineral supplementation in individuals with diabetes who do not have deficiencies.[1] Exceptions include folate for the prevention of birth defects.[1] Supplementation above the tolerable upper intake level (UL) established by the Institute of Medicine increases the risk of adverse effects and should be considered only after review of safety and efficacy determined by controlled clinical trials.[9] Routine supplementation of antioxidants such as vitamins C and E and β-carotene is not advised due to possible adverse effects and the lack of efficacy shown in large placebo-controlled clinical trials.[6,10]

There may be a need for vitamin and mineral supplementation in individuals on calorie-restricted diets, pregnant and lactating women, elderly individuals, and strict vegetarians.[1]

Chromium supplementation has been studied for its potential influence on glycemia, insulin resistance, and body weight. Current studies have not conclusively demonstrated efficacy; therefore, chromium supplementation is not recommended.[6] For information on the use of herbal preparations, see chapter 19, on biological complementary therapies in diabetes.

> With changes in lifestyle, the effect on blood glucose levels is evident almost immediately.

MNT and Glycemic Control

A primary goal in the management of diabetes is the regulation of blood glucose to achieve near-normal blood glucose levels. With changes in lifestyle, the effect on blood glucose levels is evident almost immediately. Food adjustments that limit postprandial hyperglycemia can also improve overall glycemic control and help prevent complications of diabetes.[6]

Clinical trials and outcome studies have shown that MNT can reduce A1C levels[3,4,11,12]

- A1C levels can be reduced by approximately 1% to 2% in type 2 diabetes, depending on the duration of the disease.
- A1C levels can be reduced by 1% in type 1 diabetes by adjusting insulin to planned carbohydrate intake.

Evaluation of the effectiveness of MNT on glucose should be done between 6 weeks and 3 months.[1] At that point, one can determine if the individual can achieve target goals by implementation of lifestyle strategies or if medication(s) will need to be combined with lifestyle.

Blood glucose levels following a meal are determined by the balance between nutrient intake and available insulin. Carbohydrate is the component in food that has the most effect on postprandial blood glucose. Fat slows glucose absorption, delaying the peak glycemic response, and protein does not increase plasma glucose concentrations.[13]

Dietary Carbohydrate and Glycemia

Both the amount and type of carbohydrate in a food influence blood glucose levels. For many years, sugar was assumed to be absorbed rapidly and have a much greater impact on blood glucose levels than starches. Numerous studies have since shown that some starches have more effect on blood glucose than some types of sugars and that the total amount of carbohydrate is more predictive of the glycemic response than the structure of the carbohydrate.[14] Over 20 studies have shown that when the total carbohydrate content of meals is kept the same the glucose responses are identical.[14] In a study in Great Britain, RDs taught individuals with type 1 diabetes how to adjust mealtime insulin for their planned carbohydrate intake. Without a change in total insulin, A1C levels were lowered by 1% and subjects reported a significant improvement in their quality of life despite taking more insulin injections and monitoring their blood glucose more frequently.[12] From this data, the ADA concluded that monitoring total grams of carbohydrate, whether by carbohydrate counting or using the exchange system, is a key strategy in achieving glycemic control.[13]

Spacing carbohydrate throughout the day and consistency in the amount of carbohydrate consumed at breakfast, lunch, dinner, and snacks from day to day can also improve postprandial glycemia, particularly in persons who do not adjust mealtime insulin or short-acting insulin secretagogues based on carbohydrate consumed.

A number of factors have been shown to affect the blood glucose response of carbohydrate-containing foods:

- Amount of carbohydrate
- Type of sugar or starch
- Degree of processing (grinding, rolling, pressing)
- Food preparation
- Physical form of the food (ie, juice or whole fruit, mashed or whole potato)
- Ripeness of fruit
- Specific type or variety of the food (ie, long grain or basmati rice)
- Other food components (fat, protein, fructose, fiber)

In addition, the blood glucose response to a carbohydrate-containing meal can vary based on the blood glucose level prior to the meal and the degree of insulin resistance.

Sugars. Sugars include glucose, fructose, sucrose (table sugar), and lactose (milk sugar). Glucose causes the highest glycemic peak response compared to other sugars. Fructose, sucrose, and lactose all have less effect on blood glucose peak levels than glucose and starches. This is because fructose and galactose (a component of lactose) are metabolized by the liver to glycogen and/or triglycerides (in the case of fructose) and very little is converted to glucose.[15]

Starches. The ability of digestive enzymes to break down the starch, rather than the size of the starch molecule, determines the glycemic effect of a particular starch. This depends on the structure of the starch, the type of processing and cooking, and how the starch is packaged.[16] Starches composed of higher proportions of amylopectin, such as potatoes, have more effect on blood glucose levels than starchy foods that contain more amylose, such as certain types of rice.

Achieving Glycemic Control

Monitoring total grams of carbohydrate is a key strategy. Spacing carbohydrates more evenly throughout the day also helps improve postprandial glucose.

Glycemic Index. The glycemic index (GI) is a system of ranking carbohydrate foods according to their effect on postprandial glycemia.[13] The glycemic effect of 50-g of digestible carbohydrate from a single food is measured over a 2-hour period. The food is then assigned a value compared to the response of a reference food (glucose or bread). The glycemic load of foods or meals takes into account both the quantity of food consumed and the GI value of the food. The glycemic load is determined by multiplying the GI by the amount of carbohydrate in each serving of food and then totaling the values for all foods in a meal.

The GI was first developed in 1981 and has been an area of controversy since that time. The relative importance of the type of carbohydrate on postprandial blood glucose and the variability of the GI of foods are 2 issues of debate. Although the diet books claim the GI measures how rapidly blood glucose and insulin levels increase after eating carbohydrate foods, the GI actually measures the relative area under the postprandial glucose curve of 50 g of digestible carbohydrate compared with 50 g of a standard food. A statement by the ADA on dietary carbohydrate states that both the amount and type of carbohydrate influence blood glucose and that monitoring total grams of carbohydrate remains a key strategy in achieving glycemic control.[13] A recent analysis of the randomized, controlled trials that have examined the efficacy of the GI on overall blood glucose control indicated that use of the GI can provide an additional benefit over that observed when total carbohydrate is considered alone[13] and can, therefore, be used as an adjunct to carbohydrate counting.

Persons with diabetes are encouraged to determine their individual glycemic response to various carbohydrate foods and carbohydrate-containing meals by monitoring preprandial and postprandial blood glucose levels. Staying within a target amount of carbohydrate for meals and choosing less-processed foods and foods that are naturally high in fiber (ie, whole grains, fruits, vegetables, low-fat dairy foods, legumes, nuts and seeds) can help lower the glycemic response of meals.

Fiber. The average amount of fiber a person in the United States consumes (10 to 20 g per day) does not appear to affect glycemia. Studies that have shown improved glycemia included diets containing ~50g of fiber per day, an amount that may be difficult for many

Americans to consume due to the palatability and gastrointestinal side effects.[1] Foods that are good sources of fiber are encouraged because they provide vitamins, minerals, fiber, and other nutrients important for good health.

Sweeteners. Sucrose can be used by persons with diabetes without aggravating hyperglycemia if the total carbohydrate is taken into account. Clinical studies demonstrate that isocaloric amounts of starch and sugar result in similar increases in glycemia.[1] Since many sucrose-containing foods are low in nutritional value and high in fat and calories, their use should be limited.

Food products that contain sugar alcohols impact glycemia. Studies have shown that most sugar alcohols, including erythritol, hydrogenated starch hydrolysates, isomalt, lactitol, maltitol, mannitol, sorbitol, and xylitol, produce a smaller rise in blood glucose, although there is no evidence that use of sugar alcohols improves long-term glycemia.[1] Sugar alcohols contain, on average, about half the calories of sucrose or glucose.[1] Persons counting carbohydrates can subtract one-half of sugar alcohol grams from total carbohydrate when using foods containing sugar alcohols.[17]

The addition of nonnutritive sweeteners to foods and beverages does not contribute to hyperglycemia. The carbohydrate content of other ingredients in prepared or packaged foods needs to be considered in evaluating the effect on glycemia. The Food and Drug Administration (FDA) has approved the use of acesulfame potassium, aspartame, neotame, saccharin, and sucralose for use in the United States. The FDA also determines an Acceptable Daily Intake (ADI) for each nonnutritive sweetener. The ADI is the amount that can be safely consumed on a daily basis over a person's lifetime without adverse effects and includes a 100-fold safety factor.

Low-Carbohydrate Diets. Because of the glycemic effect of carbohydrate, it may seem reasonable to restrict carbohydrate in persons with diabetes. However, many foods containing carbohydrate provide nutrients that are important in reducing the risk of chronic diseases, and severely restricting these foods would likely compromise health. In addition, the Institute of Medicine recommends not restricting carbohydrate to less than 130 g per day for adults and children due to the absolute need for glucose as an energy source in the brain and central nervous system.[8] Therefore, the ADA does not recommend low- carbohydrate diets for individuals with diabetes. [6]

Dietary Protein and Glycemia

Although 50% to 60% of ingested protein theoretically converts to glucose, studies have demonstrated that blood glucose concentrations do not increase following ingestion of protein.[1] Ingestion of protein results in stimulation of insulin secretion similar to that of carbohydrate.[13]

Several small, short-term studies in subjects with diabetes suggest that diets with protein content greater than 20% of calories may improve glucose and insulin concentrations, reduce appetite, and improve satiety.[18,19] Current recommendations caution that protein intakes in this range may be a risk factor for the development of diabetic nephropathy.[6] Furthermore, long-term adherence to high-protein diets appears difficult to achieve.[20]

Dietary Fat and Glycemia

Dietary fat alters the predicted postprandial response to a carbohydrate-containing meal. Dietary fat slows glucose absorption, delaying the peak glycemic response to the ingestion of a food than contains glucose.[13] Insulin adjustments that prolong the mealtime insulin coverage can minimize postprandial hyperglycemia following a high-fat meal (ie, splitting the bolus and taking half before the meal and half after the meal, or delivering a bolus over an extended time period in insulin pump users). (Chapter 17, on pump therapy, discusses this more.) Some studies suggest that reduced intake of fat, particularly saturated fat, may improve insulin resistance independent of energy restriction.[21]

Physical Activity and Glycemia

Physical activity can lead to improved glycemia in individuals with diabetes. In individuals at risk for diabetes and those with type 2 diabetes, physical activity/exercise increases insulin sensitivity, increases utilization of glucose, and reduces liver glucose production.[22] Studies have demonstrated that the combination of regular physical activity and weight loss in overweight persons at risk for diabetes significantly reduces the risk of developing diabetes.[23,24] Both exercise and energy restriction independently and additively reduce glucose and insulin levels in overweight and sedentary persons.[25,26] Physical activity and meal planning should be considered complementary therapies that together promote optimal glycemic control and reduced risk for chronic diseases.[22]

In type 1 diabetes, self-adjustment of insulin is required to accommodate exercise, although regular physical activity should be recommended for the overall health benefits. See chapters 14 and 30 on physical activity and the self-care behaviors related to being active.

When to Expect Results

Within 6 weeks to 3 months, both the impact of lifestyle changes on blood lipids and the effectiveness of MNT on glucose can be evaluated and observed.

Alcohol and Glycemia

Moderate amounts of alcohol (less than 1 drink per day for adult women and less than 2 drinks per day for adult men) when ingested with food have minimal, if any, effect on glucose and insulin concentrations.[6] Individuals using insulin or insulin secretagogues should consume food with alcohol to avoid hypoglycemia. Blood glucose testing should be used to determine if extra carbohydrate and/or a reduction in insulin is needed to reduce the risk of hypoglycemia during the night or the next morning following consumption of alcohol the previous evening.[27] People with a history of alcohol abuse or dependence, women during pregnancy, and people with medical problems such as liver disease, pancreatitis, advanced neuropathy, or severe hypertriglyceridemia should abstain from alcohol.

MNT and Weight Control

A major challenge to diabetes care providers is the high incidence of overweight and obesity. Weight loss is an important goal for overweight or obese persons with or at risk for type 2 diabetes because it prevents or delays onset of diabetes and reduces other risk factors for cardiovascular disease. Providers need to be alert to any weight increases and intervene to assist their patients in weight management. A moderate weight loss of 5% to 10% can reduce risk and improve glycemia, particularly in individuals who are primarily insulin resistant, including those with prediabetes and early-onset type 2 diabetes.[28,29] As individuals become more insulin deficient, weight loss may fail to significantly improve glycemia.[30,31]

Moderate weight loss also reduces the risk of cardiovascular disease by reducing blood pressure, improving lipids (increasing HDL-C and lowering total cholesterol, LDL-C, and triglycerides) and reducing markers of inflammation.[32] A sustained weight loss of ≥5% is needed to maintain a decrease in triglycerides, whereas total cholesterol and LDL-C revert toward baseline if ≥10% diet-induced weight loss is not maintained.[32]

Energy restriction, with or without weight loss, can decrease insulin resistance.[33] Weight loss strategies that use a behavioral approach, combining a reduction in energy intake with an increase in physical activity, are most effective.[34] Reducing calories by approximately 500 to 1000 per day is recommended to achieve a weight loss of about 1 to 2 lb per week.[6] However, weight loss begins to plateau at approximately 6 months after a weight loss intervention is begun. At that point, maintenance of the weight lost should become the focus of the intervention.[35]

Most of the evidence supports the fact that weight loss is primarily associated with energy deficit and diet adherence, but not with nutrient composition.[36,37] Data from intervention trials indicate that a low-fat diet (25% to 30% of calories) is effective to promote weight loss.[38] Currently

Low-Carb Diets

Low-carbohydrate diets are not generally recommended for persons with diabetes—safety and efficacy for weight loss are unproven, and nutrients from carbohydrates help reduce the risk of chronic diseases.

Case—Part 2: Improving Glycemic Control

One of LW's initial short-term goals was improving glycemic control. In evaluating her usual diet, it appeared she could make a few small changes that might make a significant difference in her blood glucose control. LW appeared to be consuming the bulk of her calories and carbohydrate later in the day, often skipping breakfast, eating a light lunch, and a heavier dinner. Studies show that eating fairly consistent amounts of carbohydrate spaced throughout the day can improve glycemia. Despite selecting "sugar-free" ice cream, LW could have been ingesting a significant amount of carbohydrate and calories after dinner, depending on the serving size.

LW could begin with a basic carbohydrate-counting meal planning approach with carbohydrate spaced throughout the day. Monitoring her blood glucose levels 2 hours after meals would reinforce the effect of varying amounts of carbohydrates on blood glucose levels. (Chapter 29, on healthy eating, provides a basic explanation of carbohydrate counting; chapter 17, on pump therapy, also discusses this topic.)

LW was encouraged to begin some type of physical activity, such as a brisk walking, to further improve her glycemic control. She was instructed to begin slowly and work toward a goal of 30 to 45 minutes, 5 times per week. A pedometer was recommended as a motivational tool to encourage more steps in a day. Her glycemic control would be evaluated initially with blood glucose records, after she had implemented her lifestyle changes, to assess whether she needed to change her diabetes medication.

available evidence does not support the long-term efficacy and safety of low-carbohydrate, high-protein/high-fat diets for weight control in individuals with diabetes.[28] The results of randomized, controlled trials showed greater short-term (6 months), but not long-term (12 months) weight loss.[39,40,41]

A single type of weight loss approach that works for everyone has not been identified. Dietary advice for reducing energy intake should be individualized to account for food preferences and the individual's preferred approach for reducing energy intake.[28] A variety of behavioral strategies can be employed that have shown to be successful.[28] (See also chapter 14, on physical activity.)

Challenges With Pharmacologic Therapy

Diabetes pharmacotherapy often presents an additional challenge to the diabetes care team—in that weight gain often accompanies diabetes pharmacologic therapy, hampering the individual's efforts at weight loss.

- Diabetes medications that can increase weight include sulfonylureas, thiazolidinediones, and insulin.
- Biguanides, alpha-glucosidase inhibitors, exenatide, and pramlintide can result in weight loss.[42,43,44]

Decisions are often made to accept some weight gain in exchange for improvement in glycemic control. See chapter 2 for information on weight and diabetes prevention.

Physical Activity and Weight Control

Physical activity is a key component of a comprehensive weight management program that enhances the rate of weight loss and greatly improves the prospects for long-term weight maintenance.[45] Guidelines for physical activity should take into account a person's ability, safety, and willingness, gradually increasing duration and frequency to 30 to 45 minutes of moderate aerobic activity, 3 to 5 days per week, when possible.[6] Greater activity levels of at least 1 hour per day of moderate activity may be needed to achieve successful long-term weight loss. [6] (Chapters 14 and 30, on physical activity and self-management behaviors related to being active, provide more information.)

Case—Part 3: Weight Loss

LW's weight put her at risk for cardiovascular disease and other comorbidities. Weight loss needed to be encouraged to improve her lipid profile and blood pressure.

A modest caloric restriction (a 500- to 1000-calorie deficit) was recommended to improve LW's blood glucose levels, even though the weight loss might not significantly improve LW's blood glucose levels, due to the duration of her diabetes and any significant beta-cell dysfunction she might have had.

MNT and the Prevention and Treatment of Cardiovascular Disease

Individuals with type 2 diabetes have a 3- to 4-fold increase in the risk of cardiovascular disease (CVD).[46] Many individuals with type 2 diabetes or prediabetes have metabolic syndrome, a cluster of risk factors including abdominal obesity, insulin resistance, hyperglycemia, dyslipidemia, and hypertension. MNT is integral to the prevention and treatment of CVD in diabetes. Lifestyle factors that reduce risk factors associated with CVD, including dyslipidemia, hypertension, poor glycemic control, and obesity, should be addressed in counseling all individuals with prediabetes or type 2 diabetes.

MNT and the Prevention and Treatment of Dyslipidemia

Dietary Factors and Dyslipidemia

The primary goal in persons with diabetes and those with prediabetes is to achieve LDL-C goals to reduce cardiovascular risk. Specific studies have not been done to determine the effect of varying the percentage of specific types of dietary fats and cholesterol on blood lipids in individuals with diabetes. Therefore, the nutrition recommendations are the same as for the general public.

Dietary Fat and Cholesterol. A fat intake of 25% to 35% of calories is recommended to provide a cardioprotective effect.[8,47] Saturated and trans fats are the major components in the diet that affect LDL-C levels. Dietary cholesterol can also raise LDL-C. Reducing saturated fat to <7% of calories, reducing dietary cholesterol to <200 mg per day, and minimizing consumption of foods with trans fat is recommended in persons with diabetes.[6,47]

Unsaturated fats, including both monounsaturated and polyunsaturated, have been shown to improve blood lipids levels.[48,49,50] Replacing calories from saturated fat with unsaturated fat or carbohydrate has been shown to lower LDL-C.[48,49,50]

Omega-3 fatty acids have been shown in epidemiological and clinical trials to reduce the incidence of CVD.[51] Dietary intake of omega-3 fatty acids from both plant sources (α-linolenic acid) and marine sources (eicosapentaenoic [EPA] and docasahexanoic [DHA] acids) is associated with a reduction in cardiac events.[51,52] Dietary recommendations by the American Heart Association include 2 or more servings of fish per week, particularly fatty fish (ie, salmon, herring, and mackerel), along with food sources of α-linolenic acid (ie, canola and soybean oil, flaxseed, and English walnuts) (English walnuts are the type most commonly sold in the United States).[52]

Soluble Fiber. The addition of soluble fiber can further reduce LDL-C levels. Studies have demonstrated that 5 to 10 g per day of viscous fiber, such as oatmeal or oatbran, apples, pears, psyllium, barley, and legumes, can decrease LDL-C levels by 5%.[53]

Plant Stanols/Plant Sterols. Stanol and sterol esters inhibit the absorption of dietary and biliary cholesterol in the intestine.[54] Use of fortified food products that provide ~2 g per day of plant stanols or sterols has been shown to reduce LDL-C and total cholesterol levels.[55] It takes about 2 to 4 servings of various foods fortified with plant stanols/sterols such as spreads, orange juice, cheese, or yogurt to provide the 2 g per day.

Alcohol and Dyslipidemia/CVD Risk

Studies show that mild to moderate alcohol consumption (≤1 to 2 drinks per day) is associated with a decreased incidence of coronary heart disease in persons with diabetes.[56] The apparent protective effect of alcohol on heart disease risk has been attributed to an increase in HDL-C, decrease in platelet aggregation, or increase in fibrinolytic activity associated with alcohol consumption.[56] Individuals with severe hypertriglyceridemia should abstain from alcohol.[1] The available evidence does not support recommending alcohol consumption in persons who do not currently drink.

Physical Activity and Dyslipidemia/CVD Risk

Strong evidence supports the role of exercise and physical activity in reducing the risk factors for CVD in adults without diabetes. Although there are limited studies investigating the effect of physical activity on CVD in individuals with diabetes, early epidemiological data suggest that individuals with diabetes benefit as do those without diabetes.[57] Improved physical fitness can reduce total cholesterol, triglycerides, and LDL-C as well as increase HDL-C, particularly in the presence of weight loss.[58] However, a number of studies report that physical fitness, independent of weight loss, is also beneficial in reducing cardiovascular events and mortality.[59,60]

Macrovascular disease prevention and treatment are further discussed in chapter 21. Pharmacologic treatment of dyslipidemia is the topic of chapter 18.

MNT and the Prevention and Treatment of Hypertension

Hypertension (blood pressure >130/80 mm Hg) increases the risk of microvascular and macrovascular complications in persons with diabetes. Management of hypertension has been demonstrated to reduce the rate and progression of diabetic nephropathy and to reduce complications of hypertensive nephropathy, CVD, and cerebrovascular disease.[61] Adoption of healthy lifestyle strategies is critical for the prevention of high blood pressure and an indispensable part of the management of those with hypertension.[62]

Lifestyle modifications effective in preventing and managing hypertension include weight loss, a Dietary Approaches to Stop Hypertension (DASH) eating plan, high potassium intake, reduced sodium intake, moderate alcohol intake, and physical activity.[62,63] Several studies have demonstrated the additive effects of combining lifestyle interventions.[63,64,65,66]

Weight Loss and Hypertension

Obesity and overweight, particularly abdominal obesity, has consistently correlated closely with increased blood pressure independent of other risk factors for hypertension.[67] In persons with diabetes, there is a general association between weight reduction and a reduction in blood pressure, but there is a great deal of variability in the response. In almost all weight-reduction studies in the general population, systemic blood pressure is reduced, even if the degree of weight loss is small.[68] The JNC 7 (Joint National Committee) summary reports that a 5- to 10-mm Hg reduction in systolic blood pressure is possible per 10 kg of weight loss.[62]

DASH Eating Plan

The Dietary Approaches to Stop Hypertension (DASH) Trial showed that a diet high in fruits, vegetables, and low-fat dairy foods and low in total fat, saturated fat, and cholesterol significantly reduced blood pressure in the absence of weight change and at sodium intakes typical of those living in the United States.[69] (See Tables 13.1 and 13.2.) The beneficial effect on blood pressure from the DASH eating plan is likely due to a combination of factors, none of which can be specifically identified from this study.

Sodium and Hypertension

Moderate sodium restriction (~2300 mg per day) has been shown to be an effective strategy in the prevention and treatment of hypertension among a general population, not specifically those with diabetes.[62] Several studies have demonstrated that reducing sodium intake significantly reduces blood pressure in hypertensive and normotensive individuals, independent of other risk factors for hyper-

TABLE 13.1 Food Group, Daily Servings, and Serving Sizes for the DASH Diet

Food and Servings	*Sample Serving Sizes*
Grains and Grain Products 7–8 daily	1 slice bread 3/4 cup dry cereal 1/2 cup cooked rice, pasta, or cereal
Vegetables 4–5 daily	1 cup raw leafy vegetables 1/2 cup cooked vegetables 6 oz vegetable juice
Fruits 4–5 daily	1 medium fruit 1/4 cup dried fruits 1/2 cup fresh, frozen, or canned fruit 6 oz fruit juice
Low-Fat or Nonfat Dairy Foods 2–3 daily	8 oz skim or 1% milk 1 cup yogurt 1 1/2 oz low-fat cheese
Meat, Poultry, and Fish ≤2 daily	3 oz cooked lean meat, poultry (skinless white meat), or fish
Nuts, Seeds, and Legumes 4–5 per week	1 1/2 oz or 1/3-cup nuts 1/2 oz (2 Tb) seeds 1/2 cup cooked legumes
Fats and Oils 2–3 daily	1 teaspoon soft margarine or butter 1 Tb low-fat mayonnaise 1 Tb salad dressing or 2 Tb light salad dressing 1 tsp oil (olive, corn, canola, safflower, flaxseed, or other)
Sweets 5 per week	1/3 cup sherbet 3 pieces of hard candy Small piece (2 oz) angel food cake

TABLE 13.2 A DASH Diet With Approximately 2000 mg Sodium and Carbohydrate Counting

DASH Menu (number of carbohydrate servings)
Breakfast: 1 small banana (1) 3/4 cup corn flakes (1) 1 cup nonfat or low-fat milk (1) 1 slice whole wheat bread (1) with 1 tsp soft margarine *Total: 4 carbohydrate servings*
Lunch: 3/4 cup chicken salad for sandwich Pita bread (2) Raw vegetables: 3–4 carrot sticks, 3–4 celery sticks, 2 lettuce leaves 1 cup nonfat or low-fat milk (1) Small apple (1) *Total: 4 carbohydrate servings*
Dinner: 3 oz roast beef, lean 1/2 large baked potato (2) 1 Tb reduced-fat sour cream 1/2 cup steamed broccoli Spinach salad: 1/2 cup raw spinach, 2 cherry tomatoes, 1/2 cup sliced cucumber 1 Tb light Italian dressing 1 small whole-wheat dinner roll (1) 1 tsp. soft margarine 1 cup melon balls (1) *Total: 4 carbohydrate servings*
Snacks (morning, afternoon, evening, or added to meals): 1/4 cup dried apricots (1) 1/2 cup orange juice or 1 orange (1) 3/4 cup unsalted mini-pretzels (1) 1 cup low-fat yogurt (1) 2 Tb unsalted mixed nuts *Total: 4 carbohydrate servings*
Total carbohydrate servings for the day: 16

Source: Adapted from the National Heart, Lung and Blood Institute. The DASH healthy eating plan. On the Internet at: www.nhlbi.nih.gov/hbp/prevent/h_eating/h_e_dash.htm. Accessed 21 Mar 2006.

tension.[62,64] The DASH-Sodium Trial showed that lower sodium intakes resulted in greater reductions in blood pressure. Combining sodium restriction and the DASH eating plan had the greatest effect on blood pressure.[64]

Physical Activity and Hypertension

Physical activity is an important strategy for the prevention and treatment of high blood pressure. Persons who are less active and less fit have a 30% to 50% greater risk for high blood pressure.[70] Several clinical trials have demonstrated that regular aerobic activity reduces blood pressure in hypertensive and normotensive persons, independent of weight loss.[71] The underlying mechanisms responsible for an exercise-induced reduction in blood pressure are unclear. Insulin resistance and hyperinsulinemia may contribute to the pathogenesis of hypertension, and physical activity reduces insulin resistance and insulin levels in individuals with hypertension.[72]

Alcohol and Hypertension

Light to moderate alcohol consumption in persons with diabetes appears to have no adverse effects on blood pressure.[1] Short-term studies with small numbers of postmenopausal women without diabetes showed beneficial effects on blood pressure.[73] However, chronic, excessive alcohol intake (3 or more drinks per day) appears to increase blood pressure in both men and women.[74]

Hypertension is also discussed within the chapter on macrovascular disease (chapter 21), and pharmacologic treatment of hypertension is the focus of chapter 18.

MNT and the Prevention and Treatment of Nephropathy

Glycemic control and effective treatment of hypertension and proteinuria have been shown to be effective in delaying the onset and progression of nephropathy in both type 1 and type 2 diabetes.[75] Dyslipidemia has also been associated with progression of nephropathy in observational data.[76]

There currently is no evidence to suggest that restricting protein to less than 15% to 20% of calories has any effect on the onset or progression of nephropathy in individuals with normal renal function.[6] The long-term effects of consuming >20% of energy as protein on the development of nephropathy have not been determined.[6]

Case—Part 4: Cardiovascular Disease

LW was at considerable risk for CVD based on her hyperglycemia, dyslipidemia, and uncontrolled hypertension. Her food history and 24-hour recall revealed that her usual diet was high in total fat and saturated fat (2 factors that increase LDL-C) and high in sodium.

The next goal was to help LW reduce her risk of CVD by improving her blood lipids and blood pressure. A major focus was on reducing her LDL-C to <100 mg/dL. In addition to her walking program and moderate caloric restriction, she could lower her blood pressure by reducing her sodium intake and adopting an eating plan similar to the DASH eating plan that incorporates more fruits, vegetables, low-fat dairy foods and reduces the total fat, saturated fat, and trans fats. This, along with adding at least 2 servings of fish each week to provide omega-3 fatty acids, would also help improve her lipid profile. The addition of a spread containing a plant sterol/stanol might further reduce her LDL-C.

Since LW did not currently drink alcoholic beverages, she was not encouraged to start despite the reported benefits of light to moderate alcohol on blood pressure and CVD risk. Alcoholic beverages add calories and may result in less attention to diabetes self-care management.

An initial strategy toward achieving her goals was to help her choose what she might be willing and able to try: eat out less frequently, eat less when eating out, or make healthier food choices. The dietitian also discussed organizational techniques to help LW with the time constraints involved in preparing more meals at home and taking lunch to work. This would allow her more low-fat, lower sodium options and more availability of fruits and vegetables.

Regular physical activity was encouraged in each of LW's visits to improve lipids, blood pressure, and glycemia. LW was encouraged to perform resistance exercises 3 times a week (she had no contraindications). She was also taught to keep a record of her physical activity along with her blood glucose values to observe the effect on glycemia.

LW was instructed to self-monitor her blood pressure, in addition to blood pressure checks on follow-up visits, to assess the effect of her lifestyle changes and any need for medication additions or changes. The dietitian told her that the impact of lifestyle changes on blood lipids could be observed in a lipid profile in just 6 to 12 weeks.

Restricting protein to 0.8 g per kilogram per day has been shown to improve the glomerular filtration rate and reduce urinary albumin excretion rates in studies with type 1 and type 2 diabetes.[77] In studies of type 1 diabetes with overt nephropathy, restricting protein to 0.8 g per kilogram per day slowed the decline in the glomerular filtration rate.

Current MNT guidelines to prevent nephropathy include lifestyle modifications to maintain glycemic control, blood pressure control, and lipid control and to limit protein intake to the RDA (0.8g per kilogram) in individuals with any degree of chronic kidney disease.[6]

For further information on diabetic kidney disease, see chapter 23.

Nutrition Interventions in Youth

Nutrition goals for youth with diabetes should focus on optimal glycemic goals, lipid and blood pressure goals, and normal growth and development.[1]

Children and adolescents with diabetes have similar nutritional needs as those without diabetes.[1] Calorie needs can be estimated based on DRIs[8] and a history of the child's or adolescent's usual food intake. Growth and weight gain should be evaluated on a regular basis by recording height and weight on pediatric growth charts.

The meal plan must be individualized based on food preferences, cultural practices, family schedules and eating patterns, age, weight, activity level, and insulin action. Macronutrient composition of the meal plan should be based on blood glucose, lipids, and requirements for growth and development.

Education in problem solving based on blood glucose monitoring results is important for all youth with diabetes.

Youth with Type 1 Diabetes

Blood glucose goals for children and adolescents with type 1 diabetes are accomplished by balancing food intake, insulin, and physical activity and should emphasize achieving glycemic goals without excessive hypoglycemia. Withholding food or having a child eat without an appetite to avoid hypoglycemia should be discouraged. A flexible insulin regimen with long-acting basal and rapid-acting boluses precludes the need for a rigid meal plan, allowing the child or adolescent more flexibility in food choices and timing of meals and snacks. Carbohydrate counting using insulin-to-carbohydrate ratios is a meal planning approach often used with youths with type 1 diabetes on physiological insulin regimens because it offers more flexibility.[78]

For more information on carbohydrate counting, see chapter 16 on pattern management, chapter 17 on insulin pump therapy, and chapter 29 on self-care behaviors related to healthy eating.

Youth With Type 2 Diabetes

The goals for youth with type 2 diabetes are to facilitate appropriate changes in eating and physical activity habits, as many are overweight or obese.[1] Since these behaviors are generally family behaviors, family involvement in the behavior change process is encouraged. A number of meal planning approaches can be used to facilitate the selection of a variety of healthy foods in appropriate portions. Emphasis on carbohydrate consistency can improve blood glucose levels.

Successful MNT is defined as the cessation of excessive weight gain with normal linear growth and near-normal fasting blood glucose values and near-normal A1C.[79]

Nutrition Interventions in Pregnancy

See chapters 11 and 12, on pregnancy with preexisting diabetes and gestational diabetes.

Nutrition Interventions in Older Adults

MNT in older adults with diabetes presents unique challenges. Nutritional status is often compromised by changes in taste and smell, appetite, poor dentition, physical disabilities, food availability, difficulty preparing food, and side effects from medications.[80] A thorough nutrition history and an assessment of psychosocial needs are necessary to determine the appropriate nutrition interventions.[14]

MNT must address adequacy of nutritional needs, glycemic control, and nutrition-related cardiovascular risk factors that are common in this age group.[81] Weight change is the most reliable indicator of poor nutritional status in older adults.[14] An unintentional weight gain or weight loss of 10 lb or 10% of body weight in less than 6 months is a major concern.[14]

Although energy needs decrease for older adults due to loss of lean body mass and less physical activity, requirements for other nutrients remain the same or increase with age.[80] Older persons can be overweight or obese due to increased fat mass, yet still malnourished.[82] A modest calorie reduction with an emphasis on nutrient-dense foods may be beneficial along with physical activity to reduce the loss of muscle mass.

Nutrition recommendations for older adults include restricting sodium to <2300 mg per day,[7] although this can result in decreased food intake if the taste is undesirable. The most common nutrient deficiencies in older adults are calcium, zinc, magnesium, vitamin A and D, vitamin B_{12}, folate, and vitamin C.[1,80] Nutrition supplements are appropriate if a person is consuming inadequate nutrients through food. A calcium supplement is often necessary to meet the 1200 mg of calcium daily that is recommended for older adults.

Physical activity should be encouraged for older adults to minimize the loss of muscle mass, decrease bone loss, decrease central adiposity, improve insulin sensitivity, and improve cardiovascular risk factors.[1,80]

The care and education of older adults is complicated by their clinical and functional heterogeneity.[6] Some individuals are limited cognitively or physically with multiple comorbidities, yet others are relatively healthy, physically active, and active learners. A thorough assessment followed by an individualized plan for educating and providing care is key to successful outcomes in the older adult.

Focus on Education: Pearls for Practice

Teaching Strategies

- **Modest weight loss.** Overweight and obese persons benefit from weight loss and increases in physical activity for the prevention and delay of type 2 diabetes. Weight loss also assists with decreasing cardiovascular risk factors and is likely to improve glycemia in individuals with newly diagnosed type 2 diabetes who are primarily insulin resistant. Glycemia is less likely to be reduced through weight loss in individuals with longer standing diabetes who are insulin deficient.

- **Monitoring.** Encourage the use of premeal and postmeal blood glucose results to reinforce understanding of the glycemic effect of carbohydrate-containing foods in both type 1 and type 2 diabetes. Monitoring blood pressure and lipid levels is as important as monitoring blood glucose.

- **Involvement.** Set and prioritize MNT goals involving each person and family member if appropriate to individualize meal plans. Encourage food records; review them, determine understanding of meal planning principles, food group choices, and portion sizes. Measure progress in behavior changes related to healthier choices, quantity, and timing of foods. Have participants use food models to portray a dinner meal, asking for feedback about choices. Teaching the principle of eating from all the food groups for healthy eating and good nutrition is important. Demonstrating meal planning, menu preparation, and selecting meals from restaurant menus during a teaching event is useful in role-playing healthy food choices.

Messages for Patients

- **Healthier choices.** Instead of focusing on weight loss, set short-term goals that will include healthier foods in place of high-fat, highly processed foods. Involve a friend or family member to assist in reviewing menus, labels, and food products.

- **Testing blood glucose.** Check blood glucose values before and after meals to observe blood glucose response to the type and amount of carbohydrate in a meal. Avoid choosing foods based solely on their effect on blood glucose; food selection to optimize glycemia should not compromise healthy eating.

- **Activity.** Take energy expenditure as seriously as food (nutritional) intake. Use a pedometer to keep track of the number of steps taken. The baseline and progressive steps provide a goal and motivation. Consider a walking program

---

References

1. American Diabetes Association. Nutrition principles and recommendations in diabetes. Diabetes Care. 2004;27 suppl 1:S35-46.
2. Lacey K, Pritchett E. Nutrition care process and model: ADA adopts road map to quality care and outcomes management. J Am Diet Assoc. 2003;103:1061-72.
3. Pastors JG, Warshaw H, Daly A, Franz M, Kulkarni K. The evidence for the effectiveness of medical nutrition therapy in diabetes management. Diabetes Care. 2002;25:608-13.
4. Pastors JG, Franz MJ, Warshaw H, Daly A, Arnold MS. How effective is medical nutrition therapy in diabetes care? J Am Diet Assoc. 2003;103:827-31.
5. Knowler WC, Barrett-Connor E, Fowler SE, et al. Reduction in the incidence of type 2 diabetes with lifestyle intervention or metformin. N Engl J Med. 2002;346:393-403.
6. American Diabetes Association: Standards of medical care in diabetes-2006. Diabetes Care. 2006; 29 suppl 1:S4-42.
7. Krauss RM, Eckel RH, Howard B, et al. AHA dietary guidelines. Revision 2000: a statement for healthcare professionals from the Nutrition Committee of the American Heart Association. Circulation. 2000;102:2284-99.
8. Institute of Medicine: Dietary Reference Intakes: Energy, Carbohydrate, Fiber, Fat, Fatty Acids, Cholesterol, Protein, and Amino Acids. Washington, DC: National Academies Press; 2002.
9. Institute of Medicine. Dietary Reference Intakes (DRI) and Recommended Dietary Allowances (RDA). Food and Nutrition Information Center. On the Internet: www.nal.usda.gov/fnic. Accessed 15 Jan 2006.
10. Hasanain B, Mooradian AD. Antioxidants and their influences in diabetes. Curr Diabetes Reports. 2002;2:2:448-56.
11. Lemon CC, Lacey K, Lohse B, Hubacher DO, Klawitter B, Palta M. Outcomes monitoring of health, behavior, and quality of life after nutrition intervention in adults with type 2 diabetes. J Am Diet Assoc. 2004;104:1805-15.
12. DAFNE Study Group. Training in flexible, intensive insulin management to enable dietary freedom in people with type 1 diabetes: dose adjustment for normal eating (DAFNE) randomized controlled trial. BMJ. 2002;325:746-52.
13. Sheard NF, Clark NG, Brand-Miller JC, et al. Dietary carbohydrate (amount and type) in the prevention and management of diabetes: a statement of the American Diabetes Association. Diabetes Care. 2004;27:2266-71.
14. Franz MJ, Bantle JP, Beebe CA, et al. Evidence-based nutrition principles and recommendations for the treatment and prevention of diabetes and related complications (technical review). Diabetes Care. 2002;25:148-98.
15. Nuttall FQ, Gannon MC. Carbohydrates and diabetes. In: American Diabetes Association Guide to Medical Nutrition Therapy for Diabetes. Franz MJ, Bantle JP, eds. Alexandria, Va: American Diabetes Association;1999:107-25.
16. Pi-Sunyer FX. Glycemic index and disease. Am J Clin Nutr. 2002;76:290S-98.
17. Warshaw HS, Powers MA. A search for answers about foods with polyols. Diabetes Educ. 1999;25:307-21.
18. Gannon MC, Nuttall FQ. Effect of a high proein, low-carbohdyrate diet on blood glucose control in people with type 2 diabetes. Diabetes. 2005;53:2375-82.
19. Gannon MC, Nuttall FQ, Saeed A, Jordan K, Hoover H. An increase in protein improves the blood glucose response in persons with type 2 diabetes. Am J Clin Nutr. 2003;78:734-41.
20. Brinkworth GD, Noakes M, Keogh JB, Luscombe ND, Wittert GA, Cllifton PM. Long-term effects of a high-protein, low-carbohydrate diet on weight control and cardiovascular risk markers in obese hyperinsulinemic subjects. Int J Obesity. 2004;28:661-70.
21. Vessby B, Unsitupa M, Hermanses K, et al. Substituting dietary saturated for monounsaturated fat impairs insulin sensitivity in healthy men and women: the KANWU Study. Diabetologia. 2001;44:312-19.
22. Hayes C. Physical activity and exercise. In: Diabetes Medical Nutrition Therapy and Education. American Dietetic Association; 2005:71-88.
23. Diabetes Prevention Research Group. Reduction in the evidence of type 2 diabetes with life-style intervention or metformin. N Engl J Med. 2002;346:393-403.
24. Tuomilehto J, Lindstrom J, Eriksson JG, et al: Finnish Diabetes Prevention Study. Prevention of type 2 diabetes mellitus by changes in lifestyle among subjects with impaired glucose tolerance. N Engl J Med. 2001:344:1343-50.
25. Cox KL, Burke V, Morton AR, Beilin LJ, Puddey IB. Independent and additive effects of energy restric-

tion and exercise on glucose and insulin concentrations in sedentary overweight men. Am J Clin Nutr. 2004;80:308-16.

26. Duncan GE, Perri MG, Teriaque DW, Hutson AD, Eckel RH, Stacpoole PW. Exercise training without weight loss increases insulin sensitivity and postheparin plasma lipase activity in previously sedentary adults. Diabetes Care. 2003;26:557-62.

27. Turner BC, Jenkins E, Kerr D, Sherwin RS, Cavan DA. The effect of evening alcohol consumption on next-morning glucose control in type 1 diabetes. Diabetes Care. 2001;24:1888-93.

28. Klein S, Sheard NF, Pi-Sunyer X, et al. Weight management through lifestyle modification for the prevention and management of type 2 diabetes: rationale and strategies. A statement of the American Diabetes Association, the North American Association for the Study of Obesity, and the American Society for Clinical Nutrition. Diabetes Care. 2004;27:2067-73.

29. UKPDS Study Group. UK Prospective Diabetes Study: responses of fasting plasma glucose to diet therapy in newly presenting type 2 diabetes patients. Metabolism. 1990;39:905-12.

30. Wolf AM, Coonaway MR, Crowther JQ, et al. Tanslating lifestyle interventions to practice in obese patients with type 2 diabetes. Diabetes Care. 2004;27:1570-6.

31. Boucher JL, VanWormer JJ. Overweight and obesity. In: Diabetes Medical Nutrition Therapy and Education. American Dietetic Association;2005:71-88.

32. Klein S, Burke LE, Bray GA, et al. Clinical implications of obesity with specific focus on cardiovascular disease: a statement for professionals from the American Heart Association Council on Nutrition, Physical Activity, and Metabolism. Circulation. 2004;110:2952-67.

33. Markovic TP, Jenkins AB, Campbell LV, Furler SM, Kraegen EW, Chisholm DJ. The determinants of glycemic responses to diet restriction and weight loss in obesity and NIDDM. Diabetes Care. 1998;21:687-94.

34. National Heart, Lung, and Blood Institute. Clinical guidelines on the identification, evaluation, and treatment of overweight and obesity in adults. Bethesda, Md: National Institutes of Health; 2000. NIH publication 98-4083.

35. Redmon JB, Reck KP, Raatz SK, Swanson JE, Kwong CA, Ji H, Thomas W, Bantle JP. Two-year outcome of a combination of weight loss therapies for type 2 diabetes. Diabetes Care. 2005;28:1311-5.

36. Bravata DM, Sanders L, Huang H, et al. Efficacy and safety of low carbohydrate diets: a systematic review. JAMA. 2003;348:2074-81.

37. Dansinger ML, Gleason JA, Griffith JL, Selker HP, Schaefer EJ. Comparison of the Atkins, Ornish, Weight Watchers, and Zone Diets for weight loss and heart disease risk reduction: a randomized trial. JAMA. 2005;293:43-53.

38. Saris WH, Astrup A, Prentice AM, et al. Randomized controlled trial of changes in dietary carbohydrate/fat ratio and simple vs complex carbohydrates on body weight and blood lipids: the CARMEN study. The Carbohydrate Ratio Management in European National diets. Int J Obes Relat Metab Disord. 2000;24:1310-8.

39. Foster GD, Wyatt HR, Hill JO, et al. A randomized trial of a low-carbohydrate diet for obesity. N Engl J Med. 2003;348:2074-81.

40. Samaha FF, Iqbal N, Seshadri P, et al. A low-carbohydrate as compared with a low-fat diet in severe obesity. N Engl J Med. 2003;348:2074-81.

41. Brehm BJ, Seeley RJ, Daniels SR, D'Alessio DA. A randomized trial comparing a very low carbohydrate diet and a calorie-restricted low fat diet on body weight and cardiovascular risk factors in healthy women. J. Clin Endocrinol Metab. 2003;88:1617-23.

42. Beebe C. Body weight issues in preventing and treating type 2 diabetes. Diabetes Spectrum. 2003;16:261-66.

43. Chapman I. Effect on pramlintide on satiety and food intake in obese subjects and subjects with type 2 diabetes. Diabetologia. 2005;48:838-48.

44. DeFronzo RA. Effects of exenatide (exendin-4) on glycemic control and weight over 30 weeks in metformin-treated patients with type 2 diabetes. Diabetes Care. 2005;28:1092-100.

45. Pronk NP, Wing RR. Physical activity and long-term maintenance of weight loss. Obes Res.1994;2:587-99.

46. Grundy SM. Approach to lipoprotein management in 2001 National Cholesterol Guidelines. Am J Cardiol. 2002;90 8 suppl 1:S11-21.

47. National Cholesterol Education Program. Third Report of the Expert Panel on Detection, Evaluation, and Treatment of High Blood Cholesterol in Adults (Adult Treatment Panel III). On the Internet: www.nhlbi.nih.gov/guidelines. Accessed 5 Jan 2006.

48. Summers LK, Fielding BA, Bradshaw HA, et al. Substituting dietary saturated fat with polyunsaturated fat changes abdominal fat distribution and improves insulin sensitivity. Diabetologia. 2002;45:369-77.

49. Salmeron J, Hu FB, Manson JE, et al. Dietary fat intake and risk of type 2 diabetes in women. Am J Clin Nutr. 2001;73:1019-26.

50. Hu FB, van Dam RM, Liu S. Diet and risk of type II diabetes: the role of types of fat and carbohydrate. Diabetologia. 2001;44:805-17.

51. Kris-Etherton PM, Harris WS, Appel LJ, American Heart Association Nutrition Committee. Fish consumption, fish oil, omega-3 fatty acids, and cardiovascular disease. Circulation. 2002;106:2747-57.

52. Mozaffarian D, Bryson CL, Lemaitre RN, Burke GL, Siscovick DS. Fish intake and risk of incident heart failure. J Am Coll Cardiol. 2005;45:2015-21.

53. Anderson JW, Hanna TH. Impact of nondigestible carbohydrates on serum lipoproteins and risk for cardiovascular disease. J Nutr. 1999;129 7 suppl: 1457S-66.

54. Karmally W, Jahnes M. Cardiovascular disease, dyslipiemia, and hypertension in diabetes. In: Diabetes Medical Nutrition Therapy and Education. American Dietetic Association. 2005:253-63.

55. Lee YM, Haastert B, Scherbaum W, Hauner H. A phytosterol-enriched spread improves the lipid profile of subjects with type 2 diabetes mellitus-a randomized controlled trial under free-living conditions. Eur J Nutr. 2003;42:111-7.

56. Howard, AA, Arnsten JH, Gourevitch MN. Effect of alcohol consumption on diabetes mellitus: a systematic review. Ann Intern Med. 2004;140:211-9.

57. Weil, W. Cardiovascular disease, diabetes and physical activity. In: On the Cutting Edge (newsletter of the American Dietetic Association Diabetes Care & Education Practice Group). 2004;25:14-7.

58. Mullooly C, Chalmers KH. Physical activity/exercise. In: Diabetes Management Therapies: A core curriculum for diabetes education. 5th ed. Chicago, Ill: The American Association of Diabetes Educators; 2003:61-92.

59. Church TS, Cheng YJ, Earnest CP, et al. Exercise capacity and body composition as predictors of mortality among men with diabetes. Diabetes Care. 2004;27:83-8.

60. Wessel TR, Arant CB, Olson MB, et al. Relationship of physical fitness vs body mass index with coronary artery disease and cardiovascular events in women. JAMA. 2004;292:1179-87.

61. Sowers JR, Epstein M. Diabetes mellitus and associated hypertension, vascular disease, and nephropathy: an update. Hypertension. 1995;26:869-79.

62. Chobanian AV, Bakris GL, Black HR, et al. The Seventh Report of the Joint National Committee on Prevention, Detention, Evaluation, and Treatment of High Blood Pressure: the JNC 7 report. JAMA. 2004;289:747-52.

63. Sacks FM, Svetkey LP, Vollmer WM, et al. DASH-Sodium Collaborative Research Group: effects on blood pressure of reduced dietary sodium and the Dietary Approaches to Stop Hypertension (DASH) diet. N Eng J Med. 2001;344:3-10.

64. Vollmer WM. Sacks FM, Ard J, et al. Effects of diet and sodium intake on blood pressure. Ann Int Med. 2001;135:1019-28.

65. Appel LJ, Champagne CM, Harsha DW, et al; Writing Group of the PREMIER Collaborative Research Group. Effects of comprehensive lifestyle modification on blood pressure control: main results of the PREMIER clinical trial. JAMA. 2003; 289:2083-93.

66. Miller ER 3rd, Erlinger TP, Young DR, et al. Results of diet, exercise, and weight loss intervention trial (DEW-IT). Hypertension. 2002;40:612-18m.

67. He J, Whelton PK, Appel LJ, Charleston J, Klag MJ. Long-term effects of weight loss and dietary sodium reduction on incidence of hypertension. Hypertension. 2000;35:544-9.

68. Kaplan NM. Lifestyle modification for prevention and treatment of hypertension. J Clin Hypertens. 2004;6:716-19.

69. Appel LJ, Moore TJ, Obarzanek E, et al: for the DASH Collaborative Research Group. A clinical trial of the effects of dietary patterns on blood pressure. N Eng J Med. 1997;336:1117-24.

70. 2000 Heart and Stroke Statistical Update. American Heart Association, Dallas, Tex: American Heart Association; 1999.

71. Whelton SP, Chin A, Xin X, He J. Effect of aerobic exercise on blood pressure. Ann Intern Med. 2002;136:493-503.

72. He J, Klag MJ, Cabellero B, Appel J, Charleston J, Whelton PK. Plasma insulin levels and incidence of hypertension in African Americans and whites. Arch Intern Med. 1999;159:498-503.

73. Davies MJ, Baer DJ, Judd JT, Brown ED, Campbell WS, Taylor PR. Effects of moderate alcohol intake on fasting insulin and glucose concentrations and insulin sensitivity in postmenopausal women: a randomized controlled trial. JAMA. 2002;287:2559-62.

74. Xin X, He J, Prontini MG, Ogden LG, Motsamai OI, Whelton PK. Effects of alcohol reduction on blood pressure: a meta-analysis of randomized controlled trials. Hypertension. 2001;38:1112-7.

75. Hill L, Goeddeki-Merickel CM. Chronic kidney disease-nondialysis. In: Diabetes Medical Nutrition Therapy and Education. American Dietetic Association; 2005:264-75.

76. Ravid M, Brosh D, Ravid-Safran D, Levy Z, Rachmani R. Main risk factors for nephropathy in type 2 diabetes mellitus are plasma cholesterol levels, mean blood pressure, and hyperglycemia. Arch Intern Med. 1998;158:998-1004.

77. Narita T, Koshimura J, Meguro H, Kitazato H, Jfuita H, Ito S. Determination of optimal protein contents for protein restriction diet in type 2 diabetic patients with microalbuminuria. Tohoku J Exp Med. 2001;193:45-55.

78. Evert A, Gerken S. Birth through adolescence. In: Diabetes Medical Nutrition Therapy and Education. American Dietetic Association; 2005:161-78.

79. American Diabetes Association. Type 2 diabetes in children and adolescents (Consensus Statement). Diabetes Care. 2000;23:381-9.

80. McLaughlin S. Diabetes in older adults. In: Diabetes Medical Nutrition Therapy and Education. American Dietetic Association; 2005:179-88.

81. Erlinger TP, Pollack H, Appel LJ. Nutrition-related cardiovascular risk factors in older people: results from the Third National Health and Nutrition Examination Survey. J Am Geriatr Soc. 2000;48:1486-9.

82. Horani MH, Mooradian AD. Management of obesity in the elderly: special considerations. Treat Endocrinol. 2002;1:387-98.

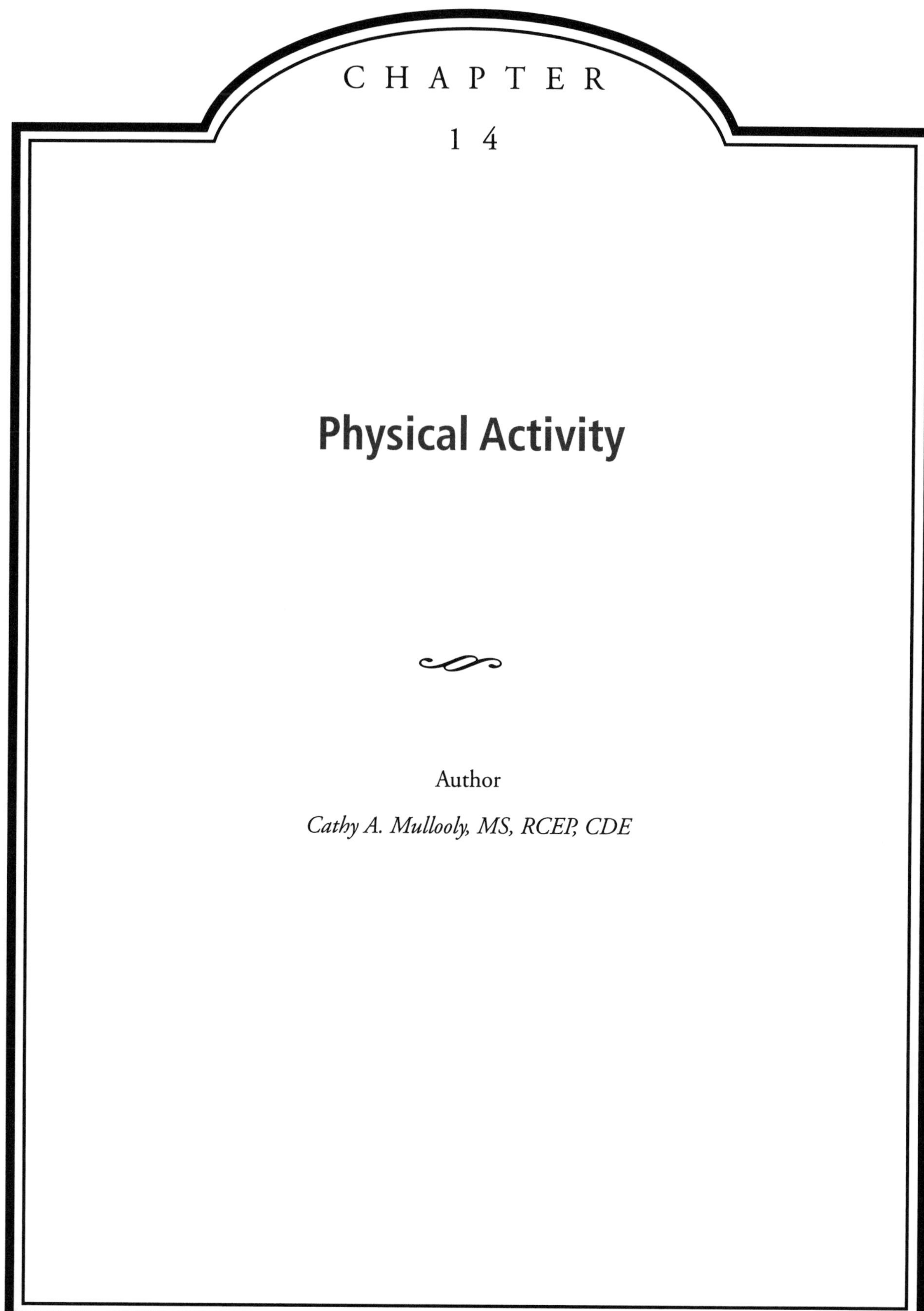

CHAPTER

14

Physical Activity

Author

Cathy A. Mullooly, MS, RCEP, CDE

Key Concepts

- Familiarity with current fitness terminology
- Understanding the role of physical fitness in diabetes prevention and treatment
- Understanding the physiological responses associated with blood glucose levels during physical activity
- Identifying the individual's risks associated with physical activity and applying clinical strategies to minimize those risks
- Recognizing 3 distinct stages in adoption and use of a fitness plan
- Implementing strategies to enable appropriately self-directed fitness plans

Introduction

A lifestyle that incorporates sufficient physical activity aids in diabetes prevention and is extremely beneficial to general health. For people with diabetes, the beneficial effects of leading a physically active lifestyle have been recognized since ancient times.[1] The discovery of insulin in the twentieth century prompted modern scientific exploration of the therapeutic effects of physical activity on the blood glucose level.[2]

Today, implementing and maintaining a health-related fitness program is regarded as a primary component of diabetes self-management. In 2003, the AADE published data identifying 7 behaviors common in the people with diabetes who are able to achieve better health outcomes; "Being Active" is 1 of those behaviors. The AADE 7 Self-Care Behaviors™ emphasize that even small changes in physical activity levels are considered beneficial.[3] More on self-care behaviors related to being active can be found in chapter 30.

To promote physical activity and help individuals implement an exercise prescription, the diabetes educator must recognize how to adjust variables within the diabetes treatment routine. The following are key aspects to be considered:

- Whether the side effect of hypoglycemia exists with the individual's diabetes medication regimen
- When the individual should perform blood glucose measurements
- How to interpret individual blood glucose responses to physical activity
- How to modify fitness guidelines and plans in light of diabetes complications and other restrictions
- How to overcome barriers limiting adequate physical activity

Learning to overcome barriers that interfere with a more physically active lifestyle is a large part of diabetes self-management education. When the diabetes complications of neuropathy, nephropathy, and retinopathy exist, certain physical movements may pose challenges and safety issues. Also, not all individuals with diabetes are capable of or willing to participate in a fitness program, regardless of the benefits they can achieve. The diabetes educator's task is to explore all the options and alternatives available for the patient so that a safe, effective, and realistic fitness plan can be designed and successfully implemented.

Current Physical Fitness Terminology

In recent years, the role of physical activity in people's daily lives has been widely examined. Western culture's rapid adaptation to sedentary lifestyles over the last few decades has been associated in this same, relatively short time span with growing rates of metabolic diseases. Unfortunately, reporting on this topic has also led to much confusion in the lay population. One part of clarifying the messages provided to the public is for health, physical fitness, and research professionals to use accepted terminology in regard to fitness. In 2000, the President's Council of Physical Fitness collected terms and definitions from many respected sources and organized them into an outline intended for common use.[4]

In that document, physical fitness is simply defined as "a set of attributes that people have or achieve relating to their ability to perform physical activity."[4] What complicates physical fitness for the layperson is that there are many different reasons to engage in a physically active lifestyle. Table 14.1 organizes the accepted terminology under 4 different categories of physical fitness: physiological fitness, health-related fitness, skill-related fitness, and sports.

While none of the categories are mutually exclusive, they are also not dependent on each other. The terminology of fitness is intended to be more inclusive and less athletic in nature when considering what affects an individual's fitness level and health outcomes. However, most laypersons believe they need to possess skill-related talents or participate in sports to achieve physiological or health-related benefits. This misperception precludes many people from considering or engaging in a physically active lifestyle.

Physiological Fitness

The physiological fitness category includes terms that have little to do with how one performs a physical activity.[4] Yet physiological fitness is influenced by the lifelong inclusion, or exclusion, of habitual physical activity. For example, the cholesterol level does not influence the ability to walk. Yet, the more one walks, the more once can expect to see an impact on the cholesterol level.

- *Metabolic Fitness:* Status of metabolic systems and variables predictive of the risk for diabetes and cardiovascular disease
- *Morphological Fitness:* Status of body compositional factors, such as body circumference, body fat content, and regional body fat distribution
- *Bone Integrity* (bone strength): Status of bone mineral density

Health-Related Physical Fitness

The health-related physical fitness category contains terms that are recognized for their direct relationship to good health.[4] These terms are also more likely to be of interest to the individual engaging in a fitness program. The layperson measures success, or lack of success, on changes seen in regard to these terms.

- *Body Composition:* Relative amounts of muscle, fat, bone, and other vital parts of the body
- *Cardiovascular Fitness:* Ability of the circulatory and respiratory systems to supply oxygen during sustained physical activity
- *Flexibility:* Range of motion available at a joint
- *Muscular Endurance:* Muscle's ability to continue to perform without fatigue
- *Strength:* Muscle's ability to exert force

Physical Activity Versus Exercise (Training)

- *Physical Activity:* Bodily movement produced by the contraction of skeletal muscle that substantially increases energy expenditure
- *Exercise (Training):* Subset of physical activity conducted with the intention of developing physical fitness; includes cardiovascular, strength, and flexibility training options

The recommendation to use the broader term "physical activity" in place of the narrower term "exercise" has also caused some confusion.[4] The intent, with evidence supported by research, is to recognize that many types of movements can have a positive impact on health-related physical fitness. It is also true that a variety of movements are required to yield measurable improvements for each of the components in the health-related fitness category. Table 14.2 provides an overview of some general categories that can be used to identify options for physical activity.

TABLE 14.2 Subcategories of Physical Activity

Physical Activity				
Exercise	Sport	Leisure Activities	Dance	Others

Source: President's Council on Physical Fitness. Definitions: health, fitness, and physical activity. Research Digest; 2000.

TABLE 14.1 Currently Accepted Terminology Regarding Physical Fitness

Physical Fitness			*Skills*
Physiological	*Health-Related*	*Skill-Related*	*Sports*
Metabolic	Body composition	Agility	Team
Morphological	Cardiovascular fitness	Balance	Individual
Bone integrity	Flexibility	Coordination	Lifetime
Other	Muscular endurance	Power	Other
	Muscle strength	Speed	
		Reaction time	
		Other	

Source: President's Council on Physical Fitness. Definitions: health, fitness, and physical activity. Research Digest, 2000.

Role of Physical Activity in Diabetes Prevention and Treatment

Physical activity is well associated with substantial improvement in insulin sensitivity.[6,7,8] Much research has been focused on understanding these physiological pathways. There are acute and long-term benefits for the individual with, or at risk for, developing diabetes. However, the beneficial effects of physical activity also diminish quickly if not performed on a regular basis.

The diabetes educator must have a basic understanding of these physiological pathways. This knowledge is of value both in the prevention of diabetes and in the care of diabetes and its complications throughout the life span. With this basis of knowledge, the educator can best assist individuals in implementing physical fitness programs.

The role of physical activity in diabetes prevention was examined in the Finnish Diabetes Prevention Study[9] and Diabetes Prevention Program.[10] Data from both studies showed that modest weight loss brought on by physical activity and nutrition strategies reduced the incidence of developing type 2 diabetes by 58%. While the studies did not determine which strategy was more effective, inclusion of moderate intensity exercise for 150 minutes a week was reported to contribute to results. Even though these results are not conclusive, much is already known about physical activity and its contribution to insulin sensitivity.

Physical activity activates a hormonal response that determines how fuel substrates will be used for metabolism (Table 14.3). Changes to the secretion of these hormones allow fuel substrates to be made available as an energy source while maintaining glucose homeostasis. An important point is that insulin secretion is decreased during physical activity. Suppression of insulin secretion is an essential step in allowing for hepatic glucose production to maintain the balance of glucose in the blood.[11]

Glycogen stores in the liver and muscle need to be replenished following each bout of physical activity. This demand is met by an increased rate of glucose uptake until the depleted glycogen stores are replenished. This activity may take 24 to 48 hours to complete. This extended recovery period is also characterized by enhanced insulin sensitivity.[11] There are also many long-term adaptations (Table 14.4) to habitual physical activity that may hold the key to the prevention of type 2 diabetes.

Promoting Lifestyle Changes Among Family Members of Those Diagnosed. Family history has long been accepted as an important determinant of who may develop type 2 diabetes. Whether the ultimate trigger is genetics or environmental factors, health statistics reveal that type 2 diabetes is occurring more often in all age and ethnic groups.[12] Therefore, the known patient with type 2 diabetes has established an increased risk of developing the disease for other family members. The challenge and opportunity for the diabetes educator is to use the research data to assist those family members in making the recommended lifestyle changes.

Effect of Physical Activity on Diabetes Management

Cardiovascular Exercise

Type 2 Diabetes

The chronic effects of performing cardiovascular exercise appear to benefit the individual with type 2 diabetes in a number of ways:[13]

- Reduces A1C level
- Improves insulin sensitivity

TABLE 14.3 Normal Hormonal Response and the Acute Metabolic Effects of Physical Activity

Hormone	*Response During Physical Activity*	*Metabolic Effect*
Insulin	Decreases	Facilitates hepatic glucose and FFA production
Glucagon	Increases	Increases hepatic glucose production; increase glucose supply available in the blood
Epinephrine	Increases	Stimulates FFA production, which provides glycerol as a substrate for gluconeogenesis
Norepinephrine	Increases	Stimulates hepatic and muscle
Growth Hormone/Cortisol	Increases	Increases lipolysis, decreases insulin-stimulated glucose uptake, increases gluconeogenic substrates

TABLE 14.4 Metabolic Adaptations to Regular Physical Activity

Hormone	*Adaptation*	*Metabolic Effect*
Proinsulin[1]	Decreases	Decreased synthesis of insulin in the pancreas
Glucokinase[1]	Decreases	Decreased secretion of insulin from the pancreas
GLUT4[2,3]	Increases	Increases the capacity for insulin-stimulated glucose transport in the muscle
PI3-Kinase[4]	Increases	Increased activity is thought to improve insulin signaling
MAP Kinase Pathway[5]	Increases	Increase activity in this pathway may be associated with changes in the muscle leading to improved glucose storage and disposal
Nonesterified Fatty Acids (NEFAs)[6]	Increases	Increased ability to store and mobilize NEFAs as a fuel source; improved muscle capacity to extract NEFAs from the blood and oxidize for energy

Sources:

1. Koranyi LI, Bourey RE, Slentz CA, Hollosky JO. Coordinate reduction of rat pancreatic islet glucokinase and proinsulin mRNA by exercise training. Diabetes. 1991;40:401-4.
2. Lee JS, Bruce CR, Tunstall RJ, Cameron-Smith D, Hugel H, Hawley JA. Interaction of exercise and diet on GLUT-4 protein and gene expression in type I and type II rat skeletal muscle. Acta Physiol Scand. 2002;175:37-44.
3. Terada S, Yokozeki T, Kawanaka K, et al. Effects of high intensity swimming training on GLUT-4 and glucose transport activity in rat skeletal muscle. J Appl Physiol. 2001;90:2019-24.
4. Kirwin JP, Aguila LFD, Hernandez JM, et al. Regular exercise enhances activiation of IRS-1-associated PI3-kinase in human skeletal muscle. J Appl Physiol. 2000;88:797-803.
5. Osman A, Hancock J, Hunt DG, Ivy JL, Mandarino LJ. Exercise training increases ERK3 activity in skeletal muscle of obese Zucker rats. J Appl Physiol. 2001;90:454-60.
6. Romijn JA, Klein S, Coyle EF, Sidossis LS, Wolfe RR. Strenuous endurance training increases lipolysis and triglyceride-fatty acid cyling at rest. J Appl Physiol. 1993;75:108-13.

- Assists in attainment and maintenance of desirable body weight
- Decreases coronary artery disease (CAD) risk factors

Several long-term studies demonstrate a sustained improvement in glucose control while a regular physical activity program is maintained.[14,15,16] Thus, remaining physically active is an essential component of diabetes self-management behavior for all individuals with type 2 diabetes. In general, there are also many benefits that can be expected with improved functioning of the cardiovascular system:[11]

- Improved strength and physical work capacity
- Decreased risk factors for CAD
- Adjunct therapy for controlling hypertension
- Reduction in plasma cholesterol, triglycerides, and low-density lipoprotein (LDL) cholesterol
- Increase in high-density lipoproteins (HDL)
- Increased insulin sensitivity
- Enhanced fibrinolysis
- Favorable changes in body composition (reduction of body fat and weight; increase in muscle mass)

Type 1 Diabetes

Physical activity should be included as part of diabetes self-management training for the individual with type 1 diabetes; however, since the literature has shown inconsistent A1C results when physical activity has been studied in this population, care must be taken when promoting this as an expected outcome of fitness. Focusing instead on the general benefits[11] listed in the previous section (type 2 diabetes) or the role physical activity plays in the prevention of insulin resistance may be best.[9,10] While more study is needed to determine how physical activity affects the disease of type 1 diabetes, throughout the life span the individual with type 1 diabetes gains much by engaging in a fitness plan.

Promote An Active Lifestyle

Remaining physically active is an essential part of self-care for all persons with type 2 diabetes. For those with type 1 diabetes, activity's health benefits are also important to emphasize.

To safely and successfully pursue a physically active lifestyle, the individual with type 1 diabetes needs to develop hypoglycemia prevention strategies. The success of a workout should not always be gauged by how much blood glucose numbers fall. In fact, large drops in the blood glucose are more likely to lead to hypoglycemia. The focus needs to be on keeping the blood glucose level from interfering with the workout or intended physical activity. Hypoglycemia prevention is discussed later in this chapter.

Resistance Exercises

This form of exercise is an important means of preserving and increasing muscular strength and endurance. Resistance exercise has been shown to improve glycemic control as well as many of the abnormalities associated with the metabolic syndrome.[17] An older adult also receives the added advantage of preventing accidental falls and increased mobility. This can allow an elderly person to remain more independent and self-sufficient.[18]

Flexibility Exercises

Stretching should be considered an option to include in the fitness plan for treatment of diabetes. While recent studies may place doubt on whether this type of exercise protects an individual from injury,[19] movements of this type can provide other fitness benefits. Research performed on tai chi[20] and yoga[21] reported improvements to the participant's cardiovascular fitness level, and a systematic review of the use of yoga suggested that it may aid in the management of cardiovascular disease and other insulin-resistant conditions.[22] Both of these modalities use basic stretching movements as part of the instruction. In addition, flexibility programs are easy to perform and may provide the perfect introduction toward a more physically active lifestyle.

Physiological Responses to Physical Activity: Understanding Changes Associated With Blood Glucose Levels

Blood glucose levels change during and after physical activity. The physiological responses associated with these changes in blood glucose readings are detailed in the paragraphs that follow.

Cases in Point: Facilitating Self-Management of Physical Activity

Type 2 Diabetes

DK was a 62-year-old mother of three. She was diagnosed with gestational diabetes mellitus during her third pregnancy. She had learned then that her risk of developing type 2 diabetes would be higher. She told herself that she would take off the 80 lb that had accumulated over 3 pregnancies. But the years went by and she found that her days were full working as a dental hygienist, being a wife, and raising 3 children and 40 more pounds were added. Thus, she was not surprised when she was diagnosed with type 2 diabetes 6 years ago when seeking treatment for recurrent vaginal yeast infections. While she had been happy to see 60 lb come off the scale over the previous year, she knew her thirst, fatigue, and blurry vision were not good signs. A blood glucose value of 370 mg/dL confirmed her suspicions. She was immediately started on metformin (Glucophage).

Type 1 Diabetes

HW was a 48-year-old telecommunications manager, married, and a father of two. Athletic throughout his life, his family time often included sports or outdoor pursuits. So everyone was shocked when he was told at age 45 that he had diabetes. He was first treated for type 2 diabetes. When his blood glucose levels did not improve on oral agents, his wife convinced him to see his healthcare provider. Hugh then had autoimmunity tests performed and was diagnosed with type 1 diabetes.

To be honest, he was somewhat relieved. Hugh had been exercising to the best of his ability, eating almost nothing, and his blood glucose levels were even higher. He had been ready to accept the fact that hiking, camping, hunting, biking, kayaking, and ice hockey refereeing were all a thing of the past. The diagnosis of type 1 diabetes explained why his blood glucose levels had stayed so high. He was immediately started on insulin therapy and hoped he could continue the active lifestyle he and his family enjoyed.

As Physical Activity Begins. The breakdown of adenosine triphosphate (ATP) by the enzyme myosin ATPase produces the energy necessary for muscle contraction. ATP needs to be replenished continuously. This process is accomplished during the breakdown of carbohydrates, fats, and proteins by muscle fibers. During the first few minutes of physical activity, intramuscular glucose is broken down anaerobically (without oxygen present). Although this pathway does not provide an abundant quantity of ATP, the pathway is important at the onset of physical activity when oxygen availability is limited. As physical activity continues, an adequate supply of oxygen becomes available for the aerobic breakdown of carbohydrates, fats, and proteins.[5]

After 5 to 10 Minutes. During sustained movement, carbohydrate, protein, and fat continually recharge the phosphate pool. After the first 5 to 10 minutes, muscle glycogen breakdown decreases, as circulating glucose from glucose being broken down in the liver becomes a major fuel source (hepatic glycogenolysis).[5]

Beyond 20 Minutes. As exercise continues beyond 20 to 30 minutes, the muscles' glycogen stores are depleted. Blood glucose is now maintained by hepatic glycogenolysis and utilization of triglycerides mobilized from adipose tissue (free fatty acids, or FFA). This marks an important transition from the beginning of exercise, when hepatic glycogenolysis was the major provider of fuel. Now, as physical exertion continues, gluconeogenesis becomes increasingly important in providing the glucose required for fuel. The main substrates for hepatic gluconeogenesis during physical exertion are lactate, amino acids, and glycerol.[5]

Longer Duration. As exercise duration increases, the contribution of FFA for fuel increases relative to glucose. Exercise of low-to-moderate intensity relies primarily on FFA as the oxidative fuel for muscle. The oxidation of fat-derived fuels cannot replace the utilization of glucose. When carbohydrate is limited, fat is not completely oxidized and ketone bodies are formed.[5]

Hypoglycemia

Assessing Risk for Hypoglycemia

Being physically active is extremely beneficial to general health, important in diabetes prevention, and an essential self-management behavior for those with diabetes. However, due to differences in pathophysiology and treatment options, physical activity affects blood glucose differently in type 1 and type 2 diabetes. Understanding these differences helps the diabetes educator identify and avoid common blood glucose concerns with physical activity.

Modern pharmacological regimens for people with diabetes vary greatly based on the individual's needs. Today, the regimens used to treat type 2 diabetes often include combinations of different classes of antihyperglycemic agents. Each class of medication has its own list of potential side effects. Since hypoglycemia is the most common concern associated with physical activity by people with diabetes, the patient must understand whether the potential of this side effect exists within the diabetes medication regimen in use.

Insulin—found in pharmacological treatment regimens for both type 1 and type 2 diabetes—is the medication that poses the greatest risk for hypoglycemia. In contrast, an individual with type 2 diabetes who is not prescribed any diabetes medications carries little risk of experiencing the symptoms associated with hypoglycemia. Even so, the degree of risk associated with hypoglycemia varies from person to person. During assessment, the educator must identify other variables that may contribute to or protect the individual from hypoglycemia (ie, elevated A1C, near-normal A1C, usual timing of activity, type or duration of diabetes, typical food preferences). At times, the best risk indicator for hypoglycemia is the individual's own personal experience. When the risk does exist, strategies to prevent hypoglycemia during physical activity need to be reviewed.

Help patients understand their individualized risk for hypoglycemia

Risk of hypoglycemia varies from person to person. Those with type 2 diabetes who take no diabetes medications have little risk and will be relieved to hear it. Those who take insulin have the greatest risk. At times, the best indicator is the individual's past experience.

When the risk of hypoglycemia *does not* exist, it is just as important to communicate this information to the patient and family members. This eliminates a perceived barrier to a physically active lifestyle. The person with diabetes will no longer harbor the fears or have concerns about what they have heard about physical activity and hypoglycemia.

Table 14.5 can be used as a reference to categorize prescription diabetes medications and identify those that place the user at risk for hypoglycemia. In addition to the medications listed in the table, diabetes educators and other clinicians must be aware of the possibility of a hypoglycemia side effect from other medications the person may be taking and from diabetes medications that are new on the market. Steroids and β-adrenergic blocking agents are just 2 other classes of prescription medications that need to be considered when interpreting an individual's blood glucose response to physical exertion.

TABLE 14.5 Risk of Hypoglycemia Side Effects With Various Diabetes Medications

Not At Risk	*At Risk*
Acarbose: Precose	Glimepiride: Amaryl
Metformin and combinations with metformin: Glucophage Avandamet (metformin/ rosiglitizone)	Glipizide and combinations with glipizide: Glucotrol, Glucotrol XL Metaglip (glipizide/ metformin)
Miglitol: Glyset Pioglitazone: Actos Rosiglitizone: Avandia	Glyburide and combinations with glyburide: Diabeta Glynase Micronase Pres Tab Glucovance (glyburide/ metformin)
	Nateglinide: Starlix
	Repaglinide: Prandin
	Insulin: All types and delivery methods

Note: Well-known brand names are listed under the generic names—read carefully. Also, consider new diabetes medications that may not be listed and medications prescribed for diabetes complications or other conditions.

Establishing Blood Glucose Goals

Once the individual understands if he or she is at risk for hypoglycemia, the next step is establishing reasonable blood glucose goals for physical activity. This process engages the individual's problem-solving skills, another of the AADE 7 Self-Care Behaviors™.[3] The educator must gear the complexity of these steps to the individual's abilities. Additional complications or circumstances that may have an effect also must be considered. For example, gastroparesis may already exist, making blood glucose levels erratic. If the individual has hypoglycemia unawareness, additional blood glucose readings may be helpful. Or if more blood glucose readings can not be performed due to finances or the individual's unwillingness to do so, other options should be explored to make sure any risk, and the risks associated with hypoglycemia, are minimized. Modifications may, for example, factor in the following: exercising after meals, shorter duration of physical activity, highest blood glucose level of the day, or exercising in the presence of trained helpers.

The personal history of the individual can help the educator establish reasonable blood glucose goals for physical activity. If none exists, these guidelines are a good starting point:

- *Using diabetes medication with hypoglycemia side effect:* Keep level above 90 mg/dL
- *Using insulin:* Keep level above 110 mg/dL
- *With other complications or circumstances:* Keep level above 120 mg/dL
- *Using oral agents that do not cause hypoglycemia or not on medication for diabetes:* No threshold is necessary

Adjusting Facets of the Diabetes Regimen to Accommodate Physical Activity

To keep the blood glucose above the goal before, during, and after the physical activity, most people will need to consider making adjustments to another part of the diabetes regimen. These adjustments are intended to either

- *Increase the amount of glucose* available through the blood glucose (additional carbohydrates), or
- *Reduce the amount of insulin* circulating during physical activity (medication adjustments)

Both strategies result in the blood glucose level "drifting" higher for a short period of time. However, once the physical activity begins, this glucose will be used to fuel the energy needs of the active muscles.

Questions to Ask. Including questions in the assessment process to determine what the person with diabetes has already tried is very helpful. Often, the person understands basic concepts, but has not implemented them correctly. The person may know to check blood glucose more often, eat a snack, or adjust the insulin dose, but still not see the desired blood glucose readings. Below are some appropriate points for discussion.

Troubleshoot hypoglycemia with questions

When are the blood glucose readings being measured? Often, the blood glucose numbers being reported were taken hours before or after the physical activity was done. The person needs to check within minutes of starting and ending to get more accurate information.

Is hypoglycemia a possibility or a concern? If so, ask for an extra reading to be taken during the physical activity. Sometimes, higher blood glucose readings after the workout are caused by unrecognized hypoglycemia during the workout. If this is the cause, discuss a plan to prevent hypoglycemia.

Was a snack eaten? If so, was it enough and was it eaten at the correct time? If not, should a snack be included in the future?

Why is the blood glucose higher after the physical exertion? There are a few possibilities for this blood glucose response:

- *How much did blood glucose increase?* Get specifics. If the level went from 105 mg/dL to117 mg/dL, that still reflects excellent results! If the level went from 209 mg/dL to 277 mg/dL, the person has an A1C of 11% and is trying to avoid insulin: this describes the other extreme.
- *Could this be the individual's normal response?* This can be a "catch 22" for some people during physical activity. While glucose is in demand as a fuel, it is also being released to keep the supply available. For some people, supply can exceed demand. This is also a normal response to very vigorous types of physical activity. Fortunately, this is short-lived and blood glucose usually drops within an hour or so. This response does not erase other fitness benefits, but the individual may feel discouraged or concerned about doing harm. The educator should direct attention to other health outcomes to help the individual recognize the benefits, which include, for example, weight loss, less medication, better A1C, and improved lipids.
- *What role does food have on the blood glucose response?* Sometimes the person does not consider a meal or snack that was eaten, or sometimes the person has eaten later or more food than usual. If this is the cause, the blood glucose reading will probably be better than it would have been if the person had not been physically active. This may not require any changes, only explanations.
- *Has this only happened once?* A single occurrence may not repeat itself. Just like many blood glucose readings, it may not be useful for clinical consideration.

Cases—Part 2: Activity's Effect on Blood Glucose

Type 2 Diabetes

When diagnosed with type 2 diabetes, DK decided to start exercising. She was motivated to lose a lot of weight (the faster, the better). She remembered when she was active and able to enjoy dancing, exercise classes, and playing games with her children. She was not sure how that person got lost, but was determined to find her again!

- She was cleared by her healthcare provider, who told her any weight loss would improve her hypertension and hyperlipidemia
- She heard from a friend that a snack was important to eat before exercise—to keep her blood glucose from going too low
- She remembered that metformin (Glucophage) did not cause low blood glucose levels, but was not sure what to do for exercise

To be safe, she ate a package of 4 peanut butter nabs before walking a mile around her neighborhood. She became frustrated when she figured out she ate 130 calories, but walked off only 100. Also, her blood glucose readings seemed higher after her walk. To her, this made no sense!

Type 1 Diabetes

HW was eager to do what he needed to take care of his diabetes. He was also happy to start back into his fitness routine. He liked to workout in the evenings. This was when he could get to the health club and when he usually refereed hockey games.

- He read that hypoglycemia would be prevented by exercising after a meal. Because eating food makes the blood glucose go higher and exercise makes it drop, he figured everything would come out even.

Twenty-five minutes into his workout, however, HW had to stop and treat blood glucose of 57 mg/dL. This was not what he expected!

Interpreting Hyperglycemia

In some circumstances, extremely high blood glucose readings can lead to other medical concerns. Higher blood glucose readings could be an indication of insulin deficiency. People with type 2 diabetes can have high blood glucose readings often from a combination of insulin resistance and inadequate insulin secretion. Extremely elevated glucose with severe dehydration can result in hyperosmolar hyperglycemia (see chapter 8, on hyperglycemia). When hyperosmolar hyperglycemia does occur, it is mitigated by other extenuating health issues (eg, dehydration, severe illness, infections). Individuals with type 2 diabetes typically do not produce ketones; if ketones do exist, often it is termed starvation ketosis, as opposed to insulin deficiency and acidosis. People with type 1 diabetes are more susceptible to insulin deficiency since they lack the ability to produce any insulin in their pancreas; therefore, they need to receive instruction on why and when to check for the production of ketones. This is especially important if the individual is using an insulin pump. If ketones are present, then the higher blood glucose levels are a result of insulin deficiency and corrective action should be taken immediately.

Based on this medical concern, most diabetes educators teach people with type 1 diabetes to check for ketones with blood glucose levels above 250 mg/dL.[23] This advice can only be followed by the individual with diabetes when a blood glucose value is measured. Most readings are performed to determine an insulin dose for a meal or snack. These are usually the lower blood glucose levels of the day. When the blood glucose is being measured for physical activity, it must be taken at different times of day. Therefore, the individual with diabetes may be seeing a normal blood glucose response to a meal and consider it too high for physical activity. In the absence of ketones, these higher readings should not pose a medical threat.[24] However, some people report headaches, blurry vision, or lack of energy with these blood glucose results, which are reasons in themselves to avoid physical activity until the level improves.

Modern insulin regimens paired with frequent blood glucose measurements greatly diminish the chance of insulin deficiency developing. Therefore, ketones are rarely found when performing blood or urine checks. In these circumstances, the blood glucose levels should not interfere with performance of the physical activity. The individual's problem-solving skills again become important. The educator must consider the ability of the individual to perform this testing and understand the complexity of the information.

On the other hand, physical activity performed at very intense aerobic levels (>80% of maximum oxygen consumption, $\dot{V}O_2max$) can result in blood glucose levels climbing higher with type 1 diabetes.[25] In this circumstance, the catecholamine response to very intense exertion results in an exaggerated release of glucose for fuel. When the activity is completed, the insulin need can double

Cases—Part 3: Learning to Make Appropriate Adjustments

Type 2 Diabetes

Snacks and Timing

DK thought about her preexercise snack and decided she did not need the peanut butter nabs before walking. However, she was still concerned about hypoglycemia and decided only to walk after she had eaten a meal. Sometimes this worked in her schedule, and sometimes it did not. When she was able to fit in a walk, DK noticed that her blood glucose levels had dropped when she finished. She was also glad she could skip all of those extra calories. Yet she was sure she would have to walk a lot more to lose weight.

Type 1 Diabetes

Insulin Dose Adjustments

HW remembered being told that he may need to reduce his insulin dose before he exercised. The next time he went to the health club, he took 1 unit away from his 10-unit dose. He thought the blood glucose of 154 mg/dL before his workout was high enough and hoped to see it drop. And did it drop—but too fast, and 15 minutes into his workout he had to stop and treat another low blood glucose. This time is was 63 mg/dL. He decided to reduce his insulin by half next time. He was alarmed, though, when his blood glucose reading the next night was 287 mg/dL before his workout. He remembered something about not exercising if his blood glucose was over 250 mg/dL and he had positive ketones. Since he did not have ketone strips with him, he skipped the workout. He went home not knowing what to do.

during the postexertion period. If not met with the correct insulin dosing, this state of hyperglycemia may last for several hours for an individual with type 1 diabetes before returning to the desired level.[26] The individual will observe and report higher meter readings at the end and for a few hours after the physical exertion ends. This pattern of hyperglycemia needs to be confirmed and be fairly predictable before suggesting that any action be taken. When appropriate, those using insulin pump therapy sometimes find it useful to bolus a small amount of insulin to address this physiological need. If the individual is injecting insulin by syringe, an additional insulin injection can also be considered. The timing and amount of insulin need careful consideration and monitoring to accomplish the desired blood glucose result. Regardless of the delivery method, this additional insulin dose can still result in hypoglycemia and may not be advisable.

Self-Management Strategies for Safe Physical Activity

Adding Carbohydrates

Snacking is the easiest adjustment for laypeople to understand and a strategy those with diabetes often implement by themselves. Unfortunately, estimating the amount of food needed can be difficult. When the snack is not sufficient, hypoglycemia can still happen. Or a snack that is larger than necessary may be eaten. When weight loss is an expectation of the fitness plan, both of these circumstances can result in more total calories being eaten, and when enough calories are consumed, weight gain will result instead of the desired weight loss.

Monitoring. Blood glucose monitoring is useful to determine if and when a snack is required to keep the glucose above the established goal.

Encourage monitoring for problem solving regarding physical activity

Blood glucose readings taken at the *start* and *end* of the exertion allow the individual to gauge the amount of change happening during physical activity and determine if additional carbohydrates are needed. For example, if blood glucose usually drops between 30 to 40 mg/dL during a physical activity and the goal is to stay above 90 mg/dL, a preexertion snack should be eaten with a reading below 130 mg/dL.

To prevent hypoglycemia, a snack containing 15 to 30 g of carbohydrate should be consumed for every 30 to 60 minutes of physical activity (see Table 14.6).

TABLE 14.6 Carbohydrate Replacement During Physical Activity

Intensity	*Duration*	*Carbohydrate Replacement*	*Frequency*
Mild-to-moderate	<30 minutes	May not be needed	—
Moderate	30 to 60 minutes	15 g	Each hour
High	60+ minutes	30 to 50 g	Each hour

Source: Franz MJ. Nutrition: can it give athletes with diabetes a boost? Diabetes Educ. 1991;17:163-72.

Type of Snack. The snack option needs to meet the fuel needs of the physical activity. Often, people with diabetes choose to consume juice or glucose tabs at the start of the physical activity; they know these options are used to treat hypoglycemic events and assume they are useful to prevent them as well. These rarely work because the glucose provided by these options is absorbed and used very quickly.

Snacks to prevent hypoglycemia should not be the same as those used to treat it

In *preventing* hypoglycemia, a snack with more fiber, fat, or protein may be a better match for the fuel requirements of physical activity than juice or glucose tabs (snacks used to *treat* hypoglycemia). For example, an apple may be a better option than apple juice, or a fruit-flavored yogurt may work better than an apple. The best snack option should be based on when the desired blood glucose level is achieved during physical activity.

Timing of Snack. The next consideration is timing: when the snack should be eaten.

- *If activity is being performed after a meal or usual snack.* No extra food may be needed. If more food is required, the amount of carbohydrate can be adjusted to achieve the desired blood glucose level.
- *If activity is being performed more than 2 hours after a meal.* The snack should be eaten within 15 minutes of beginning the physical activity. This gives the glucose sufficient time to be digested and enter the bloodstream so it can provide the fuel needed for energy in the active muscles.

Fluids. Water is also a consideration during physical exertion. Replenishing fluids is very important if the physical activity results in excessive perspiration or lasts more than 1 hour. If water is being consumed during the activity, additional carbohydrates can also be introduced as a beverage.[27] Drinks containing less than 8% carbohydrate empty from the stomach more rapidly than drinks with a concentration of carbohydrate greater than 10%. Fruit juices and most regular soft drinks contain approximately 12% carbohydrate and can lead to gastrointestinal upset, such as cramps, nausea, diarrhea, or bloating. This can often be remedied by diluting the beverage or sports drink with water. However, since the carbohydrates in beverages are absorbed quickly, every 5 to 10 minutes a few ounces must be consumed to provide the consistent supply of fuel required for the energy needs of the active muscles. This option also minimizes the total calories consumed. In a beverage, 15 g of carbohydrate equals 60 total calories, while 15 g of carbohydrate in a food option that includes fat or protein can total 150 calories.

Medication Adjustments

Oral Agents. Meglitinides are the only class of oral antihyperglycemic agents that can be adjusted for physical activity. Because repaglinide (Prandin) and nateglinide (Starlix) have short durations of action, these medications can be reduced or omitted if physical activity is planned to occur a few hours after the meal. However, if physical activity is erratic or unpredictable, this option may not be the best to implement.

Insulin Adjustments. When engaging in physical activity, the main focus for the patient using insulin is the blood glucose level.

- If circulating level of insulin is greater than physiological needs, hypoglycemia can occur
- If circulating level of insulin is insufficient, hyperglycemia can result

Problem Solving

Determining the best routine to follow during periods of physical exertion takes time—the individual with diabetes must learn, practice, and problem solve. Often, information from multiple workout sessions is needed as well as frequent blood glucose readings and patience. When appropriate, the individual can wear a continuous glucose monitoring sensor (CGMS). These devices can provide useful information about blood glucose trends before, during, and after the physical activity. The interpretation of this information can lead to a better understanding of the insulin and snacking adjustments required to support the energy needs of physical exertion.

In addition, the educator must consider that the routine will vary from person to person. Each person's responses will be different, due to the following:

- Type of diabetes
- Type and delivery method of insulin
- Time of day
- Type and duration of physical activity
- Fitness level of individual
- Many other factors contributing to the blood glucose response to physical activity

Because many of these factors can change over time for the individual, from visit to visit the educator needs to ensure the routine continues to fit the physiological needs. The following must be regularly reconsidered:

- Seasonal variations
- Weight loss or gain
- Improved or decreased fitness levels
- Changes to medication dosing

Benefits Gained Can Quickly Diminish

Beneficial effects of physical activity diminish quickly if activity does not occur on a regular basis. Support patients to ensure benefits continue.

Many strategies can be considered to prevent hypoglycemia during physical activity

- *Blood Glucose Monitoring.* Monitoring before and after a period of physical activity provides needed feedback for the individual learning to adjust insulin and/or carbohydrate while active. While readings done at the start and end of exertion are the most common to gather, to identify trends it may be necessary to check 45 minutes prior to exertion, in the midst of exercise, or for a few hours after completion.
- *Adjusting the Insulin.* Hepatic glucose production is blocked or partially inhibited by exogenous insulin.[28] The physiological decrease in circulating insulin levels that occurs with physical activity does not take place in persons treated with insulin. The person may need to reduce the rapid-acting or short-acting insulin dose administered prior to the exertion by 30% to 50%.[29,30] A dose administered within an hour after the exertion is completed may also need to be decreased.
- *Proper Administration of Insulin.* Insulin should be injected into the subcutaneous fat layer. Syringe users should be taught to avoid intramuscular injection of insulin because muscle contractions accelerate the absorption of insulin into the circulation.[31]

Although changing the injection site to a part of the body not involved in the activity was recommended based on published reports in the 1970s,[32] this has not been shown to be effective in preventing hypoglycemia. If the level of circulating insulin is elevated for any reason, hypoglycemia is likely to occur. Dose reductions should accompany any physical activity performed during the peak action of the insulin.[30]

- *Individualized Adjustments.* Adjustments should be tailored to the specific response to physical activity of each individual (Table 14.7). The choices depend on the individual's goals and may require using a combination of both strategies (additional carbohydrates and insulin adjustments).

Hypoglycemia often occurs several hours after physical exertion and is a significant concern to the individual treated with insulin. This is the result of acutely increased insulin mobilization and sensitivity, increased glucose utilization, replenishment of glycogen stores, and defective counterregulatory mechanisms.[33] When this response is recognized, these options are useful in minimizing future occurrences:

- Educate the patient about the possible cause of hypoglycemia
- Reduce insulin doses as needed following physical exertion
- Increase the amount of carbohydrate consumed after physical exertion
- Limit physical activity prior to bedtime
- Monitor blood glucose more often following physical exertion

Insulin Pump Therapy. With insulin pump therapy, basal rates and boluses can be adjusted based on the timing, duration, and type of activity performed. The amount of insulin decrease or the amount of carbohydrate supplement depends on an individual's fitness level and the duration and intensity of the activity. Insulin pump users have these options to prevent hypoglycemia during periods of physical activity:

- Reduce the basal infusion rate
- Consume additional carbohydrates
- Temporarily suspend pump use (see "Being Active" in chapter 17 for details)

TABLE 14.7 Options for Adjusting Therapy to Prevent Hypoglycemia With Physical Activity

Adjust *insulin* for:
• Weight loss (may require less insulin) • Improved control (may require more or less insulin) • Planned, regularly scheduled physical activity
Adjust with additional *carbohydrate* if:
• Preexertion blood glucose level is not sufficient • Long duration of physical activity is planned • Unplanned or erratic physical activity schedule • Oral hypoglycemic medication is prescribed

As suggested in this chapter, many strategies can be used to prevent hypoglycemia during physical activity. Table 14.7 compares the insulin and snack adjustment options and suggests when they may be best to use. While one option may be preferred by or for an individual, there will be situations when the opposite, or a combination of both of these strategies, aid in achieving the desired blood glucose results.

The Exercise Prescription

The exercise prescription is simply the plan a person is to follow to attain physical fitness. The most difficult aspect for the clinician is designing a plan that meets the desired physical fitness goals. A well-designed exercise prescription is based on technical and evidence-based research. Over the decades, the exercise prescription has been adapted as new information has been reported. Sometimes these changes can seem unreasonable or impossible for most laypersons to achieve. The true artistry of the exercise prescription is found in simplifying its core messages to realistic situations that can be performed as part of everyday life. This requires the educator to understand the 4 components of an exercise prescription:

- Intensity
- Mode
- Frequency
- Duration

Determining Acceptable Intensity

Determining the intensity of the physical activity takes the most care and attention for people with diabetes. This does not mean the harder the workout, the better the results. Rather, the intensity level of the physical activity must be matched to the individual's current fitness capabilities. An activity period that is too easy will not have the intended effect on the fitness level. If it is too hard, the individual will not be able to complete the workout.

Determining Appropriate Modes

The type of physical activity chosen by the patient is in many ways less crucial than other components of the

Cases—Part 4: Adjusting Workout Intensity

DK decided she would just have to walk longer to burn off calories and improve her blood glucose level. She decided to walk 60 minutes each day she was able to fit in her walk. She was sure this would work, until she tried it. After 40 minutes, she was not even sure she was going to make it home. When she walked into her house, she felt very shaky and checked her blood glucose. It was 104 mg/dL—the lowest number she had seen it yet. She immediately went to the freezer and pulled out the ice cream. To top off her woes, her right hip was in severe pain for days. She surely was not going to put herself through that again!

exercise prescription. While the mode of physical activity (ie, cardiovascular, strength training, flexibility exercises) is important to consider, any type of increased movement appears to initially improve the fitness level.[34] The literature consistently reports that any group of sedentary individuals participating in physical activity sees measurable results in the fitness level.

As such, a wide range of physical activities can be explored and made part of the fitness plan. All opportunities the individual can identify should be assessed and, if safe to perform, encouraged. As the individual becomes more successful and confident, options can be expanded and other types of physical activities explored. See chapter 30, on being active, for more on strategies in support of this self-management behavior.

Determining Acceptable Frequency and Duration

Physical activity sessions can be performed in a variety of combinations in terms of frequency and duration.[34]

- *Frequency.* Most research concludes that physical activity should be performed 3 to 5 days per week.
- *Duration.* Varying the duration of the fitness session has been investigated. While 20 minutes has long been the minimal recommendation to provide cardiovascular improvements, multiple shorter bouts of 10 minutes, repeated to equal 30 total minutes, have also resulted in measurable improvements.[35] Longer bouts of physical activity, lasting 60 minutes or more, may be required to achieve weight loss or to prevent weight regain.[36]

While each individual's needs and goals are varied, evidence-based research can assist in the design of a program for health-related physical fitness. Special considerations for children, teens, and the elderly are discussed below.

Expecting Progress in Stages

In the United States, most people lead sedentary lifestyles.[37] Many people do not think about, or think it even possible, to spend 60 minutes per day doing any type of physical activity. Diabetes educators must, therefore, provide realistic instruction that includes both how to start a fitness program and what to reasonably expect in terms of progress[34] (see Table 14.8). While working on fitness level improvements, the individual must understand what type of progress to expect, how much, and when. Over a period averaging at least 4 months, each individual moves through 3 distinct stages in developing and using a fitness plan:

Initial Stage
in which habits are established
↓
Improvement Stage
in which progress is seen, but habits may weaken
↓
Maintenance Stage
in which extensions are planned

Initial Stage. Most people never make it out of this critical stage. They either attempt activities too difficult for their fitness level or develop unrealistic expectations for what they will be able to accomplish. They quickly become discouraged and stop. The real success from this initial stage is for the individual to begin forming physical activity habits that integrate into his or her lifestyle.

- Help the individual understand that measurable changes may not occur during this period. Building fitness habits takes at least 4 weeks and may be longer in individuals who start with very poor fitness levels.

Improvement Stage. During this second stage, the focus shifts from developing habits to improving the fitness level. The individual now has more stamina and endurance, is able to spend longer amounts of time doing

Habit Formation: the Initial Goal

In the first 4 weeks or so of a fitness plan, the goal is not to achieve measurable changes in fitness, but rather to establish habits that will make fitness progress possible.

TABLE 14.8 Sedentary Individual's Rate of Progression in the 3 Stages of a Physical Activity Program

Program Stage	*Week*	*Frequency (per week)*	*Intensity (% HRR, heart rate reserve)*	*Duration (minutes)*
Initial	1–4	3–4	40%–60%	15–30
Improvement	5–24	3–5	60%–85%	25–40
Maintenance	24+	3–5	70%–85%	20–60

physical activity, and can begin adding to the workload or intensity of the workout. Over the 3 or more months of this stage, measurable health benefits should start to be observed. However, individuals can interpret this initial success as permanent change, which may sabotage their efforts. The individual may allow other routine parts of everyday life to take priority again and start missing workout sessions.

- Identify and seek progress in fitness goals
- Once improvements begin to show, help the person avoid slacking off; foster success beyond the first milestone and for the long term

Maintenance Stage. Once an individual has successfully met the major goals originally defined, new goals and a new plan need to be developed. The new goal may be as simply stated as "preventing weight regain" or as challenging as "training for a competitive event."

- Review goals routinely at medical and diabetes education visits
- Reassess for medication changes, new diagnosis, or progression of existing disease to ensure the fitness routine continues to be safe and effective
- Develop new goals and plans once existing ones are achieved

Special Populations

Children and Teens

Physical activity has a direct impact on weight control, cardiovascular risk factors, bone development, and mental health. A sedentary lifestyle in young people is often seen to lead to negative health consequences in the near term and later in life.

- *Frequency and Duration.* For the pediatric population, 30 minutes of physical activity performed on most days of the week is the general guideline.[38]
- *Mode.* Care should be taken to identify safe and age-appropriate options for physical activity. Options evolve as the individual undergoes normal transformations in coordination, motor skills, social development, and personal interests.
- *Assigned Responsibilities.* Responsibility for diabetes care decisions also evolves; teenagers begin to take on more of the responsibility and seek independence from parental supervision. Diabetes counseling should include clear assignment of the expected tasks to be performed and distribution of these care responsibilities.
- *Hypoglycemia Prevention.* The blood glucose changes that occur during physical activity need to be addressed for anyone at risk of hypoglycemia. This also holds true in the pediatric population. One research study confirmed lower starting blood glucose levels increased the incidence of hypoglycemia.[39] Hypoglycemia occurred in 86% of subjects performing a 75-minute physical activity session when starting blood glucose values were less than 120 mg/dL, in 13% of subjects when starting glucose was 120 to 180 mg/dL, and in 6% of subjects when starting glucose was 180 mg/dL. The study also revealed that a 15-g carbohydrate snack was often not enough to successfully treat a hypoglycemic event. This study reinforces the necessity of beginning at a blood glucose level and consuming a sufficient amount of carbohydrate in order to decrease the risk of experiencing a hypoglycemic episode during physical activity.

Elderly Adults

Elderly adults who have been primarily sedentary and may have physical limitations present a challenge for diabetes educators. Getting an elderly person to do any kind of physical activity can benefit not only blood glucose control, but also muscle tone, flexibility, and outlook. Yard work and housework are activities many people feel comfortable doing.

- *Frequency and Intensity.* Generally, what is important is that the elderly individual engage in some physical activity each day. Setting goals that this population can reach is most important. For example, a very sedentary elderly person may be able to walk for 5 minutes for 3 days a week and increase that by 1 to 2 minutes per week.

- *Safety.* Safety is an issue as well. Safety concerns may preclude someone from walking if there is a high risk for falls and subsequent fracture. Options may include using a stationary bicycle, lifting light weights, or exercising while seated. Exercise videos, classes, and routines that can be done from a chair, rather than standing, may be helpful.

Medical Considerations

Preactivity Medical Exam and Assessment

Individuals diagnosed with diabetes should consult a healthcare provider before beginning any physical fitness program. The medical examination conducted before a new physical activity or fitness program is begun has a variety of components.[40] Information gathered during this preparticipation exam, or chart review of the health information, provides the basis for outcome of this medical consultation.

Often, other comorbidities exist that affect the intended fitness regimen more than the diagnosis of diabetes. In the diabetes population, cardiovascular disease, neuropathy, nephropathy, and retinopathy are found more frequently; many clinicians, therefore, include additional consideration for these comorbidities to determine if they exist and/or the degree of progression that has occurred. Factoring in comorbidities and other relevant health considerations, the medical advice provided can contribute to the safest design of the exercise prescription. Table 14.9 lists the general categories to be considered during this examination.

TABLE 14.9 Components of the Preparticipation Medical Exam

Measurement of • Body weight (BMI, waist girth, body composition) • Apical pulse rate and rhythm • Resting blood pressure (seated, supine, standing)
Auscultation of • Lungs, with specific attention to uniformity of breath sounds in all areas (absence of rales, wheezes, and other breathing sounds) • Heart, with specific attention to murmurs, gallops, clicks, rubs • Carotid, abdominal, and femoral arteries
Palpitation of • Cardiac apical impulse, point of maximal impulse (PMI) • Carotid, abdominal, and femoral arteries • Inspection of lower extremities for edema and presence of arterial pulses
Evaluation of • Abdomen, for bowel sounds, masses, visceromegaly, and tenderness • Absence or presence of tendon xanthoma and skin xanthelasma • Tests of neurological function, including reflexes and cognition • Skin inspection, especially lower extremity in patients with diabetes
Follow-up exam related to orthopedic or other medical conditions that would limit exercise

Cases—Part 5: Obtaining Medical Clearance

DK called her healthcare provider about the hip pain she had from walking. She was sure the type 2 diabetes was now causing some other problems and was afraid she was going to lose her leg. Once her healthcare provider calmed her down, DK was scheduled to have a few medical tests. She learned that diabetes was not the reason for her hip pain; she had some arthritis in her hips. She was told that while the arthritis would cause some discomfort, weight loss could help. Now exercise was more important for her than ever.

Cardiovascular Disease

Cardiovascular disease is the major cause of morbidity and mortality for people with diabetes.[41] As such, a careful cardiac assessment is warranted prior to initiating any fitness program. Existence of any cardiac risk factors should be determined and emphasis should be placed on their treatment so cardiovascular disease can be prevented and/or slowed. When a fitness program that exceeds the demands of everyday living (more intense than brisk walking) is being considered for a previously sedentary individual, the American Diabetes Association has established criteria[24] to help determine if a graded exercise test is warranted (Table 14.10).

Neuropathy

The main forms of diabetic neuropathy present themselves as autonomic neuropathy, peripheral neuropathy, and gastroparesis.[42]

TABLE 14.10 Criteria for Graded Exercise Test, from American Diabetes Association

Age >40 years, with or without CVD risk factors other than diabetes
Age >30 years and • Type 1 or 2 diabetes of >10 years' duration • Hypertension • Cigarette smoking • Dyslipidemia • Proliferative or preproliferative retinopathy • Nephropathy, including microalbuminuria
Any of the following, regardless of age • Known or suspected CAD, cerebrovascular disease, and/or peripheral vascular disease • Autonomic neuropathy • Advanced nephropathy with renal failure

Source: Sigal RJ, Kenny GP, Wasserman DH, Castaneda-Sceppa C. Physical activity/exercise and type 2 diabetes. Diabetes Care. 2004;27:2518–39.

Autonomic Neuropathy. When the autonomic nerves of the cardiac system are affected, it represents a very serious complication. The heart rate response is abnormal at rest, when standing, and when performing a Valsalva maneuver. The blood pressure response is also abnormal when changing positions or performing isometric exercise. The individual does not have the physical stamina to perform prolonged periods of exertion. Cardiac autonomic neuropathy carries a very poor prognosis and greatly increases mortality. Therefore, care must be taken with all components of the exercise prescription.

Peripheral Neuropathy. Peripheral neuropathy, with the associated decrease in sensation, carries with it a greater risk of injury. The individual does not have the pain sensation needed to recognize that an injury has occurred. Repeated trauma to a bone or blister is not noticed. Also, sensations connected to balance and strength can be diminished. The gait can be altered, contributing to development of orthopedic issues. The individual may become fearful of falling. Walking, standing, or getting out of a chair can be difficult. Safety must be the prime consideration of the exercise prescription.

Gastroparesis. Gastroparesis produces physically uncomfortable and sometimes potentially embarrassing episodes for the individual with this complication. Common complaints are nausea, vomiting, feeling "stuffed" after eating, bloating, intestinal pain, and lack of appetite. Any of these can make physical activity difficult to perform. Medications and foods must be balanced as part of the exercise prescription to help minimize these symptoms.

Table 14.11 lists the special considerations for physical activity that should accompany each of these forms of neuropathy. When progression of these symptoms presents safety issues, a clinically supervised exercise setting may be prudent. When this option is not available, self-monitoring is important; the person must be able to make appropriate decisions independently when engaged in physical activity.

Nephropathy

The intensity of the physical activity is the main consideration of the exercise prescription when nephropathy is present.[43] This is because of the linear association of the blood pressure response to the intensity of the exertion. As the workload being performed with physical activity increases, the blood pressure response also increases. Light to moderate physical activity, with an acceptable blood pressure response, is generally considered safe and beneficial in those with incipient nephropathy or microalbuminuria (urinary albumin excretion rates >20 to 200 mcg per minute). For those with overt nephropathy or clinical albuminuria (>200 mcg per minute), strenuous physical activity (>70% maximum heart rate, HRmax, or >60% $\dot{V}O_2$max) is not prudent due to the exaggerated blood pressure response in this population.

The risk for developing specific comorbidities increases as nephropathy progresses. Often, the individual with overt nephropathy has diminished capacity for physical exertion, causing a self-limitation of strenuous physical activity. Yet, people at all stages of nephropathy can benefit from staying physically active. Table 14.12 provides information highlighting these considerations for the exercise prescription.

Retinopathy

The presence of retinopathy should be evaluated for all patients with diabetes, based on established clinical guidelines.[44] People without diabetic retinopathy or who have only mild nonproliferative diabetic retinopathy (NPDR) do not have activity limitations. Those with moderate, severe, and very severe NPDR and those with proliferative diabetic retinopathy should be educated on the limitations for activity, including exercise as well as routine activities. Macular edema and glaucoma should be evaluated by an ophthalmologist or optometrist, with activity guidelines determined by the results of the examination. More specific information is provided in Table 14.13 for the different levels of retinopathy.

TABLE 14.11 Physical Activity Considerations When Neuropathy is Present

Type of Neuropathy	*Safety Concern Associated With Type of Neuropathy*	*Action to Discuss*
Autonomic	Inability to recognize signs and symptoms of hypoglycemia	Monitor blood glucose during physical activity; set higher blood glucose goals
	Blunted heart rate response to exertion	Monitor intensity with Ratings of Perceived Exertion (RPE) or "Talk" Test
	Erratic blood pressure response during exercise, increased risk of postural hypotension	Monitor blood pressure during physical activity; determine if different positions (sitting, standing, reclining, supine) affect results
	Lack of effective thermoregulation for hot and cold environments	Monitor environment, drink fluids to prevent dehydration, wear proper clothing
Peripheral	Discomfort or pain with physical activity	Limit weight-bearing options based on level of tolerance
	Injury, infection, ulceration	Monitor feet daily for blisters, cuts, scrapes; teach proper hygiene techniques for foot and skin care; choose appropriate footwear (shoes and socks); consider need for orthotics or orthopedic shoes
Gastroparesis	Erratic emptying rate of stomach and digestion of food	Monitor blood glucose as needed; use foods absorbed in the mouth to treat hypoglycemia (eg, glucose tabs, glucose gels, hard candies); delay injection of rapid-acting insulin until after exertion
	Discomfort following consumption of a meal or specific type of food	Determine if physical activity impedes or promotes food mobility; plan timing of physical activity as symptoms tolerate

TABLE 14.12 Physical Activity Considerations When Nephropathy is Present

Increased Risk of	*Physical Activity*	*Points to Consider*
Bone disease	Strength training program	Promotes bone strength; improves balance and gait; reduces risk of falls and fractures
Hypertension or exaggerated blood pressure response to exertion	Avoid or modify physical activities that cause extreme increase to systolic blood pressure	BP should be monitored. Medications should be adjusted as needed to keep resting and exercise blood pressure in desired ranges
Edema	As tolerated	Instruction should be provided for dietary and fluid intake to minimize this condition; foot elevation or use of compression stockings may be useful
Anemia	As tolerated	Treat as needed to keep hematocrit levels between 33%–36%
Loss of independence	Promote physically active lifestyle	Increases ability to maintain Activities of Daily Living (ADLs), which may limit dependence on others as disease progresses
Depression	Promote physically active lifestyle	Shown to provide a level of protection from depression, hopelessness, and doom

TABLE 14.13 Physical Activity When Retinopathy is Present: Guidelines and Recommendations

Level of Retinopathy	*Physical Activity and Exercise Recommendations*
No diabetic retinopathy	No physical activity/exercise limitations.
Mild nonproliferative	No physical activity/exercise limitations.
Moderate nonproliferative	Avoid activities that dramatically elevate blood pressure (eg, power lifting).
Severe to very severe nonproliferative	Limit increase in systolic blood pressure (eg, Valsalva maneuvers) and avoid activities that jar the head. Heart rate should not exceed that which elicits a systolic blood pressure response greater than 170 mm Hg (eg, boxing and intense competitive sports).†
Proliferative	Avoid strenuous activity, high-impact activities, Valsalva maneuvers, and activities that jar the head (eg, weight lifting, jogging, high-impact aerobic dance, racquet sports, strenuous trumpet playing, and competitive sports).
Encourage activities that are low-impact and aerobic and stress cardiovascular conditioning (eg, swimming without diving, walking, low-impact aerobic dance, stationary cycling, and endurance exercising).*	

*Aiello LM, Cavallerano J, Aiello LP, Bursell SE. Retinopathy. In: The Health Professional's Guide to Diabetes and Exercise. Ruderman NB, Devlin JT, eds. Alexandria, Va: American Diabetes Association; 1995.

†Graham C, Lasko-McCarthey P. Exercise options for persons with diabetic complications. Diabetes Educ. 1990;16:212-20.

Case Wrap-Up: Education Aids Implementation of Exercise Prescription

Type 2 Diabetes

Identifying Activity Options

DK met with a diabetes educator. During the appointment, she learned more about her diabetes medication and how it did not place her at risk of hypoglycemia. She realized she could exercise whenever she could fit in it her day. The diabetes educator also talked about other options for exercise. They decided it would be best for her to add something else besides walking because of the pain it caused with her hip. DK had a friend who did water aerobics. Plus the diabetes educator gave her information about an exercise program for people with arthritis. She would learn more about those options.

Working Systematically in Stages

The diabetes educator also helped DK chart a plan for how much time to spend exercising. DK then understood she would need to work on her fitness plan for a few months to get her fitness level to where it should be. She would start with a small amount of exercise and add more as she could tolerate it. She promised she would return to talk to the diabetes educator before she tried to add too much. Now DK felt like she was going to be able to get her life back!

Type 1 Diabetes

Data Interpretation and Support

HW went to his follow-up appointment with the diabetes educator. He was sure the educator was going to tell him he would have to stop being active. After all, trying to workout was still making his blood glucose levels worse. The educator's response surprised him. The educator not only explained what happened to HW's blood glucose numbers, but also encouraged him to keep trying. They talked about what he should try and what he should expect to see his blood glucose numbers doing. If he had a problem he could not solve on his own, he was relieved the educator wanted him to call right away. He learned that figuring out the right balance of food, insulin, and workouts would take a little time, but could be done.

Integrating Exercise Prescription into the Education Plan

Diabetes educators are charged with providing instruction related to the various components of physical fitness in the prevention and treatment of diabetes.[45] As the individualized assessment is performed, the educator gathers information useful in addressing the role of physical activity in the self-management plan. Often, physical activity may not be one of the initial outcomes identified by the diabetes educator or individual with diabetes to implement. Many times, other skills or self-care concepts need to be covered in the best interest of the patient or are of more interest to the person with diabetes. When the time presents itself, the diabetes educator can direct the person in planning, implementing, and assessing the impact of the personalized fitness program.

Questions and Controversies

The Graded Exercise Test

A controversial topic diabetes educators often have to address is the recommendation to complete a graded exercise test prior to exercise participation. Diabetes is an independent risk factor for cardiac disease. The established ADA criteria (listed in Table 14.10) provide healthcare providers with a broad referral base upon which to determine if a graded exercise test is warranted. These criteria are more inclusive than exclusive. They can, therefore, be applied to most individuals seen in a diabetes practice. While this offers straightforward access, performing the test may not be the course of action required for each individual. The risk of a false-positive result can overshadow the benefits an otherwise healthy individual receives from starting a fitness program. Likewise, a negative test result does not guarantee the individual is protected from having a cardiac event. While careful consideration for the presence of cardiac disease should not be ignored, clinical judgment needs to be included when making the final determination on whether this test is necessary and in evaluating the results for the individual in question.

Focus on Education: Pearls for Practice

Teaching Strategies

Helping the person who hates to exercise. Many people voice this opposition. When a person makes this statement, the diabetes educator or other clinician has a huge opportunity to ask more questions. Digging deeper, the educator often finds the real root of the problem and can help prevent it from interfering again. For example:

- *Does Not Like to Sweat.* Promote lighter types of activities such as stretching, pool activities, or leisurely paced walking The individual may be surprised to find these are options in a fitness plan.
- *Had A Bad Experience.* Determine what went wrong and prepare a plan that will replace that experience with a positive one.
- *Feels Self-Conscious in Front of Others.* May be best to start with "solo" options, such as videos, home-based equipment, or a personal trainer. A group fitness class or specific fitness facility may provide support if the person feels they "fit in" with the other members.
- *Has Always "Failed" With Fitness Programs.* Help set reasonable goals, prescribe a fitness program that will meet those goals, and provide positive support to the person through each step whether the person experiences a success or a setback.

Helping the person who underestimates insulin adjustments needs. Many individuals need reassurance that a large reduction to their insulin dose is the correct action to take. They are willing to take 1 or 2 units off a dose initially, but hesitant to do more. With support, they can omit 50% to 100% of their dose if that is what is required.

Helping the person who delays or avoids snacks. Even when the blood glucose indicates a snack is needed, many individuals will wait to see if they really need a snack. This often results in hypoglycemia and the need for a larger volume of food to treat the reaction. Pointing out that a smaller snack at the right time can help them avoid consuming a larger number of calories later to treat a reaction can help.

Identifying support and assistance. Whether the individual is of school age, a working professional, a parent, or retired, support and assistance from others close to the individual is important. The person may need to ask someone to join in the fitness program to promote regularity or ask someone to take over a chore or responsibility to free up the time for physical activity. Financial resources may also need to be allocated so the individual can buy appropriate clothing and shoes or have access to exercise equipment.

Role modeling. Model a lifestyle incorporating physical activity and planned exercise to emphasize that physical activity is a lifestyle priority.

Messages for Patients

Be prepared to troubleshoot your fitness plan. Determining the best routine to follow to safely and effectively engage in physical activity takes time (frequent blood glucose readings and data from multiple physical activity sessions), patience, and problem-solving.

Monitoring provides valuable information. Recognize the need to measure blood glucose levels before and after exercise. Doing so is critical for good decision-making in the future. Decisions on snacks, timing of exercise, and the results of exercise as well as observations of blood glucose patterns and effects of exercise can be reinforced with this information.

Timing snacks appropriately can help keep calorie counts down. A smaller snack at the right time can help you avoid consuming a larger number of calories later to treat a reaction.

Insulin dose adjustments may be larger than you expect. A large reduction in your insulin dose may be the correct action to take.

References

1. Sushruta SCS. Vaidya Jadavaji Trikamji Acharia. Bombay, India: Sagar; 1938.
2. Lawrence RH. The effects of exercise on insulin action in diabetes. BMJ. 1926;1:648-52.
3. Mulcahy K, Maryniuk M, Peeples M, et al. Diabetes Self-Management Education Core Outcomes. Diabetes Educ. 2003;29(5):768-803.
4. President's Council on Physical Fitness. Definitions: health, fitness, and physical activity. Research Digest; 2000.
5. Ivy J. Exercise physiology and adaptations to training. In: Handbook of Exercise in Diabetes. Ruderman N, Devlin JT, Schneider SH, Kriska A, eds. American Diabetes Association, Alexandria, Va; 2002.
6. Wojtaszewski JFP, Hansen BF, Gade J, et al. Insulin signaling and insulin sensitivity after exercise in human skeletal muscle. Diabetes. 2000;49:325-31.
7. Cusi K, Maezono K, Osman A, et al. Insulin resistance differentially affects the PI 3-kinase and MAP kinase-mediated signaling in human muscle. J Clin Invest. 2000;105:311-20.
8. Kirwan JP, del Aguila LF, Hernandes JM, et al. Regular exercise enhances insulin activation of IRS-1-associated P13K in human skeletal tissue. J Appl Physiol. 2000;88:797-803.
9. Tuomilehto J, Lindstrom J, Eriksson JG, et al. Prevention of type 2 diabetes mellitus by changes in lifestyle among subjects with impaired glucose tolerance. N Engl J of Med. 2001;344:1343-50.
10. Diabetes Prevention Research Group. Reduction in the incidence of type 2 diabetes with lifestyle intervention or metformin. N Engl J Med. 2002;346(6):393-403.
11. McArdle WD, Katch FI, Katch VL. Essentials of Exercise Physiology. Philadelphia, Pa: Lippincott, Williams & Wilkins; 2004.
12. Koranyi LI, Bourey RE, Slentz CA, Hollosky JO. Coordinate reduction of rat pancreatic islet glucokinase and proinsulin mRNA by exercise training. Diabetes. 1991;40:401-4.
13. Schneider SH, Amorosa LF, Khachadurian AK, Ruderman NB. Studies on the mechanism of improved glycemic control during regular exercise in type II diabetes. Diabetologia. 1984;26:355-60.
14. Eriksson KF, Lindgarde F. Prevention of type II diabetes mellitus by diet and physical exercise: the 6-year Malmo Feasibility Study. Diabetologia. 1991;34:891-8.
15. Heath GW, Wilson RH, Smith J, Leonard BE. Community-based exercise and weight control: diabetes risk reduction and glycemic control in Zuni Indians. Am J Clin Nutr. 1991;53:S1642-6.
16. Schneider SH, Khachadurian AK, Amorosa LF, Clemow L, Ruderman NB. Ten-year experience with an exercise-based outpatient lifestyle modification program in the treatment of diabetes mellitus. Diabetes Care. 1992;15 suppl 4:1800-10.
17. Ivy JL. Role of exercise training in the prevention and treatment of insulin resistance and treatment of insulin resistance and non-insulin-dependent diabetes mellitus. Sports Med. 1997;24:321-36.
18. Willey KA, Fiatarone-Singh MA. Battling insulin resistance in elderly obese people with type 2 diabetes: bring on the heavy weights. Diabetes Care. 2003;26:1580-8.
19. Shier I. Stretching before exercise does not reduce the risk of local muscle injury: a critical review of the clinical and basic science literature. Clin J Sports Med. 1999;9:221-7.
20. Lan C, Lai JS, Chen SY. Tai Chi Chuan: an ancient wisdom on exercise and health promotion. Sports Med. 2002;32(4):217-24.
21. Ray US, Sinha B, Tomer OS, Pathak A, Dasgupta T, Selvamurthy W. Aerobic capacity & perceived exertion after practice of hatha yoga exercises. Indian J Med Res. 2001;114:215-21.
22. Innes KE, Bourguignon C, Taylor AG. Risk indices associated with the insulin resistance syndrome, cardiovascular disease, and possible protection with yoga: a systematic review. J Amer Board Fam Pract. 2005;18:491-519.
23. American Diabetes Association. Hyperglycemic crises in diabetes (position statement). Diabetes Care. 2004;27 suppl 1:S94-102.
24. Sigal RJ, Kenny GP, Wasserman DH, Castaneda-Sceppa C. Physical activity/exercise and type 2 diabetes. Diabetes Care. 2004;27:2518–39.
25. Mitchell TH, Abraham G, Schiffrin A, Leiter A, Marliss EB. Hyperglycemia after intense exercise in IDDM subjects during continuous subcutaneous insulin infusion. Diabetes Care. 1988;11:311-7.
26. Purdon C, Brousson M, Nyveen SL, et al. The roles of insulin and catecholamines in the glucoregulatory

response during intense exercise and early recovery in insulin-dependent diabetic and control subjects. J Clin Endocrinol Metab. 1993;76:566-73.

27. Coyle EF, Montain SJ. Benefits of fluid replacement with carbohydrate during exercise. Med Sci Sports Exerc. 1993;25:966-9.

28. Zinman B, Vranic M, Albisser AM, Leibel BS, Marliss ED. The role of insulin in the metabolic response to exercise in the diabetic man. Diabetes. 1979;28 suppl 1:76-81.

29. Tuominen JA, Karonen SL, Melamimies L, Bollie G, Koivisto VA. Exercise-induced hypoglycemia in IDDM patients treated with a short-acting insulin analogue. Diabetologia. 1995;38:106-11.

30. Schiffrin A, Parikh S. Accommodating planned exercise in type I diabetic patients on intensive treatment. Diabetes Care. 1985;8:337-42.

31. Frid A, Ostman J, Linde B. Hypoglycemia risk during exercise after intramuscular injection of insulin in thigh in IDDM. Diabetes Care. 1990;13:473-7.

32. Koivisto VA, Felig P. Effects of leg exercise on insulin absorption in diabetic patients. N Engl J Med. 1978;298:79-83.

33. American Diabetes Association. Physical activity/exercise and diabetes mellitus. Diabetes Care. 2003;26 suppl 1:S73-7.

34. Whaley MH, Brubaker PH, Otto RM, eds. American College of Sports Medicine Guidelines for Exercise Testing and Prescription, 7th ed. American College of Sports Medicine, Philadelphia, Pa: Lippincott, Williams and Williams; 2006.

35. Jakicic JM, Wing RR, Butler BA. Prescribing exercise in multiple short bouts versus one continuous bout: effect on adherence, cardiorespiratory fitness, and weight loss in women. Int J Obes Relate Metab Disord. 1995;19:893-901.

36. Centers for Disease Control and Prevention, National Center for Chronic Disease Prevention and Health Promotion. Physical activity and health: a report of the Surgeon General. US Department of Health and Human Services. Atlanta, Ga; 1996.

37. Ganley T, Sherman C. Exercise and children's health: A little counseling can pay lasting dividends. Phys Sports Med. 2000;28(2):85-92.

38. American College of Sports Medicine. Appropriate intervention strategies for weight loss and prevention of weight regain for adults (position stand). Med Sci Sports Exerc. 2001;33:2145-56.

39. Diabetes Research in Children Network (DirecNet) Study Group. Effects of aerobic exercise on glucose and counterregulatory hormone concentrations in children with type 1 diabetes. Diabetes Care. 2006;29:20-25.

40. Bickley LS. Bate's pocket guide to physical examination and history taking, 4th ed. Philadelphia, Pa: Lippincott, Williams and Wilkins; 2003.

41. Centers for Disease Control and Prevention. National diabetes fact sheet: general information and national estimates on diabetes in the United States, 2002. Atlanta, Ga: US Department of Health and Human Services, Centers for Disease Control and Prevention; 2003.

42. Vinik AI, Erbas T. Neuropathy. In: Handbook of Exercise in Diabetes. American Diabetes Association. Ruderman N, Devlin JT, Schneider SH, Kriska A, eds. Alexandria, Va: American Diabetes Association; 2002.

43. Mogensen CE. Nephropathy: early. In: Handbook of Exercise in Diabetes. Ruderman N, Devlin JT, Schneider SH, Kriska A, eds. Alexandria, Va: American Diabetes Association; 2002.

44. Aiello LP, Wong J, Cavellerano JD, Bursell SE, Aiello LM. Retinopathy. In: Handbook of Exercise in Diabetes. Ruderman N, Devlin JT, Schneider SH, Kriska A, eds. Alexandria, Va: American Diabetes Association; 2002.

45. American Association of Diabetes Educators. The scope of practice, standards of practice, and standards of professional performance for diabetes educators. Diabetes Educ. 2005;31:487–512.

CHAPTER

15

Pharmacologic Therapies for Glucose Management

Author

Condit F. Steil, PharmD, FAPhA, CDE

Key Concepts

- The pathophysiology of the different types of diabetes helps determine the appropriate therapy.
- In the treatment for people with type 2 diabetes, combination therapies are frequently used that target the different metabolic abnormalities seen in type 2 diabetes. Using multiple medication regimens can increase the risk of drug interactions.
- The goal of insulin therapy is to approach normal physiology. A variety of insulin regimens can be used to achieve this goal.
- The various insulin preparations differ in action and duration. Proper administration and storage can affect the effectiveness of insulin therapy.
- The role of the diabetes educator is to help those with diabetes understand the medications they are taking and provide guidelines for monitoring and effective use of the drug therapies.

Introduction

This chapter reviews pharmacologic therapies for glucose management in type 1 and type 2 diabetes. Options for drug therapy in type 2 diabetes, when medications are needed to supplement lifestyle change therapy, are discussed first. Insulin and newer therapies for both type 1 and type 2 diabetes are also discussed in detail as the chapter progresses. Hypoglycemia (causes, prevention, and treatment) is discussed as the chapter draws to a close.

Landmark studies published in the 1990s demonstrated that glucose management or metabolic control matters.[1,2] In all persons with diabetes, the goal should be to reach the best possible glycemic control while avoiding acute complications or problems, especially hypoglycemia. Optimal metabolic control slows the long-term complications of diabetes and improves the lives of those with diabetes.

In the past decade, several new drug therapy choices have been developed, tested, and approved for use in persons with diabetes. Five different groups of oral agents have been introduced for clinical use in the United States since 1995; also available are several new insulin preparations and a peptide substance that is usually secreted by the pancreas with insulin.[3] Technology for administration of insulin continues to be refined, with the ultimate goal of near-physiologic action of administered insulin.[4] New approaches to improving glycemic control that involve gastrointestinal enzyme alteration and use of a product that enhances insulin's actions have been introduced,[5,6] with several other potential products showing promise for clinical use.

In addition to the expanded armamentarium for treating diabetes, the person with diabetes may also be using medications for disorders related to diabetes as well as for unrelated disorders. Pharmacologic therapies for hypertension and dyslipidemia in people with diabetes are discussed in chapter 18. Because the drug regimens can be complex, the knowledgeable, up-to-date diabetes educator can be of value to the person with diabetes in ensuring the best possible use of pharmacologic therapies.

Treatment Goals

The goals of treatment for diabetes control, for both type 1 and type 2 diabetes, are stated as achieving near-normal glucose levels (A1C <7.0%). Included in these goals should be a limited incidence of abnormally high or low blood glucose swings.

Medications for Type 2 Diabetes

As this chapter's case study makes evident, type 2 diabetes is a chronic disorder with multiple defects. Type 2

Case in Point: Type 2 Diabetes

CR was a 52-year-old African American male with type 2 diabetes. When diagnosed, he had a casual glucose of 281 mg/dL and an A1C of 9.9%. Three months later, he presented to the clinic with continued, though decreased, polyuria and nocturia for the prior 2 weeks. His BP was 128/82 mm Hg. His fasting glucose was 216 mg/dL.

Past Medical History

- h/o hypertension × 3 years
- h/o hyperlipidemia × 4 months
- Obesity

Family History

- Father: h/o CVD/hypertension, deceased
- Mother: h/o type 2 diabetes, hypertension

Social History

- Tobacco: 24 pack years, currently smoked
- Illicit drug use: none
- Alcohol: occasional/socially

Current Medications

- Pravastatin (Pravachol) 40 mg daily
- Metoprolol succinate (Toprol XL) 50 mg bid
- Quinapril (Accupril) 40 mg daily
- Furosemide (Lasix) 40 mg daily

Adherence to Drug Therapy

CR picked up his prescriptions within 5 days (early or late) of the due date for his medication refills. He related taking his medications as prescribed.

Physical Exam

- Ht: 69 in
- Wt: 241 lb
- BMI: 35 kg/m^2
- Waist circumference: 42 in

Vitals

- BP: 128/82 mm Hg
- HR: 72 beats per minute
- RR: 18

Lab Data

- ALT: 24
- Serum creatinine: 1.4
- Fasting blood glucose : 201 mg/dL
- A1C: 9.3%
- Total cholesterol: 218 mg/dL
- LDL-C: 131 mg/dL
- Triglycerides: 162 mg/dL
- HDL-C: 37 mg/dL

As this case continues throughout the chapter, considerations for maximizing glycemic control by pharmacologic intervention are the focus. Control of related abnormalities is also discussed.

diabetes usually begins with insulin resistance, but progresses to an insulin secretory defect and related insulin deficiency. Interventions (medical nutrition therapy, physical activity, lifestyle changes) are the basis of initial and ongoing treatment. Today, many clinicians choose to begin a nonpharmacologic, but intensive effort at lifestyle change for achieving glycemic control prior to starting drug therapy for type 2 diabetes.[7] However, at some point in the progression of this disease, medication becomes necessary.

Pharmacologic Treatment

There are currently 5 classes of orally administered agents used for type 2 diabetes (see the complete list in Table 15.1):

- Sulfonylureas
- Meglitinides
- A biguanide
- Thiazolidinediones
- Alpha-glucosidase inhibitors

TABLE 15.1 Oral Medications for Type 2 Diabetes

Sulfonylureas	
Glyburide • Micronase • Glynase Glipizide • Glucotrol • Glucotrol XR Glimepiride • Amaryl	*Action.* Reduce glucose by increasing insulin secretion from pancreatic beta cells in persons with residual beta-cell function. *Contraindications.* Documented hypersensitivity; DKA; type 1 diabetes; pregnancy—category C. *Interactions.* Numerous possible, few clinically significant. Sulfonamides may enhance hypoglycemic effect. *Precautions.* Hypoglycemia. Caution in hepatic or renal impairment; risk factors are older age, malnutrition, and irregular eating. May cause rash, sun sensitivity, nausea, vomiting, leukopenia, agranulocytosis, aplastic anemia (rare), intrahepatic cholestasis (rare), disulfiram-like reaction, flushing, headache, and SIADH causing hyponatremia.
Meglitinides	
Repaglinide • Prandin Nateglinide • Starlix	*Action.* Short-acting insulin secretagogues; stimulate insulin release from pancreatic beta cells. *Contraindications.* Documented hypersensitivity; DKA; type 1 diabetes. *Interactions.* CYP3A4 inhibitors (eg, clarithromycin, ketoconazole, miconazole, erythromycin) decrease metabolism, increasing serum levels and effects. Thiazides, diuretics, corticosteroids, estrogens, oral contraceptives, nicotinic acid, CCBs, phenothiazines, and thyroid products may lower glycemic control. Toxicity increased with highly protein-bound drugs (eg, NSAIDs, sulfonamides, anticoagulants, hydantoins, salicylates, phenylbutazone). *Precautions.* Hypoglycemia, especially if carbohydrate not eaten after drug. Caution in hepatic impairment.
Biguanides	
Metformin • Glucophage • Glucophage XR	*Action.* Increase sensitivity of insulin by decreasing hepatic gluconeogenesis (primary effect) and increasing peripheral insulin sensitivity (secondary effect). They do not increase insulin levels or weight gain. Alone, they do not cause hypoglycemia. *Contraindications.* Serum creatinine level >1.5 (men) or >1.4 (women) mg/dL; hepatic dysfunction; acute or chronic acidosis; local or systemic tissue hypoxia; excessive alcohol intake; drug therapy for congestive heart failure. *Interactions.* Numerous possible, few (if any) clinically significant. Can cause GI upset, nausea, and diarrhea; take with food or milk to minimize GI effects. *Precautions.* Fatal lactic acidosis if given with contraindication (rare without contraindication). Discontinue before IV contrast enhancement, do not restart until creatinine level normal. Withhold in acute hypoxia. Check renal function regularly and discontinue if abnormal. Adverse effects, including GI, especially diarrhea (30%), may cause discontinuation (5%).

TABLE 15.1 Oral Medications for Type 2 Diabetes

Alpha-Glucosidase Inhibitors	
Miglitol • Glyset Acarbose • Precose	*Action.* Inhibit action of alpha-glucosidase (carbohydrate digestion), delaying and attenuating postprandial blood glucose peaks. Undigested sugars are delivered to the colon, where they are converted into short-chain fatty acids, methane, carbon dioxide, and hydrogen. They do not increase insulin levels or inhibit lactase; major effect is to lower postprandial glucose levels (lesser effect on fasting levels). They do not cause weight gain and may restore ovulation in anovulation due to insulin resistance. *Contraindications.* Documented hypersensitivity, DKA, or cirrhosis; inflammatory bowel disease; colonic ulceration; serum creatinine level >2 mg/dL; elevated liver enzyme levels; partial or predisposition to intestinal obstruction. *Interactions.* Hypoglycemia with insulin or sulfonylurea agents (give glucose as dextrose, as absorption of long-chain carbohydrates is delayed). May decrease absorption and bioavailability of digoxin, propranolol, and ranitidine. Digestive enzymes (eg, amylase, pancreatin) may reduce effects. *Precautions.* May cause GI symptoms; not recommended in significant renal dysfunction.
Thiazolidinediones	
Rosiglitazone • Avandia Pioglitazone • Actos	*Action.* Increase peripheral insulin sensitivity by increasing transcription of nuclear proteins that help increase uptake of glucose, probably with effects on free fatty acid levels. About 12-16 weeks to achieve maximal effect. May restore ovulation in anovulation due to insulin resistance. Improves target cell response to insulin without increasing insulin secretion from pancreas. Decreases hepatic glucose output and increases insulin-dependent glucose use in skeletal muscle and possibly liver and adipose tissue. *Contraindications.* Documented hypersensitivity; active liver disease; DKA; type 1 diabetes; class III or IV congestive heart failure. *Interactions.* With insulin or oral hypoglycemics (eg, sulfonylureas), may increase risk of hypoglycemia. *Precautions.* Monitor transaminases every 2 months for first year, periodically thereafter; discontinue if ALT above 3X ULN. Caution in edema and congestive heart failure. May decrease hemoglobin, hematocrit, and WBC counts (dilution). Effects on lipids neutral or beneficial (decreased triglyceride, increased HDL levels).

Source: Adapted from Votey SR. Diabetes mellitus, Type 2-A review, 2005. Available at www.emedicine.com/emerg/topic 134.htm. Accessed 15 Mar 2006.

Generally, monotherapy with any of these agents is associated with a reduction in A1C levels of approximately 0.5% to 2.0%.[8,9] When combination therapy is used (2 or more oral agents or an oral agent combined with insulin), an additive effect is observed, as demonstrated by a further decrease in the A1C level.[8] Fixed-dose combination products are available. These agents are not advised for use during preconception care or pregnancy, though some evidence of resultant uneventful use is documented.[10]

Of all the oral medications for type 2 diabetes, only metformin has been approved for use in children.[11] This presents a concern with the increase in type 2 diabetes among young people.

Today, clinicians have a variety of medication options for treating type 2 diabetes that target the specific pathophysiological defects.

Insulin, pramlintide (Symlin), and exenatide (Byetta) are injectable agents demonstrated to be effective in type 1 and type 2 diabetes. An inhalable, powdered form of recombinant human insulin (Exubera) was recently approved by the US Food and Drug Administration (FDA) that may also be effective in treating diabetes.

General Considerations

Patients should be reminded that any pharmacologic treatment for type 2 diabetes is only a supplement to lifestyle changes. These changes include adherence to a medical nutrition therapy plan, regular appropriate physical activity, and alteration of other specific health habits (eg, smoking cessation). The healthcare provider should confirm that the patient understands the proper dose, daily schedule of when to take each dose, and effects to expect. A review and emphasis of the importance of routine self-monitoring of blood glucose should be included. Patients should receive a review of the potential for side effects. This review should include a discussion of the signs and symptoms that are possible and the appropriate action needed when these changes occur.[12,13]

The pathophysiology of type 2 diabetes includes insulin resistance, eventually leading to an insulin secretory defect, of either the first- or second-phase insulin release or of both phases. The first phase is the insulin released with a meal, and the second phase is the basal, or background, release of insulin. Different medications work on different defects, and as a result, some medications are very effective used in combination.

Sulfonylureas

Sulfonylureas are classified as first- and second-generation oral hypoglycemic agents. The first-generation agents are described as rapid-acting, intermediate-acting, and long-acting products based on their onset and duration.[11] Sulfonylureas are hypoglycemic agents, and their major pharmacologic action has the potential to reduce blood glucose levels below normal (ie, cause hypoglycemia). Sulfonylurea agents are useful only in persons who still produce endogenous insulin; hence, they are used exclusively in type 2 diabetes.

Sulfonylureas are often used as either a first step or second agent in treating type 2 diabetes. A typical candidate for sulfonylurea monotherapy is an individual with type 2 diabetes without dyslipidemia who is not overweight.[13,14] Some individuals will not respond at all to sulfonylureas, and most over time will experience treatment failure with sulfonylureas as the disease progresses.

Mechanism of Action/Effects

Sulfonylureas' primary mechanism of action is to increase release of insulin from the pancreas, especially at the onset of therapy. These agents close the energy-sensitive potassium channel in the cell membrane of the beta cells. This effect causes an increase in the available insulin for action throughout the body,[15] although these agents may be less effective in those with impaired first-phase insulin release. Absorption of sulfonylureas is generally rapid, fairly complete, and unaffected by food except for short-acting glipizide. Significant variance in metabolism and excretion of these agents helps determine product choice. Most sulfonylureas are metabolized in the liver to active or inactive

Sulfonylureas: Dosage Information

Drug	*Trade Names*	*Common Dose and Available Strengths*	*Common Frequency*
First Generation			
Acetohexamide	Dymelor	250 to 1500 mg daily *Tabs:* 250 mg, 500 mg	Daily to twice daily
Chlorpropamide	Diabinese	100-250 mg to 500 mg daily *Tabs:* 100 mg, 250 mg	Daily
Tolazamide	Tolinase	100-250 mg to 1.0 g daily *Tabs:* 100 mg, 250 mg, 500 mg	Daily to twice daily
Tolbutamide	Orinase	500-2000 mg to 3.0 g daily *Tabs:* 500 mg	Three times a day
Second Generation			
Glimepiride	Amaryl	1-2 mg to 8 mg daily *Tabs:* 1 mg, 2 mg, 4 mg	Daily to twice daily
Glipizide	Glucotrol Glucotrol XL	2.5-5 mg to 40 mg daily/ max 20 mg with XL daily *Tabs:* 5 mg, 10 mg; XL 2.5 mg, 5 mg, 10 mg	Twice daily to daily
Glyburide	Diabeta Micronase	2.5-5 mg to 20 mg daily *Tabs:* 1.25 mg, 2.5 mg, 5 mg	Daily to twice daily
Glyburide, micronized	Glynase	1.5-3 mg to 12 mg daily *Tabs:* 1.5 mg, 3 mg, 4.5 mg, 6 mg	

metabolites. However, chlorpropamide is partially excreted unchanged in the urine. Biliary excretion is significant with glyburide and to a lesser extent with glipizide.[15] Caution must be exercised with liver disease or renal insufficiency.

Dosing

Sulfonylureas should be started at the lowest dose and titrated as needed to reach target blood glucose levels. Outlined in the sulfonylurea chart are the most commonly used dosages. Although first-generation sulfonylureas are rarely used, they are included.

Precautions

Persons with diabetes can experience a sulfonylurea hypersensitivity reaction.[11] This reaction does not indicate a cross-sensitivity with sulfonamide agents. Rarely, diabetic ketoacidosis, altered glucose control from a severe infection, surgery, trauma, or other severe metabolic stressors may induce toxicity in persons receiving sulfonylureas.[16] Elderly, debilitated, or malnourished persons and those with adrenal, pituitary, or hepatic insufficiency who are particularly susceptible to the hypoglycemic effects of glucose-lowering agents should be monitored closely when using a sulfonylurea.

Contraindications

Type 1 diabetes, ketoacidosis, allergy or documented hypersensitivity to these agents.

Side Effects

Perhaps the most common and most serious adverse reaction is hypoglycemia.[16] An additional complicating factor is a progressive age-related decline in renal function that alters drug clearance and predisposes the person to hypoglycemia. Weight gain probably secondary to increased insulin secretion will occur, and skin rashes can be seen in about 2% of persons using the medication. The skin rashes usually resolve and the sulfonylurea can be continued. Usually mild gastrointestinal disturbances are reported in approximately 5% of users. Metabolic disorders such as a syndrome of inappropriate antidiuretic hormone (SIADH) occurs in about 4% of persons treated with chlorpropamide, manifested by hyponatremia and hypervolemia.[17] Blood changes described with tolbutamide and chlorpropamide include abnormal hepatic function tests, thrombocytopenia, agranulocytosis, and hemolytic anemia, but are very rare with second-generation sulfonylureas.[18]

Drug Interactions

Sulfonylureas may interact with a variety of medications. These interactions may alter the effect of the sulfonylurea or the other medication or both. Commonly, it is accepted that more drug-drug interactions occur with the first-generation agents than the second-generation agents. One of the principle mechanisms of these interactions is a competition for protein binding sites. As this competition for binding sites occurs, more sulfonylurea is circulating freely in the bloodstream and capable of exerting its hypoglycemic effect. Altered hepatic enzyme activity may also alter clearance of sulfonylureas.

Monitoring

Baseline renal and hepatic function levels should be documented prior to starting sulfonylurea therapy. Persons with diabetes who use this medication should self-monitor their blood glucose daily. They should be able to detect and treat hypoglycemia episodes. The number of tests each day and timing of the tests, usually postprandial and at bedtime, should be determined by the goal of therapy and needs for access to control information.

Continued monitoring and follow-up visits should occur to assess the ongoing effectiveness of the agent. Up to 20% of persons with diabetes will not respond to sulfonylureas. This is termed a primary failure of therapy. Secondary failure is defined as a significantly diminished or missing response to the sulfonylurea following an initial therapeutic response. Persons with diabetes who experience this treatment failure should be changed to another class of medication.[12]

Instructions for Patients

Sulfonylureas may enhance a person's sun sensitivity, and use of appropriate sun screen is prudent to advise as part of patient teaching. Prevention, recognition, and treatment for hypoglycemia should be included in patient education for people taking these medications (see the section on hypoglycemia near the end of this chapter).

Meglitinides

Meglitinides are hypoglycemic agents whose major pharmacologic action has the potential to reduce the blood glucose level to below normal. Repaglinide and nateglinide are the 2 agents in this category. Repaglinide is a nonsulfonylurea agent, but shares many of the pharmacologic actions and side effects of sulfonylureas. Nateglinide is a D-phenylalanine (amino acid) derivative and is a very rapid-acting oral agent.[19]

Combination therapy, or transition to insulin monotherapy, may be considered when treatment using these medications approaches the maximum dose without achieving target blood glucose levels. Meglitinides should not be used in persons who have already experienced primary or secondary failure on a sulfonylurea.

Repaglinide or nateglinide therapy also results in better glycemic control when combined with another oral agent for glycemic control.[20] The exception to this concept is use of repaglinide or nateglinide with a sulfonylurea.

Meglitinides: Dosage Information

Drug	*Trade Name*	*Common Dose and Available Strengths*	*Common Frequency*
Repaglinide	Prandin	0.5-1.0 mg three times per day to 16 mg daily *Tabs:* 0.5 mg, 1 mg, 2 mg	Three times per day before meals
Nateglinide	Starlix	60-120 mg three times per day to 360 mg daily *Tabs:* 60 mg, 120 mg	Three times per day before meals

This results in no additional glycemic benefit and actually is a therapeutic duplication.

Meglitinides are used in treating diabetes mellitus as monotherapy only in type 2 diabetes or secondary diabetes in individuals with substantial capacity for insulin production. A typical candidate for initial repaglinide monotherapy has type 2 diabetes, without dyslipidemia, with or without renal failure, without overweight, and with fasting plasma glucose level >20 mg/dL above the target concentration.

Nateglinide can be effectively used as monotherapy in persons with type 2 diabetes with a capacity for insulin production whose hyperglycemia is not adequately controlled by nutrition therapy and physical activity and who have not been treated long-term with other oral glucose-lowering agents

Mechanism of Action

These agents increase release of insulin from the pancreas in a glucose-dependent manner and are therefore effective in helping restore first-phase insulin release. Treatment with repaglinide and nateglinide is effective in persons with well-controlled type 2 diabetes[21] or in those with type 2 diabetes whose control is suboptimal.[22] Nateglinide is a D-phenylalanine (amino acid) derivative and is a very rapid-acting oral insulin secretagogue that stimulates insulin secretion when needed (postprandial) and then allows insulin concentrations to return to normal basal concentrations.[22]

Persons treated with repaglinide or nateglinide who missed or delayed a meal had less risk of hypoglycemia compared to treatment with longer acting sulfonylurea drugs. Absorption of repaglinide from the gastrointestinal tract is rapid and complete, and food slightly decreases absorption.[23]

Dosing

The usual initial and maintenance dose of nateglinide is 120 mg taken just before meals (1 to 30 minutes before). Titration of dose is not usually necessary. The 60-mg dose may be used in those who are near their A1C goal.[24] Dose adjustment is not needed in the elderly, in persons with mild to severe renal insufficiency, or in those with mild hepatic insufficiency.[24]

Repaglinide is initiated at a low, single daily dose, with gradual increases to reach glucose goals, and taken 15 minutes (0 to 30 minutes) before each meal. The number of daily doses taken is determined by the number of meals eaten. This type of meal-based dosing frequency may offer advantages for persons who vary frequency of daily meals or for those who choose to eat only 2 meals a day and need to avoid persisting hypoglycemic activity between the meals. The initial dosage does not need to be adjusted for persons with renal dysfunction, but upward titration should proceed cautiously. The initial dose for those previously treated with glucose-lowering drugs and with an A1C level >8% is usually 1 or 2 mg with each meal. The dose may be adjusted weekly, perhaps doubling each preprandial dose until desired effect is attained. The maximum dose is 16 mg daily.

Precautions

Repaglinide and nateglinide are not indicated for use during pregnancy, for breastfeeding women, or for children.

Repaglinide should be used with caution in persons with impaired hepatic function, with careful monitoring and adjustment of dosing.

Elderly, debilitated, or malnourished persons and those with adrenal, pituitary, or hepatic insufficiency are particularly susceptible to the hypoglycemic effects of repaglinide.

Contraindications

Type 1 diabetes, diabetic ketoacidosis, severe infection, surgery, trauma or other severe stressor.

Side Effects

Side effects associated with repaglinide include gastrointestinal disturbances in approximately 4% of persons receiving the drug. Upper respiratory infection or congestion problems have been noted along with back pain. Hypoglycemia is the most common serious adverse effect. Different series document the incidence to be between 16% to 31%.[23] Also, similar to sulfonylurea use, primary or secondary treatment failure occurs when an individual is insensitive to the effects of repaglinide. No clinically significant interactions are noted with nateglinide.

Side effects associated with nateglinide include hypoglycemia, usually mild, in approximately 2.4% of patients in clinical trials. There were no reports of hypoglycemia requiring third-party assistance or nocturnal hypoglycemia in the phase III trials (2400 patients). Dizziness was reported in approximately 3.6% of users with a weight gain of <1 kg from baseline. This weight gain is lowered with concomitant use of metformin.[22]

Monitoring

Blood glucose monitoring should include some premeal and postmeal readings to assess the effectiveness of the medications. The mean time to reach maximum concentrations of nateglinide after oral administration is 0.82 hours. High-fat meals reportedly result in a 12% increase in maximum concentration and a 52% reduction in the time to reach that concentration.[24]

Instructions for Patients

Meglitinides should be taken right before eating. Due to the potential for hypoglycemia, those taking this medication should be advised to monitor blood glucose levels for confirmation and subsequent treatment with fast-acting carbohydrate.[25]

Biguanides

Biguanides are not considered hypoglycemic agents because their major pharmacologic action does not increase insulin secretion and thus does not increase the risk of hypoglycemia. Currently, only one agent is marketed in the United States: metformin. Metformin is indicated for use in type 2 diabetes as a step-one drug or adjunct to other therapy. This agent has proven to be an effective antihyperglycemic agent or an insulin sensitizer[26,27] and, as with all oral agents for diabetes, requires endogenous insulin production for its effectiveness.

Metformin is useful as monotherapy only in type 2 diabetes or secondary diabetes with substantial capacity for insulin production. A typical candidate for initial metformin monotherapy has type 2 diabetes, with dyslipidemia, with obesity or genetic factors favoring insulin resistance, and with an elevated fasting plasma glucose level.[26]

Mechanism of Action

Metformin's primary effects include reducing hepatic glucose production by reduction in glycogenolysis and enhancing insulin-stimulated glucose transport in adipose tissue and skeletal muscle. This reverses or at least partially reverses insulin resistance. A minor effect is a decrease in intestinal absorption of glucose. Metformin is approved for use in children 10 years of age or older.[26]

The oral bioavailability is 50% to 60%, and food decreases the bioavailability with a slight delay in the absorption of metformin. Metformin does not bind to liver or plasma proteins and is primarily excreted by the kidneys, largely unchanged, through an active tubular process.

Dosing

Metformin therapy is initiated at a low dose, with gradual increases to obtain desired control. The usual initial dose for the standard formulation is 500 mg or 850 mg daily or twice daily, with doses taken just prior to a meal. The extended-release (XR) formulation dose is usually adjusted every week until the goal is met, while the standard formulation is usually adjusted every 2 weeks. The maximum daily dose is 2550 mg daily (850 mg twice daily), but the maximal effective dose is achieved with 2000 mg daily. Children's therapy should be started with 250 mg twice daily and titrated slowly until treatment goals are attained.

Metformin: Dosage Information

Drug	*Trade Name*	*Common Dose and Available Strengths*	*Common Frequency*
Metformin Metformin extended release	Glucophage Fortamet Glucophage XR	500 mg twice daily to 2550 mg daily (max. effective: 2000 mg daily) *Tabs:* 500 mg, 850 mg, 1 g *XR:* 500 mg, 750 mg, 1 g	Twice daily
Metformin liquid	Riomet	500 mg twice daily *Solution:* 100 mg/mL	Twice daily

Precautions

Use of metformin is not recommended during pregnancy or for breastfeeding women. Some experience with use in pregnancy has been reported with no untoward effects; however, this remains an unlabeled use.

In acute illness or any situation that would predispose the individual to acute renal dysfunction or tissue hypoperfusion, metformin should be temporarily withheld. Included in this set of conditions are acute myocardial infarction, acute exacerbation of congestive heart failure, use of iodinated contrast media, and major surgical procedures.[28] Persons with diabetes using this medication should be instructed to stop the metformin the day of the use of the iodinated contrast media, and restart the metformin in 2 days when renal function has returned.[28] Metformin may restore ovulation in women who were previously anovulatory due to insulin resistance.

Contraindications

Metformin is contraindicated in males with serum creatinine levels >1.5 mg/dL and in females with levels >1.4 mg/dL. In 2001, a recommendation was presented to have persons 80 years of age or older undergo a 24-hour creatinine clearance for a more precise assessment of renal function.[11] Because metformin is excreted by the kidneys, it can accumulate in persons with renal dysfunction.

The presence of hepatic dysfunction can predispose persons receiving metformin to lactic acidosis because lactate metabolism is carried out in the liver. Persons with a history of hypoxic conditions (chronic obstructive pulmonary disease, history of cardiac function decline) are not good candidates due to the potential for lactate accumulation. Persons with a history of alcoholism or binges of alcohol intake are not good candidates for the therapy.

Side Effects

Metformin produces some side effects that can be beneficial for those with diabetes. Frequently, a slight (2-kg to 5-kg) weight loss is seen with metformin therapy, though the actual cause of weight loss is not known. Metformin reduces triglyceride concentrations by approximately 16%, low-density lipoprotein cholesterol (LDL-C) by approximately 8%, and total cholesterol by approximately 5%. Metformin is associated with an increase in high-density lipoprotein cholesterol (HDL-C) by approximately 2%.[29]

Metformin does not directly induce hypoglycemia, though a few persons have reported some mild symptoms as their nutrition and physical activity programs became more effective in lowering glucose levels.[1] This indicates the need to reduce the dose of medication.[30] Persons using metformin in combination with sulfonylureas, meglitinides, or insulin may experience hypoglycemia secondary to the hypoglycemic agent.[30] Gastrointestinal effects are experienced in up to 30% of users, including abdominal bloating, nausea, cramping, feeling of fullness, and diarrhea.[31] Up to 4% of persons using the medication will stop taking the drug. However, these effects are usually self-limiting, transient (7 to 14 days), and patient teaching at the start of therapy can minimize this effect by recommending the drug be taken with food, starting with a low dose, and slow upward titration of dosage. Part of this reaction will be the comment of a metallic taste.

Metformin therapy is associated with a reduction in vitamin B_{12} levels, although no cases of anemia have been reported in the United States. Lactic acidosis can occur with the administration of metformin but is rare (0.03 cases per 1000 patient years). Lactic acidosis is primarily associated with its use in persons who have contraindications to the drug or in cases of overdose.[32]

Monitoring

Metformin use over the age of 80 is not contraindicated, but due to the deterioration of renal function of the elderly, glomerular filtration rate testing should be done at the beginning of therapy and periodically after. Metformin therapy should be monitored with self-monitoring of blood glucose and follow-up visits to achieve target glycemic control. Continual review with the patient who has the potential for the aforementioned renal or hepatic effects should be undertaken, with encouragement concerning the possible gastrointestinal side effects. As with the other oral agents, combination therapy or transition to insulin monotherapy is considered when metformin therapy approaches the maximum effective dose.[30]

Drug interactions with metformin may include the effect that intravenous contrast media have on renal function, enzyme induction in the liver by cimetidine, and alcohol potentiation of lactate metabolism.

Instructions for Patients

Persons who receive metformin should be instructed to take each dose of the medication with the first bite of a meal. They should be told of the potential that a metallic taste will occur, which will subside in time. While metformin itself does not induce significant hypoglycemic reactions, the use of metformin in combination with other hypoglycemic agents (sulfonylureas, meglitinides, insulin) can be associated with hypoglycemia due to the other agents. With this in mind, persons using metformin with hypoglycemic agents should receive the same instruction as those taking only the hypoglycemic agents. Women of reproductive age should be advised of the risk of pregnancy as metformin can restore ovulation in anovulation due to insulin resistance.

Thiazolidinediones

Thiazolidinediones (TZDs) are not hypoglycemic agents; the major pharmacologic action does not increase insulin secretion and thus does not increase the risk of hypoglycemia. Currently, the 2 compounds approved for use in the United States are pioglitazone and rosiglitazone. These agents may best be described as antihyperglycemic agents or insulin sensitizers. One should note, though, that TZDs and biguanides, while termed insulin sensitizers, have distinctly different actions in the body.

Mechanism of Action

The TZDs probably reduce insulin resistance and improve blood glucose levels via the stimulation of peroxisome-proliferator-activated receptor-gamma (PPAR-γ).[33] They enhance insulin action at the receptor and postreceptor level in hepatic and peripheral tissues, thus reversing or partially reversing insulin resistance. These agents also have some cardiovascular effects that improve cardiac work efficiency, which can be beneficial in many individuals.[34] The significance of this feature and its application clinically continues to evolve when reviewing the overall cardiovascular and fluid-handling actions of TZDs. Another group of TZDs are under development though not yet marketed. These products are so-called dual-action TZDs, as they apparently stimulate both the PPAR-γ and α systems intracellularly.[35] Data indicate positive effects both with blood glucose and lipids control. However, concern for enhanced side effects has triggered an FDA recommendation for additional safety study. TZDs are used as monotherapy only in type 2 diabetes or secondary diabetes with substantial capacity for insulin production.[36] They are also used in combination therapy with other diabetes agents.

Both medications are extensively bound (>99%) to serum albumin and are extensively metabolized in the liver. Metabolites and parent compounds are eliminated primarily in the feces with minor amounts in the urine.

Dosing

Therapy is usually started at a low dose, with gradual increases to reach plasma glucose goals. TZDs should be taken with the main meal of the day, or with the 2 primary meals if 2 doses daily are needed. Several weeks (8 to 12) are necessary to assess the full benefit from a dose level for the medication secondary to its mechanism. The doses may be titrated upward until the desired therapeutic effect is reached. Dose increases are not recommended more frequently than every 4 weeks.

Both of these medications are well absorbed without regard to meals. Pioglitazone is always given once daily, whereas rosiglitazone may need to be given twice daily in many persons with type 2 diabetes.

Precautions

TZDs are not indicated during pregnancy, for breastfeeding women, or for children. However, TZDs may restore ovulation in women who are anovulatory due to insulin resistance.

TZDs cause fluid retention and carry a warning that in persons who are predisposed to heart failure they can induce an exacerbation or worsen existing heart failure. Patients should be observed for signs and symptoms of heart failure. TZDs should be used with caution in persons with hepatic dysfunction.

TZD therapy can cause elevated hepatic enzymes. Rare cases of severe idiosyncratic hepatocellular injury occurred with troglitazone. It now does not appear to be a class effect.

While the hepatic injury associated with troglitazone was generally reversible, rare cases of hepatic failure, including death, were reported, which prompted removal of this drug from the market.[33] In premenopausal anovulatory women with insulin resistance, TZD therapy may result in resumption of ovulation, with a subsequent risk of pregnancy.

Due to plasma volume expansion, small reductions in hemoglobin, hematocrit, and neutrophil counts will occur with TZD use. Weight gain appears to be a class effect of the TZDs, and both of the current TZDs have been associated with mild to moderate edema. Small increases in HDL-C and LDL-C may occur with rosiglitazone, while reductions in triglycerides and elevations of HDL-C have been reported with pioglitazone. The clinical significance of the lipid effects of this class of drugs is unclear.[37]

Thiazolidinediones: Dosage Information

Drug	*Trade Name*	*Common Dose and Available Strengths*	*Common Frequency*
Pioglitazone	Actos	15 mg to 45 mg daily *Tabs:* 15 mg, 30 mg, 45 mg	Once daily
Rosiglitazone	Avandia	2 mg to 8 mg daily *Tabs:* 2 mg, 4 mg, 8 mg	Twice daily

Contraindications

TZDs are contraindicated in persons with NYHA class III and IV heart failure[37] and active liver disease. Rosiglitazone is metabolized by CYP2C9 and CYP2C8. In vitro studies have suggested that inhibition of these isoenzymes by rosiglitazone does not occur at concentrations usually encountered clinically.[38] The isoenzyme CYP3A4, which is responsible for the metabolism of several drugs including erythromycin, calcium channel blockers, corticosteroids, and HMG-CoA reductase inhibitors, is also partially responsible for the metabolism of pioglitazone. Therefore, the possibility of altered safety or efficacy should be considered when using these agents with pioglitazone.

Monitoring

Persons who receive either of these medications should perform routine self-monitoring of blood glucose probably multiple times daily as their condition and glucose control dictates. Serum transaminase levels should be monitored every 2 months during the first year of therapy and periodically thereafter.[11] Hepatic function studies should be periodically performed and symptoms of muscular pain and flank/abdominal discomfort should be monitored. One should keep in mind that these agents can induce some weight gain, a parameter that requires close monitoring.[33] Edema, shortness of breath, and other possible signs and symptoms of heart failure should be included in assessing TZD therapy.

Instructions for Patients

Each dose should be taken with a meal and persons using this medication should be presented with a review of their complete drug regimen and how this treatment helps improve glycemic control. TZDs require several weeks to achieve the maximum benefit from a dosage level, and those taking it must be encouraged to continue the therapy. If they notice edema/swelling, shortness of breath, or muscle aches, patients should contact their healthcare provider for assessment of the side effect. Women should be cautioned regarding the risk of pregnancy as ovulation may be restored in women who have been anovulatory due to insulin resistance.

Alpha-Glucosidase Inhibitors

Alpha-glucosidase inhibitors are used as monotherapy only in type 2 diabetes or secondary diabetes with substantial capacity for insulin production.[39] A good candidate for initial alpha-glucosidase inhibitor monotherapy has type 2 diabetes, with dyslipidemia or obesity, and symptoms suggesting—or a blood glucose profile demonstrating—significant postprandial hyperglycemia. Due to their limited ceiling of effect on A1C, their limited group of candidates, and their side effect potential, these drugs are not commonly used as monotherapy but rather as an adjunct to therapy. Individuals demonstrating significant premeal hyperglycemia without a significant premeal-to-postmeal glucose rise would not be expected to respond optimally to alpha-glucosidase inhibitor monotherapy.

Mechanism of Action

Alpha-glucosidase inhibitors are not hypoglycemic agents, as their major pharmacologic action does not increase insulin secretion and thus does not increase the risk of hypoglycemia. These agents may best be described as antihyperglycemic agents. They inhibit alpha-glucosidase enzymes in the brush border of the small intestine[40] and pancreatic alpha-amylase,[41] leading to a reduction in carbohydrate-mediated postprandial blood glucose elevation. Alpha-glucosidase enzymes (maltase, isomaltase, glucoamylase, and sucrase) hydrolyze oligosaccharides, trisaccharides, and disaccharides to glucose and other monosaccharides in the brush border of the small intestine. Alpha-amylase enzymes hydrolyze complex starches to oligosaccharides in the lumen of the small intestine. This enzyme inhibition reduces the rate of digestion of starches and the subsequent absorption of glucose. These agents will induce up to a 1% improvement in A1C levels.

Dosing

Alpha-glucosidase therapy is initiated at a low dose to minimize gastrointestinal side effects, with gradual increases to reach glucose goals. The usual initial dose is 25 mg with meals, and each dose should be taken with the first bite of the meal for the drug to be effective. Titrate the dose

Alpha-Glucosidase Inhibitors: Dosage Information

Drug	*Trade Name*	*Common Dose and Available Strengths*	*Usual Frequency*
Acarbose	Precose	Start: 25 mg (25 mg to 100 mg) *Tabs:* 25 mg, 50 mg, 100 mg	Three times daily
Miglitol	Glyset	Start: 25 mg (25 mg to 100 mg) *Tabs:* 25 mg, 50 mg, 100mg	Three times daily

upward as patient tolerance (to gastrointestinal effects) allows, until desired therapeutic effect is reached. Combination therapy should be considered when the maximum dose is reached.[40]

Precautions

Due to their site of action, these compounds are not well absorbed from the gastrointestinal tract. Acarbose plasma levels can be elevated in persons with creatinine clearance <25 mL per minute, suggesting accumulation of acarbose. However, dosage adjustment in this setting is not feasible because acarbose acts locally.[42]

Contraindications

These drugs are generally not indicated during pregnancy, for breastfeeding women, or for children. Inflammatory bowel disease, colonic ulceration, obstructive bowel disorders, or chronic intestinal disorders of digestion or absorption are contraindications to use of these agents.[41] Acarbose is contraindicated in persons with cirrhosis of the liver and not recommended in persons with serum creatinine levels >2.0 mg/mL. Studies indicate increases in drug or metabolite plasma concentrations with renal dysfunction. Neither agent is recommended in persons with creatinine clearances of <25 mL per minute.

Side Effects

Gastrointestinal effects, occurring primarily at initiation of therapy or when dosage is increased, are diarrhea, abdominal pain, and flatulence (up to 78% incidence) secondary to the drugs' mechanism. These effects are usually self-limiting and transient and can be minimized by starting with a low dose and slow upward titration of dosage. Redistribution of the inhibited enzymes usually occurs after several weeks of therapy resulting in a mitigation of side effects.[41]

Monitoring

Alpha-glucosidase is often monitored by using 2-hour postprandial glucose measurements. This allows an assessment of the rapid effects and timing of the action of the medication. Alpha-glucosidase inhibitor monotherapy is not associated with hypoglycemia.[41] Persons using combination therapy with insulin or sulfonylureas may experience hypoglycemia secondary to the insulin or sulfonylurea. Hypoglycemia in this situation is best managed with oral glucose (if the person is conscious) or intravenous glucose or glucagon (if the person is unconscious). These drugs blunt the digestion of complex sugars to glucose; oral sugar sources other than glucose or lactose (eg, glucose tablets, milk) are unsuitable for rapid correction of hypoglycemia.[41] Elevation of serum transaminases (AST or ALT) has been observed in clinical trials in patients taking acarbose at a dose of 200 to 300 mg daily.[42] Liver function should be periodically monitored. Alpha-glucosidase inhibitors' effects may be altered by charcoal and may also interact with ranitidine, propranolol, and digoxin by decreasing their bioavailability.

Instructions to Patients

Persons using alpha-glucosidase inhibitors should be encouraged to maintain physical movement, especially after a meal, to limit the buildup of gastrointestinal tract gas from the fermenting carbohydrate as the drug limits carbohydrate absorption. The medication should be taken with the first bite of food at mealtime or with a large snack. While this medication will not induce hypoglycemia, those taking it should be instructed on the products of choice for hypoglycemic episodes if this agent is used in combination with one of the other agents that can induce hypoglycemia (see the section on hypoglycemia near the end of this chapter).

Combination Oral Medications for Type 2 diabetes

Several combination medications that combine 2 classes of drugs are used to treat type 2 diabetes. The benefit is that some people find it easier to take a single medication as opposed to 2 separate medications. These medications may be started after the person has already been on 1 drug without good effect; rather than starting another drug, the combination may used. However, these combinations are only available in specific dosages (see Table 15.2). In addition, when starting a combination tablet in a person who has never taken either agent separately, any side effect or allergy could be due to one or both medications. In some cases, these drugs may cost more than taking each drug separately. The clinician must weigh the risks and benefits of using combination medications.

TABLE 15.2 Combination Oral Medications for Type 2 Diabetes

Medication	*Available Dosages*	*Initial Dose*
ACTO plus met (pioglitazone/metformin)	15 mg/500 mg 15 mg/850 mg	*Already on Metformin:* 15 mg/500 mg or 15 mg/850 mg once or twice a day *Already on Pioglitazone:* 15 mg/500 mg twice a day, or 15 mg/850 mg daily *Maximum Dose:* piaglitazone 45 mg/metformin 2550 mg
Avandaryl (rosiglitazone/glimepiride)	4 mg/1 mg 4 mg/2 mg 4 mg/4 mg	*Already on Rosiglitazone or Glimepiride:* 4 mg/1mg or 4 mg/2 mg daily *Maximum Dose:* rosiglitazone 8 mg/glimepiride 4 mg
Avandamet (rosiglitazone/metformin)	1 mg/500 mg 2 mg/500 mg 4 mg/500 mg 2 mg/1000 mg 4 mg/1000 mg	*Already on Rosiglitazone:* usual rosiglitazone dose/metformin 1000 mg divided dose twice daily *Already on Metformin:* rosiglitazone 4 mg/usual metformin dose divided dose twice daily *Maximum Dose:* rosiglitazone 8 mg/metformin 2000 mg
Glucovance (glyburide/metformin) generic available	1.25 mg/250 mg 2.5 mg/500 mg 5 mg/500 mg	*As Initial Therapy:* 1.25 mg/250 mg daily or twice daily *As Second-Line Therapy:* 2.5 mg/500 mg or 5 mg/500 mg twice daily *Maximum Dose:* glyburide 20 mg/metformin 2000 mg
Metaglip (glipizide/metformin)	2.5 mg/250 mg 2.5 mg/500 mg 5 mg/500 mg	*As Initial Therapy:* 2.5 mg/250 mg daily or twice daily *Maximum for Initial Therapy:* glipizide 10 mg/metformin 2000 mg *As Second-Line Therapy:* 2.5 mg/500 mg or 5mg/500 mg twice daily *Maximum for Second-Line Therapy:* Glipizide 20 mg/metformin 2000 mg

Source: Adapted from Oral combination products for type 2 diabetes. Pharmacist's Letter/Prescriber's Letter. 2006;222(2):220206.

Incretin Mimetics: Exenatide

Over the past several years, a great deal of research and attention has been focused on the impact of incretin hormones on glycemic control. In 2005, the first of a highly anticipated group of medications (called incretin mimetics) was approved for use in persons with type 1 and type 2 diabetes with actions on glucose control through the incretin system.[43] Exenatide is a synthetic form of a protein found in the saliva of the Gila monster, a lizard that is native to Mexico and the southwestern United States. Exenatide mimics the action of incretins such as glucagon-like peptide-1 (GLP-1), while other products in development apparently block GLP-1 breakdown by blocking the effects of an enzyme (DPP). The drug is believed to bind to and activate GLP-1 receptors, resulting in a drop in fasting and postprandial glucose concentrations. Exenatide improves glycemic control in type 2 diabetes through several mechanisms including increased insulin synthesis and secretion in the presence of elevated glucose concentrations, improvement of first-phase insulin response, reduced

Case—Part 2: Pharmacologic Intervention

Despite adherence to a nutrition and physical activity plan, CR's blood glucose control was not in the recommended target range. Pharmacologic intervention was thus appropriate. Typically, an oral agent is chosen as the initial therapy for a person with type 2 diabetes, although insulin and exenatide also are rational choices for therapy. Certainly, if blood glucose is above 300 to 340 mg/dL, insulin should be strongly considered.

The choice of products is generally made by considering the individual's specific characteristics and the agents' actions and effects. Renal effects, hepatic effects, effects on lipids, effect on weight, drug interaction potential, doses required daily, age-related issues with use, and cost are important considerations. Metformin would be a good choice in CR's situation since there were no contraindications and the metformin would not promote weight gain or cause hypoglycemia when used as monotherapy and might have a favorable effect on his lipids.

After a review of CR's assessment, metformin 500 mg twice daily was initiated, with plans to titrate the dose as needed up to the maximum effective dose of 2000 mg daily.

glucagon concentrations during hyperglycemic swings, slowed gastric emptying, and reduced food intake.[44]

Concurrent use of insulin, metformin, sulfonylureas, or a combination of these drugs with exenatide is recommended. It is not a substitute or replacement for insulin therapy in type 1 diabetes. The primary goal of therapy is to improve glucose control as demonstrated with A1C levels. Significantly reduced A1C levels have been observed in persons using exenatide, with a reduction in both fasting and postprandial plasma glucose concentrations. A reduction in body weight was also noted in persons who received the higher dose (10 mcg).[45]

Dosing

Exenatide is administered by subcutaneous injection in the thigh, upper arm, or abdomen at any time within the 60 minutes before morning and evening meals. It should not be given after a meal. The initial dose should be 5 mcg twice a day for the first month, and the dose can then be increased to 10 mcg twice a day based on the response.[45] If a dose is missed, the treatment should be restarted at the next scheduled dose time.

Precautions

Due to its slowing effect on gastric emptying, the extent and rate of slowing absorption of orally administered drugs should be considered. Pain medication particularly should be administered either 2 hours or more before or after injection. Exenatide may delay and reduce the peak concentration of digoxin, but not its area under the curve. It can reduce the peak and area under the curve of both lovastatin and acetaminophen.[46]

Contraindications

Exenatide is classified in pregnancy category C and should be used during pregnancy only if the potential benefit justifies the risk.

Exenatide should not be used in persons with severe gastrointestinal disorders, including gastroparesis.[47] Presently, it is not known whether the drug is excreted in human milk, and a choice between use of the drug or continued nursing is usually required. Pediatric effectiveness and safety have not been demonstrated.

The potential for antiexenatide antibodies development must be considered. Persons who developed these antibodies in clinical trials did not experience a difference in glucose control versus the persons who did not develop a measurable level of antibodies. Exenatide is eliminated renally by glomerular filtration with proteolytic degradation. Clearance is only slightly reduced in persons with mild-to-moderate renal impairment, but exenatide is not recommended in persons with severe renal impairment (creatinine clearance <30 mL per minute).[45]

Side Effects

Common side effects include nausea, with reports up to 44%. Vomiting, diarrhea, dizziness, headache, and dyspepsia are also noted, but less frequently. Mild to moderate nausea

Exenetide: Dosage Information

Drug	*Trade Name*	*Common Dose and Available Forms*	*Common Frequency*
Exenatide	Byetta	5 mcg to 10 mcg twice daily *Pen injectors:* 1.2 mL, 2.4 mL	Twice daily

is reported most often when therapy is started, with frequency and severity decreasing as treatment is continued.

Monitoring

Careful monitoring and instruction to take orally administered medications at least 1 hour before exenatide doses is necessary. This is especially true with medications such as antibiotics, oral contraceptives, and agents with a narrow therapeutic index.[46]

Instructions to Patients

When used with a hypoglycemic agent, exenatide may cause hypoglycemia; therefore, those taking this medication should be cautioned to monitor blood glucose levels carefully.

Exenatide is supplied as a sterile solution that contains 250 mcg/mL in a glass cartridge in a pen injector. Two pens, containing 1.2 mL or 2.4 mL, are available to deliver doses of 5 mcg or 10 mcg. Each pen will provide 60 doses to give a 30-day supply. Needles are not included with the pen and are purchased separately. Proper storage and use of the pen requires patient teaching. The drug should be stored in the refrigerator and protected from light. The pen should be discarded within 30 days after its first use.[11]

Managing Type 2 Diabetes

Many different pharmacologic treatment options are currently available for treating type 2 diabetes. The healthcare professional must weigh benefits and risks of the different therapies. Table 15.3 outlines some recommended approaches to the treatment of type 2 diabetes with available agents.

TABLE 15.3 Approach to Therapy for Type 2 Diabetes
Nonpharmacologic Therapy • Lifestyle modification and patient education are essential for all treatments regardless of medication. • If target ranges are not achieved in 2 to 4 months, add medication.
Oral Monotherapy • *If Obese.* Start metformin at low dose and increase the dose over 3-4 weeks (≤2000 mg/day). Avoid using higher doses in the elderly. If metformin is contraindication or not well tolerated, consider another medication class. • *If Not Obese.* Start sulfonylurea, insulin secretagogue, or metformin and increase dose over 3 to 4 weeks as needed. If postprandial blood glucose is elevated, consider an alpha-glucosidase inhibitor or a meglitinide with metformin. Other agents that may be effective are the TZDs (effect seen in 8 to 16 weeks). If A1C targets are not met, combination therapy may be initiated.
Oral Combination Therapy Numerous combinations can be used safely: • Sulfonylureas and metformin • Sulfonylureas and TZD • Sulfonylureas and alpha-glucosidase inhibitor • Metformin and TZD • Metformin and meglitinide • Metformin and exenatide • Metformin and pramlintide • TZD and meglitinide Sulfonylureas and meglitinides should not be used together as they have no added benefit. Sometimes 3 agents are used together if in different classes.
Injectable Therapy • Exenatide is indicated for the treatment of type 2 diabetes in persons already on metformin or a sulfonylurea who have not achieved adequate glucose control. • Pramlintide can be used in persons taking insulin, with or without metformin or a sulfonylurea. If A1C targets are not met, insulin therapy may be added. There are several options (see the insulin regimens in Figure 15.1): • Bedtime insulin (NPH, or glargine or detemir) and daytime oral medication (sulfonylureas, metformin, TZD, meglitinides, or alpha-glucosidase inhibitors), *or* • Discontinuing oral agents and switching to insulin therapy 1-4 times a day

Source: Adapted from Rogier L, Downey S, Jensen B. Diabetes agents for type 2 diabetes, update 9/05. Available from www.rxfiles.ca/newsletters.htm. Accessed 24 Mar 2006.

Amylin Analog

Pramlintide

The discovery of amylin, which is produced and secreted in the pancreas beta cells in response to food intake in addition to insulin, occurred in 1987. Both insulin and amylin have similar fasting and postprandial secretion patterns.[48] But, in persons with type 1 diabetes and persons with type 2 diabetes who need insulin, secretion of both insulin and amylin is diminished due to pancreatic-cell dysfunction or damage. A recombinant form of amylin, pramlintide (Symlin), is now available for clinical use.[11] Pramlintide affects the rise of postprandial glucose by slowing gastric emptying, suppressing glucagon secretion, and reducing total caloric intake. Some research and discussion of this satiety sensation has led to the possible conclusion of a central effect.[11] Pramlintide is administered subcutaneously just before major meals and is indicated for both type 1 and type 2 diabetes therapy in persons who use mealtime insulin therapy. People with type 2 diabetes who take pramlintide may also be taking metformin or a sulfonylurea. While always used along with insulin, pramlintide cannot be mixed and must be given as a separate injection.[49]

Dosing

Persons with type 1 diabetes should receive a starting dose of 15 mcg before major meals titrated in 15-mcg increments to a dose of up to 60 mcg as tolerated with nausea. Persons with type 2 diabetes using insulin usually receive an initial dose of 60 mcg before major meals. Pending the tolerance to nausea, the dose can be titrated to 120 mcg. Adjustment of the dose occurs to reach the desired glycemic control and tolerance to nausea.[49] The bioavailability of a single subcutaneous dose is approximately 40%, and its half-life is 48 minutes with a 3-hour duration after injection. Pramlintide is primarily metabolized in the kidneys to an active metabolite with a short half-life. Clearance of the drug was not altered in persons with moderate or severe renal impairment.[50]

Precautions

Pramlintide is categorized in pregnancy category C and should be used in pregnancy only if the potential benefit justifies the risk. The major concern with pramlintide use is the risk for hypoglycemia; careful monitoring and patient instruction for monitoring this action is mandatory. This effect is not actually due to the pramlintide, but rather secondary to the pramlintide making the insulin more effective, which can induce the blood glucose swing.[50]

Contraindications

Gastroparesis is a contraindication to the use of pramlintide due to its effect in slowing gastric emptying. Further, pramlintide should not be considered for persons taking drugs that alter gastrointestinal motility (eg, anticholinergic agents) or slow absorption of nutrients (eg, alpha-glucosidase inhibitors).[51] Pramlintide can slow the rate of absorption of orally administered medications.

Side Effects

Nausea is the most common side effect noted with use of pramlintide, ranging up to 48%, though the incidence is higher at the start of therapy and decreases with time. Gradual titration to the recommended dose reduces this reaction. Other side effects can include anorexia, vomiting, fatigue, and headache.[50]

Instructions to Patients

Medications that mandate a prompt or rapid onset of action should be taken at least 1 hour before or 2 hours after a pramlintide dose.[51] The dose is adjusted to reach the desired glycemic control and tolerance to nausea.[49] Pramlintide vials require refrigeration, though the vial in use can be stored at room temperature at a temperature of less than 77°F. Opened vials must be used within 28 days and then be discarded.

Insulin

Physiology of Insulin in Diabetes

Insulin is a hormone produced in the beta cells of the islets of Langerhans in the pancreas; it is formed from a substance called proinsulin. When the pancreas is stimulated, primarily by an elevated blood glucose level, the proinsulin is cleaved at 2 sections of the molecule. When the proinsulin molecule is broken apart, insulin and the connecting peptide (C-peptide) are both secreted and enter the bloodstream in equimolar amounts.[51] Exogenous insulin is made chemically identical to human insulin by recombinant DNA technology.[52] Another polypeptide, amylin, is also produced in the pancreas and released with insulin to assist in regulating the effects of insulin and to attenuate the actions of insulin.[53]

Mechanism of Action

The physiologic actions of insulin on body tissues include the following:[54]

- Stimulates entry of amino acids into cells, enhances protein synthesis
- Enhances fat storage (lipogenesis) and prevents mobilization of fat for energy (lipolysis and ketogenesis)
- Stimulates entry of glucose into cells for use as an energy source and promotes the resultant storage of glucose as glycogen (glycogenesis) in muscle and liver cells
- Inhibits production of glucose from liver or muscle glycogen (glycogenolysis)
- Inhibits formation of glucose from noncarbohydrates, such as amino acids (gluconeogenesis)

Several hormones in the body exert antagonistic effects to the hypoglycemic actions of insulin. These hormones are collectively referred to as counterregulatory hormones. The primary counterregulatory hormones include glucagon (produced in the alpha cells of the pancreas), epinephrine, norepinephrine, growth hormone, and cortisol.[55,56] Blood glucose management in diabetes needs to take into account, and make compensation for, the release of 1 or more of these hormones throughout the day in response to a variety of stimuli.

Indications for Use

Insulin is always indicated for people with type 1 diabetes and many type 2 persons with diabetes when other forms of therapy do not effectively control glucose levels. Insulin may also be indicated in those with type 2 diabetes who may be well controlled on oral agents but experience periods of physiological stress such as surgery or infection, which cause severe hyperglycemia that is not responsive to the oral agents. Women with gestational diabetes may need insulin if medical nutrition therapy alone does not adequately control blood glucose levels. Persons receiving parenteral nutrition or high-caloric supplements to meet an increased energy need may require exogenous insulin to maintain normal glucose levels during periods of insulin resistance or increased insulin demand. Insulin is necessary in treating diabetic ketoacidosis and often needed in treating hyperosmolar hyperglycemic state.[57]

Animal insulins are no longer manufactured. Human insulin is less antigenic than beef insulin and slightly less antigenic than pork insulin. Insulin analogs and U-500 insulin all require a prescription, although other insulin preparations are available without a prescription.[11]

The concentrations of insulin currently available in the United States are U-100 and U-500, indicating 100 units/mL or 500 units/mL, respectively.[52] U-100 insulin is the insulin of choice for nearly all patients. Persons requiring large doses of insulin may benefit by using U-500 regular insulin. The onset and duration of action of U-500 is not the same as U-100 regular. It may have a slower onset and slightly longer duration of activity. U-500 regular (Humulin R) is available in the United States only by prescription.

Insulin is also classified according to onset, peak effect, and duration of action. See Table 15.4.

Short- or Rapid-Acting Insulin

The currently available rapid-acting insulins are insulin lispro, insulin aspart, and insulin glulisine.[58] The short-acting insulin is regular insulin. Administration is into the subcutaneous tissue, although regular and the rapid-acting insulin analogs also may be given intravenously.[11] Regular insulin and the insulin analogs are clear solutions; the other insulin preparations are suspensions. Insulin lispro,

TABLE 15.4 Time Action for Insulin Preparations

Insulin Preparations	*Onset of Action*	*Peak*	*Duration of Action*
Lispro Aspart Glulisine	5-15 minutes	1-2 hours	4-6 hours
Regular, human	30-60 minutes	2-4 hours	6-10 hours
NPH, human	1-2 hours	4-8 hours	10-18 hours
Glargine	1-2 hours	Flat	up to 24 hours
Detemir	1-2 hours	Flat*	up to 24 hours

*With detemir, in the initial week(s) of therapy, one may observe a peaking effect; thereafter, the activity curve is flat.

Source: Adapted from Facts and Comparisons. St. Louis, Mo: Wolters Kluwer Health, Inc; 2005:287.

aspart, and glulisine with their very rapid onset and short duration of action can generally be used in place of regular insulin to provide better coverage of postprandial glycemic excursions. Insulin lispro can be injected immediately prior to eating (generally less than 15 minutes preprandially); injecting insulin lispro 30 to 60 minutes prior to meals may result in profound hypoglycemia. Several studies show reduced hypoglycemia in patients with type 1 diabetes treated with insulin lispro compared with those treated with regular human insulin. Insulin lispro has also been shown to be a suitable pump insulin. Also, when compared to regular insulin, it reduced A1C levels in pump users; however, both reduced the incidence of hypoglycemia compared to injected insulin.[59]

Insulin aspart can improve postprandial glycemic control by reducing hyperglycemic and hypoglycemic reactions, when compared to use of human short-acting (regular) insulin.[60,61] Insulin aspart has a glucose-lowering response similar to insulin lispro, and its duration of action is shortest after abdominal subcutaneous injection.[62] Insulin aspart is also reported to be effective when used in insulin pump therapy.[60] Insulin glulisine has a more rapid dissociation rate than human regular insulin, producing a more rapid onset. The pharmacokinetic profile of insulin glulisine is comparable to insulin lispro and insulin aspart. Additionally, insulin glulisine combined with NPH produced greater reductions in A1C levels than a regimen of regular and NPH.[52]

Intermediate-Acting Insulin

The intermediate-acting insulin is NPH. NPH is an abbreviation for neutral protamine Hagedorn. It is neutral in pH, contains the protein protamine (as well as zinc), and is named for the researcher who derived the formulation. The zinc/protamine complex prolongs the duration of action. Both protamine and zinc have occasionally been implicated as the causative agents of immunologic reactions such as urticaria or other allergic type reactions at the injection site. Since protamine is the antidote for heparin toxicity, some have expressed concerns about sensitizing persons to protamine with NPH insulin, but these concerns have not proven to be warranted.

Long-Acting Insulins

Long-acting insulins are the analogs insulin glargine (Lantus) and insulin detemir (Levemir). The long-acting analogs provide a true peakless pharmacokinetic or drug effect pattern. Interestingly, the 2 agents differ greatly in terms of their mechanism or the explanation for their extended basal-type action curve.

Insulin glargine is a clear solution that is prepared in a solution with a pH of 4.0; due to its acidic nature, insulin glargine may cause a mild burning when injected. Following injection, insulin glargine forms a microcrystalline precipitate that results in a depot in the subcutaneous fat. This depot gives the glargine its duration of action. Insulin glargine can be given at bedtime or at any time of the day, but should be given consistently at the same time each day.[63] Insulin glargine must not be mixed in the same syringe with other insulins. The syringe must not contain any other medicine or residue.[63] Insulin glargine provides only basal insulin coverage and in most cases will be used in combination with other insulin preparations or oral agents.

Insulin detemir is a clear solution whose protracted action is due to increased self-aggregation and also albumin binding in the plasma and adjacent to the injection site.[64] Initially, a peak effect is reached in 6 to 8 hours; following routine administration, however, a constant rate of insulin detemir is found in the bloodstream. This results in a plateau or basal effect that approaches 24 hours.[64] Insulin detemir must not be diluted or mixed with any other insulin preparations.

Premixed Insulins

Commercially available premixed insulins and insulin analogs (70/30, 50/50, 75/25) are manufactured and stabilized by altered buffering.[62] These products may be appropriate for persons who may have difficulty mixing their own insulins or for those in whom these ratios are effective. However, for intensive insulin regimens, these insulins are usually not recommended.

Dosing

The starting dose and schedule of insulin administration is based on several factors, including the type of diabetes; the clinical assessment of insulin deficiency and suspected insulin resistance; and the individual's preferences for eating times and amounts of carbohydrate, physical activity, and waking/sleeping patterns.[65] Target blood glucose levels for before meals, after meals, and during sleep should be established with the patient. Setting targets enhances acceptance, understanding and decision making as the individual observes changes in blood glucose levels in relation to changes in food, exercise, stress, or illness. Subsequent adjustments in dose or timing of the insulin are based on self-monitoring of blood glucose results and clinical signs and symptoms of hypoglycemia or hyperglycemia. Other parameters used to refine the insulin dose and schedule include glycosylated hemoglobin levels, achievement of weight or lipid goals, and variability of lifestyle or activities from day to day.

A goal of contemporary insulin therapy is to mimic, as nearly as possible, the physiologic profile of insulin secretion (basal/bolus).[57] The evolution of insulin management in the United States for people with type 1 diabetes and many with type 2 has clearly moved from single daily injection therapy to multiple injections with multiple insulins. Such a pattern was difficult to achieve prior to the era of the insulin analogs.[58] To optimize glycemic control, the pharmacology and pharmacokinetics of insulin require that a person with type 1 diabetes receive insulin continuously (basal, also referred to as background insulin), with boluses of insulin before meals and snacks (often called mealtime insulin).[57] Physiologic insulin secretion typically occurs at a rate of 0.5 to 1 unit per hour. The metabolic balance between basal insulin, the counterregulatory hormones, hepatic glucose production, and circulating glucose normally provides the body with sufficient glucose to function between meals. Bolus insulin is rapidly released in response to nutrient intake from a meal and under normal circumstances reduces postprandial glycemic excursions back to baseline in 60 to 90 minutes.[66]

Insulin requirements for individuals with type 1 diabetes or who are within 20% of ideal body weight are usually 0.5 to 1.0 unit per kilogram of body weight per day. Insulin requirements may be higher (even double) in the presence of intercurrent illness or other metabolic instability. Insulin requirements will be less (0.2 to 0.6 unit per kilogram of body weight per day) during the honeymoon phase, the period of relative remission early in the course of the disease.

Insulin Therapy in Pregnancy

Preexisting Diabetes

Insulin requirements for women with preexisting diabetes during the second and third trimesters of pregnancy gradually increase and can be 0.9 to 1.2 units per kilogram of body weight per day (as much as twice the total daily dosage of insulin needed before pregnancy).[67] These increases in plasma insulin are opposed by diminished responsiveness to insulin action due to placental production of counterregulatory hormones. Women with preexisting diabetes should be treated with an intensive insulin regimen, 3 to 4 injections or an insulin pump, to provide the basal/bolus regimen.

Gestational Diabetes Mellitus

Approaches to insulin therapy for gestational diabetes differ greatly. Please see the discussion on taking medication in chapter 12, on gestational diabetes mellitus. A total dose of 20 to 30 units given before breakfast is commonly used to initiate therapy.[67] The total dose is usually divided into two-thirds intermediate-acting insulin and one-third rapid-acting or short-acting insulin. For obese women, a higher starting dose of insulin is usually needed due to insulin resistance. The total initial dosage may be as high as 0.8 to 1.0 unit per kilogram of body weight per day.[67]

Insulin Regimens

Insulin regimens vary and should be designed with regard to a person's meals, exercise, medications, work or activity schedule, and emotional factors. Appropriate alterations can be made in the insulin regimen to accommodate a midnight or rotating work schedule or other lifestyle preferences. Figure 15.1 shows some different types of insulin regimens using 2 to 4 or more injections a day. Although the typical split and mixed 2-injection daily regimen is often used, it may not be adequate to reach target ranges.

Multiple injections of insulin (3 or more) are components of the system called flexible or intensive insulin therapy. With 3-injection regimens, insulin is administered in the morning before breakfast, before the evening meal, and at bedtime, or before each meal. Before breakfast, a combination of rapid-acting or short-acting and intermediate-acting insulin is often used. Before the evening meal, rapid-acting or short-acting insulin is often used alone. At bedtime, intermediate-acting insulin is then often used. This type of therapy can reduce the risk of nocturnal (2 to 4 AM) hypoglycemia, allows better insulin coverage for early morning (5 to 10 AM) hyperglycemia from the release of cortisol and growth hormone (the dawn phenomenon), and, in some cases, may accommodate sleeping in.[68]

With 4-injection regimens, a long-acting insulin such as insulin glargine or insulin detemir is administered once a day, and at mealtimes a rapid-acting or short-acting insulin is administered. If snacks contain more than 15 g of carbohydrate, an injection of rapid-acting insulin may be needed before a snack. This regimen is illustrated in Figure 15.1. The rapid-acting or short-acting insulin provides postmeal glycemic control, while the long-acting insulin dose ensures a low, steady rate of insulin throughout the day. This type of regimen or use of an insulin pump can best duplicate normal physiologic insulin action.[69] In persons with type 1 diabetes, physiologic replacement using basal insulin and a mealtime rapid-acting insulin improves A1C levels and results in fewer episodes of hypoglycemia than previous regimens.[70] This regimen can provide individuals with diabetes the flexibility in insulin doses necessary for busy and active lifestyles.

Pump therapy is a continuous basal amount of insulin (0.5 to 1.0 units per hour) that is usually administered in addition to bolus doses given prior to meals.[69] See chapter 17 on intensifying insulin therapy and insulin pump therapy for more information.

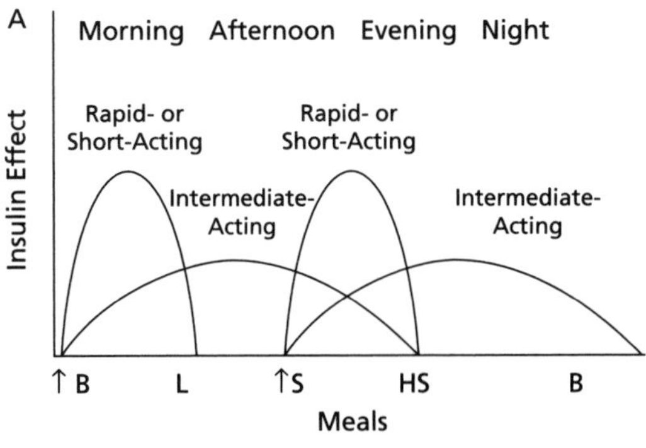

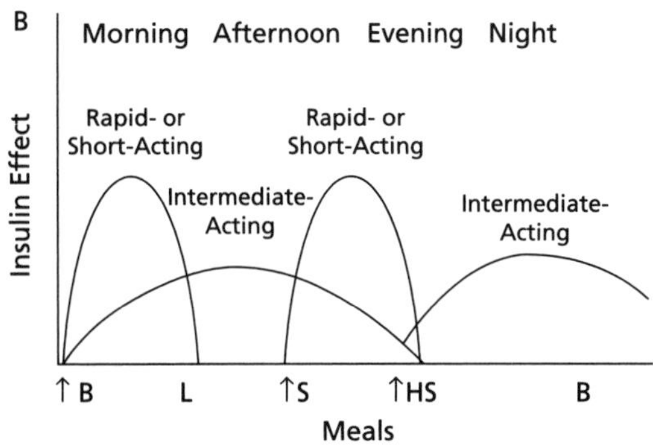

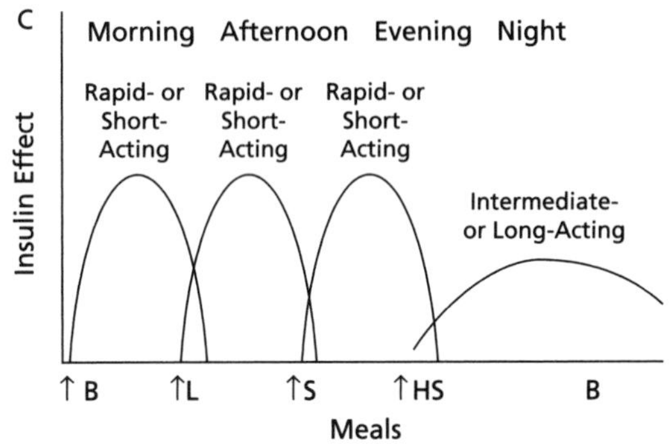

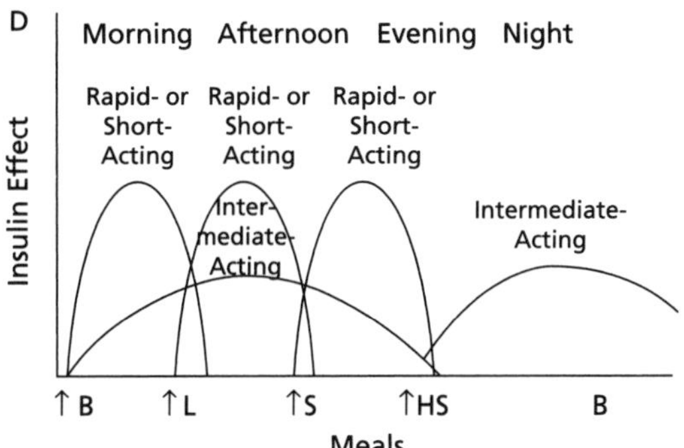

FIGURE 15.1 Potential Multiple-Injection Insulin Regimens

Parts A, B, C, and D represent options for insulin injection scheduling.

Source: Reprinted with permission from the American Diabetes Association. Copyright © 1998 American Diabetes Association. Lebovitz HE. Therapy for Diabetes Mellitus and Related Disorders, 3rd ed. Alexandria, Va.

Insulin Therapy in Type 2 diabetes

For type 2 diabetes, insulin therapy may be used in 2 ways. First, insulin may be a supplement or additional agent added to an oral agent or multiple oral agents. Typically, single daily injections are used, commonly starting at 10 to 20 units per dose. Single daily injection regimens for type 2 diabetes dictate that insulin is administered in the morning or at bedtime. Due to the insulin resistance seen in type 2 diabetes, the dose of insulin as monotherapy in persons with type 2 diabetes is higher (0.7 to 2.5 units per kilogram per day). An intermediate-acting or a long-acting insulin is usually used, but could include a combined dose of a rapid-acting or short-acting and intermediate-acting insulin product.[71]

Type 2 diabetes can also be treated with insulin as the sole pharmacological agent. This requires at least a 2-injection regimen, or a multiple-injection (3 or greater) regimen. In 2-injection regimens, insulin is administered in the morning before breakfast and before the evening meal or at bedtime. This regimen may include only intermediate-acting insulin, or doses of regular or rapid-acting insulins mixed with long-acting or intermediate-acting insulin, or premixed formulations (ie, mixtures such as Humalog Mix 75/25 or Novolog Mix 70/30) at 1 or both injection times. Using mixed doses in the morning and before the evening meal is often called a split-mixed regimen and is considered fixed or conventional insulin therapy. Usually two-thirds of the total daily dose of insulin is given before breakfast (using a ratio of 1 part rapid-acting or short-acting insulin to 2 parts intermediate-acting insulin) and one-third is given before the evening meal (using a ratio of 1:1 or 1:2, rapid-acting or short-acting to intermediate insulin).[71]

Insulin Delivery Devices

Syringe

Disposable insulin syringes with attached needles for U-100 insulin are available in different syringe sizes, chosen according to the dose of insulin to be injected: 0.25 cc (for doses <25 units), 0.3 cc (for doses <30 units), 0.5 cc (for doses <50 units), or 1 cc (for doses 50 to 100 units). Needle length may be 5/16-in or 1/2-in. The "short needle" (5/16-in length) is appropriate only for individuals with normal or near-normal body mass index (BMI) (<27 kg/m^2) to assure subcutaneous injection. In most situations, syringes and needles may be safely reused; however, reuse may carry an increased risk of infection for some individuals.[52] Advise those who choose to reuse syringes that the markings on the syringe may rub off and that the needle becomes dull with repeated use. Instruct patients to safely recap the needle and store at room temperature.

Pump

Continuous subcutaneous insulin infusion (CSII) pumps became available in 1974. An insulin pump consists of a reservoir filled with insulin, a small battery-operated pump and a computer chip that allows the user to control the insulin delivery (see chapter 17, on intensifying insulin therapy, for more on insulin pump therapy).

Jet Injector

Jet injectors are a novel, needle-free system that delivers insulin transcutaneously. Jet injectors release a fine stream of insulin at high speed and under high pressure to penetrate the skin.

Pen Device

Pen devices have been a popular insulin delivery option in Europe for years. They were introduced in the United States in 1987. They combine the insulin container and the syringe into a single modular unit that allows for convenient insulin delivery. Insulin pens are available in a variety of types and styles. Pens may be reusable or prefilled. Reusable pens and prefilled pens both hold cartridges of insulin. With the reusable pen, the patient must first load an insulin cartridge. This step is eliminated with prefilled pen devices.[72]

Inhalation Device

Pulmonary delivery of insulin (inhaled insulin) is discussed later in the chapter.

Future Possibilities

In the future, insulin may be delivered by implantable insulin pumps or transdermal systems. Two types of implantable pumps exist: a closed-loop system and an open-looped system.

Insulin Use

Monitoring

Self-monitoring of blood glucose and periodic A1C levels (every 3 months until goal level is attained, then every 6 months) should be the primary long-term monitors for insulin therapy, although blood glucose readings can be valuable in day-to-day blood glucose management. Inquiries about hypoglycemic episode severity and frequency should also be included in the assessment. Normal daily insulin secretion in a healthy, nonpregnant adult who is not obese is approximately 0.5 to 0.7 units of insulin per kilogram of body weight per day. Since insulin and C-peptide are jointly secreted, a measurement of C-peptide level is used as a clinical monitor of endogenous insulin production and can be used to determine type of diabetes. Direct measurement of insulin secretion is difficult, except under controlled or research conditions, because insulin is rapidly removed from the blood as it exerts its pharmacologic action.[73] Because insulin and C-peptide have different biologic durations, a measurement of C-peptide level may not accurately reflect the endogenous insulin level at that period of time.

Precautions

Insulin is the drug treatment of choice for glycemic control during pregnancy. The major adverse effect of insulin therapy is hypoglycemia. Virtually all persons who inject insulin will experience hypoglycemia at some time. Common causes of hypoglycemia include excessive doses of insulin; delayed, missed, or insufficient food intake; or too much (unplanned) physical activity.[54]

Contraindications

Evaluate drug allergies to avoid acute allergic reaction to some of the preparations.

Side Effects

Various problems or complications may arise from insulin characteristics. Insulin impurity can cause lipodystrophies (atrophy and/or hypertrophy). Atrophy, which is a concavity or pitting of the fatty tissue, is an immune phenomenon that occurs in a small number of persons and is related to species/source or purity. Use of highly purified insulins such as human insulin or purified pork reduces the occurrence of atrophy. Persons who develop this problem may benefit from injecting human or highly purified insulin around the periphery of the atrophied areas.[74] Many clinicians recommend a review of the person's insulin dose and injection technique when lipodystrophy occurs. Hypertrophy, which is a fatty thickening of the lipid tissue, is best prevented by rotating injection sites.

Allergies to insulin are possible but rare. Insulin allergy may occur as local reactions (rash, urticarial cutaneous reaction) or systemic reactions (serum sickness, anaphylaxis). Prior to insulin purification, local cutaneous reactions were more common. Zinc or protamine in the insulin, preservatives, and rubber or latex stoppers have all been implicated in inducing allergic reactions. Both local and systemic reactions appear to be immunologically mediated through induction of high titers of IgG and IgE antibodies. If a systemic reaction occurs, desensitization to the insulin will be necessary. If desensitization is needed, the attending physician should be encouraged to contact the insulin manufacturer for the desensitization kit and the procedure to follow.[75]

Instructions for Patients

Insulin mixing standards are based on published data.[52] Varying the time delay for injecting after mixing may result in a different insulin action. As a general rule, the 2 insulins to be mixed should be of the same brand. Rapid-acting or regular insulin is usually drawn up first, followed by the intermediate-acting insulin. This practice limits the potential for contamination, which may result in dose variance.

All insulin mixtures must be thoroughly resuspended immediately prior to an injection or after storage for any time period. Those using these products should be instructed to gently roll the vial or prefilled syringe or pen device between the palms several times to thoroughly mix the component insulins.

Strategies to reduce the risk of hypoglycemia include performing routine self-monitoring of blood glucose levels and observing for and responding quickly to early symptoms of hypoglycemia. Insulin users are instructed to ingest appropriate quantities and choices of a preexercise carbohydrate supplement and apply a consistent food/meal plan and pattern.[55]

Those using insulin should be instructed to take extra supplies when traveling to foreign countries, as some countries may still use U-40 insulins. Insulin users should be taught to store insulin according to the manufacturer's recommendations. Generally, insulin should be refrigerated at 36°F to 46°F (2C° to 8°C). Unopened insulin products may be stored under refrigeration until the expiration date noted on the product label. Injecting a cold insulin preparation can produce local irritation and increased pain at the injection site; to bring the insulin to room temperature, the prepared syringe should be rolled between the palms of the hands. Other options include returning the vial of insulin to room temperature before withdrawing the dose or storing the insulin at room temperature. Opened or unopened vials of insulin may be stored at a controlled room temperature of 59°F to 86°F (15°C to 30°C) for a period of 1 month; unused insulin should be discarded after that time.[52] Storage guidelines differ for used (punctured) or unused cartridge insulin and disposable prefilled insulin pens:

- Used or unused insulin cartridges or regular prefilled insulin pens may be kept unrefrigerated for 28 days (1.5-mL or 3.0-mL cartridges).
- Humalog Mix 75/25 may be used for 10 days capped at room temperature (72°F) and out of direct sunlight; unused can be stored without refrigeration for 28 days, but should be stored in the refrigerator to preserve its effectiveness until the labeled expiration.
- 70/30 insulin cartridges or prefilled insulin pens may be kept and used unrefrigerated for 10 days, unused units should be refrigerated or if unrefrigerated, discarded in 10 days.
- NPH insulin cartridges or prefilled insulin pens may be kept and used unrefrigerated for 14 days, unused units should be refrigerated or if unrefrigerated, discarded in 14 days.

Manually prefilled syringes of either single formulations or mixtures of insulins are to be refrigerated and used within 21 to 30 days.[52] Availability of insulin and supplies may vary; teach patients to carry insulin and supplies when traveling. Due to the variance of temperature, insulin should not be left in a car or checked through in airline baggage. Instruct those using insulin to examine vials of insulin for sediment or other visible changes before withdrawing the insulin into the syringe. Cloudiness or discoloration of clear insulin, clumping of insulin suspensions, or flocculation (frosting) of insulin suspensions indicates that the insulin has lost potency and should not be used but returned to the pharmacy for exchange. The incidence of frosting may be minimized if temperature is stabilized through refrigeration and if agitation or shaking of the vial is minimized.

Teach persons using insulin to follow a specific routine for insulin injections, including consistent technique, accurate dosage, and site rotation. Injections are given into the subcutaneous tissue. Most individuals are able to lightly grasp a fold of skin and inject at a 90-degree angle. Thin individuals or children may need to pinch the skin and inject at a 45-degree angle to avoid intramuscular injection.[52] Insulin may be injected into the subcutaneous tissue of the upper arm, the anterior and lateral aspects of the thigh, the buttocks, and the abdomen (with the exception of a circle with a 2-in radius around the navel).[52] These sites are chosen because of general patient acceptability and accessibility.

Areas for injection must be determined individually, allowing for scar tissue, areas with less subcutaneous fat, and individual preference. Both the person with diabetes and the health professional need to examine injection areas at regular intervals to detect bruising, redness, infection, lipoatrophy, or lipohypertrophy. Teach patients to rotate injection sites to prevent local irritation. Rotating within a single area is recommended (eg, rotating injections systematically within the abdomen) rather than rotating to a different area with each injection. This practice may decrease variability in absorption from day to day.[52] Insulin absorption may vary depending on several parameters. Abdominal injection provides the most rapid absorption, followed by the arms, thighs, and buttocks. [52] However, note that insulin glargine does not display this difference of absorption rates at different sites.[58] Deeper intramuscular injections induce faster absorption and shorter duration of action. High levels of insulin antibodies can also inhibit insulin action following injection. Exercise or massage of the injection site may induce more rapid absorption.

Pulmonary Insulin

Recent technological advances have made it feasible to deliver insulin to the alveolar space, where it is rapidly absorbed into the alveolar capillaries and disbursed throughout the systemic circulation.[76] A powdered form of human recombinant-DNA insulin (Exubera) is the first insulin preparation approved for use via inhalation. This product's use provides a rapid-acting form of insulin, but does not replace basal insulin therapy.[77] Insulin administered via the pulmonary route in human studies has a soluble, rapid-acting formulation.

Exubera is a fine-powdered formulation of insulin. The particle size is less than 5 μm in diameter. Particles of this size are able to reach the deep lung with slow, deep inhalation, and they then pass a single cellular layer into the circulation. Insulin from this system will be available in "blister packs" and will remain stable at room temperature for up to 2 years. The device used to deliver the insulin is about the size of a mechanical flashlight.

Other systems of accessing the body with insulin through the pulmonary system are being researched.[78] Clinical trials have demonstrated the effectiveness, safety, and acceptability of inhaled insulin in persons with type 2 and type 1 diabetes.[79] Persons using Exubera should monitor their blood glucose similarly to persons receiving bolus doses by injection.

Drug Interactions

Other drugs can interact with medications used for diabetes control. Certain drugs or foods can have an effect on blood glucose levels by altering the action, the effect, or the outcome from a particular drug regimen. These actions are generally categorized as follows:

- Drug-drug (or pharmacokinetic) interaction
- Drug-disease (or pharmacodynamic) interaction
- Drug-food interaction

A drug-drug interaction is said to occur when a medication is added to an individual's regimen that alters the effect of another medication the person is taking. Some of these interactions are listed in Table 15.5. This type of interaction can occur with changes anywhere along the map of drug transport through the body.[81] Specifically, a drug can have its absorption into the body, distribution through the body, metabolism by the body—usually the liver or kidneys, and elimination from the body changed by another agent. The effect may be an increase or decrease in the rate of a particular step or an altered level of protein binding in the bloodstream, resulting in either a decreased or increased net action by the medication. This type of interaction is also termed a pharmacokinetic interaction, since the alteration is on the flow of the drug through its normal kinetic movement through the body.[82]

A drug-disease interaction has an intrinsic physiologic effect as a particular medication may alter the level of control of a particular disorder. The interaction can either improve or worsen the level of control of a particular problem and is termed a pharmacodynamic interaction.

Case—Part 3: Combining Agents

CR returned to the diabetes clinic 1 year after his metformin dose was increased to 1000 mg twice daily. His A1C was still elevated at 8.8%, and he continued to have fasting glucose levels over 200 mg/dL. He had lost about 10 lb in the past year with increased physical activity and more attention to his eating. He reported that he had some tingling in his hands and feet and wanted better control of his diabetes. There were several options.

Combining agents was a logical step in providing optimal treatment for CR's type 2 diabetes. A combination of more than 1 agent would provide up to 1.8% further improvement of A1C than use of a single agent.[80] Appropriate monitoring of each agent would be necessary with use of any combination of products. Adding a sulfonylurea, TZD, insulin, or exenatide were all viable options.

After discussion with the diabetes team, CR decided to try a bedtime injection of NPH insulin to help lower his fasting glucose. He received diabetes education regarding prevention, recognition, and treatment of hypoglycemia; proper injection technique; and proper storage. A plan for the frequency of self-monitoring of blood glucose was agreed upon, and monthly follow-up was scheduled with the diabetes educator. CR's target was to achieve an A1C of < 7%.

TABLE 15.5 Drug-Disease and Drug-Drug Interactions

Interacting Drug	*Drug-Disease (Intrinsic Effect)*	*Drug-Drug Interaction**	*Net Effect on Blood Glucose*	*Notes*
Allopurinol	No	Sulfonylureas and Meglitinide	↓	• Decreased renal tubular secretion of chlorpropamide
Androgens/ anabolic steroids	Yes	—	↓	• Mechanism unknown
Anticoagulants, oral (Dicumarol)	No	Sulfonylureas and Meglitinide		• Interfere with metabolism of tolbutamide, chlorpropamide
Asparaginase I	Yes	—	↑[1] ↓[2]	1. Hyperglycemia associated with inhibition of insulin synthesis 2. Hypoglycemia reported occasionally
Aspirin	Yes[3]	Sulfonylureas[4] and Meglitinide	↓	3. Large daily doses (~4 g/d): Increased basal and stimulated release of insulin 4. Displace sulfonylurea from protein binding; decrease urinary excretion of sulfonylurea
β-Adrenergic antagonists	Yes	—	↑↓	• Both hypoglycemic and hyperglycemic response has been reported; may alter physiologic response to, and subjective symptoms of, hypoglycemia; may reduce hyperglycemia-induced insulin release or decrease tissue sensitivity to insulin
Calcium channel blockers	Yes	—	↑↓	• Hypoglycemia reported with verapamil • Hyperglycemia reported with diltiazem, nifedipine
Cholestyramine	No	TZD[5] and Acarbose[6]	↑[5] ↓[6]	5. Cholestyramine reduces absorption of coadministered drugs 6. Cholestyramine may enhance effects of acarbose; interactions may be avoided by administering cholestyramine 2 hours apart from other medications
Chloramphenicol	No	Sulfonylureas and Meglitinide		• Decreased hepatic metabolism and/ or protein binding displacement of tolbutamide, chlorpropamide
Chloroquine	Yes	—	↓	• Mechanism unknown

(continued)

TABLE 15.5 Drug-Disease and Drug-Drug Interactions

Interacting Drug	*Drug-Disease (Intrinsic Effect)*	*Drug-Drug Interaction**	*Net Effect on Blood Glucose*	*Notes*
Cimetidine/ possible other H2 antagonists	No	Sulfonylureas,[7] Meglitinide, and Metformin[8]	↓	7. Increased absorption and/or decreased clearance of glipizide, glyburide, tolbutamide 8. Decreased renal tubular secretion of metformin; other drugs excreted via renal tubular transport *may* similarly interfere with metformin clearance
Clofibrate	Yes[9]	Sulfonylureas[10] and Meglitinide	↓	9. Intrinsic hypoglycemic effect: mechanism unknown 10. Displace certain sulfonylureas from protein binding
Corticosteroid	Yes		↑	• Increased gluconeogenesis; transient insulin resistance
Cyclosporine	Yes	—	↑	—
Diazoxide	Yes		↑	• Inhibition of insulin secretion
Dicumarol	No	Sulfonylureas and Meglitinide	↓	• Inhibits hepatic metabolism of tolbutamide, chlorpropamide
Disopyramide	Yes	—	↑	• Most susceptible: elderly or patients with renal or liver impairment
Diuretics	Yes	—	↑	—
Estrogen products	Yes	—	↑	• Mechanism unknown
Ethanol	Yes	Sulfonylureas[11] and Meglitinide	↑[12] ↓[13]	11. Disulfiram-like reaction may also occur, especially with chlorpropamide; not noted with second-generation sulfonylureas 12. Chronic alcohol ingestion may increase metabolism of sulfonylurea; alcohol ingestion, especially with carbohydrate-based drink (beer, mixed drink), has caloric effect. 13. Intrinsic hypoglycemic effect; impairs gluconeogenesis and increases insulin secretion; effect is potentiated if alcohol consumed without food or in fasting state
Fluoxetine	Yes	—	↑↓	• Hypoglycemia and hyperglycemia have been reported
Fluconazole	No	Sulfonylureas and Meglitinide	↓	
Gemfibrozil	Yes	—	↑	• Reported interaction with glipizide

(continued)

TABLE 15.5 Drug-Disease and Drug-Drug Interactions

Interacting Drug	*Drug-Disease (Intrinsic Effect)*	*Drug-Drug Interaction**	*Net Effect on Blood Glucose*	*Notes*
Glyburide	Yes	Acarbose and Miglitol[14]	↑	14. Miglitol reduces the area under the curve (AUC) and peak concentration of glyburide
Guanethidine	Yes	Sulfonylureas[15] and Meglitinide	↓[16]	15. Protein-binding displacement of certain sulfonylureas 16. Intrinsic glycemic effect
NSAID (nonsteroidal anti-inflammatory drugs)	Yes[17]	Sulfonylureas[18] and Meglitinide	↑	17. Possible intrinsic hypoglycemic effect 18. Protein-binding displacement (tolbutamide, tolazamide)
Isoniazid	Yes	—	↑	• Increases glycogenolysis
Ketoconazole	Yes	Pioglitazone	↑	• In vitro studies suggest that ketoconazole inhibits the metabolism of pioglitazone
Metformin	No	Alpha-glucosidase inhibitors	↑	• Acarbose reduces metformin bioavailability by ~35% when separate doses to avoid coadministered; separate doses to avoid
Monoamine oxidase inhibitors	Yes[19]	Sulfonylureas[20] and Meglitinide	↓	19. May stimulate insulin secretion (beta-adrenergic stimulation) or may be secondary to hepatotoxicity 20. May interfere with metabolism of sulfonylurea
Nicotinic acid (niacin)	Yes	—	↑	• Dose dependent, when lipid-lowering doses are used • Insignificant effect at vitamin supplement dose
Octreotide	Yes	—	↑↓	• Hypoglycemia and hyperglycemia have been reported
Oral contraceptives	Yes	Pioglitazone[21] and Rosiglitazone[22]	↑	21. Pioglitazone has not been evaluated; however, caution should be used 22. No clinically significant effect on ethinyl estradiol or norethindrone
Pancrelipase/ pancreatic enzymes	Yes	—	↑	• Do not administer these agents concurrently with acarbose
Pentamidine	Yes	—	↑↓	• Initially, hypoglycemia; hyperglycemia may occur days or even months after initiation of therapy

(continued)

TABLE 15.5 Drug-Disease and Drug-Drug Interactions

Interacting Drug	*Drug-Disease (Intrinsic Effect)*	*Drug-Drug Interaction**	*Net Effect on Blood Glucose*	*Notes*
Phenothiazines	Yes	—	↑↓	• Hypoglycemia observed with some phenothiazines, hyperglycemia with others
Phenytoin	Yes	—	↑	• Decreased insulin secretion
Probenecid	Yes[23]	Sulfonylureas[24] and Meglitinide	↓	23. Intrinsic glycemic effect 24. Decrease urinary excretion of chlorpropamide
Protease inhibitors	Yes	—	↑	—
Rifampin	Yes[25]	Sulfonylureas[26] and Meglitinide	↑[26] ↓[25]	25. Possible intrinsic hypoglycemic effect 26. Increased metabolism of chlorpropamide, glyburide, tolbutamide
Salicylates	Yes[27]	Sulfonylureas[28] and Meglitinide	↓	27. Large daily doses (~4 g/d): Increase basal and stimulated release of insulin 28. Displace sulfonylurea from protein binding; decrease urinary excretion of sulfonylurea
Sulfonamides, highly protein-bound	No	Sulfonylureas and Meglitinide	↓	• Various effects upon chlorpropamide, tolbutamide kinetics: displacement from protein binding, decreased urinary excretion, and/or altered metabolism
Tacrolimus	Yes	—	↑	—
Thyroid products	Yes	—	↑	• Once euthyroid status is achieved, diabetes medications may need to be adjusted to compensate for glycemic effect of thyroid product
Urinary acidifiers	No	Sulfonylureas and Meglitinide	↓	• Interfere with chlorpropamide excretion

• This listing is not intended to be inclusive. Before any new medication is initiated, consult the package labeling (insert) or other reference. In general, these interactions are based on moderate to severe clinical significance and/or possible or established documentation.

• Interactions with sulfonylureas, meglitinide, metformin, pioglitazone, and rosiglitazone (both thiazolidinediones), alpha-glucosidase inhibitors, and insulin are listed.

Source: White JR, Campbell RK. Pharmacologic therapy of diabetes mellitus. In: A Core Curriculum for Diabetes Education: Diabetes Management Therapies, 5th ed. Franz MJ, ed. Chicago, Ill: American Association of Diabetes Educators; 2003: 120-3.

Drug actions can also be altered by concurrent ingestion of certain foods. A common mechanism of this interaction is to alter the absorption of a medication from the gastrointestinal tract, although other mechanisms of interactions (eg, effect on enzymes) have also been identified with other specific agents.

Medication Side Effects:

Self-Management Considerations

Certain drug side effects have an impact on diabetes self-management.[82] Persons with diabetes who are taking medication must be taught to be attentive to particular signs and symptoms that may indicate impending hypoglycemia or hyperglycemia.

In addition, certain procedures and aspects of diabetes care require the person with diabetes to be alert, coordinated, and capable of making self-management decisions. A drug that mimics an individual's usual warning signs of hypoglycemia or hyperglycemia, or one that impairs a person's ability to perform necessary self-care tasks, may adversely affect glycemic control.

Hypoglycemia

Defining hypoglycemia on the basis of a specific plasma glucose level is difficult. Absolute blood glucose levels cannot be used to describe the severity of hypoglycemic episodes because glycemic thresholds for the onset of symptoms, as well as symptom magnitude, differ greatly among individuals and from episode to episode, depending on various mediating variables. Some individuals remain alert with only a few symptoms at a plasma glucose level of 50 mg/dL (2.8 mmol/L), while others become stuporous at the same glucose concentration. Even the same person may tolerate low glucose levels differently on different occasions. Therefore, hypoglycemia is better defined based on symptoms:

- *Mild hypoglycemia* is characterized by symptoms such as sweating, trembling, difficulty concentrating, lightheadedness, and a lack of coordination. These symptoms are usually alleviated quickly by drinking or eating foods containing carbohydrates.
- *Severe hypoglycemia* is characterized by an inability to self-treat due to mental confusion, lethargy, or unconsciousness. Because the individual is unable to self-treat, others must provide treatment to raise the blood glucose level out of a dangerously low range.

Causes of Hypoglycemia

All hypoglycemic episodes are caused by an excess of the medications used to lower blood glucose (insulin, sulfonylureas, or insulin secretagogues) relative to food intake and activity level.

The first step in determining what is causing frequent hypoglycemia is a careful examination of the treatment *regimen*. Insulin excess and hypoglycemia are more likely to occur at those times of the day when insulin action is peaking. Some of the newer insulin analogs, including rapid-acting insulins (eg, insulin lispro or aspart) and long-acting (glargine or detemir) insulins, appear to reduce some of the problems with hypoglycemia, but still carry risk.

Hypoglycemia is more of a risk when an individual has taken insulin or a medication that promotes insulin secretion and has not eaten for several hours or when an individual takes medication and has significantly increased physical activity. Alcohol consumption, without food intake, may result in hypoglycemia.

Prevention of Hypoglycemia

Prevention is the best intervention. Treatment regimens should be developed that include intake of carbohydrate at peak times of the insulin or medications if necessary and snacks for increased physical activity. In addition, the individual should understand that foods high in fat or protein and very low in carbohydrate will not prevent hypoglycemia.

Treatment of Hypoglycemia

Treatment for hypoglycemia is to eat or drink 10 to 15 g of *glucose* or any form of carbohydrate that contains glucose, such as the following:

- 3-4 glucose tablets
- 8-10 lifesaver candies
- 2 tablespoons of raisins
- 4-6 oz nondiet soft drink
- 4-6 oz fruit juice
- 1 piece of fruit
- 1 cup of lowfat or nonfat milk

The challenge is to treat, but not overtreat. Overtreating hypoglycemia causes posttreatment hyperglycemia. Overtreating hypoglycemia is relatively common. The person may continue eating until all symptoms disappear. Some people may be so fearful of the symptoms (often feeling like they are losing control) that they overeat. It is sometimes difficult to prevent people from overtreating hypoglycemia. Using commercially available, portion-controlled glucose products may help individuals avoid overtreatment.

The choice of glucose or carbohydrates containing glucose should be based on choosing one that will raise the blood glucose levels rise quickly. Drinks or foods that are high in fat content slow gastric emptying and absorption of carbohydrate and, therefore, take longer to raise blood glucose levels. Adding protein to the treatment of hypoglycemia does not raise blood glucose levels and does not prevent subsequent hypoglycemia.

If possible, blood glucose levels should be tested before treatment, then 15 to 20 minutes after initiating treatment. If the blood glucose level is still low (less than 70 mg/dL), then treatment should be repeated whether or not the symptoms have disappeared. If not scheduled to eat a meal or snack within the next hour, the person should be cautious about additional hypoglycemia. Patients should be instructed that their blood glucose level may fall again if food is not eaten within the next hour. The blood glucose level should be tested again and treated if low.

General guidelines for treating hypoglycemia:

- Do not keep eating after the initial treatment; wait 15 to 20 minutes, then test blood glucose level to determine whether further treatment is needed
- Do not keep eating until symptoms disappear
- Avoid using high-fat foods for treatment
- Always carry some type of carbohydrate
- Keep something at your bedside to treat nocturnal hypoglycemia
- Keep something in the car at all times to treat episodes of hypoglycemia that might occur while driving
- Always wear diabetes identification

Treatment for hypoglycemia may need to be given by others. A person with type 1 diabetes who is experiencing hypoglycemia often has to be treated by others because hypoglycemia may affect the individual's judgment and behavior. Family members and significant others should be taught how to cope with episodes of severe hypoglycemia and what to expect in terms of the person's behavior (eg, stupor or possible resistance). Coworkers, friends, and teachers also need to know how to respond to symptoms of hypoglycemia, which can be a problem if individuals do not want to reveal their diabetes to others. In cases in which others may be too anxious or frightened to treat the hypoglycemia, they should be instructed to call 911.

Severe hypoglycemia treatment guidelines:

Severe hypoglycemia occurs when the individual is unable to self-treat. The following basic guidelines are recommended for treating severe hypoglycemia.

- *Able to Swallow.* Persons who are able to swallow without risk of aspiration may be coaxed into drinking juice or a soft drink. If this is not possible, place some glucose gel, honey, syrup, or jelly inside the individual's cheek.
- *Unable to Swallow.* Persons who are unable to swallow without risk of aspiration can be given glucagon by subcutaneous or intramuscular *injection*. See Table 15.6. Glucagon is a hormone that stimulates hepatic glucose production. Glucagon will produce substantial hyperglycemia, but its effects are very short lived, and as soon as the individual is able to swallow, liquid carbohydrates should be given to maintain normoglycemia.

The person with diabetes and those likely to be involved in treatment need to know that glucagon may cause nausea and vomiting.

Frequent *blood glucose monitoring* is needed over the next several hours to detect blood glucose levels that are falling again or to detect hyperglycemia due to overtreatment.

Family and significant others should be taught how and when to administer glucagon. Patients should keep glucagon in their homes at all times. Individuals who may be required to administer the injection need to know how to use the *glucagon kit*; this may include a teacher, coworker, roommate, friend, or neighbor. Glucagon kits can be obtained by prescription. Patients also need to be aware of the expiration date on their glucagon.

Treating Hypoglycemia in Type 2 Diabetes

Persons with type 2 diabetes who are taking oral glucose-lowering medication also need to be taught about hypoglycemia, even though they appear to be at less risk for severe hypoglycemia.

TABLE 15.6 Recommended Doses for Glucagon
Adults and Children >20 kg: 1 mg subcutaneously or intramuscularly*
Children <20 kg: 0.5 mg subcutaneously or intramuscularly, or 20 to 30 mcg per kilogram (9.1 to 13.6 mcg per pound) of body weight*

* If necessary, the dose may be repeated after 15 minutes.

Source: Banion C, Chase HP. Hypoglycemia. In: Understanding Diabetes, 11th ed. Chase HP, ed. Denver, Colo: SFI; 2006.

Persons who are changing from oral medications to insulin may have considerable fears and concerns about hypoglycemia and need to be taught to monitor themselves for warning symptoms, especially at those times of the day when they are at most risk (eg, just before lunch). These persons may also need to increase the frequency of self-monitoring of blood glucose.

Many persons with type 2 diabetes are not adequately educated about hypoglycemia and are not aware of the risks that hypoglycemia can impose. Knowledge about hypoglycemia, including warning symptoms, needs to be assessed even in persons who have been taking medication for a long period of time. Hypoglycemia is treated by carbohydrate consumption, following the guidelines prescribed for persons with type 1 diabetes.

Persons with diabetes also need to be educated about the risk of hypoglycemia in other potentially dangerous situations, such as when caring for young children or when using heavy tools (eg, electric saws, lawn mowers).

Summary

Treatment Plan for Diabetes

Diabetes management requires prompt attention to the needs of the particular person with diabetes in achieving glycemic control in a timely manner. Each person's treatment must be individualized for his or her needs. Consideration should be given to the ability and willingness of the individual to actively participate in care and to the history of drug allergies, renal and/or hepatic function, and the cost of medications. Return to desired levels of blood glucose in a shorter time frame appears to predict a more positive long-term outcome for the person with diabetes.[83] Sound patient teaching and support for good nutrition and physical activity habits are necessary components to this plan, in addition to continual monitoring. With a good understanding of the effects of drug therapy and the characteristics and needs of the person, a plan to maximize glycemic control while limiting the intrusion on a person's lifestyle is possible.

Rather than waiting for long periods of time for a drug regimen to be effective, clinicians should advance drug therapy with multiple agents or additional dosing to achieve the desired goal. The effectiveness of any regimen and nutrition/physical activity plan should be assessed in at least 3 months. One study found the average time for a regimen to be used was 35 months.[84] Using this approach, chronic complications can be slowed by attaining the reduction in blood glucose levels.

Questions and Controversies

- What will be the proper place in therapy for pramlintide and incretin compounds?
- What are the risks and benefits of using TZDs in persons with cardiovascular disease?
- What safety and effectiveness will the dual-action TZDs demonstrate?
- Which agents will be included as safe and effective for use in children (oral agents for type 2 diabetes)?
- What therapy choices will evolve as viable choices during pregnancy?
- Will inhaled insulin prove to be effective therapy?

Focus on Education: Pearls for Practice

Teaching Strategies

- **Multiple medications.** Emphasize the unique function of each drug—oral agents, injection therapies, and insulin—and the options available for best control. Encourage documentation of blood glucose and monitoring of premeal and postmeal levels as often as prescribed to observe changes and determine the usefulness of the medication.

- **New medicines.** Many new products are available. Know the dosing, side effects, and potential issues that affect use of the drugs to individualize to the population served.

- **Involvement in decision making.** Empowering good decision making is based on factual information, discussion of pros and cons for medications, and good detective work in documenting results as a team helps determine proper medication advice and prescription. In addition, prompt attention to achieving glycemic control plays a role in long-term diabetes success.

Patient Education

- **Lifestyle change considerations.** First make every attempt to plan for good nutritional intake, meal planning, portion control, a wide variety of foods as well as scheduled physical activity and modest lifestyle adjustments, as these will assist in weight control and blood glucose management.

- **Consider all the options.** Seek information about each medication and its function and side effects. Ask for specific instructions as to the timing of medications; their effect on blood glucose, kidneys, and bodily functions; and the timing of blood glucose testing. Knowing these enables you to make judgments on the effects of taking the medication.

- **Follow prescribed medication plan.** All medicines have a timed action. Many of them rely on consistency and take time to build up in the system in order to work. Some require laboratory monitoring to make certain they are tolerated by the body. The importance of following "the Plan" can not be stressed enough.

References

1. The Diabetes Control and Complications Trial Research Group. The effect of intensive treatment of diabetes on the development and progression of long-term complications in insulin dependent diabetes mellitus. N Engl J Med. 1993;329:977.
2. UK Prospective Diabetes Study Group. UK Prospective Diabetes Study 16: overview of 6 years' therapy of type II diabetes, a progressive disease. Diabetes. 1996;44:1249.
3. Ryan GJ, Jobe LJ, Martin R. Pramlintide in treatment of type 1 and type 2 diabetes mellitus. Clin Ther. 2005;27:1500.
4. Mouser JF. New Drugs for management of diabetes: insulin analogues, inhaled insulin, pramlintide, and novel peptides. Nutr Clin Pract. 2004;19:172.
5. Young A. Amylin's physiology and its role in diabetes. Curr Opin Endocrinol Diab. 1997;4:282.
6. Trecroci D. Byetta now available for type 2. Diabetes Health. 2005;14:36.
7. Binder C, Brange J. Insulin chemistry and pharmacokinetics. In: Ellenberg's and Rifkin's Diabetes Mellitus, 5th ed. Porte D Jr, Sherwin R, eds. Stamford, Conn: Appleton and Lange; 1997:689.
8. Nathan DM. Clinical Practice: initial management of glycemia in type 2 diabetes mellitus. N Engl J Med. 2002;347:1342.

9. Langer O, Conway DL, Berkus MD, Xenakis EM, Gonzales O. A comparison of glyburide and insulin in women with gestational diabetes mellitus. N Engl J Med. 2000;343:1134.
10. DeFronzo RA. Pharmacologic therapy for type 2 diabetes mellitus. Ann Intern Med. 1999;131:281.
11. Facts and Comparisons. St. Louis, Mo: Wolters Kluwer Health, Inc; 2005:287.
12. DeFronzo RA. Pharmacologic therapy for type 2 diabetes mellitus. Ann Intern Med. 1999;131:281.
13. Burden M. Culturally sensitive care: managing diabetes during Ramadan. Br J Commun Nurs. 2001;6:581.
14. Groop LC. Sulfonylureas in NIDDM. Diabetes Care. 1992;15:737.
15. Melander A, et al. Sulfonylureas: why, which, and how? Diabetes Care. 1990;13 suppl 3:18.
16. Zimmerman BR. Sulfonylureas. Endocrinol Metab Clin North Am. 1997;26:511.
17. Stenman S, Melander A, Groop PH, Groop LC. What is the benefit of increasing the sulfonylurea dose? Ann Intern Med. 1993;118:169.
18. American Diabetes Association. The pharmacological treatment of hyperglycemia in NIDDM. Diabetes Care. 1996;19 suppl:S54.
19. Bailey CJ. Drug on horizon for diabesity. Curr Diab Rep. 2005;5:353.
20. Kalbag JB, Walter YH, Nedelman JR, McLeod JF. Mealtime glucose regulation with nateglinide in healthy volunteers. Diabetes Care. 2001;24:73.
21. Heinemann L, Sinda K, Weyer C, Loftager M, Hirschberger S, Heise T. Time-action profile of the soluble, fatty acid acylated, long-acting insulin analogue NN304. Diabet Med. 1999;16:332.
22. Dunn CJ, Faulds D. Nateglinide. Drugs. 2000;60:607.
23. Hatorp V. Clinical pharmacokinetics and pharmacodynamics of repaglinide. Clin Phamacokinet. 2002;41:471.
24. Lebovitz HE. Insulin secretagogues and repaglinide. In: Therapy for Diabetes Mellitus and Related Disorders, 3rd ed. Lebovitz HE, ed. Alexandria, Va: American Diabetes Association; 1998:160.
25. Inzucchi SE. Oral antihyperglycemic therapy for type 2 diabetes: scientific review. JAMA. 2002;287:360.
26. Bailey CJ, Turner RC. Metformin. N Engl J Med. 1996;334:574.
27. Bell PM, Hadden DR. Metformin. Endocrinol Metab Clin North Am. 1997;26:523.
28. Kirpichnikov D, McFarlane SI, Sowers JR. Metformin: an update. Ann Intern Med. 2002;137:25.
29. UK Prospective Diabetes Study Group. Effect of intensive blood-glucose control with metformin on complications in overweight patients with type 2 diabetes (UKPDS 34). Lancet. 1998;352:854.
30. Klepser TB, Kelly MW. Metformin hydrochloride: an antihyperglycemic agent. Am J Health Syst Pharm. 1997;54:893.
31. Aviles-Santa L, Sinding J, Raskin P. Effects of metformin in patients with poorly controlled, insulin-treated type 2 diabetes. Ann Intern Med. 1999;131:182.
32. Stacpoole PW. Metformin and lactic acidosis: guilt by association? Diabetes Care. 1998;21:1587.
33. Yale JF, Valiquett TR, Ghazzi MN, et al. The effect of a thiazolidinedione drug, troglitazone, on glycemia in patients with type 2 diabetes mellitus poorly controlled with sulfonylurea and metformin: a multimember, randomized, double-blind, placebo-controlled trial. Ann Intern Med. 2001;134:737.
34. Spiegelman BM. PPAR-gamma: radiogenic regulator and thiazolidinedione receptor. Diabetes. 1998;47:507.
35. Nissan S, Woolskin K, Tool E. Effect of muraglitazar on death and major adverse cardiovascular events in patients with type 2 diabetes mellitus. JAMA. 2005;249:20.
36. Henry RR. Thiazolidinediones. Endocrinol Metab Clin North Am. 1997;26:553.
37. Mudaliar S, Henry RR. New oral therapies for type 2 diabetes mellitus: the glitazones for insulin sensitizers. Annu Rev Med. 2001;52:239.
38. Hussar DA. New drugs: exenatide, pramlintide acetate, and micafungin sodium. J Am Pharm Assoc (Washington DC). 2005;45:524.
39. Campbell LK, Baker DE, Campbell RK. Miglitol: assessment of its role in the treatment of patients with diabetes mellitus. Ann Pharmacother. 2000;34:1291.
40. Lebovitz HE. Alpha-glucosidase inhibitors. Endocrinol Metab Clin North Am. 1997;26:539.

41. Alpha-glucosidase inhibitors. In: Medications for the Treatment of Diabetes. White J, Campbell RK. Alexandria, Va: American Diabetes Association; 2000:57.

42. Yee HS, Fong NT. A review of the safety and efficacy of acarbose in diabetes mellitus. Pharmacotherapy. 1996;16:792.

43. Vilsboll T, Krarup T, Deacon CF, Madsbad S, Holst JJ. Reduced postprandial concentrations of intact biologically active glucagon-like peptide in type 2 diabetic patients. Diabetes. 2001;50:609.

44. Zander M, Madsbad S, Madsen JL, Holst JJ. Effect of 6-week course of glucagons-like peptide 1 on glycaemic control, insulin sensitivity, and beta-cell function in type 2 diabetes: a parallel-group study. Lancet. 2002;359:824.

45. DeFronzo RA, Ratner RE, Han J, Kim DD, Fineman MS, Baron AD. Effects of exenatide (synthetic exendin-4) on glycemic control and weight over 30 weeks in metformin-treated patients with type 2 diabetes. Diabetes Care. 2005;28:1092.

46. Barnett AH. Exenatide. Drugs Today. 2005;41:563

47. Rosak C. The pathophysiologic basis of efficacy and clinical experience with the new oral antidiabetic agents. J Diabetes Complications. 2002;16:123.

48. Nolte MS, Karam JH. Pancreatic hormones and antidiabetic drugs. In: Basic and Clinical Pharmacology, 8th ed. Katzung B, ed. New York, NY: Lange Medical Books/McGraw Hill; 2001:711.

49. Weyer C, Fineman MS, Strobel S, Shen L, Data J, Kolterman OG, Sylvestri MF. Properties of pramlintide and insulin upon mixing. Am J Health Syst Pharm. 2005;62:816.

50. Schmitz O, Brock B, Rungby J. Amylin agonists: a novel approach in treatment of diabetes. Diabetes. 2004;53 suppl:S233.

51. Hussar DA. New drugs: exenatide, pramlintide acetate, and micafungin sodium. J Am Pharm Assoc (Washington DC). 2005;45:524.

52. American Diabetes Association. Insulin administration (position statement). Diabetes Care. 2004 suppl 1;27:S106.

53. McQueen J. Pramlintide acetate. Am J Health Syst Pharm. 2005;62:2363-72.

54. Guyton AC, Hall JE, eds. Textbook of Medical Physiology, 10th ed. Philadelphia, Pa: WB Saunders; 2000:884.

55. American Diabetes Association. Nutrition recommendations and principles for people with diabetes mellitus. Diabetes Care. 2001;24 suppl 1:S44.

56. Palmer J, Lernmark A. Pathophysiology of type 1. In: Ellenberg's and Rifkin's Diabetes Mellitus, 5th ed. Porte D Jr, Sherwin R, eds. Stamford, Conn: Appleton and Lange; 1997:455.

57. Hirsch IB. Implementation of intensive insulin therapy for IDDM. Diabetes Review. 1995;3:288.

58. Comparison of insulins. Pharmacist's Letter/Prescriber's Letter. 2006;22(3):220309.

59. Pickup J, Keen H. Continuous subcutaneous insulin infusion at 25 years: evidence base for the expanding use of insulin pump therapy in type 1 diabetes. Diabetes Care. 2002;25:593.

60. Oki JC, Isley WL. Diabetes mellitus. In: Pharmacotherapy: A Pathophysiologic Approach, 5th ed. DiPiro JT, Talbert RL, Yee GC, Matzke GR, Wells BG, Posey LM, eds. New York, NY: McGraw-Hill; 2002:1335.

61. Burge MR, Schade DS. Insulins. Endocrinol Metab Clin North Am. 1997;26:575.

62. Guyton AC, Hall JE, eds. Textbook of Medical Physiology, 10th ed. Philadelphia, Pa: WB Saunders; 2000:884.

63. Takiya L, Dougherty T. Pharmacist's guide to insulin preparations: a comprehensive review. Pharmacy Times. 2005;71:90.

64. Culy CR, Jarvis B. Repaglinide: a review of its therapeutic use in type 2 diabetes mellitus. Drugs. 2001;61:1625.

65. Bouldin MJ, et al. Quality of care in diabetes: understanding the guidelines. Am J Med Sci. 2002;324:196.

66. Strowig S, Raskin P. Intensive management of insulin-dependent diabetes mellitus. In: Ellenberg's and Rifkin's Diabetes Mellitus, 5th ed. Porte D Jr, Sherwin R, eds. Stamford, CT: Appleton and Lange; 1997:709.

67. American Diabetes Association. Gestational diabetes mellitus. Diabetes Care. 2001;24 suppl 1:S77.

68. Saudek CD. Novel forms of insulin delivery. Endocrinol Metab Clin North Am. 1997;26:599.

69. Lenhard MJ, Reeves GD. Continuous subcutaneous insulin infusion: a comprehensive review of insulin pump therapy. Arch Intern Med. 2001;161:2293.

70. Ratner RE, Hirsch IB, Neifing JL, Garg SK, Mecca TE, Wilson CA. Less hypoglycemia with insulin glargine in intensive insulin therapy for type 1 diabetes: U.S. study group of insulin glargine in type 1 diabetes. Diabetes Care. 2000;23:639.

71. DeWitt DE, Hirsch IB. Outpatient insulin therapy in type 1 and type 2 diabetes mellitus: scientific review. JAMA. 2003;289:2254-64.

72. Cefalu WT. Evolving strategies for insulin delivery and therapy. Drugs. 2004;64:1149.

73. DeFelippes M, et al. Insulin Chemistry and Pharmacokinetics. In: Ellenberg's and Rifkin's Diabetes Mellitus, 6th ed. Porte DS, Baron A, eds. New York, NY: McGraw-Hill; 2003:481.

74. Griffin ME, Feder A, Tamborlane WV. Lipoatrophy associated with lispro insulin in insulin pump therapy: an old complication, a new cause? Diabetes Care. 2001;24:174.

75. Bodtger U, Wittrup M. A rational clinical approach to suspected insulin allergy: status after five years and 22 cases. Diabet Med. 2005;22:102.

76. Trubo R. Interest in inhaled insulin grows. JAMA. 2005;294:1195.

77. Rosenstock J, Zinman B, Murphy LJ, et al. Inhaled insulin improves glycemic control when substituted for or added to oral combination therapy in type 2 diabetes: a randomized controlled trial. Ann Intern Med. 2005;143:549.

78. Skyler JS, Weinstock RS, Raskin P, et al. Use of inhaled insulin in a basal/bolus insulin regimen in type 1 diabetic subjects. Diabetes Care. 2005;28:1630.

79. Skyler JS, Cefalu WT, Kourides IA, et al. Efficacy of inhaled insulin in type 1 diabetes mellitus: a randomized proof-of-concept study. Lancet. 2001;357:324.

80. Chipkin SR. How to select and combine oral agents for patients with type 2 diabetes mellitus. Am J Med. 2002;118:4S.

81. Gibaldi M, Perrier D. Pharmacokinetics, 2nd ed. New York, NY: Marcel Dekker; 1980.

82. Davies D, ed. Textbook of Adverse Drug Reactions, 3rd ed. Oxford, England: Oxford University Press;1985.

83. Krentz AJ, Bailey CJ. Oral hypoglycemic agents: current role in type 2 diabetes mellitus. Drugs. 2005;65:385.

84. Gaede P, Vedel P, Larsen N, Jensen GV, Parving HH, Pederson O. Multifactorial intervention and cardiovascular disease in patients with type 2 diabetes. New Engl J Med. 2003;348:383.

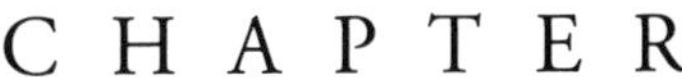

CHAPTER

16

Combating Clinical Inertia with Pattern Management

Authors

Debbie A. Hinnen, ARNP, BC-ADM, CDE, FAAN
Belinda P. Childs, ARNP, BC-ADM, CDE
Diana W. Guthrie, PhD, ARNP, CDE
Richard A. Guthrie, MD, FAAP, FACE, CDE
Susan D. Martin, RD, LD, CDE

Key Concepts

- Pattern management is a way to combat clinical inertia and promote self-management.
- A diabetes educator's assessment of the cognitive function, knowledge, and ability of the individual to perform diabetes self-care skills and problem solving is a necessary prerequisite for pattern management.
- Blood glucose monitoring is necessary to provide data for pattern management.
- Specific schedules for glucose monitoring are necessary to interpret the relationships and effect that food, physical activity, and medication have on glycemic control.
- Pattern management takes a proactive approach to diabetes management.

Introduction

Improving diabetes self-management starts with educating and empowering people with diabetes to make adjustments in their own treatment plan. This includes adjustments in medication doses, physical activity, and eating habits. Diabetes self-management is critical to attaining metabolic control and preventing complications of diabetes. The reduction in microvascular and macrovascular complications with good glycemic control, hypertension management, and lipid management have clearly been documented with landmark studies including the Diabetes Control and Complications Trial (DCCT), UK Prospective Diabetes Study (UKPDS), Scandinavian Simvastatin Survival Study (4S), and Care and Recurrent Event Trial (CARE).[1-4] In spite of this overwhelming evidence, the translation of research to clinical practice and outcomes has been slow, has never reached optimal levels, and has been deteriorating.

Several organizations have developed guidelines to help improve the quality of care for people with diabetes. These guidelines also help ensure that all people with diabetes receive standard and uniform care. Great emphasis has been placed on assuring that the American Diabetes Association Standards of Medical Care in Diabetes are met.[5] The Diabetes Quality Improvement Project is one set of national clinical guidelines that are measured to recognize and evaluate diabetes management in the United States. While clinicians are held accountable for improvement in diabetes care, this process has not necessarily translated into adequate metabolic control.[6-8] Comparisons of aggregate data from the 1988 to 1994 National Health and Nutrition Examination Survey to the 1999 to 2000 Survey showed a deterioration in A1C and blood pressure control.[9] The National Committee for Quality Assurance (NCQA) showed approximately a 9.5% decrease in poor metabolic control (defined as an A1C >9%) from 2000 to 2005 (NCQA, 2005), which is believed to be due to increased A1C monitoring.[10]

Diabetes self-management education (DSME), including medical nutrition therapy, plays a large role in good glycemic control. However, medication initiation and titration may play a larger role. Lack of medication adjustment by healthcare professionals in patients not meeting therapeutic goals has been termed "clinical inertia." Clinical inertia is associated with poor outcomes and risk factor control.[11,12] Even in academic medical centers around the United States, fewer than half of the patients with A1C's above target had changes in diabetes medication therapy.[13] Despite growing scientific evidence, more technologically advanced glucose monitoring systems, insulin delivery devices, and a plethora of sophisticated medications, clinicians today are doing a poorer job managing diabetes and the comorbid diseases.[13]

Diabetes educators have an opportunity to help facilitate self-management in the person with diabetes through empowerment and problem solving. This can be done through the process of pattern management. Pattern management is a comprehensive approach to blood glucose management that includes all aspects of current diabetes therapy.[14] It is the review of several days of blood glucose readings to identify patterns of recurring problems. It involves looking not only at blood glucose values, but also at food intake, activity, insulin doses, illness, and other factors that can contribute to changes in blood glucose values. Pattern management promotes diabetes self-management by teaching the person with diabetes to recognize patterns, identify problems, and modify the treatment plan or resolve issues that can restore glucose levels to their target levels. Although pattern management tends to be used more frequently in those treated with insulin, persons with all types of diabetes can benefit from DSME on pattern management.

Prerequisites to Pattern Management

There are generally 3 prerequisites that a person with diabetes needs to effectively perform pattern management:

- Cognitive function
- Sound knowledge of diabetes self-care skills
- Problem-solving skills

Cognitive Function

Several studies have determined that cognitive impairment may be present in people with type 1 and type 2 diabetes. A meta-analysis of 33 studies on neuropsychological functioning in type 1 diabetes[15] concluded there is a relationship between type 1 diabetes and cognitive dysfunction. The type of dysfunction is difficulty applying acquired knowledge in a new situation. Learning and memory do not appear to be affected.[15] In type 2 diabetes, there may be some cognitive dysfunction that manifests as impaired information processing, working memory, and attention associated with acute hyperglycemia.[16] Cognitive dysfunction in individuals over 65 years of age with type 2 diabetes (as evidenced by a low score on mental status examinations) may be seen as less involvement in self-care, specifically blood glucose monitoring, than in individuals without diabetes.[17] However, cognitive impairment was found not to adversely affect diabetes self-management in a study with uncomplicated type 2 diabetes in older adults.[18] The diabetes educator, therefore, should be alert to any cognitive impairment and should assess the individual for his or her knowledge of diabetes before beginning pattern management education.

Self-Care Skills

Self-care skills for diabetes self-management include healthy eating, physical activity, taking medications, monitoring, problem solving, reducing risks, and healthy coping. Assuring the necessary knowledge and skills can present a challenge for diabetes educators. Educators need to use teaching strategies that implement adult teaching principles, such as making the education problem centered and outcome centered as opposed to subject oriented, integrating diabetes education in the individual's own personal experience, and helping ensure that the person with diabetes is an active participant in the learning process. Other key principles are to repeat key information, assure hands-on interactive teaching, slow down the pace of presentation, and verify the participants understanding of the information and skills presented.[19] Using a variety of teaching and learning strategies enhances the individual's understanding of pattern management.

Problem Solving

The ability to problem solve is a critical skill necessary for pattern management. Reviewing blood glucose records with the person while using interactive questioning and role playing will enhance the person's understanding. Practicing and rehearsing for anticipated problems or circumstances enhances the individual's self-efficacy and helps demonstrate progress in problem-solving abilities.

Facilitating Pattern Management in the Person With Diabetes

Pattern management is a process that takes work, concentration, and commitment by both the diabetes educator and the person with diabetes. Small, incremental steps and continued learning are necessary to master self-management. There are several things the diabetes educator can do to facilitate this process:

- Motivate the person with diabetes to become an active participant in his or her own care. People may be more motivated if they feel confident in their abilities.
- Negotiate individualized blood glucose goals—goals that are established by the person with diabetes and the care team. Current acceptable targets by the American Diabetes Association[5] and American College of Endocrinology[20] are as shown in Table 16.1. However, adjustments may need to be made based on an individual's medical status, abilities, and desires.
- Help empower the individual through education for decision making and problem solving.
- Facilitate goal setting to help promote the individual's long-term motivation.

TABLE 16.1 Blood Glucose Targets

	American Diabetes Association	*American College of Endocrinology*
Fasting	90 to 130 mg/dL	<110 mg/dL
2-Hour Postmeal Glucose		<140 mg/dL
1-Hour Postmeal Glucose	<180 mg/dL	

Sources: American Diabetes Association. Standards of Medical Care in diabetes, 2006. Diabetes Care. 2006;29 suppl:S4-42. American College of Endocrinology consensus development conference on guidelines for glycemic control. Endocr Pract Suppl. Nov/Dec 2001.

- Explain the purpose, strategies, and value of pattern management for intensive therapy to achieve blood glucose goals.
- Help the individual articulate his or her own personal belief system related to the value of health and intensive diabetes management.
- Promote frequent interaction between the person with diabetes and the diabetes care team. This may include use of the telephone, fax, and e-mail to discuss glucose patterns between visits.
- Identify support systems to provide emotional and clinical management support.
- Provide a diabetes care team with on-call clinical support.
- Provide ongoing learning opportunities such as suppport groups and hospital-based DSME (ie, hospital, education center).

Knowledge Necessary for Diabetes Self-Management

The knowledge base needed for self-management education includes the following:

- Relationship of glucose levels, food, activity, and medications
- Prevention of hypoglycemia or hyperglycemia
- Sick day management
- How to access diabetes and health-related supplies

Use of the AADE 7 Self-Care Behaviors™ aids the diabetes educator in assessment and teaching plan management, specifically the self-care behaviors related to Monitoring, Healthy Eating, Taking Medication, and Problem Solving.

Monitoring

The schedule and frequency of self-monitoring of blood glucose (SMBG) may change based on the information needed to find patterns. SMBG results should be written in a record book, or downloaded electronically, to provide data for making adjustments. Glucose monitoring provides the data for adjustment in the treatment plan for all people with diabetes. Since the value of glycemic control is clearly demonstrated for all people with diabetes, it is logical to request glucose monitoring of everyone with diabetes, albeit with different frequencies of testing. The value and frequency of glucose monitoring for people with type 2 diabetes continues to be a topic of debate.[21-23] However, increasing glucose monitoring frequency for those requiring insulin results in reductions in A1C levels.[5,24-26]

The frequency of glucose monitoring should be based on the treatment plan and availability of testing supplies. For pattern management purposes, this would suggest testing could be done at different times of day several days per week. The Centers for Medicare and Medicaid Services (CMS) reimburses 100 test strips per month for the person on insulin and 100 test strips for 3 months for the person on oral medications or whose diabetes is successfully controlled by diet, unless the health professional prescribes and documents the reason for increased glucose testing.[27] For pattern management purposes, the educator must be creative in negotiating a weekly testing schedule that will provide several blood glucose readings at consistent times of the day.

Healthy Eating

The person with diabetes should have a food/meal plan to follow that may include basic skills of consistency in calorie and carbohydrate intake. This includes a plan for weight loss and/or weight maintenance. The person trying to maintain or lose weight may choose to do carbohydrate budgeting (maintaining a consistent amount of carbohydrate at meals) rather than adjusting the insulin-to-carbohydrate ratio at each meal. Some individuals use a calorie point system, where 1 point equals 75 calories, which allows for counting all the calories of intake. Counting all calories, not just carbohydrate, is of value for people with type 2 diabetes who are trying to manage their weight. Adjusting meal insulin based on carbohydrates only helps attain glycemic control, and not monitoring overall calorie levels may lead to weight gain. Adjusting meal insulin based on carbohydrates is focused on glycemic control and needs to be accompanied by monitoring of overall calories.

Taking Medication

To interpret blood glucose patterns, the person with diabetes must understand the action of insulin or other diabetes medication. The person must have advanced skill in adjusting insulin based on carbohydrate intake. Insulin-to-carbohydrate ratios are developed by determining the amount of insulin needed to cover usual carbohydrate intake.[28-29]

Problem Solving

Advanced skills necessitate an understanding of complex medication protocols. Since most of these protocols are a combination of basal and bolus insulin therapy, the person must understand why the basal/bolus regimen is useful and how it works. The regimen may involve multiple injections of insulin, insulin pump therapy, or combinations of oral agents and insulin.

Basal/bolus therapy provides a rapid-acting insulin before each meal and a long-acting insulin with 24-hour coverage. Additional therapies to enhance basal/bolus therapy might include either of the following:

- Symlin (pramlintide) with insulin
- Byetta (exenatide) with multiple oral agents

Problem solving also includes self-adjustments of the treatment regimen. The person must adjust a single parameter at a time to evaluate how changes in food intake, physical activity, or medication affect blood glucose levels.

Process of Pattern Management

Information Required

The process of pattern management involves reviewing a record of the following:

- *Glucose:* At least 3 to 4 days of glucose records
- *Food:* Type, quantity, and timing of food eaten
- *Physical Activity:* Any physical activity that occurred
- *Events:* Any other event that could affect blood glucose values

Obtaining information on all parameters is necessary to get a complete picture. Such information is difficult to obtain if the only data collected is what was downloaded from the blood glucose meter. Therefore, the individual should be instructed to keep detailed diaries of food intake (amounts and time eaten); time, intensity, and duration of physical activity; timing and dosing of medications; and other any factors that may affect blood glucose levels.

A Proactive Approach

Being proactive is key to pattern management. The critical concept of pattern management is to evaluate the "big picture" by looking for patterns and/or trends that have occurred in the previous few days. This is in stark contrast to the concept of sliding scale insulin, which involves obtaining a single elevated glucose reading and adjusting medication at that time. The sliding scale is a one-time reaction to a single elevated blood glucose. Adding supplemental or sliding scale insulin at the time of a single elevated glucose level solves the problem only for that particular point in time, but does not prevent the problem from occurring again. The use of sliding scale insulin is reactive—treating the problem "after the fact"—rather than being proactive.

Being proactive entails anticipating when the glucose will be too high or too low and making changes in the regimen to prevent it from happening again. Pattern management involves a problem-solving approach in which the person with diabetes and the practitioner attempt to discover the reasons for vacillations or changes in blood glucose levels. This requires knowledge of all the factors that may increase or decrease blood glucose levels.

When an elevated glucose is obtained, it has occurred from events that happened earlier. The person with diabetes and the healthcare practitioner must look to the earlier block of time. For example, an elevated prelunch blood glucose may be occurring because the morning rapid-acting insulin or basal insulin is not enough *or* because the breakfast meal included too many calories or carbohydrates. If insulin is given when the high blood glucose occurs at the prelunch time, the person is "chasing his tail"; that is, he or she is not correcting the problem in a way that prevents it from recurring on subsequent days.

To determine patterns, food intake, physical activity, and insulin or other medications must initially be as consistent as possible. If daily variability exists in all areas, resulting blood glucose fluctuations can occur. Any change in meal patterns, the amount of physical activity, or stress levels should be noted in the logbook to explain highs and lows in persons using insulin.

Reviewing all variables that affect blood glucose levels—food, physical activity, stress, and illness—and not just insulin or other medication adjustments is necessary for pattern management.[30] A common problem among people who are new to pattern management is focusing only on insulin doses. It is important to emphasize the other factors that can be modified as well.

Data Interpretation and Organization

Understanding the data is mandatory to decision making. A logbook that includes information on all these factors is important. Simply downloading a meter may not provide the details needed to use pattern management; however, it does provide some helpful information.

Whether data is documented in a logbook or downloaded from the meter, the glucose values must be organized in a fashion so that all glucose values that occur at the same time of day can be seen and reviewed together.

For example, the fasting blood glucose readings need to be reviewed together. Downloaded data usually allows for averaging, thus allowing even more finely tuned assessments of numbers. Nearly all the meter companies have software to help aggregate the data into *like* times of day over several weeks. Whether done via technology or manually, this step is necessary to analyze data. Glucose values at specific times of day provide information on a block of time. Understanding what contributes to each block of time is key to problem solving; this is critical to the concept of pattern management.

Consider the following 4 points:

1. *Premeal glucose measurements* are needed to evaluate basal (or background) insulin dose(s)—such as NPH, glargine (Lantus), or detemir (Levemir). If fasting or premeal readings are out of target range, consider adjusting basal insulin doses. For the person on oral agents, the fasting blood glucose is an indication of the hepatic glucose release during the night. If meal planning is well regulated, a pattern of elevated fasting glucoses may indicate that the meal plan needs to be adjusted or that the dosing of metformin (Glucophage) or other diabetes medication needs to be added or increased. The pattern may be an indication for initiation of metformin (or increasing the metformin dose).
2. *Premeal glucose data* compared to postmeal values from the same meal provide specific glycemic excursion information from the meal. This helps determine whether enough insulin has been taken for the carbohydrate eaten and can help determine insulin-to-carbohydrate ratios. The insulin-to-carbohydrate ratio is how much insulin is needed for a specific amount of carbohydrate. The common starting point is 1 unit of short- or rapid-acting insulin for 10 to 15 g of carbohydrate. (See chapter 17, on intensifying insulin therapy, for a more complete discussion of calculating insulin-to-carbohydrate ratios.)
3. *Two-hour postprandial glucose readings* are needed to adjust rapid-acting insulin—such as insulin lispro (Humalog), insulin aspart (Novolog), or glulisine (Apidra)—for mealtime injections. Postmeal readings are also used to evaluate the effect of food on blood glucose as well as the effectiveness of insulin secretagogues; glipizide, glyburide, repaglinide (Prandin), and nateglinide (Starlix) as well as exenatide (Byetta), pramlintide (Symlin), and drugs that delay carbohydrate metabolism: alpha-glucosidase inhibitors (Acarbose); and other glucose-lowering agents. For the person using insulin, the postprandial glucose reading can help determine whether the insulin-to-carbohydrate ratio is adequate.
4. *Elevated fasting glucose levels may require 3 AM testing* and recording at least once a week to determine the cause. High fasting glucose levels can be caused by the following:
   - Overnight hypoglycemia that triggers the liver to release glucose (Somogyi or rebound effect)
   - Normal hormonal changes that trigger the liver to release excessive glucose in the early morning (dawn phenomenon)
   - Insufficient basal or background insulin
   - In youth, growth hormone secreted at night during the growth spurt
   - Excessive hepatic glucose release, which is a defect in type 2 diabetes
   - Eating a snack in the middle of the night

> In pattern management, comparing blood glucose levels from *like* times of day and understanding what contributed to each block of time is critical.

Questions to Ask

Evaluating Blood Glucose Readings for Pattern Management

- Is there a repeating pattern when evaluating 3 to 5 days of blood glucose readings?
- Does something happen at the same time every day, such as an insulin reaction or a high glucose after breakfast?
- Are there blood glucose readings representing key "times" of the day, ie, fasting, premeal, post meal? (See below for information from each test.)
- Are there blood glucose readings representing the "peak" times of each medication (insulins and/or oral agents)?
- Are there readings to represent peak glucose readings after all meals?
- Are there "other notes" or "changes" such as meal times, carbohydrate or calorie variances, exercise changes, unusual hours of work or school, stress, or illness?
- Is prevention of weight gain or weight loss important for this person? If so, consideration should be given to careful titration of the hypoglycemic medications (ie, insulin or insulin secretagogues). If doses are too high and hypoglycemia occurs frequently, eating extra calories will likely lead to subsequent weight gain.
- Does this person have a history of weight loss? Is the weight loss caused by poor glycemic control?[1]

Case in Point: Pattern Management

CV had type 2 diabetes of 5 years' duration. An Hispanic woman with good English language skills, CV had completed 1 year of community college. She was married to José, who worked in construction. CV had 2 children who were in the public high school; her oldest daughter was married, and CV was a new grandmother. CV made most of the family healthcare decisions. She worked at a call center and sat most of the time at her job. She had completed 10 hours of diabetes self-management education and demonstrated good self-care skills. Recently, CV had converted to an intensive basal/bolus, 4-shot regimen. CV was motivated to be in good health because she had a new grandchild whom she wanted to watch grow up. CV's glucose goals were fasting plasma glucose less than 110 mg/dL and 2-hour postprandial less than 140 mg/dL.

During a follow-up visit one day, the educator made sure that CV's blood glucose monitor was functioning properly and assessed her self-care skills, including blood glucose monitoring technique and her understanding of carbohydrates, proteins, and fats in meal planning. After self-injecting saline and reviewing the time actions and doses of insulin with the educator, CV asked, "How do I know if my insulin is the right dose?" This question provided the educator an opportunity to empower CV to learn to adjust her own insulin. The pattern management classes were offered to CV, and she was scheduled for the sessions that began in 2 weeks.

Clinical Data

- Height: 66 in
- Weight: 248 lb
- A1C: 8.4%
- Mild peripheral neuropathy in the feet
- No visual changes
- No microalbuminuria

CV's starting insulin dosages were as follows:

- Breakfast: 3 units insulin lispro (Humalog)
- Lunch: 5 units insulin lispro (Humalog)
- Supper: 6 units insulin lispro (Humalog)
- Bedtime: 16 units insulin glargine (Lantus)

Choosing an Appropriate Meal Plan

CV wanted to lose weight so an appropriate amount of calories had to be determined. One way of doing this was to assign a daily caloric intake that provided enough calories, but would still result in weight loss. Because CV wanted to lose weight, her caloric intake was set at 1600 calories per day. This was divided into 3 meals and a bedtime snack, which was her desired meal plan. Half of the total daily calories would come from carbohydrates. The table below shows how the number of daily carbohydrate (CHO) servings, or choices, were determined for CV.

CV was thus to have 14 daily total of carbohydrate servings, and she would divide them among her 3 meals and snack as follows:

- *Breakfast:* 3 carbohydrate servings
- *Lunch:* 5 carbohydrate servings
- *Dinner:* 5 carbohydrate servings
- *Evening Snack:* 1 carbohydrate serving

Estimating Daily Amount of Carbohydrate: 50% of Total Calories

Formula	*As Determined for CV*
Total daily calories ÷ 2 = CHO calories	1600 calories ÷ 2 = 800 calories of CHO
CHO calories ÷ 4 calories (4 calories in each gram of carb) = grams of CHO per day	800 calories ÷ 4 = 200 g of CHO per day
grams of CHO ÷ 15 g per serving = servings per day	200 g ÷ 15 = ~13-14 CHO servings per day

Matching Insulin to Carbohydrates

CV was taking 12 units of long-acting insulin (glargine) as a basal insulin after supper and insulin lispro 1 unit for every 15 g of carbohydrate as the rapid-acting insulin with meals. The educator was not sure if the amount of insulin lispro CV was taking with her meals was the proper amount for the amount of carbohydrate CV was eating, nor whether CV was accurately counting her carbohydrates. To adequately evaluate this, the educator asked CV to monitor her blood glucose levels for several days and to record her food intake, insulin doses, and any activity in her logbook. (See "week 1" log.)

(continued)

Case in Point: Pattern Management (continued)

Pattern Management

In reviewing CV's logbook, the educator and CV found a pattern: CV had high blood glucose every morning after breakfast. There were several possible causes for this pattern, the educator explained, and the educator and CV reviewed them to find the problem:

- Too much carbohydrate or calories at breakfast for the current insulin (see food notes)
- Not enough insulin before breakfast
- Insulin-to-carbohydrate ratio was wrong, needed to be recalculated
- CV might not be counting the carbohydrate correctly

CV decided there were several possible solutions to correct the elevated midmorning glucose elevations. She knew she must change something in her routine to impact and prevent the high tests and lose weight. Since her fasting glucose values were near normal, she decided to focus on other areas. She could choose to do one of the following:

- Decrease total carbohydrate or calories at breakfast
- Increase insulin lispro before breakfast by 10%
- Recalculate the insulin-to-carbohydrate ratio; for example, increase the insulin-to-carbohydrate ratio at breakfast to 1 unit insulin lispro per 10-g carbohydrate serving (1:10)
- Include exercise after breakfast, as it was effective on Sunday after lunch
- Eat the exact same amount of carbohydrate for breakfast every morning

CV decided to recalculate her insulin-to-carbohydrate ratio for breakfast. The ratio was changed to 1 unit per 10 g of carbohydrate (rather than the 1 unit per 15 g of carbohydrate she was taking), thus increasing the breakfast dose to 5 units of insulin lispro.

CV's testing values after another week (3 more days of data) showed much improvement (see "week 2" log). She had been counting her carbohydrates and using an insulin-to-carbohydrate ratio of 1 unit for 10 g of carbohydrate for breakfast and 1 unit for every 15 g of carbohydrate at lunch and supper.

Week 1 Logbook Entries

Day	*Before Breakfast*	*After Breakfast*	*Before Lunch*	*After Lunch*	*Before Supper*	*After Supper*
Wed.						
Blood glucose *Insulin dose* *Food eaten* Breakfast meal	103 3 units insulin lispro Two 4-inch waffles, 2 Tb low-cal syrup	315	208 5 units insulin lispro	269	6 units insulin lispro	144 12 units insulin glargine
Fri.						
Blood glucose *Insulin dose* *Food eaten* Breakfast meal	110 3 units 1/2 cup juice, 2 tortillas	315	292 5 units	133	6 units	149 12 units insulin glargine
Sun.						
Blood glucose *Insulin*	100 3 units	248	5 units	149	6 units	137 12 units insulin glargine
Notes:				walked		

Week 2 Logbook Entries						
Day	*Before Breakfast*	*After Breakfast*	*Before Lunch*	*After Lunch*	*Before Supper*	*After Supper*
Mon.						
Blood glucose *Insulin dose*	103 5 units insulin lispro	147	132 5 units insulin lispro	169	6 units insulin lispro	129
Tues.						
Blood glucose *Insulin dose*	108 5 units insulin lispro	133	128 5 units insulin lispro	158	126 5 units insulin lispro	171
Thurs.						
Blood glucose *Insulin dose*	99 5 units insulin lispro	141	5 units insulin lispro	149	5 units insulin lispro	137

Correction Factor

The educator explained to CV that just taking insulin for the amount of carbohydrate eaten works fine when the premeal blood glucose is within the target range. However, when the premeal blood glucose level is too high, the same amount of insulin will not keep the blood glucose within the target range. To fine-tune the insulin dose to keep the glucose within target range, a correction factor can be calculated. Calculating a correction factor was an additional, more advanced approach. The correction factor, or Insulin Sensitivity Factor (ISF), would add extra insulin *at the time* of the glucose elevation in an attempt to bring the blood glucose level in a desired range. (See chapter 11, on intensifying insulin therapy, for a more complete discussion, including ISF calculation.)

CV's correction factor was calculated. It was determined that 1 unit of rapid-acting insulin would bring her blood glucose level down 50 mg/dL. CV's target glucose level before her meal was 100 mg/dL.

On Wednesday, CV's prelunch glucose was 208 mg/dL. So, she subtracted her glucose target (100 mg/dL) from that number, 208. The result, 108 mg/dL, equalled the amount of glucose elevation to be corrected for with extra insulin. Since 1 unit of rapid-acting insulin should theoretically drop the glucose an estimated 50 mg/dL, the next step was to divide 108 by 50 mg/dL (108 ÷ 50 mg/dL = 2 units). This yielded the number of additional units of rapid-acting insulin that needed to be added to the usual 5 units at lunch on Wednesday. Thus, CV's total premeal insulin dose should be 7 units.

To calculate for Thursday's prelunch insulin dose:

292 mg/dL - 100 mg/dL = 192 mg/dL
192 mg/dL ÷ 50 mg/dL = 4 units

The amount of additional insulin needed to correct for the high blood glucose level was 4 units.

Important Note: Do not confuse this with the sliding scale. To apply this concept to pattern management, the next step would be to to add that additional amount of insulin (correction factor) to the amount of insulin that CV took the day before (Thursday) for breakfast. Since CV took only 3 units of insulin lispro on Thursday, she would add the 2 units of correction to Friday's breakfast insulin dose. The new breakfast dose for CV on Friday would be 3 units (the usual dose) plus 2 units (the correction factor), for a total of 5 units of insulin lispro.

Sometimes, the meal insulin is not the problem. If premeal glucose elevations persist, the long-acting insulin may not be enough. An increase of 10% is often suggested as the amount to increase an insulin dose at any given time. If a 10% addition is made to the long-acting insulin dose basal, the fasting *and* premeal glucose values will be the determining factor on whether enough of a dose increase was made. It is important when making insulin adjustments with long-acting insulin to maintain the dose change for about 3 or 4 days before making any additional adjustments to the dose. Since long-acting insulin has such a long duration of action, it may take a few days to see the results of the increase or decrease in the dose.

Pattern Management in Children

When using pattern management for children, the same concepts apply. If, for example, a preschooler is given 5 units of insulin lispro with meals, a 10% (or lower) adjustment is appropriate. The adjustments are based on the current insulin dose for that individual. Percentage adjustments account for variations in dosing, insulin resistance, calorie/carbohydrate levels, body size, and so on. Percentage adjustments personalize the dose adjustment. Preset formulas, in comparison, may suggest giving 3 units if the blood glucose is 150 mg/dL and 5 units if the blood glucose is 200 mg/dL, for example. The sliding scale or preset doses may nearly double the current dose, for example if the preschooler is on 5 units of insulin lispro before meals.

Pattern Management for Hypoglycemia

If hypoglycemia is noticed for several days, adjustment of the dose should occur before a week goes by. Glucose targets may be more lenient in the preschooler since the central nervous system is not fully developed until about 5 years of age. Severe hypoglycemia should be avoided.

Pattern management is more of a challenge in young children, especially if they are picky eaters. Ensuring consistency in calorie/carbohydrate intake in young children is difficult, and avoiding hypoglycemia is paramount. One method to prevent hypoglycemia may be to calculate the dose based on the amount eaten and then give the insulin after the meal.

Common Patterns and Possible Solutions

Low Blood Glucose After Exercise

A low blood glucose level after exercise may occur in people on insulin or oral agents. If this is documented more than once, the problem solving should begin with evaluation of the block of time in which hypoglycemia occurs. For example, if the student has physical education on Monday, Wednesday, and Friday at 10:00 AM, hypoglycemia at 10:45 AM is likely a result of increased activity on those days. The student may include a snack before physical education on those days or decrease the morning analog insulin by 10%. Adults on oral agents will not want to increase calories routinely. That would likely result in weight gain. If exercise can be placed after a meal, the calories/carbohydrates from the meal may help prevent hypoglycemia. See chapter 14, on physical exercise, for more information.

Elevated Fasting Glucose

In type 2 diabetes, elevated fasting glucose levels are a very common and frustrating finding. People who are being very careful to not eat after dinner are confused with a bedtime glucose reading of 125 mg and a fasting glucose of 186 mg. The hepatic glucose release in type 2 diabetes occurs primarily at night, thus causing an elevated fasting glucose. Possible solutions might include the following:

- Exercising in the evening
- Adding (or increasing) metformin (Glucophage) at supper (to counteract the hepatic glucose release overnight)
- Adding insulin glargine (Lantus)/detemir (Levemir) in the evening
- A low dose of a long-acting secretagogue (1 mg glimiperide at supper) may also be considered

Normal Fasting Glucose With Elevated Glucose After Meals

This is another common pattern. Metformin (Glucophage) is one of the most commonly prescribed drugs for monotherapy in type 2 diabetes. If fasting glucose levels are near normal, the metformin is successfully suppressing nocturnal hepatic glucose release. Elevated glucose levels after meals indicates that the endogenous insulin is not sufficient to "cover" the amount of carbohydrate/calories eaten at the meal. This may be an indication for including exenatide (Byetta), an insulin secretagogue, or analog insulin at mealtime. Eating little or no carbohydrate is a strategy commonly employed by those with diabetes, in hopes of preventing the need for additional medication. Most clinicians agree this is *not* a healthy strategy.

Pattern Management With Incretin Mimetics or Amylin Analogs

These medications can work with insulin to lower blood glucose levels, and often the insulin dose needs to be readjusted. When initiating pramlitide (Symlin), the recommendation is to give pramlitide with the first bite of food and insulin with the last bite eaten. This allows a more accurate correlation of the food and the insulin dose. After stabilization, the bolus insulin can be given with the food. To implement pattern management, the glucose and food records are reviewed weekly with the same strategies implemented as mentioned above. If exenatide (Byetta) is part of the therapeutic treatment plan, the same concepts apply for pattern management as above.

Summary

The steps of problem solving outlined in this chapter, when put together in an organized fashion, make flexibility and good glycemic control much more possible for people with diabetes. Self-management is a patient-driven empowerment tool that the diabetes educator can facilitate in people with diabetes. Given the clinical inertia that is beginning to be documented in practitioners, it is incumbent for those involved in diabetes education to help those with diabetes help themselves to make therapeutic changes to attain glycemic control.

Questions and Controversy

Optimal Frequency

The optimal frequency for blood glucose monitoring remains a controversial topic, especially in people with type 2 diabetes. The DCCT demonstrated that more frequent blood glucose monitoring was associated with lower A1C. In clinical practice, this has been extended to include people using insulin, not just people with type 1 diabetes. However, there are no studies that specify the number of times someone with type 2 diabetes should test. Common practice for pattern management requires that in a week's time, several blood glucose readings are available for each time of day. People on oral agents may test twice per day, at staggered times, or 4 times per day several days per week, for example. This is an item often negotiated between patient and practitioner. Insurance reimbursement for test strips may dictate the frequency as well.

Not Sliding Scale

Pattern management is a "big picture" approach that reviews recent glucose monitoring history and tries to problem solve to *prevent* problems. Sliding scale is still used in many practices and institutions. This practice only serves to react to high blood glucose levels after the fact rather than taking the proactive approach. People have reported that the "roller coaster" effect experienced with sliding scale affects their feeling of well-being due to the dramatic swings in glucose readings.

Weight Control

Carbohydrate counting versus total calorie counting has implications for pattern management and weight control. Studies in this area would be useful for clarifying management strategies.

Communication Technologies

Technologies such as telephonic and e-mail communication are being more widely used for assistance with case management and self-management. However, issues of privacy (including regulations for the Health Insurance Portability and Accountability Act, HIPAA) and accountability of the healthcare provider for response and intervention must be carefully considered and effectively addressed. More studies in this area are needed to refine strategies and reassure traditional providers of care of the implications of these interventions.

Knowledge Is Not Enough

How do we change behaviors? By increasing self-confidence and empowering people? To facilitate self-management by the person with diabetes, data are emerging to direct providers to address the perceptions of those with diabetes regarding barriers to self-care and to evalauate values, motivations, and goals.[31-35] The strategies emerging need to be more clearly defined, targeted, and implemented at all levels of diabetes care.

Pearls for Practice: Focus on Education

Teaching Strategies

- **Pattern management.** This is an organized process of glucose review and problem solving. Identifying patterns by time of day, activity, and food practices helps in adjusting insulin. Create examples of common glucose patterns using logbooks for teaching tools.

- **Implementing adult teaching principles with interactive participation.** Repetition and role-playing will increase individuals' ability to problem solve. Questions from the educator help "role play" identification of the problem and the solutions.

- **Offer opportunties for decision making.** Empowering individuals to observe patterns and "experiment" within modest medication change parameters will increase their independence in decision making.

Patient Education

- **Documentation takes on a new role.** Instead of just doing blood glucose readings to show the medical staff, take the opportunity to review for "patterns" and offer an opinion on how to make changes in behavior, insulin, or oral medication. Work with the healthcare team to know what kinds of medication changes to make safely on your own. Software packages for downloading to the computer could offer new ways to analyze the blood glucose data.

- **Continue learning.** There are many new skills, new technologies, and newer approaches to diabetes care available. In fact, now more than ever technology and research are offering new information. Change is constant. Find classes, computer programs, journals, and memberships in organizations such as the American Association of Diabetes Educators or the American Diabetes Association. These offer opportunties for updating information. Ask your healthcare team about the newest meters and medications and how they might affect you.

References

1. Diabetes Control and Complications Trial Research Group. The effect of intensive treatment of diabetes on the development and progression of long-term complications in insulin-dependent-diabetes mellitus. New Engl J Med. 1993;329;997-86.
2. UK Prospective Diabetes Study Group. Tight blood pressure control and risk of macrovascular and microvascular complication in type 2 diabetes: UKPDS 38. BMJ. 1998;317:703-13.
3. Pyorala K, Pedersen TR, Kjekshus J, Faergeman O, Olsson AG, Thorgeirsson F. Cholesterol lowering with simvastatin improves prognosis of diabetic patients with coronary heart disease: a subgroup analysis of the Scandinavian Simvastatin Survival Study (4S). Diabetes Care. 1997;20:614-20.
4. Goldberg RB, Mellies MJ, Sacks FM, et al. Cardiovascular events and their reduction with pravastatin in diabetic and glucose intolerant myocardial infarction survivors with average cholesterol levels: subgroup analyses in the cholesterol and recurrent events (CARE) trial: the Care Investigators. Circulation. 1998;98:2513-9.
5. American Diabetes Association. Standards of Medical Care in Diabetes, 2006. Diabetes Care. 2006;29 suppl 1:S4-42.
6. Saaddine JB, Engelgau MM, Beckles GL, Gregg EW, Thompson TJ, Venkat Narayan KM. A Diabetes Report Card for the United States: quality of care in the 1990's. Ann Intern Med. 2002;136;565-74.
7. Chin MH, Auerbach SB, Cook S, et al. Quality of diabetes care in community health centers. Am J Pub Health. 2000;90:431-4.

8. Saydah SH, Fradkin J, Cowie CC. Poor control of risk factors for vascular disease among adults with previously diagnosed diabetes. JAMA. 2004;291:335-42.

9. Koro CE, Bowlin SJ, Bourgeois N, Fedder DO. Glycemic control from 1988 to 2000 among US adults diagnosed with type 2 diabetes. Diabetes Care. 2004;27:17-20.

10. National Committee for Quality Assurance. Comprehensive diabetes care: State of Health Care Quality 2005. 2005; 38-9.

11. Phillips LS, Branch WT, Cook CV, et al. Clinical inertia. Ann Int Med. 2001;135:825-34.

12. Grant RW, Caliero E, Dubey AK, et al. Clinical inertia in the management of type 2 diabetes metabolic risk factors. Diabet Med. 2004;21:150-5.

13. Grant RW, Buse JB, Miegs JB, for the University Health System Consortium (UHC) Diabetes Benchmarking Project Team. Quality of diabetes care in US academic medical centers. Diabetes Care. 2005;28:2; 337-42.

14. Hinnen D, Guthrie D, Childs B, Guthrie RA. Pattern management of blood glucose. In: A Core Curriculum for Diabetes Education. Diabetes Management Therapies, 5th ed. Franz MJ, ed. Chicago, Ill: American Association of Diabetes Educators; 2003.

15. Brands A, Biessels GJ, Haan E, Kappelle LJ, Kessels RP. The effects of type 1 diabetes on cognitive performance: a meta-analysis. Diabetes Care. 2005;28:726-35.

16. Sommerfield, AJ, Deary, IF, Grier, BM. Acute hyperglycemia alters mood and impairs cognitive performance in people with type 2 diabetes. Diabetes Care. 2004;27:2335-40.

17. Sinclair AJ, Girling AJ, Bayer A. Cognitive dysfunction in older subjects with diabetes mellitus: impact on diabetes self-management and use of care services. Diabetes Res Linc Pract. 2000;50:203-12.

18. Asimakopoulou K, Hampson SE. Cognitive functioning and self-management in older people with diabetes. Diabetes Spectrum. 2002;5(2):116-21.

19. Redman BK. The Practice of Patient Education, 9th ed. St Louis, Mo: Mosby, Inc.; 2001.

20. American College of Endocrinology consensus development conference on guidelines for glycemic control. Endocr Pract Suppl. Nov/Dec 2001.

21. Welschen LMC, Bloemendal E, Nijpels G, Deller JM, Hein RJ, Stalman WAB, Bouter LM. Self-monitoring of blood glucose in patients with type 2 diabetes mellitus who are not using insulin: a systematic review. Diabetes Care. 2004;28:1510-7.

22. Davidson MB. Counterpoint: self-monitoring of blood glucose in type 2 diabetic patients not receiving insulin. Diabetes Care. 2005;28: 1531-3.

23. Harris MI. Frequency of blood glucose monitoring in relation to glycemic control in patients with type 2 diabetes. Diabetes Care. 2001;24:979-82.

24. Strowig SM, Raskin P. Improved glycemic control in intensively treated type 1 diabetic patients using blood glucose meters with storage capability and computer-assisted analysis. Diabetes Care.1998;21:1694-98.

25. Evans JMM, Newton RW, Ruta DA, MacDonald TM, Stevenson RJ, Morris AD. Frequency of blood glucose monitoring in relation to glycaemic control: observational study with diabetes database. BMJ. 1999;319:83-6.

26. Karter AJ, Ackerson LM, Darbinian JA, et al. Self-monitoring of blood glucose levels and glycemic control: the Northern California Kaiser Permanente Diabetes Registry. Am J Med. 2001;111:1-9.

27. US Department of Health and Human Services, CMS. Medicare coverage of diabetes supplies and services, CMS #11022, Sep 2004.

28. American Dietetic Association. Medical Nutrition Therapy. Evidence-Based Guides for Practice: Nutrition Practice Guidelines for Type 1 and Type 2 Diabetes. Chicago, Ill: American Dietetic Association; 2001.

29. Franz MJ, Bantle JP, Beebe CA, et al. Evidence-based nutrition principles and recommendations for the treatment and prevention of diabetes and related complications. Diabetes Care. 2002;25:148-98.

30. Davidson J, Reader D, Rickheim O. Blood Glucose Patterns. A Guide to Achieving Targets. Minneapolis, Minn: International Diabetes Center Park Nicollet Institute, 2003.

31. Norris SL, Engelgau MM, Narayan KM. Effectiveness of self-management training in type 2 diabetes: a systematic review of randomized controlled trials. Diabetes Care. 2001;24:561-87.

32. Heisler M, Piette J, Spencer M, Kieffer E, Vijan S. The relationship between knowledge of recent HbA1c values and diabetes care understanding and self-management. Diabetes Care. 2005;28:816-22.

33. Glasgow RE, Funnell MM, Bonomi AE, Davis C Beckham V Wagner EH. Self-management aspects of the improving chronic illness care breakthrough series: implementation with diabetes and heart failure teams. Ann Behav Med. 2002;24:80-7.

34. Brown SA. Interventions to promote diabetes self-management: state of the science. Diabetes Educ. 1999;25:52-61.

35. Holman H, Lorig K. Patients as partners in managing chronic disease: partnership is a prerequisites for effective and efficient health care. BMJ. 2000;320:526-7.

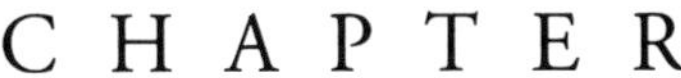

CHAPTER

17

Intensifying Insulin Therapy: Multiple Daily Injections to Pump Therapy

Authors

Donna M. Tomky, MSN, APRN, C-ANP, CDE
Karmeen Kulkarni, MS, RD, BC-ADM, CDE

Key Concepts

- Understanding the benefits, risks, and limitations of intensive therapy is extremely important in counseling and assisting patients in the use of multiple daily injections and continuous subcutaneous insulin infusion.
- Not all individuals who express interest are good candidates for these more intense forms of therapy. Candidates should be selected based on a detailed assessment of patient characteristics, resources, and self-care behaviors.
- To be considered an appropriate candidate for intensive therapy, via multiple daily injection or an insulin pump, an individual must reliably demonstrate and thereafter continue to employ certain safe, consistent self-care behaviors. These include frequent blood glucose monitoring, insulin injections, carbohydrate counting, and problem solving for high and low blood glucoses and sick day management. These behaviors cannot be abandoned once intensive therapy is begun; they must persistently continue for as long as intensive therapy is employed.
- Preparing the patient and support persons in problem-solving skills with intensive insulin therapy prior to pump therapy initiation is critical to using an insulin pump safely and effectively.
- Pump therapy requires a healthcare team that is knowledgeable about the unique and special requirements of those using insulin pumps.
- To ensure best practice, professionals involved in the care of pump patients must keep pace with rapidly advancing technological enhancements and developments.
- Understanding obstacles and the needs of special populations (such as youth and those with impaired vision) is important for intensive insulin therapy and the continuum of care.
- Pump therapy is most commonly used by persons with type 1 diabetes, but may also be of value for people with type 2 diabetes, older adults with profound insulin deficiency, and pregnant women with diabetes.

State of Disease

Pivotal studies in the early 1990s revealed that blood glucose control matters.[1,2] The goal for individuals, with either type 1 or type 2 diabetes, who are willing and able to actively participate in management of their disease should be to achieve the best possible level of glycemic control without experiencing undue short-term crises, including avoiding hypoglycemia.[3,4] Meticulous metabolic control minimizes the long-term complications of diabetes and improves the quality and length of life for individuals with diabetes.[4] To achieve this kind of glycemic control, insulin therapy often needs to be intensified. Intensification of insulin therapy can occur in either of the following ways:

- Multiple daily injections of insulin (MDI)
- Continuous subcutaneous insulin infusion (CSII), also known as insulin pump therapy

Since the first insulin pumps in 1978, insulin pump therapy has gained popularity. By 2002, more than 162,000 persons with diabetes had used CSII therapy.[5,6] Pump therapy is a realistic alternative for intensive insulin delivery in both pediatric and adult populations, including older adults.[7-12] Insulin pumps have allowed persons with diabetes who desire intensive insulin management and can be successful in self-management to achieve as close to euglycemia as possible with minimal hypoglycemia.[13]

There are, however, many different approaches to insulin therapy, ranging from various conventional regimens to intensive therapies. Viable treatment options for those seeking improved glycemic control include basal-bolus insulin regimens, MDI, and CSII. With the development of analog insulins (both rapid-acting and long-acting), intensive insulin therapy is more accessible and excellent glycemic control is more achievable, particularly among those who prefer MDI to CSII. This chapter focuses on the skills needed for intensive insulin therapy, particularly those needed for CSII. (More on analog insulin regimens can be found in chapter 15, on pharmacologic therapies for glucose control.) Another option, inhaled insulin therapy, has recently been added, and this may have an effect on the number of patients interested in using CSII and patient satisfaction in relationship to other options. Since inhaled insulin has only recently been FDA approved, experience with it will determine whether it is preferred over CSII, or simply another intensive therapy option.

Principles of Insulin Physiology and Pump Delivery

Both MDI and insulin pump delivery are designed to more closely mimic pancreatic function. For optimal glycemic control, insulin delivery should closely simulate the "normal" pattern of insulin secretion (shown in Figure 17.1). As shown in Figure 17.2, continuous or "basal" insulin levels are thus required throughout the day to cover hepatic glucose output and glucose disposal in the fasting state, while brief increases in insulin levels ("boluses") are needed to coincide with ingestion of food or meals.[3] For many patients, this approach is counter to the behavior they learned in using treatment regimens that predominantly employ intermediate or long-acting insulin.

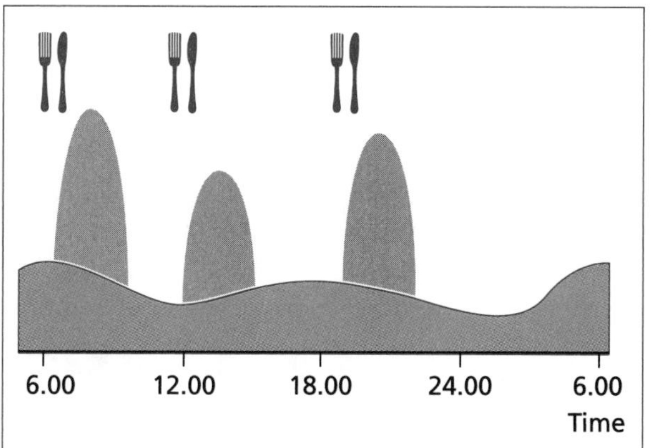

FIGURE 17.1 Insulin Secretion in Persons Without Diabetes

Source: Copyright © 2005 American Diabetes Association. Tomky D. Continuous subcutaneous insulin infusion (insulin pump therapy). In: Complete Nurses Guide to Diabetes Care. Childs AB, Cypress M, Spollett G, eds. American Diabetes Association: Alexandria, Va; 2005; 262. Reprinted with permission form the American Diabetes Association.

> ***Gaining Flexibility With Foods***
>
> Individuals who can (*a*) determine the carbohydrate content of foods and anticipate the food's glycemic effect and (*b*) understand the action of mealtime insulin can "mimic" endogenous insulin secretion. The ultimate result is flexibility in food choices and mealtimes.

- *In MDI,* a long-acting insulin analog, such as glargine (Lantus) or insulin detemir (Levemir), is used as a basal insulin analog, and a rapid-acting insulin is given with meals or when carbohydrates are ingested.
- *In pump therapy,* basal and bolus insulin doses are preprogrammed by the wearer and delivered through a small portable device that is designed to give doses precisely calculated for an individual's requirements.

One of the unique features of CSII is the ability to preprogram changes in basal insulin delivery.[14] This feature is especially useful during the night when insulin pharmacokinetics and the dawn phenomenon may change basal insulin requirements.[15]

Multiple Daily Injections of Insulin

A variety of choices exist for MDI; however, a common regimen, sometimes referred to as the "poor man's pump,"

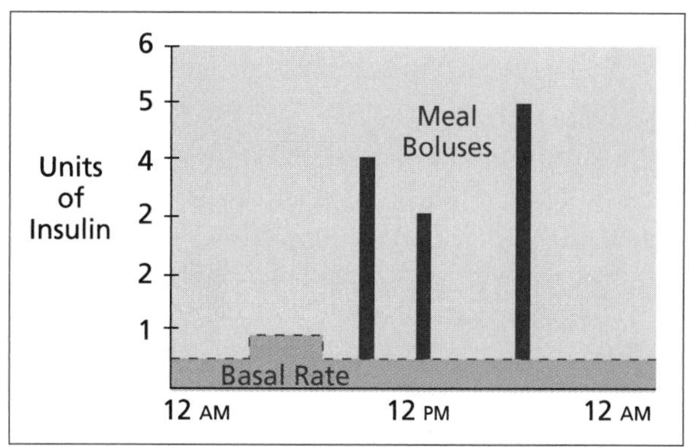

FIGURE 17.2 Pump Insulin Delivery

Source: Copyright © 2005 American Diabetes Association. Tomky D. Continuous subcutaneous insulin infusion (insulin pump therapy). In: Complete Nurses Guide to Diabetes Care. Childs AB, Cypress M, Spollett G, eds. American Diabetes Association: Alexandria, Va; 2005; 262. Reprinted with permission form the American Diabetes Association.

is to use a long-acting basal insulin, usually once a day, with injections of rapid-acting insulin when eating carbohydrates. The injections coinciding with food are administered at least twice a day or several times more during the day, depending on the individual's eating schedule. Additional injections, referred to as correction boluses, may become necessary if the blood glucose value is too high, in which case an injection of rapid-acting insulin is needed to lower the blood glucose to the target level. Some individuals may prefer using regular insulin (also known as short-acting insulin) for the correction and meal bolus dose. One example is if the individual has problems with delayed gastric emptying. A short-acting insulin will take longer to become effective, as it has a later peak and longer duration than rapid-acting insulin. Care must be taken, however, to prevent hypoglycemia when using short-acting or rapid-acting insulin, as the next paragraph explains.

Hypoglycemia can result from "stacked" correction doses

Short-acting insulin, because of its longer duration of action, can cause hypoglycemia several hours after food is eaten. The effect of the short-acting insulin combines with that of the long-acting or basal insulin. An MDI regimen poses the risk for hypoglycemia, particularly when the individual administers additional injections to bring an elevated glucose level back into the target range. Most people want to see their glucose level in their target range quickly; they may not wait long enough for the insulin to work before taking additional injections. The effect of the insulins overlap, a phenomenon referred to as *stacking*, which causes hypoglycemia. Diabetes educators should anticipate this practice and caution their patients to avoid repeated injections to correct glucose levels.

How Pumps Work

An insulin pump is a small, battery-operated mechanical device that contains a reservoir or syringe that is filled with rapid-acting insulin (and only rapid-acting insulin). The reservoir attaches to a plastic tube, called an infusion set. At the end of the infusion set is a detachable 25- or 27-gauge needle or soft Teflon catheter. The catheter (or needle) is inserted into the subcutaneous tissue and stays in place with self-adhesive tape or a biocclusive dressing. The person wearing the insulin pump operates the device. Every 48 to 72 hours, the pump wearer changes the infusion site, using aseptic technique.

Initially, insulin pumps weighed just under 1 lb and allowed simple delivery of basal and bolus insulin. Current models weigh as little as 3 oz and can be worn discretely under clothing or on a belt, like a pager or cell phone. Newer models contain miniature computers that provide an array of basal and bolus functions for more accurate calculations. Several pumps now connect via infrared ports to blood glucose monitors. This enables direct download of blood glucose data to facilitate more accurate and easy bolus calculations. The pump wearer must always, however, verify the data for further decision making before delivering recommended insulin doses. Most pumps connect (via infrared or cable) to computers or handheld devices so that insulin doses and blood glucose levels can be reviewed. Availability of these results allows the healthcare professional and wearer to analyze the data for pattern recognition to intensify diabetes management.

Other advanced features include tracking the amount of "insulin on board"—ie, the amount of insulin that is still active in the tissues from previous carbohydrate-based insulin boluses or correction boluses. Before this feature was developed, pump wearers often delivered boluses too frequently, trying to correct for elevated blood glucoses, instead of waiting for the full duration of insulin action before administering another bolus. This stacking of

Case in Point: Young Woman With Type 1 Diabetes

KT was a 23-year-old Mexican American female referred by her internist for consultation about pump therapy. She was diagnosed with type 1 diabetes at age 10 and presented with background diabetic retinopathy. Her glucose control was mediocre, as demonstrated by a recent A1C of 8.3%. Her regimen was NPH and Humalog insulin administered before breakfast and supper. She had recently spent 2 weeks as a counselor at summer camp for teenagers with diabetes. Most all of the other counselors wore an insulin pump and told her she had to get one!

Issues in KT's case will be discussed throughout the chapter to provide readers with insight into careful and appropriate candidate selection and the extensive preparation and training required for successful insulin pump therapy.

insulin resulted in low blood glucoses several hours after repeated boluses, as described earlier. Other advanced features offered by newer pumps include site change reminders, blood glucose and missed bolus alerts, calculation of food bolus based on preset insulin-to-carbohydrate ratios (also known as insulin:carb ratios or ICRs), alerts to recheck blood glucose (BG) if previous level was below or above target, and preprogrammed insulin sensitivity factors (ISFs) that allow for accurate calculation of required boluses to correct elevated BG. Some pumps include a food database that can be individualized for commonly consumed foods. Over time, pumps are getting smarter, but currently the wearer still needs to perform self-monitoring of blood glucose (SMBG) and make appropriate decisions based on that information.

Candidate Selection

Evidence Versus Practice: Appropriate Candidates for Pump Therapy

Prerequisite Skills and Experience

Pumps are considered safe and effective for a variety of populations; however, changing directly to pump therapy without previous experience using intensified insulin therapy (ie, MDI) is inappropriate. Individuals interested in using pump therapy first need to learn and develop a variety of skills. The following are important to master as prerequisites to pump therapy:

- Frequent blood glucose monitoring
- Carbohydrate counting
- Calculating bolus insulin
- Problem solving through interpretation of blood glucose pattern
- Adjusting insulin

Only individuals who have mastered these skills should be considered for insulin pump therapy. Note also that these are just the prerequisites; other skills need to be taught and developed.

Importance of Experienced, Multidisciplinary Team

One of the important considerations for successful pump therapy is using a team for education, training, and treatment that is both multidisciplinary and familiar with insulin pump therapy.[13,16,17] Ideally, insulin pump therapy should be prescribed, implemented, and followed by a skilled diabetes care team that is familiar with the therapy and capable of supporting the patient 24 hours a day, 7 days a week.[18]

Other Key Elements

The following are also key elements for implementing pump therapy:

- Appropriate patient selection
- Adequate preparation with sufficient education and training
- Ongoing follow-up

Traits and Clinical Indicators

Patients with unrealistic expectations of CSII therapy can be identified with an established screening protocol.[19] Although the clinical indications for pump therapy are still being debated, pump experts agree that the following are clear justifications:[5,18]

- Frequent, unpredictable hypoglycemia or a marked dawn phenomenon
- Condition persists after attempts to improve control with intensive insulin injection regimens

The AADE and American Diabetes Association (ADA) position statements highlight clinical indications and desirable traits in selecting CSII hopefuls;[13,18] these are summarized in the sidebar on the next page.

Evidence Versus Practice: Success Rates

Despite the initial interest expressed by patients, the literature suggests that about 50% of individuals who start pump therapy discontinue it within 2 years.[11,19] Whether this is because they have not been properly prepared to deal with the challenges of intensifying therapy or because these individuals experienced problems specifically with insulin pump therapy is unknown. Preparing patients for pump therapy by first using MDI and problem solving may, however, increase the chances for success.

Using a Saline Trial. Sandfield et al showed that a structured screening protocol with a saline pump trial was effective in decreasing the cost of CSII initiation while increasing continuation of CSII therapy.[19] A saline trial allows the prospective insulin pump user to experience daily management (eg, showering, bathing, sleeping, sexual intimacy) before proceeding further in the screening process.[20]

> ***Best Preparation for CSII***
>
> Preparing patients for pump therapy by first using multiple daily injection therapy and problem solving helps increase the chance these individuals will reach their goal and succeed with this therapy.

Clinical Indications for Insulin Pump Therapy

Clinical indications for insulin pump therapy that have been identified in position statements by the AADE and ADA include the following:[13,18]

- Unpredictable hypoglycemia
- Marked dawn phenomenon
- Failure to obtain optimal glycemic control using 3 to 4 daily injections of insulin
- Patient desires greater lifestyle flexibility, particularly with regard to meal schedules and travel
- Patient is motivated and daily schedule makes conventional therapy less effective
- Pregnancy requiring improved metabolic control

Traits Desired

Most pump experts agree the following are desirable traits for a pump user to have:[13,18]

- Is motivated to improve glucose control
- Accepts day-to-day self-care responsibilities
- Has realistic expectations about CSII therapy
- Is able to understand and demonstrate use of the insulin pump and self-monitoring of blood glucose (including documentation of the results and use of the data)
- Demonstrates effective coping patterns and problem solving
- Has support systems available and financial resources

Benefits and Limitations: MDI and Pump Therapy

Multiple Daily Injections

Benefits of MDI

MDI more closely mimics normal insulin secretion than conventional therapy (ie, NPH and regular insulin or NPH insulin and a rapid-acting analog). MDI provides for more dietary flexibility; with this therapy, the individual can calculate bolus insulin based on food intake. There is less hypoglycemia overnight than with conventional therapy, and the person is not forced to eat when not hungry to prevent hypoglycemia at peak times of insulin.

Limitations of MDI

Basal insulin is given once or twice a day and is a steady amount of insulin. It cannot be quickly changed for exercise or other activities that may require more or less basal coverage. Frequent and multiple injections of insulin may be difficult to fit into an individual's lifestyle.

Insulin Pump Therapy

Benefits of Pump Therapy

Evidence shows that using pump therapy to maintain normal or near-normal glycemia can improve health and reduce the long-term complications of diabetes.[1] Improvement in blood glucose levels is possible with pumps. Pumps do not use long-acting insulin, but instead use short- or rapid-acting insulin that provides more predictable physiologic delivery of insulin. Dosing of insulin is precisely delivered within one-hundredth of a unit. Insulin absorption is more predictable from a continuous insulin depot.

Case—Part 2: Selection Criteria

KT was engaged to be married soon and stated she wanted an insulin pump to improve her glucose control for eventual pregnancy. She had occasional hypoglycemia episodes, but was able to recognize and treat it (sometimes she overtreated it). Her blood glucoses fluctuated widely, with blood glucose patterns revealing elevated fasting blood glucoses that suggests a dawn phenomenon. She was covered by her parents' insurance while finishing her college degree and expected continuous coverage from her fiancé's health insurance.

As with any potential pump candidate, KT's reasons for desiring a pump needed to be explored to determine whether CSII was an appropriate treatment for her. Was peer pressure her primary reason for requesting pump therapy? What were her true motivations?

A full assessment of her self-care behaviors needed to be completed to fully understand if she fit the criteria that predicted improved glycemic control and had the determination to persist with the daily demands of intensive insulin therapy. The AADE 7 Self-Care Behaviors™ would be useful in assessing for desired outcomes.

Dawn phenomenon effects are easier to manage; a variable basal rate can be set to accommodate fluctuations in insulin requirements overnight. Basal rates can be quickly changed to accommodate growth spurts in children or increased insulin needs during pregnancy, stress, illness, and/or physical activity.

Pump therapy can help reduce the frequency and severity of hypoglycemia. Pumps offer an improved safety profile by reducing the basal rate during periods of low physiological requirements, which can minimize nocturnal or daytime hypoglycemia. Using a temporary basal rate that meets the short-term physiologic needs can accommodate for sick days or anticipated physical activity.

Insulin pump therapy offers an improvement in lifestyle flexibility and patient satisfaction by allowing meals and snacks to be customized to fit the individual's schedule and preferences in timing, size of meal, and type of food. Using ICRs to count carbohydrates is one method of matching appropriate amounts of insulin in bolus doses to intake of food (described later in this chapter). Weight loss may be achieved more easily in motivated individuals, although initial improved glycemia may promote weight gain if there is no alteration in caloric intake.[21,22]Another benefit of a pump is the ability to tailor insulin needs to changes in schedules related to travel or work.

Limitations of Pump Therapy

Risks and limitations of pump therapy must be fully understood by the wearer, family or support person, and healthcare team. Pumps are not for everyone, and the person using one must maintain a high degree of motivation before and after pump initiation![23] The person must be willing to maintain habitual and frequent self-monitoring of blood glucose. Some people with diabetes struggle with self-care behaviors and applying appropriate problem-solving skills. Being connected to a pump is a constant reminder of having diabetes. Technical or mechanical failure is possible and if not corrected quickly can lead to diabetic ketoacidosis within a few hours in individuals with type 1 diabetes. Skin irritations and infections are possible, although these are avoidable with proper technique, including skin care and site rotation. Some patient populations, such as children or people who are visually impaired, may require assistance from a caregiver.

Many healthcare professionals are unfamiliar with pump therapy and may not provide the needed training and support. The cost of insulin pumps is often over $6000 and supplies (not including blood glucose monitoring supplies) cost more than $400 per month. Insurance companies typically cover only 80% of pump expenses, and coverage varies from state to state and plan to plan. Reimbursement for diabetes education to support the patient also varies.

Contraindications to Pump Therapy

Individuals who unrealistically expect that pump therapy will automatically control the diabetes are not appropriate candidates for CSII. Severe depression or other serious behavioral health disorders may distract the person from paying attention to details that are critical to successful pump therapy. A history of poor self-care behaviors and healthcare practices, such as failure to perform SMBG, keep appointments, give consistent insulin doses, or appropriately apply problem-solving skills, is a predictor of a poor outcome.[21] Lack of financial resources for initiating and maintaining optimal pump therapy practices also present barriers.

Self-Care Behaviors and Behavior Change

The AADE 7 Self-Care Behaviors™ framework provides structure for assessment, intervention, and the evaluation process before, during, and after pump initiation. Evidence shows that a multidisciplinary team with pump experience is most effective at educating, training, and managing pump therapy patients. The "dream team" from the Diabetes Control and Complications Trial (DCCT) consisted of a diabetes nurse, dietitian, behaviorist, and diabetologist.[1] At minimum, CSII therapy teams usually consist of a nurse, dietitian, and endocrinologist. A pump therapy team member should always be available for emergency contact.

Healthy Eating

Core competence in diabetes medical nutrition therapy (MNT) is essential for successful implementation of intensified insulin therapy. To maximize the benefits and minimize the risks associated with intensive therapy, the pump wearer needs knowledge of meal planning and the ability to plan meals, modify food choices, and determine insulin doses.

The DCCT provided an opportunity to look at various nutrition strategies to counsel patients to attain normoglycemia. The MNT strategies employed included healthy food choices based on the food pyramid, exchange lists, carbohydrate counting, and total available glucose. The nutrition interventions were used along with behavior management approaches and intensive insulin therapy.[24] MNT studies have looked at both the glycemic response to total carbohydrate in specific foods as well as glycemic response to specific forms of the carbohydrate in foods, such as simple or complex carbohydrates. From these studies evolved the ultimate recommendation for persons with diabetes in regard to the selection of carbohydrates for inclusion in their meal plan. The total amount of carbohydrate in meals or snacks is more important than the source or type and is the first priority in planning meals and snacks.[25] This has led to the implementation of carbohydrate counting, in which foods are listed as carbohydrate choices based on the amount and not the source of the carbohydrate.[25]

Whether using MDI or insulin pump therapy, carbohydrate counting is a meal planning approach that supports either basal-bolus therapy. Carbohydrate counting enables a flexible eating schedule and more dietary freedom for people on an intensive insulin regimen.[26] To succeed, individuals using this approach need to understand the relationship of carbohydrates to both their basal and bolus insulin.

Early research on CSII demonstrated that while basal insulin could be adjusted based on fasting blood glucose levels, premeal insulin boluses were related solely to carbohydrate intake.[27] Additional research documented the relationship of insulin doses to carbohydrate.[28,29] Mixed meals (carbohydrate plus protein and fat) were shown to have very little effect on carbohydrate-based bolus insulin doses.[26]

The amount of carbohydrate in the meal helps determine the mealtime bolus dose of insulin.[29-31] Algorithms based on the amount (in grams) of carbohydrate eaten are effective.[30] In general the glycemic index, fiber, fat, and caloric content of the meal do not affect the bolus insulin doses.[30,31] This finding is further supported by the DCCT, which demonstrated that individuals on intensive therapy who adjusted their meal insulin doses based on carbohydrate intake lowered their A1C by 0.5% (P <.03).[24,31]

Dose adjustment for normal eating (DAFNE) is a method that includes the skills of matching insulin doses to carbohydrate intake in an effort to maintain blood glucose levels close to normal.[32] In clinical studies, DAFNE was shown to improve quality of life and glycemic control in people with type 1 diabetes without worsening hypoglycemia.[32] Thus, research has provided evidence that matching insulin to the amount of carbohydrate intake, known as using an ICR, is effective.[33]

Carbohydrate-Counting Skills

Carbohydrate counting can be taught in levels:[34]

- Basic carbohydrate counting
- Advanced carbohydrate counting

Basic Carbohydrate-Counting Skills. Basic skills include learning to determine the amount of carbohydrates in foods, by reading food labels, and weighing and measuring food portions. Individuals learn to identify carbohydrates as starches, fruit, milk, and desserts. Emphasis is placed on developing consistency in the timing, variety, and amount of carbohydrate-containing foods consumed.[34] Another basic skill is understanding the relationship among food, diabetes medications, physical activity, and blood glucose level. Basic skills training introduces the steps needed to manage these variables based on patterns of blood glucose levels.

Advanced Carbohydrate-Counting Skills. Advanced skills training teaches the person using MDI or CSII how to use ICRs to match short-acting or rapid-acting insulin to carbohydrate consumption.[33] Basic carbohydrate-counting skills are expanded by analyzing portions, types, and effect of foods on blood glucose values and learning to use food scales to accurately quantify portions. The individual also develops an understanding of the principles of the basal-bolus insulin concept to achieve target blood glucose levels. The individual learns to look for patterns in glucose values over time to interpret blood glucose levels.

Case—Part 3: Assessing Skills

To evaluate whether KT was an appropriate candidate for CSII, her diabetes educator assessed her knowledge about the effect of food on blood glucose, sources of carbohydrates, and meal planning.

KT was given resources to assist in making food choices to aid in building her skills in meal planning, weighing and measuring food, carbohydrate counting, and label reading. As KT learned these skills, her diabetes educator assessed for environmental triggers, emotional status, cultural preferences, and financial barriers that might interfere with KT meeting her clinical goals.

KT's eating behaviors were frequently evaluated. The educator reviewed her food records, blood glucose records, and 24-hour food recall; observed her skills; and listened for self-reports (eg, on the amount of food eaten, timing of meals, alcohol intake, effect of food on glucose) to assess KT's ability to problem solve in special situations.[37]

Both basic and advanced carbohydrate-counting require that the individual have an understand the target blood glucose levels and the difference between basal and bolus insulin. Most importantly, the person must be willing and able to keep adequate records, including blood glucose monitoring and food intake records. Individuals wishing to learn carbohydrate counting should be encouraged to work with a registered dietitian or diabetes educator experienced in teaching these skills. Excellent patient education materials are available to supplement learning.[35,36]

Correction Boluses and the Insulin Sensitivity Factor. An important and advanced skill in carbohydrate counting is using both the ICR and the insulin sensitivity factor (ISF) for correction bolus. Correction-dose insulin therapy is an important adjunct to the scheduled insulin that is usually given before meals.[38] The ISF is used to calculate the amount of insulin needed to bring the blood glucose level into target range and is used to as a correction or supplemental amount of insulin when glucose levels are too high or too low before meals. Calculating the ISF also helps the individual make adjustments for special situations.[39] Both the ICR, which is based on matching the rapid-acting insulin to the carbohydrate content of food to be eaten, and the ISF need to be individualized (see the later section on taking medication). Newer "smart" pumps have dose calculators built in to assist with accurate dosing of both the ICR and correction bolus.

Determining Insulin-to-Carbohydrate Ratios

The ICR is based on the principle that 1 unit of rapid-acting insulin is needed to cover or match a specified amount of carbohydrate. The ratio is determined by the individual's sensitivity to insulin. An adult who is not obese may have an ICR of 1 unit of insulin to "cover or match" 10 to 15 g of carbohydrate. The ratio can vary—from toddlers (who are typically very sensitive to insulin) requiring 1 unit of rapid-acting insulin for every 30 g of carbohydrate to overweight adults requiring 1 unit of rapid-acting insulin for every 5 g of carbohydrate consumed.

There are different approaches and methods for determining the ICR for an individual (see Table 17.1 for starting adult dose calculations). Bolus or mealtime insulin doses can be based on the total number of grams of carbohydrate to be eaten or on the total number of grams of carbohydrate or choices consumed at a meal. In calculating a meal bolus, insulin dose is based on the total amount of grams of carbohydrate to be eaten.[34]

Food Records. Food records are used to help determine the total amount of carbohydrate at each meal and snack for at least 3 days. It is helpful to also look for situations that may have interfered with eating consistent amounts of carbohydrate, such as eating out or not knowing how to count the carbohydrate in combination foods. The best way to begin to decide how much insulin is needed with meals is for the patient to keep records of food intake and the amount of insulin generally taken.

To determine the total units of bolus insulin, the total number of grams of carbohydrate for the anticipated meal is divided by the number of units of rapid-acting insulin taken for the meal.

Challenges and Advantages of Carbohydrate Counting

Avoiding Weight Gain. Bode et al followed over 800 CSII patients for approximately 15 years and found that these patients experienced a reduction in insulin requirements and less weight gain with greater flexibility in food intake.[21] In contrast, in the DCCT, intensive therapy resulted in significant weight gain.[40] Carbohydrate counting does not guarantee weight management. Individuals using intensive insulin therapy still need to maintain a balance of healthy food choices and caloric intake.[25]

Maintaining Healthy Eating Behaviors. Most individuals using pump therapy enjoy the increased flexibility in selecting a variety of foods and the timing of their meals that intensive insulin therapy coupled with carbohydrate counting offers.[6] Carbohydrate counting does, however, present some individuals with challenges in weight management.[25] Some individuals are tempted with eating as desired and to forget about general nutrition principles of healthy eating behaviors. These concerns should be discussed with patients before they begin using carbohydrate counting and monitored at subsequent visits.[39]

Adjusting for Fat, Fiber, and Unique Responses. High-fat meals can cause a delay in gastric emptying, and, therefore, problems in unpredictable food absorption. Patients eating high-fat foods may require an adjustment in their bolus insulin amount or in the timing of their mealtime insulin to avoid early postprandial hypoglycemia and later hyperglycemia (see more in gastric motility section, toward the end of this chapter). Similarly, dietary fiber is not usually digested. Patients need to be taught that if a food contains more than 5 g of fiber per serving, the total amount of fiber must be subtracted from the total amount of carbohydrate before calculating an insulin dose. Some individuals may also notice their own unique responses to certain carbohydrate foods and may need to adjust their bolus doses accordingly.[39]

Carbohydrate counting is not a perfect system; it presents many challenges and concerns.[39] Most people find weighing and measuring foods tedious and often impractical when eating out. Keeping a food record is initially

TABLE 17.1 Starting Adult Dosage Calculations

Basal Rate Calculations Generally, a single basal rate is recommended; multiple basal rates are sometimes programmed based on individualized requirements (eg, prednisone doses or well-documented, distinct dawn phenomenon)	
Method 1:	1. Determine TDD* of insulin with injections; reduce by 25%-30% 2. Divide TDD by 50% = total basal dose in units 3. Divide total basal dose by 24 hours = starting basal rate (unit/hour)
Method 2:	1. Multiply 0.5 × patient's weight (kg) = TDD, then reduce by 20%-25% 2. Divide TDD by 50% = total basal dose in units 3. Divide total basal dose by 24 hours = starting basal rate (unit/hour)
Method 3:	Optimally controlled basal-bolus MDI patients may convert total dosage of glargine divided by 24 hours = starting basal rate (unit/hour) *Note:* Reducing by 10%-15% for the first 24 hours allows for "wash out" of glargine
Bolus Calculations See chapter's section on carbohydrate counting	
Method 1:	TDD is divided into 450 or 500 to determine how many grams of carbohydrate are covered by 1 unit of insulin *Example:* 500 ÷ 50 unit/day (TDD) = 1 unit per 10 g of carbohydrate
Method 2:	1. Based on weight and TDD 2. 2.8 × weight (lb) ÷ TDD = ICR
Method 3:	Optimally controlled basal-bolus MDI patients may convert from previous ICR
Correction Bolus Calculations or Insulin Sensitivity Factor	
Method:	1. Determine the correction dose for elevated glucose levels to determine the mg/dL that 1 unit of insulin decreases the blood glucose value 2. Divide 1500 when using regular insulin or 1700 when using lispro or aspart insulin by the TDD *Example:* 1700 ÷ TDD = insulin sensitivity factor

*TDD is the total daily dose

Sources: Bode BW. Tamborlane WV, Davidson PC. Insulin pump therapy in the 21st century. Postgrad Med. 2002;111(5):69-78.

Wolpert, H. Smart pumping: a practical approach to mastering the insulin pump. Alexandria, Va: American Diabetes Association; 2002.

challenging, and maintaining ongoing food records can be burdensome. Monitoring blood glucose before and after meals can be challenging, but such monitoring is necessary and proven effective for identifying appropriate dose of insulin to achieve and maintain euglycemia.[21] Still, carbohydrate counting offers several advantages. It focuses on a single nutrient, provides a more precise method of matching food and mealtime insulin, allows flexibility in meal planning, improves blood glucose control, and is empowering to those who use it.[34] Understanding the need to adjust insulin for meal sizes, individualizing premeal and postmeal blood glucose targets, using pattern management skills, and calculating bolus and basal insulin doses is helpful for people with diabetes to be successful with healthy eating behaviors.[35]

Patients should be encouraged to try to learn the carbohydrate content of their commonly consumed foods. Remind them that most people with and without diabetes eat very similar foods day after day. Most patients are able to determine the carbohydrate content of their commonly consumed foods in 1 to 2 weeks. There are now many carbohydrate-counting resources available online, as software programs for personal digital assistants (PDAs), and as small reference books.

Case—Part 4: Obtaining Skills

Once KT understood her basal needs and mastered the basic skills of carbohydrate counting, she was ready to move on to the advanced skills she would need to be able to adjust her insulin based on the amount of carbohydrate she would eat. KT wanted more flexibility in her eating schedule and to intensify her regimen as a means to improve her glycemic control. This was also a good time to introduce MDIs so KT could begin to use all her new carbohydrate-counting skills.

KT was instructed to eat a consistent amount of carbohydrate at meals. In addition, she was asked to record where she ate, what types of food she ate (including approximate amounts), her premeal and postmeal blood glucose levels, and how much bolus insulin she took for each meal and snack. When she brought these records in, the diabetes educator reviewed them and determined both the average intake of carbohydrate and the average range for each meal and snack.

KT's records indicated she was eating an average of 64 g of carbohydrate per meal. Her blood glucose levels before and after meals varied, but she had several instances in which her premeal and postmeal glucose values were in her target range.

Intensive insulin therapy includes adjusting premeal insulin not only for carbohydrate intake, but also based on blood glucose levels. To determine KT's ICR, the diabetes educator chose to focus on the meals in which both premeal and postmeal glucose levels were in her target range. The educator then calculated KT's ratio by looking at KT"s records, which showed that she ate 64 g of carbohydrate and took 8 units of insulin. Since KT's premeal and 2-hour postmeal blood glucose were in her target blood glucose range, the educator divided KT's total grams of carbohydrate by total units of insulin:

64 g of carbohydrate/8 units of
insulin = 8 g/1 unit = 8

KT's ratio was thus determined to be 1:8 (1 unit of insulin per 8 g of carbohydrate). Therefore, on days when KT was planning to eat 64 g of carbohydrate, she would take 8 units of bolus insulin. However, if she would be eating more or less carbohydrate, she would adjust her bolus dose by 1 unit for every 8 g of carbohydrate. If KT planned to eat an additional 16 g of carbohydrate, she would take an extra 2 units of insulin (10 units). If she were going to eat approximately 16 g less of carbohydrate, she would take 2 units less of insulin (6 units). KT thus had a simplified formula to adjust insulin that would give her flexibility in the amounts and types of food she desired to eat.

The educator told KT that other circumstances such as illness or physical activity stress might require KT to make additional adjustments to the premeal insulin dose. The educator explained that finding the ratio that works sometimes takes time. KT was taught to calculate her basal needs, bolus needs, and insulin sensitivity factors. She was told to try her calculated ICR for several weeks, while closely monitoring her blood glucose levels (preferably premeal and 2 hours postmeal) as well as her food intake, physical activity, and any other factors that might affect her blood glucose level. Doing so would ensure that the basal-bolus regimen was effective in keeping her blood glucose in her target range.

Other Carbohydrate Counting Methods

Another method would have been for KT to adjust her mealtime or snack insulin based on her carbohydrate intake. If KT planned to eat 80 g of carbohydrate, she could use her ICR:

1 unit for every 8 g of carbohydrate =
10 units of insulin for 80 g of carbohydrate

Some people are more comfortable using the carbohydrate choice method as an indicator of how much insulin to take for meals or snacks.[36] The carbohydrate choice method is similar to the method discussed above. Since 1 carbohydrate choice is the amount of food containing 15 g of carbohydrate, KT could determine the total number of carbohydrate choices from meals and snacks per day by dividing the total daily insulin dose by the number of carbohydrate choices. This would be her ICR. For example, if KT took a total of 20 units of bolus insulin per day and ate a total of 13 carbohydrate choices (4 at breakfast, 3 at lunch, 4 at dinner, and 2 at bedtime), the ICR would be as follows:

20 units of bolus insulin per day/
13 carbohydrate choices per day = 1.5 units

Therefore, KT's breakfast bolus would be 6 units (4 carbohydrate choices × 1.5 units), her lunch bolus 4.5 units, her dinner bolus 6 units, and the bedtime snack bolus 3 units. After 3 to 5 days, KT might need to recalculate her doses based on glucose monitoring data.

Being Active

A person using an insulin pump who increases his or her physical activity often experiences a decreased need for, or better utilization of, insulin; the result may be a decrease in insulin required to reach glucose goals.[41] Acute effects of being physically active generally cause a reduction in plasma glucose.[42] Ongoing participation in a physically active lifestyle results in improved insulin sensitivity and glucose tolerance because of changes in body composition and the additive effects of daily physical exertion. The hormonal response to an episode of increased physical activity depends on the degree of diabetes control, insulin dose, time and content of last meal, fitness level, and type of activity performed.[43] Hypoglycemia is the most commonly encountered problem in individuals with diabetes when they are physically active and are on an insulin pump.[41,44] On the other hand, some research involving intense exercise with CSII use has shown it produces hyperglycemia.[45]

The type of insulin adjustment depends on when the person is going to engage in physical activity relative to his or her mealtime boluses. In MDI, the person may need to anticipate the physical activity and decrease the basal insulin. If the physical activity will occur within 3 hours after the premeal bolus, then that bolus can be adjusted. If physical activity will be between meals, then the basal rate needs adjusting. Some parameters are given below:[46]

- *Light Activities.* For light activities such as housework or yard work, a 10% to 20% reduction in insulin requirements 1 hour preceding and 1 hour after the activity usually works well in keeping the blood glucose stable.
- *Activities of Moderate Intensity and Short Duration.* Moderate intensity and short duration (1 to 2 hours) of activity such as tennis, brisk walking, running, or biking requires a 30% to 50% reduction for the 1 hour preceding and the 1 hour after the activity, in addition to the duration of the activity itself.
- *Isometric Exercises.* Isometric exercises such as weightlifting usually require no adjustment.
- *Prolonged Activity.* Prolonged activity requires a sustained reduction for the duration of activity and may require extended reduction to avoid nocturnal hypoglycemia.

Pump wearers are advised not to remove the pump during exercise unless basal insulin is replaced, as a bolus prior to removal or as depot long-acting insulin (see section on switch back therapy later in this chapter). Schmulling et al found several strategies helpful in preventing hypoglycemia during a short workout, including reducing the premeal bolus or consuming quickly absorbable carbohydrates just before the workout. Monitoring blood glucose before and after exercise is vital to understanding individual responses.[42] See chapters 14 and 29 for more information on physical activity and the self-care behaviors related to being active.

Case—Part 5: Adjusting the Insulin Pump for Physical Activity

KT joined a gym. Her basal dose of insulin seemed to be working well in keeping her blood glucose levels in her target range, and her ICR ratio was working well for her meals. The first time she tried walking on the treadmill, though, she experienced hypoglycemia and became frustrated.

Increased physical activity is often one of the primary goals of self-management education. Even small changes are considered beneficial. With the help of a diabetes educator, KT was guided to incorporate physical activity into her daily routine.

During assessment, the educator gathered information to understand the type of physical activity KT liked and the anticipated duration and intensity of her workouts. KT, of course, needed to understand safety precautions and special considerations as she might experience hypoglycemia even during her other activities (activities such as house cleaning, gardening, or shopping). Skills she needed to learn involved developing an appropriate activity plan and adjusting her premeal bolus if exercising after a meal or adding a snack if spontaneously exercises. If she planned on a consistent workout time, intensity, and duration of physical activity, she could then use a basal rate of long-acting insulin analog to match her needs. She would also need to learn to balance her food and insulin during her active periods.[37]

KT was taught to monitor her blood glucose levels both before and after exercise to help determine whether she needed to adjust her basal or her bolus insulin on exercise days to prevent hypoglycemia.

KT's diabetes team provided guidance on how to safely exercise based on her blood glucose levels. By measuring the type of activity, frequency, duration, and intensity (with a pedometer) and by examining blood glucose records and using observation and self-report, KT could better adjust her bolus or basal insulin needs.

Monitoring

Evidence from the DCCT and others showed that a minimum consistency of SMBG 3 or more times per day is required to achieve lowering of mean A1C and glucose.[21,47] Pump patients who monitor blood glucose levels 3 or more times a day achieved a lower average A1C level than patients who monitored levels once or twice daily (7.2% versus 8%). Of patients who self-reported that they monitored blood glucose levels 5 or more times a day, 62% had an average A1C level of less than 7%.[21]

Each day's additional glucose measurement corresponds to a 0.2% reduction in A1C[5]

Experience in structured and frequent monitoring should begin with the initiation of intensive insulin therapy and maintained indefinitely.[13] Methods of measuring monitoring behavior include reviewing the logbook, meter memory review or printout, and self-report. To help understand problem areas in behavior, the following can be reviewed: frequency of missed tests, schedule of testing, planned or unplanned testing, and, if needed, pharmacy refill record.[37] Further evidence shows that reduction in a pump patient's A1C values of 0.4% to >1% correlates to the recording of insulin doses and blood glucose values in a logbook.[5]

Frequency and Timing of SMBG in Intensive Therapies

The optimal frequency and timing of the SMBG schedule is as follows:

- Fasting
- Premeal
- 2-Hour postprandial
- Bedtime
- An occasional 3 AM

Continuous Glucose Monitoring. A new technology poised to network with insulin pump therapy is continuous glucose monitoring (CGM). A retrospective data collection system is currently available, known as continuous glucose monitoring system (CGMS) technology (from Medtronic). Real-time data systems are under development. CGMS measures subcutaneous interstitial glucose levels and continuously records values on average every 5 minutes within a range of 40 to 400 mg/dL.[48] The retrospective, collected data is uploaded to a computer for analysis. Kaufman et al describe their experience using CGMS information to alter insulin regimens of selected pump patients because of glucose management problems for decreasing A1C.[49] Real-time CGM systems are anticipated to attach directly to an insulin pump, giving patients the option to accept or modify the suggested dose for direct dose administration.[50] With this anticipated technology, closed-loop systems will be closer to reality.

Taking Medication

Persons on an NPH and regular insulin regimen are not candidates for pump therapy, unless they have tried a more intensive insulin regimen. Pregnancy can be an exception because glycemic control is critical to achieve very rapidly (see discussion toward end of chapter). The insulin pump is a more expensive and invasive method of insulin delivery.[18,19] Some insurance companies may require a period of intensive injected insulin therapy before approving an insulin pump.

Albright et al showed a lowering of A1C (8.1% to 7.4%) by switching type 1 patients on twice-daily NPH insulin and lispro/aspart to once- or twice-daily glargine (Lantus) with lispro/aspart, basal-bolus regimens.[51] Since introduction of analog bolus and basal insulin (glargine with aspart/lispro), glycemic control differences between MDI and CSII are not as great as those seen in the past. Apparently as a result, fewer patients are now starting insulin pump therapy;[52] although, a short-term cross-over trial of MDI using glargine and aspart compared to CSII using

Case—Part 6: Monitoring Behavior

KT was monitoring her blood glucose 2 to 4 times daily. Initial assessment of KT's current monitoring behaviors included her knowledge about the testing schedule, target values, disposal of sharps, and interpretation of results. The educator knew it was important to review KT's skills to ensure adequacy of technique, recording of BG results, and use of equipment.

If KT's monitoring behavior was suboptimal to maintain optimal glycemia, then barriers such as financial, physical, cognitive, time, inconvenience, or emotional factors would need to be explored and resolved. Monitoring behaviors are directly linked to problem solving that involves the prevention, detection, and treatment of high or low blood glucoses and dealing with sick days.

aspart showed a reduction in fructosamine levels in the CSII group.[53] Doyle et al found similar results in lowering A1C levels by studying randomly assigned type 1 children to either CSII or MDI using glargine and aspart.[54] They concluded that inadequate insulin coverage for between-meal snacks may be problematic with MDI users; experienced clinicians frequently see this.

Several clinical trials involving type 1 and 2 individuals comparing CSII to MDI showed no difference in A1C.[55-58] Raskins et al showed MDI using NPH and aspart to be comparable to CSII in type 2 individuals.[57] Herman et al looked at older individuals with type 2 diabetes (mean age 66 years) and demonstrated no difference in A1C, frequency or severity of hypoglycemia, or treatment satisfaction results.[56]

Another benefit of implementing an intensive insulin therapy plan consisting of 3 or more daily injections is that the patient learns and advances necessary skills—namely, frequent SMBG, carbohydrate counting and matching bolus insulin, problem solving by adjusting insulin for high or low blood glucoses, and using appropriate monitoring of urine ketones during illness.[13]

The time line from beginning intensive insulin therapy to initiating insulin pump therapy is program defined. The literature does not describe an accepted universal preparation protocol, although several themes emerge for allowing enough time (3 to 6 months) to ensure competent self-care behaviors and clinical indications are detected. Exception to the rule for using MDI prior to initiating insulin pump therapy is generally seen in pediatrics with young children as well as with pregnancy, where rapid improvement in control is needed.[5,49]

Elevated Fasting Blood Glucoses

Observing changes in overnight blood glucoses from bedtime until dawn can assist in making the correct diagnosis, thus facilitating further treatment. Inadequate coverage of food with mealtime insulin can be corrected by changing the bolus ratio for supper or snacks. Basal insulin can be increased if blood glucoses slowly rise overnight. If blood glucoses fall below 70 mg/dL by 3 AM, then reducing the basal rate would be appropriate. A marked rise in blood glucose concentration from bedtime to dawn has come to be known as the "dawn phenomenon."[59]

Dawn Phenomenon. The most agreed-upon reason for using CSII is controlling the dawn phenomenon.[6,21,60,61] There are several reasons for blood glucose elevations in the early morning hours before breakfast. One possibility—a simple decline in insulin levels—is seen in many individuals using NPH or Lente insulin as the basal insulin at supper or bedtime. This usually results in routinely elevated morning glucose because a peak effect during the early night hours is responsible for a high risk of nocturnal hypoglycemia. The hormonal basis for the dawn phenomenon is thought to be due mainly to overnight growth

Case—Part 7: Clinical Indicators

When KT first began discussing pump therapy with the diabetes educator, she was on a conventional insulin therapy plan. She weighed 140 lb, her height was 68 in, and her regimen was 20 units of NPH and 5 units of regular insulin twice daily. Her last A1C had been 8.3%. She reported frequent mild hypoglycemic episodes and a severe nocturnal episode within the last year.

Before she could be considered for pump therapy, she needed to start on a basal-bolus analog-based insulin injection regimen. After 3 months of MDI with glargine and aspart, KTs frequent blood glucose records revealed consistent elevated fasting blood glucoses of at least 50 to 100 mg/dL higher than bedtime levels.

The educator considered all possible reasons to explain these results: the possibility of not covering a bedtime snack with adequate doses of aspart, a late supper consisting of high-fat foods or large portions of food, inadequate basal insulin, the Somogyi effect, or the occurrence of the dawn phenomenon. Sorting out the problem required several adjustments with food, insulin, and blood glucose monitoring.

The simplest strategy, and the first one used, was to eliminate all food intake within 4 to 5 hours of bedtime. Then KT was asked to increase the frequency of blood glucose monitoring to evaluate 2-hour postsupper, bedtime, 3 AM, and 6 AM results.

After 6 months of MDI therapy, KT was dosing with 25 units of glargine at bedtime and 1 unit of aspart for every 10 g of carbohydrate, for a total daily dosage of 50 units per day. Her A1C had decreased to 7.2%. Sorting out the reasons for her fasting hyperglycemia revealed a modest dawn phenomenon of a 50-mg/dL increase in her blood glucose from bedtime levels. Given this clinical indication, the educator planned for KT to initiate pump therapy using aspart insulin and wondered if preprogramming a basal rate profile to correct for anticipated dawn phenomenon was indicated.

hormone (GH) secretion and cortisol and increased insulin clearance.[62,63] It is a normal physiologic process seen in most individuals with diabetes, who compensate with more insulin output.[63] An individual with type 1 diabetes cannot compensate; declining insulin levels if using evening NPH or Lente insulin may exacerbate the problem. The dawn phenomenon is usually recurrent and modestly elevates most morning glucose levels. Nocturnal surges in plasma GH levels are higher in type 1 individuals with suboptimal control and correlate with the overnight glucose increase. Individuals with diabetes who work shift rotations or experience jet lag often have difficulty maintaining glycemic control due to changes in circadian rhythms. This requires careful adjustment of insulin therapy. CSII therapy provides the means to enhance the required flexible insulin delivery.

Somogyi Phenomenon. Rarely, high morning glucose is due to the Somogyi phenomenon, a theoretical rebound from hypoglycemia late at night or in the early morning, which is thought to be due to an exaggerated counterregulatory response. The existence of this phenomenon is controversial. It is unlikely to be a common cause, in that most individuals with diabetes remain hypoglycemic once nighttime glucose levels decline.[63]

Use of CGM may allow clarification of puzzlingly elevated morning glucose levels.

Which Insulin to Use?

Atlanta Diabetes Associates[5] reported, based on 20 years of experience, that when using rapid-acting insulin analog versus short-acting regular human insulin, A1C values in adults were reduced to 7.3% with lispro versus 7.7% with buffered regular insulin. In a comparison study, aspart, lispro, and buffered regular insulin were shown to be equally efficacious and well tolerated in CSII therapy.[64] The rapid-acting insulin analogs (aspart and lispro) offer greater flexibility for mealtime insulin needs because the bolus can be administered immediately before meals. The use of rapid-acting insulin analog in pump therapy has demonstrated improved postprandial glucose control and allowed for fine-tuning of basal rates, with better control of dawn phenomenon. For these reasons, using rapid-acting analog insulin in insulin pumps is acceptable and preferred practice.

Calculating Starting Doses

Several methods of calculating starting doses of insulin for CSII were described in the literature for adults and children. Methods to calculate dosage for basal, bolus, and correction doses are listed in Table 17.1 (for adults) and 17.2 (for children). See also the sidebar on the next page for ways to fine-tune basal rates and bolus ratios.

TABLE 17.2 Starting Pediatric Dosing Calculations*

Basal and Bolus Calculations for Pediatric Patients
1. Determine how much insulin to use in the pump by averaging the total units of insulin used per day for 2 weeks. Decrease by 20% for hypoglycemia, by 10% for euglycemia, and make no reduction for hyperglycemia for children.
2. Divide the total dosage in half: 50% for basal and 50% bolus.
3. Divide the portion for bolus by 3. Divide the portion for basal by 24 to determine the hourly basal rate.
4. Check midnight and 3 AM blood glucose levels for 2 weeks before pump placement for evidence of night or early-morning abnormalities of glycemia. For hypoglycemia, reduce the nighttime basal rate by 10%. For hyperglycemia, increase the 3 AM by 10%.
5. Determine the insulin:carb ratio. (Divide 450 or 500 rule by the total units per day to determine the number of grams of carbohydrate for 1 unit of insulin.)
6. Determine the correction dose for elevated glucose levels. (Divide 1800 for insulin aspart or lispro by the total units of insulin per day to determine the mg/dL that 1 unit of insulin decreases the blood glucose value.)

*Childrens Hospital Los Angeles methods (Kaufman et al, 2001)

Sources: Bode BW, Tamborlane WV, Davidson PC. Insulin pump therapy in the 21st century. Postgrad Med. 2002;11(5):69-78.

Kaufman, FR, Halvorson M, Carpenter S, Devoe D. Pump therapy for children: weighing the risks and benefits: view 2: insulin pump therapy in young children with diabetes. Diabetes Spectrum. 2001;14(2):84-89.

Common Problems With Intensive Insulin Regimens: Medication Taking Behaviors

Some of the medication dosing issues that emerge in follow-up relate to accuracy of carbohydrate counting. Often patients are unable to estimate their bolus doses.

Fine-Tuning Basal Rates and Bolus Ratios

Adults

- Basal and bolus doses are adjusted according to SMBG measurements taken fasting, before meals, 2 hours after meals, at bedtime, at midnight, and at 3 AM.
- The basal rate is increased or decreased by 0.1 unit per hour to keep the premeal and overnight blood glucose levels within a 30-mg glucose excursion from baseline. Newer pumps offer 0.05 unit per hour increments that may be ideal to fine-tune basal doses.
- If the glucose level raises more than 30 mg/dL (1.7 mmol/L) from the 3 AM measurement to the prebreakfast measurement, a second basal rate is added for 4 to 6 hours, starting 2 to 3 hours before the usual breakfast time. This basal rate may be 10% to 50% more than the first basal rate, although basal rate adjustments can vary from 10% to 100% depending on the rise in the glucose.[21]
- Testing the overnight basal rate requires the patient to eat an early meal and avoid snacking 3 to 4 hours before retiring for bed. SMBG measurements at midnight, 3 AM, 6 AM, and before breakfast can provide information to determine if further basal refinement is needed.
- Asking the patient to fast during a scheduled meal with frequent (hourly) SMBG measurements helps further fine-tune daytime basal rates. However, missing multiple meals changes basal insulin requirements and is not recommended.
- Adjusting bolus ratios depends on accuracy in carbohydrate counting and matching bolus insulin. The ideal method is for the patient to accurately measure carbohydrate for the selected mealtime and engage in the same activity for several days. The desired 2-hour postmeal rise of blood glucose is less than 60 mg/dL or ideally less than 140 to 160 mg/dL.
- IRCs can vary throughout the day. For example, a patient's ratio can be 1:10 at breakfast, 1:12 at lunch, and 1:8 at dinner.
- Newer pumps are equipped with varying bolus features. Carbohydrates are covered by a normal or standard bolus (delivered immediately). An extended, or square wave, bolus is delivered over a length of time chosen by the patient. A combination, or dual wave, bolus combines the normal and extended bolus. Type of bolus can vary based on the amount of carbohydrate or fat and gastric emptying; this is not readily measured and relies on patient experience. (See more in the healthy eating, carbohydrate counting, and gastric motility sections of chapter.)

Children

- Patients/families monitor glucose levels 8 times per day and call for help with management issues daily until the desired glycemic pattern is achieved.
- On average, patients/families need to call daily for 2 to 3 weeks, after which weekly contact is maintained for 3 months.
- At 3 months, a follow-up A1C level is obtained to ensure that pump therapy has maintained or improved glycemic outcome.
- Once the efficaciousness of CSII has been validated for the patient, blood glucose monitoring can be done 4 to 6 times a day.
- Some pump manufacturers have software programs that allow a wealth of information about basal and bolus doses to be downloaded. Such information clearly shows the family and healthcare provider how the pump is being used at all times.

Any time a patient experiences widely fluctuating blood glucoses, basic skills must be reassessed. The educator may need to verify portion sizes and the accuracy of carbohydrate counting (weighing food with food scales and using measuring cups or spoons ensures accuracy of portions). Missed mealtime or snack insulin injections for boluses seem to also be a major cause of suboptimal glycemic control. [65] Often, small snacks or "just a little taste of food" can be problematic and cause blood glucose excursions when not accounted for with precisely matched insulin dosing.

Review basic and advanced skills before considering changes in insulin doses

The diabetes educator must review basic and advanced skills of intensive insulin therapy before considering changes to insulin doses. All patients need periodic reeducation and reevaluation of skills. This is sometimes overlooked by clinicians.

Problem Solving

Successful insulin pump therapy requires the patient and the patient's family members to have the requisite skills, knowledge, and self-management capabilities.[13,18,49,66] Problem-solving activities applied with all of the diabetes self-care behaviors are effective in preventing, detecting, and treating acute fluctuations in glucose control and acute complications. Problem-solving measures have been shown to be effective predictors of dietary, exercise, and medication self-care.[66] Problem-solving skills are critical for helping individuals manage chronic illness regimens. Potential acute problems associated with CSII include hypoglycemia, diabetic ketoacidosis (DKA), and skin infections.[21,23,37,67] Table 17.3 lists the emergency supplies needed by pump wearers.

TABLE 17.3 Emergency Pump Supplies

- Glucose meter and monitoring supplies
- Ketone test strips (preferably individually foil-wrapped)
- Pump supplies: insulin, reservoirs, infusion sets, batteries, site preparation supplies
- Back-up insulin syringe or pen with needles
- Carbohydrates to treat hypoglycemia and glucagon emergency kit in case of severe hypoglycemia
- Written record of basal rates and an alternative insulin injection regimen if pump fails
- Emergency contact numbers for pump manufacturer, physician, diabetes educator, and family member to contact in an emergency

Hypoglycemia

Hypoglycemia is the main side effect of insulin, regardless of delivery method. Insulin pump therapy does not seem to have any higher rate of hypoglycemia than MDI. Pickup and Keen's review of 25 years of CSII results found the incidence of hypoglycemia to be 30% to 60% less in insulin pump therapy compared to MDI.[6] Initial reports of severe hypoglycemia may have been due to unfamiliarity with management of tight control.[1] The decrease in severe hypoglycemia may be due to better pharmacokinetic delivery of insulin and better understanding that lower insulin requirements are needed at the time of pump initiation.[5,68]

> *Type 1 Diabetes:* Keep a glucagon 1-mg injectable kit available to treat low blood sugars with unresponsiveness.
>
> *Type 1 and 2 Diabetes:* Consider a brief (30") pump suspension for milder low blood sugar.

Intensive insulin therapy can pose a threat of severe hypoglycemia resulting in loss of consciousness. Not everyone gets warning signs of low blood glucose (hypoglycemia unawareness); therefore, reinforcing frequent blood glucose monitoring (especially before driving or when operating equipment) to patients following an intensive insulin regimen is essential. SMBG is the state-of-the-art method for verifying the blood glucose level at any time of day.

Frequent blood glucose monitoring is necessary to safely use a pump. The patient must be instructed to always check a blood glucose before giving insulin. Patients need to be taught and reminded to carry rapidly absorbable carbohydrate at all times, to treat hypoglycemia if and when it occurs. Family, friends, and coworkers must be educated and trained to recognize hypoglycemia and administer glucagon when appropriate.

Hyperglycemia and Diabetic Ketoacidosis

The absence of depot long-acting insulin with CSII puts patients at greater risk for rapid development (within 2 hours of interruption of basal insulin delivery) of (DKA). Elevated blood glucoses can occur for numerous reasons, including infection, illness, stress, menstrual cycle, pump battery failure, infusion set or catheter occlusion, leaking

Case—Part 8: Education

The diabetes educator reminded KT that she needed to carry a rapidly absorbable carbohydrate at all times for treatment of mild hypoglycemia. Her family members, friends, and coworkers received education and training on how to administer intramuscular glucagon and learned where KT kept a glucagon emergency kit for them to use if she experienced a severe hypoglycemic event.[23]

The educator emphasized that the basic rule KT needed to follow was this:

- Always check the blood glucose level before giving insulin

KT was also instructed to carry with her or have readily accessible emergency supplies. She was reminded that although people tend not to consider a day trip without supplies to be of any real importance, it only takes a couple of hours with interrupted insulin delivery to be in DKA.

connection, inadequate or missed meal bolus, or poor absorption of insulin from site.[23] Patient education about how to detect and treat high blood glucose is key in preventing DKA.[21] Patients should be instructed to check urine ketones with unexplained hyperglycemia or if experiencing nausea or flu-like symptoms. When hyperglycemia is present, the wearer must have a list at hand, such as that shown in Table 17.4, to quickly review possible explanations and respond promptly to correct the problems.[69]

Persons using CSII need to be taught ***5 important steps*** for detecting, treating, and preventing DKA. If blood glucose levels remain elevated after a correction dose is given, the patient should follow these steps:[46]

1. Check urine for ketones. If positive, proceed with step 2. If ketones are absent but blood glucose continues to be elevated, check for pump malfunction.
2. Give supplemental insulin with a conventional insulin syringe.
3. Correct known problems immediately.
4. If source of problem is not readily identified, change the site, using a new reservoir or cartridge, infusion set, and catheter.
5. Contact healthcare provider if unable to resolve problems within 2 to 3 hours.

TABLE 17.4 Problem Solving for Hyperglycemia With Insulin Pump Therapy

- Red, tender, and swollen catheter site
- Leakage, breakage, or kinking of tubing
- Battery failure
- Empty reservoir or cartridge
- Improper positioning of reservoir or piston rod
- Improper basal rate programming
- Air in tubing
- Illness
- Menstrual cycle fluctuations
- Omitted bolus or improper amount given
- Ineffective insulin (expired date, exposure to heat or cold)
- Crimped catheter or needle not penetrating skin
- Change in usual routine
- Suspect site not absorbing if no other apparent reason for high blood glucose

BEWARE! Any of these can occur even though the site was recently changed.

Source: Tomky D. Continuous subcutaneous insulin infusion (insulin pump therapy). In: Complete Nurses Guide to Diabetes Care. Childs AB, Cypress M, Spollett G, eds. American Diabetes Association: Alexandria, Va; 2005; 261.

Evidence shows that with proper education and attention to details, the frequency of ketoacidosis is the same on insulin pump therapy as injection therapy.[6] Problem-solving skills should be in place prior to initiating pump therapy, including knowing when and how to correct high blood glucoses. Supplemental insulin can now be preprogrammed within the pump to accurately adjust doses of insulin. Correction bolus or insulin sensitivity factor is derived from the previously discussed formula (Tables 17.1 and 17.2). Patients still are required to check capillary blood glucoses for direct entry from the meter to the pump or input of the result into the pump by the patient. "Smart" pumps with these newer features prevent the patient from frequently bolusing to correct elevated blood glucose. When unexplained hyperglycemia does occur, pump wearers need to problem solve appropriately to correct elevated glucoses. Urine ketostix prescriptions are essential supplies for those on insulin pumps. Often, catheter occlusion or pump malfunction is the culprit. For patients who frequently experience problems, Johansson et al recommend shorter intervals between infusion set changes.[70] The diabetes educator should always inspect the patient's subcutaneous tissue during follow-up visits to check for lipodystrophy.

Problem Solving for Sick Days

Providers and patients should not automatically assume illness or flu-like symptoms are the cause of elevated blood glucoses. Nausea, vomiting, or dehydration often herald the onset of DKA. Patients always need to go through the troubleshooting checklist (see Table 17.4) and the 5 important steps (listed at left) and then decide if illness is causing the elevated glucoses.

Temporary basal rate increases are particularly useful in treating insulin resistance due to intercurrent illness or use of steroids. During these times, patients often need reminding to maintain adequate fluid intake with salted broth, water, or noncaloric beverages. If liquid carbohydrates are used for fluid replacement, appropriate boluses must be given. Often, bolus ratios need to be temporary increased, as does the basal rate until the condition is resolved. When blood glucoses are within target range, and nausea and urine ketones are present, the patient needs to sip on carbohydrate-containing beverages and give appropriate boluses based on ICR to eliminate ketones.[71] Patients are often reluctant to use additional carbohydrates in this situation, but to reverse ketosis both insulin and carbohydrates are necessary.

Special Situations

When elective surgery, medical procedures, or delivery of a baby is scheduled, patients need to discuss options with their anesthesiologist and/or surgeon. The patient must clarify in advance the anesthesiologist's comfort level about continuing CSII during procedure. If the patient is well controlled on insulin pump therapy, then basal rates should be adequate to maintain euglycemia during surgery.[72] It is critical to ensure the pump is not discontinued before intravenous insulin or a subcutaneous injection of long-acting insulin is given. If the pump is to be worn during surgery, the patient must be instructed to insert a new catheter 12 to 24 hours in advance to establish adequate infusion of insulin. The catheter should be inserted in a site away from the planned surgical field and the tubing secured with additional tape.

Depending on the institution's policy and procedures, patients admitted to the hospital with normal mentation and capabilities should be allowed to work the pump if they have previously demonstrated good glycemic control. A diabetes consult is a good idea if any concerns arise.[72] Often, the hospital can provide insulin and syringes if injection therapy is used, but patients should be prepared to provide their own pump supplies during their stay.

Infection at Site of Infusion. Another potential complication, but seen less so with advancing years of pump therapy, is infection at the infusion site. The patient should be taught to change the infusion site every 48 to 72 hours and to follow recommended skin preparation.[13] Johansson and colleagues surveyed pump patients about real-life practices with daily management. They showed more catheter occlusions and bleeding at the infusion site than patients using insulin lispro. Surveyed patients with those problems changed the infusion set less frequently than they were taught and less frequently than recommended in insulin analog clinical trials. The survey showed that patients became relaxed in technique and violated recommendations and advice given for routine use of pump and accessories.[70] Newer pumps can be set to remind wearers of routine site changes. One way to help patients avoid this problem is to advise the patient to hang a calendar in the bathroom to mark site-change days. Patients should also be advised to avoid overfilling the pump cartridge or reservoir; this prevents the patient from wearing the pump until it literally runs out of insulin.

Healthy Coping

CSII therapy is being increasingly used because of its proven efficacy, improvements in pump technology, and increased patient preference for it.[53] In general, CSII allows patients to have a more normal lifestyle by simplifying irregular meal schedules and other unplanned activities.

Improved quality of life and advantages of insulin pump therapy may explain why more than 50% of healthcare professionals with type 1 diabetes who are members of the AADE and ADA,[73] as well as many athletes, use insulin pumps. As a result of these benefits, the rate of long-term continuation with CSII is greater than 97%.[5] In contrast, Sandfield et al, in a review of the literature on long-term CSII use, noted a 50% rate of discontinuing CSII within 2 years of initiation. They found that using a structured screening protocol was effective at identifying individuals who would initiate CSII and continue the therapy for at least 2 1/2 years. Their protocol not only evaluated candidacy for metabolic criteria, but also reviewed psychosocial stability and support, adequate financial resources, and cognitive or psychomotor abilities.[19] The importance of proper patient selection for effective CSII cannot be overemphasized.[19]

Longitudinal studies of patients who have switched from MDI to CSII have shown that when there are reductions in A1C and hypoglycemia, patients generally report increased treatment satisfaction and improved quality of life.

Case—Part 9: Problem Solving With KT on the Phone

KT became ill and contacted the diabetes educator about her blood glucose of 406 mg/dL and symptoms of nausea and headache. The educator asked her the following to determine the next step for her.

- What are your symptoms (how do you feel)?
- How long have you been ill?
- What have you already done?
- What have your blood glucoses been the last few days?
- Do you have ketones in your urine?
- How much insulin have you given? When and by what method (syringe or pump)?
- What are your basal rates?
- Any signs or symptoms of illness, such as fever, gastrointestinal changes, dysuria, or others?
- Is the pump working? Have any alarms gone off? Is there any possibility of kinking or dislodging of the catheter?
- Are you able to keep liquids down without vomiting?
- Any dietary changes or excessive alcohol consumption?

However, there is a lack of randomized trials that support this.[74] Peyrot and Rubin reported promising reliability and validity results of the Insulin Delivery System Rating Questionnaire that maybe useful in identifying the factors that contribute to users' preferences for different insulin delivery systems.[75] Regardless of screening appropriately, the desire to discontinue CSII may occur. Patients do "burn out" with chronic illness and need to be frequently assessed for depression or coping difficulty with self-care behaviors. If CSII adds to the patient's distress level or unhealthy coping puts the patient at risk for acute complications, then providing a temporary holiday from the pump may be warranted.

Switching Back to Injection Therapy. The easiest way to switch back to injections or inhaled doses from CSII is by converting the person's total daily basal rate of rapid-acting insulin to a long-acting basal insulin such as glargine (Lantus).[76] With the glargine, pump premeal bolus and correction doses are continued; the rapid-acting insulin is given with a syringe, pen, or inhalation device. If no long-acting insulin is immediately available, a rapid-acting insulin will suffice for a short period of time. The patient would take the rapid-acting insulin every 2 to 3 hours, making the calculation based on the basal rate. For example:

2 hours × 0.8 units per hour basal rate = 1.6 units*

*or round up to 2 units to replace 2 hours of basal insulin

Reducing Risks

Pregnancy

Pump therapy is an effective means of managing diabetes during pregnancy, but pregnant patients using CSII, as a group, do not achieve better control than those using MDI.[6] CSII is a viable option for motivated and capable patients who fail to achieve excellent control with MDI. Keep in mind that the potential risk of DKA with interrupted insulin flow is not tolerated in pregnancy and must be carefully considered before starting this kind of therapy in a woman with type 1 diabetes. Hieronimus et al concluded that fetal prognosis is not overall significantly different with an insulin pump compared with intensified conventional therapy.[77] The benefit-to-risk ratio of CSII must be assessed and result in a tailored prescription that is based on individual needs. Preferably, this option is discussed before conception, as planned pregnancy is a main prognostic factor. Diabetes duration and complications remain key factors for the prognosis for best pregnancy outcomes.[77] Simmons et al reviewed charts of mothers with type 2 diabetes or gestational diabetes who were using insulin injections or insulin pump therapy. They found that the mothers using insulin pumps had greater insulin requirements than patients not using pumps (median maximum 246 versus 130 units per day). They also experienced greater weight gain (10.6 versus 5.0 kg). Their babies were more likely to be admitted to the pediatric intensive care unit, but the babies were neither significantly heavier nor experienced greater hypoglycemia than control subjects. They concluded that insulin pump therapy seems safe and effective for maintaining glycemic control in pregnancies complicated by gestational or type 2 diabetes and requiring large doses of insulin.[78] Ronsin et al looked at factors for CSII discontinuation rates and found end of pregnancy to be a key factor for discontinuation.[79]

Absolute requirements for CSII therapy to be successful in pregnancy are patient education, motivation by an experienced team, and preconception counseling.[80] For more information on managing pregnancies complicated by diabetes, see chapters 11 and 12.

Gastric Motility

When gastric motility is slowed from autonomic neuropathy, (ie, gastroparesis diabeticorum), medications (such as tricyclic antidepressants, opioids, anticholinergics, or pramlintide), or high-fat meals, rapid-acting insulin is often mismatched with food digestion. Using an extended bolus or combination bolus allows for a slower delivery of rapid-acting insulin that can match reduced gastric motility.

Often pump wearers notice high-fat meals (ie, pizza) cause problems with blood glucoses, usually resulting in an elevated fasting glucose. Jones et al's research evaluated insulin pump dosing and postprandial glycemia following a pizza meal using the continuous glucose monitoring system. Their results showed that using a 50% immediate release and 50% extended release bolus delivered over an 8-hour period following a pizza meal provided significantly less postprandial hyperglycemia in the late postprandial period (8 to 12 hours) with no increased risk of hypoglycemia.[81]

There is a dearth of literature regarding insulin pump dosing for gastroparesis diabeticorum or synthetic amylin (pramlintide). However, clinical observations may support the use of extended or combination bolus features in matching rapid-acting insulin with individual response to food absorption. For more information on gastroparesis, see chapter 24 on neuropathy.

Practice Environment

The practice environment has changed for initiating pump therapy from hospitalization to almost exclusively an outpatient setting. The following summarizes visits generally required for insulin pump therapy.

- *Initial Training.* Most of the training on the technical aspects of using the new, improved pump systems can be accomplished in 1 or 2 60- to 90-minute outpatient visits,[5] although this can vary.
- *Clinical Follow-Up.* Clinical follow-up consists of having patients monitor blood glucose levels 4 or more times a day (including 3 AM) and report to the provider's office daily for the first few days via fax, e-mail, or phone on blood glucoses, insulin doses, and carbohydrate amounts and then once or twice a week until normal blood glucose levels are achieved.
- *Diabetes Education Follow-Up.* Follow-up visits with a diabetes educator or provider providing dietary, pump dosing adjustment, and technical support are scheduled in 1 to 2 weeks and as needed thereafter.
- *Medical Management Follow-Up.* A follow-up visit for medical management of the diabetes is also scheduled in 2 to 4 weeks, and once the patient's condition is stable, visits are scheduled on a quarterly basis.
- *Every Visit.* At each visit, a healthcare professional should review hypoglycemia troubleshooting, hyperglycemia and ketoacidosis prevention, sick day management, site rotation, and all other self-care behaviors as needed. If the pump has a download feature, reviewing this data is important clinically, as this information yields a true picture of how the pump is being used by the patient.

Special Populations Using Pump Therapy

Older Adults

Lepore et al reported their clinical observation of 25 patients in poor glycemic control retrospective CSII study was more advantageous, with a lowering of A1C by 1.45% in patients older than 50 years of age compared to patients under 20 years of age by 0.5%.[82] A similar observation suggested that insulin pump therapy is useful and safe in older adults with type 1 diabetes.[10] All previously discussed screening criteria would apply to any selected population. Goals of therapy should, as usual, be individualized (eg, addressing the individual's living situation and comorbid conditions).

Type 2 Diabetes

Experience with insulin pump therapy in patients with type 2 diabetes is limited but encouraging.[5] In older subjects with insulin-treated type 2 diabetes, both CSII and MDI achieved excellent glycemic control with good safety and patient satisfaction.[56,57] Davidson showed in a cohort of 11 type 2 patients who failed to control blood glucose levels with use of MDI that the average A1C level fell from 9.2% at baseline to 7.5% 6 months after the start of pump therapy and to 7.2% 18 months after the start of pump therapy.[83] Other investigators[84,85] have confirmed the benefits of pump therapy for type 2 diabetes. Differences in the pathophysiology of type 1 and type 2 diabetes affect pump selection. Certain features better suit the needs of those with type 2 diabetes. People with type 2 diabetes often have higher insulin needs due to insulin resistance, so reservoir capacity and frequency for refilling it are a concern. Other key concerns for the patient with type 2 diabetes, as compared to those with type 1, are needs for a higher basal rate, larger premeal boluses, and battery life.[69] People with type 2 diabetes often have greater insulin needs than people with type 1, due to insulin resistance, a common characteristic of type 2 diabetes.

There is some concern about the potential increased number of type 2 patients using pump therapy. At this point in time, Medicare has limitations on paying for CSII for type 2 diabetes. All patients requesting benefits from Medicare for pump therapy must prove to be insulinopenic by requesting verification of complete absence of insulin production.[69] Private insurance coverage varies from plan to plan.

Pediatric Patients

In 2002, Bloomgarden reviewed the literature and concluded that insulin pump therapy did not yet clearly offer benefit in the pediatric population, although it might play a role in the patient with difficult-to-manage hypoglycemia.[86] Since then, large pediatric diabetes clinics report more encouraging outcomes with CSII use.[21,49] Willi et al concluded that CSII is effective in lowering A1C and the occurrence of severe nocturnal hypoglycemia without excessive weight gain in most children with type 1 diabetes. They also found that preadolescents' response to CSII is poorer than in young children or teenagers.[87] Since the DCCT recommendations for strict metabolic control and improvements in pump technology, the United States reports an increase in 1997 from 500 users to more than 7500 in 2001.[21]

In 2002, the Yale Pediatric Diabetes Clinic reported data from the first 161 patients (aged 18 months to 18 years) to start pump therapy in their pediatric diabetes clinic, since 1997. Across all age groups, A1C levels were consistently lower by 0.6% to 0.7%. The Yale Clinic also reported a fewer number of severe hypoglycemic events while maintaining a continuation rate of 98%.[21] Kaufman et al reported similar positive findings with insulin pump therapy in their pediatric population.[49] The following are attributes cited by successful pump programs:[6,21,49]

- Appropriate patient selection criteria
- Standardized methodology
- Protocols for initiating, following, and supporting patients and their families
- Employing a sufficient number of experienced diabetes educators to take daily phone calls and to perform ongoing teaching/validation over the weeks to months required to achieve stable glycemia

In Summary

Intensive insulin therapy, whether achieved through MDI or CSII therapy, can be a safe and effective therapeutic tool in highly motivated and capable individuals with diabetes. Selection of appropriate candidates is one of the most important factors in determining whether an individual will be successful, and extensive preparation through self-management training can reduce discontinuation rates. Potential candidates must demonstrate their ability to follow an intensive regimen of blood glucose monitoring, carbohydrate counting, and problem solving before being considered for insulin pump therapy. Appropriate training and ongoing support by an experienced pump team is critical to achieving desired learning, behavioral, and clinical outcomes. Using the AADE 7 Self-Care Behaviors™ framework provides a comprehensive approach for assessment, intervention, and monitoring outcomes for all patients using intensive insulin therapy.

Questions and Controversies

The main controversies discussed among experienced diabetes educators and practitioners revolve around pump choices and clinical reasons for starting pumps. Fortunately, pumps and CSII therapy are continuing to evolve for the better. Scientific evidence assists in making wiser therapeutic choices with patients. In some cases financial or medical insurances drive decisions on whether to pump or not to pump and which pump to use.

Newer pumps offer advanced pumping features for calculating a bolus dose based on a predetermined insulin-to-carbohydrate ratio, food databases, insulin on board, insulin sensitivity factors, extended or combination boluses, multiple basal programming features, and various alerts. Pump selection should be based on an individual's needs and the provider/educator's experience and comfort level in providing training and support to the pump wearer. Some pump manufacturers offer pump training by diabetes educators who are employed or contracted by the manufacturer. In some instances, providing basic or additional training is a good thing, but often physicians without an experienced and available pump team can leave the patient without continuity of care. Caution must also be taken as there is a risk for some inappropriate pump initiations, especially when patients are referred by inexperienced practitioners who may not be aware of the issues surrounding appropriate and safe patient candidate selection. In contractual relationships, pump practices must review liability issues and who is to provide needed emergency services.

Pickup and Keen reviewed 25 years of evidence for expanding use of pump therapy in type 1 individuals. They found the evidence suggests that the expanding use of CSII is justified. They also found that unwillingness to fund pump therapy in some countries arises in part from the erroneous belief that this therapy is indicated for a large proportion of those with type 1 diabetes, opening a floodgate of cost implications. They proposed reaching an agreement about some simple clinical guidelines for CSII to benefit those who could be greatly helped at an affordable cost. Finally, they recommend a continued audit of the clinical reasons for starting pump therapy, its metabolic effectiveness, possible side effects, impact on long-term tissue complications, quality of life, and patient choice of treatment methods in type 1 diabetes.[6]

Focus on Education: Pearls for Practice

Teaching Strategies

Using the AADE 7 Self-Care Behaviors™ provides a conceptual framework for assessing and applying interventions related to use of insulin pump therapy.

Successful intensive insulin therapy. Preparation is the key. The professional skills required are in-depth knowledge of blood sugar interpretation (patterns), pump equipment and functions, the calculation and use of correction factors, onboard insulin, and carbohydrate counting. Discussion, demonstration, and role-playing strategies enhance the patient's understanding. Wearing a pump for several days, or using saline injections, and testing blood sugars with meal and activity plans in mind is useful to "get a feel" for the demands of this regimen.

Candidate screening and selection. Advance review and assessment of potential candidates (using Table 17.5) during educational events and clinic visits, problem-solving using MDI, follow-up visits, and phone interventions offer opportunities for just-in-time (teachable moments) teaching. This sets up experiential learning and practice time. Establishing the time and personal commitment to intensive therapy as a part of clinical, educational practice is critical.

TABLE 17.5 Criteria for Insulin Pump Use

Medical/Metabolic Indications	*Cognitive/Psychomotor Criteria*
• Suboptimal glycemic control • Wide blood glucose excursions • Dawn phenomenon with elevated fasting blood glucose levels • Frequent severe hypoglycemia • Nocturnal hypoglycemia • Pregnant or planning contraception • Variable daily schedule not well managed with injections • Insulin sensitivity and requires low doses of insulin	• Has sound rationale for pursuing and realistic expectation of CSII therapy • Learns technical and cognitive components of the pump • Applies appropriate problem-solving skills to troubleshoot hyper/hypoglycemia events and sick days • Is able to match carbohydrate with insulin using carbohydrate-counting skills • Modifies treatment plan upon outcome evaluation
Motivational Ability	*Technical/Physical Ability*
• Performs frequent blood glucose monitoring as a lifetime behavior • Complies with recommendations for safe insulin pump use • Pays attention to details as to the insulin regimen and needed adjustments • Anticipates insulin needs as situations changes	• Performs blood glucose monitoring accurately and frequently, greater than 4 to 6 times daily • Performs the technical components of insulin pump use or has necessary support if visually impaired • Free from serious disease that would impair technical performance • Provider observes set change technique and site rotation on a regular basis
Financial Resources	
• Adequate financial resources to cover initial and ongoing costs of CSII therapy	

Source: Tomky D. Continuous subcutaneous insulin infusion (insulin pump therapy). In: Complete Nurses Guide to Diabetes Care. Childs AB, Cypress M, Spollett G, eds. American Diabetes Association: Alexandria, Va; 2005; p. 261.

Messages for Patients

Benefits and risks. Take time to investigate all the facts about the benefits, risk, and limitations of intensifying insulin, whether considering a new intensive insulin treatment plan using multiple daily injections or an infusion pump. Read information and ask questions. Think about what signs and symptoms to look for if the blood sugar goal is to be near-normal. This target may mean more blood sugar testing and more sugar readings in the low range. Persons using intensive therapy need to be able to recognize, treat, and prevent very low or elevated blood sugar.

Realistic expectations—you are not alone. Recognize that this approach may require new skills, more intense observation of food intake and activity expenditure, and medication adjustments. Accepting the self-care and informed decision-making that are needed with this therapy could be new and a bit overwhelming. Plan to experiment and discuss options with others, including the healthcare team. You will also have the opportunity to use new techniques and equipment and to meet different people who can serve as resources (eg, pump manufacturer representatives and mail-order suppliers). Most importantly, transitioning to intensive insulin therapy can be accomplished with support and help from your healthcare team, friends, and family. Expect that all of this may take time and practice.

References

1. The Diabetes Control and Complications Trial Research Group. The effect of intensive treatment of diabetes on the development and progression of long-term complications in insulin-dependent diabetes mellitus. N Engl J Med. 1993;329(14):977-86.
2. UK Prospective Diabetes Study Group. UK Prospective Diabetes Study 16: overview of 6 years' therapy of type II diabetes: a progressive disease. Diabetes. 1995;44(11):1249-58.
3. Sherwin, R. Diabetes mellitus. In: Cecil Textbook of Medicine. Arend WP, Armitage JO, Drazen JM, Gill GN, Griggs RC, Scheld WM, eds. St. Louis, Mo: WB Saunders Co; 2004; 1433-5.
4. Pickup JC, Keen H, Parson JA, Alberti KG. Continuous subcutaneous insulin infusion: an approach to achieving normoglycaemia. Br Med J. 1978;1(6107): 204-7.
5. Bode BW. Tamborlane WV, Davidson PC. Insulin pump therapy in the 21st century. Postgrad Med. 2002;111(5):69-78.
6. Pickup J, Keen H. Continuous subcutaneous insulin infusion at 25 years: evidence base for the expanding use of insulin pump therapy in type 1 diabetes. Diabetes Care. 2002;25(3):593-8.
7. Weinzimer SA, Ahern JH, Doyle EA, et al. Persistence of benefits of continuous subcutaneous insulin infusion in very young children with type 1 diabetes: a follow-up report. Pediatrics. 2005;115(2):518.
8. Nathan DM, Lou P, Avruch J. Intensive conventional and insulin pump therapies in adult type I diabetes: a crossover study. Ann Intern Med. 1982;97(1):31-6.
9. Plotnick LP, Clark LM, Brancati FL, Erlinger T. Safety and effectiveness of insulin pump therapy in children and adolescents with type 1 diabetes. Diabetes Care. 2003;26(4):1142-6.
10. Siegel-Czarkowski L, Herold KC, Goland RS. Continuous subcutaneous insulin infusion in older patients with type 1 diabetes. Diabetes Care. 2004;27(12):3022-3.
11. Ronsin O, Jannot-Lamotte MF, Vague P, Lassman-Vague V. Factors related to CSII compliance. Diabetes Metab, 2005;31(1): 90-5.
12. Pickup JC, Keen H, Parsons JA, Alberti KG. Continuous subcutaneous insulin infusion: an approach to achieving normoglycaemia. Br Med J. 1978;1(6107):204-7.
13. American Association of Diabetes Educators. Education for continuous subcutaneous insulin infusion pump users (position statement). Diabetes Educ. 2003;29(1):97-9.
14. King AB, Armstrong D. A Comparison of basal insulin delivery: continuous subcutaneous insulin infusion versus glargine. Diabetes Care. 2003;26(4):1322.
15. Heller SR, Amiel SA, Mansell P. Effect of the fast-acting insulin analog lispro on the risk of nocturnal hypoglycemia during intensified insulin therapy. UK Lispro Study Group. Diabetes Care. 1999;22(10):1607-11.

16. Tamborlane WV, Frederickson LP, Ahern JH. Insulin pump therapy in childhood diabetes mellitus: guidelines for use. Treat Endocrinol. 2003;.2(1):11-21.

17. Tucker C. The insulin pump specialty. Diabetes Educ. 2004;30(2):232-4.

18. Continuous subcutaneous insulin infusion. Diabetes Care. 2004;27:S110.

19. Sanfield JA, Hegstad M, Hanna RS. Protocol for outpatient screening and initiation of continuous subcutaneous insulin infusion therapy: impact on cost and quality. Diabetes Educ. 2002;28(4):599-607.

20. Wredling R, Lins PE, Adamson U. Factors influencing the clinical outcome of continuous subcutaneous insulin infusion in routine practice. Diabetes Res Clin Pract. 1993;19:59-67.

21. Bode BW, Tamborlane WV, Davidson PC. Insulin pump therapy in the 21st century: strategies for successful use in adults, adolescents, and children with diabetes. Postgrad Med. 2002;111(5):69-77; quiz 27.

22. Purnell JQ, Hokanson JE, Marcovina SM, Steffes MW, Cleary PA, Brunzell JD. Effect of excessive weight gain with intensive therapy of type 1 diabetes on lipid levels and blood pressure: results from the DCCT. Diabetes Control and Complications Trial. JAMA. 1998;280(2):140-6.

23. Tomky D. Continuous subcutaneous insulin infusion (insulin pump therapy). In: Complete Nurses Guide to Diabetes Care. Childs B, Cypress M, Spollett G, eds. Alexandria, Va; American Diabetes Association; 2005:260-9.

24. Anderson EJ, Richardson M, Castle G, et al. Nutrition interventions for intensive therapy in the Diabetes Control and Complications Trial. The DCCT Research Group. J Am Diet Assoc. 1993; 93(7):768-72.

25. Franz MJ. Carbohydrate and diabetes: is the source or the amount of more importance? Curr Diab Rep, 2001;1(2):177-86.

26. Franz MJ. 2002 Diabetes nutrition recommendations: grading the evidence. Diabetes Educ. 2002;28(5):756-66.

27. Hamet P, Abarca G, Lopze D, et al. Patient self-management of continuous subcutaneous insulin infusion. Diabetes Care. 1982;5(5):485-91.

28. Slama G, Klein JC, Delage A, et al. Correlation between the nature and amount of carbohydrate in meal intake and insulin delivery by the artificial pancreas in 24 insulin-dependent diabetics. Diabetes. 1981;30(2):101-5.

29. Rabasa-Lhoret R, Garon J, Langelier H, Poisson D, Chiasson JL. Effects of meal carbohydrate content on insulin requirements in type 1 diabetic patients treated intensively with the basal-bolus (ultralente-regular) insulin regimen. Diabetes Care. 1999;22(5):667-73.

30. Lafrance L, Rabasa-Lhoret R, Poisson D, Ducros F, Chiasson JL. Effects of different glycaemic index foods and dietary fibre intake on glycaemic control in type 1 diabetic patients on intensive insulin therapy. Diabet Med. 1998;15(11):972-8.

31. Delahanty LM, Halford BN. The role of diet behaviors in achieving improved glycemic control in intensively treated patients in the Diabetes Control and Complications Trial. Diabetes Care. 1993;16(11):1453-8.

32. Training in flexible, intensive insulin management to enable dietary freedom in people with type 1 diabetes: dose adjustment for normal eating (DAFNE) randomised controlled trial. BMJ. 2002;325(7367):746.

33. Gillespie SJ, Kulkarni KD, Daly AE. Using carbohydrate counting in diabetes clinical practice. J Am Diet Assoc. 1998;98(8):897-905.

34. Kulkarni, KD. Carbohydrate counting: a practical meal-planning option for people with diabetes. Clin Diabetes. 2005; 23(3):120-22.

35. Daly A, Bolderman K, Franz M, Kulkarni K. Basic Carbohydrate Counting. Alexandria, Va and Chicago, Ill: American Diabetes Association and American Dietetic Association; 2003.

36. Daly A, Bolderman K, Franz M, Kulkarni K. Advanced Carbohydrate Counting. Alexandria, Va and Chicago, Ill: American Diabetes Association and American Dietetic Association; 2003.

37. Mulcahy K, Maryniuk M, Peeples M, et al. Diabetes self-management education core outcomes measures. Diabetes Educ. 2003; 29(5):768-70, 773-84, 787-8 passim.

38. Clement S, Braithwaite SS, Magee MF, et al. Management of diabetes and hyperglycemia in hospitals. Diabetes Care. 2004;27(2):553-91.

39. Brooks A, Kulkarni K. Insulin pump therapy and carbohydrate counting for pump therapy: insulin-to-carbohydrate ratios. In: A Core Curriculum for Diabetes Education: Diabetes Management Therapies. Franz MJ, ed. Chicago, Ill: American Association of Diabetes Educators; 2003.

40. The Diabetes Control and Complications Trial Research Group. Influence of intensive diabetes treatment on body weight and composition of adults with type 1 diabetes in the Diabetes Control and Complications Trial. Diabetes Care. 2001;24(10):1711-21.

41. Tamborlane WV, Fredrickson LP, Ahern JH. Insulin pump therapy in childhood diabetes mellitus: guidelines for use. Treat Endocrinol. 2003;2(1):11-21.

42. Schmulling RM, Jakober B, Pfohl M, Overkamp D, Eggstein M. Exercise and insulin requirements. Horm Metab Res Suppl. 1990;24:83-7.

43. Oskarsson PR, Lins PE, Wallberg Henriksson J, Adamson UC. Metabolic and hormonal responses to exercise in type 1 diabetic patients during continuous subcutaneous, as compared to continuous intraperitoneal, insulin infusion. Diabetes Metab. 1999;25(6):491-7.

44. Admon G, Weinstein Y, Falk B, et al. Exercise with and without an insulin pump among children and adolescents with type 1 diabetes mellitus. Pediatrics. 2005;116(3):348-55.

45. Mitchell TH, Abraham G, Schiffrin A, Leiter LA, Marliss EB. Hyperglycemia after intense exercise in IDDM subjects during continuous subcutaneous insulin infusion. Diabetes Care. 1988;11(4):311-7.

46. Wolpert H. Smart Pumping: A Practical Approach to Mastering the Insulin Pump. Alexandria, Va: American Diabetes Association; 2002.

47. Group TDR. The effect of intensive treatment of diabetes on the development and progression of long-term complications in insulin-dependent diabetes mellitus. N Engl J Med. 1993;329:977-86.

48. Mostrototoro J. The MiniMed continuous glucose monitoring system (CGMS). J Pediatr Endocrinol Metab. 1999;12suppl.3:751-8.

49. Kaufman FR, Halvorson M, Carpenter S, Devoe D, Pitukcheewanont P. Pump therapy for children: weighing the risks and benefits: view 2: insulin pump therapy in young children with diabetes. Diabetes Spectrum. 2001;14(2):84-89.

50. Valentine V. Continuous glucose monitoring has left the station: are you onboard? Diabetes Educ. 2005;31(5):649-62.

51. Albright ES, Desmond R, Bell DSH. Efficacy of conversion from bedtime nph insulin injection to once- or twice-daily injections of insulin glargine in type 1 diabetic patients using basal/bolus therapy. Diabetes Care. 2004;27(2):32-633.

52. Hirsch IB. Treatment of patients with severe insulin deficiency: what we have learned over the past 2 years. Am J Med. 2004;116(3A):S17S-S22.

53. Hirsch IB, Bode BW, Garg S, et al. Continuous subcutaneous insulin infusion (CSII) of insulin aspart versus multiple daily injection of insulin aspart/insulin glargine in type 1 diabetic patients previously treated with CSII. Diabetes Care. 2005;28(3):533-8.

54. Doyle EA, Weinzimer SA, Steffen AT, Ahern JA, Vincent M, Tamborlane WV. A randomized, prospective trial comparing the efficacy of continuous subcutaneous insulin infusion with multiple daily injections using insulin glargine. Diabetes Care. 2004;27(7):1554-8.

55. Alemzadeh R, Palam-Sisto P, Parton EA, Holzum MK. Continuous subcutaneous insulin infusion and multiple dose of insulin regimen display similar patterns of blood glucose excursions in pediatric type 1 diabetes. Diabetes Technol Ther. 2005;7(4):587-96.

56. Herman WH, Ilag LL, Johnson SL, et al. A clinical trial of continuous subcutaneous insulin infusion versus multiple daily injections in older adults with type 2 diabetes. Diabetes Care. 2005;28(7):1568-73.

57. Raskin P, Bode BW, Marks JB, et al. Continuous subcutaneous insulin infusion and multiple daily injection therapy are equally effective in type 2 diabetes: a randomized, parallel-group, 24-week study. Diabetes Care. 2003;26(9):2598-603.

58. Weintrob N, Benzaquen H, Galatzer A, et al. Comparison of continuous subcutaneous insulin infusion and multiple daily injection regimens in children with type 1 diabetes: a randomized open crossover trial. Pediatrics. 2003;112(3):559-64.

59. Schmidt MI, Hadji-Georgopoulos A, Rendell M, Margolis S, Kowarski A. The dawn phenomenon, an early morning glucose rise: implications for diabetic intraday blood glucose variation. Diabetes Care. 1981;4(6):579-85.

60. Carroll MF, Schade DS. The dawn phenomenon revisited: implications for diabetes therapy. Endocr Pract. 2005;11(1):55-64.

61. Schade DS, Valentine V. To pump or not to pump. Diabetes Care. 2002;25(11):2100-2.

62. Alemzadeh R, Wyatt DT. Diabetes in children. In: Nelson Textbook of Pediatrics. Behrman R, Klieg-

man, RM, Jenson, HB, eds. Philadelphia, Pa: WB Saunders Co; 2004:1947-72.

63. Van Cauter E, Polonsky KS, Scheen AJ. Roles of circadian rhythmicity and sleep in human glucose regulation. Endocr Rev. 1997;18(5):716-38.

64. Bode B, Tamborlane WV, Davidon PC. Comparison of insulin aspart with buffered regular insulin and insulin lispro in continuous subcutaneous insulin infusion: a randomized study in type 1 diabetes. Diabetes Care. 2002;25(3):439-44.

65. Burdick J, Chase HP, Slover RH, Knievel K, Scrimgeous L, Maniatis AK, Klingensmith GJ. Missed insulin meal boluses and elevated hemoglobin A1c levels in children receiving insulin pump therapy. Pediatrics. 2004;113(3):e221-e224.

66. Mulcahy K, Maryniuk M, Peeples M, et al. Diabetes self-management education core outcomes measures. Diabetes Educ. 2003;29(5):768-803.

67. Johansson UB, Adamson U, Lins PE, Wredling R. Patient management of long-term continuous subcutaneous insulin infusion. J Adv Nurs. 2005;51(2):112-8.

68. Hanaire-Broutin H, Melki V, Bessieres-Lacombe S, Tauber JP. Comparison of continuous subcutaneous insulin infusion and multiple daily injection regimens using insulin lispro in type 1 diabetic patients on intensified treatment: a randomized study. The Study Group for the Development of Pump Therapy in Diabetes. Diabetes Care. 2000;23(9):1232-5.

69. Tomky D. Continuous subcutaneous insulin infusion (insulin pump therapy). In: Complete Nurses Guide to Diabetes Care. Childs B, Cypress M, Spollett G, eds. Alexandria, Va: American Diabetes Association; 260-69.

70. Johansson UB, Adamson U, Lins PE, Wredling R. Patient management of long-term continuous subcutaneous insulin infusion. J Adv Nurs. 2005;51(2):112-8.

71. Sherwin RS. Diabetes mellitus. In: Cecil Textbook of Medicine. Arend WP, Armitage JO, Drazen JM, Gill GN, Griggs RC, Scheld WM, eds. St Louis, Mo: WB Saunders Co; 2004: p. 1433-1435.

72. Lee SI, Im R, Magbual R. Current perspectives on the use of continuous subcutaneous insulin infusion in the acute care setting and overview of therapy. Crit Care Nurs Q. 2004;27(2):172-184.

73. Graff MR, Rubin RR, Walker EA. How diabetes specialists treat their own diabetes: findings from a study of the AADE and ADA membership. Diabetes Educ. 2000;26(3):460-7.

74. de Galan, BE. Insulin pump therapy, should we consider it more often? J Med. 2004;62(10):341-3.

75. Peyrot M, Rubin RR. Validity and reliability of an instrument for assessing health-related quality of life and treatment preferences: The Insulin Delivery System Rating Questionnaire. Diabetes Care. 2005;28(1):53-8.

76. Bode BW, Steed RD, Schleusener DS, Strange P. Switch to multiple daily injections with insulin glargine and insulin lispro from continuous subcutaneous insulin infusion with insulin lispro: a randomized, open-label study using a continuous glucose monitoring system. Endocr Pract. 2005;11(3):157-64.

77. Hieronimus S, Cupelli C, Bongain A, Durand-Reville M, Beertheir F, Fenichel P. Pregnancy in type 1 diabetes: insulin pump versus intensified conventional therapy. Gynecol Obstet Fertil. 2005;33(6):389-94.

78. Simmons D, Thompson CF, Conroy C, Scott DJ. Use of insulin pumps in pregnancies complicated by type 2 diabetes and gestational diabetes in a multiethnic community. Diabetes Care. 2001;24(12):2078-82.

79. Ronsin O, Jannot-Lamotte MF, Vague P, Lassman-Vague V. Factors related to CSII compliance. Diabetes Metab. 2005;31(1):90-5.

80. Vanhaverbeke G, Mertens A, Mathieu C. Diabetic management in high risk patients (pregnancy, insulin pumps). Acta Clin Belg. 2004;59(4):173-81.

81. Jones SM, Quarry JL, Caldwell-McMillan M, Mauger DT, Gabbry RA. Optimal insulin pump dosing and postprandial glycemia following a pizza meal using the continuous glucose monitoring system. Diabetes Technol Ther. 2005;7(2):233-40.

82. Lepore G, Dodesiniar, Noseri I, Trevison R. Age and A1C Are important clinical predictors of continuous subcutaneous insulin infusion efficacy in type 1 diabetic patients. Diabetes Care. 2005; 28(7):1834-5.

83. Davidson J. Should postprandial glucose be measured and treated to a particular target? yes. Diabetes Care. 2003;26(6):1919-21.

84. Jennings AM, Lewis KS, Murdoch S, Talbot JF, Bradley C, Ward JD Randomized trial comparing continuous subcutaneous insulin infusion and conventional insulin therapy in type II diabetic patients poorly controlled with sulfonylureas. Diabetes Care. 1991;14(8):738-744.

85. Wainstein J, Metzger M, Wexler ID, Cohen J, Raz I. The use of continuous insulin delivery systems in severely insulin-resistant patients. Diabetes Care. 2001;24(7):1299.

86. Bloomgarden, ZT. Treatment issues in type 1 diabetes. Diabetes Care. 2002;25(1):230-6.

87. Willi SM, Planton J, Egede L, Schwarz S. Benefits of continuous subcutaneous insulin infusion in children with type 1 diabetes. J Pediatr. 2003;143(6):796-801.

CHAPTER

18

Pharmacologic Therapies: Dyslipidemia and Hypertension in Persons With Diabetes

Authors

Susan Cornell, BS, PharmD, CDE, CDM
Christopher J. Vito, PharmD

Key Concepts

- Pharmacotherapy for management of dyslipidemia and hypertension in people with diabetes is complex and continually evolving.
- When developing strategies for managing diabetes, equal emphasis should also be given to dyslipidemia and hypertension. These need to be treated as aggressively as hyperglycemia.
- Treatment strategies for diabetic dyslipidemia and for hypertension may require combination therapies that provide different mechanisms of action to obtain optimal levels of lipid and blood pressure control.
- Patients on multiple medications should be monitored frequently for adverse events and possible drug or food interactions.
- Patient education should include medication safety, proper dosing, and timing medications for optimum effect.

Introduction

Cardiovascular disease (CVD) has been identified as the most common cause of morbidity and mortality for people with diabetes. More alarming is that CVD and its effects may be present for many years prior to the diagnosis, particularly in type 2 diabetes.[1]

Diabetes is associated with a 2- to 4-fold increased risk for CVD and is recognized as a coronary heart disease (CHD) risk equivalent.[2,3] Risk factors for CHD include hypertension, dyslipidemia, obesity, and smoking.

Persons with diabetes who have a myocardial infarction (MI) are likely to have an increased risk of death from that MI. Results from one Finnish study showed that the 1-year mortality rate following an MI was higher in men and women with diabetes (44% and 37%, respectively) compared to those without diabetes (33% and 20%).[4,5] A Swedish study examined patients hospitalized for an MI who had not been diagnosed with type 2 diabetes and found that one-third had prediabetes and one-third had newly diagnosed diabetes.[6,7] Additionally, cardiovascular complications are the most significant cause of healthcare expenditures in people with diabetes.

Therefore, prioritizing and treating CVD risk factors in patients with diabetes is crucial. When developing strategies for managing diabetes, equal emphasis must thus also be given to dyslipidemia and hypertension. These must be treated as aggressively as hyperglycemia (the subject of chapter 8; pharmacotherapy for glucose management is discussed in chapter 15).

The focus of this chapter is on describing the medications used to treat hypertension and diabetic dyslipidemia; information on promoting appropriate self-care behaviors related to taking medication can be found in chapter 31. For a thorough discussion of macrovascular disease, including screening guidelines, diagnostic criteria, and risk-reduction, see chapter 21.

Diabetic Dyslipidemia

Triglycerides (TG) and cholesterol are water-insoluble lipids that are derived from dietary sources (exogenous system) and hepatic synthesis (endogenous system). Lipids other than TG and cholesterol that are involved in these systems and are routinely scrutinized include very low-density lipoproteins (VLDL), low-density lipoproteins (LDL-C), and high-density lipoproteins (HDL-C).[8–10] Figure 18.1 depicts the exogenous and endogenous lipid transport system.

Diabetic dyslipidemia is typically composed of elevated TG and decreased HDL-C, with LDL-C elevations comparable to that of persons without diabetes. However, the particle size of the LDL-C in persons with diabetes tends to be smaller and denser, which can increase atherogenicity.[11-13]

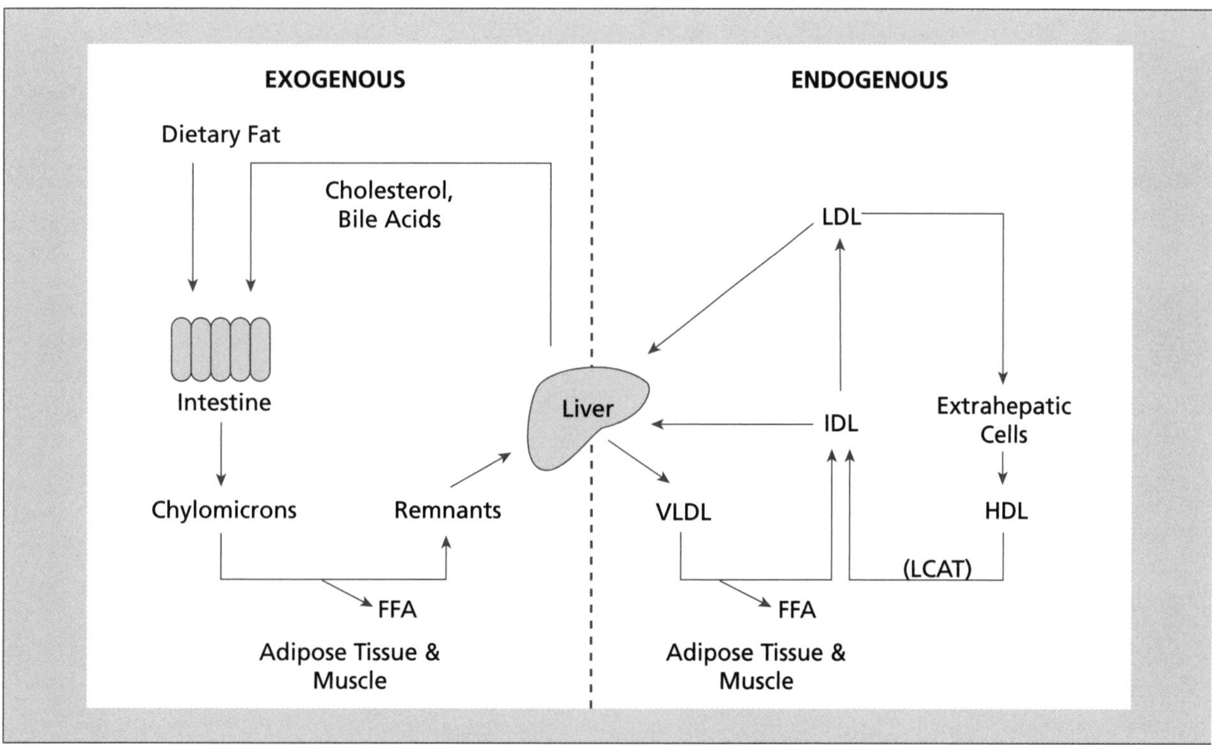

FIGURE 18.1 Exogenous and Endogenous Lipid Transport System

Key: FFA = free fatty acids; IDL = intermediate-density lipoprotein cholesterol; LCAT = lecithin cholesterol acyltransferase; LDL = low-density lipoprotein cholesterol; TC = total cholesterol; TG = triglycerides; VLDL = very low-density lipoprotein cholesterol

The small, dense LDL-C particles often seen with diabetes raise the risk for heart disease:

The abnormalities in the small, dense LDL-C composition are partially due to hypertriglyceridemia and are associated with a 3-fold increased risk of CHD.[12]

This increased risk is caused by the particles' ability to enter blood vessel walls faster than the normal, large, and less-dense LDL-C particles; thus, endothelial function is impaired and susceptibility to thrombosis increases.[13]

Elevated triglycerides are a key contributor to low HDL-C:

Elevated TG levels can result from 2 abnormalities: overproduction of VLDL and/or impaired lipolysis of TG. Persons with type 2 diabetes overproduce triglyceride-rich VLDL, a result of elevated free fatty acids levels, hyperglycemia, obesity, and insulin resistance.[14] Impaired lipolysis of VLDL triglycerides is thought to be due to a reduction in lipoprotein lipase activity.[3]

HDL-C is the major lipoprotein responsible for removing excess cholesterol from peripheral tissues, which is known as reverse cholesterol transport. Therefore, suboptimal levels of HDL-C can result in increases in TG, VLDL, and LDL-C.[8,9]

Treatment Goals: Diabetic Dyslipidemia

Dyslipidemia may be secondary to poorly controlled diabetes, and in some cases improved control of hyperglycemia may reduce dyslipidemia. Some glucose-lowering agents will lower triglyceride levels and may have a modest effect on raising HDL levels; however, complete reversal of dyslipidemia by improved control of hyperglycemia is usually unachievable and treatment with lipid-lowering agents is warranted.

The American Diabetes Association (ADA) and the National Cholesterol Education Program (NCEP) Expert Panel on Detection, Evaluation and Treatment of High Blood Cholesterol in Adults [Adult Treatment Panel III (ATP III)] recommend targeting the LDL-C first. The groups differ, however, on the secondary target: the ADA, focused on people with diabetes, supports treatment to raise HDL-C as the secondary target, whereas the ATP III's secondary target is to lower TG.[2,15] Table 18.1 lists these

Case in Point: An African American With Type 2 Diabetes

DC is a 64-year-old African American male who was diagnosed with type 2 diabetes 2 years ago. He presented at the clinic one day for a follow-up visit (from his appointment 2 weeks earlier) to recheck his blood pressure and obtain the results of his recent lab work. At his last visit, his BP was 138/86 mm Hg.

Past Medical History:
Seasonal allergic rhinitis
Obesity
Type 2 diabetes

Family History:
Father: history of CVD, MI, deceased
Mother: history of type 2 diabetes, HTN, deceased

Social History:
(-) tobacco
(-) illicit drug use
(+) alcohol (socially)

Vital Signs:
BP: 146/88 mm Hg
HR: 76
RR: 14

Physical Exam:
Ht: 70 in
Wt: 235 lb
BMI:34 kg/m^2
Waist circumference: 43 in

Current Medications:
Metformin (Glucophage) 2000 mg daily
Pioglitazone (Actos) 15 mg daily
Multiple vitamin daily
Aspirin 81mg daily
Fexofenadine (Allegra) 60 mg twice daily as needed

Adherence to Pharmacologic Therapy:
DC picks up most of his medications consistently every 30 days at his pharmacy. However, pharmacy computer records indicate he purchased his metformin (Glucophage) every 45 days instead of every 30 days. Initially, DC denies missed doses, but upon further interviewing he admits to forgetting occasional doses of medications because he "does not like to take too many pills."

Laboratory Data:
TC: 235 mg/dL
LDL-C: 143 mg/dL
TG: 287 mg/dL
HDL-C: 35 mg/dL
FBG: 160 mg/dL
A1C: 7.2%
Liver function test:
AST: 16 U/L (reference range: 10-42)
ALT: 12 U/L (reference range: 10-40)

Diagnosis
DC is diagnosed with both diabetic dyslipidemia and hypertension. His LDL-C level is above the target of less than 100 mg/dL, his HDL-C level is below the target of greater than 40 mg/dL, and his TG level is above the target of less than 150 mg/dL. DC's past and current blood pressure readings indicate his blood pressure is also above the target goal of 130/80 mm Hg for a person with diabetes. Since 2 readings have been obtained from 2 separate clinic visits and DC was seated for more than 5 minutes prior to having his blood pressure taken, his condition classifies as stage 1 hypertension

The case study progresses throughout the chapter. Considerations for the risk of CVD need to be addressed as well as appropriate treatment options for dyslipidemia and hypertension with diabetes.

treatment goals. According to the ATP III guidelines, the intensity of treatment depends on the degree of risk. Since diabetes is a CHD risk equivalent, more aggressive therapy is necessary.[16] For people with prediabetes, using this table requires identifying their risk factors and current laboratory values and implementing the indicated therapies. Table 18.2 depicts LDL-C treatment goals.

Most hyperglycemic treatment strategies include use of multiple medications that target different organs to lower blood glucose. Treatment strategies for diabetic dyslipidemia may also require combination therapy that targets different mechanisms and lipoproteins to obtain optimal levels in diabetic dyslipidemia.

Lifestyle modification, including medical nutrition therapy (MNT) and physical activity, should always be a standard treatment for dyslipidemia in addition to pharmacologic treatment. More information on these interventions can be found in the following: chapters 13 and 14,

TABLE 18.1 Dyslipidemia Treatment Goals

	NCEP ATP III: All People		*ADA: People With Diabetes*	
Target	*Lipid*	*Goal (mg/dL)*	*Lipid*	*Goal (mg/dL)*
Primary	LDL-C	<100	LDL-C	<100
Secondary	TG	≤150	HDL-C	>40 (men) >50 (women)
Tertiary			TG	<150

Key: ADA = American Diabetes Association; HDL-C = high-density lipoprotein cholesterol; LDL-C = low-density lipoprotein cholesterol; NCEP ATP III = National Cholesterol Education Program (NCEP) Adult Treatment Panel III; TG = triglycerides

Sources: American Diabetes Association. Standards of medical care in diabetes. Diabetes Care. 2006; 29(Suppl):S4-S42; Expert Panel on Detection, Evaluation, and Treatment of High Blood Cholesterol in Adults (Adult Treatment Panel III). JAMA. 2001; 285:2486-97.

TABLE 18.2 LDL-C Treatment Goals

Risk Category	*LDL-C Goal (mg/dL)*	*Initiate TLC (mg/dL)*	*Consider Drug Therapy (mg/dL)*
High Risk: CHD or CHD risk equivalents* (10-y risk >20%)	<100 Optional goal <70	≥100	≥100 (consider drug options when <100)
Moderate High Risk: 2+ risk factors (10-y risk 10%-20%)	<130	≥130	≥130 (consider drug options when 100-129)
Moderate Risk: 2+ risk factors (10-y risk <10%)	<130	≥130	≥160
Lower Risk: 0-1 risk factor	<160	≥160	≥190 (consider drug options when 160-189)

* Diabetes is a CHD risk equivalent; people with diabetes require treatment as designated for the high-risk category.

Key: CHD = coronary heart disease; LDL-C = low- density lipoprotein cholesterol; TLC = therapeutic lifestyle changes

Source: Grundy SM, Cleeman JI, Merz CN et al, for the Coordinating Committee of the National Cholesterol Education Program. Implications of recent clinical trials for the National Cholesterol Education Program Adult Treatment Panel III Guidelines. NCEP Report. Circulation. 2004; 110:227-39.

on medical nutrition therapy and physical activity, and chapters 29 and 30, on the self-management behaviors for healthy eating and being active.

Standard Treatment

Dyslipidemia—Lifestyle modification, including MNT and physical activity, should always be a standard treatment for dyslipidemia in addition to pharmacotherapy

Children and Adolescents

Children with diabetes should be screened and monitored for dyslipidemia; see chapter 21 for specific recommendations. The ADA does not recommend initiation of pharmacotherapy for dyslipidemia in children.[2]

Pharmacologic Treatment: Diabetic Dyslipidemia

There are currently 6 classes of lipid-lowering agents prescribed in the treatment of dyslipidemia. These categories include the following:

- HMG-CoA reductase inhibitors (statins)
- Selective intestinal absorption inhibitors
- Fibric acid derivatives (fibrates)
- Bile acid resins
- Niacin
- Omega-3 fatty acids

Plant stanols and sterols, although not considered pharmacotherapy, play a role in the management of dyslipidemia as well; see chapter 13, on MNT, for more information.

HMG-CoA Reductase Inhibitors (Statins)

HMG-CoA reductase inhibitors, commonly referred to as statins, are the most widely used lipid-lowering agent and often the first choice for treatment of diabetic dyslipidemia.[17,18] Their primary lipoprotein effect is in lowering LDL-C, with secondary beneficial effects of decreased TG and increased HDL-C. Additionally, statins may increase the buoyancy or particle size of LDL-C, thereby reducing the amount of small, dense LDL-C in circulation.[12,13]

Mechanism of Action

Statins primarily reduce LDL-C, by competitively inhibiting HMG-CoA reductase, the enzyme that converts HMG-CoA to melvalonate in the hepatic synthesis of cholesterol, resulting in reduced endogenous cholesterol. Statins will reduce but not totally block cholesterol synthesis. The decreased endogenous cholesterol production activates LDL-C receptor synthesis, resulting in enhanced clearance of circulating LDL-C particles.[9,18,19]

Dosing

Statins are generally administered once daily, often in the evening since cholesterol synthesis occurs at night. The dosage is dependent on the percentage of lipid lowering needed to achieve target goals. However, initial therapy commonly starts with a lower dose and can be titrated up every 4 to 6 weeks as needed to reach the necessary or maximum dosage and to minimize adverse effects.[19-21] Table 18.3 allows comparison of the lipid-lowering agents and their effects on the various lipoproteins.

Pregnancy, Precautions, and Contraindications

Statins are contraindicated in pregnancy and in women who are breastfeeding; they should be used cautiously in those with impaired renal or hepatic function.[19,22,23]

Adverse Effects

Overall, statins are well tolerated with minimal side effects, especially if monitored appropriately. The more common adverse reactions include headache, nonspecific muscle and joint pain, and gastrointestinal complaints, such as nausea, diarrhea, constipation, flatulence, or abdominal pain.[19, 22, 23]

Significant elevations of liver enzymes can occur. There have been reports of hepatic toxicity associated with statins: from 0.1% to 0.4% in persons on usual daily doses and up to 2% in persons on maximum dosage.[19] Discontinue treatment when liver enzymes are greater than 3 times the upper limit of normal.[22] The frequency of monitoring at baseline and during therapy varies with each drug in the family of statins; see package inserts for the most current monitoring guideline for each compound.

Myopathy, a disease of the muscle, and rhabdomyolysis, the breakdown of striated muscle, have been reported in 1% to 5% of patients and in 1 in 2000 patients, respectively. Therefore, patients should be instructed to report any experience of muscle weakness, tenderness, pain, or fever. Laboratory testing of serum creatinine kinase can confirm or rule out rhabdomyolysis.[22] An increase in creatinine kinase to 3 to 10 times the upper limits of normal

HMG-CoA Reductase Inhibitors (Statins): Dosage Information

Drug	*Trade Names*	*Common Dose*	*Common Frequency*
Atorvastatin	Lipitor	10 to 80 mg	Once daily
Fluvastatin	Lescol Lescol XL	20 to 40 mg 80 mg	Once to twice daily Once daily
Lovastatin	Mevacor Altoprev	10 to 40 mg 10 to 60 mg extended-release	Once to twice daily Once daily
Pravastatin	Pravachol	10 to 80 mg	Once daily
Rosuvastin	Crestor	5 to 40 mg	Once daily
Simvastatin	Zocor	10 to 80 mg	Once daily

TABLE 18.3 Lipid-Lowering Comparison

Drug	Daily Dose	*Effect on Lipoprotein (% Change from Baseline)*			
		TC	*LDL-C*	*TG*	*HDL-C*
Atorvastatin (Lipitor)	10 mg 20 mg 40 mg 80 mg	-29 -33 -37 -45	-39 -43 -50 -60	-19 -26 -29 -37	6 9 6 5
Fluvastatin (Lescol)	20 mg 40 mg 40 mg bid XL 80 mg	-17 -19 -27 -25	-22 -25 -36 -35	-12 -14 -18 -19	3 4 6 7
Lovastatin (Mevacor)	10 mg 20 mg 40 mg 40 mg bid	-16 -17 -22 -29	-21 -24 -30 -40	-10 -10 -14 -19	5 6 7 9
Pravastatin (Pravachol)	10 mg 20 mg 40 mg 80 mg	-16 -24 -25 -27	-22 -32 -34 -37	-11 -15 -20 -19	7 12 15 3
Rosuvastin (Crestor)	5 mg 10 mg 20 mg 40 mg	-33 -36 -40 -46	-45 -52 -55 -63	-35 -10 -28 -28	13 14 8 10
Simvastatin (Zocor)	5 mg 10 mg 20 mg 40 mg 80 mg	-19 -23 -28 -31 -36	-26 -30 -38 -41 -47	-12 -15 -19 -18 -24	10 12 8 9 8
Fenofibrate (Tricor)	145 mg	-18	-20	-29	11
Gemfibrozil (Lopid)	600 mg bid	-10	± 10	-20-50	10-15
Niacin 500-mg tablet	1 g/d 1.5 g/d 2 g/d		-6 -12 -16		
Extended-release niacin (Niaspan)	500 mg 1000 mg 1500 mg 2000 mg	-2 -5 -11 -12	-3 -9 -14 -17	-5 -11 -28 -35	10 15 22 26
Colesevelam (Welchol)	3.8 g (6 tabs)	-7	-15	10	3
Cholestyramine (Questran) 4 g/9 g pwd 4 g/5 g pwd	4-8 g bid max 24g/d		-15-30	5-10	3-5

(continued)

TABLE 18.3 Lipid-Lowering Comparison

		Effect on Lipoprotein (% Change from Baseline)			
Drug	*Daily Dose*	*TC*	*LDL-C*	*TG*	*HDL-C*
Colestipol (Colestid) 5g/7.5g pwd 1-g tabs	max 30g/d max 16 g/d		-15-30	5-10	3-5
Ezetimibe (Zetia)	10 mg	-13	-18	-8	+1
Omega 3 (Omacor)	1 g 4 g		+10 +31	-3.5 -45	+13
Plant Stanols (Benecol)	3 servings daily	-10	-14		
Plant Sterols (Take Control)	2 servings daily		-17		

Key: HDL-C = high-density lipoprotein cholesterol; LDL-C = low-density lipoprotein cholesterol; TC = total cholesterol; TG = triglycerides

Note: Generic names of drugs are listed first; brand names are in parentheses for reader convenience.

Sources: Lexi-Drugs Platinum for Palm OS. www.lexi.com/downloads; Worz CR, Bottorff M. Treating dyslipidemic patients with lipid-modifying and combination therapies. Pharmacotherapy. 2003;23:625-37; Jones P, Kafonek S, Laurora I, et al. Comparative dose efficacy study of atorvastatin versus simvastatin, pravastatin, lovastatin, and fluvastatin in patients with hypercholesterolemia (the CURVES study). Am J Cardiol. 1998;81:582-7; Antilipidemic agents. In: Monthly prescribing guide: November. Montvale, NJ. Thompson PDR. 2005:89-95; Cardiovascular system: hyperlipoproteinemias. In: Monthly prescribing reference: Nov. www.prescribingReference.com. Accessed 7 Nov 2005.

(450 to >1000) can be observed in myopathy or myositis, respectively. The degree of muscle pain associated with myopathy and myositis, an inflammation of the voluntary muscles, can vary among individuals. Rhabdomyolysis, a more severe adverse affect, typically presents with additional signs and symptoms that include weight gain from fluid retention, fever, nausea, tachycardia, and dark or colored urine.

Drug Interactions

Most statins are metabolized through the cytochrome P-450 3A4 pathway in the liver. Concurrent medications and foods (such as grapefruit juice) that are also metabolized through this system should be used cautiously and monitored for increased levels and risks of adverse reactions.[19,24]

Statins typically are the drug that is affected by inhibitors or inducers of the CYP-450 pathway, thereby delaying or enhancing their elimination from the body and resulting in increased or decreased statin serum concentration. Monitoring adverse effects and lipid profiles can help identify potential drug interactions and reduce the risk of toxicity, myopathy, and/or rhabdomyolysis. Table 18.4 lists common drugs that interact with statins.

Monitoring

A baseline lipid profile, CPK enzyme, liver function, and renal function tests should be conducted prior to initiating statin therapy. Monitoring lipid profiles and liver function tests should be done every 12 weeks in the first 6 months of treatment and periodically thereafter. CPK levels should be monitored if complaints of muscle pain or discomfort are mentioned.[19,22,23]

Instructions

Statins are best dosed in the evening, either with supper or at bedtime. They can be taken with or without food in most cases. Monitoring for cholesterol reduction and liver enzyme elevation should be done every 12 weeks within the first 6 months of initial treatment and periodically thereafter. Patients should also be educated on the signs and symptoms of myopathy, such as persistent muscle or joint pain. Patients should disclose all medications, prescribed and over-the-counter, to their healthcare provider to reduce the risk of potential drug interactions with statins. Caution patients on consuming large amounts of grapefruit juice (greater than 8 oz per day).

TABLE 18.4 Statin Use: Selected Interactions Between Cytochrome P-450 Isoenzymes and Common Drugs

Isoenzyme	*Substrate*	*Inhibitor*	*Inducer*
CYP3A4	Amlodipine (Norvasc) **Atorvastatin (Lipitor)** Diltiazem (Cardizem) Felodipine (Plendil) **Fluvastatin (Lescol)** Glyburide (DiaBeta; Micronase; Glynase)* **Lovastatin (Mevacor)** Nifedipine (Procardia) **Pravastatin (Pravachol)** Repaglinide (Prandin)* **Simvastatin (Zocor)** Verapamil (Calan) R-Warfarin (Coumadin)	Clarithromycin (Biaxin) Diltiazem (Cardizem) Erythromycin Fluconazole (Diflucan) Fluoxetine (Prozac) Grapefruit juice Ketoconazole (Nizoral) Miconazole Norfloxin (Noroxin) Verapemil (Calan) Zafirlukast (Accolate)	Carbamazepine (Tegretol) Dexamethasone (Decadron) Phenytoin (Dilantin) Primidone (Mysoline) Rifampin Pioglitazone (Actos)*
CYP2C9	Glimepiride (Amaryl)* Losartan (Cozaar) S-Warfarin (Coumadin)	Amiodarone (Cordarone) Cimetidine (Tagamet) Fluconazole (Diflucan) Fluoxetine (Prozac) **Fluvastatin (Lescol)** Isoniazid Ketoconazole (Nizoral) Metronidazole (Flagyl) Nateglitinide (Starlix)* Omeprazole (Prilosec) Sertraline (Zoloft) Sulfonamides Zafirlukast (Accolate)	Carbamazepine (Tegretol) Phenytoin (Dilantin) Pioglitazone (Actos)* Rifampin Rosiglitazone (Avandia)

**Note:* Drugs in bold are statins. Drugs marked with an asterisk (*) are common oral glucose-lowering medications.

Sources: Lexi-Drugs Platinum for Palm OS. www.lexi.com/downloads; Antilipidemic agents. In: Monthly prescribing guide: November. Montvale, NJ. Thompson PDR. 2005:89-95; Cardiovascular system: hyperlipoproteinemias. In: Monthly prescribing reference: Nov. www.prescribingReference.com. Accessed 7 Nov 2005; Lexi-Interact Platinum for Palm OS. www.lexi.com/downloads.

Bile Acid Sequestrants

The primary lipoprotein affected by bile acid sequestrants is LDL-C, with a secondary effect of a modest increase in HDL-C. Bile acid sequestrants are not commonly prescribed in the treatment of diabetic dyslipidemia. They can often increase TG, which are often elevated in persons with diabetes; thus, bile acid sequestrants should not be used as monotherapy in cases with high TG (>250).

Mechanism of Action

Bile acid sequestrants bind to bile acids in the intestinal lumen, thereby decreasing cholesterol production. They also inhibit enterohepatic circulation of bile acids and increase elimination of fecal acidic steroids, resulting in a decrease in LDL-C.[9,19]

Bile Acid Sequestrants: Dosage Information

Drug	*Trade Names*	*Dose Range*	*Preparation*
Cholestyramine	Questran	4 to 16 g per day	1-g tablets, powder (1 scoop = 4 g)
Colesevelam	Welchol	3.8 to 4.5 g per day	625-mg tablets
Colestipol	Colestid	2 to 16 g per day	1-g tablets, powder (1 scoop = 5 g)

Bile acid sequestrants may increase TG due to an increased production of VLDL from the up-regulation of cholesterol synthesis.

Dosing

Bile acid sequestrants are available as a tablet and as a powder for dilution. Dosing can be once or twice daily. Lower doses are recommended for initial therapy and can be titrated up every 4 to 8 weeks as necessary to reach optimal or maximum dose.[19,22,23]

Pregnancy, Precautions, and Contraindications

Bile acid sequestrants' safety in pregnancy varies with the different agents. Colesevelam is listed as category B, indicating no evidence of risk in humans, whereas cholestyramine and colestipol are listed as category C, indicating risk cannot be ruled out.[19,22]

Bile acid sequestrants are contraindicated when the TG level is >400 mg/dL and in primary biliary cirrhosis. As noted above, they should not be used as monotherapy when the TG level is above 250 mg/dL.

Caution should be used in persons with renal insufficiency, volume depletion, and chronic constipation. Bowel and biliary obstructions are contraindications.[22,23]

Adverse Effects

The adverse affects reported with bile acid sequestrants are mostly gastrointestinal in nature, due to the lack of systemic absorption. The most common complaints are headache, unpalatable taste, nausea, bloating, flatulence, and constipation.[22,23]

Drug Interactions

Bile acids sequestrants can bind to other medications, resulting in decreased absorption and clinically significant drug interactions. Therefore, it is recommended to separate bile acid sequestrants from other medications by administering them 1 hour before or 4 hours after the bile acid sequestrants.[19,24]

Prolonged use of bile acid sequestrants may result in a decrease in absorption of fat-soluble vitamins and folic acid.[9,19]

Monitoring

Baseline lipid profiles with a follow-up at 4 to 6 weeks for efficacy are recommended for bile acid sequestrants. This medication is not systemically absorbed and is considered safe overall, except, as noted above, in cases of high TG. Electrolytes should be routinely checked as imbalances have been reported. Prolonged use of bile acid sequestrants may produce hyperchloremic acidosis.[19,22,23] Due to the gastrointestinal discomfort associated with bile acid sequestrants, patient compliance should be reviewed at each visit.

Instructions

Tablets should be swallowed whole and taken with plenty of liquid. Powder packets must be diluted in liquid thoroughly prior to consuming. Bile acid sequestrants should be taken separately from other medications, either 1 hour after or 4 hours before.

Cholesterol Absorption Inhibitors

The primary effect of cholesterol absorption inhibitors is observed in the reduction of LDL-C; however, slight decreases in TG and increases in HDL-C may be noticed. Cholesterol absorption inhibitors are often prescribed in combination with statins for persons with diabetic dyslipidemia to enhance the lowering of LDL-C.

Mechanism of Action

Cholesterol absorption inhibitors reduce cholesterol by selectively inhibiting the absorption of cholesterol from the small intestine. This results in a decreased delivery of cholesterol to the liver and a reduction of hepatic cholesterol stores, with an overall lowering of cholesterol, primarily LDL-C.[19]

Cholesterol Absorption Inhibitors: Dosage Information

Drug	*Trade Name*	*Common Dose*	*Common Frequency*
Ezetimibe	Zetia	10 mg	Once daily

Dosing

Initial and maintenance dosage is 10 mg once daily and may be used in conjunction with statins or bile acid sequestrants.[19,22,23]

Pregnancy, Precautions, and Contraindications

Ezetimibe (Zetia) is listed as category C for pregnancy and should be avoided to reduce risks. Caution should be used in persons with hepatic dysfunction.[19,22]

Adverse Effects

Ezetimibe (Zetia) is generally well tolerated with minimal adverse effects. The more common complaints are gastrointestinal, such as diarrhea and abdominal pain, as well as back pain, arthralgia, and sinusitis.[19,22]

Drug Interactions

Bile acid sequestrants may interfere with absorption. Therefore ezetimibe (Zetia) should be administered 1 hour before or 4 hours after the bile acid sequestrants if used concurrently. Fibrates can increase cholesterol excretion into the bile; concurrent use is not recommended. International Normalized Ratios (INR) should be monitored in those on warfarin.[19,22,24]

Monitoring

Baseline lipid profiles and liver function tests should be conducted prior to initiating therapy. When used concurrently with statins, liver enzymes should be monitored prior to initiating statin therapy and every 12 weeks in the first 6 months of treatment and periodically thereafter.[19,22]

Information

Tablets can be taken with or without food. Statins can be taken at the same time as ezetimibe (Zetia); however, bile acid sequestrants must be separated, either 1 hour after or 4 hours before ezetimibe (Zetia).

Fibrates

Fibrates exert their lipoprotein-lowering effects on TG, with additional benefits of increasing HDL-C. These agents are more commonly prescribed when elevations in TG are present. They are also useful in combination with statins to cover the entire spectrum of lipoprotein abnormalities in diabetic dyslipidemia. However, close monitoring is warranted with combination therapy.

Mechanism of Action

Fibrates are most effective for decreasing VLDL and TG levels while raising HDL-C levels.[9,19] Although the mechanism of action is not clear, these agents can increase lipoprotein lipase, resulting in the breakdown of VLDL. Fibrates also decrease hepatic VLDL synthesis while enhancing the removal of triglyceride-rich lipoproteins.[9]

Fibrates: Dosage Information

Drug	*Trade Name*	*Common Dose*	*Common Frequency*
Fenofibrate	Tricor	48 to 145 mg	Once daily
Gemfibrozil	Lopid	600 mg	Twice daily

Dosing

Fibrates are generally administered once to twice daily, often prior to or with a meal. The dosage depends on the percentage of lipid lowering needed to achieve target goals. However, initial therapy commonly starts with a lower dose and can be titrated up every 4 to 8 weeks as necessary to reach the optimal or maximum dosage and to minimize adverse effects.[19,22,23]

Pregnancy, Precautions, and Contraindications

Fibrates are listed as category C for pregnancy and should be avoided to reduce risks.[19,22]

Caution and lower dosages should be used for patients with renal dysfunction and the elderly.

Preexisting gallbladder disease, hepatic dysfunction, and severe renal dysfunction are contraindications.[22,23]

Adverse Effects

Fibrates are generally well tolerated with minimal adverse reactions. The more common adverse effects are gastrointestinal and include indigestion, nausea, diarrhea, flatulence, and abdominal pain. Rare side effects that have been reported are rash, fever, weight gain, muscle weakness, drowsiness, decreased potassium levels, anemia, and low white blood cell count.[19,22] Myopathy and rhabdomyolysis have been seen in monotherapy but are more common in conjunction with HMG-CoA reductase inhibitors.[19,23]

Drug Interactions

Fibrates are highly protein bound and can increase the adverse reactions of medications that are also highly protein bound. Common protein-bound medications include warfarin, sulfonylureas, and meglitinides.[19,24]

Bile acid sequestrants may impair absorption. Fibrates should be administered 1 hour before or 4 hours after the bile acid sequestrants.

Monitoring

TG and cholesterol levels should be measured prior to initiating fibrate therapy and at 3- to 6-month intervals. Liver function tests and complete blood cell counts should also be monitored at baseline and 6-month intervals. Discontinue treatment when liver enzymes are greater than 3 times the upper limit of normal. Monitor for hematologic changes such as decreased hemoglobin and hematocrit, thrombocytopenia, and neutropenia.[9,19,22]

If concurrent therapy includes statins, sulfonylureas, warfarin, or bile acid sequestrants, close monitoring for enhanced adverse reactions is warranted, especially for hypoglycemia and increased INR.

Instructions

Gemfibrozil (Lopid) should be taken 30 minutes prior to a meal. Fenofibrate (Tricor) can be administered with or without regard to meals. Patients should also be educated on the signs and symptoms of myopathy, such as persistent muscle or joint pain, especially if they are concurrently on an HMG-CoA reductase inhibitor.

Niacin

The primary lipoprotein effect of niacin is an increase in HDL-C, with a modest reduction in TG and LDL-C. Although niacin can be useful in increasing HDL-C levels, it can also increase blood glucose levels, especially in prediabetes or newly diagnosis patients.

Mechanism of Action

Niacin reduces the catabolism of HDL and selectively decreases the excretion of HDL apo-A-1, stimulating reverse cholesterol transport in hepatic cells.[9,19] Additionally, niacin reduces hepatic VLDL production, resulting in a reduction of LDL–C, thereby lowering TG and LDL-C levels.[9]

Niacin: Dosage Information

Drug	*Trade Name*	*Common Dose*	*Common Frequency*
Niacin sustained release	Niaspan	500 to 1000 mg	Once daily
Nicotinic acid immediate release	Niacin	100 to 1000 mg	1 to 3 times daily
Nicotinic acid sustained release	Slo-Niacin	250 mg	Once to twice daily

Dosing

Niacin is available in an immediate-release, sustained-release, and extended-release dose; these formulations should not be interchanged.

Immediate-release nicotinic acid often is preferred over sustained release for initial treatment, due to unfavorable adverse drug effects. Therapy should be started with small doses and titrated up as necessary and tolerable. Doses as low as 100 mg 3 times daily can be gradually increased to the maximum dose of 3 g per day in divided doses.[19,22,23]

Sustained-release nicotinic acid can be initiated at 250 mg twice daily and titrated up as tolerated to a maximum dose of 2 g per day, administered in a single or divided dose. Single doses can be given at bedtime with a low-fat snack.[19,22,23,25]

Pregnancy, Precautions, and Contraindications

Niacin is listed as category C for pregnancy and should be avoided to reduce risks.[22]

Caution should be used in persons with preexisting gout, heavy alcohol use, or renal dysfunction.

Liver dysfunction, active peptic ulcer disease, and arterial bleeding are contraindications.[19, 22]

Adverse Effects

The adverse effects of niacin can be a drawback. The more common effects include headache; hypotension; gastrointestinal discomfort, such as nausea, vomiting, and diarrhea; as well as the more notorious dermatological reactions of flushing, pruritis, and rash.[9,19,22,25] Flushing typically decreases with continuous use and can be reduced by taking niacin with meals. Aspirin taken once daily, 30 minutes prior to the niacin dose, can also minimize flushing.[19]

Patients on large doses of niacin, greater than 2 g per day, may be at increased risk of hepatotoxic effects. Significant elevations of liver enzymes can occur. Discontinue treatment when liver enzymes are greater than 3 times the upper limit of normal.[19,22]

Drug Interactions

Niacin is known to inhibit the release of insulin from the beta cell, resulting in hyperglycemia. This is especially notable in newly diagnosed type 2 diabetes patients and those with prediabetes, in whom beta-cell production of insulin has not been diminished or exhausted. The benefits of increasing HDL-C levels must outweigh the risks of increased blood glucose levels with niacin therapy.

Alcohol and hot drinks can increase flushing and pruritis effects. Rhabdomyolysis may occur when used in combination with HMG-CoA reductase inhibitors.[19,22]

Monitoring

A baseline lipid profile, liver function, uric acid, and blood glucose levels should be performed prior to initiating niacin therapy and repeated at 6-week intervals while adjusting the dosage. Lipid profiles should be reviewed at 3- to 6-month intervals. Blood glucose levels should be monitored regularly, especially in those newly diagnosed or with prediabetes. Liver enzymes should also be monitored at 12-week intervals during the first year of treatment.[19,22,25]

Instructions

Niacin should be taken 30 minutes after an aspirin or with a low-fat snack to minimize flushing effects. Advise patients to avoid taking niacin with hot beverages or alcohol. Blood glucose levels need to be monitored to identify glycemic elevations. Patients should also be educated on the signs and symptoms of myopathy, such as persistent muscle or joint pain, especially if they are concurrently on an HMG-CoA reductase inhibitor.

Omega-3 Fatty Acids

Lower TG is the primary effect observed with omega-3 fatty acids. Increasing HDL-C is a secondary benefit; however, this occurs only when higher doses are used. LDL-C levels tend to increase, and the increase is dose related.

Mechanism of Action

Omega-3 fatty acids are effective at lowering elevated TG through a reduction in hepatic VLDL production. Omega-3 fatty acids reduce the quantity of free fatty acids available for TG synthesis, subsequently lowering VLDL synthesis and increasing lipoprotein lipase activity, which results in TG clearance.[19,26-28]

Omega-3 Fatty Acids: Dosage Information			
Drug	*Trade Name*	*Common Dose*	*Common Frequency*
Omega-3-acid ethyl esters 90	Omacor	1000 mg	Once daily

Dosing

The initial dose of omega-3 fatty acids as Omacor is 1 to 2 1000-mg capsules daily and can be titrated up to a maximum dosage of 4 g per day. Omacor should be taken with food to minimize gastrointestinal adverse effects.[19,26,27]

Pregnancy, Precautions, and Contraindications

There are no adequate studies with pregnant women; therefore, omega-3 fatty acids should be avoided during pregnancy. Caution should be used in persons with renal or hepatic dysfunction, elderly patients, and those at high risk of hemorrhage.[19]

Adverse Effects

The more common adverse effects are dizziness and gastrointestinal, such as, dyspepsia, nausea, and abdominal pain. Rare adverse effects of headache, pruritis, and hyperglycemia have been reported.[19,26-28]

Drug Interactions

Omega-3 fatty acids may decrease the production of thromboxane A_2, resulting in an increase in bleeding time. INR can increase in concurrent use with warfarin. Limited studies have been done with other lipid-lowering therapies and other medications.[19,26-28]

Monitoring

A baseline lipid profile and liver function tests should be performed prior to initiating omega-3 fatty acids therapy and repeated at regular intervals, especially while adjusting dosage. Patients on anticoagulant therapy should have their INR monitored for increases in bleeding time.[26-28]

Instructions

Omega-3 fatty acids should be taken with food to minimize adverse effects.

Combination Drugs

When designing treatment strategies in diabetes management, often multiple agents are necessary to achieve desired blood glucose goals. The same holds true for designing a treatment strategy for diabetic dyslipidemia. Since multiple lipoproteins are involved, often multiple agents must be used to reach optimal lipid levels.

For ease of use and improved adherence to medication regimens, combination drugs can be useful. It is important to recognize which lipoproteins need to be targeted and the benefits each component of the combination product has on the various lipoproteins.

Combination drugs available include 1) Vytorin, which contains ezetimibe (a cholesterol absorption inhibitor) and simvastatin (an HMG-CoA reductase inhibitor) and 2) Advicor, which contains lovastatin (an HMG-CoA reductase inhibitor) and niacin.[19,22]

Considerations in Diabetic Dyslipidemia Therapy

Treatment goals and strategies for diabetic dyslipidemia must be given equal emphasis and be as aggressive as those developed for hyperglycemia.

Primary target:

The primary lipoprotein target is the LDL-C; however, TG, HDL-C, and particle size of the LDL-C must be addressed in the treatment plan. Achieving optimal levels of these lipoproteins should be considered when choosing drug therapy. Combinations of lipid-lowering agents are often necessary to accomplish this.

Adding medication to existing regimens requires behavior change by the patient. Thus, the person's readiness to change, conviction, and confidence levels require assessment. The use of precombined medications can be beneficial for persons who are reluctant to take more medication.

First-line therapy:

Statins are traditionally the initial drug of choice in diabetic dyslipidemia. However, the addition of a cholesterol absorption inhibitor can enhance the LDL-C lowering, and a fibrate can reduce TG levels and raise HDL-C. Two or more lipid-lowering agents may be necessary for some patients.

Lipid profiles, liver enzymes, and adverse effects as well as patient adherence must be routinely monitored.

Hypertension

Blood pressure is the product of cardiac output (CO) and total peripheral resistance (TPR), where CO is the result of stroke volume and heart rate. The pathophysiology of hypertension in most people is a multifactorial process that occurs due to the body's inability to maintain the homeostasis between CO and TPR.[29]

Two important systems exist that work to maintain normal blood pressure: the autonomic nervous system and the renin-angiotensin-aldosterone system (RAAS).[29] Recent evidence suggests that the RAAS is part of the multifactorial progression of diabetes, CVD, and renal disease. Through RAAS inhibition, blood pressure is reduced and albuminuria can be reversed. Studies have also shown that RAAS inhibition can decrease CVD and slow progression of diabetes.[30,31]

Renin-Angiotensin-Aldosterone System (RAAS)

Understanding of the RAAS has evolved over the decades and continues to do so. The RAAS regulates the balance of fluid volume, electrolyte balance, and blood volume in the body. Changes in the RAAS result in changes in vascular tone and sympathetic nervous system activity.

Stimulation of the RAAS leads to vasoconstriction, sodium retention, smooth muscle proliferation, and increased antidiuretic hormone in the vasculature.[32-34] In the kidney, activation of the RAAS is associated with intraglomerular hypertension, a precursor of proteinuria. Endothelial cells line the glomerulus as well as the blood vessels and function as the gatekeeper for cardiovascular and renal systems.[33,34] Abnormal RAAS activity can impair endothelium-dependent vasodilation in persons with type 2 diabetes, resulting in decreased acetylcholine stimulation and enhanced oxidative stress.[33,34] These changes lead to insulin resistance, endothelial dysfunction, and microalbuminuria.

To briefly review, the RAAS begins with a release of renin, an enzyme synthesized in the kidney, in response to changes within or outside the kidney. Renin then acts on angiotensinogen, a hepatic peptide, to create angiotensin-I (AT-I). Angiotensin-converting enzyme (ACE), located in the pulmonary and vascular endothelium, converts AT-I to angiotensin-II (AT-II).[32-34] ACE converts approximately 30% of circulating AT-I to AT-II. Other enzymes, such as chymase, tonin, and cathepsin-G, are responsible for the remaining 70% of AT-II production.[34,35] This peptide, AT-II, binds to AT-I receptors, which are primarily in vascular and myocardial tissue, to increase vasoconstriction, sympathetic activity, and aldosterone secretion. These increases result in peripheral vascular resistance, vasoconstriction and increased heart rate, and fluid retention, respectively, which contribute to the development of hypertension.[33-35] Figure 18.2 summarizes this process.

Treatment Goals: Hypertension

The Seventh Report of the Joint National Committee on Prevention, Detection, Evaluation, and Treatment of High Blood Pressure (JNC 7 Report) identifies evidence-based treatment strategies for the management of hypertension.[36]

Blood pressure has been classified into 4 stages; normal, prehypertension, stage 1 hypertension, and stage 2 hypertension.[36] Table 18.5 lists the criteria for each stage. Diagnosis and classification of hypertension is determined from the average of 2 blood pressure readings obtained from 2 separate clinic visits; it is measured with the person in a seated position, after a 5- to 10-minute rest.

Hypertension goal:

In adults with diabetes, the blood pressure goal is less than 130 mm Hg systolic and less than 80 mm Hg diastolic; however, depending on the presence of comorbid conditions, such as nephropathy, the goal may be even lower.[36-38]

Treatment strategies for hypertension often require combination therapy that targets different mechanisms to obtain optimal levels in blood pressure.

TABLE 18.5 Classification of Hypertension in Adults

Stage	*Systolic Pressure (mm Hg)*	*Diastolic Pressure (mm Hg)*
Normal	<120 *and*	<80
Prehypertension	120-139 *or*	80-89
Stage 1 hypertension	140-159 *or*	90-99
Stage 2 hypertension	≥160 *or*	≥100

Source: Chobanian AV, Bakris GL, Black HR, et al. The Seventh Report of the Joint National Committee on Prevention, Detection, Evaluation, and Treatment of High Blood Pressure: the JNC 7 report. JAMA. 2003;289:2560-72.

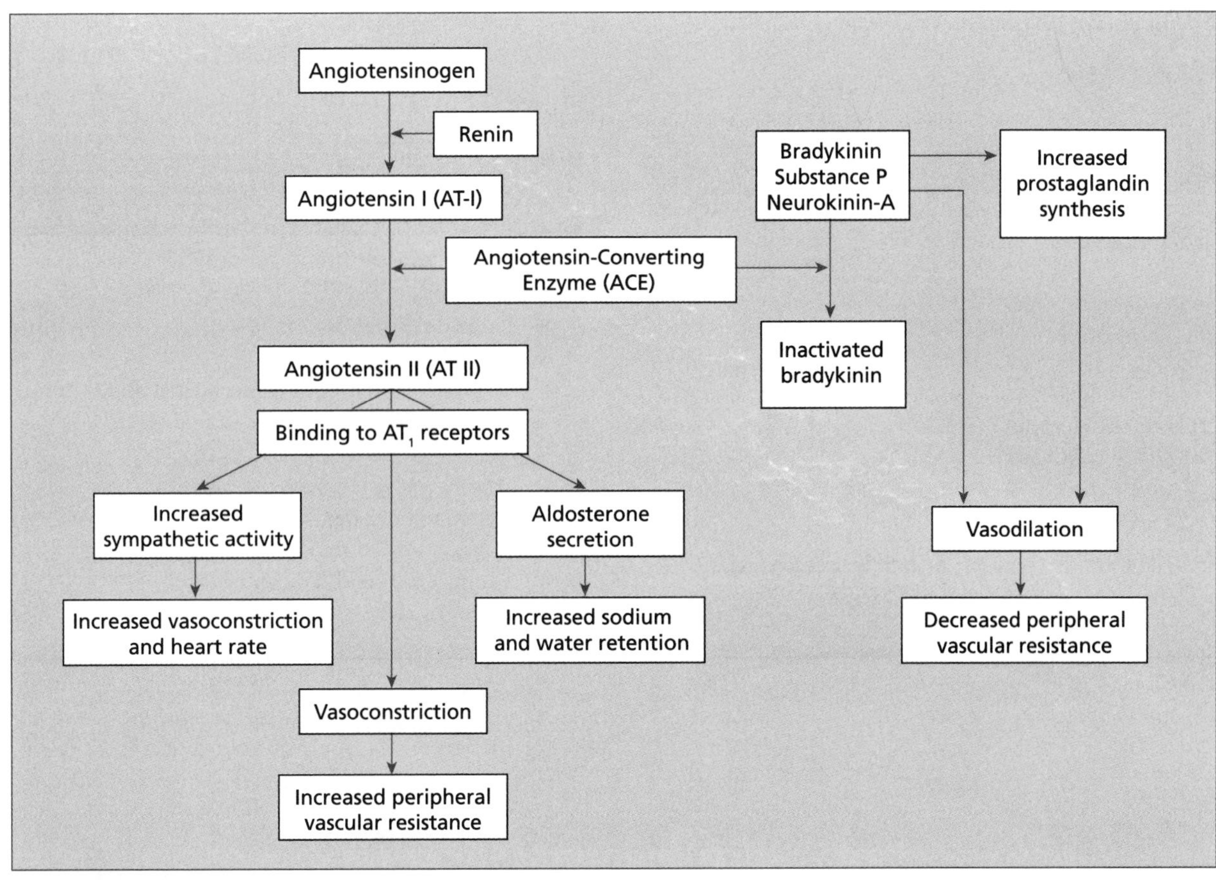

FIGURE 18.2 Renin-Angiotensin-Aldosterone System

Sources: Carter BL, Saseen JJ. Hypertension. In: Pharmacotherapy: A Pathophysiologic Approach, 6th ed. Dipiro JT, Talbert RL, Yee GC, Matzke GR, Wells BG, Posey LM, eds. New York: McGraw Hill Companies, Inc; 2005; Carter BL. Management of essential hypertension. In*:* Pharmacotherapy Self-Assessment Program Book 1: Cardiovascular I, 4th ed. Kansas City, Mo. American College of Clinical Pharmacy;2001:1-39; Jacobsen EJ. Hypertension: update on use of angiotensin II receptor blockers. Geriatrics. 2001;56(2):25-8.

Children and Adolescents

The 2006 ADA Standards for Medical Care in Diabetes make the following recommendations on screening and treating hypertension in children.[2] Hypertension in childhood is defined as an average systolic or diastolic blood pressure ≥95th percentile for age, sex, and height percentile measured on at least 3 separate days. "High-normal" blood pressure is defined as an average systolic or diastolic blood pressure ≥90th but <95th percentile for age, sex, and height percentile measured on at least 3 separate days. Normal blood pressure levels for age, sex, and height and appropriate methods for determinations are available online at www.nhlbi.nih.gov/health/prof/heart/hbp/hbp_ped.pdf.

Treatment in Children and Adolescents

Lifestyle Intervention. Treatment of high-normal blood pressure (systolic or diastolic blood pressure consistently above the 90th percentile for age, sex, and height) should include dietary intervention and exercise, aimed at weight control and increased physical activity, if appropriate.

Pharmacologic Therapy. If target blood pressure is not reached within 3 to 6 months of lifestyle intervention, pharmacologic treatment should be initiated. Pharmacologic treatment of hypertension (systolic or diastolic blood pressure consistently above the 95th percentile for age, sex, and height or consistently greater than 130/80 mmHg, if 95% exceeds that value) should be initiated as soon as the diagnosis is confirmed. ACE inhibitors should be considered for the initial treatment of hypertension. These pharmacotherapy recommendations from the ADA are based on expert consensus or clinical experience.

Pharmacologic Treatment: Hypertension

Lifestyle modification should always be a standard treatment for hypertension in addition to pharmacologic treatment. MNT, increased activity, moderation of alcohol consumption, and modest weight reduction can have beneficial effects on blood pressure.[37,38] See chapter 13's discussion of the role of MNT in hypertension prevention and management.

> *Standard Treatment*
>
> *Hypertension*—Standard treatment for hypertension includes pharmacotherapy plus lifestyle modifications: MNT, increased activity, moderation of alcohol consumption, and modest weight reduction

Classes of Antihypertensive Agents

There are multiple classes of antihypertensive agents prescribed in the treatment of hypertension. Categories are listed below.[39,40] Of the various classes, several are preferred when treating hypertension in persons with diabetes (those are listed in bold), and others should be avoided unless the benefits outweigh the risks.[36-38]

- **Thiazide diuretics**
- **β-Blockers**
- **Angiotensin-converting enzyme (ACE) inhibitors**
- **Angiotensin II receptor blockers (ARB)**
- Calcium channel blockers (CCB)
- Central-acting α-adrenergic agonists
- Diuretics other than thiazides
- α_1-Receptor blockers
- Combined α- and β-receptor blockers
- Vasodilators

Any of these classes can be used as monotherapy or in combination for the treatment of hypertension. Not uncommonly, 2 or more medications from different classes

Case—Part 2: What pharmacologic treatment for dyslipidemia, if any, is appropriate?

Provided DC's CPK levels and renal and hepatic function are within normal limits, a statin could be added to his medications. Statins are the first-line treatment option in diabetic dyslipidemia. Choice of statin should be based on the percentage of LDL-C lowering needed to obtain his lipoprotein goals.

Dosage. The initial dosage of the statin should be on the lower end and titrated up if necessary and tolerated. Liver enzymes should be checked 12 weeks after the start of therapy, and DC's lipid profile should be reviewed in 3 months.

Three-Month Follow-Up

If in 3 months, DC has not reached optimal lipoprotein levels, consideration of an increase in dosage of current therapy or addition of a second lipid-lowering agent is warranted.

Pharmacotherapy Options. Options for DC at that point would then include an increase in his current statin dose or use of a precombined lipid-lowering agent, such as Vytorin or Advicor. (Advicor contains a statin plus niacin, whereas Vytorin has a statin plus a cholesterol adsorption inhibitor.) Since DC was diagnosed with type 2 diabetes 2 years ago, consideration of the function of his pancreatic beta cells must be considered. The addition of niacin may inhibit release of insulin, resulting in elevated blood glucose levels. Therefore, Vytorin may be the preferred choice for DC at this time.

A bile acid sequestrant would not be preferred, since its use in persons with diabetes is not recommended.

Behavior Change Considerations. DC's readiness to change, conviction, and confidence in regard to adding another medicine should be assessed. Based on a possible adherence problem with his metformin (Glucophage), the addition of another medication may not be the best therapy plan. If adherence to pharmacologic therapy is not determined to be a problem, the addition of a fibrate would be an acceptable consideration.

Patient empowerment, education, close monitoring, and follow-up are needed to obtain and maintain the lipoprotein levels necessary to reduce this man's risk of CVD and cardiac events.

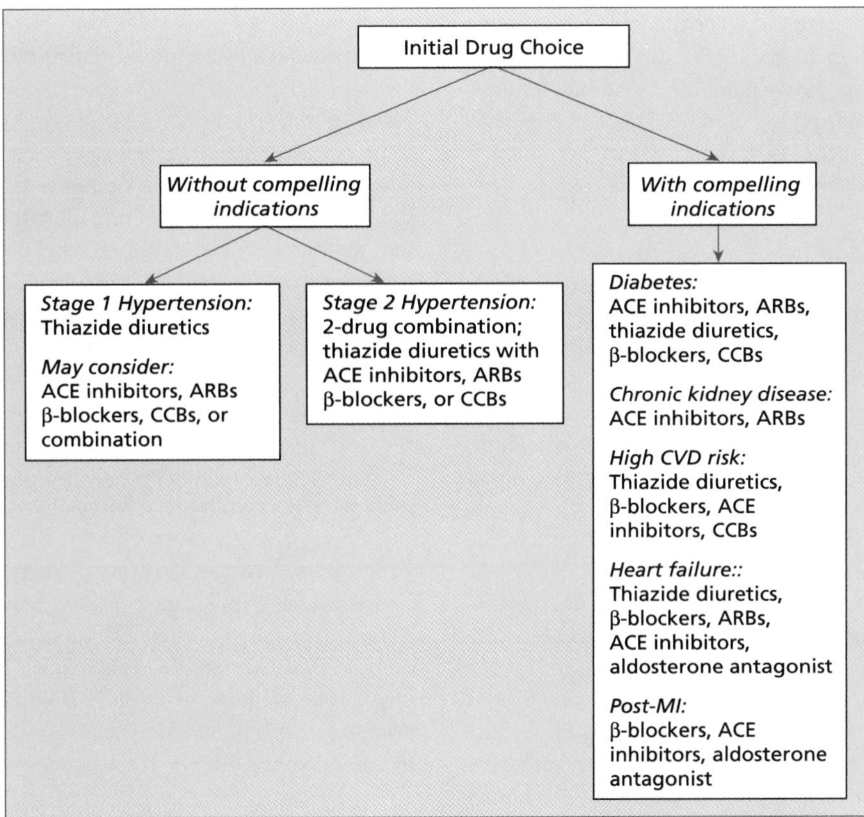

FIGURE 18.3 Hypertension: Pharmacologic Treatment Recommendations

Sources: Cardiovascular system: antihypertensives. In: Monthly prescribing reference: Nov. www.prescribingReference.com Accessed 28 Nov 2005; Black HR. The evolution of low-dose diuretic therapy: the lessons from clinical trials. Am J Med. 1996;101(3A):47S-52S.

are required to attain the goal of optimal blood pressure. Figure 18.3 outlines pharmacologic treatment for hypertension based on recommendations in the JNC 7 Report.

Diuretics

Diuretics are clinically classified based on their mechanism and/or site of action. There are 4 types: thiazide-type, loop, potassium-sparing, and carbonic anhydrase inhibitors; carbonic anhydrase inhibitors are not, however, used in the treatment of essential hypertension. Baseline renal function and serum potassium are important factors in determining the initial choice of diuretic. Typically, diuretics are not the first-line therapy for hypertension in persons with diabetes.[37] However, thiazide diuretics are often used for their additive effects with other preferred antihypertensive agents when treating hypertension in those with diabetes.[36]

Thiazide-Type Diuretics. The JNC 7 Report recommends thiazide-type diuretics as first-line therapy for uncomplicated hypertensive patients.[36] Hydrochlorothiazide (HCTZ) is the most frequently prescribed diuretic for the treatment of hypertension alone. In fact, many hypertensive drugs have HCTZ coformulations, in which HCTZ is combined with a drug from the same or another class, such as an ACE inhibitor or an ARB. Some examples of coformulations include Hyzaar (ARB with HCTZ), Prinizide (ACE inhibitor with HCTZ), and Aldactazide (potassium-sparing diuretic with HCTZ).

Thiazide diuretics are also used when treating hypertension with compelling indications. They can be used as monotherapy and in combination in the treatment of heart failure, recurrent stroke prevention, and high-risk CVD, such as diabetes.[36]

Loop Diuretics. Loop diuretics are often employed when the person's glomerular filtration rate (GFR) falls below 30 mL/min or the person needs greater diuresis due to another disease state (eg, heart failure). Thiazide-type diuretics (except metolazone) are relatively ineffective when GFR falls below 30 mL/min. Reduced GFR allows more opportunity for sodium and water reabsorption to occur.[29]

Potassium-Sparing Diuretics. As their name implies, potassium-sparing diuretics are the only diuretics that increase serum potassium; other diuretics lower it. Clinically, potassium-sparing diuretics are combined with a thiazide-type diuretic to balance serum potassium.[29] Alone, they do little to lower blood pressure.

Mechanisms of Action

The various types of diuretics exert their effects on different areas of the kidney. Thiazide-type diuretics inhibit the Na^+/Cl^- symporter on the distal convoluted tubule of the nephron, whereas loop diuretics inhibit the $Na^+/K^+/2Cl^-$ symporter on the ascending limb of the loop of Henle.[29,32] These inhibitions increase the urinary excretion of sodium, chloride, potassium, and water. Initially, the drop in blood pressure from diuretics is due to a decreased cardiac output as a result of decreased blood volume. With chronic use, the blood pressure reduction is not a result of diuresis. Cardiac output normalizes and the blood pressure reduction becomes a result of decreased peripheral vascular resistance.[29,32]

The mechanism of potassium-sparing diuretics is more complicated. Potassium-sparing diuretics inhibit the absorption of Na^+ and the excretion of K^+ in the principal cells of the late distal tubule and collecting duct.[29] Amiloride and triamterene inhibit the luminal Na^+ channels of the principal cell. Spironolactone and eplerenone are antagonists at aldosterone receptors on the principal cell.[29]

Dosing

Diuretics are generally taken once daily in the morning. The rationale for morning dosing is that people tolerate the increased frequency of urination from diuretics during waking hours, but oppose the disruption of sleep from frequent urination with evening dosing. Some potassium-sparing and loop diuretics may be dosed up to twice daily to increase diuresis for conditions other than hypertension.[39,40] Lower doses are recommended for the initial therapy and can be titrated up if necessary. When solely treating hypertension, larger doses, >25mg, have not shown any additional benefit of further decreasing blood pressure when compared to lower dosages.[36,41]

Pregnancy, Precautions, and Contraindications

Diuretic safety in pregnancy varies with the different agents. Most are category C, where risk cannot be ruled out; however, HTCZ, torsemide, eplerenone, indapamide, and metolazone are listed as category B, indicating there is no evidence of risk in humans. Reference to the packet insert of the individual diuretic is always recommended.[39,40]

Thiazide-Type Diuretics: Dosage Information

Drug	*Trade Name*	*Common Dose*	*Common Frequency*
Hydrochlorothiazide	HydroDIURIL Microzide	12.5 to 50 mg	Once daily
Chlorthalidone	Clorpres	12.5 to 25 mg	Once daily
Metolazone	Zaroxolyn	2.5 to 5 mg	Once daily
Indapamide	Lozol	1.25 to 2.5 mg	Once daily

Loop Diuretics: Dosage Information

Drug	*Trade Name*	*Common Dose*	*Common Frequency*
Furosemide	Lasix	20 to 40 mg	Twice daily
Torsemide	Demadex	5 to 10 mg	Once daily
Bumetanide	Bumex	0.5 to 2 mg	Twice daily

Potassium-Sparing Diuretics: Dosage Information

Drug	*Trade Name*	*Common Dose*	*Common Frequency*
Amiloride	Midamor	5 to 10 mg	Once daily
Triamterene	Dyrenium	37.5 to 75 mg	Once daily
Spironolactone	Aldactone	25 to 50 mg	Once to twice daily
Eplerenone	Inspra	50 mg	Once to twice daily

Caution should be used when treating persons with preexisting gout or uric acid stone disease, severe renal impairment, hepatic dysfunction, and/or electrolyte imbalances.[39]

Thiazide-type diuretics (except metolazone) are contraindicated in persons with a known hypersensitivity to sulfonamides. The absolute risk of cross-sensitivity in a sulfa-allergic patient is not well established. However, extreme caution is advised in patients with a documented allergic reaction.[40,42]

Adverse Effects

Adverse effects associated with diuretics are often associated with changes in serum electrolytes, such as hypokalemia, hypomagnesemia, hyperuricemia, hyperglycemia, hyperlipidemia, and hyper/hypocalcemia. Signs and symptoms of these imbalances are muscle cramps, fatigue, dizziness, and cardiac arrthymias.[19,39,40] Other common adverse effects include headache, photosensitivity, dry mouth, taste alterations, nausea, vomiting, impotence, and orthostatic hypotension.[39]

Drug Interactions

Since diuretics increase the excretion of sodium and potassium, many drug interactions stem from changes in electrolytes. Some of significance include nonsteroidal anti-inflammatory drugs (NSAIDS), which can decrease the antihypertensive efficacy of diuretics. Evidence suggests that this might occur more often with ibuprofen and indomethacin.[39] Diuretics can substantially increase lithium levels by decreasing lithium's elimination; therefore, lithium levels should be monitored 5 to 7 days after starting or discontinuing a diuretic.[24] Also, high sodium intake can decrease the effectiveness of diuretics.

Thiazide diuretics are known to inhibit the release of insulin from the beta cell, resulting in hyperglycemia. This is especially notable in persons newly diagnosed with type 2 diabetes or with prediabetes, where beta-cell production of insulin has not been diminished or exhausted. In general, this disease interaction is clinically insignificant at lower doses, such as less than 25 mg of HCTZ daily.[43,44]

Monitoring

Baseline blood pressure, serum electrolytes, uric acid, glucose, and lipids should be measured prior to initiating therapy and periodically thereafter. A regimen with diuretic therapy is often supplemented with potassium and magnesium.[39,40] When diuretics are combined with other antihypertensive agents, monitoring for hypotension is warranted.

Instructions

Diuretics should be taken in the morning with or without food. Intake of foods high in potassium, such as bananas or strawberries, can help maintain adequate potassium levels. Blood pressure must be monitored daily to identify elevations and patterns. Blood glucose levels need to be monitored to identify possible glycemic elevations from the diuretic. Patients should be educated on signs and symptoms of hypokalemia, such as muscle cramps and fatigue. To avoid episodes of orthostatic hypotension, patients should be reminded to rise slowly from lying or seated positions.

Angiotensin-Converting Enzyme (ACE) Inhibitors

ACE inhibitor or an ARB is traditionally used as first-line or preferred therapy for hypertension and renal protection in persons with diabetes.[30,32,34] ACE inhibitors can delay the progression of microalbuminuria to macroalbuminuria.

ACE inhibitors are also beneficial in the treatment of hypertension with compelling indications, such as heart failure, post-MI, recurrent stroke prevention, and chronic kidney disease.[30]

Mechanism of Action

ACE inhibitors inhibit the formation of AT-II by blocking the conversion of AT-I to AT-II. Additionally, ACE inhibitors block the action of kininase, the enzyme that converts bradykinin, substance P, and neurokinin-A to inactive

ACE Inhibitors: Dosage Information

Drug	*Trade Name*	*Common Dose*	*Common Frequency*
Benazepril	Lotensin	10 to 40 mg	Once daily
Captopril	Capoten	12.5 to 50 mg	2 to 3 times daily
Enalapril	Vasotec	2.5 to 20 mg	Once to twice daily
Fosinopril	Monopril	10 to 40 mg	Once daily
Lisinopril	Prinivil Zestril	10 to 40 mg	Once daily
Moexipril	Univasc	7.5 to 30 mg	Once daily
Perindopril	Aceon	4 to 8 mg	Once daily
Quinapril	Accupril	10 to 80 mg	Once daily
Ramipril	Altace	2.5 to 20 mg	Once daily
Trandolapril	Mavik	1 to 4 mg	Once daily

ingredients, thereby increasing their concentrations. The increase in bradykinin stimulates release of nitric oxide, a vasodilator.[30,32,34]

Dosing

ACE inhibitors are generally administered 1 to 3 times daily with or without food. Once-daily dosing can be in the morning or evening, based on patient preference and adverse effects, such as drowsiness. However, taking the medication at the same time every day is important. The presence of food may affect the absorption of captopril and moexipril and dosing prior to a meal may be warranted. The effects of blood pressure lowering can be seen within 1 hour of administration, with maximum effects after 6 to 8 hours. Initial therapy often starts with a lower dose and can be titrated as tolerated.[39,40] Addition of a thiazide diuretic is usually more beneficial at lowering blood pressure than increasing dosage of the ACE inhibitor. ACE inhibitors are often coformulated with low-dose hydrochlorothiazide (6.25 to 25 mg) to enhance blood pressure reduction and improve patient adherence in taking medication.

Pregnancy, Precautions, and Contraindications

ACE inhibitors are contraindicated during pregnancy. Use in the second or third trimesters can lead to fetal injury or death.

ACE inhibitors are also contraindicated in persons with bilateral renal artery stenosis or unilateral stenosis of a single, functional kidney. ACE inhibitors cause dilation of the efferent arteriole in the renal circulation, which can substantially reduce GFR and result in acute renal failure.

Caution should be used in patients with renal and/or hepatic dysfunction, angioedema, congestive heart failure (CHF), and hyperkalemia.[39]

ACE inhibitors are often less effective at lowering blood pressure and may increase risk of angioedema in African Americans.[39,45]

Adverse Effects

Overall, ACE inhibitors are well tolerated with few side effects, especially if monitored appropriately. The most notorious adverse effect and often the reason for discontinuation of ACE inhibitors is cough. This adverse effect is primarily due to the increase in bradykinin activity that increases prostaglandin synthesis. An estimated 10% to 20% of persons taking ACE inhibitors will develop a cough.[19,39]

Other adverse effects commonly associated with ACE inhibitors include fatigue, headache, dizziness, drowsiness, hyperkalemia, acute hypotension, and gastrointestinal problems, such as diarrhea, nausea, and vomiting. Skin rash, taste disturbances, angioedema, and hematologic effects, such as neutropenia and agranulocytosis, have also been reported.[39,40]

Drug Interactions

Concurrent use of NSAIDS, potassium-sparing diuretics, and potassium supplements may increase potassium levels significantly. ACE inhibitors can increase lithium levels, due to decreased fluid volume and loss of sodium ions; therefore, close monitoring of lithium levels is recommended.[24]

Monitoring

Blood pressure, serum electrolytes, and renal function should be measured at baseline and periodically throughout treatment. Potassium levels should be monitored within the first month of initial therapy and periodically thereafter due to the rapid onset of hyperkalemia.[39]

Changes in renal function can occur with use of ACE inhibitors, and this is more common in patients with preexisting renal dysfunction. Close monitoring of kidney function should be done throughout treatment and especially during dose titration. Discontinuation of the ACE inhibitor is not always necessary, provided the patient is being monitored and assessed closely.[39]

Instructions

ACE inhibitors should be taken at the same time daily. If the patient experiences drowsiness or dizziness, taking the medication in the evening can minimize these effects in the waking hours. Monitor blood pressure daily to identify elevations and patterns. Patients who develop a persistent cough within the first few months of initial therapy should discuss this with their healthcare provider at their next clinic visit. To avoid episodes of orthostatic hypotension, patients should be reminded to rise slowly from lying or seated positions.

Angiotensin Receptor Blockers (ARBs)

ARBs can be beneficial for persons with diabetes because these medications lower blood pressure and have renoprotective ability. ARBs are traditionally prescribed when ACE inhibitor therapies are not tolerated. However, they have been used as first-line therapy in some cases and are preferred over other antihypertensive agents for persons with diabetes. Additional compelling indications for which ARBs are used as monotherapy or in combination include heart failure and chronic kidney disease.[30,35]

ARBs and ACE inhibitors lower blood pressure and protect kidneys:

Due to their renoprotective ability, ARBs and ACE inhibitors are preferred over other antihypertensive agents for persons with diabetes.

Mechanism of Action

ARBs inhibit AT-II release by blocking the AT-I receptor. This leads to a reduction in aldosterone secretion, vasoconstriction, and sympathetic activity.[29,34]

Angiotensin Receptor Blockers (ARBs): Dosage Information

Drug	*Trade Name*	*Common Dose*	*Common Frequency*
Candesartan	Atacand	8 to 32 mg	Once daily
Eprosartan	Teveten	600 mg	Once daily
Irbesartan	Avapro	150 to 300 mg	Once daily
Losartan	Cozaar	25 to 100 mg	Once daily
Olmesartan	Benicar	20 to 40 mg	Once daily
Telmisartan	Micardis	20 to 80 mg	Once daily
Valsartan	Diovan	80 to 320 mg	Once daily*

*Dose divided and given 2 times daily if patient also has heart failure

Dosing

ARBs are generally administered once daily and can be dosed in the morning or evening, based on patient preference and adverse effects, such as drowsiness. However, taking the medication at the same time every day is important. Fluid volume or sodium depletion must be corrected prior to initiating therapy with ARBs.[39,40] Initial therapy often starts with a lower dose and can be titrated as tolerated. Addition of a thiazide diuretic is usually more beneficial at lowering blood pressure than increasing dosage of ARBs.

ARBs are often coformulated with low-dose HCTZ (6.25 to 25 mg) to enhance blood pressure reduction and improve patient adherence in taking medication.

Pregnancy, Precautions, and Contraindications

ARBs are listed as category C for the first trimester of pregnancy and category D for the second and third trimesters; therefore, ARBs should be avoided in pregnancy.

ARBs are also contraindicated in persons with bilateral renal artery stenosis or unilateral stenosis of a single, functional kidney.[39]

Caution should be used in persons with renal and/or hepatic dysfunction, angioedema, and/or CHF. Severe hypotension can occur in patients with CHF.[39,40]

Adverse Effects

ARBs are generally well tolerated with minimal side effects. The more common adverse effects associated with this class of antihypertensive agents include dizziness, drowsiness, diarrhea, dyspepsia, hyperkalemia, headache, and upper respiratory complaints, such as infection, pharyngitis, rhinitis, and cough. However, the frequency of cough associated with ARBs is significantly less than that with ACE inhibitors.[19,39,40]

Drug Interactions

Concurrent use of potassium-sparing diuretics, potassium supplements, or salt substitutes may increase serum potassium levels significantly. Increases in serum creatinine in persons with heart failure have also been reported. Use of ACE inhibitors and/or β-blockers with ARBs should be avoided in patients with heart failure.[24] ARBs can increase lithium levels due to decreased fluid volume and loss of sodium ions; therefore, close monitoring of lithium levels is recommended.[24]

Monitoring

Similar to ACE inhibitors, blood pressure, serum electrolytes, and renal function should be measured at baseline and periodically throughout treatment. Potassium levels should be monitored within the first month of initial therapy and periodically thereafter due to the rapid onset of hyperkalemia.[39,40]

Changes in renal function can occur with use of ARBs and tend to be more common in persons with preexisting renal dysfunction. Renal impairment can occur soon after initiating therapy. Close monitoring of kidney function should be done throughout treatment and especially during dose titration.[19,39]

Instructions

ARBs should be taken at the same time daily. If the patient experiences drowsiness or dizziness, taking the medication in the evening can minimize these effects in the waking hours. Blood pressure needs to be monitored daily to identify elevations and patterns. To avoid episodes of orthostatic hypotension, patients should be reminded to rise slowly from lying or seated positions.

β-Blockers

β-Blockers are commonly prescribed as an addition to an existing hypertension treatment plan for persons with diabetes. They are traditionally not first-line or preferred treatment for persons with diabetes, but may typically be a second or third option. β-Blockers are beneficial for persons with concurrent cardiac problems. In addition to reducing hypertension, β-blockers are indicated for persons

β1-Selective Receptor Blockers: Dosage Information				
Drug	*Trade Name*	*Common Dose*	*Common Frequency*	*Lipid Solubility*
Acebutolol*	Sectral*	200 to 400 mg	Twice daily	Low
Atenolol	Tenormin	25 to 100 mg	Once daily	Low
Betaxolol	Kerlone	5 to 20 mg	Once daily	Low
Bisoprolol	Zebeta	2.5 to 10 mg	Once daily	Low
Metoprolol tartrate	Lopressor	25 to 50 mg	Once to twice daily	Moderate
Metoprolol succinate	Toprol XL	25 to 100 mg	Once daily	Moderate
*Agents with intrinsic sympathomimetic activity				

Nonselective β-Receptor Blockers: Dosage Information				
Drug	*Trade Name*	*Common Dose*	*Common Frequency*	*Lipid Solubility*
Nadolol	Corgard	40 to 120 mg	Once daily	Low
Penbutolol*	Levatol*	20 mg	Once daily	High
Pindolol*	Visken*	5 to 20 mg	Twice daily	Low
Propanolol	Inderal	40 to 120 mg	Twice daily	High
Propanolol extended release	Inderal LA	80 to 160 mg	Once daily	High
Timolol	Blocadren	10 to 30 mg	Twice daily	Low to moderate
*Agents with intrinsic sympathomimetic activity				

Combined α- and β-Receptor Blockers: Dosage Information			
Drug	*Trade Name*	*Common Dose*	*Common Frequency*
Carvedilol	Coreg	6.25 to 25 mg	Twice daily
Labetalol	Normodyne	100 to 300 mg	Twice daily

with high risk for coronary disease and for prevention of a second MI and heart failure.

Mechanism of Action

There are 2 main types of β-receptors in human physiology, β1 and β2. β1 Receptors are located on the heart, where activation causes an increase in heart rate, contractility, and conduction velocity. Blockade of these receptors reduces cardiac output.[46]

β-Receptors also have a wide range of functions in the body outside the heart. Activation of β1 receptors located in the juxtoglomerular cells of the kidney affect the RAAS by stimulating the release of renin.[47] Activation of β2 receptors in the liver increases hepatic-mediated glucose output.[48] Activation of β2 receptors in the lungs induces bronchodilation.[46] β2-receptor activation also causes an increase in intraocular pressure and relaxation of skeletal muscle vessels.[47] β-Receptor blockade opposes all these effects. In some of these cases, β-receptor blockade is beneficial and others it is not.

As for differences with β-blocker drugs, some are β1-receptor selective and preferentially inhibit the β1 receptor. Others are nonselective and inhibit both the β1 and β2 receptors with equal affinity. It is important to remember that when higher doses of a β1-selective blocker are given, selectivity diminishes.[46] β-receptor blockers also differ in lipid solubility. Highly lipid-soluble β-receptor blockers cross the blood brain barrier (BBB) readily and increase the risk of central nervous system (CNS) adverse effects. Some β-blockers also have intrinsic sympathomimetic activity (ISA). ISA β-blockers act as a partial agonist at β receptors while blocking physiological β-agonists such as epinephrine. The net effect is some preservation of β-receptor function and a potential decrease in side effects.[46] These agents are used infrequently, however, due to inferior clinical trial data in post-MI patients.[49]

Dosing

β-Blockers are administered once to twice daily and given without regard to meals. If drowsiness is experienced, daily doses can be given in the evening to minimize this adverse effect during waking hours. However, administration should occur at a consistent time. Initial therapy often starts with a lower dose and can be titrated as tolerated.

Pregnancy, Precautions, and Contraindications

Most β-blockers are classified as pregnancy category C. Atenolol is classified as pregnancy category D. Atenolol crosses the placental barrier and has resulted in the birth of infants small for their gestational age. β-Blockers should be used with caution in pregnancy, if at all, and used only if the benefit clearly outweighs the risk.[46]

β-Blockers are contraindicated in persons with sinus bradycardia.[46] Nonselective β-blockers are contraindicated in persons with asthma, due to the blockade of β2-mediated bronchodilation.[46]

β1-Selective agents should be used cautiously and with the lowest possible dose.[50] Additionally, caution must be used with β-blockers in older adults who have preexisting ventricular dysfunction.[46]

Persons with diabetes must also exercise caution when using β-blockers. β-Blockers may inhibit the release of insulin from the pancreas, resulting in increased blood glucose levels in persons with type 2 diabetes. Additionally, all β-blockers have the potential to mask hypoglycemic-induced tachycardia, which can decrease the individual's awareness of hypoglycemia.[46,48] Dizziness and sweating induced by hypoglycemia are typically unaffected by β-blockers.[46] Nonselective β-blockers can reduce β2-mediated hepatic glucose output.[48] Normally, this would be a beneficial effect, but during an episode of hypoglycemia, it may delay the body's ability to return to normoglycemia.[51]

Adverse Effects

The more common adverse effects associated with this class of antihypertensive agents are CNS-related, such as sedation, dizziness, drowsiness, lightheadedness, fatigue, and headache. Other notable adverse effects include bradycardia, hypotension, depression, and sexual dysfunction, especially in older adults. Gastrointestinal effects of constipation, diarrhea, and nausea are reported but less frequent.[46]

Drug Interactions

β-Blockers have additive effects with nondihydropyridine calcium channel blockers (Diltiazem and Verapamil), amiodarone, and digoxin.[46] Concurrent use of these agents may cause heart block; therefore, extreme caution should be used when combining these agents. Typically, persons taking β-blockers need to be tapered off the drug and should not abruptly discontinue.[46] Diphenhydramine and hydrochloroquine may increase the plasma concentrations of some β-blockers through inhibition of the cytochrome P-450 isoenzyme CYP2D6, resulting in enhanced adverse effects including hypotension.[46] NSAIDs may decrease the antihypertensive effects of β-blockers.[46]

Monitoring

Baseline blood pressure, heart rate, lipid profile, and blood glucose levels should be conducted. Since β-blockers can decrease heart rate, patients should have their heart rate assessed at each clinician visit.[46] Generally, the β-blocker dose is adjusted if the heart rate falls below 50 beats per minute. β-Blockers also have the potential to increase total cholesterol, LDL-C, and triglycerides and decrease HDL-C, although these effects are transient and usually of little clinical significance.[52] Nevertheless, serum lipids should be monitored regularly, especially when coadministered with other agents that increase serum lipids, such as thiazide diuretics.[46] Blood glucose levels should be monitored regularly, especially in those newly diagnosed with diabetes or with prediabetes.

Instructions

Patients should be educated not to stop β-blockers abruptly unless directed by their healthcare provider. Abrupt withdrawal could lead to increased blood pressure and worsening of preexisting angina and possibly lead to MI. Blood pressure and heart rate need to be monitored daily to identify changes, elevations, and patterns. Patients with diabetes should be encouraged to monitor their blood glucose levels more frequently. Patients should be educated on signs and symptoms of hypotension and CHF, such as edema and difficulty in breathing during activity.

Calcium Channel Blockers

CCBs are usually not used as first-line therapy for lowering blood pressure in persons with diabetes. Although they can be used in those with diabetes, typically they are a second or third option, since they have less of an impact on CVD when compared to other antihypertensive agents, such as ACE inhibitors, ARBs, diuretics, and β-blockers. Nondihydropyridine CCBs can be considered for persons who have not tolerated ACE inhibitor or ARB therapy. Data are conflicting, but nondihydropyridine CCBs may have antiproteinuric effects.[53-56]

Mechanism of Action

Calcium channel blockers (CCBs) are classified into nondihydropyridine and dihydropyridine, based on their chemical structure. CCBs block the L-type calcium channel, which results in vasodilation. Nondihydropyridine CCBs primarily cause vasodilation within coronary vessels and have a more depressive effect on cardiac conduction. Thus, blood pressure reduction is due to decreased CO.[57,58] Dihydropyridine CCBs primarily cause vasodilation in the

Nondihydropyridine CCBs: Dosage Information			
Drug	*Trade Name*	*Common Dose*	*Common Frequency*
Diltiazem sustained release	Cardizem SR	60 to 180 mg	Twice daily
Diltiazem extended release	Cardizem CD Tiazac Cardizem LA	120 to 360 mg	Once daily
Verapamil immediate release	Calan	40 to 80 mg	Three times daily
Verapamil sustained release	Calan SR	120 to 360 mg	Once daily
Verapamil extended release	Covera-HS Verelan PM	120 to 360 mg 100 to 300 mg	Once daily

vascular smooth muscle. Thus, blood pressure reduction is due to decreased TPR.[57]

Dosing

CCBs are dosed 1 to 3 times daily and can be taken with food to minimize adverse effects. Initial dosage should be at the low range and titrated every 2 weeks based on patient tolerance, blood pressure, and heart rate. An immediate-release dosage form is rarely used for the treatment of hypertension. All once-daily formulations are dosed in the morning except Verapamil extended-release products, which are dosed at bedtime.[57]

Dihydropyridine CCBs: Dosage Information			
Drug	*Trade Name*	*Common Dose*	*Common Frequency*
Amlodipine	Norvasc	2.5 to 10 mg	Once daily
Felodipine	Plendil	2.5 to 20 mg	Once daily
Isradipine controlled release	DynaCirc CR	5 to 10 mg	Once daily
Nicardipine sustained release	Cardene SR	30 to 60 mg	Twice daily
Nifedipine long-acting	Adalat CC Procardia XL	30 to 60 mg	Once daily
Nisoldipine	Sular	10 to 40 mg	Once daily

Dihydropyridine CCBs are dosed once daily and can be given without regard to time of day. However, administration should be at a consistent time. Initial dosage should be at the low range and titrated gradually based on patient tolerance, blood pressure, and heart rate.[57]

Pregnancy, Precautions, and Contraindications

All CCBs are pregnancy category C and should be avoided unless the benefit outweighs the risk.

CCBs are also contraindicated in persons with sick sinus syndrome or a heart block without a pacemaker. Verapamil, specifically, is contraindicated in persons with moderate-to-severe CHF.

Caution should be used in persons with renal and/or hepatic dysfunction, ventricular dysfunction, and CHF.[57]

Adverse Effects

CCBs have a wide range of adverse effects, which can include headache, dizziness, nausea, dyspepsia, flushing, and constipation. Nondihydropyridine CCBs are associated with cardiac adverse effects including cardiac conduction abnormalities and bradycardia, which are typically found in persons with preexisting cardiac conditions. Dihydropyridine CCBs have adverse effects related to their relaxing of vascular tone. Peripheral edema occurs more frequently in these agents; however, all CCBs have the potential to cause peripheral edema.[57]

Drug Interactions

Most CCB drug interactions stem from the cytochrome P-450 enzyme system. All inducers and inhibitors of the CYP3A4 isoenzyme affect the metabolism of CCBs, thereby delaying or enhancing their elimination from the body and resulting in increased or decreased CCB concentration.[57] Concurrent medications and foods (such as grapefruit juice) that are also metabolized through this system should be used cautiously and monitored for increased levels and risks of adverse reactions. Additionally, diltiazem and verapamil can inhibit other CYP3A4 substrates, such as statins and theophylline.[57] Monitoring adverse effects and blood pressure can help identify potential drug interactions and reduce the risk of toxicity. See Table 18.4 for a list of common drugs that interact with CCBs.

CCBs may also inhibit platelet function, resulting in an increased risk for bleeding if used concurrently with anticoagulants, such as warfarin or aspirin. Although this interaction is usually not clinically significant, caution is warranted.[57] Concurrent use of diuretics, β-blockers, and ACE inhibitors may increase risk of hypotension. Additive effects may occur with agents that affect cardiac contractility.[57]

Monitoring

Blood pressure, heart rate, liver enzymes, and cardiac function should be measured at baseline and periodically throughout treatment, especially when titrating doses of CCBs and/or other medications metabolized by the cytochrome P-450 system.[57] Monitor for CHF, edema, angina, and changes in heart rate. INR and risk of bleeding assessments should be done regularly for patients on anticoagulation therapy.

Instructions

CCBs should be taken at the same time daily. For once-daily dosed CCBs, patients can take the medication in the evening if they experience drowsiness or dizziness. Taking CCBs with meals can minimize gastrointestinal adverse effects and can often increase adherence. Blood pressure needs to be monitored daily to identify changes, elevations, and patterns. Patients should be educated on signs and symptoms of CHF, such as edema and difficulty in breathing at rest or during activity.

α_1-Receptor Blockers

Although indicated for the treatment of hypertension, α_1-receptor blockers are rarely prescribed for this indication, especially in persons with diabetes. They are most beneficial in persons with benign prostatic hyperplasia (BPH). α_1-Receptor blockers can be a treatment option for persons with both diabetes and BPH.

Mechanism of Action

The α_1-receptor blockers inhibit the binding of norepinephrine to vascular α_1 receptors. Activation of the α_1 receptor by norepinephrine leads to vasoconstriction, resulting in an increase in TPR. In addition, inhibition of the α_1 receptor in the prostate causes a decrease in urethral resistance and improvement in symptoms in persons with BPH.[59]

Dosing

The α_1-receptor blockers are preferably dosed at bedtime to minimize the risk of postural hypertension often observed within hours after administration. Initial therapy often starts with a lower dose and can be titrated as tolerated.[59]

α_1-Receptor Blockers: Dosage Information

Drug	*Trade Name*	*Common Dose*	*Common Frequency*
Doxazosin	Cardura	1 to 16 mg	Once daily
Prazosin	Minipress	1 to 5 mg	2 to 3 times daily
Terazosin	Hytrin	1 to 10 mg	Once to twice daily

Pregnancy, Precautions, and Contraindications

All α_1-blockers are classified as pregnancy category C and should be avoided unless the benefit outweighs the risk. Animal studies indicated possible risk, and no human studies exist.

The α_1-receptor blockers also cause a mild decrease in neutrophils and white blood cell counts. In most persons, the decrease is clinically insignificant. Caution should be exercised in immunocompromised patients.[59]

Adverse Effects

Adverse effects commonly associated with α_1-receptor blockers include fatigue, malaise, dizziness, shortness of breath, hypotension, edema, and weight gain. Blurred vision, palpitations, and sexual dysfunction have also been reported. Thrombocytopenia has been observed in patients on terazosin.[59]

Drug Interactions

The α_1-blockers have relatively few drug interactions. Alcohol increases the risk of hypotension with these agents, and coadministration of verapamil increases the serum concentrations of prazosin and terazosin. Concurrent use of other antihypertensive agents with α_1-blockers may increase the risk of hypotension.[59]

Monitoring

Blood pressure and heart rate should be monitored at baseline and frequently after initiating treatment. If antihypertensive agents are added, the patient should be assessed for first-dose syncope and postural hypotension.[59] Syncope is usually prevented when dosing is started low and increased slowly. Interruptions in therapy increase the risk; thus, nonadherent patients are not good candidates for this drug. Syncope is managed by having the patient lie down, rest, and receive supportive care as necessary. Dizziness and lightheadedness are more common than loss of consciousness.[59]

Instructions

Patients should be educated that α_1-blockers have the potential to cause syncope and postural hypotension.

Alcohol, exercise, long periods of standing, and hot weather can increase the risk.[59] Patients and their family should be educated on management of syncope in case it occurs. Advise patients to avoid driving or operate machinery after the first dose, an increase in dose, or the addition of another antihypertensive agent until they can tolerate treatment. Lastly, male patients should also be advised to go immediately to the emergency room if a prolonged erection, lasting 4 hours or more, occurs.

Central-Acting α-Adrenergic Agonists

Although indicated for the treatment of hypertension, central-acting α-adrenergic agonists are rarely prescribed for this indication, especially in persons with diabetes.

Mechanism of Action

Central-acting α-adrenergic agonists stimulate α_2 receptors in the brain, inhibiting the production of serotonin, dopamine, norepinephrine, and epinephrine. This inhibition results in a decrease in heart rate and TPR.[60]

Central-Acting α-Adrenergic Agonists: Dosage Information

Drug	*Trade Name*	*Common Dose*	*Common Frequency*
Clonidine tablets	Catapres	0.1 to 0.8 mg	Twice daily
Clonidine patch	Catapres-TTS	0.1- to 0.3-mg per day patch	Once weekly
Methyldopa	Aldomet	250 to 1000 mg	2 to 3 times daily

Dosing

Central-acting α-adrenergic agonists are available in tablets and a transdermal patch. Tablets are taken in daily divided doses, preferably at consistent times. Patches are applied once weekly.[61] When methyldopa is administered with any other antihypertensive agent, other than thiazide-type diuretics, limit the initial dose to no more than 500 mg per day in divided doses.[60]

Pregnancy, Precautions, and Contraindications

Clonidine is classified as pregnancy category C and should be avoided.[61] Methyldopa is pregnancy category B and therefore can be used in pregnancy. It is converted to α-methylnorepinephrine, a natural byproduct of catecholamine breakdown. There are no documented fetal adverse effects despite wide use, and it does not reduce maternal cardiac or fetal blood flow.[62] Although it can be used during pregnancy, methyldopa presents with many adverse effects to the mother that often lead to discontinuation (see adverse effects below).

The use of a monoamine oxidase inhibitor (MAOI) is contraindicated in persons taking methyldopa. Although the mechanism is unknown, there are numerous reports of hypertensive crisis in persons taking both medications.[60]

Central-acting α-adrenergic agonists are contraindicated in persons with severe coronary insufficiency, recent MI, cerebrovascular disease, and renal or hepatic dysfunction.[60-62]

Adverse Effects

Although methyldopa can be used in pregnancy, it presents with many adverse effects to the mother and to the general patient. Some of these include nausea, vomiting, constipation, dry mouth, and CNS-related effects, such as sedation, weakness, nervousness, dizziness, and drowsiness. Hypotension, blood dyscrasia, sexual dysfunction, and hair thinning or loss have been reported.[60]

Drug Interactions

The use of an MAOI is contraindicated in persons taking methyldopa. Although the mechanism is unknown, there are numerous reports of hypertensive crisis in persons taking both medications.[60]

Iron can decrease the absorption of methyldopa up to 66%. Therefore, iron should be separated by at least 2 hours from methyldopa administration.[60] Methyldopa also increases the risk of lithium toxicity, even in the presence of normal lithium levels. Signs and symptoms of lithium toxicity, such as lethargy and muscle weakness, should be monitored.[62] Patients should also exercise caution when taking entacapone (Comtan) and methyldopa. Entacapone is a catechol-O-methyltransferase (COMT) inhibitor, and methyldopa is metabolized by COMT.[62]

The over-the-counter drug products pseudoephedrine and ma huang (ephedra, ephedrine) can increase blood pressure. This is greatly enhanced for persons takingmethyldopa and clonidine.[60-62] Tricyclic antidepressants—eg, amitriptyline (Elavil) and imipramine (Janimine, Tofranil)—may antagonize central α_2 receptors, limiting nists. Clonidine and methyldopa should also be used with caution with β-blockers, since withdrawal of these agents in persons concurrently on β-blockers has led to life-threatening increases in blood pressure.[60-62]

Monitoring

Blood pressure and heart rate should be monitored at baseline and frequently after initiating treatment. Patients should be monitored for signs of depression at clinician visits. Clinicians who wish to discontinue a central-acting α-adrenergic agonist should taper the dose gradually over 2 to 4 days to prevent withdrawal.[60-62] Monitoring for tachycardia, rebound hypertension, nausea, vomiting, and flushing should also be conducted. Patients on methyldopa also should undergo liver function testing at periodic intervals.[60]

Instructions

Patients must be educated to never abruptly discontinue their medication and should be aware of the signs and symptoms of withdrawal. Since these agents affect catecholamine and aldosterone levels, remind patients with diabetes to monitor blood glucose levels more frequently as greater fluctuation can occur.[60-62] Drowsiness is common, so patients should exercise caution when driving or operating heavy machinery until the medication is tolerated.[60] Dry mouth can occur during the first 2 weeks of therapy. Ice chips, hard candy, or chewing gum can minimize problems with dry mouth.[60] The clonidine patch should be applied every 7 days on a hairless part of the upper arm or torso. Patients should be educated to apply the adhesive overlay over the system for proper adhesion. Patients taking methyldopa should be aware that urine may darken in color after exposure to air.[60]

Considerations in Hypertension Therapy in Persons With Diabetes

Treatment goals and strategies for hypertension in persons with diabetes must be given equal emphasis and treated as aggressively as hyperglycemia. Most likely, 2 or more antihypertensive agents will be necessary to lower and maintain blood pressure to the goals of the ADA and JNC 7 Report, of 130/80 mm Hg.[2,36]

When using combination therapy for hypertension in persons with diabetes, medication adherence must be reviewed at each patient visit. Adding medication to existing regimens requires behavior change on the part of the patient; thus, the person's readiness to change, conviction, and confidence levels require assessment. Use of precombined medications can be beneficial for individuals who are reluctant to take more medication.

ACE inhibitors or ARBs are traditionally the initial drug of choice for hypertension in persons with diabetes. The addition of a thiazide diuretic can enhance the blood-pressure lowering effects of ACE inhibitors and ARBs. However, monitoring for hypotension and electrolytes changes, especially potassium, must be conducted routinely.

Case—Part 3: What pharmacologic treatment for hypertension, if any, is appropriate?

Provided that DC's electrolytes, primarily potassium, and renal and hepatic function are within normal limits and he has no signs or symptoms of CHF, DC may be prescribed ACE inhibitors or ARBs. ACE inhibitors or ARBs are the first-line treatment option in hypertension for persons with diabetes. However, because DC is African American, caution must be used if an ACE inhibitor is chosen, due to an increased risk of angioedema; an ARB may thus be a better choice to start with for DC.

Dosage. Initial dosage should be on the lower end and titrated up if necessary and tolerated. Blood pressure, electrolytes, and renal function should be testing within the first month of initiating ARB therapy.

Three-Month Follow-Up

If after 3 months of therapy, DC has not reach optimal blood pressure goals, consideration of an increase in dosage of current therapy or addition of a second antihypertensive agent is warranted.

Pharmacotherapy Options. Options for DC at this point might include an increase in his current ARB dose or use of a precombined ARB with low-dose HCTZ agent.

Self-Management Considerations. DC's readiness of change, conviction, and confidence in regard to the addition of another medicine should be assessed. As mentioned earlier, DC may have a possible adherence problem with his medications; therefore, adding another medication may not be the best therapy plan.

Patient empowerment, education, close monitoring, and follow-up with the patient are necessary to ensure that optimal blood lipids and blood pressure goals are met and to decrease CVD risks and events.

Focus on Education: Pearls for Practice

Teaching Strategies

- **First acknowledge the need for lifestyle change.** Pharmacologic treatment is always in addition to lifestyle change. Teach patients to recognize and make realistic changes in activity and food intake as a first step.

- **Dosing starts small and builds.** Initiation of medication therapy is an important change in treatment and health management. Titration of medications to achieve targets is essential for effective and comprehensive diabetes care management.

- **Combining medications.** Achieving optimal levels of LDL-C, TG, and HDL-C should be considered when choosing drug therapy. Combinations of lipid-lowering agents are often necessary to achieve target goals. Describe each medication's unique function and effect. For example, achieving optimal blood pressure control often requires a combination of medications with different mechanisms of action rather than more of a single medication.

- **Resisting medications.** Adding medication to existing regimens is a behavior change. Readiness to change, conviction, and confidence levels affect adherence to the regimen. Discuss and plan for accommodation into existing lifestyle. Identify and help diminish barriers to effective pharmacotherapy.

Messages for Patients

- **Treatment goals.** Identify target goals for dyslipidemia and hypertension. Put as much emphasis on these and be as aggressive as you are with blood sugar goals. Be certain you are aware of the target blood levels your healthcare team identifies for lipids, blood pressure, and blood sugars.

- **Consistency.** Work with the healthcare team and pharmacist to know all the medications you are taking (prescription and over the counter). Know their interactions and side effects. Always carry a list of medications. Never abruptly discontinue medication; be aware of the signs and symptoms of withdrawal. Have a handout of resources to call if questions.

References

1. Haffner SM. Dyslipidemia management in patients with diabetes and the metabolic syndrome. Fam Pract. 2005;27:49-64.
2. American Diabetes Association. Standards of medical care in diabetes. Diabetes Care. 2006;29suppl: S4-42.
3. Bierman EL. Atherogenesis in diabetes. Arterioscler Thromb. 1992;12:647-56.
4. Miettinen H, Lehto S, Salomaa V, et al, for the FINMONICA Myocardial Register Study Group. Impact of diabetes on mortality after the first myocardial infarction. Diabetes Care. 1998;21:69-75.
5. Kannel WB, McGee DL. Diabetes and cardiovascular disease: The Framingham Study. JAMA. 1979;241:2035-8.
6. Haffner SM, Lehto S, Ronnemaa T, et al. Mortality from coronary heart disease in subjects with type 2 diabetes and in nondiabetic subjects with and without prior myocardial infarction. N Engl J Med. 1998;339:229-34.
7. Norhammar A, Tenerz A, Nilsson G, et al. Glucose metabolism in patients with acute myocardial infarction and no previous diagnosis of diabetes mellitus: a prospective study. Lancet. 2002;359:2140-4.
8. Ganong WF. Review of Medical Physiology, 17th ed. Norwalk, Conn: Appleton & Lange;1995:277-81, 436-8.

9. Sisson EM, Tisdel KA. Hyperlipidemias. In: Pharmacotherapy Self-Assessment Program Book 1: Cardiovascular I, 4th ed. Kansas City, Mo: American College of Clinical Pharmacy; 2001:45-83.
10. Luscher TF. Endothelial dysfunction in atherosclerosis. J Myocardial Ischemia. 1995;7suppl:15-20.
11. Ginsberg HN. Lipoprotein physiology in nondiabetic and diabetic states: relationship to atherogenesis. Diabetes Care. 1991;14:839-55.
12. Lamarche B, Lemieux I, Despres JP, et al. The small, dense LDL phenotype and the risk of coronary heart disease: epidemiology, pathophysiology and therapeutic aspects. Diabetes Med. 1999;25:199-211.
13. Tribble DL, Holl LG, Wodd PD, et al. Variations in oxidative susceptibility among six low density lipoprotein subfractions of differing density and particle size. Atherosclerosis. 1992;93:189-99.
14. Garg A, Grundy SM. Management of dyslipidemia in NIDDM. Diabetes Care. 1990;13:153-69.
15. Expert Panel on Detection, Evaluation, and Treatment of High Blood Cholesterol in Adults. Executive Summary of the Third Report of the National Cholesterol Education Program (NCEP) Expert Panel on Detection, Evaluation, and Treatment of High Blood Cholesterol in Adults (Adult Treatment Panel III). JAMA. 2001;285:2486-97.
16. Grundy SM, Cleeman JI, Merz CN, et al, for the Coordinating Committee of the Recent Clinical Trials for the National Cholesterol Education Program Adult Treatment Panel III Guidelines. Circulation. 2004;110:227-39.
17. American Diabetes Association. Management of dyslipidemia in adults with diabetes. Diabetes Care. 2003;26suppl:S83-6.
18. Jones PH. A clinical overview of dyslipidemias: treatment strategies. Am J Med. 1992;93:187-98.
19. Lexi-Drugs Platinum for Palm OS. Hudson, Ohio: Lexi-Comp Inc; 2004.
20. Worz CR, Bottorff M. Treating dyslipidemic patients with lipid-modifying and combination therapies. Pharmacotherapy. 2003;23:625-37.
21. Jones P, Kafonek S, Laurora I, et al. Comparative dose efficacy study of atorvastatin versus simvastatin, pravastatin, lovastatin, and fluvastatin in patients with hypercholesterolemia (the CURVES study). Am J Cardiol. 1998;81:582-7.
22. Antilipidemic agents. In: Monthly Prescribing Guide: November. Montvale, NJ: Thompson PDR; 2005:89-95.
23. Cardiovascular system: hyperlipoproteinemias. In: Monthly Prescribing Reference. Nov 2005. On the Internet: www.prescribingReference.com Accessed 7 Nov 2005.
24. Lexi-Interact Platinum for Palm OS. Hudson, Ohio: Lexi-Comp Inc; 2004.
25. McKenney JM, Proctin JD, Harris S, et al. A comparison of the efficacy and toxic effects of sustained versus immediate release niacin in hypercholesterolemia patients. JAMA. 1994;271:672-7.
26. Oh R. Practical applications of fish oil (omega-3 fatty acids) in primary care. J Am Board Fam Pract. 2005;18:28-36.
27. Studer M, Briel M, Leimenstoll B, et al. Effect of different antilipidemic agents and diets on mortality: a systematic review. Arch Intern Med. 2005;165:725-30.
28. Brown M. Do vitamin E and fish oil protect against ischaemic heart disease? Lancet. 1999;354:441-2.
29. Carter BL, Saseen JJ. Hypertension. In: Pharmacotherapy: A Pathophysiologic Approach, 6th ed. Dipiro JT, Talbert RL, Yee GC, Matzke GR, Wells BG, Posey LM, eds. New York: McGraw Hill Companies, Inc; 2005.
30. Sowers JR, Haffner SM. Treatment of cardiovascular and renal risk factors in the diabetic hypertensive. Hypertension. 2002;40:781-8.
31. Higashi Y, Sasaki S, Nakagawa K, et al. Endothelial function and oxidative stress in renovascular hypertension. N Engl J Med. 2002;346:1954-62.
32. Carter BL. Management of essential hypertension. In: Pharmacotherapy Self-Assessment Program Book 1: Cardiovascular I, 4th ed. Kansas City, Mo: American College of Clinical Pharmacy; 2001:1-39.
33. Jacobsen EJ. Hypertension: update on use of angiotensin II receptor blockers. Geriatrics. 2001;56(2):25-8.
34. Ramahi TM. Expanded role for ARBs in cardiovascular and renal disease. Postgrad Med. 2001;109(4):115-22.
35. Willenheimer R, Dahlof B, Rydberg E, et al. AT-1 receptor blockers in hypertension and heart failure: clinical experience and future directions. Eur Heart J. 1999;20(14):997-1008.

36. Chobanian AV, Bakris GL, Black HR, et al. The Seventh Report of the Joint National Committee on Prevention, Detection, Evaluation, and Treatment of High Blood Pressure: the JNC 7 report. JAMA. 2003;289:2560-72.

37. American Diabetes Association. Treatment of hypertension in adults with diabetes. Diabetes Care. 2003;26suppl:S80-2.

38. Kidney Disease Outcomes Quality Initiative (K/DOQI). K/DOQI Clinical Practice Guidelines: Hypertension and Antihypertensive Agents in Chronic Kidney Disease. Am J Kidney Dis. 2004;435 suppl 1: S1-290.

39. Hypertension/heart failure agents. In: Monthly Prescribing Guide: November. Montvale NJ: Thompson PDR; 2005:99-126.

40. Cardiovascular system: antihypertensives. In: Monthly Prescribing Reference. Nov 2005. On the Internet: www.prescribingReference.com Accessed 28 Nov 2005.

41. Black HR. The evolution of low-dose diuretic therapy: the lessons from clinical trials. Am J Med. 1996;101(3A):47S-52S.

42. Sullivan TJ. Cross-reactions among furosemide, hydrochlorothiazide, and sulfonamides. JAMA. 1991;265(1):120-1.

43. Fries ED. The efficacy and safety of diuretics in treating hypertension. Ann Intern Med. 1995;122(3):223-6.

44. Siegel D, Saliba P, Haffner S. Glucose and insulin levels during diuretic therapy in hypertensive men. Hypertension. 1994;236 pt 1:688-94.

45. ALLHAT Officers and Coordinators for the ALLHAT Collaborative Research Group. The Antihypertensive and Lipid-Lowering Treatment to Prevent Heart Attack Trial. Major outcomes in high-risk hypertensive patients randomized to angiotensin-converting enzyme inhibitor or calcium channel blocker vs diuretic: The Antihypertensive and Lipid-Lowering Treatment to Prevent Heart Attack Trial (ALLHAT). JAMA. 2002;288(23):2981-97.

46. Beta-Adrenergic Blocking Agents. Drug Facts and Comparisons. eFacts [online]. Wolters Kluwer Health, Inc; 2005. Accessed 9 Dec 2005.

47. Propranolol (drug monograph). In: DRUGDEX® System (electronic version). Klasco RK, ed. Greenwood Village, Colo: Thomson Micromedex. On the Internet: www.thomsonhc.com. Accessed 7 Dec 2005.

48. Verschoor L, Wolffenbuttel BH, Weber RF. Beta-blockade and carbohydrate metabolism: theoretical aspects and clinical implications. J Cardiovasc Pharmacol. 1986;8suppl 11:S92-5.

49. Freemantle N, Cleland J, Young P, et al. Beta blockade after myocardial infarction: systematic review and meta regression analysis. BMJ. 1999;318(7200):1730-7.

50. Salpeter S, Ormiston T, Salpeter E. Cardioselective beta-blockers for reversible airway disease. Cochrane Database Syst Rev. 2002;(1):CD002992.

51. Kleinbaum J, Shamoon H. Effect of Propranolol on delayed glucose recovery after insulin-induced hypoglycemia in normal and diabetic subjects. Diabetes Care. 1984;7(2):155-62.

52. Lakshman MR, Reda DJ, Materson BJ, et al. Diuretics and beta-blockers do not have adverse effects at 1 year on plasma lipid and lipoprotein profiles in men with hypertension. Department of Veterans Affairs Cooperative Study Group on Antihypertensive Agents. Arch Intern Med. 1999;159(6):551-8.

53. Ruggenenti P, Fassi A, Bergamo Nephrologic Diabetes Complications Trial (BENEDICT) Investigators. Preventing microalbuminuria in type 2 diabetes. N Engl J Med. 2004;351(19):1941-51.

54. Smith AC, Toto R, Bakris GL. Differential effects of calcium channel blockers on size selectivity of proteinuria in diabetic glomerulopathy. Kidney Int. 1998;54(3):889-96.

55. Bakris GL, Mangrum A, Copley JB, et al. Effect of calcium channel or beta-blockade on the progression of diabetic nephropathy in African Americans. Hypertension. 1997;29(3):744-50.

56. Hemmelder MH, de Zeeuw D, de Jong PE. Antiproteinuric efficacy of verapamil in comparison to trandolapril in non-diabetic renal disease. Nephrol Dial Transplant. 1999;14(1):98-104.

57. Calcium Channel Blocking Agents. Drug Facts and Comparisons. eFacts [online]. Wolters Kluwer Health, Inc; 2005. Accessed 9 Nov 2005.

58. Diltiazem (drug monograph). In: DRUGDEX® System (electronic version). Klasco RK, ed. Greenwood Village, Colo: Thomson Micromedex. On the Internet: www.thomsonhc.com. Accessed 9 Dec 2005.

59. Alpha-1-adrenergic blockers. Drug Facts and Comparisons. eFacts [online]. Wolters Kluwer Health, Inc; 2005. Accessed 9 Nov 2005.

60. Methyldopa (monograph). Drug Facts and Comparisons. eFacts [online]. Wolters Kluwer Health, Inc; 2005. Accessed 9 Dec 2005.

61. Clonidine (drug monograph). In: DRUGDEX® System (electronic version). Klasco RK, ed. Greenwood Village, Colo: Thomson Micromedex. On the Internet: www.thomsonhc.com. Accessed 9 Dec 2005.

62. Methyldopa (drug monograph). In: DRUGDEX® System (electronic version). Klasco RK, ed. Greenwood Village, Colo: Thomson Micromedex. On the Internet: www.thomsonhc.com. Accessed 9 Dec 2005.

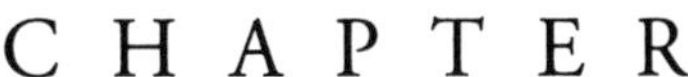

CHAPTER

19

Biological Complementary Therapies in Diabetes

Author

Laura Shane-McWhorter, PharmD, BCPS, FASCP, BC-ADM, CDE

Key Concepts

- Biological complementary therapies include botanical, vitamin, and mineral products; these are sometimes referred to as "dietary supplements" and "over-the-counter" (OTC) products
- The Dietary Supplement Health and Education Act (DSHEA) of 1994 provides a specific definition of dietary supplements
- Many persons with diabetes use dietary supplements to lower blood glucose or treat diabetes-related comorbidities or diabetes-related complications
- There are a number of reasons for concern with the use of biological complementary therapies
- Biological complementary or CAM therapies have various chemical ingredients and varying theorized mechanisms of action
- As with other pharmacologically active agents, CAM therapies may produce side effects and drug interactions
- Those involved in diabetes care and education should develop a clear understanding of biological complementary therapies to be able to provide unbiased, nonjudgmental information to patients about these therapies
- Evidence-based references should be used to answer questions about CAM products

Introduction

This chapter reviews information on biological complementary therapies of interest for use in diabetes care, including therapies aimed at the complications of diabetes. Before looking at specific therapies that patients may propose, we frame the issue in broader terms so those on the care team can discuss safety, evaluation, and information-gathering strategies with patients.

The increased numbers of persons with diabetes has precipitated an interest in use of many therapeutic modalities for treatment, ranging from medical nutrition therapy to increased physical activity and use of pharmacological agents. However, along with traditional medications, some persons with diabetes have turned to use of nontraditional therapies, including complementary and alternative medicine (CAM). There is a broad range of therapeutic modalities that are considered CAM treatments. A landmark study of "alternative medicine" use stated that these therapies included acupuncture, relaxation techniques, massage, chiropractic, and spiritual healing as well as consumption of herbal medicine and megavitamins.[1]

The National Center for Complementary and Alternative Medicine (NCCAM) has provided a definition of complementary and alternative medicine. According to the NCCAM, complementary and alternative medicine covers a broad range of healing philosophies, approaches, and therapies. CAM is generally defined as treatments and healthcare practices not widely taught in medical schools, not generally used in hospitals, and not usually reimbursed by insurance companies. In many therapies, the healthcare practitioner considers the whole person, including physical, mental, emotional, and spiritual aspects—hence, the term "holistic." Some of these therapies are used alone and referred to as "alternative," while some are used in combination with other alternative or conventional therapies and referred to as "complementary."[2]

Reasons for Concern Regarding CAM Use

No large survey currently available evaluates how many persons with diabetes use CAM, but a survey indicated that persons with diabetes are 1.6 times more likely than persons without diabetes to use CAM.[3] Commonly used therapies included nutritional advice and lifestyle diets (such as Ayurvedic diets, naturopathic or homeopathic nutrition diets, melatonin, vitamin megadoses, and magnesium) administered by CAM practitioners, spiritual healing, herbal remedies, massage therapy, and meditation training. Other surveys indicate that 17% to 57% use CAM.[4-6] Certain ethnic groups such as Hispanics, Native Americans, and certain Asian populations may use CAM

Case in Point: Patient Inquires About Complementary Therapies

A 69-year-old male with type 2 diabetes, hypertension, hyperlipidemia, atrial fibrillation, and depression is seen for diabetes education.

- The patient is taking a combination of glipizide and metformin (Metaglip) for diabetes; a combination of losartan and HCTZ for hypertension (Hyzaar); simvastatin (Zocor) for hyperlipidemia; digoxin (Lanoxin) for rate control in atrial fibrillation; warfarin (Coumadin), a blood thinner, to prevent thromboembolic events associated with the atrial fibrillation; and sertraline (Zoloft) for depression.
- He has heard that some complementary therapies may be useful for diabetes and his other diseases. Products he has heard are useful for diabetes include gymnema sylvestre, cinnamon, fenugreek, ginseng, and chromium. He has also heard that garlic may be useful for hypertension and hyperlipidemia and St John's wort may be useful for depression. In addition, he would like to take ginkgo biloba because he is starting to have some short-term memory problems and forgetfulness, such as where he placed his keys.

This individual is concerned about taking so many prescription products. He is hopeful that he may be able to discontinue some of these drugs and substitute them with "natural" products that have no side effects and are more holistic. He asks his diabetes educator to help select some products that may be better alternatives to all the drugs he has to take.

- What products mentioned by the patient may be useful? Which ones should be avoided?
- What other "natural" products may this or another patient consider taking for diabetes or diabetes-related conditions?
- What sources of information may be useful for a diabetes educator to answer the questions this individual has raised?

This chapter helps diabetes educators answer some of the questions raised in this case. Diabetes educators must be knowledgeable about products that individuals may consider for diabetes or related conditions.

more often.[7-9] Summarized below are reasons for concern regarding CAM use. The paragraphs that follow provide the details.

Summary of reasons for concern with CAM use:

- Potential side effects
- Drug interactions
- Variability of products
- Lack of product standardization
- Possibility of contamination
- Possibility of misidentification
- Delay in using more effective interventions
- Additional costs for medical care

Side Effects and Drug Interactions. Side effects and drug interactions are the 2 largest issues that arise with use of CAM therapies. Less than 40% of patients tell their healthcare provider they are using these treatments,[1,10] and a patient may experience a side effect that the provider may attribute to another medication. Many serious side effects have been experienced by persons taking complementary therapies.[11,12] Another concern is potential drug interactions.[13,14] Since persons with diabetes often have to take other medications, concomitant use of complementary therapies may result in toxicity secondary to exaggerated or subtherapeutic effects from their medications. Additionally, many persons with diabetes may take several different complementary therapies concomitantly and the potential for interactions between these agents and with standard medications may dramatically increase. For instance, a person may be taking garlic along with ginkgo biloba and fenugreek, in which case the potential for bleeding reactions secondary to the intrinsic antiplatelet activity of these agents may provide an additive danger to the individual.

Cultural Competence Alert

Certain ethnic groups may use CAM more often, such as Hispanic, Native American, and certain Asian populations.

Product Variability. Product variability is another reason for concern. Products are available as capsules and tablets as well as other forms including water extracts (also called decoctions or infusions), tinctures (hydroalcoholic extracts), and glycerites (glycerin-extracted preparations that are alcohol-free). The quality of botanical products may depend on what part of the plant was used, how it was grown and stored, length of storage, processing technique, and how the extract was prepared.[12] Contamination of CAM products used to treat diabetes has been reported.[15,16] Some products are available in a form that is standardized for pharmacologic activity.

Lack of Standardization. Standardization should guarantee consistency from batch to batch and stability of the active ingredients. However, standardization is not a simple process because the active constituents are unknown for many agents. A product that is standardized for certain markers may show consistency, but the marker may not be the active ingredient. Pharmacologic action may be due to additive or synergistic effects of several ingredients, but the individual ingredients found separately may not have the same activity as the whole plant.[17] Active constituents in extracts or dried botanicals may vary secondary to differences in geographic location and/or soil; exposure to sunlight and/or rainfall; harvest time; and methods of drying, storage, and processing. These variables may affect pharmacologic activity.[18]

Other Concerns Regarding Ingredients. Other factors involve potential misidentification, mislabeling, and possibly the addition of unnatural toxic substances, such as adulteration with heavy metals or steroids and contamination with microbes, pesticides, fumigants, and radioactive products.[18] An example is a dietary supplement found in American stores and available through mail order where the product was found to contain an unlabeled ingredient, glyburide, a prescription sulfonylurea.[19]

Increased Costs. Another concern is the potential increased indirect costs of diabetes because persons with diabetes may substitute ineffective complementary therapies or delay treatment with proven therapeutic agents. These costs may include increased hospitalizations, acute complications such as ketoacidosis, acute hyperglycemia, or chronic complications such as retinopathy.[20] Other potential costs include decreased work productivity and diminished ability to function in a social or occupational setting.

> ***Points for Education***
>
> Discuss with interested patients how biological complementary therapies are vulnerable to product contamination, substitution, and variability.

Dietary Supplement Health and Education Act of 1994

Biological complementary therapies are classified as dietary supplements. Prior to 1994, these products were classified as foods or drugs, depending on their intended use. In 1994, Congress passed the Dietary Supplement Health and Education Act (DSHEA). This legislation created a separate category for botanicals and other products that classifies them as dietary supplements.[21] Under this legislation, these products are not required to undergo the same stringent approval process that is required for drugs and, hence, do not require proof of safety and effectiveness to be marketed. The reclassification has resulted in a serious dilemma. Sometimes contaminants or substitutes have been found in the products. For instance, diabetes products have been contaminated with lead.[15,16]

A possible solution would be the use of standardized products. Standardization guarantees that each dose provides a consistent level of the active ingredient. However, proponents of biological complementary therapies argue that standardized extracts may not always contain all of the therapeutic ingredients found in the natural product.

The DSHEA allows manufacturers of biological complementary therapies to make claims regarding the ability to maintain "structure and function" of the body, but not regarding diagnosis, treatment, cure, or prevention of disease.[21] If a manufacturer makes a claim stating the product affects body structure or function, the label must include the following statement: "This statement has not been evaluated by the Food and Drug Administration (FDA). This product is not intended to diagnose, treat, cure, or prevent any disease." The manufacturer must also notify the FDA within 30 days after a product is on the market if it bears such a label.

The FDA has implemented regulations that ban implied as well as expressed disease claims.[21] For example, claims made by a manufacturer that a consumer could misconstrue as a treatment or prevention of a disease are no longer allowed. The Dietary Supplement Strategy (Ten Year Plan)[22] is a plan that sets the year 2010 as the goal for when FDA will have a "science-based regulatory program that fully implements DSHEA, in an effort to provide consumers with a high level of confidence in the safety, composition, and labeling of dietary supplement products." This program will assist diabetes educators in providing better information to persons with diabetes who use complementary therapies.

Testing of Dietary Supplements

Resources are now available that enable consumers and healthcare professionals to verify the accuracy and purity of ingredients listed on the label of a dietary supplement. However, no resources are available that evaluate product efficacy.

Some organizations have established certification programs for dietary supplements. The US Pharmacopoeia (USP) has a program called the Dietary Supplement Verification Program.[23] A product showing the "USP-verified mark" on the label indicates the label's product ingredients are accurate, the product is pure and will dissolve properly, and the product has been manufactured using good manufacturing practices (GMPs). The USP Web site also lists manufacturers that have gone through the evaluation process.[23] NSF International (formerly known as the National Sanitation Foundation) also verifies products for label and content accuracy, checks purity and contaminants, and audits the manufacturing process for GMP compliance.[24] Consumer Lab also tests supplements;[25] it tests certain classes for accuracy of ingredient content and purity. All 3 entities require manufacturers to pay for testing.[26] Consumer Reports also tests different groups of products and reports findings in their publication.[27] The National Nutritional Foods Association (NNFA) has also launched a GMP program; more information may be obtained at the NNFA Web site.[28]

Evaluating Claims From Manufacturers of Dietary Supplements

Diabetes educators should be aware of and instruct patients about deceptive marketing tactics manufacturers may use to promote their products. A source of information is the article on the FDA Web site "How to Spot Health Fraud."[29] Other resources are discussed below.

Warn consumers to be wary of products making claims such as these:

- Product claims to have benefit in a variety of unrelated diseases (eg, problems ranging from menstrual problems to asthma to rheumatology complaints)
- Product for which the evidence of benefit is based on personal testimonials
- Product claiming an unusually rapid benefit
- Meaningless phrases of benefit that sound scientifically impressive, but for which a consumer is unable to determine veracity

Questions to ask manufacturers:

- Has the product been evaluated in clinical studies that were published in peer-reviewed journals? If so, can the company share these studies?

Resources

The Web site of the FDA Center for Food Safety and Applied Nutrition helps consumers evaluate information about dietary supplements. Healthcare professionals can read and direct patients to the Center's article "Tips for the Savvy Supplement User: Making Informed Decisions and Evaluating Information" at www.cfsan.fda.gov/~dms/ds-savvy.html. The Web site includes basic points to consider such as these:

- Check with a healthcare provider before using a supplement
- Understand that some supplements may interact with prescription or over-the-counter medicines
- Supplements can have unwanted effects during surgery
- How to report adverse effects of dietary supplements
- How to search the World Wide Web for information on dietary supplements, such as finding out who operates the site, the purpose of the site, information source and references, and whether the information is current

The following information, which includes excerpts published in *The Health Professional's Guide to Popular Dietary Supplements,*[30] also may be helpful.

- Remind consumers that nationally known companies are more likely to have strict quality control and good manufacturing practices (GMP). Some companies import products tested in Europe. A list of these is included in *The Complete German Commission E Monographs: Therapeutic Guide to Herbal Medicines.*[31]
- Encourage those considering using supplements to contact manufacturers. Asking the questions featured on this page may yield useful information.[30]

- Can the manufacturer explain the pharmacologic mechanism? Is there research to support this mechanism?
- Does the company complete an analysis on the active and inert ingredients?
- Does the company complete an analysis on the final product to ensure that contents in the package match what is on the label?
- Does the product meet bioavailability standards for disintegration dissolution?
- Are there any storage or stability issues?
- What are the contraindications for product use?

Review of CAM Therapies

Patients with diabetes may inquire most often about alternative and complementary therapies to achieve two main goals: lowering blood glucose and decreasing the complications of diabetes. Not all products proposed for these uses can be recommended as safe supplements, therapies, or food, as this part of the chapter will show. The sections that follow describe characteristics of (1) botanical products used to lower blood glucose, (2) nonbotanical products used to lower blood glucose, and (3) products, both botanical and nonbotanical, used to treat diabetes complications. These kinds of products are often incorrectly categorized as "herbal"; the botanical and nonbotanical origins are worth noting. Patients may also call them "nutraceuticals." Tables 19.1, 19.2, and 19.3 provide specific information regarding each entity's chemical constituents, mechanism of action, side effects, and drug interactions.

Lowering Blood Glucose. Patients may have heard about the following products for use in lowering blood glucose. Not all are safe or effective. Each is discussed in detail in the paragraphs that follow.

- Cinnamon
- Gymnema
- Fenugreek
- Bitter melon
- Ginseng
- Nopal
- Aloe vera
- Banaba
- Caiapo
- Bilberry*
- Milk thistle*
- Chromium
- Vanadium
- Nicotinamide

Decreasing Diabetes Complications. Patients may also inquire about the following products for use in decreasing diabetes complications. Again, not all are safe or effective. Each is discussed separately in the paragraphs that follow.

- Gamma linolenic acid
- Ginkgo biloba
- Garlic
- Alpha-lipoic acid
- St John's wort

Botanical Products Used to Lower Blood Glucose

Cinnamon, fenugreek, bitter melon, ginseng, nopal, aloe, banaba, caiapo, bilberry, and milk thistle are among the botanical products patients may inquire about for lowering blood glucose levels. Each of these 10 products is reviewed separately below.

Cinnamon

Cinnamon (*Cinnamomum cassia*) comes from an evergreen tree that grows in tropical climates, and the aromatic bark is removed in short lengths and dried.[32] Cinnamon has been used for type 2 diabetes and for gastrointestinal (GI) complaints such as dyspepsia or flatulence. Cinnamon is a popular flavoring agent in different foods and beverages. Information regarding chemical constituents, mechanism of action, side effects, and drug interactions is found in Table 19.1.[33,34]

Evidence. Randomized controlled trial in persons with type 2 diabetes taking sulfonylureas found that cinnamon improved glucose and lipids.[34] Fasting blood glucose declined by 18% to 29% after 40 days in all 3 groups. After cinnamon was withheld for the next 20 days, fasting glucose was still lower than at baseline, indicating that cinnamon may have a sustained benefit.

Summary. Research is currently underway to evaluate the effects of cinnamon in type 1 diabetes. The active ingredient is thought to be hydroxychalcone, which may enhance insulin sensitivity.[33] Cinnamon has been found to decrease fasting glucose, total cholesterol, low density lipoprotein (LDL), and triglycerides. Doses used in the available study were 1, 3, or 6 g per day in divided doses.[34] Although blood glucose was decreased, effects on hemoglobin A1C (A1C) were not reported, thus indicating there is still a paucity of information on this product. However, as a food, the amount that may be used is equivalent to approximately a half teaspoonful a day. Overall, cinnamon used as a food is safe.

*Claims have been made for bilberry and milk thistle (*Silybum marianum*), but there is less evidence for these two and for other products not mentioned here.

TABLE 19.1 Botanical Products Used to Lower Blood Glucose

Botanical Product	*Chemical Constituents*	*Mechanism of Action*	*Side Effects & Drug Interactions*
Cinnamon	Hydroxychalcone[33]	• ↑ insulin sensitivity • ↑ cell/tissue glucose uptake • Promotes glycogen synthesis[33]	*Side effects:* • No side effects reported; may cause irritation or dermatitis if used topically[31] *Drug interactions:* • May ↓ blood glucose if used with secretagogues[36]
Gymnema	• Gymnemosides • Saponins • Stigmasterol • Amino acid derivatives –betaine –choline –trimethylamine (Reference 37)	• Impairs ability to discriminate "sweet" taste • ↑ enzymes promoting glucose uptake • May stimulate beta cells • May ↑ beta cell number • May ↑ insulin release (Refs. 35-36, 38-40)	*Side effects:* • None reported • May cause hypoglycemia[35,36] *Drug interactions:* • Possible hypoglycemia if combined with secretagogues[35,36]
Fenugreek	• Saponins • Glycosides • Seeds contain: –alkaloids –4-hydroxyisoleucine –fenugreekine (Refs. 35-37, 43-45)	• Delayed gastric emptying • Slowed carbohydrate absorption • Glucose transport inhibition • ↑ insulin receptors • Improved peripheral glucose utilization • Possible stimulation of insulin secretion (Refs. 36, 43-45)	*Side effects:* • Diarrhea, gas • Uterine contractions • Allergic reactions (Refs. 35, 46) *Drug interactions:* • May ↑ anticoagulant effects of warfarin or herbs with anticoagulant activity (boldo, garlic, ginger)[36,47]
Bitter melon	• Momordin • Charantin • Polypeptide P • Vicine (Refs. 35-36, 52)	• Hypoglycemic action • Tissue glucose uptake; glycogen synthesis • Inhibition of enzymes involved in glucose production • Enhanced glucose oxidation of Glucose-6-phosphate-dehydrogenase (G6PDH) pathway (Refs. 35, 52-53)	*Side effects:* • Gastrointestinal discomfort • Hypoglycemic coma • Favism • Hemolytic anemia in persons with G6PDH deficiency • Contains known abortifacients (α and β momorcharin) • Seeds have produced vomiting, death in children (Refs. 35, 52) *Drug interactions:* • Hypoglycemia when used with sulfonylureas[54]

(continued)

TABLE 19.1 Botanical Products Used to Lower Blood Glucose

Botanical Product	*Chemical Constituents*	*Mechanism of Action*	*Side Effects & Drug Interactions*
Ginseng	Ginsenosides[35,59]	• May ↓ carbohydrate absorption in portal circulation • May ↑ glucose transport and uptake • Modulation of insulin secretion (Refs. 35-36, 59-60, 62-65)	*Side effects:* • Insomnia, headache, restlessness • ↑ blood pressure or heart rate • Mastalgia • Mood changes, nervousness (Refs. 35-36, 66) *Drug interactions:* • ↓ warfarin effectiveness • ↓ diuretic effectiveness • Additive estrogenic effects • Possible ↑ effects of certain analgesics and antidepressants • Possible additive hypoglycemia with secretagogues (Refs. 35-36, 59)
Nopal	• Mucopolysaccharide fibers • Pectin (Refs. 35-36)	• Slows carbohydrate absorption • ↓ lipid absorption • Possibly ↑ insulin sensitivity (Refs. 35-36, 74)	*Side effects:* • Diarrhea, nausea, abdominal fullness • ↑ stool volume (Refs. 35-36, 75) *Drug interactions:* • Improved blood glucose and insulin with sulfonylureas (without hypoglycemia) (Refs. 35-36, 76)
Aloe	• Aloe gel contains glucomannan (polysaccharide similar to guar gum and glycoprotein) (Refs. 35, 78)	• Fiber may promote glucose uptake[35,78]	*Side effects:* • None reported *Drug interactions:* • Possible hypoglycemia if combined with secretagogues • Intraoperative blood loss in surgery patients where sevoflurance was used[79]
Banaba	Corsolic acid and ellagitannin called lagerstroemin[82,83]	• Ellagitannins bind to protein kinase A subunit • May stimulate glucose uptake and have insulin-like activity (secondary to activation of insulin receptor tyrosine kinase or inhibition of tyrosine phosphatase) (Refs. 82-83)	*Side effects:* • None reported *Drug interactions:* • Possible hypoglycemia if combined with secretagogues

TABLE 19.1 Botanical Products Used to Lower Blood Glucose

Botanical Product	*Chemical Constituents*	*Mechanism of Action*	*Side Effects & Drug Interactions*
Caiapo	Acidic glycoprotein[85,86]	• Improved insulin sensitivity • ↓ insulin resistance (Refs. 85, 87)	*Side effects:* • Constipation, gastrointestinal pain, meteorism[84] *Drug interactions:* • Possible hypoglycemia if combined with secretagogues
Bilberry	• Anthocyanosides (bioflavonoids) • Chromium in bilberry leaf (Refs. 36, 89)	• May ↓ vascular permeability and redistribute microvascular blood flow (Refs. 36, 89)	*Side effects:* • Mild gastrointestinal distress • Skin rashes (Refs. 35, 36) *Drug interactions:* • None known
Milk thistle	• Silymarin, containing silybin, silychristine, and silidianin (Refs. 91-92)	• Inhibition of hepatotoxin binding to hepatocyte membrane receptors • ↓ glutathione oxidation (may then replenish diminished glutathione levels in liver and intestines) (Reference 91)	*Side effects:* • Diarrhea, weakness, sweating • Possible allergic reactions if also allergic to ragweed, marigolds, daisies, chrysanthemums (Refs. 35, 91) *Drug interactions:* • No adverse interactions known • Beneficial interactions with hepatotoxic agents such as acetaminophen, antipsychotics, alcohol[91]

Gymnema

A member of the milkweed family, gymnema (*Gymnema sylvestre* R.Br.) is a woody climbing plant that is found in the tropical forests of India and also in Africa.[35,36] Gymnema leaf has been used for centuries to treat diabetes and as a digestive system stimulant, as an antimalarial, and for other purposes. Information regarding chemical constituents, mechanism of action, side effects, and drug interactions is found in Table 19.1.[35-40]

Evidence. There are only a few human studies, but no randomized controlled trials studying gymnema. Uncontrolled trials conducted in persons with type 1 and type 2 diabetes reported decreases in levels of A1C, fasting blood glucose, and lipids.[41,42] However, these studies did not report important details of study design, such as blinding and randomization. In a study in type 1 diabetes, only 27 subjects were followed for 6 to 30 months. A1C declined from 12.8% at baseline to 9.5% after 6 to 8 months ($P < .001$). At the end of 30 months, only 6 individuals remained, and A1C was 8.2% (P values not reported). In the study of 22 individuals with type 2 diabetes, A1C declined from 11.9% to 8.5% ($P < .001$) after 18 to 20 months.

Summary. There is limited evidence of efficacy of gymnema in humans, although studies are being done. Gymnema has been studied for up to 2 years in type 1 and type 2 diabetes. The gymnemosides may help stimulate glucose uptake and utilization as well as stimulate beta cell function.[35-40] In studies, subjects did not achieve target goals for A1C. If used, a standardized extract should be used. Typical doses are 400 mg per day, standardized to contain 24% gymnemic acids.[36] The product should not be used without medical supervision because of potential hypoglycemia. Doses of secretagogues may have to be adjusted if gymnema is used. Hence, overall safety of gymnema may be a concern when combined with other diabetes medications.

Fenugreek

Fenugreek *(Trigonella foenum-graecum)* is a member of the Leguminosae family, along with other plants such as chickpeas, peanuts, and green peas.[35,36] The plant grows in India, Egypt, and other parts of the Middle East. It has been used as a cooking spice and flavoring agent for centuries.[36] Seed extracts are used to flavor imitation maple syrup. It has also been used as a medicinal agent to treat diabetes, constipation, and hyperlipidemia. Although there are no studies evaluating this, fenugreek has been used postpartum with a substance called jaggery to promote lactation. Since the taste and odor resemble maple syrup, it has been used to mask the taste of medicines. Information regarding chemical constituents, mechanism of action, side effects, and drug interactions is found in Table 19.1.[35-37,43-47]

Evidence. There are few human studies on fenugreek. Most are short term involving few patients, and details of the study design are not well reported. Most studies have used unusual forms of fenugreek, such as defatted seed powder in chapati (unleavened bread) or powdered fenugreek seed. Although clinical studies have been done in both type 1 and type 2 diabetes, details of the study design are often sketchy or missing.[48-50] A recent study indicated that in 25 newly diagnosed patients with type 2 diabetes, a hydroalcoholic fenugreek seed extract improved area under the curve blood glucose, insulin levels, and hypertriglyceridemia.[51]

Summary. Although fenugreek has been categorized by the FDA as Generally Recognized as Safe (GRAS), the quality of studies evaluating this agent is suboptimal. Fenugreek contains a variety of alkaloids, coumarin-like ingredients, and other components that may affect carbohydrate absorption and glucose transport.[35-37,43-45] Most side effects are uncomfortable GI effects.[35] Pregnant women should avoid fenugreek since uterine contractions may occur.[35] Fenugreek has been used as a galactogogue, and it may appear in breast milk and, thus, adversely affect the breastfeeding infant. Individuals who are on antiplatelet agents should avoid fenugreek. The recommended dose is variable, although a typical dose is 10 to 15 g per day (as a single dose or divided with meals) or 1 g per day of a hydroalcoholic extract.[36,51] Medical supervision is warranted with fenugreek use. Women of childbearing age, persons on anticoagulants, and those who have asthma or are highly allergic to different foods or substances may not be candidates for fenugreek use. Hence, fenugreek has limited overall safety.

Bitter Melon

Bitter melon *(Momordica charantia)* is also known by other names such as bitter gourd, bitter apple, bitter cucumber, karolla, and karela. It is a vegetable cultivated in tropical areas, including India, Asia, South America, and Africa. The vegetable is yellow-orange, resembles a gherkin, and is bitter but edible. It has been used as an ingredient in certain curries.[35,36] Bitter melon has been used to treat diabetes and for cancer, HIV, and psoriasis. Women have used it to help induce menstruation and as an abortifacient.[52] Information regarding chemical constituents, mechanism of action, side effects, and drug interactions is found in Table 19.1.[35-36,52-54]

Evidence. Most studies of bitter melon in humans involve few patients, are of short duration, and provide only vague details of the study design, including blinding and randomization. Studies have been done primarily in type 2 diabetes,[55-57] although a small study using injectable polypeptide-P, an insulin-like polypeptide, included persons with both type 1 and type 2 diabetes.[56] Results from these various studies have shown that there are responders as well as nonresponders. Long-term studies have not been done, but a trial in a small number of patients demonstrated a decline in A1C levels after 7 weeks.[58]

Summary. There is insufficient information to recommend a reliable dose of bitter melon.[52] Various forms have been used in research, including powdered, extract, juice, and the cooked vegetable. Some sources recommended eating 1 small unripe melon daily or drinking 50 to 100 mL of fresh juice daily with food.[52] Tinctures and oral forms are starting to become available. Bitter melon contains a variety of ingredients that may produce hypoglycemic effects and affect glucose uptake.[35,36,52,53] Bitter melon may inhibit enzymes involved in glucose production and glucose oxidation, which may be of importance in persons of Mediterranean ancestry.[35,36,52,53] Medical supervision is always necessary when using bitter melon, due to the possibility of adverse effects, especially in certain populations such as those of Mediterranean ancestry or women of childbearing age. As a food, bitter melon is a safe agent; as a supplement, bitter melon may not be safe to use in certain populations.

Ginseng

Two main ginseng products are used in diabetes: Asian or Korean ginseng (*Panax ginseng* CA *Meyer*) and American ginseng (*Panax quinquefolius L*). The root is the part used.[35,36,59,60] Korean and American ginseng belong to the plant family *Araliaceae* and the genus *Panax*. Ginseng has been described as an adaptogen, an agent that may increase resistance to adverse influences such as infection and stress.[59,60] Individuals use ginseng to enhance physical or psychomotor performance and cognitive function and for immunomodulation, infections, sexual dysfunction, and diabetes.[59-61] Information regarding chemical constituents, mechanism of action, side effects, and drug interactions is found in Table 19.1.[35,36,59,60,62-66]

Evidence. Ginseng has been studied extensively. A recent meta-analysis evaluated the effects of ginseng on physical or psychomotor performance, cognitive function, immunomodulation, and other miscellaneous uses.[61] This analysis, which comprised only randomized, placebo-controlled studies, showed suboptimal efficacy of ginseng. In persons with newly diagnosed type 2 diabetes, ginseng 100 mg or 200 mg daily was compared to placebo. Although baseline values for glucose and A1C levels were not stated, lower A1C values were reported.[67] However, the A1C level in the 200-mg ginseng group was 6%, and the value was 6.5% in the 100-mg and placebo groups. Hence, there may have been an issue with the accuracy of diagnosis or the study population. In 2 other studies, American ginseng was reported to acutely lower postprandial glucose levels, when patients were given a 25-g oral glucose tolerance test (OGTT).[62,68] In a double-blind crossover trial, Korean red ginseng has been shown to improve erectile dysfunction, which may be of importance to men with diabetes.[69]

Ginseng products have been found to be adulterated with other substances, including mandrake root or phenylbutazone (a nonsteroidal anti-inflammatory drug); 1 case even led to a positive doping test in an athlete.[70] Furthermore, there has been inconsistency between the actual amount of active ginsenosides contained in ginseng products and the amount stated on the label.[71] The amount actually found in the products ranged from 12% to 137% of what was stated on the label.

Summary. Ginseng is a complex product that contains several ginsenosides with varying effects on blood pressure and the central nervous system.[35,36] Patients should be aware that there are 2 main types of ginseng used for diabetes (Asian and American); hence, doses may vary. Ginseng has been studied only in type 2 diabetes. Ginseng may affect glucose transport and insulin secretion.[35,36,59,60,62-65] Furthermore, there are a variety of side effects and drug interactions that may occur, particularly with antihypertensives, antidepressants, estrogens, and warfarin.[35,36,59,60,62-66] Asian ginseng is dosed at 200 mg per day.[67] American ginseng is dosed at 3 g per day,[62,68] right before and up to 2 hours before a meal. Other forms of ginseng used range from fresh and dried roots to extracts, solutions, sodas, teas, and cosmetics. Length of use should be limited to 3 months, due to concerns about hormone-like effects.[31] Also, blood pressure and mood should be carefully monitored. The overall safety of ginseng may be somewhat questionable due to potential side effects and drug interactions.

Nopal

Nopal (*Opuntia streptacantha*), also known as prickly pear, is a member of the cactus family.[35] Multiple species are known as *Opuntia*, including *Opuntia megacantha*, *Opuntia ficus indica*, and *Opuntia fuliginosa*. Research has focused on *Opuntia streptacantha Lemaire* to lower blood glucose. Nopal originated as a food source in Mexico; the stems, flowers, and fruit are used. Leaves and stems are also used to treat diabetes and hyperlipidemia. Nopal has also been used for benign prostatic hyperplasia[72] and alcohol hangover.[73] Information regarding chemical constituents, mechanism of action, side effects, and drug interactions is found in Table 19.1.[35,36,74-76]

Evidence. Most trials with nopal have been small and published in Spanish only, although abstracts are available in English. In 2 small trials in persons with type 2 diabetes, the acute glucose response of nopal, water, and zucchini or nopal and water were compared.[74,77] A decrease in the postprandial glucose response from nopal was noted.

Summary. Nopal may help lower blood glucose when cooked or taken as a supplement. Although some individuals may prepare a blended shake using raw nopal, the raw stems may not lower glucose. Nopal may decrease carbohydrate absorption due to the fiber and pectin content.[35,36,74] Major side effects relate to GI upset.[35,36,75] The dose used is 100 to 500 g of broiled nopal stems taken with meals.[36] However, ideal doses and the optimal preparation have not been established. Nopal is a high-fiber, low-calorie functional food that may be useful for diabetes and hyperlipidemia. There are no known risks, but long-term studies with good study design of nopal in supplement form have not been done. Hence, as a food, nopal is safe.

Aloe

Aloe (*Aloe vera L*) is a desert plant with a cactus-like appearance that belongs to the family *Liliaceae*.[35] There are over 500 species of aloe plants, but the most familiar form is aloe vera. Two products come from the plant: dried juice (latex), which is taken from pericyclic cells just below the leaf skin, and aloe gel, which comes from the center of the leaf and is of interest in treating diabetes.[35] Aloe gel is used topically for burns, sunburn, wound healing, moisturizing, and other skin problems, including psoriasis and seborrhea. Orally, it has also been used to enhance the immune system and to treat asthma and diabetes. Information regarding chemical constituents, mechanism of action, side effects, and drug interactions is found in Table 19.1.[35,36,78,79]

Evidence. In a small, uncontrolled study in 5 persons with type 1 diabetes, improvements in fasting blood glucose and A1C levels were reported when aloe was given for 4 to 14 weeks.[80] In a 6-week study of 40 persons with newly diagnosed type 2 diabetes, aloe decreased fasting glucose and triglycerides ($P = .01$).[78] Another study showed that aloe added to glibenclamide (a sulfonylurea) resulted in a decline in fasting glucose and triglycerides, without hypoglycemia.[81]

Summary. Doses of aloe are variable, ranging from 50 to 200 mg per day of aloe gel.[36] In 2 studies, 15 mL twice daily of aloe leaf gel was used.[78,80] Aloe gel contains glucomannan, a polysaccharide that is high in fiber and may promote glucose uptake. However, the aloe juice contains cathartics, and there is concern that there may be inadvertent inclusion of these components in aloe products. Aloe is highly used by Hispanic people; the Spanish word for aloe is savila. There is a case report of prolonged bleeding in a person undergoing surgery when the anesthetic agent sevoflurane was used.[79] There is insufficient evidence for use of aloe as an oral product in diabetes. Supplementation is not recommended, especially due to the potential contamination of cathartic ingredients and problems with fluid and electrolyte disturbances. Hence, this product may not be safe to use.

Banaba

Banaba (*Lagerstroemia speciosa L*) is a type of crepe myrtle that grows in the Philippines, India, Malaysia, and Australia. A tea made from the leaves is used to treat diabetes.[82] Banaba has been used for diabetes and weight loss. Information regarding chemical constituents, mechanism of action, side effects, and drug interactions is found in Table 19.1.[82,83]

Evidence. A 15-day randomized control trial was done in 10 patients with type 2 diabetes and fasting glucose levels between 140 and 250 mg/dL, using a soft or hard gel formulation.[82] The trial used a 1% corsolic acid extract called Glucosol™. There was a significant dose-related decrease in blood glucose that was greater with the soft gel product. Blood glucose decreased 11% and 30% with the 32-mg and 48-mg soft gel formulations, respectively, after 15 days of treatment ($P \leq .01$ and $P \leq .002$, respectively). The hard gel did not produce as great a decline in blood glucose.

Summary. Banaba is a tropical plant with promising use in type 2 diabetes. The active ingredients (corsolic acid and the ellagitannins lagerstroemin, flosin B, and reginin A) are thought to stimulate cell glucose uptake by insulin-like activity.[36,82,83] In 1 small study, there were no adverse effects or drug interactions reported.[82] However, the authors only reported the lowering of blood glucose only in percentages, not with the actual numbers. The dose is 48 mg per day of the 1% corsolic acid extract, using a soft gel formulation.[82] There is no long-term information available, and the effect on hemoglobin A1C has not been reported. Safety has not been proven due to the dearth of available information.

Caiapo

Caiapo (*Ipomoea batatas*) is a form of white sweet potato cultivated in a mountainous region of Kagawa Prefecture, Japan. An extract of the skin of the root has been used as a dietary supplement for type 2 diabetes in Japan.[84] Caiapo has also been eaten raw in the belief that it may help diabetes, hypertension, and anemia. Caiapo also grows in the mountains of South America. It has also been used by Native Americans to decrease "thirst and weight loss," possible symptoms of diabetes.[85] Information regarding chemical constituents, mechanism of action, side effects, and drug interactions is found in Table 19.1.[84-87]

Evidence. A 6-week pilot study of 18 patients with type 2 diabetes compared 2 g and 4 g of caiapo to placebo.[87] Fasting glucose decreased with both doses, but hemoglobin A1C decreased from 7.1% to 6.8% with the higher dose (P value not significant). Total and LDL cholesterol also decreased in patients on the higher dose. A 3-month randomized double-blind placebo-controlled trial was conducted in 61 patients with type 2 diabetes.[84] A1C declined from 7.2% to 6.7% ($P < .001$). Fasting, postprandial glucose, and cholesterol also declined significantly. Weight decreased by 3.7 kg in the caiapo group ($P < .0001$ vs. baseline) after 3 months.

Summary. There is preliminary information that caiapo taken once a day before breakfast may help treat diabetes, lower cholesterol, and decrease weight. Caiapo contains an acidic glycoprotein that may improve insulin sensitivity and decrease insulin resistance. Adverse effects are mostly related to GI upset. The dose of caiapo is 4 g per day.[84] Information regarding long-term human use is not available. Overall, caiapo is a promising agent, but long-term safety is not known.

Bilberry

Bilberry (*Vaccinium myrtillus*) is a plant related to the American blueberry, cranberry, and huckleberry.[35] Two forms of bilberry are used: the dried fruit and the leaf. The dried fruit is used to treat diarrhea and improve night vision, cataracts, and varicose veins.[31,35,36] A dried fruit extract has been used for diabetes and hypertension-related retinopathy.[88] The leaf is used for diabetes, arthritis, and circulatory disorders.[31,35] In folk medicine, bilberry is used as a blood-sugar-reducing drug and is therefore a common constituent in antidiabetic teas. Information regarding chemical constituents, mechanism of action, side effects, and drug interactions is found in Table 19.1.[35,36,89]

Evidence. During World War II, bilberry preserves were speculated to improve night vision in Royal Air Force pilots.[35] However, this effect has not been demonstrated in controlled trials.[90] Although bilberry has been used in teas for diabetes, there is no evidence from clinical studies that support this use. It is thought that perhaps the chromium content of the leaf may be responsible for a benefit in diabetes.[88]

Summary. Bilberry contains anthocyanosides, which may be helpful for vision and vascular-related claims.[36] Standard doses of the ripe berries are 20 g to 60 g daily. Decoctions are prepared by placing mashed berries in cold water and simmering for several minutes. The liquid is then strained and consumed. The leaf is prepared as a tea. Bilberry extract, 160 mg twice daily, has been used in retinopathy.[89] Although bilberry has not been reported to cause side effects other than GI upset,[35,36] there are no trials in humans to document efficacy in diabetes.[36] Bilberry may be a safe agent to use, but efficacy is not well established.

Milk Thistle

Milk thistle (*Silybum marianum*) is a member of the aster family (*Asteraceae* or *Compositae*), which also includes daisies and thistles.[91] Milk thistle has been used extensively for various hepatic disorders. It is used for uterine complaints and stimulating menstrual flow. In Europe, it is also used as a vegetable. Chemical constituents are found in the fruit, seeds, and leaves of the plant. Information regarding chemical constituents, mechanism of action, side effects, and drug interactions is found in Table 19.1.[35,91,92]

Evidence. The studies that have been done evaluating milk thistle have had serious problems with study design. Several studies have evaluated effects of milk thistle on hepatic disease with inconclusive results.[92] Milk thistle was evaluated in a randomized, open-label trial in a small number of type 2 diabetes patients with cirrhosis.[93] Improved glucose and liver function and lower insulin requirements were reported.

Summary. Use of milk thistle has been proposed in diabetes to diminish insulin resistance.[93] Side effects include GI upset and possible allergies to members of the daisy family.[36,91] No adverse drug interactions have been noted, but milk thistle may attenuate hepatotoxicity associated with acetaminophen, antipsychotics, halothane, and alcohol.[91] The typical dose of milk thistle for liver disease is 200 mg 3 times daily. Milk thistle extract should be standardized to contain 70% silymarin (140 mg of silymarin). Since phosphatidylcholine enhances oral absorption, preparations containing this ingredient may be dosed at 100 mg per day.[91] Doses differ from those used in clinical studies, which ranged from 280 mg to 800 mg per day. Overall, milk thistle may be safe to use, but long-term safety and exact doses are unknown.

Nonbotanical Products Used to Lower Blood Glucose

Chromium, vanadium, and nicotinamide are 3 nonbotanical products patients may inquire about for lowering blood glucose. Each is reviewed separately below.

Chromium

Chromium is a trace element found as a trivalent or hexavalent form. The hexavalent form is a carcinogen with toxicity occurring only in industrial exposure. The benign trivalent form is found in certain foods such as brewer's yeast, oysters, mushrooms, liver, potatoes, beef, cheese, and fresh vegetables.[35,36] Chromium has been used for weight loss, for its ergogenic properties, and to improve lipid and glycemic control.[35,36] Since increased chromium excretion may occur with steroid use, chromium supplementation has been used to reverse corticosteroid-induced diabetes.[94] Information regarding chemical constituents, mechanism of action, side effects, and drug interactions is found in Table 19.2.[35,36,96]

Chromium deficiency may occur if a person is on total parenteral nutrition (TPN); during pregnancy; or if the person has a poor diet, high glucose intake, or poor glucose control. There is currently no evidence to show that chromium deficiency rates are different in persons with diabetes versus the general population.

The Food and Nutrition Board of the Institute of Medicine determined there was not sufficient evidence to set an estimated average requirement for chromium.[95] An adequate intake (AI) was set based on estimated mean intakes. The AI for young men is 35 mcg per day (30 mcg per day for age 51 and older) and 25 mcg per day for young women (20 mcg per day for age 51 and older). Because few serious adverse effects are reported from excess intake of chromium from food, no tolerable upper level was established. Since there is no accurate assay for body chromium stores, it is difficult to determine when an individual has chromium deficiency and how supplementation may affect the deficiency.

TABLE 19.2 Nonbotanical Products Used to Lower Blood Glucose

Nonbotanical Product	*Chemical Constituents*	*Mechanism of Action*	*Side Effects & Drug Interactions*
Chromium	Trivalent chromium (Refs. 35-36)	• May enhance cellular effects of insulin • May ↑ number of insulin receptors • May ↑ insulin binding or insulin activation (Reference 96)	*Side effects:* • Related to excessive intake and include renal toxicity (Reference 96) *Drug interactions:* • May ↓ blood glucose if used with secretagogues (Reference 36)
Vanadium	Trace element (Refs. 36, 104)	• May function in various parts of the insulin signaling pathway • May have insulin-mimetic activity and ↑ tissue sensitivity to insulin (Refs. 104, 106-107)	*Side effects:* • GI upset • Animal research shows potential for accumulation (Refs. 36, 108) *Drug interactions:* • May potentiate anticoagulant effects of antiplatelet agents • May potentiate therapeutic or toxic effects of digoxin (Refs. 35-36)
Nicotinamide	Vitamin B_3 (Refs. 35-36)	• May improve and preserve beta-cell function • May inhibit an enzyme (poly[ADP-ribose]polymerase or PARP) responsible for depletion of NAD+, thereby preventing islet cell destruction via apoptosis (Reference 114)	*Side effects:* • Headache • Skin reactions, allergies • GI upset • May trigger gout and peptic ulcer disease • May adversely affect liver function—monitor LFTs and platelet function (Refs. 35-36) *Drug interactions:* • May ↑ serum concentrations of certain anticonvulsants (Reference 36)

Evidence. Positive effects of chromium have been shown in persons with type 1 and type 2 diabetes, gestational diabetes, and impaired glucose tolerance.[97-100] Studies have shown variable benefits for diabetes and hyperlipidemia. Lower toenail chromium concentration was shown in persons with increased risk of diabetes.[101] Studies have demonstrated the safety of large doses of chromium III.[97] Trials with negative results used less bioavailable forms of chromium, such as chromium chloride or chromium-rich yeast.

In a randomized, double-blind, placebo-controlled trial in 180 Chinese persons, fasting blood glucose and A1C levels decreased significantly in the group taking 1000 mcg per day of chromium picolinate compared with the group taking 500 mcg per day and the placebo group.[97] However, these individuals may have significantly different dietary chromium intake compared with the US population and may be leaner than many obese persons with type 1 diabetes in the United States. Effects were dose-dependent and were seen within 2 months and 4 months. A recent meta-analysis of randomized, controlled trials evaluated the effects of chromium use on insulin and glucose; it reported that data are inconclusive and more studies are needed to evaluate the role of chromium supplementation in diabetes.[102] Another review evaluated several studies, including those with long-term administration of chromium with higher doses.[100]

Summary. Although higher doses of chromium have been studied and shown to be more effective, a typical dose is 200 mcg per day.[36] Short-term, dose-related responses have been shown, and doses up to 1000 mcg per day for 64 months have not shown adverse effects,[100] but more study is needed. Results from chromium research are not conclusive, particularly in light of the lack of information regarding the most appropriate biomarkers for chromium or the most appropriate formulation. If used, the picolinate salt appears to be the most appropriate form. Supplements containing chromium picolinate in combination with biotin are undergoing extensive study.[103] Chromium is a promising agent, but, it is difficult to comment on its safety.

Vanadium

Vanadium is a trace element found in several foods, including condiments such as black pepper, parsley, and dill seeds; certain vegetables such as mushrooms and spinach; and shellfish.[104] Vanadium has been used for diabetes and for bodybuilding, although it has not been found effective for bodybuilding[105] and has limited evidence of efficacy in diabetes. Information regarding chemical constituents, mechanism of action, side effects, and drug interactions is found in Table 19.2.[36,104,106-108]

Vanadium intake is reported to range from 6.5 mcg to 11 mcg per day for infants, children, and adolescents and from 6 mcg to 18 mcg per day for adults and the elderly.[95] Indicators for establishing an adequate intake for vanadium are not currently available. The estimate of tolerable upper level for vanadium for adults is 1.8 mg per day.

Evidence. Vanadium use in humans has only been evaluated in small studies. It has been studied in type 1 and type 2 diabetes. Improvements include decreased fasting plasma glucose and A1C levels. Other effects include decreased insulin requirements in patients with type 1 diabetes and enhanced insulin sensitivity in patients with type 2 diabetes.[107,109-110] Vanadium has been studied only in small numbers of humans and for a maximum period of a few weeks.[105]

Summary. Vanadium has not yet been shown to be essential in the diet. It has been administered to humans as the sodium metavanadate and vanadyl sulfate salts.[95] There is no established recommended daily allowance for vanadium. The estimate of tolerable upper level for adults is 1.8 mg per day,[95] and studies in persons with diabetes used doses far exceeding this amount (100 mg to 125 mg per day). Although vanadium may function in various parts of the insulin signaling pathway with insulin-mimetic activity, it is an agent for which issues have been raised from animal research, with the potential for accumulation and possible toxicity. Studies have been done only in small numbers of patients; therefore, vanadium supplementation is not recommended. Vanadium is not considered a safe agent to use.

Nicotinamide

Nicotinamide is one form of vitamin B_3,[36] which is necessary for appropriate functioning of more than 50 enzymes in the body. Dietary sources of nicotinamide include yeast, bran, nuts, wild or brown rice, and certain grains.[36] Nicotinamide has been studied in diabetes prevention[111] and has been used to improve blood glucose control.[112,113] The vitamin is available in 2 major forms: nicotinic acid (niacin) and nicotinamide (niacinamide). Both forms have similar effects in low doses. In high doses, they have differing effects: nicotinic acid is used as a treatment for dyslipidemia, and nicotinamide for diabetes and diabetes prevention.[36] Information regarding chemical constituents, mechanism of action, side effects, and drug interactions is found in Table 19.2.[35,36,114]

Evidence. Nicotinamide trials in diabetes have focused on treatment and prevention. A meta-analysis of 10 randomized trials in recently diagnosed persons with type 1 diabetes reported higher C-peptide levels in nicotinamide-treated patients, but no differences in insulin doses and A1C levels after 1 year.[112] A small, single-blind trial in persons with type 2 diabetes reported improved C-peptide levels in the groups receiving nicotinamide.[113] A large, nonrandomized, population-based trial in high-risk children in New Zealand showed promise of decreasing the incidence of type 1 diabetes by administering nicotinamide.[115] A long-term trial, the European Nicotinamide Diabetes Intervention Trial (ENDIT), evaluated diabetes prevention with regular use of nicotinamide.[115] This trial evaluated relatives (with positive islet cell antibodies) of persons with a first-degree family member with type 1 diabetes. Of the 552 participants, 159 developed diabetes; of these, 82 had been given nicotinamide and 77 had been given placebo. Another 2-year trial in children with recent-onset type 1 diabetes found that nicotinamide alone or combined with vitamin E preserved C-peptide levels for 2 years in certain children.[116]

Summary. A variety of doses of nicotinamide have been used; in the ENDIT trial, a dose of 1.2 g/m^2 was used, and the dose used in the IMDIAB IX trial, in which C-peptide levels were preserved, was 25 mg per kilogram per day.[115,116] Nicotinamide is a B vitamin and is theorized to help protect beta cell function by inhibiting enzymatic activity involved in islet cell destruction. For side effects, mostly GI disturbances have been reported, and nicotinamide may increase levels of certain anticonvulsants. Although nicotinamide may have potential merit in diabetes, caution should be exercised until long-term trial results are known and more information is obtained. Nicotinamide may be relatively safe for use, although efficacy is in question.

Products (Botanical and Nonbotanical) Used to Treat Diabetes Complications

Alpha-lipoic acid, gamma linolenic acid, gingko biloba, garlic, and St John's wort are 5 of the CAM products patients may inquire about to reduce the complications of diabetes.

Alpha-Lipoic Acid

Alpha-lipoic acid (ALA), a vitamin-like substance that is also known as thioctic acid, is a disulfide compound that is synthesized in the liver. ALA functions as a cofactor in enzyme complexes such as pyruvate dehydrogenase and assists in the conversion of pyruvic acid to acetyl-coenzyme A in oxidative glucose metabolism.[117] Information regarding chemical constituents, mechanism of action, side effects, and drug interactions is found in Table 19.3.[35,36,118,119]

Alpha-lipoic acid is readily converted to the reduced form, dihydrolipoic acid (DHLA). ALA and DHLA are both potent antioxidants.[118] ALA may increase insulin sensitivity.[119] In vitro and animal research has shown that elevated glucose may increase free radical–mediated oxidation, which in turn is implicated in the pathogenesis of diabetic neuropathy.[120] Since ALA may decrease oxidative stress (caused by increased blood glucose), it may potentially help to minimize symptoms of neuropathy.[36] ALA has been widely used in Germany to treat peripheral neuropathy.[36]

Evidence. ALA has been studied in a series of Alpha-Lipoic Acid in Diabetic Neuropathy (ALADIN) trials.[121-123] The first trial in type 2 diabetes patients with symptomatic peripheral neuropathy reported improvements in symptoms of neuropathy after 3 weeks of intravenous (IV) ALA.[121] ALADIN II was a trial in patients with type 1 or type 2 diabetes with polyneuropathy symptoms.[122] ALA was administered intravenously for 5 days and then orally for 2 years. Improvements were again noted in symptoms of neuropathy. ALADIN III was a trial in patients with type 1 diabetes.[123] Both IV and oral ALA were studied: IV treatment for 3 weeks, then oral for 6 months. Improvements in symptoms were significant only after 19 days.

The NATHAN I (Neurological Assessment of Thioctic Acid in Neuropathy) trial is an ongoing, long-term, multicenter trial in North America and Europe that is assessing the role of ALA given orally in prevention and treatment of diabetic neuropathy.[124] NATHAN II addressed the use of an intravenous agent for relief of painful neuropathy symptoms, but this has not yet been published. The SYDNEY trial[125] was a randomized, controlled trial in 120 patients in which ALA was given intravenously or placebo was given 5 days a week for a total of 14 treatments. Total symptom scores declined significantly.[125] A meta-analysis of 1258 persons in trials that used IV ALA or placebo (ALADIN I and III trials, the NATHAN II and SYDNEY trials) found that 52.7% of patients on ALA versus 36.9% on placebo had improved total symptom scores.[126]

Summary. ALA is a much-studied agent that may potentially help with peripheral neuropathy. Hyperglycemia has been theorized to result in complications by the production of free radicals, and ALA may help attenuate the damaging activity of these chemicals by its antioxidant activity. No serious side effects have been reported, even though it has been used intravenously and in long-term trials. Minor GI side effects may occur. Decreases in A1C levels have not been significant.[121-123] Typical doses of oral ALA are 600 mg to 1200 mg per day.[36] Although ALA has been used for decades in Germany, long-term trials are necessary to determine whether ALA slows the progression of neuropathy versus only improving the neuropathy symptoms. The American Diabetes Association does not recommend use of unproven therapies, but ALA is a relatively safe agent to use.

Gamma Linolenic Acid

Gamma linolenic acid (GLA) is an omega-6 fatty acid. The main source used in nutritional supplements is evening primrose oil,[35,36] which is extracted from the small seeds of the plant. GLA is used as a nutritional supplement or as an ingredient in food products in many countries. GLA has been used to treat diabetic neuropathy, hyperlipidemia, mastitis, premenstrual syndrome (PMS), eczema, rheumatoid arthritis, and multiple sclerosis.[35] Linolenic acid conversion to GLA is thought to be impaired in neuropathy, potentially leading to problems with nerve function. Supplementation with GLA may alleviate these problems.[127] Information regarding chemical constituents, mechanism of action, side effects, and drug interactions is found in Table 19.3.[35,36,127,128]

Evidence. Clinical trials have evaluated GLA use in peripheral neuropathy in both type 1 and type 2 diabetes. A small trial in persons with type 1 and type 2 diabetes reported improvements in neuropathy scores.[127] In a 1-year, multicenter trial in persons with type 1 and type 2 diabetes

TABLE 19.3 Products (Botanical and Nonbotanical) Used to Treat Diabetes Complications

Product	*Chemical Constituents*	*Mechanism of Action*	*Side Effects & Drug Interactions*
Alpha-lipoic acid	Disulfide compound synthesized in the liver (Refs. 117-119)	• ↑ insulin sensitivity • Functions as antioxidant to: –scavenge free radicals –regenerate endogenous antioxidants (Vitamins C & E, glutathione) –metal chelating activity (Refs. 118-120)	*Side effects:* • May cause GI upset • Possible skin allergies (Reference 118) *Drug interactions:* • Possible hypoglycemia if combined with secretagogues (Reference 118)
Gamma linolenic acid (GLA)	Omega-6 essential fatty acid (Refs. 35-36)	GLA is converted to dihomo-gamma-linolenic acid and arachidonic acid; these are prostaglandin precursors that: • Regulate platelet aggregation • Maintain blood flow in small blood vessels (Refs. 35-36, 127)	*Side effects:* • Headache, GI upset • Case reports of bleeding time prolongation • Case report of seizures (Refs. 35-36) *Drug interactions:* • Theoretical interaction with phenothiazines with result in seizure activity (Refs. 35-36)
Ginkgo biloba	• Flavonoids (ginkgo-flavone glycosides) • Terpenoids –ginkgolides –bilobalides (Reference 129)	• Flavone glycosides have antioxidant activity and inhibit platelet aggregation • Ginkgolides may improve circulation and inhibit platelet activating factor • Bilobalides are thought to be neuroprotective (Reference 129)	*Side effects:* • Headache • GI upset • Bleeding reactions • Seizures if handling or eating the seeds (Refs. 35-36, 130-131) *Drug interactions:* • Bleeding reactions if combined with drugs or complementary products having antiplatelet properties[36] • May slightly increase serum concentrations of certain drugs including some antipsychotics, cardiac medications, warfarin, and caffeine[36] • Coma when combined with trazodone[132]

(continued)

TABLE 19.3 Products (Botanical and Nonbotanical) Used to Treat Diabetes Complications

Product	*Chemical Constituents*	*Mechanism of Action*	*Side Effects & Drug Interactions*
Garlic	• Alliin –Must be converted to allicin (active form) by the enzyme allinase • Ajoene (formed by acid-catalyzed reaction from 2 allicin molecules • Allylpropyl disulfide (Refs. 35-36)	• Antioxidant activity • Allicin may ↑ levels of catylase and glutathione peroxidase activity • Ajoene ↓ the activity of factors needed for lipid synthesis by reducing the thiol group in coenzyme A and HMG CoA reductase and by oxidizing NADPH • Ajoene has antiplatelet activity and interferes with thromboxane synthesis and ↓ platelet activity • Allopropyl disulfide may ↓ blood glucose and ↑ insulin • ↑ serum insulin and improved hepatic glycogen storage (Refs. 35-36, 137)	*Side effects:* • ↑ gastrointestinal upset[35,36] • Bleeding reactions[138-140] *Drug interactions:* • Additive antiplatelet effects when combined with drugs or complementary products having antiplatelet properties[35,36]
St John's wort	• Hypericin • Hyperforin (Refs. 35-36)	• Serotonergic activity as well as possible effects on other neurotransmitters (Refs. 35-36)	*Side effects:* • Phototoxicity • Gastrointestinal upset, anxiety • ↑ thyroid stimulating hormone • Withdrawal symptoms when discontinued abruptly (Refs. 35-36, 144-146) *Drug interactions:* • Induces metabolism of certain drugs, thereby decreasing their serum concentrations (certain antihypertensives, certain statins, warfarin, digoxin, oral contraceptives, cyclosporine, protease inhibitors)[36,147] • Serotonin syndrome if combined with serotonergic drugs such as paroxetine or fluoxetine[36,147]

who were given 480 mg of GLA, significant improvements were reported in 13 of 16 parameters of neuropathy.[128]

Summary. GLA is a product that has been highly used for a variety of therapeutic purposes. This agent is relatively benign; most adverse effects are mild and include headache and GI discomfort. There are reports of prolonged bleeding time and 1 case of seizure activity, although these have been only case reports.[35,36] Since A1C levels do not improve with GLA, the beneficial effects on symptoms of neuropathy are not secondary to blood glucose control.[127,128] Doses of GLA used to treat neuropathy are 360 mg to 480 mg per day.[36,127,128] For maximal absorption, GLA should be taken with food. The role of GLA in treating neuropathic complications is unknown at this time. Overall, GLA is a safe agent to use.

Gingko Biloba

Gingko biloba is one of the world's oldest living tree species, dating back over 200 million years.[36] Extracts from dried leaves of younger trees are used in complementary therapies. Gingko biloba is one of the most widely used drugs in Germany, where it is widely used for cerebrovascular insufficiency and dementia.[129] In diabetes, gingko biloba may be useful for peripheral circulatory problems (such as intermittent claudication) and retinopathy.[35,36] Information regarding chemical constituents, mechanism of action, side effects, and drug interactions is found in Table 19.3.[35,36,129-132]

Evidence. A meta-analysis evaluated the effect of gingko biloba on intermittent claudication and reported an increase in pain-free walking distance.[133] The weighted mean difference was 34 meters. A 3-month study in 25 persons with type 2 diabetes and retinopathy found that 240 mg per day of a ginkgo biloba extract improved retinal capillary circulation without increasing blood glucose.[134]

Summary. Ginkgo biloba is a highly used product, both by persons with and without diabetes. It contains different flavonoids and terpenoids that may improve circulation and have antioxidant activity.[35,36] However, one of the biggest issues with ginkgo biloba is the antiplatelet activity. There are many case reports of bleeding reactions; thus, the possibility of interactions with drugs or complementary therapies with antiplatelet activity warrants caution. Hence, ginkgo biloba should not be used with warfarin, aspirin, COX-2 inhibitors, or CAM therapies (ginger, garlic, feverfew, as well as many other CAM therapies). Also, ginkgo biloba may inhibit metabolism of drugs that are metabolized by various cytochrome P450 (CYP450) pathways, including 2D6,1A2, and 2C9.[36] Hence, ginkgo biloba may slightly increase serum concentrations of some antipsychotics, cardiac medications, theophylline, and warfarin.[36] Doses of gingko biloba are variable: 120 mg to 240 mg per day for dementia,120 mg to 160 mg per day for peripheral vascular disease, and 240 mg per day for retinopathy.[35,36,133,134] Gingko biloba is administered in divided doses, usually 2 to 3 times daily. Administration for 6 to 8 weeks is required to determine the benefit. Although it may help in retinopathy, the role of gingko biloba in diabetes for lowering blood glucose is unknown; thus, close monitoring of blood glucose and A1C are warranted. Safety of ginkgo biloba use is in question due to the high likelihood of drug interactions and its intrinsic antiplatelet activity.

Garlic

Garlic (*Allium sativum*), a member of the lily family, has been used in cooking for thousands of years.[36] Garlic is used for hyperlipidemia, hypertension, cancer prevention, and antibacterial activity. Garlic has been reported in the past to reduce blood glucose in animals and humans,[135] but reviews of trials using garlic have not shown a beneficial effect on lowering blood glucose.[136] Information regarding chemical constituents, mechanism of action, side effects, and drug interactions is found in Table 19.3.[35,36,137-140]

Evidence. A review of trials that have evaluated garlic use for cardiovascular risk factors has indicated a small, short-term benefit on lipids; an insignificant effect on blood pressure; and no effect on glucose levels.[136] A recently published meta-analysis of garlic reported that garlic reduced total cholesterol modestly (15.7 mg/dL).[141] Therefore, patients should be told that garlic may be of benefit only in mild hyperlipidemia. Persons with diabetes generally need more aggressive lipid-lowering agents to insure that LDL cholesterol is less than 100 mg/dL. A meta-analysis of the effect of garlic on mild hypertension indicated a modest decrease in systolic blood pressure (7.7 mm Hg) and diastolic blood pressure (5 mm Hg) compared with placebo.[142] Persons with diabetes may need more aggressive antihypertensive effects than garlic can provide.

Summary. Garlic contains the sulfur-based chemical constituent alliin, which must be converted to the active form, allicin, by the enzyme alliinase. This reaction occurs when the garlic bulb is chewed or crushed.[35] Commercial preparations of garlic usually contain alliin, not allicin or ajoene. Conversion requires alliinase, which is unstable in stomach acids. Dried garlic preparations may be effective only if the product is enteric-coated to prevent gastric acid breakdown and permit release in the small intestine. Fresh garlic is effective.[35,36] For fresh garlic, the dose is 1 clove daily.[36] Dried garlic powder preparations standardized to 1.3% allicin content have been used in studies. Dried garlic preparations should be enteric-coated to prevent breakdown by stomach acids. Although researchers have noted that garlic use may be associated with increased serum insulin and improved hepatic glycogen storage,[137] studies have not shown there is a benefit on glucose levels.[136] In hyperlipidemia and hypertension studies, garlic extracts, 600 mg to 1200 mg per day in divided doses, have been used. Overall, garlic has shown only modest effects on hyperlipidemia and hypertension. It is important for patients to be instructed that antiplatelet activity is a serious potential problem and that the person may experience bleeding reactions, especially if using drugs or CAM therapies with antiplatelet properties. As a food, garlic is safe; however, when used as a supplement, very close monitoring is required due to the potential for bleeding reactions.

St John's Wort

St John's wort (*Hypericum perforatum*) is a perennial that grows throughout the United States, Canada, and Europe. Its bright flowers bloom in late June, and the flowering top is used in the product.[35] It has been used to treat depression, anxiety, and insomnia. Many persons with diabetes suffer from depression, and this has been considered a complication of diabetes. Information regarding chemical constituents, mechanism of action, side effects, and drug interactions is found in Table 19.3.[35,36,143-47]

Evidence. St John's wort has been compared with placebo and traditional antidepressants. The Cochrane Review assessed randomized controlled studies.[148] In about half of the studies, more patients responded to St John's wort than placebo, and fewer side effects were reported. Another study reported greater efficacy of St John's wort than placebo, but equal efficacy when compared to the tricyclic antidepressant imipramine.[149] St John's wort has been found equal in efficacy to the antidepressants fluoxetine[150] and sertraline.[151] Another study, however, reported no benefits for major depression.[152] Numerous studies continue to be published—some confirm the efficacy of St John's wort in mild to moderate depression; other trials do not corroborate this effect, particularly for severe depression.[153]

Summary. St John's wort is a unique botanical product that has been used for centuries to treat depression. This product is an example of the dilemma mentioned earlier regarding CAM therapies—2 of the chemical constituents, hypericin and hyperforin, have been used as standardized extracts, although it is unknown which of the constituents is responsible for the pharmacological activity. This is also a product whose use may have significant consequences because of the potential for serious drug interactions. St John's wort is a CYP450 enzyme inducer of important drugs that persons with diabetes may be using, such as certain statins, calcium channel blockers, angiotensin receptor blockers, oral contraceptives, warfarin, and cyclosporine. It may also reduce serum concentrations of digoxin and interact adversely with serotonergic drugs (such as fluoxetine, sertraline, or paroxetine) or narcotics and result in toxicity. Doses of St John's wort are 300 to 600 mg 3 times daily.[36] Standardized extracts used in studies include 0.3% hypericin and the hyperforin-stabilized version of this extract. Patients should always inform their healthcare providers if they are taking St John's wort, particularly because of the potential for drug interactions with medications they may be using. Overall, St John's wort may not be considered a safe agent to use in diabetes due to the potential for drug interactions. Moreover, if a person is depressed, use of a traditional antidepressant should be encouraged.

> ***Recommended Resources***
>
> See the FDA's consumer tips on using supplements on the World Wide Web. Educators wanting to know more can also consult the review by Yeh et al, the resources listed in the case discussion, and the ADA statement on unproven therapies.

Other Biological Complementary Products

A recent systematic review of herbs and dietary supplements for glycemic control by Yeh et al provides a comprehensive review.[154] Most of the products included in this chapter are discussed in that publication, but the review also includes other products such as *Coccinia indica*, *Bauhinia forficata*, *Myrcia uniflora*, magnesium, vitamin E, L-Carnitine, and certain combination products. The diabetes educator may find the article by Yeh et al a valuable resource. Quality of evidence for products reviewed was assessed using the US Preventive Services Task Force criteria[155] and the American Diabetes Association evidence grading system[156] for clinical practice recommendations.

The diabetes educator is also directed to the statement by the American Diabetes Association on unproven therapies that acknowledges the widespread use of alternative therapies and the need for cautious evaluation of these products.[157]

For More Information

Below are references healthcare professionals may wish to use to obtain more information:

- *Natural Medicines Comprehensive Database*[36]
- National Institutes of Health NCCAM Web site[2]
- *The Health Professional's Guide to Popular Dietary Supplements*[30]

> ***Research Watch***
>
> Major research is underway on CAM therapies. Look for the ACCORD Trial and similar large, well-done studies.

Case Wrap-Up

All of the complementary therapies that the person in the case has heard about—cinnamon, gymnema, fenugreek, ginseng, and chromium—may have an effect in lowering blood glucose.

Regarding the specific products, these comments can be made:

- The patient may be advised that a half teaspoonful of ground cinnamon may be used in his foods (for instance, in cereal or oatmeal).
- The other products, particularly gymnema and fenugreek, may produce side effects such as hypoglycemia and interact with the sulfonylurea that he is taking to result in additive hypoglycemia. Fenugreek also may produce allergic reactions and adverse GI effects.
- Chromium may be a relatively benign agent and may help as an insulin sensitizer, although there are still unknown consequences with long-term use.
- Ginseng may cause edema, increase blood pressure, and produce anxiety.
- Another concern is that fenugreek, ginseng, garlic, and ginkgo biloba may interact with warfarin with the possible resultant effect of increased bleeding.
- St John's wort may lower serum concentrations of the statin, digoxin, and warfarin and result in subtherapeutic effects of these drugs. In combination with his antidepressant, St John's wort may result in serotonin syndrome.

Self-Care Implications

The patient needs to be made aware that if complementary therapies are used, self-care behaviors should include the following:

- Closely monitor products' effect(s) on blood glucose and A1C levels
- Inform healthcare provider of products used so appropriate monitoring will be done
- Consider that the complementary therapy may have no impact whatsoever on blood glucose or A1C levels; seek to evaluate results in a defined time period

Other Therapies

There are many other therapies that persons with diabetes may be tempted to use. For instance, many persons are treated for depression with SSRIs, such as fluoxetine and sertraline, which may cause them to have difficulty sleeping. Agents such as valerian or kava may sometimes be used to address this problem. There are intrinsic problems in that these agents may interact with prescription sedative-hypnotic medications or with alcohol. Furthermore, kava has the potential for hepatotoxicity and may interact with agents such as statins or glitazones and result in additive toxicity.

Questions and Controversy

The entire content of this chapter is controversial. CAM therapies are not approved for use for diabetes treatment. These are pharmacologically active products that may have a benefit in diabetes treatment. However, it is important to note that many have side effects or may interact in adverse ways with other concurrent disease states or with prescription products the individual is taking. For instance, although ginseng may benefit postprandial glucose values, it may also increase blood pressure and attenuate the antihypertensive effects of blood pressure medications the person is taking. Another equally important issue is that some of the products may have contaminants or subtherapeutic or supratherapeutic amounts of the active ingredients. Strides are, however, being made in this area with different verification programs and with use of standardized extracts.

Those working on the diabetes care team must bear in mind that persons with diabetes are more prone to use complementary therapies than other persons. Certain individuals should not, however, use these products—children, pregnant or lactating women, and elderly people, for example. Those involved in diabetes care and education should not turn their backs on the use of these products. We must acknowledge and respect the healthcare beliefs of patients if they decide to use these products and collaborate with patients who come to us so that we may improve all aspects of their care.

Focus on Education: Pearls for Practice

Teaching Strategies

- **Be a knowledgeable resource.** Because of the increasing popularity of complementary alternative medicines, diabetes educators may find themselves serving as a resource for persons with diabetes who are interested in using such therapies. Strive to familiarize yourself with current research in this area. Develop an open-minded, yet evidence-based approach.

- **Support patients' efforts at self-care.** Individuals with diabetes who are considering use of these therapies are likely to be very actively involved in their own health care—congratulate them for their initiative and interest. Be aware, however, that many individuals are reluctant to inform their healthcare providers of complementary therapy use. Work in partnership with your patients to (1) encourage open communication about complementary therapy use, (2) provide safety and efficacy information about supplements, and (3) discourage use of dangerous or ineffective products and those for which there is little evidence of efficacy.

- **Help patients share information about their use of supplements and OTC products.** Encourage patients to keep healthcare providers informed about any dietary supplements they may be taking. Complementary therapies are not benign; they have side effects and may interact with concomitant diseases, drugs, nutrients, or other complementary therapies. Healthcare providers should know the entire spectrum of products the patient is using to provide the best possible care.

- **Identify patient's goals.** A key role of educators is to help patients identify what they hope to achieve when using a biological complementary therapy, keep records of the effects, and evaluate the impact on diabetes care.

- **Discuss importance of local pharmacist.** Local pharmacist can help patient keep a medication history, check for drug interactions, and so on.

Messages for Patients

- **Make safety a priority.** Complementary therapies are not necessarily safer than other products just because they are "natural." Because most natural agents are not subject to rigorous government safety and efficacy testing, they may be potentially more dangerous than conventional forms of medication.

- **Get the facts first.** Conduct background research on a product before starting to take it, particularly since many products are very expensive and may provide questionable health benefits. Note that there is less published evidence for use of complementary therapies than for conventional diabetes medications and insufficient information to support universal use of these products by persons with diabetes. The American Diabetes Association has published a statement on unproven therapies.[157] Excellent information for supplement users is available from the FDA Web site; see the article *Tips for the Savvy Supplement User* article, at www.cfsan.fda.gov/~dms/ds-savvy.html.

- **Shop smart.** Read labels carefully and use the manufacturer's contact information (phone, Web site, address) so you can ask questions of the manufacturer. Note also the product expiration date. Purchase only standardized products, whenever possible. To ensure purity and safety, buy products from companies that invest in research and meet good manufacturing practice (GMP) guidelines, as noted on the product label. Recent problems have included contamination of products with ingredients that were not listed on the label. Buy products that have been evaluated through DSVP by the USP or NSF International.

- **Check with healthcare team before use.** Before using complementary medicines or over-the-counter products, discuss with appropriate diabetes care team member(s).

- **Don't neglect essential elements of care plan.** If using supplements, use them only in addition to the essential elements of the diabetes care regimen, such as meal planning, physical activity, and medications. Do not use these products as replacements for prescribed modalities. Remember that taking pills does not make up for an unhealthy lifestyle or unhealthy behaviors.

- **Start with small doses and single ingredients.** Starting with single-ingredient products is usually better than starting with multiple-ingredient products because if there is an adverse effect or a worsening of blood glucose, it is easier to determine which ingredient is responsible. Start with a small dose of a product and work up to the recommended dose to determine whether the supplement has any effect on blood glucose levels. Some products take several weeks to determine whether there is efficacy or any effect on blood glucose.

- **Monitor blood glucose levels frequently** when taking any type of nutritional supplement, and share any concerns about changes in blood glucose with the healthcare team.

- **Maintain records** to assess progress toward desired effects such as improvements in blood glucose, lipid profile, blood pressure, weight, neuropathy symptoms, and other aspects of diabetes care.

- **Evaluate effect.** Start by using the product for a specified time period to evaluate the effect. If there is no benefit, discontinue use. Consider saving a few pills in the bottle should the need arise to perform an assay of the product (in case of adverse effects).

References

1. Eisenberg DM, Kessler RC, Foster C, Norlock FE, Calkins DR, Delbanco TL. Unconventional medicine in the United States: prevalence, costs, and patterns of use. N Engl J Med. 1993;328:246-52.
2. What is Complementary and Alternative Medicine? National Center for Complementary and Alternative Medicine, National Institutes of Health, US Department of Health and Human Services. Last modified 2005 Jul 12. On the Internet at: http://nccam.nih.gov/health/whatiscam. Accessed 2005 Sep.
3. Egede LE, Ye X, Zeng D, Silverstein MD. The prevalence and pattern of complementary and alternative medicine use in individuals with diabetes. Diabetes Care. 2002;25:324-29.
4. Leese GP, Gill GV, Houghton GM. Prevalence of complementary medicine usage within a diabetes clinic. Pract Diabetes Int. 1997;14:207-8.
5. Ryan EA, Pick ME, Marceau C. Use of alternative medicines in diabetes mellitus. Diabet Med. 2001;218:242-5.
6. Yeh GY, Eisenberg DM, Davis RB, Phillips RS. Use of complementary and alternative medicine among persons with diabetes mellitus: results of a national survey. Am J Public Health. 2002;92:1648-52.
7. Noel PH, Pugh JA, Larme AC, Marsh G. The use of traditional plant medicines for non-insulin dependent diabetes mellitus in South Texas. Phytother Res. 1997;11:512-17.
8. Kim C, Kwok YS. Navajo use of native healers. Arch Intern Med. 1998;158:2245-49.
9. Mull DS, Nguyen N, Mull JD. Vietnamese diabetic patients and their physicians: what ethnography can teach us. West J Med. 2001;175:307-11.
10. Eisenberg DM, Davis RB, Ettner SL, et al. Trends in alternative medicine use in the United States, 1990-1997: results of a follow-up national survey. JAMA. 1998;280:1569-75.
11. Shaw D, Leon C, Koley S, Murray V. Traditional remedies and food supplements: a 5-year toxicological study (1991-1995). Drug Safety. 1997;17:342-56.
12. Boullata JI, Nace AM. Safety issues with herbal medicine. Pharmacotherapy. 2000;20:257-69.
13. Miller LG. Herbal medicinals: selected clinical considerations focusing on known or potential drug-herb interactions. Arch Intern Med. 1998;158:220-22.
14. Fugh-Berman A. Herb-drug interactions. Lancet. 2000;355:134-8.
15. Keen RW, Deacon AC, Delves HT, Moreton JA, Frost PG. Indian herbal remedies for diabetes as a cause of lead poisoning. Postgrad Med J. 1994;70:113-14.
16. Beigel Y, Ostfeld I, Schoenfeld N. Clinical problem-solving: a leading question. N Engl J Med. 1998;339:827-30.
17. Bonati A. How and why should we standardize phytopharmaceutical drugs for clinical validation? J Ethnopharmacol. 1991;32:195-7.
18. Grant KL. Patient education and herbal dietary supplements. Am J Health Syst Pharm. 2000;57:1997-2003.
19. Liqiang 4 Dietary Supplement Capsules. FDA Talk Paper. 2005 Jul 21. On the Internet at: http://www.fda.gov/medwatch/SAFETY/2005/safety05.htm#liqiang. Accessed 2005 Sep.
20. Gill GV, Redmond S, Garratt F, Paisey R. Diabetes and alternative medicine: cause for concern. Diabet Med. 1994;11:210-3.
21. US Food and Drug Administration. Regulation on statements made for dietary supplements concerning the effect of the product on the structure or function of the body. Fed Register. 2000;65:1000-50.
22. US Food and Drug Administration. Dietary supplement strategy (ten year plan). Center for Food Safety and Applied Nutrition. Washington, DC. 2000 Jan. On the Internet at: http://www.cfsan.fda.gov/~dms/ds-strat.html. Accessed 2005 Sep.
23. USP dietary supplement verification program overview. US Pharmacopoeia. On the Internet at: http://www.usp.org/USPVerified/dietarySupplements. Accessed 2005 Sep.
24. NSF dietary supplements certification program. NSF International. Ann Arbor, Mich. On the Internet at: http://www.nsf.org/consumer/dietary_supplements. Accessed 2005 Sep.
25. ConsumerLab.com. White Plains, NY. On the Internet at: http://www.consumerlab.com. Accessed 2005 Sep.
26. Peterson A. New seals of approval certify unregulated herbs, vitamins. The Wall Street Journal. July 10, 2002.
27. What's in this stuff? Consumer Reports. March 1999.
28. NNFA GMP Program. National Nutritional Foods Association. On the Internet at: http://www.nnfa.org/

site/PageServer?pagename=ic_gmp. Accessed 2005 Dec.

29. Kurtzweil P. How to Spot Health Fraud. FDA Consumer Magazine. 1999 Nov-Dec. On the Internet at: www.fda.gov/fdac/features/1999/699_fraud.html. Accessed 2005 Dec.

30. Sarubin Fragakis A. The Health Professional's Guide to Popular Dietary Supplements, 2nd ed. Chicago, Ill: American Dietetic Association; 2003.

31. Blumenthal M, Busse WR, Goldberg A, et al, eds. The Complete German Commission E Monographs: Therapeutic Guide to Herbal Medicines. Klein S, trans. Boston, Mass: American Botanical Council; 1998.

32. Encyclopedia of spices: Cassia (Cinnamomum cassia). The Epicentre. On the Internet at: http://www.theepicentre.com/Spices/cassia.html. Accessed 2005 Sep.

33. Jarvill-Taylor KJ, Anderson RA, Graves DJ. A hydroxychalcone derived from cinnamon functions as a mimetic for insulin in 3T3-L1 adipocytes. J Am Coll Nutr. 2001;20:327-36.

34. Khan A, Safdar M, Ali Khan MM, et al. Cinnamon improves glucose and lipids of people with type 2 diabetes. Diabetes Care. 2003;26:3215-18.

35. The Review of Natural Products by Facts and Comparisons. St Louis, Mo: Wolters Kluwer Co; 1999.

36. Jellin JM and Therapeutic Research Faculty staff, eds. Pharmacist's Letter/Prescribers Letter Natural Medicines Comprehensive Database, 8th ed. Stockton, Ca: Therapeutic Research Faculty; 2006. (available in book and electronic PDA formats)

37. Kapoor LD. Handbook of Ayurvedic Medicinal Plants. Boca Raton, Fla: CRC Press; 1990:200-1.

38. Shanmugasundaram ER, Panneerselvam C, Samudram P, Shanmugasundaram ERB. Enzyme changes and glucose utilization in diabetic rabbits: the effect of gymnema sylvestre. J Ethnopharmacol. 1983;7:205-34.

39. Persaud SJ, Al-Majed H, Raman A, Jones PM. Gymnema sylvestre stimulates insulin release in vitro by increased membrane permeability. J Endocrinol. 1999;163:207-12.

40. Shanmugasundaram ERB, Gopinath KL, Radha Shanmugasundaram KR, Rajendran VM. Possible regeneration of the islets of langerhans in streptozotocin-diabetic rats given gymnema sylvestre leaf extracts. J Ethnopharmacol. 1990;30:265-79.

41. Shanmugasundaram ERB, Rajeswari G, Baskaran K, et al. Use of gymnema sylvestre leaf extract in the control of blood glucose in insulin-dependent diabetes mellitus. J Ethnopharmacol. 1990;30:281-94.

42. Baskaran K, Kizar B, Ahamath K, Radma Shanmugasundaram K, Shanmugasundaram ERB. Antidiabetic effect of a leaf extract from gymnema sylvestre in noninsulin-dependent diabetes mellitus patients. J Ethnopharmacol. 1990;30:295-306.

43. Madar Z. Fenugreek (trigonella foenumgraceum) as a means of reducing postprandial glucose levels in diabetic rats. Nutr Rep Int. 1984;29:1267-73.

44. Raghuram TC, Sharma R, Sivakumar D, Sahay BK. Effect of fenugreek seeds on intravenous glucose disposition in non-insulin dependent diabetic patients. Phytotherapy Res. 1994;8:83-6.

45. Flammang AM, Cifone MA, Erexson GL, Stankowski LF JR. Genotoxicity testing of a fenugreek extract. Food Chem Toxicol. 2004;42:1769-75.

46. Patil SP, Niphadkar PV, Bapat MM. Allergy to fenugreek (trigonella foenum graecum). Ann Allergy Asthma Immunol. 1997; 78:297-300.

47. Lambert JP, Cormier A. Potential interaction between warfarin and boldo-fenugreek. Pharmacotherapy. 2001;21:509-12.

48. Sharma RD, Raghuram TC, Sudhakar Rao N. Effect of fenugreek seeds on blood glucose and serum lipids in type 1 diabetes. Eur J Clin Nutr. 1990;44:301-6.

49. Madar Z, Abel R, Samish S, Arad J. Glucose-lowering effect of fenugreek in non-insulin dependent diabetics. Eur J Clin Nutr. 1988;42:51-4.

50. Sharma RD, Sarkar A, Hazra DK, et al. Use of fenugreek seed powder in the management of non-insulin-dependent diabetes mellitus. Nutr Res. 1996;16:1331-9.

51. Gupta A, Gupta R, Lal B. Effect of Trigonella foenum-graecum (fenugreek) seeds on glycaemic control and insulin resistance in type 2 diabetes mellitus: a double blind placebo controlled study. J Assoc Physicians India. 2001;49:1057-61.

52. Basch E, Gabardi S, Ulbricht C. Bitter melon (*Momordica charantia*): a review of safety and efficacy. Am J Health-Syst Pharm. 2003;60:356-9.

53. Ali K, Khan AK, Mamum MI, et al. Studies on hypoglycaemic effects of fruit pulp, seed, and whole plant of momordica charantia on normal and diabetic model rats. Planta Med. 1993;56:408-12.

54. Aslam M, Stockley IH. Interaction between curry ingredient (karela) and drug (chlorpropamide). Lancet. 1979;i:607.

55. Ahmad N, Hassan MR, Halder H, Bennoor KS. Effect of momordica charantia (karolla) extracts on fasting and postprandial serum glucose levels in NIDDM patients. Bangladesh Med Res Counc Bull. 1999;25:11-13.

56. Khanna P, Jain SC, Panagariya A, Dixit VP. Hypoglycemic activity of polypeptide p from a plant source. J Nat Prod. 1981;44:648-55.

57. Akhtar MS. Trial of momordica charantia linn (karela) powder in patients with maturity-onset diabetes. J Pak Med Assoc. 1982;32:106-7.

58. Srivastava Y, Venkatakrishna-Bhatt H, Verma Y, Venkaiah K. Antidiabetic and adaptogenic properties of Momordica charantia extract: an experimental and clinical evaluation. Phytother Res. 1993;7:285-289.

59. Raman A, Houston P. Herbal products—ginseng. Pharm J. 1995;255:150-2.

60. Kiefer D, Pantuso T. Panax ginseng. Am Fam Physician. 2003;68:1539-42.

61. Vogler BK, Pittler MH, Ernst E. The efficacy of ginseng, a systematic review of randomized clinical trials. Eur J Clin Pharmacol. 1999;55:567-75.

62. Vuksan V, Sievenpiper JL, Koo VY, et al. American ginseng (Panax quinquefolius L) reduces postprandial glycemia in nondiabetic subjects and subjects with type 2 diabetes mellitus. Arch Intern Med. 2000;160:1009-13.

63. Yuan CS, Wu JA, Lowell T, Gu M. Gut and brain effects of American ginseng root on brainstem neuronal activities in rats. Am J Chin Med. 1998;26:47-55.

64. Ohnishi Y, Takagi S, Miura T, et al. Effect of ginseng radix on GLUT2 protein content in mouse liver in normal and epinephrine-induced hyperglycemic mice. Biol Pharm Bull. 1996;19:1238-40.

65. Kimura M, Waki I, Chujo T, et al. Effects of hypoglycemic components in ginseng radix on blood insulin level in alloxan diabetic mice and on insulin release from perfused rat pancreas. J Pharmacobiodyn. 1981;4:410-17.

66. Siegel RK. Ginseng abuse syndrome: problems with the panacea. JAMA. 1979;241:1614-15.

67. Sotaniemi EA, Haapakoski E, Rautio A. Ginseng therapy in non-insulin dependent diabetic patients. Diabetes Care. 1995;18:1373-5.

68. Vuksan V, Stavro MP, Sievenpiper JL, et al. Similar postprandial glycemic reductions with escalation of dose and administration time of American ginseng in type 2 diabetes. Diabetes Care. 2000;23:1221-6.

69. Hong B, Ji YH, Hong JH, Nam KY, Ahn TY. A double-blind crossover study evaluating the efficacy of korean red ginseng in patients with erectile dysfunction: a preliminary report. J Urol. 2002;168:2070-3.

70. Cui J, Garle M, Eneroth P, Bjorkhem I. What do commercial ginseng preparations contain? [letter]. Lancet. 1994;344:134.

71. Harkey MR, Henderson GL, Gershwin ME, Stern JS, Hackman RM. Variability in commercial ginseng products: an analysis of 25 preparations. Am J Clin Nutr. 2001; 73:1101-6.

72. Palevitch D, Earon G, Levin I. Treatment of benign prostatic hypertrophy with Opuntia ficus-indica (L.) Miller. Int J Comp Alt Med. 1994;Sept 21-2.

73. Wiese J, McPherson S, Odden MC, Shlipak MG. Effect of Opuntia ficus indica on symptoms of the alcohol hangover. Arch Intern Med. 2004;164:1334-40.

74. Frati-Munari AC, Gordillo BE, Altaminrano P, Ariza CR. Hypoglycemic effect of opuntia streptacantha lemaire in NIDDM. Diabetes Care. 1988;11:63-6.

75. Rayburn K, Martinez R, Escobedo M, et al. Glycemic effects of various species of nopal (Opuntia sp) in type 2 diabetes mellitus. Texas J Rural Health. 1998;26:68-76.

76. Meckes-Lozyoa M, Roman-Ramos R. Opuntia streptacantha: a coajutor in the treatment of diabetes mellitus. Am J Chin Med. 1986;14:116-8.

77. Frati AC, Gordillo BE, Altamirano P, Ariza CR, Cortes-Franco R, Chavez-Negrete A. Acute hypoglycemic effect of opuntia streptacantha lemaire in NIDDM [letter]. Diabetes Care. 1990;13:455-6.

78. Yongchaiyudha S, Rungpitarangsi V, Bunyapraphatsara N, Chokechaijaroenporn O. Antidiabetic activity of Aloe vera L juice I: clinical trial in new cases of diabetes mellitus. Phytomedicine. 1996;3:241-3.

79. Lee A, Chui PT, Aun CST, et al. Possible interaction between sevoflurance and Aloe vera. Ann Pharmacother. 2004;38:1651-4.

80. Ghannam N. The antidiabetic activity of aloes: preliminary clinical and experimental observations. Horm Res. 1986;24:288-94.

81. Bunyapraphatsara N, Yongchaiyudha S, Rungpitarangsi Chokechaijaroenporn O. Antidiabetic activity of Aloe vera L Juice II: clinical trial in diabetes mellitus patients in combination with glibenclamide. Phytomedicine 1996;3:245-8.

82. Judy WV, Hari SP, Stogsdill WW, et al. Antidiabetic activity of a standardized extract (Glucosol™) from *Lagerstroemia speciosa* leaves in type II diabetics: a dose-dependence study. J Ethnopharmacol. 2003;87:115-7.

83. Hattori K, Sukenobu N, Sasaki T, et al. Activation of insulin receptors by lagerstroemin. J Pharmacol Sci. 2003;93:69-73.

84. Ludvik B, Neuffer B, Pacini G. Efficacy of *Ipomoea batatas* (Caiapo) on diabetes control in type 2 diabetic subjects treated with diet. Diabetes Care. 2004;27:436-40.

85. Ludvik B, Waldhausl W, Prager R, et al. Mode of action of *Ipomoea batatas* (Caiapo) in type 2 diabetic patients. Metabolism. 2003;52:875-80.

86. Kusano S, Abe H, Tamura H. Isolation of antidiabetic components from white-skinned sweet potato (*Ipomoea batatas L*) Biosci Biotechnol Biochem. 2001;65:109-14.

87. Ludvik BH, Mahdjoobian K, Waldhaeusl W, et al. The effect of *Ipomoea batatas* (Caiapo) on glucose metabolism and serum cholesterol in patients with type 2 diabetes. Diabetes Care. 2002;25:239-40.

88. Perossini M, Guidi G, Chiellini S, Siravo D. [Diabetic and hypertensive retinopathy therapy with Vaccinium myrtillus anthocyanosides (Tegens): double blind, placebo-controlled clinical trial] [Article in Italian]. Ann Ottalmol Clin Ocul. 1987;113:1173-7.

89. Gruenwald J, Brendler T, Jaenicke C, eds. PDF for Herbal Medicines, 2nd ed. Montvale, NJ: Thomson Medical Economics; 2000.

90. Muth ER, Laurent JM, Jasper P. The effect of bilberry nutritional supplementation on night visual acuity and contrast sensitivity. Alternative Med Rev. 2000;5:164-173.

91. Pepping J. Alternative therapies—milk thistle: silybum marianum. Am J Health Syst Pharm. 1999;56:1195-7.

92. Flora K, Hahn M, Rosen H, Benner K. Milk thistle (silybum marianum) for the therapy of liver disease. Am J Gastroenterol. 1998;93:139-143.

93. Velussi M, Cernigoi AM, De Monte A, Dapas F, Caffau C, Zilli M. Long-term (12 months) treatment with an anti-oxidant drug (silymarin) is effective on hyperinsulinemia, exogenous insulin need and malondialdehyde levels in cirrhotic diabetic patients. J Hepatol. 1997;26:871-9.

94. Ravina A, Slezak L, Mirsky N, Bryden NA, Anderson RA. Reversal of corticosteroid induced diabetes mellitus with supplemental chromium. Diabet Med. 1999;16:164-7.

95. Food and Nutrition Board. Institute of Medicine. Dietary Reference Intakes for Vitamin A, Vitamin K, Arsenic, Boron, Chromium, Copper, Iodine, Iron, Manganese, Molybdenum, Nickel, Silicon, Vanadium, and Zinc. Washington, DC: National Academy Press; 2005. On the Internet at: www.nap.edu/books/0309072794/html. Accessed 2005 Sep.

96. Anderson R, Polansky M, Bryden N, Canary J. Supplemental chromium effects on glucose, insulin, glucagon, and urinary chromium losses in subjects consuming controlled low-chromium diets. Am J Clin Nutr. 1991;54:909-16.

97. Anderson RA, Cheng N, Bryden NA, et al. Elevated intakes of supplemental chromium improves glucose and insulin variables in individuals with type 2 diabetes. Diabetes. 1997;46:1786-91.

98. Cefalu WT, Bell-Farrow AD, Stegner J, et al. Effect of chromium picolinate on insulin sensitivity in vivo. J Trace Elem Exp Med. 1999;12:71-83.

99. Jovanovic L, Gutierrez M, Peterson CM. Chromium supplementation for women with gestational diabetes mellitus. J Trace Elem Exp Med. 1999;12:91-107.

100. Cefalu WT, Hu FB. Role of chromium in human health and in diabetes. Diabetes Care. 2004;27:2741-51.

101. Rajpathak S, Rimm EB, Li T, et al. Lower toenail chromium in men with diabetes and cardiovascular disease compared with healthy men. Diabetes Care. 2004;27:2211-6.

102. Althuis MD, Jordan NE, Ludington EA, Wittes JT. Glucose and insulin responses to dietary chromium

supplements: a meta analysis. Am J Clin Nutr. 2002;76:148-155.

103. Diachrome. Nutrition 21. Purchase, NY. On the Internet at: www.diachrome.com. Accessed 2005 Sep.

104. Srivastava AK, Mehdi MZ. Insulino-mimetic and anti-diabetic effects of vanadium compounds. Diabet Med. 2005;22:2-13.

105. Fawcett JP, Farquhar SJ, Walker RJ, Thou T, Lowe G, Goulding A. The effect of oral vanadyl sulfate on body composition and performance in weight-training athletes. Int J Sport Nutr. 1996;6:382-90.

106. Fantus IG, Tsiani E. Multifunctional actions of vanadium compounds on insulin signaling pathways: evidence for preferential enhancement of metabolic versus mitogenic effects. Mol Cell Biochem. 1998;182:109-19.

107. Cohen N, Halberstam M, Shlimovich P, Chang CJ, Shamoon H, Rossetti L. Oral vanadyl sulfate improves hepatic and peripheral insulin sensitivity in patients with noninsulin-dependent diabetes mellitus. J Clin Invest. 1995;95:2501-9.

108. Domingo JL, Gomez M, Liobet JM, Corbella J, Keen CL. Oral vanadium administration to streptozotocin-diabetic rats has marked negative side effects which are independent of the form of vanadium used. Toxicology. 1991;66:279-287.

109. Boden G, Chen X, Ruiz J, van Rossum GDV, Turco S. Effects of vanadyl sulfate on carbohydrate and lipid metabolism in patients with non-insulin dependent diabetes mellitus. Metabolism. 1996;45:1130-5.

110. Goldfine AB, Simonson DC, Folli F, Patti ME, Kahn CR. Metabolic effects of sodium metavanadate in humans with insulin-dependent and non-insulin-dependent diabetes mellitus: in vivo and in vitro studies. J Clin Endrocrinol Metab. 1995;80:3311-20.

111. Elliott RB, Pilcher CC, Fergusson DM, et al. A population-based strategy to prevent insulin-dependent diabetes using nicotinamide. J Pediatr Endocrinol Metab. 1996;501-9.

112. Pozilli P, Browne PD, Kolb H, and the Nicotinamide Trialists. Meta-analysis of nicotinamide treatment in patients with recent-onset IDDM. Diabetes Care. 1996;19:1357-63.

113. Polo V, Saibene A, Pontiroli AE. Nicotinamide improves insulin secretion and metabolic control in lean type 2 diabetic patients with secondary failure to sulphonylureas. Acta Diabetol. 1998;35:61-4.

114. Head KA. Type 1 diabetes: prevention of the disease and its complications. Alternative Med Rev. 1997;2:256-81.

115. Gale EA, Bingley PJ, Emmett CL, Collier T, European Nicotinamide Diabetes Intervention Trial (ENDIT) Group. European Nicotinamide Diabetes Intervention Trial (ENDIT): a randomized controlled trial of intervention before the onset of type 1 diabetes. Lancet. 2004;363:925-31.

116. Crino A, Schiaffini R, Manfrini S, et al, IMDIAB group. A randomized trial of nicotinamide and vitamin E in children with recent onset type 1 diabetes (IMDIAB IX). Eur J Endocrinol. 2004;150:719-24.

117. Nichols TW. Alpha-lipoic acid: biological effects and clinical implications. Alternative Med Rev. 1997;2:177-183.

118. Packer L. Antioxidant properties of lipoic acid and its therapeutic effects in prevention of diabetes complications and cataracts. Ann NY Acad Sci. 1994; 738:257-64.

119. Evans JL, Goldfine ID. Alpha-lipoic acid: a multifunctional antioxidant that improves insulin sensitivity in patients with type 2 diabetes. Diabetes Technol Ther. 2000;2:401-13.

120. Giugliano D, Ceriello A, Paolisso G. Oxidative stress and diabetic vascular complications. Diabetes Care. 1996;19:257-67.

121. Ziegler D, Hanefeld M, Ruhnau K-J, et al, and the ALADIN Study Group. Treatment of symptomatic diabetic peripheral neuropathy with the anti-oxidant alpha-lipoic acid: a 3-week multicentre randomized controlled trial (ALADIN Study I). Diabetologia. 1995;38:1425-33.

122. Reljanovic M, Reichel G, Rett K, et al, and the ALADIN II Study Group. Treatment of diabetic polyneuropathy with the antioxidant thioctic acid (alpha-lipoic acid): a two year multicenter randomized double-blind placebo controlled trial (ALADIN II). Alpha Lipoic Acid in Diabetic Neuropathy. Free Radic Biol Med. 1999;31:171-9.

123. Ziegler D, Hanefeld M, Ruhnau K-J, et al, and the ALADIN III Study Group. Treatment of symptomatic diabetic polyneuropathy with the antioxidant alpha-lipoic acid: a 7-month multicenter randomized controlled trial (ALADIN III Study). Diabetes Care. 1999;22:1296-1301.

124. Ziegler D, Reljanovic M, Mehnert H, Gries FA. Alpha-lipoic acid in the treatment of diabetic

polyneuropathy in Germany: current evidence from clinical trials. Exp Clin Endocrinol Diabetes. 1999;107:421-30.

125. The SYDNEY Trial Study Group. The sensory symptoms of diabetic polyneuropathy are improved with lipoic acid. Diabetes Care. 2003;26:770-6.

126. Ziegler D, Nowak H, Kemplert P, et al. Treatment of symptomatic diabetic polyneuropathy with the antioxidant lipoic acid: a meta-analysis. Diabet Med. 2004;21:114-21.

127. Jamal GA, Carmichael H. The effect of gamma-linolenic acid on human diabetic peripheral neuropathy: a double-blind placebo-controlled trial. Diabetic Med. 1990;7:319-323.

128. Keen H, Payan J, Allawi J, et al. Treatment of diabetic neuropathy with gammalinolenic acid. The Gamma-Linolenic Acid Multicenter Trial Group. Diabetes Care. 1993;16:8-15.

129. Kleijnen J, Knipschild P. Ginkgo biloba. Lancet. 1992;340:1136-9.

130. Kudolo GB. The effect of 3-month ingestion of Gingko biloba extract (Egb 761) on pancreatic beta-cell function in response to glucose loading in individuals with non-insulin-dependent diabetes mellitus. J Clin Pharmacol. 2001;41:600-11.

131. Granger AS. Gingko biloba precipitating epileptic seizures. Age Ageing. 2001;30: 523-5.

132. Galluzzi S, Zanetti O, Binetti G, Trabucchi M, Frisoni GB. Coma in a patient with Alzheimer's disease taking low dose trazodone and gingko biloba. J Neurol Neurosurg Psychiatry. 2000;68:679-80.

133. Pittler MH, Ernst E. Ginkgo biloba extract for the treatment of intermittent claudication: a meta analysis of randomized trials. Am J Med. 2000;108:276-81.

134. Huang SY, Jeng C, Kao SC, et al. Improved haemorrheological properties by Ginkgo biloba extract (Egb 761) in type 2 diabetes mellitus complicated with retinopathy. Clin Nutr. 2004;23:615-21.

135. Castleman M. The Healing Herbs. Emmaus, Penn: Rodale Press; 1991.

136. Ackermann RT, Mulrow CD, Ramirez G, Gardner CD, Morbidoni L, Lawrence VA. Garlic shows promise for improving some cardiovascular risk factors. Arch Intern Med. 2001;161:813-4.

137. Pareddy SR, Rosenberg JM. Does garlic have useful medicinal purposes? Hosp Pharm Rep. 1993;8:27.

138. Rose KD, Croissant PD, Parliament CF, Levin MB. Spontaneous spinal epidural hematoma with associated platelet dysfunction from excessive garlic ingestion: a case report. Neurosurgery. 1990;2:880-2.

139. German K, Kumar U, Blackford HN. Garlic and the risk of TURP bleeding [letter]. Br J Urol. 1995;76:518.

140. Burnham BE. Garlic as a possible risk for postoperative bleeding [letter]. Plast Reconstr Surg. 1995;95:213.

141. Stevinson C, Pittler MH, Ernst E. Garlic for treating hypercholesterolemia, a meta-analysis of randomized clinical trials. Ann Intern Med. 2000;133:420-9.

142. Silagy CA, Neil HA. A meta-analysis of the effect of garlic on blood pressure. J Hypertens. 1994;12:463-8.

143. Gulick RM, McAuliffe V, Holden-Wiltse J, et al. Phase I studies of hypericin, the active compound in St John's wort, as an antiretroviral agent in HIV-infected adults. Ann Intern Med.1999;130:510-14.

144. Beckman SE, Sommi RW, Switzer J. Consumer use of St John's wort: a survey on effectiveness, safety, and tolerability. Pharmacotherapy. 2000;20:568-74.

145. Ferko N, Levine MA. Evaluation of the association between St John's wort and elevated thyroid-stimulating hormone. Pharmacotherapy. 2001;21:1574-8.

146. Hauben M. The association of St John's wort with elevated thyroid-stimulating hormone. Pharmacotherapy. 2002;22: 673-5.

147. Public Health Advisory: Risk of drug interactions with St John's Wort and Indinavir and other drugs. Washington, DC: US Food and Drug Administration Center for Drug Evaluation and Research. 2000 Feb 10. Available on the Internet at: www.fda.gov/cder/drug/advisory/stjwort.htm. Accessed 2003 Jun 14.

148. Linde K, Mulrow CD. St John's wort for depression. Cochrane Rev [computer software]. In: The Cochrane Library. Oxford: Update software; 2000.

149. Woelk H. Comparison of St John's wort and imipramine for treating depression: randomized controlled trial. BMJ. 2000;321:536-9.

150. Shrader E. Equivalence of St John's wort (ZE117) and fluoxetine: a randomized, controlled study in mild-moderate depression. Int Clin Psychopharmacol. 2000;15:61-8.

151. Brenner R, Azbel V, Madhusoodanan S, Pawlowska M. Comparison of an extract of hypericum (LI 160) and sertraline in the treatment of depression: a double-blind, randomized pilot study. Clin Ther. 2000;22:411-9.

152. Selton RC, Keller MB, Gelenberg A, et al. Effectiveness of St John's wort in major depression: a randomized control trial. JAMA. 2001;285:1978-86.

153. Hypericum Depression Trial Study Group. Effect of Hypericum perforatum (St John's wort) in major depressive disorder: a randomized controlled trial. JAMA. 2002;287:1807-14.

154. Yeh GY, Eisenberg DM, Kaptchuk TJ, Phillips RS. Systematic review of herbs and dietary supplements for glycemic control in diabetes. Diabetes Care. 2003;26:1277-94.

155. US Preventive Services Task Force. Guide to Clinical Preventive Services: an Assessment of the Effectiveness of 169 Interventions. Baltimore, Md: Williams and Wilkins, 1989.

156. American Diabetes Association. Standards of medical care for patients with diabetes mellitus (position statement). Diabetes Care. 2002;25 Suppl 1: S33-49.

157. American Diabetes Association. Unproven therapies (position statement). Diabetes Care. 2003;26:S142.

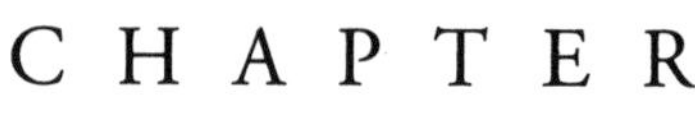

CHAPTER

20

Chronic Complications

Author

Edna Gail Johnson-Gutierrez, RN, MSN, ANP-BC, CDE

Key Concepts

- With the rising incidence of diabetes, the diabetes healthcare community must make prevention, delay, and reduction of chronic complications a major focus.
- Chronic complications of diabetes include cardiovascular disease, neuropathy, nephropathy, retinopathy, and foot complications.
- Combinations of multiple risk factors are responsible for the development of the chronic complications in people with diabetes; some are modifiable and some are not.
- Modifiable risk factors including hyperglycemia, hypertension, dyslipidemia, obesity, physical activity, smoking cessation, and excessive alcohol consumption are the target for diabetes treatment and self-management education.
- Some complications can be minimized and even avoided when attention is given to underlying causes, such as inadequate blood glucose, poorly controlled or uncontrolled blood pressure, and dyslipidemia.
- Dental and skin problems are often-neglected complications. Encourage routine exams and follow-up.

State of the Problem

Chronic complications of diabetes mellitus were unheard of prior to the discovery of insulin in 1921 because most persons died within a few years of diagnosis. Descriptions of renal disease, neuropathy, and retinopathy did not appear until the 1930s and 1940s. It was not clear whether these complications were related to the disease of diabetes or the effect of long periods of elevated blood sugars.[1] Studies such as the Diabetes Control and Complications Trial (DCCT)[2] for individuals with type 1 diabetes, the UK Prospective Diabetes Study (UKPDS)[3] for individuals with type 2 diabetes, and the Kumamoto Study[4] from Japan have demonstrated that these complications can be minimized or avoided with adequate glucose control.

Chronic Complications Can Be Divided Into 2 Classes:	
Microvascular Includes diabetic eye disease, nephropathy, neuropathy, foot ulcers, and skin and dental problems	*Macrovascular* Includes coronary artery disease, cerebrovascular disease, and peripheral vascular disease

Costs, Both Economic and Human. Diabetes mellitus is often referred to as the "silent killer" because it annually contributes to approximately 18% of all deaths and is the sixth leading cause of death in the United States among patients who are age 25 or older.[5] Chronic complications of diabetes are costly not only in terms of human life; the economic expenditures are also great. Direct and indirect expenditures attributable to diabetes were estimated to be $132 billion in 2002.[6] The economic burden of diabetes will become greater over time.

Projected Increases. Between 2000 and 2050, the number of cases of diabetes diagnosed is expected to increase 225%; this estimate is based on age-, sex-, and race-specific rates from the 1984 to 2000 National Health Interview Survey and census projections. Across all ages, the number of diagnosed persons is expected to increase from 12 million to 39 million cases, and prevalence is expected to increase 120%, from 4.4% to 9.7%. By age group and impact, the projected increases are as follows:

- *Persons 75 years of age and older:* Expected to increase 460%, the largest increase in terms of the number of persons affected
- *Persons 65 to 74 years old:* Expected increase 241%
- *Persons 45 to 64 years old:* Expected increase 159%
- *Persons 0 to 19 years old:* Expected increase 97%

Among racial and ethnic groups, the prevalence is expected to increase as follows:

- *Hispanics*: Expected increase 149%
- *Blacks:* Expected increase 118%
- *Whites:* Expected increase 104%

These increases are due to expected demographic changes in the population (26%), population growth (20%), and, mostly, changes in prevalence (54%).[7] Increasing prevalence among younger age groups and the start of type 2 diabetes in children may worsen these predictions in the future.

A Heavy Burden, but an Opportunity. Much of the blame for the economic impact of diabetes can be traced to chronic complications of the disease. Direct medical expenditures alone totaled $91.8 billion and comprised $23.2 billion for diabetes care, $24.6 billion for chronic complications attributable to diabetes, and $44.1 billion for excess prevalence of general medical conditions in 2002. People older than age 65 incurred 51.8% of direct medical expenditures.[8] Once glucose is controlled to a sufficient degree to avoid the acute effects of hyperglycemia or hypoglycemia, the ultimate goal of diabetes treatment is to prevent the chronic complications of this disease and thus reduce the physical and financial burdens.

Multiplicity of Causes. The effects of diabetes complications have been studied over the years to determine if a single etiology or multiple origins cause complications. A combination of complex factors, including hyperglycemia and risk factors, have been found to play roles in the causative factors of chronic complications. In some individuals, a single risk factor may be most important, while in others, multiple risk factors may need to be present to initiate the development of a chronic complication over a span of years.

Education must emphasize prevention and modifiable risk factors:

Those responsible for diabetes education can help prevent chronic complications by emphasizing the following in patient education:

- Modifiable risk factors
- Behavior and lifestyle modifications
- Pharmacologic and nonpharmacologic options for care

All identified risk factors for chronic complications of diabetes must be fully discussed with and understood by persons with diabetes so they can make the best decisions about their lifestyles and participation in care. In any standard diabetes program, educators are expected to emphasize the need to reduce the acute complications resulting from hyperglycemia. As well, patient self-management education must stress methods to reduce modifiable risk factors for chronic complications.

Prevent, Delay, Reduce

These are the 3 main goals in avoiding and minimizing effects from chronic complications of diabetes.

Cardiovascular Complications

The chronic macrovascular complications of diabetes include coronary artery disease, peripheral vascular disease, myocardial infarction, hypertension, heart failure, and cerebral vascular accident. Cardiovascular disease (CVD) is the leading cause of death in individuals with type 1 and type 2 diabetes. Individuals with diabetes are 2 to 3 times more likely to develop CVD than people without diabetes, and women with diabetes are at especially high risk.[9] In 2003, 38.1% of individuals with diabetes age 35 years and older reported receiving a diagnosis of CVD.[10]

The pathophysiology of CVD in individuals with diabetes remains a complex phenomenon. Development of CVD involves the interaction of both modifiable and nonmodifiable risk factors:

- *Nonmodifiable Risk Factors:* Including duration of diabetes, age, gender, race, and genetics
- *Modifiable Risk Factors:* Including hyperglycemia, hypertension, dyslipidemia, smoking, eating habits, obesity, exercise habits, type A personality, increased platelet adherence, increased insulin levels, and increased homocysteine levels

Nonmodifiable Risk Factors

These risk factors are somewhat less easily understood in terms of their relationship to cardiovascular disease.

- *Age.* There appears to be a linear relationship between duration of diabetes and cardiovascular disease and possibly age. Obviously, the older individual with long-standing diabetes is at higher risk for cardiovascular problems than a younger, newly diagnosed individual with diabetes.
- *Genetics and Ethnicity.* Genetics plays a role in development of complications of CVD; however, specific predictive factors have not yet been determined. For example, African American individuals with diabetes have a higher incidence of macrovascular disease than Caucasians,[11] and Mexican American

individuals with diabetes have an increased risk for peripheral vascular disease.[12]

- *Gender.* Prior to menopause, there is a gender-protective factor for females without diabetes for CVD and CVD events; however, there is no gender-protective advantage for females with diabetes. Females with diabetes have an equal risk for CVD as males with diabetes.[13]

Modifiable Risk Factors

Among individuals with diabetes, educators, and providers of care, much attention is paid to hypertension, hyperglycemia, dyslipidemia, smoking, diet, obesity, exercise, and personality types as modifiable risk factors. This, for example, is known:

- *Blood Pressure.* The importance of adequate blood pressure control, defined as <130/80[14] for individuals with diabetes, was demonstrated in the UK Prospective Diabetes Study.[15]
- *Lipids.* Abnormal lipid levels (elevated cholesterol, decreased high-density lipoprotein levels, increased low-density lipoprotein, and elevated triglyceride levels) significantly increase the risk of atherosclerotic cardiovascular disease. Lipid levels are influenced by many different factors, including glucose control, obesity, exercise, alcohol, medications, and genetics.
- *Smoking.* Although the hazards of cigarette smoking have been widely published, many individuals continue to smoke. If individuals are successful with smoking cessation, the change can impact health and longevity as much as reduction of other risk factors.
- *Obesity.* Obesity (defined as >20% over ideal body weight), particularly central obesity, represents increased intra-abdominal fat and is associated with a high risk of cardiovascular disease.[16]
- *Other Factors.* Diet (high in fats), lack of exercise, and certain high-strung personality types also have been linked to an increased cardiovascular risk.[17]

To prevent and delay CVD:

Prevention of CVD in individuals with diabetes must be a top priority. Identify underlying CVD and aim to slow its progression, especially among those with diabetes of long duration. Education and self-management topics include blood pressure and lipid management.

Published treatment guidelines are somewhat inconsistent regarding goals for blood pressure and lipid management, which has caused confusion and inconsistency among educators and providers. Regardless, goals and multifaceted approaches to achieve reductions in risks must become a regular part of the educational process of individuals with diabetes. See chapter 21 for further information on macrovascular disease.

Diabetic Neuropathy

Diabetic neuropathy has a large effect on the health and quality of life for many individuals with diabetes. Several distinct syndromes of neuropathy have been identified, each demonstrating different clinical manifestations, anatomical distributions, course, and pathophysiology. Factors associated with neuropathy include the following:[18]

- Age
- Hypertension
- Height
- Microvascular disease
- Abnormal high-density lipoprotein cholesterol
- Smoking
- Cardiovascular disease

There is no data to suggest that diabetes medications, specific diets, obesity, exercise, or increased insulin levels are linked to development of neuropathy. Complete understanding of neuropathy remains somewhat of a mystery. Thus, neuropathy poses a clinical challenge to providers and those affected.

Neuropathies Are Usually Divided into 2 Types:	
Diffuse Peripheral Neuropathies Including symmetrical polyneuropathies and autonomic neuropathy	***Focal Neuropathies*** Involving single or multiple peripheral nerves and including mononeuropathies, radiculopathy, and entrapment neuropathy

Peripheral Neuropathies

Distal symmetrical polyneuropathies are the most common neuropathy. Presentation usually begins with a sensory loss (numbness or paresthesia) in the toes or fingers, which then moves upward, forming a "stocking" or "glove" pattern. Clinical assessment of sensitivity to touch, reflexes, vibratory sensation, and use of a monofilament to determine sensation is mandatory for individuals presenting with symptoms.

Symptoms related to other peripheral neuropathies include the following:

- Pain
- Decreased deep tendon reflexes
- Cold feet
- Motor weakness

- Impaired balance
- Diminished proprioception
- Ataxia
- Muscle cramping
- Cranial nerve palsy
- Carpal and tarsal tunnel syndrome

Education aids in managing neuropathy:

Treatment consists of control of hyperglycemia, decreased alcohol use, smoking cessation, and analgesic medication, all of which should be topics of diabetes self-management education.

Autonomic Neuropathies

These most often affect the cardiovascular system, gastrointestinal tract, genitourinary system, sweat glands, adrenal medulla, and ocular pupil. Symptoms seen with this type of neuropathy include the following:[19]

- Tachycardia
- Hypotension
- Decreased exercise tolerance
- Heat intolerance
- Esophageal dysfunction
- Gastroparesis
- Alterations in bowel habits
- Incontinence
- Impaired bladder sensitivity
- Erectile dysfunction
- Dyspareunia
- Neurogenic bladder
- Gustatory sweating
- Symmetrical distal anhidrosis
- Hypoglycemia unawareness
- Decreased diameters of the pupils at rest

Autonomic neuropathy often goes unnoticed due to its slow onset. If patients have peripheral neuropathy, approximately 50% will also have asymptomatic autonomic neuropathy.[20] A detailed health history is important to obtain to determine if symptoms or problems are related to neuropathy. See chapter 24 for more detail.

Diabetic Foot Complications

As a result of the increasing diagnosis and prevalence of diabetes in the United States, the number of nontraumatic lower amputations and chronic foot problems has also increased. Approximately 85% of all lower extremity amputations result from a previous foot ulceration.[21] By 1999, the economic impact of diabetic foot complications was skyrocketing, with management of foot ulcers estimated to cost approximately $27,000 per occurrence for the 2 years following diagnosis.[22] Diabetic foot complications also affect quality of life, function, and emotional well-being in individuals with diabetes.

Associated Risks

Several complications of diabetes play important roles in the development of diabetic foot problems. Other associated risks are also listed below. See also chapter 24, on neuropathy.

- *Peripheral vascular disease* as manifested by poor tissue oxygenation and impaired blood flow may cause poor healing, ischemia, and ultimately gangrene
- *Sensory neuropathy* is seen as a contributory factor due to the lack of a protective factor; thus, the foot is at increased risk for undetected trauma or foot stressors
- *Neuropathies* may also lead to deformities, pressure points, and trauma leading to an increased predisposition to foot ulcers
- *Other associated risks* include improperly fitting shoes, nail abnormalities, visual problems, and lack of self-management skills

Helping avoid foot ulcers and amputations:

Reinforce information and instruction on foot care so patients routinely inspect and attend to problems affecting their feet.

The goal of management and prevention of foot complications can be addressed with patient education and self-management skills. Potential complications and preventive strategies should emphasize the following:

- Proper care of nails, calluses, and injuries
- Proper fitting footwear
- Daily inspection of feet
- Follow-up care as recommended

Education of individuals and their families about foot care, enrollment in self-management education sessions, detailed written instructions, and evaluation of the individual's capability to perform self-care will enhance compliance and reduce complications.

Diabetic Nephropathy

Diabetic nephropathy is a complication of diabetes that is characterized by albuminuria, hypertension, and a progressive loss of renal function. It occurs in 20% to 40% of individuals with diabetes and is the most common cause of end-stage renal disease if not treated adequately. The earliest clinical indicator of nephropathy is microalbuminuria, which indicates microvascular involvement of the kidney.

Persistent microalbuminuria in the range of 30 to 299 mg per 24 hours has been shown to be the earliest stage of diabetic nephropathy in type 1 diabetes and a marker of development of nephropathy in type 2 diabetes.[23] By the time the urinary albumin exceeds 300 mg per gram of creatinine, the cutoff point of macroalbuminuria, it is a matter of years before end-stage renal disease begins. In individuals with type 1 diabetes, the development of nephropathy can begin after only 5 years of duration, increasing over the next 10 to 15 years.

As with other complications of diabetes, the pathogenesis of diabetic nephropathy is complicated and involves direct effects by high plasma glucose concentrations on vascular, glomerular, tubular, and interstitial cellular function of the kidney. Changes in renal blood flow brought about by diabetes lead to increased glomerular pressure gradients and cause damage to the glomeruli and defects in glomerular permeability, which lead to end-stage renal disease.

Screening and Diagnosis

Diabetic renal disease is diagnosed by detecting microalbuminuria. Screening is conducted using the measurement of the albumin-to-creatinine ratio on first AM urine or random spot urine and a creatinine clearance rate, which includes a serum creatinine and 24-hour urine collection. Because certain factors can influence the albumin excretion (urinary tract infections, illness, exercise, hypertension, hyperglycemia, or heart failure), at least 2 of the 3 tests measured should show an elevation within a 6-month period. The ADA has guidelines for interpretation of microalbuminuria for each test:[24]

- *Screening of Type 1 Diabetes Patients:* Begin at puberty or after 5 years' duration of the disease and conduct yearly thereafter
- *Screening of Type 2 Diabetes Patients:* Begin at the time of diagnosis and conduct at least yearly thereafter

Risk Factors

There are similar risk factors for individuals with type 1 and type 2 diabetes, including the following:

- *Nonmodifiable:* Duration of disease, age, genetics, race
- *Modifiable:* Poor glycemic control, hypertension, smoking, diet, dyslipidemia

Ethnicity. Certain ethnic groups such as African Americans, Hispanics, and Native Americans have a greater prevalence of diabetic nephropathy than whites with diabetes.

Delaying Onset and Advancement

Management of known factors that influence the development and progression of nephropathy can help to delay onset and advancement of the disease.

Evidence that the control of blood pressure can significantly reduce the development of nephropathy was demonstrated in the UKPDS study.[25] Both systolic and diastolic hypertension accelerates the progression of renal complications. Blood pressure measurements should be part of each visit. The goal, as determined by the ADA Standards of Medical Care in Diabetes, is to maintain blood pressure below 130/80.[26]

If blood pressure is not at goal, an angiotensin-converting enzyme (ACE) inhibitor or angiotensin receptor blocker (ARB) should be initiated if there are no contraindications. In a head-to-head comparison of the renoprotective effects of an ACE inhibitor and ARB in individuals with type 2 diabetes, the primary end-point of change in the glomerular filtration rate was similar in both groups. The 2 treatments had similar effects on the secondary endpoints, including annual changes in glomerular filtration rate, serum creatinine levels, urinary albumin excretion rate, blood pressure, end-stage renal disease, cardiovascular events, and all cause mortality.[27] If renal disease progresses further after other measures are taken, restriction of dietary protein may be initiated.

Self-management important in protecting kidney health:

Encourage individuals to self-monitor blood pressure and emphasize the importance and benefits of adequate control of blood glucose. Promote healthy eating and smoking cessation.

For individuals with type 2 diabetes, the presence of microalbuminuria doubles the risk of cardiovascular morbidity and mortality. For these reasons, early identification and subsequent renoprotective therapy are essential parts of quality care. In addition, patients and their families should be monitored for signs of depression, anxiety, and increased levels of stress associated with renal complications, with referral or treatment initiated as appropriate. See chapter 23 for more information on nephropathy.

Diabetic Retinopathy and Other Ocular Conditions

Diabetic retinopathy is the most frequent cause of new cases of blindness among adults aged 20 to 74 years. During the first 2 decades of disease, nearly all patients with type 1 diabetes and greater than 60% of patients with type 2 diabetes have retinopathy.[28] The 20-year prevalence rate of retinopathy is approximately 80% in individuals who required insulin and approximately 20% in those who did not require insulin.[30]

- *Blindness.* Retinopathy is the leading cause of blindness (defined as visual acuity <20/200) in individuals age 20 to 64 years and accounts for 12% of all new cases of blindness.
- *Visual Impairment.* Visual impairment is more common than blindness and accounts for reduced functional status. A national survey found that 25% of all individuals with diabetes had considerable visual impairment.[29]
- *Other Conditions.* Other ocular conditions not thought to be caused by diabetes but occurring more commonly in individuals with diabetes include cataracts and glaucoma.

Diabetic retinopathy develops as the result of several processes, and it can progress from mild nonproliferative disease to proliferative disease to diabetic macular edema.

- *Nonproliferative Disease.* Nonproliferative disease can be classified from mild to very severe and usually has no symptoms. Ocular characteristics at this stage include dot hemorrhages, microaneurysms, cotton wool spots, intraretinal microvascular abnormalities, hard exudates, and venous caliber abnormalities.
- *Proliferative Disease.* The proliferative stage is usually characterized by reduced vision and accompanying floaters. Characteristics usually seen include vascular proliferation, fibrous tissue proliferation, preretinal hemorrhage, and vitreous hemorrhage.
- *Diabetic Macular Edema.* This stage is characterized by blurred vision and distortion of straight lines and results from leakage of fluid from retinal vessels that accumulates in the macula of the eye. The macula is responsible for color vision and sharp visual effects. Characteristics consist of macular hard exudates and retinal thickening in the macula.[31]

Vision Loss

Vision loss from diabetes may be caused by multiple factors. Macular edema or nonprofusion of the retina may impair central vision. New vessels may grow on the optic disc and, due to their fragile nature, may rupture and bleed. When this occurs, fibrous tissue grows and contracts, causing retinal detachment. If not treated immediately, a detached retina can result in irreversible loss of vision.[32]

Risk Factors

A number of risk factors, both nonmodifiable and modifiable, are associated with diabetic retinopathy, including the following:

- Duration of diabetes
- Age
- Race
- Glycemic control
- Hypertension
- Proteinuria and renal disease
- Hyperlipidemia
- Smoking

Cornerstones of retinopathy treatment and prevention:

As with other complications of diabetes, adequate glycemic control, control of hypertension, and recognition of problems with regular follow-up are the cornerstones of treatment and prevention of retinopathy.

Patient education strategies for retinopathy include the following. For more detail on eye disease, see chapter 22.

- *Recommend Dilated Eye Exams.* At the time of diagnosis for individuals with type 2 diabetes, recommend yearly exams. Individuals with type 1 diabetes should have an eye exam at puberty, if diabetes is diagnosed by then, and within 3 to 5 years of diagnosis. If visual changes occur, more frequent exams may be necessary. Help pregnant women with preexisting diabetes undergo examinations at regular intervals during pregnancy. Discussion with all patients can include asking, "Does your health insurance cover eye exams?"
- *Discuss Self-Management Techniques and Aggressive Medical Management.* Emphasize glycemic control, hypertension, hyperlipidemia, and proteinuria.
- *Explain Treatment Strategies.* Describe laser photocoagulation and encourage this therapy when recommended by an ophthalmologist.
- *Discuss Services for the Visually Impaired.* If significant vision loss occurs, make individuals and families aware of such services and provide referrals.

Dental and Oral Disease

Individuals with diabetes are more likely than others to suffer from dental problems and periodontal diseases. Oral health complications of diabetes include the following: severe periodontitis and subsequent tooth loss, gingivitis, and dental abscesses. In addition, diabetes increases the risk of xerostomia and soft tissue lesions of the tongue and oral mucosa, such as candidiasis. Other commonly seen oral lesions in individuals with diabetes include lichen planus, angular cheilitis, and burning mouth syndrome. Prolonged hyperglycemia and the accumulation of advanced glycation endproducts in gingival tissue of individuals with diabetes are thought to be primarily responsible for oral and other complications of diabetes.[33] Severe periodontal disease associated with diabetes has been considered the sixth complication of diabetes.[34]

Risk Factors

The following are risk factors for periodontal disease:

- *Nonmodifiable:* Duration of diabetes, age
- *Modifiable:* Glycemic control, smoking

Smoking. Smoking has been associated with aggravated periodontal breakdown, poorer standards of oral hygiene, and premature tooth loss and is a major risk factor in periodontal disease; it is responsible for more than half of the cases of periodontitis among adults.[35]

Difficulty in treatment involves increased susceptibility to infection, impaired wound healing, increased inflammatory response, vascular changes, neuropathies, and gingival changes.[36]

Routine Dental Exams

Although the ADA Standards of Medical Care in Diabetes offer no guidelines on dental examinations beyond the initial oral cavity exam, the Centers for Disease Control and Prevention's recommendation is this:[37]

- Individuals with diabetes should see a dentist every 6 months and more often if periodontal disease is present

In a study by Tomar and Lester,[33] individuals with diabetes were less likely than those without diabetes to have had a recent dental examination. These individuals did not understand the need for dental care or the relationship between oral health and overall general health. When compared with other preventive services, dental care visits were the least likely to have occurred. Dental visits are also related to socioeconomic status. Among subjects with an annual income of $50,000 or more, 81.6% had seen a dentist within the past year, compared with only 41.2% of those with an income of less than $10,000 per year.

Avoiding oral disease complications:

Not only tooth care, but also stopping smoking, following the proper diet, and maintaining good glycemic control aid in reducing oral health complications.

Patient and family education issues related to diabetic dental complications include the following:

- Diabetes and oral health
- Adequate glycemic control
- Discontinuing use of cigarettes and oral tobacco
- Proper diet
- Proper brushing and flossing
- Dental examination, at least annually

Prevention of oral disease is important in the individual with diabetes because oral compromise can affect nutrition and adequate glycemic control. Educators should promote dental examinations as an important component of diabetes management and overall health of individuals with diabetes. Discussion can include asking "does your health insurance cover dental exams?"

Skin Changes With Diabetes

The skin can be affected by the microvascular changes known to occur in diabetes. Also, certain diabetes medications and autoimmune diseases associated with diabetes can lead to dermatological problems. Below are some of the most common skin conditions seen in individuals with diabetes:

- Diabetic dermopathy
- Diabetic bullae
- Acanthosis nigricans
- Diabetic thick skin
- Xanthoma
- Vitiligo

Diabetic Dermopathy

Also known as shin spots, diabetic dermopathy is the most common skin manifestation of diabetes. Although it can be present in individuals without diabetes, this condition is present in as many as 70% of individuals with diabetes and occurs most frequently in males.[38] Pigmented spots, seen on the extensor surfaces of the lower extremities, eventually become hyperpigmented macules. The lesions are asymptomatic, heal over time and leave scars, but require no specific treatment.

Diabetic Bullae

These distinctive markers for diabetes are usually seen in adults with long-standing diabetes and neuropathy. They are usually on the hands and feet and consist of either sterile and fluid-filled, hemorrhagic, or multiple bullae. They usually resolve in several weeks, but may return. There is no particular treatment, but prevention of infection is important.[39]

Acanthosis Nigricans

This skin change is usually related to insulin resistance or obesity and ranges in appearance from a thickened, velvety-brown streaking to a leathery-type hyperpigmented plaque. The condition commonly occurs around the neck or in skin folds in the axilla, under the breast, around the belt line, and in the groin, but may develop elsewhere on the body. Patients may state they have a dirty area that cannot be cleaned.[40] Microscopically, acanthosis nigricans is characterized by an increasing number of melanocytes, with papillary hypertrophy and hyperkeratosis.[41] Associated hypertrophy and hyperkeratosis cause acanthosis nigricans to be palpable rather than macular.

Recognizing acanthosis nigricans is important because the condition can be associated with insulin resistance. Type 2 diabetes is increasing in incidence in the United States, especially among African American and Hispanic children; 60% to 92% of these children have acanthosis nigricans.[42] According to a study[43] that compared 50 children with type 2 diabetes and 50 children with type 1 diabetes, acanthosis nigricans was present in 86% of the children with type 2 diabetes, but in none of the children with type 1 diabetes. Treatment of acanthosis nigricans is aimed at determining the underlying cause. If insulin resistance is present, it should be managed appropriately and screening for lipid disorders should be considered.

Diabetic Thick Skin

This condition is characterized by an abnormal collagen collection, which causes a thickness that usually occurs on the hands, knuckles, and fingers. Improved glycemic control and use of steroid preparations are sometimes helpful.

Xanthoma

These result from extracellular deposits of lipid in the form of cholesterol or triglycerides in the dermis or subcutaneous fat and usually occur when triglycerides levels exceed 800 mg/dL.[44] Lesions may be individual or form a cluster. Treatment is aimed at correcting elevated lipid levels.

Vitiligo

Vitiligo causes hypopigmentation of the skin and sometimes is seen in patients with autoimmune type disorders such as type 1 diabetes. Lesions are white in color and usually seen over joints or around orifices. Individuals usually develop new lesions over the course of their life. There is no known treatment.

Recognize skin complications early:

Self-care routines are important, and swift treatment of underlying causes can help prevent skin complications.

> ***Address Underlying Causes***
>
> Keeping blood pressure and blood glucose in control can help minimize chronic complications, as these are sometimes underlying causes.

Patient education regarding skin complications is based on early recognition and treatment of underlying causes such as glycemic control and metabolic conditions. Proper methods of rotating insulin injection sites, identification of secondary infections, vigilant monitoring for lesions not associated with diabetes, and use of sunscreen are also components that will help prevent any skin complications associated with diabetes.

Depression

Although not a direct complication of diabetes, depression screening should be initiated and monitoring should be ongoing due to the chronic nature of diabetes and the likelihood of complications. People with diabetes have twice the risk of suffering from depression when compared with people without diabetes.[45] The following all have a depressive effect on the course of diabetes:[46]

- Obesity
- Physical inactivity
- Tobacco use
- Hyperglycemia
- Autonomic neuropathy
- Inflammation

Because they can mimic the symptoms of hyperglycemia, the symptoms of depression can be overlooked. Also, depression can be looked upon with shame. Typical symptoms may include the following:[46]

- Substance abuse
- Feelings of sadness, guilt, worthlessness, and helplessness
- Loss of interest in previously pleasurable activities
- Fatigue and low energy
- Sleep problems
- Memory problem
- Thoughts of death or suicide

All healthcare professionals need to be aware of the signs of depression, screen patients, and treat or refer as needed. See chapters 4 and 34 for further information on depression.

Standards of Care

The chronic complications of diabetes are not inevitable. Addressing modifiable risk factors can help improve the prognosis for many with diabetes. The ADA Standards of Care in Diabetes outline specific guidelines for complication screening examinations.[24] The earlier these complications are detected and treated, the less people with diabetes may have to suffer devastating illness.

Questions and Controversy

The diabetes healthcare community is currently being challenged to respond to a number of issues related to the development of chronic complications. The emergence of early-onset type 2 diabetes is particularly important to recognize and respond to, as is the growing prevalence of obesity that is contributing to the problem. To improve educational strategies aimed at preventing, delaying, and minimizing the effect of chronic complications in people of all ages, research can also assist in the following areas: facilitating behavior change; defining best practices; and controlling blood pressure and blood glucose, which are underlying causes of some chronic complications.

Type 2 Diabetes in Children and Adolescents. The emergence of younger individuals (children and adolescents) with type 2 diabetes has created the need for new research regarding diabetes complications. Topics on which more information is needed include the following:

- Effects of hormonal changes, psychological development, and early assessment of individuals at risk
- Role of dietary influences, sedentary lifestyles, and genetic factors in development of early-onset diabetes (ie, in childhood and adolescence)

Obesity. Obesity, which is known to influence the development of diabetes, continues to increase in children and various ethnic groups. Obesity is now the most chronic condition of childhood.[47] The prevalence of obesity (body mass index >95th percentile) is 10% among children 2 to 5 years of age and 15% among children 6 to 19 years old. When children at risk for obesity (body mass index in 85th to 94th percentile) are included, the values increased to 20% and 30% respectively. At least 1 of every 4 children is either obese or at risk for becoming obese.[48] Prevalence of obesity varies greatly among ethnic groups, but African American youths are known to be at higher risk than the white population.[49]

Responses to these growing trends in early-onset diabetes and childhood obesity may very well include the following:

- *New Specialties.* New specialties will most likely emerge to deal with the metabolic, psychological, and emotional needs of this emerging group. Diabetes educators and providers who specialize in children will be especially needed, and research will focus on how best to educate the individuals and their families based on developmental stages.
- *Prevention Focus.* Efforts to prevent type 2 diabetes during childhood may concentrate on early intervention in school systems to address nutrition, exercise, and screening.

Behavior Change. Research is also needed in the areas of goal setting, problem solving, and behavioral changes. Methods to determine how to best assist individuals to maintain changes and modify lifestyle need to be further developed.

Best Practices. More research is needed in the area of best practices for providers, recommended treatment goals, and education interventions that help the individuals with diabetes and their families make informed choices regarding care and prevention of complications.

Blood Pressure and Blood Glucose Control. Methods to assist individuals and their families to realize control of hypertension and hyperglycemia can significantly reduce risks for long-term complications. More research is needed to assist in this.

Medications. Research will be needed to develop new medications as well as to determine what combinations of current drug therapy might be most beneficial for diabetes and its long-term complications. The issue of which medications, both current and new, can be used safely in adolescents and children needs exploration.

Focus on Education: Pearls for Practice

Teaching Strategies

- **Emphasize modifiable risk factors.** Help patients prevent, delay, and decrease complications by emphasizing modifiable risk factors. Strive for control of hyperglycemia, hypertension, and dyslipidemia.

- **Present clear information on risk factor management.** Include risk factor information as part of educational content. Discuss obesity, physical inactivity, unhealthy eating, and alcohol and tobacco use and excess. Provide clear information on how to vigorously manage.

- **Do not overlook oral and skin hygiene as educational topics.** Include oral and skin assessment and hygiene information in self-management education.

- **Promote dental health and exams.** Promote dental examinations, and participate in the assessment of dental problems.

- **Support screening for complications.** Ensure that patients are aware of and receive the complication screening examinations.

- **Use the Diabetes Care Card.** Promote use of the ADA Standards of Medical Care "Diabetes Care Card." The card, which fits in a patient's wallet, helps patients and healthcare professionals keep track of screening examinations and progress towards decreasing the risk of complications.

Messages for Patients

- **Screening exams are your opportunity to gather important information.** If your healthcare provider does not discuss the following topics as part of a physical exam or routine visit, ask what you need to know about 5 topics important in diabetes management: meal habits, weight management, use of alcohol and tobacco, skin and dental care, and physical activity.

- **Prevent, delay, and reduce the complications of diabetes by scheduling routine healthcare services.** Make regular and timely appointments for dental, eye, and skin exams. Ask members of your care team to help you identify resources that can better meet your needs. When a problem emerges, obtain care promptly and follow up thoroughly to minimize complications and costs.

- **Build up your self-monitoring skills.** Make it a habit to test your blood pressure and blood glucose levels, inspect and care for your feet, and schedule routine lab tests such as A1Cs and lipids. Consider a reward system that fosters good health.

References

1. Andrus M, Leggett-Frazier N, Pfeifer MA. Chronic complications of diabetes: an overview. In: A Core Curriculum for Diabetes Education: Diabetes and Complications, 5th ed. Franz MJ, ed. Chicago, Il: American Association of Diabetes Educators; 2003:45.
2. The DCCT Research Group. The effect of intensive treatment of diabetes on the development and progression of long-term complications in insulin-dependent diabetes mellitus. N Engl J Med. 1993;329:977-86.
3. UK Prospective Diabetes Study Group. Intensive blood glucose control with sulphonylureas or insulin compared with conventional treatment and risk complications in patients with type 2 diabetes (UKPD 33). Lancet. 1998;352:837-53.
4. Ohkubo Y, Kishikawa H, Araki E, et al. Intensive insulin therapy prevents the progression of diabetic microvascular complications in Japanese patients with non insulin diabetes mellitus: a randomized prospective 6 year study. Diabetes Research in Clinical Practice.1995;28:103-17.
5. Bailes BK. Diabetes mellitus and its chronic complications. AORN. 2002;76(2):265-82.
6. Centers for Disease Control and Prevention. National diabetes fact sheet: general information and national estimates on diabetes in the United States, 2005. Atlanta, Ga: US Department of Health and Human Services, Centers for Disease Control and Prevention; 2005.
7. Engelgau MM, Geiss LS, Saaddine JB, et al. The evolving diabetes burden in the United States. Ann Intern Med. 2004;140(11):945-50.
8. American Diabetes Association. Economic costs of diabetes in the US in 2002 (position statement). Diabetes Care. 2003;26:917-32.
9. Chyun DA, Young LH. Cardiovascular complications. In: Complete Nurse's Guide to Diabetes. Childs BP, Cypress M, Spollett G, eds. Alexandria, Va: American Diabetes Association; 2005:91.
10. Centers for Disease Control and Prevention. Diabetes Surveillance System. Atlanta, Ga: U.S. Department of Health and Human Services; 2005. On the Internet at: www.cdc.gov/diabetes/statistics/index.htm. Accessed 15 Oct 2005.
11. Tull ES, Roseman JM. Diabetes in African Americans. In: Diabetes in America. 2nd ed. National Diabetes Data Group, eds. Bethesda, Md: National Institute of Diabetes and Digestive and Kidney Diseases; 1995. NIH publication 95-1468:613-30.
12. Stern MP, Mitchell BD. Diabetes in Hispanic Americans. In: Diabetes in America, 2nd ed. National Diabetes Data Group, eds. Bethesda, Md: National Institute of Diabetes and Digestive and Kidney Diseases; 1995. NIH publication 95-1468:631-60.
13. Kuhn F, Rackley C. Coronary artery disease in women: risk factors, evaluation, treatment, and prevention. Arch Intern Med. 1993;143:2626-36.
14. American Diabetes Association. Hypertension management in adults with diabetes (position statement). Diabetes Care. 2004;27 Suppl 1:S65-7.
15. UK Prospective Diabetes Study Group. Tight blood pressure control and risk of macrovascular and microvascular complications in type 2 diabetes (UKPDS 38). BMJ. 1998;317:703-13.
16. Kannel, WB, Cupples, LA, Ramaswami R, Stokes J, Kreger BE, Higgins M. Regional obesity and risk of cardiovascular disease; the Framingham study. J Clin Epidemiol. 1991;44(2):183-90.
17. Lee CD, Blair SN, Jackson AS. Cardiorespiratory fitness, body composition, and all cause and cardiovascular disease mortality in men. Am J Clin Nutr. 1999;69:373-80.
18. Vinik AI, Newlon P, Milicevic Z, McNitt P, Stansberry KB. Diabetic neuropathies: an overview of clinical aspects. In: Diabetes Mellitus: A Fundamental and Clinical Text. LeRoith D, Taylor SI, Olefsky JM, eds. Philadelphia, Pa: Lippincott-Raven; 1996:727-51.
19. Kushion W. Peripheral and autonomic neuropathy. In: Complete Nurse's Guide to Diabetes. Childs BP, Cypress M, Spollett G, eds. Alexandria, Va: American Diabetes Association; 2005:155-65.
20. Vinik AI, Newlon P, Milicevic Z, McNitt P, Stansberry KB. Diabetic neuropathies: an overview of clinical aspects. In: Diabetes Mellitus: A Fundamental and Clinical Text. LeRoith D, Taylor SI, Olefsky JM, eds. Philadelphia, Pa: Lippincott-Raven; 1996:727-51.
21. Pecoraro RE, Reiber GE, Burgess EM. Pathways to diabetic limb amputation: basis for prevention. Diabetes Care. 1990;13:513-21.
22. Ramsey SD, Newton K, Blough D, et al. Incidence, outcomes, and cost of foot ulcers in patients with diabetes. Diabetes Care. 1999;22:382-7.
23. American Diabetes Association. Diabetic nephropathy (position statement). Diabetes Care. 2004;27 Suppl 1:S79-83.

24. American Diabetes Association: Standards of medical care in diabetes (position statement). Diabetes Care. 2005;28 Suppl 1:S4-36.

25. UK Prospective Diabetes Study Group: Tight blood pressure control and risk of macrovascular and microvascular complications in type 2 diabetes: UKPDS 38. BMJ. 1998;317:703–13.

26. American Diabetes Association: standards of medical care in diabetes (position statement). Diabetes Care. 2005;28 Suppl 1:S4-S36.

27. Yu N, Milite, CP, Inzucchi, SE. Evidence-based treatment of diabetic nephropathy. Practical Diabetology. 2005;24(4):36-41.

28. American Diabetes Association: Retinopathy in diabetes (position statement). Diabetes Care. 2004;27 Suppl 1:S84-7.

29. Saaddine JB, Narayan KM, Engelgau MM, Aubert RE, Klein R, Beckles,GL. Prevalence of self-rated visual impairment among adults with diabetes. Am J Public Health. 1999;89:1200-5.

30. Ferris FL, Davis MD, Aiello LM. Review article-drug therapy: treatment of diabetic retinopathy. N Engl J Med. 1999;341:667-78.

31. Beaser RS, ed. Microvascular complications. In: Joslin's Diabetes Deskbook, revised ed. Beaser RS and Joslin Diabetes Center staff, eds. Boston, Ma: Joslin Diabetes Center; 2003.

32. American Diabetes Association: Retinopathy in diabetes (position statement). Diabetes Care. 2004; 27 Suppl 1:S84-S87.

33. Tomar SL, Lester A. Dental and other health care visits among U.S. adults with diabetes. Diabetes Care. 2000;23(10):1505-10.

34. Loe, H. Periodontal disease. The sixth complication of diabetes mellitus. Diabetes Care. 1993;16:329-34.

35. Tomar, SL, Asma S. Smoking attributable periodontitis in the United States: findings from the NHANES III. Journal of Periodontol. 2000;71:743-51.

36. Spollett, G, Crape CA. Dental issues in patients with diabetes. In: Complete Nurse's Guide to Diabetes. Childs BP, Cypress M, Spollett G, eds. Alexandria, Va: American Diabetes Association; 2005:139.

37. Centers for Disease Control and Prevention. The prevention and treatment of complications of diabetes. U.S. Department of Health and Human Services, Public Health Service. Atlanta, Ga: 1991.

38. Ferringer T, Miller OF. Cutaneous manifestations of diabetes mellitus. Derm Clin North Am 2002;20:483-93.

39. Spollett, G, ed. Complete Nurses Guide to Diabetes Care: Dermatological Changes Associated with Diabetes. Alexandria, Va: American Diabetes Association 2005.

40. Stulberg DL, Clark N, Tovey D. Common hyperpigmentation disorders in adults: part II. Am Fam Physician 2003;68(10):1963-8.

41. Paron NG, Lambert PW. Cutaneous manifestations of diabetes mellitus. Prim Care. 2000;27:371-83.

42. Dabelea D, Pettitt DJ, Jones KL, Arslanian SA. Type 2 diabetes mellitus in minority children and adolescents: an emerging problem. Endocrinol Metab Clin North Am. 1999;28:709-29.

43. Scott CR, Smith JM, Cradock MM, Pihoker C. Characteristics of youth-onset noninsulin-dependent diabetes mellitus and insulin-dependent diabetes mellitus at diagnosis. Pediatrics. 1997;100:84-91.

44. Reeves JRT. Skin changes associated with diabetes. In: Medical Management of Diabetes Mellitus. Leahy JL, Clark NG, Cefalu WT, eds. New York: Marcel Dekker; 2000:539-58.

45. Anderson RJ, Freedland, KE, Clouse RE, Lustman, PJ. The prevalence of comorbid depression in adults with diabetes: a meta-analysis. Diabetes Care 2001:24(6),1069-78.

46. Lustman, PJ, Clouse RE. Practical considerations in the management of depression in diabetes. Diabetes Spectrum 2004:17(3),160-166

47. OBrien SH. Identification, evaluation, and management of obesity in an academic primary care center. Pediatrics. 2004;114(2):154-9.

48. Troiano RP, Flegal KM. Overweight children and adolescents: description, epidemiology, and demographics. Pediatrics. 1990;101:497-503.

49. Ogden CL, Flegal KM, Carroll MD, Johnson CL. Prevalence and trends in overweight among US children and adolescents. JAMA. 2002;288:1728-32.

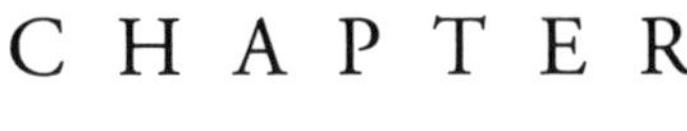

CHAPTER

21

Macrovascular Disease in Diabetes

Author

Daniel Lorber, MD, FACP, CDE

Key Concepts

- Insulin resistance, glucose intolerance, and diabetes affect multiple aspects of vascular health.
- Increased cardiovascular risk is the result of the synergy of effects on the vascular endothelium and the vessel wall.
- Macrovascular disease includes coronary artery disease (CAD), cerebrovascular disease, and peripheral vascular disease.
- Coronary artery disease occurs earlier and is more extensive in people with diabetes. It presents as angina or acute myocardial infarction, sometimes with atypical symptoms.
- People with diabetes and peripheral arterial disease are more prone to limb ischemia and increased risk of amputation.
- Macrovascular disease is multifactorial. Its reduction requires addressing all risk factors, not just glucose. Risk factor reduction includes control of hypertension and lipids, therapeutic lifestyle, smoking cessation, and use of antiplatelet therapy.
- There are many unanswered questions regarding effective treatment strategies and targets for control to prevent cardiovascular disease (CVD) in people with diabetes.

Scope of the Problem

More than 18 million Americans over 20 years of age have diabetes mellitus,[1] and the number is steadily increasing. For people born in the year 2000, the lifetime risk of developing diabetes is estimated to be 1 in 3 Americans, 2 of 5 African Americans and Hispanic Americans, and half of Hispanic American women. Diabetes affects 8.7% of people over 20 years of age and 18.3% of those over age 60. Diabetes is the sixth leading cause of death in the United States, and the leading cause of death in people with diabetes is macrovascular disease. Sixty-five percent of deaths in diabetes are due to either coronary artery disease (CAD) or cerebrovascular events. People with diabetes are 2 to 4 times more likely to have a stroke, myocardial infarction (MI), or sudden death, and those who have had a stroke are 2 to 4 times more likely to have another.

This ratio has been consistent over the past 5 decades in spite of significant decreases in cardiovascular death in the general population. Women with diabetes have over 7 times the rate of peripheral vascular disease as those without diabetes. The risk of cardiac death for women with diabetes has increased by 23% since 1950 while decreasing by 27% in women without diabetes. For men, the rate of cardiac death in the same time period has decreased slightly (13%), but much less than the decrease in men without diabetes (36%).[2,3]

These risk ratios are not limited to the United States. A recent study in the Asia-Pacific region found that the hazard ratio for fatal and nonfatal cardiovascular disease (CVD) was similarly increased in the largely European populations of Australia and New Zealand and the ethnically diverse areas of China, Korea, Japan, and southeast Asia. Furthermore, the hazard ratios were significantly higher in younger than older individuals. "The rapidly growing prevalence of diabetes in Asia heralds a large increase in the incidence of diabetes-related death in the coming decades."[4]

Data from the Framingham cohort are a bit more optimistic, showing that the incidence of cardiovascular events in both the diabetic and nondiabetic population has diminished by 54% and 35%, respectively, between a cohort studied from 1950 to 1966 and one studied from 1977 to 1995. The improvement in mortality rate has followed a highly significant improvement in control of blood pressure and cholesterol. Nonetheless, people with diabetes remain at 2 to 3 times the risk of cardiovascular events as those without diabetes.[5]

These encouraging data must be viewed in the context of the simultaneous dramatic increase in the absolute number of people with diabetes not just in the United States, but all over the world.

There are many subjects to cover in a chapter on macrovascular disease and diabetes education. This chapter focuses especially on reducing risks for macrovascular disease as an important facet of diabetes education. To approach this topic with patients, diabetes educators must first know about the macrovascular conditions of particular concern in persons with diabetes—what they are, how they present, and how they are treated, for example. In this chapter, readers learn about each of the following:

- Coronary artery disease (CAD)
- Cerebrovascular disease
- Peripheral arterial disease
- Congestive heart failure
- Cardiac autonomic neuropathy

After each condition and its treatment are summarized, opportunities for instruction by the diabetes educator are delineated, and topics pertinent to risk factors and prevention are highlighted.

Next, the chapter focuses on strategies known to be effective in reducing an individual's risk for CVD, including the cornerstones: lifestyle modifications, nutrition, physical activity, and appropriate medication. Modifiable risk factors, both those that are widely understood to have an impact as well as those of which we are less certain, are discussed next. This section looks first at the traditional risk factors:

- Glycemia
- Hypertension
- Lipid abnormalities

Newer risk assessment and treatment modalities are also given attention. Readers learn about the following:

- Interest in and use of other risk markers
- Use of inflammatory markers (C-reactive protein, cellular adhesion molecules, and fibrinogen) for clinical decision making
- Measurement of homocysteine levels and use of related supplements
- Use of insulin-resistance therapies for prevention of CVD
- Antithrombotic therapies (aspirin and clopidogrel)

Hospitalization is such a critical time for those admitted for CVD who also have diabetes. Issues and challenges in hospital disease management are emphasized as the chapter draws to a close. Some closing comments on the important unknowns are made. The chapter concludes with pearls for practice, a worthwhile to-do list for diabetes educators.

Why is there more vascular disease in diabetes?

To understand the causes of increased macrovascular disease in people with diabetes, one must start with the vascular endothelium, the lining tissue of blood vessels. For many years, the vascular endothelium was thought to be merely a passive lining tissue. Current research, however,

Case in Point: Coronary Artery Disease

PH was diagnosed with type 1 diabetes at age 10 in 1960. When first seen by the diabetes educator in 1996, PH had a history of hypertension and proteinuria. He had been treated with an angiotensin-converting enzyme (ACE) inhibitor, but was not taking this medication at the time of his first visit. His diabetes control was difficult because of social and intellectual problems. He had no history of coronary disease and no family history of coronary disease. On his initial visit, he was hypertensive with a blood pressure of 150/90 and had bilateral background retinopathy and evidence of peripheral neuropathy. Laboratory data revealed total cholesterol of 151, LDL-C 105, HDL-C 27, and triglycerides 95. Urine microalbumin was 17 mg/g of creatinine.

Over the next 8 years, PH was treated with an ACE inhibitor and a multiple dose insulin regimen with fair-to-poor glycemic control. Urine remained negative for microalbumin. Repeat cholesterol in 2004 was 135, with triglycerides of 54, HDL-C of 29, and LDL-C of 96. PH recently complained of some substernal chest pain radiating to his left arm and shoulder upon walking. Physical examination at that time revealed evidenced of peripheral neuropathy and diabetic retinopathy. Cardiac exam was unremarkable and his peripheral pulses were intact. Electrocardiogram was within normal limits.

PH was referred to the emergency room for admission. Cardiac catheterization demonstrated severe triple vessel CAD with good ventricular function. He underwent a triple coronary artery bypass. At the time of surgery, his internal mammary artery was clear of atherosclerosis, but the peripheral arteries showed significant evidence of atherosclerosis.

PH was discharged from the hospital 3 days after surgery and continued to do well with no further chest pain. At that time, in addition to multiple dose insulin, his therapy included low-dose aspirin, a statin, and continued ACE inhibitor.

has shown that the vascular endothelium is an active endocrine organ, playing a critical role in normal function of the vasculature. Vascular endothelial cells secrete a number of factors that modulate vascular function, including smooth muscle tone, nutrient delivery, inflammation, coagulation, and thrombosis. Under normal circumstances, the endothelium provides an environment that inhibits adhesion of leukocytes and platelets, enhances fibrinolysis, inhibits vasospasm, and inhibits vascular smooth muscle growth.

This is accomplished by synthesis of a number of important bioactive substances, including nitric oxide (NO), prostacycline, bradykinin, and other vasoactive substances.

The best studied and most important of these is NO.

- Nitric oxide is a potent vasodilator that mediates much of the endothelium's regulation of vasodilatation
- It reduces leukocyte adhesion and migration into the vascular wall; thus inhibiting inflammation
- It diminishes smooth muscle proliferation and migration

These effects, taken together, inhibit atherogenesis and vasospasm. Healthy endothelium also provides resistance to thrombosis, functioning as a barrier between procoagulant blood contents (platelets, clotting factors) and subendothelial substances that can activate them. In addition to its barrier function, the endothelium generates both antiplatelet factors, such as NO and prostacycline, and anticoagulant factors, such as tissue-type plasminogen activator (tPA) and heparan sulfate.

In disease states, however, endothelial function is altered in ways that accelerate atherosclerotic change, including increased vasospasm, enhanced thrombosis, and increased local inflammatory responses.

Known cardiovascular risk factors, such as hyperlipoproteinemia, smoking, diabetes, and hypertension disturb endothelial function in a variety of ways. Further, it appears the effects of these factors may be synergistic, rather than just additive.

Increasing evidence suggests that diabetes may impact on vascular function both through hyperglycemia and insulin resistance. When both are present, the effects are much greater than when either is present alone.

Endothelial Dysfunction in Diabetes

The normal metabolic response to a glucose load is an increase in glucose, free fatty acids (FFAs), and insulin. These changes result in a transient decrease in endothelium-derived NO production and, thus, in endothelium-mediated vasodilatation. In the presence of normal glucose tolerance, endothelial NO production and vasodilatation returns to normal by 2 hours after a glucose load. In the presence of impaired glucose tolerance (IGT) or diabetes, endothelium-mediated vasodilation is prolonged. Thus, the diabetic endothelium is dysfunctional for hours after each meal.

A similar effect is seen after a high-fat meal; after a mixed meal high in carbohydrate and fat, endothelial dysfunction is present for up to 4 hours. Since most people spend 10 to 12 hours a day in the postprandial state, vascular function may be abnormal for the majority of the day in individuals with glucose intolerance.

Increases in glucose, low-density lipoprotein cholesterol (LDL-C), and insulin after a meal may also trigger increased expression of vasoconstrictor substances, including endothelin-1 and angiotensin II. Chronic hyperglycemia may also enhance the production of endothelin-1 by the presence of advanced glycation endproducts (AGEs) in the vessel wall.

Enhanced Inflammation in Diabetes

Inflammatory responses and immune function play a major role in both the formation of atheromatous plaques and their rupture, often the final step in a thrombotic event.

In glucose intolerance and diabetes, a number of the metabolic derangements that are present enhance the inflammatory responses present in atherogenesis. Increased oxidative stress, diminished NO production, presence of AGEs, and postprandial increases in FFAs all activate transcription factors that increase endothelial production of inflammatory mediators. These inflammatory mediators enhance leukocyte adhesion and monocyte migration into the vessel wall, leading to their transformation into macrophages and eventually into foam cells.

Inflammation also decreases plaque stability by cytokine inhibition of collagen production in the plaque's fibrous cap. This effect weakens the cap, particularly at the "shoulder" where it attaches to the vessel wall. As a result, the plaque is more likely to rupture, releasing the contents of its lipid-rich necrotic core into the bloodstream, triggering an acute thrombotic event.

Enhanced Thrombosis in Diabetes

Diabetes, insulin resistance, and glucose intolerance are associated with a state of enhanced thrombosis, both platelet hyperaggregability and inhibition of fibrinolysis. Glucose enters platelets in an insulin-independent manner, decreasing platelet production of NO, activating the mediator protein kinase C, enhancing the production of reactive oxygen species, and enhancing platelet activation. Hyperglycemia also affects the endothelium to decrease antiaggregant production and increase production of procoagulant factors, including thrombin and von Willebrand factor. Insulin resistance, obesity, and diabetes lead to increased production of plasminogen activator inhibitor

(PAI-1), an inhibitor of fibrinolysis. PAI–1 is also increased in the vessel wall of people with diabetes. This increase in PAI-1 activity leads to increased persistence of thrombi, which may also increase the severity of stenosis.

Increased Arterial Stiffness in Diabetes

A number of components of diabetes lead to increased stiffness and decreased compliance of the arterial wall.[7] Arterial stiffness is associated with chronic hyperglycemia, probably through increased formation of AGEs in the vessel wall. Endothelial dysfunction and inflammation, discussed above, also contribute. Other risk factors for decreased arterial compliance include age and hypertension, presence of components of the metabolic syndrome, microalbuminuria, central fatness, and cardiopulmonary fitness.

As a result of stiffer arterial walls with decreased compliance, arteries lose their elastic effect of damping pulse pressure. This results in higher systolic and lower diastolic blood pressure. These changes lead to increased vascular disease by a variety of mechanisms. Increased pulse pressure places increased shear stress on the endothelium, enhancing the pathophysiologic effects described above.

The clinical associations with diminished compliance include increased risk of cardiovascular events. In type 2 diabetes, increased systolic blood pressure is associated with cerebrovascular events and left ventricular hypertrophy. Decreased diastolic pressure decreases coronary arterial flow, which thus enhances ischemia.

Increased arterial stiffness is present in early type 1 diabetes. The effect is more pronounced in the presence of microvascular disease. In type 1, increased pulse pressure and its individual components (systolic hypertension, diastolic hypotension) are all associated with increased risk of cardiovascular events.

Impact of Glucose

There are extensive epidemiologic data supporting the role of glycemia in CVD. The UK Prospective Diabetes Study (UKPDS) found that people in the upper tertile of A1C had a 50% increase in cardiovascular risk.[8] The EPIC-Norfolk study found that not only did men with diabetes have increased cardiovascular morbidity and mortality, but those without diabetes had a 28% greater risk of cardiovascular events for a 1% increase in hemoglobin A1C—even within the normal range.[9] A similar effect was found for peripheral arterial disease.[10]

A number of epidemiologic studies[11,12] and studies of glycemic interventions[13] suggest that postprandial spikes in blood glucose and triglycerides[14] may each play a greater role in CVD than either average or fasting glucose.[15]

Macrovascular Diseases

Coronary Artery Disease
Myocardial infarction
Congestive heart failure

Cerebrovascular Disease
Cerebrovascular accident (stroke)
Multi-infarct dementia
Transient ischemic attack

Peripheral Vascular Disease
Lower extremity ischemia
Mesenteric ischemia, including ischemic colitis and mesenteric infarction

Key Terms

Arteriosclerosis. General term that describes the condition in which the walls of blood vessels (both arteries and veins) are thick, hard, and nonelastic.

Atherosclerosis. Specific term referring to the process of materials being deposited along and within blood vessel walls (especially arterial).

Macrovascular disease. Refers to both arteriosclerotic and atherosclerotic changes in moderate-sized to large-sized arteries and veins. Coronary, cerebral, and peripheral macrovascular diseases are particularly significant because of the associated frequency, morbidity, and mortality and because of their economic consequences.[6]

Is risk increased with type 1 diabetes?

People with type 1 diabetes are at a fivefold increased risk for cardiovascular events between 20 and 39 years of age.[16] In most studies, duration of diabetes is the best predictor of CVD. Since most of these patients do not have classic risk factors, it would imply that abnormal glucose is the major causative factor in this population.

But the data on causation are not so clear. As obesity increases in the United States and other countries, there is an alarming increase in the prevalence of the same risk factors seen in type 2 diabetes, including dyslipidemia, hypertension, elevated inflammatory markers, and endothelial dysfunction.[17] In a 10-year follow-up of the Pittsburgh Epidemiology of Diabetes Complications study, these classic risk factors were shown to be predictive of cardiac mortality and morbidity.[18] Physical inactivity and depressive symptoms also predicted risk for CAD. In addition, the same study showed that A1C level did not predict subsequent CAD events.

Several studies of endothelial dysfunction[19,20] and of early atherosclerosis[21,22] show a strong correlation of traditional risk factors, including hypertension, smoking, and dyslipidemia with these early harbingers of CAD. Clarkson et al[20] also showed that duration of diabetes was a predictor of abnormal vascular reactivity in young adults with type 1 diabetes.

What are the implications of the rise in early-onset type 2 diabetes?

As recently as the early 1990s, over 95% of newly diagnosed childhood diabetes was type 1. By 2001, nearly half of newly diagnosed adolescent diabetes was type 2 in areas with high-risk populations. The implications of this increase are staggering. A tenfold increase in the number of young people with type 2 diabetes will lead to a massive increase in microvascular and macrovascular disease over the next 3 decades.[23]

Although the data are preliminary, it appears that young people with type 2 diabetes or the components of the metabolic syndrome are also at increased risk of CVD.[24-26] The converse is certainly true. Children with low levels of body mass index, insulin resistance, dyslipidemia, and systolic blood pressure have a significantly decreased risk for CVD.[27] Autopsy studies on children and adolescents dying from accidents, suicide, or homicide showed that early atherosclerotic lesions were correlated with many of the same risk factors (lipids, hypertension, obesity, and hyperglycemia) as in adults. In the group with A1C greater than 8%, the rate of early atherosclerosis was doubled between 15 and 25 years of age and 8 times greater between 30 and 35 years of age.[28,29]

CVD risk factors should be aggressively addressed in youth with diabetes

A number of authorities have outlined treatment implications in response to the early evidence of increased risk for CVD in young people with diabetes. In general, the recommendation is that classical risk factors—particularly dyslipidemia, smoking, and hypertension—should be addressed aggressively in young people with both type 1 and type 2 diabetes.[30,31]

Pathology of an Atheroma

The normal vascular wall consists of 3 layers. The innermost layer, called the intima, consists of a single layer of endothelial cells. The media consists primarily of smooth muscle cells that regulate vascular tone. The adventitia includes supportive fibroelastic tissue, nutrient vessels, and nerves.

The earliest lesion in atherosclerosis is the fatty streak. Lipid-laden macrophages and monocytes are present in the subendothelial layer, along with activated T-lymphocytes.

As the plaque progresses, the subintimal space is occupied by an enlarging collection of foam cells, cholesterol crystals, and necrotic cellular debris. Smooth muscle cells migrate from the intima to stabilize the atheroma, forming a fibrous cap, made up of smooth muscle cells and collagen. As the atheromatous plaque continues to grow, it occludes an increasing amount of blood flow, eventually leading to ischemia. This is the primary phenomenon in angina pectoris and intermittent claudication. Ulcerated plaques may lead to transient ischemic attacks (TIAs) or embolic stroke.

Case in Point: Coronary Artery Disease and Hyperglycemia

JH was a 62-year-old man with no prior history of cardiac symptoms who presented with crushing substernal chest pain radiating to his jaw, associated with nausea, diaphoresis, and shortness of breath. He was seen in the emergency room, where an electrocardiogram was performed and acute transmural myocardial infarction (MI) was diagnosed. Thrombolytic therapy was begun, and he was stabilized over the next few hours. He denied a history of diabetes or prior CVD.

Laboratory evaluation on admission revealed a glucose of 210 mg/dL and a total cholesterol of 247 mg/dL. Urine protein was negative. Cardiac enzymes were consistent with MI.

He was initially treated with an intravenous insulin drip; his glucose rapidly fell to normal. Subsequent attempts to discontinue the insulin resulted in recurrent hyperglycemia, and an endocrinology consultation was requested.

JH was begun on a multidose insulin regimen consisting of rapid-acting analog insulin before meals and insulin glargine (Lantus) at hour of sleep. When he objected to being discharged on insulin, the cardiology nurse practitioner explained the significance of the DIGAMI study. JH was then willing to remain on insulin for the next 3 months, following the protocol.

For many years, the assumption was that MI and thrombotic stroke were the result of progressive occlusion of coronary or cerebral vessels. More recent research has shown that it is the vulnerable 40% to 50% occluding plaques that often lead to acute coronary and cerebral thrombosis.[32] Inflammation weakens the "shoulder" of the fibrous cap, where the cap attaches to the vessel wall. This weakened area ruptures, allowing the release of highly thrombogenic plaque contents into the vessel lumen. The interaction of these lipid and necrotic substances with platelets and coagulation factors triggers an acute thrombosis.

Coronary Artery Disease

CAD occurs earlier and is more extensive in people with diabetes. The incidence of early-onset coronary disease is similar in men and women with diabetes; this is in contrast to the nondiabetic population, in which CAD is much more common in men. CAD accounts for 56% to 60% of all deaths in people with diabetes.

CAD most commonly presents with either of 2 syndromes: angina pectoris or MI. Chest pain is a common symptom that may or may not be angina or an MI. Persons with diabetes are at very high risk for CAD and should be educated regarding the warning signs (listed in Table 21.1).

Treatment of Acute Myocardial Infarction in Diabetes

Revascularization is the treatment of choice for those with acute MI, whether or not they have diabetes. The outcomes, however, are worse with diabetes. Diabetes doubles the risk of death after an MI despite advances in cardiac care over the past 4 decades.[33] This result is likely due to the same factors (described above) that cause increased morbidity and mortality in people with diabetes and MI. Acute revascularization is most commonly performed by percutaneous transluminal coronary angioplasty (PTCA) with placement of a drug-eluting stent in an artery that has been dilated by intra-arterial balloon at the site(s) of obstruction.

Treatment with thrombolytic agents has also been shown to be effective in persons with an acute MI. Individuals with diabetes do benefit from thrombolytic therapy, but do less well than those without diabetes. This is likely due to greater age and concomitant hypertension, prior MI and coronary artery bypass graft, and more congestive heart failure (CHF).[34]

Once the patient is stable, the cardiologist may perform further testing to evaluate short-term risk and therapies.

TABLE 21.1 Warning Signs of Coronary Artery Disease

	Angina	*Myocardial Infarction*
Etiology	Coronary ischemia; partial occlusion of coronary artery (may be caused by 70%-80% narrowing of 1 or more coronary vessels); usually gradual onset	Sudden total occlusion of a coronary artery; often caused by 40%-50% occlusion; vulnerable soft plaque with thin fibrous caps that rupture and release necrotic, lipid-filled material into the artery, which can initiate a thrombus and occlude an artery
Quality	Squeezing, tightness, pressure or heavy weight on the chest; more discomfort than pain	Intense, severe squeezing or crushing pain
Location	Diffuse over chest; radiating to neck, lower jaw, or left arm	Midsternal radiating to arms, neck, and jaw; epigastric pain
Timing	Rarely lasts more than 5 minutes; remits when stopping activity that precipitated it (may be triggered by exercise, sexual intercourse, cold weather, cocaine)	30-60 minutes
Associated Symptoms	Dyspnea, diaphoretic, cold clammy skin, fatigue, syncope	Diaphoresis, nausea, vomiting, weakness, dyspnea, sense of impending doom, pale
Notes	Elderly and those with diabetic autonomic neuropathy may have no pain	Autonomic neuropathy may result in loss of pain sensation; may present with onset of diabetic ketoacidosis in type 1 patients; in patient suspected of having myocardial infarction, advise to chew a full-strength aspirin and call 911

These may include exercise stress testing, echocardiogram, or coronary angiogram. In some cases, the decision may be made to perform further revascularization—either additional PTCA or a coronary artery bypass.

Risk factor management and education begin in the hospital as well. Diabetes control should be stressed, and the patient prepared for postdischarge lifestyle change and risk factor reduction. A statin, angiotensin-converting enzyme (ACE) inhibitor, β-adrenergic blocking agent (β-blocker), and antiplatelet agent should be instituted as soon as possible if there are no contraindications. Intensive modification of risk factors[35] including use of statins, ACE inhibitors, and antiplatelet agents has been shown to be effective in decreasing cardiovascular events in people with type 2 diabetes. Although β-blockers are effective in improving survival among most populations with MI, their role is controversial in diabetes.[36]

Coronary Artery Bypass Graft and Percutaneous Transluminal Coronary Angioplasty

Revascularization for CAD is considered in 2 groups of patients:

- Those whose activity is significantly limited in spite of maximal medical therapy
- Those for whom revascularization has a proven benefit on survival

The decision to choose coronary artery bypass graft surgery (CABG) versus percutaneous transluminal coronary angioplasty (PTCA) depends on a number of factors. Chief among these is the location and number of involved vessels. The more extensive the disease, the more likely is the person to have CABG. PTCA is generally limited to those with 1- or 2-vessel disease with smaller amounts of myocardium at risk.

A large number of clinical trials published in the last decade compared CABG to PTCA. In general, these trials found that survival is similar with both interventions in the general population.[37] The Bypass Angioplasty Revascularization Investigation (BARI) found that those with diabetes had a different outcome. This study, conducted in the early 1990s, compared coronary bypass with coronary angioplasty in the era before stents. There was no difference between PTCA and CABG in the nondiabetic population. However, in the diabetes population, coronary bypass grafting was found to reduce the 5-year risk of death by 50% when compared to angioplasty.[38] At the 5-year follow-up point, death rates were 20% in the subjects with diabetes and 8% in those without diabetes. Eight percent of people with diabetes had an additional Q-wave (transmural) MI. CABG reduced the risk of death after a second MI by over 90%.[39]

New developments, including the use of drug-eluting stents, have greatly modified the technology of coronary angioplasty in the last decade. These advances, combined with newer data showing the benefits of aggressive medical management of coronary disease, have raised the question as to whether the BARI conclusions are still valid for use. The Bypass Angioplasty Revascularization Investigation in Type 2 Diabetes (BARI 2D)[40] is a program to study whether, in patients with type 2 diabetes, initial treatment with angioplasty or bypass surgery is better than initial treatment with an aggressive medical program of risk factor management. At the same time, BARI 2D will compare 2 approaches to control blood sugar: providing insulin-stimulating medication or providing medication that sensitizes the body to the available insulin. Patients are randomized to intensive medical (lipid, glucose, blood pressure) management with or without anatomical (PTCA or CABG) intervention. The choice between PTCA and CABG is based on clinical judgment of the cardiologist. All patients are also randomized to initial therapy with insulin-providing medications (insulin or secretagogues) or insulin-sensitizing medications (thiazolidinediones and/or metformin). BARI 2D will not answer whether PTCA or CABG is better; it is designed to determine if surgery or angioplasty is necessary in the presence of aggressive risk factor management.

Instruction Opportunities

Education Topics After Myocardial Infarction

Persons who experienced an MI have undergone a major psychological trauma. They are often discharged from the hospital within 4 or 5 days after an uncomplicated MI, usually with a myriad of unanswered and unasked questions. The following are important education topics:

- *Importance of Follow-Up Care*—With the physician, educator, mental health counselor, and cardiac rehabilitation team, as needed.
- *Medications*—Most people with an MI go home with many new medications, including a statin, ACE inhibitor, β-blocker, aspirin, and possibly another antiplatelet agent. This is in addition to their diabetes medication, which may well be intensified at this time (see section on diabetes management after MI).
- *Exercise*—Some people with a recent MI may be afraid to exercise, and some, in the throes of denial, may overdo it. Cardiac rehabilitation programs enable the individual to work with a trained clinical team to carefully increase exercise in a supervised setting.

- *Therapeutic Lifestyle Change*—Including smoking cessation and medical nutrition therapy.
- *Psychosocial Issues*—Up to one-third of people who have had an MI have significant depressive symptoms afterward, and major depression occurs in nearly one-fifth.[41] Depression, which is more common in diabetes, is associated with a twofold to threefold increase in risk of death in the first 6 months after an MI.[42] Another study of highly stressed individuals post-MI found that home nursing visits were associated with a significant reduction in fatal and nonfatal cardiac events.[43]
- *Sexual Activity*—Many patients are concerned about when it is safe to resume sexual activity. Sexual dysfunction may be common, and its treatment should be discussed with the patient and physician.

Management of Diabetes With an Acute Myocardial Infarction

Hyperglycemia in a person with an MI increases the risk of death and of CHF whether or not the person had a diagnosis of diabetes before admission.[44] There is increasing evidence that MI may be the initial presentation of diabetes.[45] The Diabetes Mellitus Insulin Glucose Infusion in Acute Myocardial Infarction (DIGAMI) trial instituted aggressive diabetes control in the immediate post-MI period with an intravenous insulin-glucose drip, followed by 3 months of a 4-shot regimen. Patients randomized to the intensive protocol had a significant reduction in mortality. The risk reduction was greatest in those classified as low risk who had not been previously treated with insulin.[46]

Preparing Patients for Cardiac Catheterization and Angioplasty

Issues to discuss with the patient and physician include the following:

- Timing of procedure and food consumption
- Diabetes medications
- Hyperglycemia and hypoglycemia
- Hydration
- Pretreatment with steroids

Timing and Food Consumption. Whenever possible, elective cardiac catheterization should be scheduled in the morning for people taking insulin. In most cases, the patient is fasting after midnight for an early morning procedure. If the procedure is later in the day, a light meal may be allowed up to 2 to 4 hours before.

Diabetes Medications. Decisions need to be made and the patient needs to be advised on whether to decrease or withhold certain diabetes medications.

- In general, there is no reason to change evening or bedtime insulin or oral agents if the morning self-monitored glucose is acceptable.
- Persons on insulin pumps should continue their normal basal insulin infusion.
- Sulfonylureas, secretagogues, and acarbose should be held on the morning of the procedure and resumed when the person is eating normally.
- Metformin is held the morning of the procedure and resumed when there is certainty there have been no adverse renal effects of the angiogram dye.
- TZDs can be held or given, as they are long-acting drugs.

Hyperglycemia and Hypoglycemia. Planning must include how hyperglycemia and hypoglycemia will be addressed before and during the procedure.

- *Hypoglycemia* can be managed with glucose tablets or small amounts of clear sugar-containing fluid up to 2 hours before the procedure. Upon arrival in the angiography suite, the unit nurses may elect to begin an intravenous dextrose infusion.
- *Hyperglycemia* is common in people about to undergo surgery or similar procedure. Significant hyperglycemia with ketosis is an indication to delay the procedure until the patient is metabolically stable. Lesser degrees of hyperglycemia should be treated cautiously, as the patient will be sedated during the procedure and may not be able to respond to subsequent hypoglycemia.

Hydration. Patients must be instructed to increase fluid intake to enhance excretion of the angiogram dye.

Steroid Pretreatment. In patients with a history of or risk of allergy to the angiogram dye, prednisone, 20 mg 3 times a day, may be given the day before and day of the procedure. Most patients will note a significant increase in their glucose for 2 to 3 days after beginning prednisone. Preparing the patient for this effect is important so the person can be guided in appropriate medication adjustment.

Cerebrovascular Disease

Atherosclerosis

Atherosclerosis affecting the central nervous system presents in 3 characteristic ways:
Transient ischemic attack (TIA)
Vascular dementia
Cerebrovascular accident (CVA, stroke)

- *Ischemic:* Thrombotic, embolic, or systemic hypotension
- *Hemorrhagic:* Intracranial or subarachnoid

Cerebrovascular Accident (CVA)

Approximately 80% of strokes are ischemic in cause; the remainder are hemorrhagic. By definition, a CVA is tissue death resulting from either disruption by hemorrhage or from ischemic infarction. Ischemic CVA may be caused by atherosclerotic disease in either intracranial or extracranial arteries. The process may be intrinsic to the affected artery, as in atherosclerotic thrombi, or the result of embolus from either the heart or extracranial arteries. The clinical presentation depends upon the area of the brain served by the affected arteries.

In persons with diabetes (versus those without), ischemic strokes are more likely to occur at a younger age, in African Americans, when hypertension is present, and when there is a history of an MI.[47] Most thrombotic and embolic strokes occur in persons over 40 years of age. This is the result of the low rate of atherosclerosis in the younger age group. Given the accelerated atherosclerosis of type 2 diabetes and the epidemic of type 2 diabetes in adolescence, this age-specific guideline may be less predictive in the future as today's youth with type 2 diabetes reach their forties with almost 30 years of diabetes.

Risk factors for stroke:

Hypertension, including isolated systolic hypertension, is the most important risk factor in stroke. Diabetes and smoking contribute to stroke risk as well. Smoking increases the prevalence of extracranial occlusive arterial disease and more than doubles the risk of stroke. Diabetes is also associated with a doubling of stroke risk, affecting both small and large arteries. In contrast to coronary disease, hyperlipoproteinemia has not been shown to be a major risk factor for stroke in the general population.[48] In people with diabetes and ischemic stroke, however, hypercholesterolemia is more common than in stroke victims without diabetes.

Effective antihypertensive therapy and smoking cessation have both been shown to decrease stroke risk.[49,50]

Transient Ischemic Attack

Transient ischemic attack (TIA), sometimes called "mini stroke" by laypeople, is classically defined as the sudden onset of a neurologic deficit that lasts less than 24 hours and is not associated with a permanent residual defect. TIA is presumably caused by a transient decrease in blood supply, causing focal ischemia in the area of the brain that produces the symptoms.

The syndromes caused by a TIA depend on the pathogenesis and location. TIAs may be caused by decreased flow in a large artery, either intracranial or extracranial. Less commonly, an embolus from a larger artery or from the heart may result in transient ischemia. Transient ischemia may result from lesions in either the anterior (carotid) or posterior (vertebral) circulation. The symptoms of ischemia differ significantly as these vascular beds supply areas of the brain with markedly different functions.

Assessment

The initial evaluation of a person with a suspected TIA starts with a careful history. In most cases, the episode will have passed by the time the person is seen by an educator.

Case in Point: Cerebrovascular Disease

VE was a 76-year-old man with a 30-year history of type 2 diabetes. He had moderate peripheral neuropathy, but no microalbuminuria or retinopathy. A1C had been consistently below 7% on combination oral agents. LDL-C was 84, HDL-C 46, triglycerides 140 on a statin. On routine annual physical examination, VE was noted to have a loud left carotid bruit. Carotid Doppler examination revealed a 90% stenosis of the left carotid. VE denied any symptoms of cerebral ischemia; he underwent an elective carotid endarterectomy with an excellent outcome. Preoperative evaluation included a normal nuclear stress test. Four years later, his carotids remained patent.

> ***Suddenness of TIA***
>
> TIAs come on suddenly but, more importantly, require urgent referral. Strokes are known to occur within 2 days in many cases.

It is important to differentiate an ischemic event from a metabolic event, such as hypoglycemia. Seizure disorders, syncope, and migraine auras may also mimic a TIA. Physical assessment focuses on the cardiovascular system to identify carotid artery stenosis or atherosclerotic plaques that may cause local occlusion or may be the source of emboli to intracranial arteries. Further testing will involve Doppler studies of the intracranial and extracranial arteries. If a lesion is suspected in the carotid or vertebral circulation, a magnetic resonance angiogram may be performed to confirm the diagnosis and plan for possible surgery.

Urgent Referral. Patients who have had a TIA require urgent referral for further evaluation. Between 11% and 20% of patients with a TIA had a CVA in the subsequent 90 days; one-half of the strokes occurred in the first 2 days.[51,52]

Management of Carotid Disease

When deciding between medical and surgical management of carotid disease, there are 3 major decision points. First, how severe is the stenosis? Second, is the patient symptomatic; has he or she had a TIA or a CVA? Third, is the patient a good candidate for vascular surgery?

Surgery may be indicated in the following situations:

- Symptomatic patients with a 50% or greater carotid stenosis (this would include most patients with documented TIA)
- Asymptomatic patients with a 60% or greater stenosis

In both situations, the patient's coexisting disease may modify the decision. Patients with carotid atherosclerosis often have significant CAD as well and are at increased risk for perioperative MI. The presence of diabetic autonomic neuropathy increases surgical risk as well.

Whether or not a person has surgery for carotid stenosis, long-term medical management is essential. This includes management of the traditional cardiovascular risk factors:

- Treatment of hypertension has been shown to be an effective risk-reducer for stroke
- Tobacco smoking contributes to as many as 40% of strokes; smoking cessation diminishes this risk
- Antiplatelet therapy is effective in reducing the risk of stroke in those with high risk
- Treatment of dyslipidemia and hyperglycemia are more controversial, although important in the prevention of other cardiovascular events in those with cerebrovascular disease

Vascular Dementia

Vascular dementia includes those dementias caused by ischemic or hemorrhagic cerebrovascular disease.[53] It is the second most-common cause of dementia in adults, after Alzheimers disease, and may coexist with Alzheimers disease. Vascular dementia may be caused by a single infarction, or, most commonly, by the summation effect of multiple, smaller infarctions.

Risk Factors

Although diabetes is a risk factor for stroke, it has not been identified as an independent predictor of vascular dementia. The most important risk factors for vascular dementia are these:

- Older age
- Lower educational level
- Recurrent stroke
- Dominant hemisphere stroke

Patients who have had complicated stroke (pneumonia, arrhythmia, seizure) are at greater risk for vascular dementia.

> ***Preventing vascular dementia:***
>
> The best way to prevent vascular dementia is to prevent stroke. Thus, risk factor management—particularly hypertension and statin use—have been associated with decreased incidence of dementia.

Instruction Opportunities

Education Topics Regarding Cerebrovascular Disease

The diabetes educator can play an important role in the prevention, detection, and referral of patients with cerebrovascular disease.

- *Lifestyle:* Reinforcing a healthy lifestyle, including diet and appropriate exercise, is essential to cardiovascular risk management.
- *Medications:* Appropriate medication regimens may be complex and confusing. The educator can help the patient adhere to these regimens.

Early Identification. The diabetes educator is often the first professional to detect early vascular dementia. When an older person shows early signs of dementia, it is not always Alzheimer disease and may be an indicator of underlying atherosclerotic cerebrovascular disease. Prevention of further ischemic insults may stabilize the person's cognitive function.

Symptoms of cerebrovascular disease may mimic those of hypoglycemia with neuroglycopenia. See the early warning symptoms of stroke listed in Table 21.2. Current therapeutic approaches to thrombotic CVA (the most common form in diabetes) call for early institution of thrombolytic agents. TIA may be an early warning of an impending CVA. Thus, early identification is essential. Educating the person with diabetes about the difference between a hypoglycemic episode and a TIA or early CVA is clearly important.

Many of these symptoms are similar to the symptoms of hypoglycemia; there is no perfect way to distinguish between them other than to test glucose.

Peripheral Arterial Disease

Peripheral arterial disease (PAD) is the third most-important manifestation of atherosclerosis (after coronary and cerebral disease). An estimated 12 million people in the United States have PAD, although estimates of its prevalence are difficult to make, as more than half of those with PAD are asymptomatic or have atypical symptoms. Approximately one-third have classical symptoms of intermittent claudication and about one-sixth have more severe ischemia. Data from the Framingham study suggest that approximately 20% of people with PAD have diabetes; these data are likely to be an underestimate, given the frequency of asymptomatic PAD. A survey of people with diabetes over 50 years of age found the prevalence of PAD by ankle-brachial index determination to be almost 30%.[54] People with long-standing diabetes and PAD may have atypical symptoms due to neuropathy and may not present for medical care until they develop a neurogenic or ischemic ulcer or gangrene.

TABLE 21.2 Early Warning Symptoms of Stroke

The Stroke Association has publicized the following early warning symptoms of stroke and recommended that the person or witness call 911 if they occur:

- Sudden numbness or weakness of the face, arm, or leg, especially on one side of the body
- Sudden confusion, trouble speaking, or understanding
- Sudden trouble seeing in one or both eyes
- Sudden trouble walking, dizziness, or loss of balance or coordination
- Sudden, severe headache with no known cause

Source: Stroke Association. Warning signs. On the Internet: www.strokeassociation.org. Accessed 3 Mar 2006.

The increased risk of PAD in diabetes is likely to be caused by the same etiologic factors as in other vascular beds, including hypertension, dyslipidemia, tobacco, and endothelial dysfunction. Thus, the clinical diagnosis of PAD should raise concern about other vascular beds, including the coronary arteries, renal arteries, and cerebral vessels. Patients with PAD have increased risk of cardiovascular events, including stroke, renovascular hypertension, MI, and sudden death.

Risk Factors

Tobacco use and diabetes are the most important risk factors for PAD. As in other atherosclerotic diseases in diabetes, important risk factors include diabetes duration, age, hypertension, and dyslipidemia. PAD prevalence is greater in African Americans and Hispanics with diabetes.

Modifiable risk factors for PAD:

Tobacco use is the most important modifiable risk factor for PAD. Hypertension and dyslipidemia are also important.

Presentation in Those With Diabetes

The pattern of PAD is different in those whose primary risk factor is diabetes when compared to other risk factors, such as smoking and hypertension. In the presence of diabetes, PAD is more commonly present in the distal arteries—those below the knee (femoral-popliteal and tibial). Other risk factors, such as hypertension and smoking, are associated with a more proximal (aortic, iliac, and proximal femoral) arterial distribution.

The effects of PAD are determined by its progression, presence of symptoms, and associated cardiovascular risk. Although most patients with PAD remain stable, more than one-fourth have progression of symptoms over 5 years, with amputation occurring in approximately 4%. One-fifth will have a cardiovascular event in the next 5 years. Severe ischemia carries a greater risk. Thirty percent will have an amputation, and fatality rates approach 20% in 6 months. Although these data are in the general population and there have been no long-term follow-up studies of people with diabetes, event rates are likely to be even higher in people with diabetes.

Screening and Diagnosis

Screening for and diagnosing PAD is important for 2 reasons. First, the presence of PAD indicates that the person is at increased risk for other events, including stroke and MI. Second, PAD contributes to disability, particularly in those with diabetes. Much of the difference between people with PAD with and without diabetes can be explained by peripheral neuropathy.[55] Adverse effects of PAD include diminished walking ability, with slower walking and shorter walking distances. This leads to deconditioning, which contributes to diminished quality of life and progressive disability.

People with diabetes and PAD are more prone to sudden events, including an arterial thrombosis, neuroischemic ulceration, and infection. These events will lead to critical limb ischemia and increased risk of amputation. By diagnosing PAD in its earlier stages, preventive measures can be instituted to diminish PAD progression or arrange for elective revascularization in a threatened limb before amputation is necessary.

The evaluation for PAD begins with a careful history and physical assessment. The classical symptom of PAD is *intermittent claudication*. The patient will complain of pain, cramping, or aching in the calves, thighs, or buttocks. This pain will recur with walking and is relieved by rest. This pattern differs from that of diabetic peripheral neuropathy, which classically is exacerbated by rest and relieved by walking. The pain of spinal stenosis also increases with walking and may be confused with claudication.

As PAD progresses, it may present with ischemic pain at rest, tissue loss, or gangrene. The combination of PAD and peripheral neuropathy places the person with diabetes at greater risk for lower-limb amputation.

Verbal Assessment. The educator should query the patient for symptoms of claudication, rest pain, and limitations to walking. A careful exercise history will often uncover symptoms of claudication; patients will often not volunteer this information so it is important to seek it out. The pattern of the pain will help differentiate PAD from neuropathy. PAD may present with a wide variety of symptoms, ranging from asymptomatic to severe leg pain at rest. It is also important to identify patients with risk factors, such as smoking and hypertension, in addition to their diabetes. Since the person with PAD is at increased risk for other vascular events, eliciting a history of chest pain or atypical angina symptoms is important. Unfortunately, a stroke history is usually self-evident, but a history of TIAs may indicate atherosclerosis in the cerebral circulation.

Physical Assessment. The physical assessment for diabetic foot problems is part of every diabetes visit. "Shoes and socks off" should be the rule. The ischemic foot may be pale or have "dependent rubor," a deep red color when down and pallor on elevation. There is a loss of hair on the distal foot and toes; cool, dry, atrophic skin; and dystrophic toenails.

The dorsalis pedis and posterior tibial pulses are palpated; if these are absent, the popliteal pulse is palpated as well. It is important to note that palpating pulses is a learned skill. This skill takes practice and has a high rate of false-negative and false-positive examinations.

Ankle-Brachial Index. The Ankle-Brachial Index (ABI) is a ratio of the systolic pressure at the ankle (posterior tibial or dorsalis pedis pulses) and the brachial artery. The ABI has been found to be a reasonably accurate, reproducible measure for the screening and detection of PAD and its severity.

The ABI is determined by placing the blood pressure cuff just above the ankle and inflating it to above systolic pressure. A simple, handheld Doppler device is used to detect the systolic pulse in the dorsalis pedis and posterior tibial arteries as the cuff is slowly deflated. The same procedure is used in both feet and in one arm. To obtain a ratio, the systolic pressure in each of the 4 lower limb arteries is divided by the brachial systolic pressure. The higher value in each limb is the ABI for that limb. See Table 21.3 for diagnostic criteria.

Who should receive ABI screening:

A screening ABI should be performed in people over 50 years of age who have diabetes and should be considered at an earlier age in those with other risk factors (smoking, hypertension, dyslipidemia, more than 10 years of diabetes), according to American Diabetes Association (ADA) guidelines. If the test is normal, the ADA recommends repeat screening every 5 years.

An abnormal ABI is indicative but not diagnostic of PAD and should engender a referral to a vascular laboratory for more formal testing. In addition, those with poorly compressible arteries should be considered for formal vascular testing if there is a high degree of suspicion for PAD.

TABLE 21.3 Ankle-Brachial Index Diagnostic Criteria

- *Normal:* 0.91 to 1.30
- *Mild Obstruction:* 0.7 to 0.9
- *Moderate Obstruction:* 0.4 to 0.7
- *Severe:* <0.4

Note: Elevated pressures (>1.30) may indicate poorly compressible arteries and the presence of arterial calcification. In this case, the ABI may not be representative of the true degree of obstruction.

Imaging Tests. If revascularization is considered (as in a threatened limb or in the presence of a nonhealing ulcer), the next step would be a magnetic resonance angiogram (MRA). This is a noninvasive test, and the magnetic contrast dye used does not increase the risk of renal impairment or allergy (as may be seen with iodinated X-ray or computed tomography dyes). Thus, there will be no need for steroid pretreatment.

Although the MRA provides useful information about vascular anatomy, the "gold standard" test for planning lower extremity arterial reconstruction/bypass is the arteriogram. This examination requires the injection of iodinated dye, with a higher risk of renal impairment or allergy. The patient should be well hydrated before and after the test and consideration given to the glycemic effects of steroids that may be used in the presence of iodinated dye allergy.

Treatment of Peripheral Arterial Disease

Treatment for PAD should include medical therapies either alone or in combination with surgical procedures. Medical therapies are similar to the preventive measures taken for other atherosclerotic diseases, including coronary and cerebrovascular diseases, and include the following:

- Antihypertensives
- Lipid-lowering drugs
- Glucose control
- Smoking cessation
- Aspirin therapy
- Exercise

Antihypertensives. In the UKPDS hypertension treatment arm, a lowering of blood pressure by 10/5 reduced the rate of stroke, but had no effect upon the risk of amputation in PAD. In the HOPE trial, use of ramipril (Altace) lessened the risk of cardiovascular death in participants with PAD, but the impact of ACE inhibition on PAD and amputations was not studied.

Lipid-Lowering Drugs. Lipid-lowering agents have been studied extensively in the primary and secondary prevention of coronary disease. There are limited data on their effect upon PAD. In the 4S (Scandinavian Simvastatin Survival Study), lipid lowering was associated with a nearly 40% reduction in new or worsening symptoms of PAD.[56]

Glucose Control. As in other atherosclerotic diseases, glycemic control has not been shown to have an effect upon PAD progression. However, a large clinical trial with 10,000 participants, the Action to Control Cardiovascular Risk in Diabetes (ACCORD) trial, is testing the effects on major CVD events of intensive glycemic control, intensive lipid management, and intensive blood pressure control.[57] See the questions and controversies section at the end of this chapter for more on this study, which is designed to continue through 2010.

> ***Smoking, PAD, and Stroke***
>
> Smoking cessation is the most important element of risk factor management in peripheral arterial disease. Stopping smoking also reduces stroke risk.

Smoking Cessation. Every educator visit with a smoker is another opportunity to address smoking cessation. Smoking cessation is the most important element of risk factor management in PAD. Tobacco use is associated with increased progression of PAD and increased amputation number.[58]

Aspirin Therapy. Aspirin therapy is recommended for people with diabetes at risk for CVD.[59] The American Diabetes Association recommends that persons with diabetes should be on an antiplatelet agent. Aspirin is discussed further in the section on risk reduction, later in this chapter.

Exercise. For the person with intermittent claudication, supervised exercise training programs have been shown to be of benefit in improving walking. Unsupervised exercise programs have been shown to have no such benefit. All patients with PAD should undergo regular preventive foot care and be educated in self-care of the feet as well.

Instruction Opportunities

Role in Prevention and Screening for Peripheral Arterial Disease

- A careful history and simple physical assessment are all that is needed to screen for PAD and provide referral for appropriate testing and intervention.
- For patients with PAD, the educator's role is to be a guide and coach in preventive maintenance of the affected foot.

Congestive Heart Failure

Congestive heart failure (CHF) is a major contributor to morbidity and mortality in the United States, affecting an estimate 5 million people. People with diabetes, particularly women, have an increased risk of CHF, even in the absence of CAD or hypertension. A number of candidate mechanisms for these effects have been identified, including advanced glycosylation endproducts (AGEs). AGEs are thought to alter ventricular compliance (elasticity) by cross-linking collagen, increased release of proinflammatory cytokines, and activation of oxidative stress. Other factors that may contribute to the increased rate of diastolic dysfunction in people with diabetes include hypertension, diseased microcirculation, the effects of insulin resistance and hyperglycemia on growth factors, the renin-angiotensin-aldosterone system, and vascular endothelial function. These effects result in myocardial hypertrophy, fibrosis, and cellular dysfunction, leading to loss of the normal compliance of the ventricular wall and impaired relaxation. As a result, the ventricle does not relax normally during diastole, leading to impaired diastolic filling and CHF.[60,61]

Treatment

The mainstays of treatment for CHF for everyone, regardless of diabetes, are β-blockers, ACE inhibitors, and sodium restriction. CHF has been considered a relative contraindication to use of metformin (Glucophage) and TZDs,[62] primarily due to sodium retention (TZDs, especially with insulin), and possible risk for lactic acidosis (metformin).

Recent articles, however, have suggested that TZDs and metformin may improve outcomes in patients with heart failure.[63,64] As data continue to accumulate, the choice to use metformin or TZDs in people with CHF must be made based on the balance between risk and benefit.[65]

Screening and Diagnosis

There are several important questions to be answered when considering screening for CVD in people with diabetes:

- Who should be screened?
- Why screen?
- How to screen?

Since some studies suggest that everyone with type 2 diabetes should be considered to have CVD,[66] should everyone with type 2 be screened? Since there are almost 20 million people in the United States with type 2 diabetes, that would entail an immense expense. So, how do clinicians decide who should be screened? There are a number of different "risk engines" to calculate risk. The Framingham[67] and UKPDS[68] risk engines are 2 of the best known.

It is important to differentiate between screening tests and diagnostic tests:

- *Screening tests* usually refer to testing of asymptomatic people
- *Diagnostic tests*, on the other hand, are used when a clinical indication exists that disease may be present

According to the ADA Standards of Medical Care in Diabetes,[69] patients can be subdivided into those without clear or suggestive symptoms and those with those symptoms. Those with typical or atypical cardiac symptoms (chest pain, episodic dyspnea, unexplained nausea, and diaphoresis) and abnormal electrocardiogram (ECG), should be referred to a cardiologist for diagnostic evaluation. Candidates for screening include those with evidence of peripheral or carotid arterial disease, sedentary lifestyle (over age 35) and planning to begin vigorous exercise, and those with 2 or more major risk factors (listed in Table 21.4).

The ADA grades these recommendations as "E," which means they are based on expert consensus, rather than on epidemiologic or clinical trials. Other candidates for screening include patients who are to undergo high-risk vascular procedures, such as bypass surgery for peripheral vascular disease and carotid atherectomy.

Exercise ECG. In most cases, the initial screening or diagnostic test is an exercise ECG. The patient is usually fasting. ECG leads are placed in the standard locations for a 12-lead ECG. He or she then begins to walk on a level treadmill at a slow pace. The speed and incline of the treadmill are gradually increased until symptoms or ECG abnormalities occur.

Case In Point: Screening and Referral

EG was a 68-year-old Hispanic man with hypertension and a 10-year history of type 2 diabetes who was referred for diabetes management. On initial evaluation, his blood pressure was well controlled on a combination of ACE inhibitor and low-dose hydrochlorothiazide. LDL-C was 106 on a statin. Mr. G's physical examination was unremarkable, but his ECG showed nonspecific abnormalities suggestive of ischemia. He was referred to a cardiologist and underwent an exercise stress test, which was normal.

TABLE 21.4 Major Risk Factors for Cardiovascular Disease

- Dyslipidemia
- Hypertension (or use of antihypertensive medication)
- Smoking
- Microalbuminuria or macroalbuminuria
- Family history of premature CVD

Stress Echocardiogram. Another functional test is the stress echocardiogram, in which the myocardium is imaged by sonography during exercise. Areas of abnormal motion indicate ischemia.

Instruction Opportunities

Preparing the Patient for the Initial Test

Patients are usually fasting for exercise stress testing. Significant hyperglycemia or hypoglycemia may interfere with the ability to exercise to an appropriate level. Although the stress test is usually limited to 12 to 15 minutes, it may be enough to precipitate hypoglycemia during or shortly after the exercise in people taking long-acting insulins or sulfonylureas.

- The educator should discuss the possibility of hypoglycemia with the patient. This hypoglycemia is usually short-lived and can be treated with oral carbohydrate. Sulfonylureas and short-acting insulins should be held until the first posttest meal.

Preparing the Patient for Follow-Up Testing

If the exercise test is indicative of ischemia, the next step is usually radionuclide cardiac imaging, to assess myocardial perfusion, and if necessary, coronary angiogram.

- Patients are usually able to eat a light breakfast several hours before elective coronary angiography. It is important to recommend appropriate insulin modifications.
- Although the injection and movement of the angiogram catheter are not painful, the dye injection often results in transient angina-type chest pain and a feeling of warmth and flushing.

Prednisone. Many individuals have a history of allergic reactions to intravenous contrast dye. Pretreatment for these allergies includes pharmacologic doses of prednisone for 1 to 2 days before the procedure. This pretreatment will uniformly elevate blood glucose in people with diabetes. It is important to prepare the patient appropriately. In some cases, patients successfully treated with oral agents may require a brief course of insulin. Those on insulin will require significant increases in their dose, particularly in the insulins acting during the day, as corticosteroid therapy tends to increase postprandial glucose more than fasting glucose.

Other Imaging Techniques

Newer imaging techniques that are receiving increased publicity include electron beam computed tomography (EBCT), in which the amount of coronary calcification correlates with coronary atherosclerosis; computed tomography (CT); and magnetic resonance imaging (MRI) angiography. Although attractive because they are less invasive than standard angiography, these techniques require further evaluation before they can be recommended.

What about noncardiac cardiovascular disease?

The Cardiovascular Health Study[70] investigated the rate of clinical and subclinical CVD in almost 6000 people over 65 years of age. Three vascular beds—the heart, carotid arteries, and legs—were evaluated for clinical or subclinical disease. People with diabetes had increased clinical disease, primarily in the heart. Subclinical disease, on the other hand, was much more prevalent in the carotid arteries (determined by carotid ultrasound testing) than in either the heart or the leg.

Screening for peripheral or cerebral atherosclerosis begins with the physical examination. Carotids are palpated for pulse and auscultated for bruits. If the carotid pulse is weakened or a bruit is heard, the patient should be referred for carotid ultrasound Doppler examination. Results of this test are expressed as mild, moderate, or severe stenosis. Moderate-to-severe stenosis should be evaluated further with a magnetic resonance angiogram (MRA) for consideration of carotid endarterectomy.

Screening for PAD begins with determination of the ABI, as described earlier. If the ankle systolic pressure is less than 90% of the brachial pressure, PAD is likely.

Presence of carotid atherosclerosis should raise the clinician's index of suspicion that coronary disease is present as well, as Barzilay[70] found that approximately 30% of those with carotid disease had coronary disease as well. Surprisingly, PAD was much less common than either carotid or cardiac disease in both those with and without diabetes. When PAD was present, however, most patients had concomitant carotid or cardiac disease.

Cardiac Autonomic Neuropathy

Diabetic autonomic neuropathy affecting the heart is present in from 30% to 70% of persons with long-standing diabetes. Autonomic dysfunction is associated with an increased risk of mortality in people with diabetes,[71,72] in those with CVD,[73,74] and in the middle-aged and elderly population.[75,76]Autonomic neuropathy may influence function of a number of organ systems. In the cardiovascular system, autonomic neuropathy may increase the risk of silent myocardial ischemia and silent MI. Cardiac neuropathy is associated with a greater risk of sudden death, possibly due to increased arrhythmia risk. See chapter 24 for a discussion on autonomic neuropathy.

Instruction Opportunities

Persons with diabetic cardiac autonomic neuropathy should be educated about the following topics:

- Decreased exercise tolerance
- Silent ischemia and anginal equivalent symptoms such as nausea, diaphoresis, shortness of breath
- Postural hypotension, particularly after exercise
- The need for cardiologic evaluation on a regular basis

Risk-Reduction Strategies

The causes of CVD are multifactorial, including abnormalities of glucose metabolism, lipid metabolism, blood pressure, coagulation, and inflammation. Thus, programs to reduce the impact of CVD in diabetes must be multifactorial as well. Effective interventions include the following:

- Lifestyle modification
- Lipid therapy
- Blood pressure control
- Glycemic control
- Antiplatelet therapy

Other interventions that have had recent attention include vitamin supplementation with vitamins E, B_6, and folate. Key points relevant to some of these interventions are summarized below.

Therapeutic Lifestyle Change

The US population has become more obese as a result of less healthy eating patterns and decreased physical activity. Thus, the benefits of therapeutic lifestyle change go well beyond reducing CVD in people with diabetes. As a result, the ADA, American Heart Association, and American Cancer Society have joined in a collaborative effort to impact on lifestyle changes that affect diabetes, heart disease, and cancer.[77]

Smoking Cessation

Nearly 20% of deaths from CVD can be directly linked to cigarette smoking. Stopping smoking can reduce the risk of coronary death by 50% within 1 year.[78] There are numerous sources of information for smoking cessation available on the Web sites of the Centers for Disease Control and Prevention (CDC) and the US Department of Health and Human Services: www.cdc.gov and www.hhs.gov.

Nutrition

There are little data from randomized, controlled clinical trials to evaluate the effect of changes in nutrition on cardiovascular events, but it is clear that following a healthy eating pattern will improve some risk factors for both diabetes and CVD. The effects of a healthy diet have been shown to include improvement in weight, blood pressure,[79] and dyslipidemia.[80]

Vitamin Supplementation

Vitamin B_6 and Folic Acid. Data associating cardiovascular risk with higher levels of homocysteine have led to programs to reduce the level of homocysteine by supplementation with folic acid and vitamin B_6. Although these supplements effectively lower homocysteine levels, the NORVIT study[81] found that this change was not associated with an improvement in overall cardiovascular risk. More importantly, combined supplementation with pyridoxine and folate increased the risk of MI by 21%.

Vitamin E and Antioxidants. Endothelial dysfunction is associated with oxidative stress at the endothelial cell. Thus, antioxidant therapy, particularly with vitamin E, has been touted as a cardiovascular risk-reduction strategy. The SEARCH study revealed that addition of vitamin E to simvastatin (Zocor), the HMG-CoA reductase inhibitor, actually increased the risk of cardiovascular events.[82] A more recent analysis of data from the HOPE and HOPE-TOO studies found that vitamin E supplementation in people with diabetes or CVD did not reduce the rate of major cardiovascular events and may increase the risk of heart failure.[83] Brown[82] concludes that, "antioxidant vitamins E and C and beta-carotene . . . do not protect against cardiovascular disease. . . . they are potentially harmful. . . . [and] should rarely, if ever, be recommended for cardiovascular protection." Inappropriate use of antioxidant vitamins not only blunts the protective effects of other therapies, but often creates false hope that "natural" therapies are better than drugs, diverting the patient from proven therapies.

Physical Activity

A number of prospective epidemiologic studies have shown the benefits of physical activity on reducing cardiovascular events.[84] More recent data indicate the same effect is present in people with diabetes. A prospective study of over 1700 patients with type 2 diabetes found that moderate-to-high levels of exercise decreased total and cardiovascular mortality. Although smoking and higher levels of blood pressure, body mass index, and cholesterol were associated with higher risk of death from CVD, the effect of exercise was independent of these risk factors.[85] Another study showed that older adults benefit from physical activity. When sedentary adults 55 to 75 years of age initiated a program of regular supervised physical training, there was a significant reduction in metabolic markers of cardiovascular risk and a lower rate of abnormal exercise stress test results or angina pectoris.[86]

Intensive Lifestyle Therapy

A multifactorial disease requires multifactorial interventions. Intensive lifestyle therapy in the Diabetes Prevention Program not only reduced the risk of diabetes significantly, but also reduced cardiovascular risk factors.[87] (See chapter 2 for more information on this and other studies.) Intensive lifestyle modification therapy to reduce weight and increase exercise was found to improve high-density lipoprotein cholesterol (HDL-C) levels and decrease levels of the more atherogenic, small, dense LDL-C. On a more clinically practical level, lifestyle modification reduced the need for antihypertensive medication by 27% to 28% and lipid-lowering medication by 25%.

There are many known and potential contributors to the increased rate of macrovascular disease in people with diabetes. Thus, the best approach to reducing this devastating group of complications is probably to try to improve as many known risk factors as possible. The STENO-2 Study instituted intensive behavioral and pharmacologic therapy to target hyperglycemia, hypertension, dyslipidemia, and microalbuminuria for 80 patients with type 2 diabetes and microalbuminuria. Most patients were also treated with aspirin. Glycemic therapy included metformin (Glucophage) and a sulfonylurea; insulin was added when needed. Atorvastatin (Lipitor) was used for hypercholesterolemia and fibrates for hypertriglyceridemia. All patients were placed on an ACE inhibitor or an angiotensin II receptor blocker (ARB); other antihypertensive agents and combination ACE inhibitor and ARB were used when needed. Target values at the end of the study were an A1C of 6.5%, blood pressure of less than 130/80 mm Hg, total cholesterol of 175 mg/dL, and triglycerides of less than 150 mg/dL. Patients in the aggressive intervention group had significant reductions in CVD, retinopathy, nephropathy, and autonomic neuropathy.

At this time, defining which of the many available interventions are necessary and in which combinations they are effective is not possible. Answers may come from a number of ongoing studies.

Glycemia and CVD

The literature has extensively demonstrated the impact of glycemia and glycemic control on the microvascular complications of diabetes. The relationship between glucose and macrovascular disease is less clear. This was found in both cross-sectional and longitudinal studies.[88]

A number of large epidemiologic studies have shown that chronic hyperglycemia is an independent risk factor for CVD.[89] In most cases, however, these studies were limited to evaluating fasting blood glucose or A1C.

The ARIC (Atherosclerosis Risk in Communities) study found that increased levels of A1C were directly related to increased carotid intimal-medial thickness (IMT), a measure of early atherosclerosis.[90] Pooled data from a recent meta-analysis suggest that a 1% increase in A1C is associated with a 1.2- to 1.3-fold increased risk of CVD, including coronary events, stroke, and PAD.[91]

Although the UKPDS found that A1C was a good predictor of CVD,[92] intervention to lower glucose did not affect macrovascular outcomes except in the case of obese patient treated with metformin (Glucophage) alone. It is likely that this effect was the result of the impact of that medication on other risk factors, such as lipids and obesity, rather than glucose.

There is an increasing interest in the role of postprandial glucose's role in macrovascular disease. Epidemiologic data support the association of postprandial hyperglycemia and increased cardiovascular risk.[93,94] Type 2 diabetes is characterized by rapid increases in postprandial blood glucose. That these "hyperglycemic spikes" may play a role in the pathophysiology of microvascular and macrovascular complications of diabetes is an area of great research interest at this time.

Postprandial hyperglycemia was shown to be associated with increased risk of MI in the Diabetes Intervention Study.[95]

Glycemic Interventions: Type 2 Diabetes

Although there are extensive data to support the concept that glycemic control can reduce the risk of microvascular complications of diabetes, evidence is less compelling for its effect on macrovascular events, particularly in type 2 diabetes.[96]

The UKPDS intensive group had 16% fewer MIs than the control group, but this effect just missed statistical significance.[97] Secondary analyses of the UKPDS data did show a statistically significant 12% decrease in rate of MI for each 1% reduction of A1C. This effect is much less than the effect of controlling hypertension or hyperlipidemia.

Results of a study of acarbose treatment for impaired glucose tolerance[98] and a subsequent meta-analysis[99] support the hypothesis that reducing postprandial glucose excursions may decrease cardiovascular risk in people with prediabetes and with diabetes. Additional support was provided by a study comparing the short-acting secretagogue repaglinide with a glyburide, one of the long-acting sulfonylureas.[100] A1C decreased by 0.9% in both groups, but postprandial glucose was significantly lower in the repaglinide group than the glyburide group. Carotid IMT and C-reactive protein decreased in both groups with a greater effect in subjects treated with repaglinide.

Important questions remain in the management of glycemia in people with type 2 diabetes. Research is needed to determine the impact of different levels of glycemic control and the role of targeting A1C versus targeting postprandial glycemia.

Glycemic Interventions: Type 1 Diabetes

The major predictor of CVD in people with type 1 diabetes appears to be duration of disease.[101] Several lines of evidence support the long-term effects of glycemic control on reducing macrovascular risk. Pancreas transplantation normalizes glucose and has been shown to reduce increased carotid IMT to normal within 2 years of successful transplantation.[102] In a study of kidney transplant patients who received a subsequent islet transplant, the kidney-islet group had improvement of cardiac function and stabilization of carotid IMT when compared to the kidney-alone group.[103]

Long-term follow-up of the DCCT cohort has provided interesting new data about the impact of intensive control on the development of macrovascular disease in type 1 diabetes. After completion of the DCCT in 1992, most of the participants were enrolled in a long-term follow-up study, the Epidemiology of Diabetes Interventions and Complications (DCCT/EDIC) study. Glycemic control as determined by A1C between the 2 groups remained minimally different for 4 years, but by the fifth year after the end of the DCCT, there was no difference between the 2 groups. Carotid IMT was measured in 1994 to 1996 and again 4 years later. Progression of carotid IMT was associated with a number of conventional risk factors, including age, systolic blood pressure, smoking, LDL-C/HDL-C ratio, and albuminuria. Most important, progression of carotid IMT 6 years after the end of the DCCT was closely associated with allocation to the intensive therapy during the 6.5 years of the DCCT.[104]

Subsequent data from the same group were presented at the ADA Scientific Sessions: Late-Breaking Clinical Trials Session in June 2005, by Nathan.[105] Early intensive control of glycemia reduced all CV events by 42% and reduced nonfatal MI, CVA, and cardiovascular death by 57%. These effects were mediated by control in A1C during the DCCT. Thus, the combined DCCT/EDIC studies prove that early intensive control of type 1 diabetes decreases the risk of both microvascular and macrovascular complications.

Insulin-Resistance Therapies

Although insulin resistance as a component of type 2 diabetes has been recognized for many years, only in the last 2 decades has the clustering of insulin resistance, type 2 diabetes, and increased cardiovascular risk been unified and expanded, beginning with the seminal work of Reaven in 1988.[106] With the release of troglitazone (Rezulin), the first TZD, came an onslaught of research to determine if modifying insulin resistance by activators of the receptor would modify cardiovascular risk. It rapidly became apparent that not only do PPARγ agonists enhance glycemic control, but they also have pleiotropic effects on other cardiovascular risk factors, including endothelial dysfunction, coagulopathy, and dyslipidemia.[107,108]

These effects suggest that treatment with TZDs may reduce cardiovascular risk. This hypothesis was recently tested in the PROactive[109] study, in which pioglitazone (Actos) was added in addition to glucose-lowering and other medications. There was no statistical difference in the primary end-point of combined cardiovascular events and revascularization. Pioglitazone therapy did result in a statistically significant 16% reduction in a secondary endpoint consisting of death, MI, and stroke. Pioglitazone therapy resulted in an increased incidence of edema and nonfatal CHF.

Inzucchi and colleagues[110] reviewed data on almost 25,000 Medicare beneficiaries with diabetes discharged after an MI. Of 8872 patients discharged on a diabetes drug, 819 were prescribed a TZD, 1273 were prescribed metformin (Glucophage), and 139 received both drugs. Prescription of a TZD was associated with a 17% higher rate of readmission for heart failure. There was no difference in 1-year mortality in those prescribed either drug, but the combination group had a 48% reduction in 1-year mortality.

TZDs may prove to be indicated for the prevention of cardiovascular disease in adults, but not yet. More research is needed to determine who may benefit from these interesting drugs. In an editorial accompanying the PROactive report,[111] Yki-Jarvinen concludes that the PROactive study does not help determine who should be treated with pioglitazone except for "patients with type 2 diabetes and preexisting macrovascular disease who do not develop heart failure."

Control of Hypertension

Hypertension is present in over 50 million Americans[79] and is 2 to 3 times more common in people with type 2 diabetes than in the nondiabetic population. Table 21.5 lists the classification criteria for hypertension in adults. Other known cardiovascular risk factors, including age, obesity, and renal disease, all contribute to the increased prevalence of coexistent diabetes and hypertension. As the obesity epidemic continues, health professionals will continue to see more concomitant hypertension and diabetes, with the combined effect leading to a marked increase in CVD.[112] In persons with type 1 diabetes, hypertension commonly develops only after renal disease is present.[113]

Hypertension is a cardiovascular risk factor in the general population as well as a significant additive risk factor for CVD in diabetes.[113-115] Cardiovascular risk increases in a linear fashion with increased blood pressure; a 20-mm Hg systolic increase, or a 10-mm Hg diastolic increase doubles the risk of CVD.[116] Prehypertension, as defined as 120 to 139 mmHg systolic or 80 to 89 mm Hg diastolic, has also been associated with increased risk for CVD.[117]

Numerous studies have shown that blood pressure reduction in people with diabetes and hypertension can reduce overall cardiovascular mortality and, in particular, the incidence of stroke. This effect is shown even with modest reductions in blood pressure, as in the UKPDS, in which the "intensive" group reached a mean blood pressure of 144/82 mm Hg, compared to the control group's 154/87. Diabetes-related death was reduced by 32% and stroke by 44%. There was a nonsignificant 21% reduction in MI with blood pressure control. Most studies have shown the same pattern: a dramatic reduction in stroke and total cardiovascular mortality with a less dramatic effect on MI.[113]

The ADA[11,118] and JNC 7[79] report recommend a target blood pressure level of <130/80 mm Hg for adults with diabetes. Although there appears to be no threshold effect for the effect of blood pressure on cardiovascular risk, more aggressive treatment will increase the cost of care and the risk of medication side effects.

Children and Adolescents

The 2006 ADA Standards of Medical Care in Diabetes discuss screening and management of hypertension for children and adolescents with type 1 diabetes and make the following recommendations.[69] Hypertension in childhood is defined as an average systolic or diastolic blood pressure ≥95th percentile for age, sex, and height percentile measured on at least 3 separate days. "High-normal" blood pressure is defined as an average systolic or diastolic blood pressure ≥90th but <95th percentile for age, sex, and height percentile measured on at least 3 separate days. Normal blood pressure levels for age, sex, and height and appropriate methods for determinations are available online at www.nhlbi.nih.gov/health/prof/heart/hbp/hbp_ped.pdf.

TABLE 21.5 Classification of Hypertension in Adults

Stage	*Systolic Pressure (mm Hg)*	*Diastolic Pressure (mm Hg)*
Normal	<120 *and*	<80
Prehypertension	120 to 139 *or*	80 to 89
Stage 1 hypertension	140 to 159 *or*	90 to 99
Stage 2 hypertension	≥160 *or*	≥100

Source: Chobanian AV, Bakris GL, Black HR, et al. The Seventh Report of the Joint National Committee on Prevention, Detection, Evaluation, and Treatment of High Blood Pressure: the JNC 7 report. JAMA. 2003;289:2560-72.

Lifestyle Intervention in Children. Treatment of high-normal blood pressure (systolic or diastolic blood pressure consistently above the 90th percentile for age, sex, and height) in children should include dietary intervention and recommendations, based on expert consensus and clinical experience, consist of diet, exercise aimed at weight control, and increased physical activity.

Pharmacologic Therapy in Children. If target blood pressure is not reached within 3 to 6 months of lifestyle intervention, pharmacologic treatment should be initiated. Pharmacologic treatment of hypertension (systolic or diastolic blood pressure consistently above the 95th percentile for age, sex, and height or consistently greater than 130/80 mm Hg, if 95% exceed that value) in children should be initiated as soon as the diagnosis is confirmed. These ADA recommendations on pharmacologic treatment for children are based on expert consensus or clinical experience. See chapter 18 for more on pharmacologic interventions for hypertension in children and adolescents.[69]

Patient Evaluation

Evaluation of the patient with hypertension and diabetes begins by addressing lifestyle factors that may contribute to hypertension and cardiovascular risk. This is clearly in the purview of the diabetes educator. The patient is then evaluated for secondary causes of hypertension, such as renal artery stenosis, kidney disease, pheochromocytoma, or Cushing syndrome. In most cases, the secondary causes can be ruled out by a careful history and physical examination combined with appropriate laboratory testing. End-organ damage, including renal disease; left ventricular hypertrophy; or CHF, may modify the therapy and is included in an initial assessment.

Interventions for Hypertension In Adults

Therapeutic Interventions

In general, addressing systolic blood pressure will result in control of diastolic pressure as well, particularly in the type 2 population. Therapy, thus, should be targeted at systolic control. (Chapter 18 provides more detail.)

Lifestyle Modification. Lifestyle modification is an essential part of the management of hypertension. Both the JNC 7 report and ADA recommend a combination of dietary modification and moderate exercise as the initial step in hypertension management. Lifestyle change may be adequate to lower blood pressure to the target range in people with systolic blood pressure between 130 and 140 mm Hg, as the major interventions have the potential to lower systolic blood pressure between 4 and 20 mm Hg.[79] A 10-kg weight loss can lower systolic pressure between 5 and 20 mm Hg; adoption of the DASH[119] eating plan may result in an 8- to 14-mm Hg decrease; sodium restriction will result in between a 2- and 8-mm Hg reduction, and moderate aerobic activity in a 4- to 9-mm Hg reduction. See the information on hypertension in chapter 13, on medical nutrition therapy.

Pharmacologic Intervention. When a 3-month trial of lifestyle change is not adequate, or if the initial blood pressure is ≤140 mm Hg systolic or ≤90 mm Hg diastolic, pharmacologic intervention is usually necessary. The initial drug choice is dictated by the presence or absence of diabetes complications or other end-organ damage. In general, however, more than 1 drug is needed for blood pressure control, with the average in most studies being between 2 and 3. Presence of nephropathy would mandate initiating with an ACE inhibitor or an ARB. A history of MI is an indication for β-blocker therapy. As hypertension in diabetes commonly has a volume component, a low-dose thiazide diuretic is often necessary to adequately control blood pressure, particularly systolic pressure. The Antihypertensive and Lipid-Lowering Treatment to Prevent Heart Attack Trial (ALLHAT)[120] compared chlorthalidone, a long-acting thiazide diuretic, with the calcium channel blocker amlodipine, and the ACE inhibitor lisinopril. There was no significant difference in cardiovascular events between diuretic and amlodipine or between diuretic and lisinopril. This was true in subjects with and without diabetes.

In the UKPDS hypertension substudy, there was no difference in outcome between the ACE inhibitor captopril and the β-blocker atenolol.[121] Importantly, by the end of the UKPDS study, more than two-thirds of the subjects were on 2 or more drugs for blood pressure control and between 27% and 31% were on 3 or more. Given that the achieved control (144/82 mm Hg) was still higher than the JNC 7 report and ADA recommended target of 130/80 mm Hg, it is likely that even more drugs would have been necessary to achieve the lower goals.

See chapter 18 for thorough information on pharmacologic therapy for hypertension in persons with diabetes.

Instruction Opportunities

Hypertension is a major additive cardiovascular risk in people with diabetes. Its therapy, similar to that of diabetes, includes lifestyle modification and appropriate drug choices. The benefits of reaching lower blood pressure goals have been demonstrated for people with diabetes.

Lifestyle Modification. Lifestyle modification is essential in the management of hypertension with or without diabetes. Suggested changes include the following:

- Weight reduction
- Adoption of the DASH eating plan
- Dietary sodium restriction
- Increased physical activity
- Moderation of alcohol consumption

Medication Regimen, Adherence, and Safe Use. Pharmacologic regimens for hypertension are complex, involving multiple medications.

- The educator has an important role in helping the person with diabetes keep track of their medication schedule and adhere to the medication plan. Tables of medications, their purpose, and times of day to take them can facilitate adherence.
- The educator should also review potential side effects and drug interactions of antihypertensive medications with the patient. For example, over-the-counter NSAID analgesics such as ibuprofen and naproxen can interact with ACE inhibitors and ARBs to cause significant renal damage and dangerous hyperkalemia.

Chapter 18 provides much valuable information for educators on hypertension topics.

Lipid Abnormalities

Dyslipidemia is a major problem in people with type 2 diabetes; lipid abnormalities are present in more than 95% of those with type 2 diabetes.[122] See Table 21.6 for dyslipidemia screening information. The most common pattern of dyslipidemia is a combination of high triglycerides and low HDL-C. Concentration of LDL-C is similar to that of the nondiabetic population. However, the character of the LDL-C is different, with an increase in the smaller, denser, more atherogenic fraction.[123] Numerous studies have found that each of the lipoprotein abnormalities of diabetes (LDL-C, HDL-C, and triglycerides) are CVD risk predictors.[124] Treatment to lower LDL-C and triglycerides or raise HDL-C has been shown to reduce macrovascular events and mortality in the general at-risk population and, in particular, in people with diabetes.[125,126] Chapter 18 provides extensive information on this topic.

Children and Adolescents. Children with diabetes should be screened and monitored for dyslipidemia. For prepubertal children, a fasting lipid profile is recommended in all children over the age of 2 at the time of diagnosis if there is a family history of hypercholesterolemia, a family history of a cardiovascular event before the age of 55, or if the family history is unknown. If there are no family history risk factors present, the first lipid screening should be performed at puberty. The ADA does not recommend initiation of pharmacotherapy in children.[69]

Measurement of Lipid Levels

Lipid levels should be measured after an overnight fast, as postprandial triglyceride elevations may interfere with evaluation of the lipid profile. Calculation of LDL-C is often inaccurate with elevated triglycerides, and most laboratories will not report the LDL-C if the triglyceride level is greater than 400 mg/dL. In this case, either the direct LDL-C assay or calculation of the non-HDL-C may be useful. The ADA recommends calculation of the non-HDL-C in cases in which the triglyceride level is above 200 mg. Target levels for non-HDL-C are 30 mg/dL greater than LDL-C targets. Although a measurement of lipoprotein size is commercially available, there are little data to support its use in clinical practice.[123]

Lipid Goals

The National Cholesterol Education Program Adult Treatment Panel III guidelines suggest lipid treatment goals based on relative risk for cardiovascular events. See Table 21.7.

- *High Risk.* People with type 2 diabetes and others with >20% 10-year risk of cardiovascular events are considered at high risk for cardiovascular events.
- *Very High Risk.* Those with concomitant diabetes and diagnosed CVD are considered at very high risk. Others considered at very high risk include those with established CVD plus multiple major risk factors, severe or poorly controlled risk factors (especially continued tobacco smoking), multiple risk factors of the metabolic syndrome (especially high triglycerides with low HDL-C), or acute coronary syndrome.

The primary approach to lipid therapy is to lower LDL-C to levels associated with risk reduction.[126] See chapter 18 for thorough information on pharmacologic therapy for diabetic dyslipidemia.

Lipids and Blood Pressure

To prevent and delay macrovascular disease and life-threatening cardiovascular events in people with diabetes, keep lipid levels and blood pressure under control.

TABLE 21.6 Screening for Dyslipidemia for People With Diabetes

- The ADA recommends screening for lipid abnormalities annually in most adults with diabetes
- Monitoring of lipid levels should occur more often if necessary to modify treatment to reach goals
- The low-risk patient (LDL-C <100 mg/dL, HDL-C >50 mg/dL, triglycerides <150 mg/dL; no evidence of CVD) may only need lipid levels every 2 years

TABLE 21.7 Lipid Levels Associated With Risk Reduction for Cardiovascular Disease Among People With Diabetes

All People With Diabetes	*High Risk*	*Very High Risk*
Triglycerides <150 mg/dL	LDL-C <100 mg/dL	LDL-C <70 mg/dL
HDL-C Men >40 mg/dL Women >50 mg/dL	Non-HDL-C <130 mg/dL	Non-HDL-C <100 mg/dL

Children and Adolescents

The 2006 ADA Standards of Medical Care in Diabetes make the following recommendations regarding screening children and adolescents for dyslipidemia.[69]

Prepubertal Children. A fasting lipid profile should be performed on all children >2 years of age at the time of diagnosis for diabetes (after glucose control has been established) if there is a family history of hypercholesterolemia (total cholesterol >240 mg/dL), if there is a history of a cardiovascular event before age 55 years, or if family history is unknown. If family history is not of concern, then the first lipid screening should be performed at puberty (>12 years). If values are within the accepted risk levels—that is, LDL-C <100 mg/dL (2.6 mmol/L)—a lipid profile should be repeated every 5 years.

Pubertal Children (>12 years of age). A fasting lipid profile should be performed at the time of diagnosis (after glucose control has been established). If values fall within the accepted risk levels—that is, LDL-C <100 mg/dL (2.6 mmol/L)—the measurement should be repeated every 5 years.

If lipids are abnormal, annual monitoring is recommended in both age groups. These ADA recommendations are based on expert consensus or clinical experience.

Dyslipidemia Treatment

Therapeutic interventions for dyslipidemia include lifestyle change and pharmacologic therapy. The following approach is suggested:

- *Lifestyle Change.* Both the ADA and the NCEP ATP III recommend therapeutic lifestyle change (TLC) as an initial therapeutic step in the management of people with hyperlipoproteinemia.[80] Persons with clinical evidence of CVD should be considered for pharmacologic lipid-lowering therapy starting concomitantly with TLC.
- *Pharmacologic Intervention.* If after a 6-week trial of TLC, the person has not reached LDL-C goals, the NCEP ATP III recommends pharmacologic intervention.

TLC should allow some persons to reach lipid goal levels. Goals of TLC are listed in Table 21.8. Any person at high risk who had other modifiable risk factors (obesity, sedentary lifestyle, tobacco smoking) should be a candidate for TLC in addition to other therapies.

TABLE 21.8 Goals of Therapeutic Lifestyle Change

Reduce . . . • Saturated fats, trans fats, and cholesterol • Weight
Increase . . . • Dietary fiber and plant stanols/steroids • Physical activity

Omega-3 Fatty Acids

Increased intake of omega-3 fatty acids has been shown to reduce cardiovascular risk. Two servings a week of salmon or other fatty fish provide adequate supplementation for people without documented CVD. Higher amounts have been recommended for people with coronary disease. In general, dietary fish intake is not adequate for lowering triglycerides, and supplementation with omega-3 therapy is necessary.[127,128]

Pharmacologic Intervention: Lower LDL-C

It has been 30 years since publication of the MRFIT study, which attempted to prove that lowering total cholesterol by diet would reduce cardiovascular events.[129] Since that time, there have been a plethora of articles investigating the role of lipid lowering by statin or fibrate therapy, beginning with the landmark Scandinavian Simvastatin Survival Study (4S).[130] Although these studies were not exclusively of people with diabetes, most included a large diabetes subgroup. Studies have shown benefit from statin therapy in both secondary prevention in patients with established coronary disease[131] and primary prevention in people with diabetes in whom there is no evidence of preexisting CVD.[132]

Statins. A meta-analysis of 6 primary prevention studies and 8 studies of secondary prevention showed relative risk reductions of 22% and 24% by use of statins in people with type 2 diabetes.[133] Based on this analysis, the American College of Physicians published a Clinical Practice Guideline[134] with the recommendations shown in the sidebar on the following page.

Statin Use Recommendations

From the American College of Physicians Clinical Practice Guideline[134]

Recommendation: "Lipid-lowering therapy should be used for secondary prevention of cardiovascular mortality and morbidity for all patients (both men and women) with known coronary artery disease"

Comment: The NCEP ATP III and ADA consider the persons described in this first recommendation to be at very high risk and suggest lowering LDL-C to a target level of 70 mg/dL.

Recommendation: "Statins should be used for primary prevention against macrovascular complications in patients (both men and women) with type 2 diabetes and other cardiovascular risk factors"

Comment: In the group described in this second recommendation, the NCEP ATP III and ADA recommend treating to a goal LDL-C of 100 mg/dL.

Recommendation: "Once lipid-lowering therapy is initiated, patients with type 2 diabetes should be taking at least moderate doses of a statin"

Comment: The lowest dose of most statins on the market will lower LDL-C by 30% to 35%.

Recommendation: "For those patients with type 2 diabetes who are taking statins, routine monitoring of liver function tests or muscle enzymes is not recommended except in specific circumstances"

Comment: The specific circumstances described in this recommendation include prior abnormalities of these tests, symptoms of myopathy, or potential drug interactions that may increase the risk of myopathy.

Options After Statins. For those who cannot tolerate statins, or when statins alone do not achieve the target LDL-C level, there are several additional options that decrease intestinal absorption of cholesterol. These include ezetimibe (Zetia), colesevelam (Welchol), and bile-acid binding resins. In each case, these medications can potentiate the LDL-C lowering effect of statins.

Pharmacologic Intervention: Lower Triglycerides, Raise HDL-C

- Fibrates
- Niacin
- Fish oil

Fibrates. Several outcomes studies have investigated the effect of triglyceride lowering with fibrates on cardiovascular mortality. The Veterans Affairs High-Density Lipoprotein Cholesterol Intervention Trial (VA-HIT)[135] showed that gemfibrozil (Lopid) therapy resulted in a 24% reduction in CVD events in diabetic men with prior CVD, low HDL-C, and modestly elevated triglycerides. The more recent FIELD trial[136] found that fenofibrate (Tricor) treatment resulted in fewer nonfatal MI and coronary revascularizations, but no significant difference in total coronary mortality. An added side benefit to fenofibrate therapy was a decrease in urinary microalbumin and in retinopathy needing laser therapy.

Niacin. Niacin is the most potent pharmacologic agent available to raise HDL-C.[137] Its use can raise HDL-C by as much as 29%, while lowering triglycerides and shifting LDL-C from small, dense particles to the less atherogenic larger particles.

There have been a number of niacin preparations available over the years. The most commonly used today is extended-release niacin (Niaspan). Patients started on niacin should be aware of 2 significant side effects. Niacin's effect on prostaglandins may result in vasodilation and an uncomfortable flush several hours after the dose. This effect can be reduced by taking a full strength aspirin 30 to 45 minutes before the niacin dose and by giving niacin at hour of sleep. Patients who get up at night should be cautioned about postural hypotension during the period of vasodilatation. Niacin can increase insulin resistance and cause modest hyperglycemia. This effect is rare in doses $\leq$2 g per day.

Fish Oil. Supplementation with fish oil capsules or liquid to provide 2 to 4 g per day of EPA (eicosapentanoic acid) and DHA (docosahexanoic acid) can lower triglyceride levels by 20% to 30%, with a concomitant rise in HDL-C. Fish oil supplementation may raise LDL-C by as much as 5%. Thus, statin doses may need adjustment after addition of fish oil supplements.

Nontraditional Risk Factors

The use of traditional risk factors such as diabetes, hypertension, smoking, and dyslipidemia is generally understood to explain only about 50% to 60% of the variability in cardiovascular risk. Thus, the past decade has seen a concerted effort to identify other risk factors that might enhance the ability to predict cardiovascular events in an individual. In addition, more accurate risk assessment would improve therapeutic decision making. Newer risk markers include measures of the following:[138]

- Systemic inflammation
- Oxidative stress
- Coagulation
- Ventricular function

- Homocysteine
- Lipid subtypes

Inflammatory Markers

An increasing number of inflammatory markers have been identified in the past decade, including the following:

- C-reactive protein (CRP)
- Cellular adhesion molecules (ICAM, VCAM)
- Fibrinogen

These inflammatory markers are subjects of considerable research interest at this time. CRP has been shown to be a marker of coronary risk in both acute coronary syndrome and in men with hypercholesterolemia but no prior evidence of coronary disease.[139] The availability of a reliable, easy-to-perform assay for CRP (the high-sensitivity CRP, or hs-CRP, assay) has resulted in a flood of articles assessing its utility in cardiovascular risk assessment in otherwise-healthy individuals.

There are a limited number of prospective studies of CRP's predictive value in diabetes, but the data are somewhat conflicting. Because of the controversy, the CDC and American Heart Association developed recommendations for the use of inflammatory markers in cardiovascular risk assessment.[140] These recommendations state that hs-CRP is a cardiovascular risk marker that may be useful in the assessment of persons with intermediate risk (10-year risk of 10% to 20%) for cardiovascular events. Whether this additional knowledge should direct changes in risk-factor management remains controversial and highlights the need for further research. At this time, the other inflammatory markers are not appropriate for clinical decision-making because they may not have adequately standardized assays or have not been adequately studied. The assay for CRP may be useful in motivating patients to improve their lifestyle behaviors.[140]

Homocysteine Levels

Plasma levels of the amino acid homocysteine have been shown to be a marker for increased cardiovascular risk in the nondiabetic population.[141] This effect was not only present as an isolated risk factor, but elevated homocysteine levels multiplied the effects of smoking or hypertension. Homocysteine levels are usually low or normal in people with diabetes unless nephropathy is present.[142] In a large cross-sectional study of type 1 diabetes, homocysteine was associated with proteinuria, decreased GFR, and hypertension. In a smaller study of type 2 diabetes, patients with diabetes and CAD had significantly higher homocysteine levels than the group with diabetes without history of CAD.[143]

The homocysteine level can be reduced by vitamin supplementation with B_6 and folate,[144] but supplementation with these 2 compounds did not prove to reduce cardiovascular risk.[145]

Measures of Endothelial Function

Measures of endothelial function, such as microalbuminuria, may also be useful in predicting cardiovascular events. Persons with diabetes and microalbuminuria have between 2 and 8 times the risk of cardiovascular events of persons with diabetes who do not have microalbuminuria.[146] Both the presence of microalbuminuria and its progression predict increased coronary mortality in type 2 diabetes.[147]

Antithrombotic Therapy

Diabetes is recognized as a prothrombotic state, with activation of coagulation factors, decreased fibrinolysis, and platelet dysfunction. Agents that decrease platelet function have the potential to decrease cardiovascular events. The first of these agents and the most widely studied is aspirin.

Aspirin

One of the earliest studies of antiplatelet agents, the Early Treatment Diabetic Retinopathy Study (ETDRS),[148] was primarily designed to determine the effect of aspirin therapy on retinopathy. The study found that aspirin had no significant effect on retinopathy, but found, fortuitously, that aspirin decreased the rate of MI by 28%.[149] Subsequent studies confirmed and expanded understanding of the effect of aspirin on cardiovascular risk, as reviewed in the 2004 ADA position statement.[150,151]As evidence accumulates that atherosclerosis is mediated in large part by activation of the inflammatory system at the vessel wall, there has been an increasing focus on aspirin's anti-inflammatory effects as well.

Aspirin therapy recommendations:

- *As Secondary Prevention:* The ADA recommends use of aspirin (75 to 162 mg per day) as a secondary prevention strategy in people with type 2 diabetes and a history of CVD, including MI, revascularization, and other manifestations of CVD
- *As Primary Prevention:* The ADA also recommends use of aspirin (75 to 162 mg per day) as a primary prevention strategy in people with type 1 or type 2 diabetes who are at increased cardiovascular risk, as defined by age >40 years or the presence of additional risk factors

At this point, the ADA, American Heart Association, and US Preventive Services Task Force all recommend aspirin therapy for the primary prevention of CVD in those at moderate-to-high risk. In spite of these long-standing recommendations, the use of aspirin by high-risk individuals has been shown to be suboptimal. Results from the Behavioral Risk Factor Surveillance System (BRFSS) report aspirin use by only 37% of those with CVD and only 13% of those with other risk factors. The numbers are somewhat higher in those with diabetes: 83% of men and 65% of women with diabetes and known CVD reported regular aspirin use. Use of regular aspirin by men and women with diabetes but without known CVD has been reported as 42% and 34%, respectively.[152]

Clopidogrel

Another antiplatelet agent, clopidogrel (Plavix), has been shown to reduce cardiovascular events in patients with PAD. Clopidogrel decreased cardiovascular events in this group by 24% compared with aspirin. The US Food and Drug Administration has approved clopidogrel for the reduction of ischemic events in patients with PAD.

- The ADA recommends that people with diabetes take an antiplatelet agent.

Instruction Opportunities

Aspirin is an inexpensive intervention for cardiovascular risk reduction. Although clinical outcomes data are somewhat conflicting, the major health organizations recommend use of 75 to 162 mg per day of aspirin as part of a preventive program. Aspirin is underused in the at-risk population; its use should be encouraged. Health professionals have a significant role in enhancing appropriate aspirin use among their at-risk patients.

Hospital Diabetes Management

Persons with diabetes are more likely to be hospitalized for CVD than those without diabetes. Unfortunately, this often results in poor diabetes control due to a number of circumstances. These may include erratic nutritional intake, the effects of the underlying illness, concomitant medications, and, most problematic, the use of inappropriate sliding-scale insulin regimens.[153]

Hyperglycemia in the hospital is associated with increased morbidity and mortality.[154] Patients with diabetes undergoing cardiac surgery had a markedly increased risk of deep sternal wound infections in the early 1990s. The advent of more aggressive diabetes management in the perioperative and postoperative period dramatically reduced the rate of these infections[155] and the increased mortality risk in cardiac surgery for patients with diabetes.[156] Intensive insulin therapy reduced mortality and morbidity in an intensive care unit (ICU) population that was primarily postoperative cardiac surgical patients.[157] As a result of these studies and others, the ADA[158] and American College of Endocrinology[159] published guidelines for diabetes management in the hospital.

A number of different protocols for titrating intravenous insulin have been published. Developing these protocols for an individual institution depends on the collaboration of all departments involved, including administration, quality improvement, nutrition, pharmacy, nursing, and physicians.[160]

Instruction Opportunities

- The hospital-based diabetes educator has the expertise to be a leader in the effort to improve diabetes management in the hospital. For an intravenous insulin protocol to be effective, it must be nurse implemented.
- As the Yale University group showed, for a protocol to be implemented properly, nurses must be involved not only in its implementation, but also in its development.[161]
- Start with the intensive and postoperative care units. Progress to the general floors. Not only will the postoperative cardiac patients benefit; but benefits will also extend to overall diabetes care within the institution.

Questions and Controversy

The question, "how low is low enough?" is applicable to every aspect of cardiovascular risk reduction. Below is a brief summary of important questions remaining to be answered.

How low is low enough for blood glucose?
The only intervention studies of type 2 diabetes achieved little or no improvement in cardiac risk with an achieved A1C of 7%. Secondary analyses and epidemiologic studies suggest that achieving a lower A1C may result in decreased cardiovascular risk. To date, however, there are no randomized, controlled trials indicating that a lower target A1C is better.

How low is low enough for blood pressure?
Current data suggest there is no threshold for blood pressure's effect on cardiovascular risk. It is important to note, however, that most studies of blood pressure treatment show a significant decrease in stroke risk with little or no effect on MI. The ACCORD study will help answer this question, by comparing treatment to achieve a target systolic pressure of 140 with 120 mm Hg.

How low is low enough for LDL-C?
Recommendations from the ADA and NCEP ATP III suggest that a LDL-C of under 100 is an effective goal for most people with type 2 diabetes. People with type 2 diabetes and established CVD are at very high risk; the suggestion for this group is a target LDL-C of <70 mg/dL. But whether 60 mg/dL, for example, is better or whether 80 or 85 mg/dL is satisfactory is not known. More research is needed.

The ACCORD trial, a randomized multicenter trial, may help answer some of these questions. The study will examine the effects of 3 treatment strategies on major CVD events in persons with type 2 diabetes. The 3 treatments are intensive glycemic control, treatment to increase HDL-C and lower triglycerides (in the context of good LDL-C and glycemia control), and intensive blood pressure control (in the context of good glycemia control). The study will address these questions by targeting an A1C of 6% in intensive participants and a systolic pressure of less than 120 mm Hg versus a systolic blood pressure of less than 140 mm Hg. Data will be gathered for 4 to 7 years, with results expected in 2010.

Are insulin sensitizing therapies better than insulin providing therapies?
There are extensive research data to show that reduction of insulin resistance will reduce many cardiac risk factors. However, there are little data to prove that this effect will also reduce cardiovascular outcomes. The PROactive study is a good start, but more research is needed.

Should fibrates be used to raise HDL-C in patients whose LDL-C is already at target?
The VA-HIT study would argue yes. The FIELD study would argue no. In the ACCORD trial, 5800 subjects are randomized to fenofibrate or placebo to answer this question.

Focus on Education: Pearls for Practice

Teaching Strategies

- **Think macrovascular.** Macrovascular disease is prevalent in people with diabetes. Always keep it in mind when developing therapeutic plans for individuals.

- **Go after the risk factors.** Macrovascular disease is multifactorial. Its reduction requires addressing all risk factors, not just glucose. The biggest "bang for the buck" is lipid lowering, followed by blood pressure control. Glucose control, although essential for preventing microvascular complications, has minimal, if any, effect on macrovascular complications.

- **Intervene early to reduce the threat of PAD.** People with diabetes and PAD are more prone to sudden events, including an arterial thrombosis, neuroischemic ulceration, and infection. These events will lead to critical limb ischemia and increased risk of amputation. By diagnosing PAD in its earlier stages, it is possible to institute preventive measures to diminish PAD progression or arrange for elective revascularization in a threatened limb before amputation is necessary.

- **Review and individualize instructions.** Care, treatment, and educational needs are highly individualized. When preparing for education and planning care, spend time preparing and specifically individualizing the treatment options, including consideration of side effects and alternatives. Have appropriate descriptive materials, take-home handouts, and available media for viewing in the clinical setting and reviewing in the home setting.

Patient Education

- **Keys to care.** Information, individualization, decision making, skill building, and follow-up are the keys to care. Important details and factual discussions offer guided decision making and care planning. (Information in the "Instruction Opportunities" throughout the chapter can be a subject guide.)

Internet Resources

www.nhlbi.nih.gov/health/public/heart/index.htm#chol
Information for patients and the public on heart and vascular disease.

From the National Heart, Lung, and Blood Institute of the National Institutes of Health, US Department of Health and Human Services.

www.nhlbi.nih.gov/chd
Information about the National Cholesterol Education Program.

From the National Heart, Lung, and Blood Institute of the National Institutes of Health, US Department of Health and Human Services.

www.diabetes.org/makethelink
Information for patients, the public, and health professionals on the relationship between diabetes, heart disease, and stroke.

"Make the Link: Diabetes, Heart Disease, and Stroke" is an initiative cosponsored by the American Diabetes Association and the American College of Cardiology.

www.ndep.nih.gov
Extensive information for health professionals, patients, and those in school, business, and managed care organizations on diabetes and its complications. Patient brochures and pamphlets on the link between cardiovascular disease and diabetes can be downloaded.

From the National Diabetes Education Program, a partnership of the National Institutes of Health and the Centers for Disease Control.

To order NDEP publications: www.ndep.nih.gov/diabetes/pubs/catalog.htm.

www.acc.org/outreach/diabetes/diabetes.htm
Offers reproducible patient education handouts as components of a comprehensive Diabetes-Cardiovascular Disease Toolkit.

From the American College of Cardiology. Also links to the "Make the Link" Web site cosponsored by the ACC and ADA.

www.s2mw.com/heartofdiabetes/index.html
Information for patients, the public, and healthcare professionals on lowering health risks from diabetes, from the American Heart Association.

This is the home page for the AHA's "Heart of Diabetes" program, which aims to lower people's risk for heart disease and stroke.

www.nhlbi.nih.gov/health/public/heart/hbp/dash
Describes the DASH eating plan (from the Dietary Approaches to Stop Hypertension study).

From the National Institutes of Health, US Department of Health and Human Services. Download or order publications.

www.cdc.gov
www.cdc.gov/doc.do/id/0900f3ec802723eb
www.cdc.gov/diabetes/about/index.htm
An excellent source for diabetes statistics, the first address is the home page for the Centers for Disease Control, of the US Department of Health and Human Services. Also of interest is the CDC's diabetes index page (the second address), the entry to a large body of data. The third address is for the Division of Diabetes Translation, which is part of the National Center for Chronic Disease Prevention and Health Promotion, Centers for Disease Control and Prevention (CDC), US Department of Health and Human Services (DHHS).

References

1. Centers for Disease Control and Prevention. Diabetes: disabling, deadly and on the rise, at a glance 2005. On the Internet at: www.cdc.gov/nccdphp/aag/aag_ddt.htm. Accessed 27 Feb 2006.
2. Centers for Disease Control and Prevention. National Diabetes Fact Sheet, 2005. On the Internet at: www.diabetes.org/uedocuments/NationalDiabetesFactSheetRev.pdf. Accessed 27 Feb 2006.
3. American Diabetes Association. Complications of diabetes in the United States. On the Internet at: www.diabetes.org/diabetes-statistics/complications.jsp. Accessed 27 Feb 2006.
4. Asia Pacific Cohort Studies Collaboration. The effects of diabetes on the risks of major cardiovascular diseases and death in the Asia-Pacific region. Diabetes Care. 2003;26:360-6.
5. Fox CS, Coady S, Sorlie PD, et al. Trends in cardiovascular complications of diabetes. JAMA. 2004;292:2495-9.
6. Vinicor F. Macrovascular disease. In: A Core Curriculum for Diabetes Education: Diabetes Management Therapies, 5th ed. Franz MJ, ed. Chicago, Ill: American Association of Diabetes Educators; 2003.
7. Stehouwer C. The many faces of vascular dysfunction in diabetes. Paper presented at: 20th Camillo Golgi Lecture: delivered at European Association for the Study of Diabetes. 13 Sep 2005.

8. Turner RC, Millns H, Neil HAW, et al. Risk factors for coronary artery disease in non-insulin dependent diabetes mellitus: United Kingdom Prospective Diabetes Study (UKPDS 23). BMJ. 1998;316:823-8.

9. Khaw K-T, Warehan N, Luben R, et al. Glycated haemoglobin, diabetes, and mortality in men in Norfolk cohort of European Prospective Investigation of Cancer and Nutrition (EPIC- Norfolk). BMJ. 2001;322:1-6.

10. Muntner P, Wildman RP, Reynolds K. Relationship between HbA1c level and peripheral arterial disease. Diabetes Care. 2005;28:1981-7.

11. The DECODE study group: glucose tolerance and cardiovascular mortality: comparison of fasting and 2-h diagnostic criteria. Arch Intern Med. 2001;161:397-404.

12. Fodriguez BL, Lau N, Burchfield CM, et al. Glucose intolerance and 23-year risk of coronary heart disease and total mortality: the Honolulu Heart Program. Diabetes Care. 1999;22:1262-5.

13. Bonora E. Postprandial peaks as a risk factor for cardiovascular disease: epidemiological perspectives. Int J Clin Practice. 2002;suppl 129:5-11.

14. Ceriello A, Taboga C, Tonutti L. Evidence for an independent and cumulative effect of postprandial hypertriglyceridemia and hyperglycemia on endothelial dysfunction and oxidative stress generation. Circulation. 2002;106:1211-8.

15. Ceriello A. Postprandial hyperglycemia and diabetes complications: is it time to treat? Diabetes. 2005;54: 1-7.

16. Miller M, Silverstein J. Risk factors for cardiovascular disease in children with diabetes. Practical Diabetology. 2004;23(2):13-8.

17. Thorn LM, Forsblom C, Fagerudd J. Metabolic syndrome in type 1 diabetes: association with diabetic nephropathy and glycemic control (the FinnDiane study). Diabetes Care. 2005;28:2019-24.

18. Orchard TJ, Olson JC, Erbey JR, et al. Insulin resistance-related factors, but not glycemia, predict coronary artery disease in type 1 diabetes. Diabetes Care. 2003;26:1374-9.

19. Johnstone MT, Creager SJ, Scales KM. Impaired endothelium-dependent vasodilation in patients with insulin-dependent diabetes mellitus. Circulation. 1993;88:2510-6.

20. Clarkson P, Celermajer DS, Donald AE. Impaired vascular reactivity in insulin-dependent diabetes mellitus is related to disease duration and low density lipoprotein cholesterol levels. J Am Coll Cardiol. 1996;28:573-9.

21. Jarvisalo MK, Putto-Laurilla A, Jartti L. Carotid artery intima-media thickness in children with type 1 diabetes. Diabetes. 2002;51:493-8.

22. Epidemiology of Diabetes Interventions and Complications (EDIC) Research Group. Effect of intensive diabetes treatment on carotid artery wall thickness in the Epidemiology of Diabetes Interventions and Complications. Diabetes. 1999;48:383-90.

23. Dean H, Flett B. Natural history of type 2 diabetes diagnosed in childhood: long term followup in young adult years. Diabetes. 2002;51suppl 2:A24.

24. Gungor N, Thompson T, Sutton-Tyrell K. Early signs of cardiovascular disease in youth with obesity and type 2 diabetes. Diabetes Care. 2005;28:1219-21.

25. Reaven P, Traustadottir T, Brennan J. Cardiovascular risk factors associated with insulin resistance in children persist into late adolescence. Diabetes Care. 2005;28:148-150.

26. Apedo MT, Sowers JR, Banerji MA. Cardiovascular disease in adolescents with type 2 diabetes. J Ped Endo Metab. 2002;15:519-23.

27. Chen W, Srinivasan SR, Li S, et al. Metabolic syndrome variables at low levels in childhood are beneficially associated with adulthood cardiovascular risk: the Bogalusa Heart Study. Diabetes Care. 2005;28:126-31.

28. McGill HC, Hederick EE, McMahan CA, et al. Atherosclerosis in youth. Minerva Pediatrica. 2002;54:437-47.

29. McGill HC, McMahan CA, Malcom GT, et al. Relation of glycohemoglobin and adiposity to atherosclerosis in youth. Arterioscler Thromb Vasc Biol. 1995;15:431-40.

30. American Diabetes Association. Management of dyslipidemia in children and adolescents with diabetes. Diabetes Care. 2003;26:2194-7.

31. Orchard TJ, Forrest KY-Z, Kuller LH, et al. Lipid and blood pressure treatment goals for type 1 diabetes. Diabetes Care. 2001;24:1053-9.

32. Libby P. The macrophage and atherosclerotic process. In: Atlas of Atherosclerosis: Risk factors and treatment, 2nd ed. Wilson PWF, ed. Philadelphia, Pa: Current Medicine; 2000.

33. Braunwald E. Shattuck lecture: cardiovascular medicine at the turn of the millennium: triumphs, concerns, and opportunities. N Engl J Med. 1998;337:1360-9.

34. Mak KH, Moliterno DJ, Granger CB, et al. Influence of diabetes mellitus on clinical outcome in the thrombolytic era of acute myocardial infarction. J Am Coll Cardiol. 1997;30:171-9.

35. Gaede P, Vedel P, Larsen N. Multifactorial intervention and cardiovascular disease in patients with type 2 diabetes. N Engl J Med. 2003;348;383-93.

36. McDonald CG, Majumdar SR, Mahon JL, et al. The effectiveness of beta-blockers after myocardial infarction in patients with type 2 diabetes. Diabetes Care. 2005;28:2113-7.

37. van Domburg RT, Foley DP, Breeman A, et al. Coronary artery bypass graft surgery and percutaneous transluminal coronary angioplasty: twenty-year clinical outcome. Eur Heart J. 2002;23:543-9.

38. The Bypass Angioplasty Revascularization Investigation (BARI) Investigators. Comparison of coronary bypass surgery with angioplasty in patients with multivessel disease. N Engl J Med. 1996;335(4):217-25.

39. Detre KM, Lombardero MS, Brooks MM. The effect of previous coronary-artery bypass surgery on the prognosis of patients with diabetes who have acute myocardial infarction. N Engl J Med. 2000;342:989-97.

40. Bypass Angioplasty Revascularization Investigation (BARI) 2 Diabetes: a clinical study. On the Internet at: www.bari2D.org. University of Pittsburgh, Epidemiology data center, 2006. Accessed 27 Feb 2006.

41. Ziegelstein RC. Depression in patients recovering from a myocardial infarction. JAMA. 2001;296:1621-7.

42. Carinci F, Nicolucci A, Ciampi A, et al. Role of interactions between psychological and clinical factors in determining 6-month mortality among patients with acute myocardial infarction. Eur Heart J. 1997;18:835-45.

43. Frasure-Smith N. In-hospital symptoms of psychological stress as predictors of long-term outcome after acute myocardial infarction in men. Am J Cardiol. 1991;67:121.

44. Wahab NN, Cowden EA, Pearce NJ, et al. Is blood glucose an independent predictor of mortality in acute myocardial infarction in the thrombolytic era? J Am Coll Cardiol. 2002;40:1748-54.

45. Norhammer A, Tenerz A, Nilsson G, et al. Glucose metabolism in patients with acute myocardial infarction, and no previous diagnosis of diabetes mellitus: a prospective study. Lancet. 2002;359:2140-4.

46. Malmberg K. Prospective randomized study of intensive insulin treatment on long term survival after acute myocardial infarction in patients with diabetes mellitus BMJ. 1997;314:1512-5.

47. Kissela BM, Khoury J, Kleindorfer D, et al. Epidemiology of ischemic stroke in patients with diabetes: The Greater Cincinnati/Northern Kentucky Stroke Study. Diabetes Care. 2005;28:355-9.

48. Gorelick PB, Mazzone T. Plasma lipids and stroke. J. Cardiovasc Risk. 1999;6:217-21

49. UK Prospective Diabetes Study Group. Tight blood pressure control and risk of macrovascular and microvascular complications in type 2 diabetes: UKPDS 38. BMJ. 1998;317:703-13.

50. Kawachi I, Colditz GA, Stampfer MJ, et al. Smoking cessation and the decreased risk of stroke in women. JAMA. 1993;269:232-6.

51. Johnston SC, Gress DR, Browner WS, et al. Short-term prognosis after emergency department diagnosis of TIA. JAMA. 2000;284:2901-6.

52. Streifler JY, Eliasziw M, Benavente OR, et al. The risk of stroke in patients with first-ever retinal vs hemispheric transient ischemic attacks and high-grade carotid stenosis. Arch Neurol. 1995;52:246-9.

53. Roman GC. Vascular dementia revisited: diagnosis, pathogenesis, treatment, and prevention. Med Clin N Am. 2002;86:477-99.

54. Hirsch AT, Criqui MH, Treat-Jacobson D, et al. Peripheral arterial disease detection, awareness, and treatment in primary care. JAMA. 2001;286:1317-24.

55. Dolan NC, Liu K, Criqui MG, et al. Peripheral artery disease, diabetes, and reduced lower extremity functioning. Diabetes Care. 2002;25:113-20.

56. Kjekshus J, Pedersen TR. Reducing the risk of coronary events: evidence from the Scandinavian Simvastatin Survival Study (4S). Lancet. 1994;344:1383-9.

57. Wake Forest University School of Medicine's Public Health Science Department. Action to Control Cardiovascular Risk in Diabetes (ACCORD). On the

Internet at: www.accordtrial.org. Accessed 27 Feb 2006.

58. Lassila R, Lepantalo M. Cigarette smoking and the outcome after lower limb arterial surgery. Acta Chir Scand. 1988;154:635-640.

59. American Diabetes Association. Aspirin therapy in diabetes (position statement). Diabetes Care. 2003;26:S87-8. http://care.diabetesjournals.org/cgi/content/full/26/suppl_1/s87.

60. Sobel BE, Schneider DJ. Cardiovascular complications in diabetes mellitus. Curr Opin in Pharmacol. 2005;5:143-8.

61. Piccini JP, Klein L, Gheorghiade M. New insights into diastolic heart failure: role of diabetes mellitus. Am J Med. 2004;116suppl5A:64S-75S.

62. Nesto RW, Bell D, Bonow RO. Thiazolidinedione use, fluid retention, and congestive heart failure. Diabetes Care. 2004;27:256-63.

63. Masoudi FA, Inzucchi SE, Wang Y, et al. Thiazolidinediones, metformin, and outcomes in older patients with diabetes and heart failure. Circulation. 2004;111:583-90.

64. Eurich DT, Majumdar SR, McAlister FA, et al. Improved clinical outcomes associated with metformin in patients with diabetes and heart failure. Diabetes Care. 2005;28:2345–51.

65. Inzucchi SE. Metformin and heart failure: innocent until proven guilty. Diabetes Care. 2005;28:2585-7.

66. Haffner SM, Lehto S, Ronnemaa T, et al. Mortality from coronary heart disease in subjects with type 2 diabetes and in nondiabetic subjects with and without prior myocardial infarction. N Engl J Med. 1998;339:229-34.

67. National Cholesterol Education Program. Risk assessment tool for estimating 10-year risk of developing hard CHD (myocardial infarction and coronary death). Third report of the Expert Panel on Detection, Evaluation, and Treatment of Blood Cholesterol in Adults (Adult Treatment Panel III). On the Internet at: http://hin.nhlbi.nih.gov/atpiii/calculator.asp?usertype=prof. Accessed 7 Oct 2005.

68. University of Oxford, Oxford Centre for Diabetes, Endocrinology and Metabolism. UKPDS risk engine. 26 Feb 04. On the Internet at: http://www.dtu.ox.ac.uk/index.html?maindoc=/riskengine/FAQ.html. Accessed 27 Feb 2006.

69. American Diabetes Association. Standards of medical care in diabetes. Diabetes Care. 2006;29suppl 1: S4-42.

70. Barzilay JI, Spiekerman CF, Kuller LH, et al. Prevalence of clinical and isolated subclinical cardiovascular disease in older adults with glucose disorders. Diabetes Care. 2001;24:1233-9.

71. O'Brien IA, McFadden JP, Corrall RJ. The influence of autonomic neuropathy on mortality in insulin-dependent diabetes. Q J Med. 1991;79:495-502.

72. Rathmann W, Ziegler D, Jahnke M, et al. Mortality in diabetic patients with cardiovascular autonomic neuropathy. Diabet Med. 1993;10:820-4.

73. Gerritsen J, Dekker JM, TenVoorde BJ. Impaired autonomic function is associated with increased mortality, especially in subjects with diabetes, hypertension, or a history of cardiovascular disease. Diabetes Care. 2001;24:1793-8.

74. La Rovere MT, Bigger JT Jr, Marcus FI, et al. Baroreflex sensitivity and heart rate variability in prediction of total cardiac mortality after myocardial infarction. Lancet. 1998;351:478-84.

75. Dekker JM, Schouten EG, Klootwijk P, et al. Heart rate variability from short electrocardiographic recordings predicts mortality from all causes in middle-aged and elderly men: the Zutphen Study. Am J Epidemiol. 1997;145:899-908.

76. Tsuji H, Venditti FJ Jr, Manders ES, et al. Reduced heart rate variability and mortality risk in an elderly cohort: the Framingham Heart Study. Circulation. 1994;90:878-83.

77. Eyre H, Kahn R, Robertson RM. Preventing cancer, cardiovascular disease, and diabetes. Diabetes Care. 2004;27:1812-24.

78. US Department of Health and Human Services. The health benefits of smoking cessation: a report of the Surgeon General. Centers for Disease Control and Prevention, Office on Smoking and Health; 1990.

79. Chobanian AV, Bakris GL, Black HR, et al and the National High Blood Pressure Education Program Coordinating Committee. The Seventh Report of the Joint National Committee on Prevention, Detection, Evaluation, and Treatment of High Blood Pressure. JAMA. 2003;289:2560-72.

80. Expert Panel on Detection, Evaluation and Treatment of High Blood Cholesterol in Adults. Executive Summary of the third report of the National

Cholesterol Education Program (NCEP) Expert Panel on Detection, Evaluation and Treatment of High Blood Cholesterol in Adults (Adult Treatment Panel III). JAMA. 2001;285:2486-97.

81. Graham IM. NORVIT: randomized study of homocysteine lowering with B-vitamins for secondary prevention of cardiovascular disease after acute myocardial infarction. Available on the Internet at: www.escardio.org/knowledge/OnlineLearning/slides/ESC_Congress_2005/GrahamFP1335. Sept 2005. Accessed 14 Oct 2005.

82. Brown BG, Cheung MC, Lee AC. Antioxidant vitamins and lipid therapy: end of a long romance? Arterioscler Thromb Vasc Biol. 2002;22(10):1535-46.

83. Lonn E, Bosch J, Yusuf S. Effects of long-term vitamin E supplementation on cardiovascular events and cancer: a randomized controlled trial. JAMA. 2005;293:1338-47.

84. Sigal RJ, Kenny GP Wasserman DH, et al. Physical activity/exercise and type 2 diabetes. Diabetes Care. 2004;27:2518-39.

85. Hu G, Jousilahti P, Barengo NC. Physical activity, cardiovascular risk factors, and mortality among Finnish adults with diabetes. Diabetes Care. 2005;28:799-805.

86. Petrella FJ, Lattanzio CN, Demeray A. Can adoption of regular exercise later in life prevent metabolic risk for cardiovascular disease? Diabetes Care. 2005;28:694-701.

87. The Diabetes Prevention Program Research Group. Impact of intensive lifestyle and metformin therapy on cardiovascular disease risk factors in the Diabetes Prevention Program. Diabetes Care. 2005;28:888-94.

88. Laakso M. Hyperglycemia and cardiovascular disease in type 2 diabetes. Diabetes. 1999;48:937-42.

89. Coutinho M, Gerstein HC, Wang Y, et al. A metaregression analysis of published data from 20 studies of 95,783 individuals followed for 12.4 years. Diabetes Care. 1999;22:233-40.

90. Selvin E, Coresh J, Golden SH, et al. Glycemic control, atherosclerosis, and risk factors for cardiovascular disease in individuals with diabetes. Diabetes Care. 2005;28:1965-73.

91. Selvin E, Marinopoulos S, Berkenblit G. Meta-analysis: glycosylated hemoglobin and cardiovascular disease in diabetes mellitus. Ann Intern Med. 2004;141:421-31.

92. Stratton IM, Adler AI, Neil HAW, et al. Association of glycaemia with macrovascular and microvascular complications of type 2 diabetes [UKPDS 35]: prospective observational study. BMJ. 2000;321:405-12.

93. Bonora E, Muggeo M. Postprandial blood glucose as a risk factor for cardiovascular disease in type II diabetes: the epidemiological evidence. Diabetologia. 2001;44:2107-14.

94. Ceriello A. Postprandial hyperglycemia an diabetes complications: is it time to treat? Diabetes. 2005;54:1-7.

95. Hanefeld M, Fischer S, Julius U, et al. Risk factors for myocardial infarction and death in newly detected NIDDM: the Diabetes Intervention Study, 11-year follow-up. Diabetologia. 1996;39:1577-83.

96. Huang ES, Meigs JB, Singer DE. The effect of interventions to prevent cardiovascular disease in patients with type 2 diabetes mellitus. Am J Med. 2001;111:633-42.

97. UK Prospective Diabetes Study Group. Intensive blood-glucose control with sulphonylureas or insulin compared with conventional treatment and risk of complications in patients with type 2 diabetes (UKPDS 33). Lancet. 1998;352:837-53.

98. Chiasson JL, Josse RG, Gomis R, et al. Acarbose treatment and the risk of cardiovascular disease and hypertension in patients with impaired glucose tolerance: the STOP-NIDDM trial. JAMA. 2003;290:496-4.

99. Hanefeld M, Cagatay M, Petrowitsch T, et al. Acarbose reduces the risk for myocardial infarction in type 2 diabetic patients: meta-analysis of seven long-term studies. Eur Heart J. 2004;25:10-16.

100. Esposito K, Giugliano D, Nappo F, et al. Regression of carotid atherosclerosis by control of postprandial hyperglycemia in type 2 diabetes. Circulation. 2004;110:214-9.

101. Krolewski AS, Kosinski EJ, Warram JH, et al. Magnitude and determinants of coronary artery disease in juvenile-onset, insulin dependent diabetes mellitus. Am J Cardiol. 1987;59:750-5.

102. Larsen JL, Colling CW, Ratanasuwan T. Pancreas transplantation improves vascular disease in patients with type 1 diabetes. Diabetes Care. 2004;27:1706-11.

103. Fiorina P, Gremizzi C, Maffi P. Islet transplantation is associated with an improvement of cardiovascular

function in type 1 diabetic kidney transplant patients. Diabetes Care. 2005;28:1358-65.

104. The Diabetes Control and Complications Trial/Epidemiology of Diabetes Interventions and Complications Research Group. Intensive diabetes therapy and carotid intima-medial thickness in type 1 diabetes mellitus. N Engl J Med. 2003;348:2294-2303.

105. Nathan DM, Cleary PA, Backlund JY, Genuth SM, Lachin JM, Orchard TJ, Raskin P, Zinman B; Diabetes Control and Complications Trial/Epidemiology of Diabetes Interventions and Complications (DCCT/EDIC) Study Research Group. Intensive diabetes treatment and cardiovascular disease in patients with type 1 diabetes. N Engl J Med. 2005;353(25):2643-53.

106. Reaven GM. Role of insulin resistance in human disease. Diabetes. 1998;37:1595-1607.

107. Davidson MB. Is treatment of insulin resistance beneficial independent of glycemia? Diabetes Care. 2003;26:3184-6.

108. Pfutzner A , Marx N, Lubben G, et al. Improvement of cardiovascular risk markers by pioglitazone is independent from glycemic control: results from the Pioneer study. J Am Coll Cardiol. 2005;45:1925-31.

109. Dormandy JA, Charbonnel B, Eckland DJ, et al. Secondary prevention of macrovascular events in patients with type 2 diabetes and pre-existing cardiovascular disease in the PROactive Study (PROspective pioglitAzone Clinical Trial In macroVascular Events): a randomised controlled trial. Lancet. 2005;366:1279-89.

110. Inzucchi SE, Masoudi FA, Wang Y. Insulin-sensitizing antihyperglycemic drugs and mortality after acute myocardial infarction. Diabetes Care. 2005;28:1680-9.

111. Yki-Jarvinen H. The PROactive study: some answers, many questions. Lancet. 2005;366:1241-2.

112. McLaughlin T. Obesity, insulin resistance, and cardiovascular disease. Pract Diabetol. 2004;23(3):6-11.

113. Sowers J. Treatment of hypertension in patients with diabetes. Arch Intern Med. 2004;164:1850-7.

114. Stamler J, Vaccaro O, Neaton JD, et al. Diabetes, other risk factors and 12-yr cardiovascular mortality for men screened in the Multiple Risk Factor Intervention Trial. Diabetes Care. 1993;16:434-44.

115. Davis SN, Sowers JF, Vaughan DE, et al. Managing major cardiovascular risk factors in patient with diabetes. Pract Diabetol. 2004;23:(3)28-35.

116. Lewington S, Clarke R, Quizibash N, et al. Age-specific relevance of usual blood pressure to vascular mortality. Lancet. 2002;360:1903-13.

117. Liszka HA, Mainous AG III, King DF, Everett CJ, Egan BM. Prehypertension and cardiovascular morbidity. Ann Fam Med. 2005;3(4)294-299

118. American Diabetes Association. Hypertension management in adults with diabetes. Diabetes Care. 2004;27suppl 1:S65-7.

119. Sacks FM, Svetkey LP, Vollmer WM, et al. Effects of blood pressure of reduced dietary sodium and the Dietary Approaches to Stop Hypertension (DASH) diet. N Engl J Med. 2001;344:3-1

120. The ALLHAT officers and coordinators for the ALLHAT collaborative research group. Major outcomes in high-risk hypertensive patients randomized to angiotensin-converting enzyme inhibitor or calcium channel blocker vs diuretic. JAMA. 2002;288:2981-97.

121. UK Prospective Diabetes Study Group. Efficacy of atenolol and captopril in reducing risk of macrovascular and microvascular complications in type 2 diabetes. BMJ. 1998;317:713-20.

122. Fagot-Campagna A, Rolka DB, Beckles GLA, et al. Prevalence of lipid abnormalities, awareness, and treatment in US adults with diabetes. Diabetes. 2000;49suppl 1:A78-9.

123. American Diabetes Association. Dyslipidemia management in adults with diabetes. Diabetes Care. 2004;27suppl 1:S68-70.

124. Turner RC, Millns H, Neil HA, et al. Risk factors for coronary artery disease in non-insulin dependent diabetes mellitus (UKPDS 23). BMJ. 1998;316:823-8.

125. Haffner SM. Management of dyslipidemia in adults with diabetes (technical review). Diabetes Care. 1998;21:160-78.

126. Grundy, SM, Cleeman JI, Merz CNB, et al. Implications of recent clinical trials for the national cholesterol education program adult treatment panel III guidelines. Circulation. 2004;110:227-39.

127. Mukherjee SK, Golding E. Of Inuits and Americans: Omega-3s in diabetes treatment. Pract Diabetol. 2003;22(3):28-32.

128. Kris-Etherton PM, Harris WH, Appel LJ, et al. Fish consumption, fish oil, Omega-3 fatty acids, and cardiovascular disease. Circulation. 2002;106:2747-57.

129. The Multiple Risk Factor Intervention Trial (MRFIT): a national study of primary prevention of coronary heart disease. JAMA. 1976;235:825-827.

130. Scandinavian Simvastatin Survival Study Group. Randomized trial of cholesterol lowering in 4444 patients with coronary heart disease: the Scandinavian Simvastatin Survival Study (4S). Lancet. 1994;344:1383-9.

131. Pyorala K, Pedersen TR, Kjelshus J, et al. Cholesterol lowering with simvastatin improves prognosis of diabetic patients with coronary heart disease: a subgroup analysis of the Scandinavian Simvastatin Survival Study (4S). Diabetes Care. 1997;20:614-20.

132. Colhoun HM, Betteridge DJ, Durrington PN. Primary prevention of cardiovascular disease with atorvastatin in type 2 diabetes in the Collaborative Atorvastatin Diabetes Study (CARDS): multicentre randomized placebo-controlled trial. Lancet. 2004;364:685-96.

133. Vijan S, Hayward RA. Pharmacologic lipid-lowering therapy in type 2 diabetes mellitus: background paper for the American College of Physicians. Ann Intern Med. 2004;140: 650-8.

134. Snow V, Aronson MD, Hornbake ER. Lipid control in the management of type 2 diabetes mellitus: a clinical practice guideline from the American College of Physicians. Ann Intern Med. 2004;140:644-9.

135. Rubins HB, Robins SJ, Collins D. Gemfibrozil for the secondary prevention of coronary heart disease in men with low levels of high-density lipoprotein cholesterol: Veterans Affairs High-Density Lipoprotein Cholesterol Intervention Trial Study Group. N Engl J Med. 1999;341:410-8.

136. National Health and Medical Research Council Clinical Trials Centre, University of Sydney. Fenofibrate intervention and event lowering in diabetes. Dec 2005. On the internet at: http://www.thefield-trial.org. Accessed: 10 Dec 2005.

137. Shepherd J, Betteridge J, van Gaal L. Nicotinic acid in the management of dyslipidemia associated with diabetes and metabolic syndrome: a position paper developed by a European Consensus Panel. Curr Med Res Opinion. 2005;21:665-82.

138. Hernandez C, Francisco G, Chacon P, et al. Lipoprotein(a) as a risk factor for cardiovascular mortality in type 2 diabetic patients. Diabetes Care. 2005;28:931-3.

139. Rader DJ. Inflammatory markers of coronary risk. N Engl J Med. 2000;343:1179-82.

140. Smith SC, Anderson JL, Cannon RO, et al. CDC/AHA workshop in markers of inflammation and cardiovascular disease: application to clinical and public health practice. Circulation. 2004;110:e550-3.

141. Graham IM, Daly LE, Refsum HM, et al. Plasma homocysteine as a risk factor for vascular disease. JAMA. 1997;277:1775-81.

142. Audelin MC, Genest J. Homocysteine and cardiovascular disease in diabetes mellitus. Atherosclerosis. 2001;159:497-511.

143. Rudy A, Kowalska I, Straczkowski M, Kinalska I. Homocysteine concentrations and vascular complications in patients with type 2 diabetes. Diabetes Metab. 2005;31:112-7.

144. Villa P, Perri C, Suriano R. L-folic acid supplementation in healthy postmenopausal women: effect on homocysteine and glycolipid metabolism. J Clin Endocrinol Metab. 2005;90:4622-9.

145. Bonaa KH. NORVIT: Randomised trial of homocysteine-lowering with B-vitamins for secondary prevention of cardiovascular disease after acute myocardial infarction, slide set. 5 Sep 2005. On the Internet at: www.escardio.org/knowledge/onlinelearning/slides/ESC_Congress_2005/BonaaFP1334. Accessed 22 Oct 2005.

146. Park HY, Schumock GT, Pickard AS, et al. A structured review of the relationship between microalbuminuria and cardiovascular events in patients with diabetes mellitus and hypertension. Pharmacotherapy. 2003;23:1611-6.

147. Spoelstra-de Man AM, Brouwer CB, Stehouwer CDA. Rapid progression of albumin excretion is an independent predictor of cardiovascular mortality in patients with type 2 diabetes and microalbuminuria. Diabetes Care. 2001;24:2097-101.

148. Early Treatment Diabetic Retinopathy Study Research Group. Effects of aspirin treatment on diabetic retinopathy: ETDRS report number 8. Ophthalmology. 1991;98:757-65.

149. Early Treatment Diabetic Retinopathy Study Investigators. Aspirin effects in mortality and morbidity in patients with diabetes mellitus. JAMA. 1992;268:1292-1300.

150. American Diabetes Association. Aspirin therapy in diabetes (position statement). Diabetes Care. 2004;27suppl 1:S72-3.

151. Antithrombotic Trialists' Collaboration. Collaborative meta-analysis of randomized trials of

antiplatelet therapy for prevention of death, myocardial infarction, and stroke in high risk patients. BMJ. 2002;324:71-86.

152. Persell SD, Baker DW. Aspirin use among adults with diabetes. Arch Intern Med. 2004;154:2492-9.

153. Trett DL, Kelly JL, Hirsch IB. The rationale and management of hyperglycemia for in-patients with cardiovascular disease: time for change. J Clin Endocrinol Metab. 2003;88:2430-7.

154. Krinsley JS. Association between hyperglycemia and increased hospital mortality in a heterogeneous population of critically ill patients. Mayo Clin Proc. 2003;78:1471-8.

155. Furnary AM, Zerr KJ, Grunkmeier GL, et al. Continuous intravenous insulin infusion reduces the incidence of deep sternal would infection in diabetic patients after cardiac surgical procedures. Ann Thorac Surg. 1999;67:352-60.

156. Furnary AP, Gao G, Grunkmeier GL, et al. Continuous insulin infusion reduces mortality in patients with diabetes undergoing coronary artery bypass grafting. J Thorac Cardiovasc Surg. 2003;125:1007-21.

157. Van den Berghe G, Wouters P, Weekers F, et al. Intensive insulin therapy in the critically ill patients. N Engl J Med. 2001;345:1359-67.

158. Clement S, Braithwaite SS, Magee MF, et al. Management of diabetes and hyperglycemia in hospitals. Diabetes Care. 2004;27:553-91.

159. Garber AJ, Moghissi ES, Bransome ED Jr, et al. American College of Endocrinology position statement on inpatient diabetes and metabolic control. Endocr Pract. 2004;10:77-82.

160. Courtney L, Gordon M, Romer L. A clinical path for adult diabetes. Diabetes Educ. 1997;23:664-71.

161. Goldberg PA, Siegel MD, Sherwin RS, et al. Implementation of a Safe and Effective Insulin Infusion Protocol in a Medical Intensive Care Unit. Diabetes Care. 2004;27:461-7.

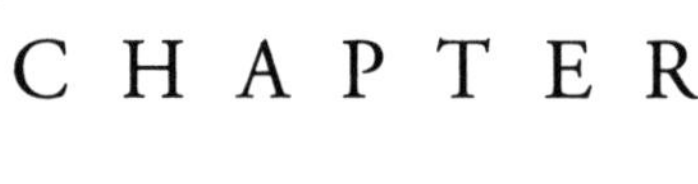

CHAPTER

22

Diabetic Eye Disease

Authors

Victor H. Gonzalez, MD
Rodolfo M. Banda, MD

Key Concepts

- The diabetic population is susceptible to a considerable number of eye problems that can lead to blindness. These generally occur more frequently and at a younger age than the norm.
- With early diagnosis, much can be done to prevent or delay these eye diseases and treat them when they occur.
- Diabetic retinopathy, the leading cause of blindness in the United States, is often present even before the person notices any visual changes.
- Tight control of blood glucose levels helps prevent severe vision loss due to diabetic retinopathy.
- The diabetes educator should encourage everyone with diabetes to have a retinal evaluation even if they do not have any ocular symptoms.
- "The sooner the better"—early treatment of diabetic retinopathy can prevent severe vision loss.

Introduction

Diabetes is the leading cause of visual loss in the United States. The literature suggests that 8,000 to 23,000 new cases of legal blindness associated with diabetes present annually.[1-5] Various ocular conditions are 25 times more common among people with diabetes than in the general population.[3] Of people with diabetes who are on work disability, 15% to 20% have some visual impairment.[6]

As people advance in age, they are more at risk for certain eye conditions, such as glaucoma and cataracts. People with diabetes have an even greater risk for these conditions, which often present earlier in age than in the general population. Uncontrolled, poorly managed diabetes creates a more serious condition called diabetic retinopathy. Retinopathy is any noninflammatory degenerative disease of the retina. Within 1 year of developing retinopathy, 5% to 10% of cases will progress to a more advanced stage.[7]

This chapter focuses on eye diseases associated with diabetes mellitus. For each ocular condition, the epidemiology, risk factors, clinical findings, stages of the disease, and appropriate treatments are outlined.

- *Common Eye Diseases.* Common eye diseases are discussed first, including cataracts, glaucoma, and other ocular manifestations that occur more frequently in people with diabetes.
- *Diabetic Retinopathy.* Information on diabetic retinopathy is presented next. Major clinical studies and current treatment strategies for diabetic retinopathy are outlined. The text emphasizes how appropriate and timely therapy can prevent severe visual loss in up to 90% of cases.[8]

Diabetic retinopathy is a disorder of the retinal vasculature that develops in varying degrees in almost all people with diabetes. The retina is the light-sensitive nerve tissue that converts images from the eyes' optical system into electrical impulses that are sent along the optic nerve to the brain to interpret as vision. Figure 22.1 identifies parts of the eye that are discussed in this chapter.

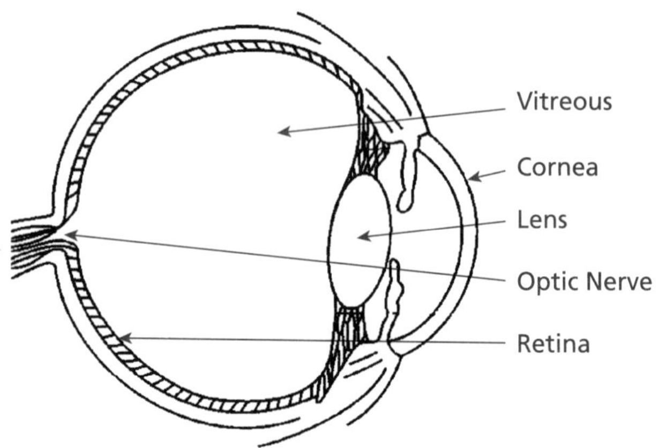

FIGURE 22.1 Normal Eye

Source: Copyright © 2004 American Diabetes Association. Modified with permission from the American Diabetes Association. Life With Diabetes.

Case in Point: Reluctance in Self-Care Leads to Vision Loss

MG was a 50-year-old male, who was diagnosed with type 2 diabetes 10 years ago. His blood glucose levels had ranged from 100 to 355 mg/dL in the last 3 months. He insisted, however, that he was doing fine because he did not "feel" that his diabetes was causing any problems. He was using oral medications to control his diabetes and lived a sedentary lifestyle; he came referred to the retina service from his family physician to rule out diabetic retinopathy. Findings from the initial examination were as follows:

- Best-corrected visual acuity was 20/40 in the right eye and 20/20 in the left eye. Since MG had never checked his vision one eye at a time before, he had never noticed the difference in visual acuity between both eyes.
- Intraocular pressure (IOP) was 19 mm Hg and 22 mm Hg on the right and left eye, respectively.
- Slitlamp biomicroscopy revealed a 2+ posterior subcapsular cataract in the right eye and mild cataract changes in the left eye.
- The fundus examination revealed a 0.5 cup-to-disc ratio (C/D) of the optic nerves.
- A few retinal microaneurysms were also noted without macular edema or neovascularization at this point.

Diagnosis

Because of the fundus examination finding and the IOP measurement, MG was considered a glaucoma suspect. He was diagnosed as follows:

- Mild nonproliferative diabetic retinopathy in both eyes
- Posterior subcapsular cataract in the right eye
- Glaucoma suspect

The findings and the importance of ocular follow-up were explained to MG. The ophthalmologist discussed the presence of cataract changes and explained that since these changes did not interfere with MG's daily activities, they did not warrant surgery at this time. MG was advised to schedule a follow-up visit within 8 to 12 months. He was also referred to a glaucoma specialist for evaluation of possible glaucoma.

Cataracts

Cataracts are one of the leading causes of blindness in the world today and at least 300,000 to 400,000 new, visually disabling cataracts occur annually in the United States. With early detection, close monitoring, and timely surgical intervention, visual impairment due to cataracts is reversible. Cataracts are a vision-impairing disease characterized by a gradual, progressive thickening and opacification of the lens. The lens is the eye structure in charge of focusing images on the retina. The lens' transparent intraocular tissue helps bring rays of light to focus on the retina.

The most common patient complaint is a gradual decrease in visual acuity, but patients may complain of a decrease in contrast sensitivity in brightly lit environments, disabling glare during the day, and/or glare with oncoming headlights at night. The progression of cataracts may frequently result in a mild-to-moderate degree of myopic shift or increase in nearsightedness. Consequently, presbyopic patients report an increase in their near vision and less need for reading glasses as they experience the so-called "second sight." Patients must be told that this change is temporary and that they will eventually lose the "second sight." In some cases, patients with cataracts may present with monocular diplopia that is not corrected with use of spectacles or prisms. These cases can usually be solved with cataract surgery.

How do cataracts form?

When the blood glucose level is high, there is also an elevation of the aqueous glucose levels. The glucose diffuses through the lens capsule and increases its concentration within the crystalline lens. This results in a glycosylation of lens proteins. Some of the glucose is converted by the intracellular enzyme aldose reductase into sorbitol. This causes alterations in lens permeability and results in cataract formation.[9]

Cortical Cataract. A special type of cortical cataract is seen in many diabetic patients. It has a "snowflake" appearance with bilateral, widespread subcapsular changes. Often, it has an abrupt onset and an acute course. These cataracts are seen most often in the younger person whose diabetes is not controlled. These lens changes mature rapidly and result in total opacification over a period of a few weeks with very significant visual loss. This "true diabetic cataract" is becoming rarer as better programs to control diabetes have been available.

Common Senile Cataract. Common senile cataracts (nuclear sclerotic cataracts and posterior subcapsular cataracts) occur more frequently, at younger ages, and progress more rapidly in persons afflicted with diabetes.[10]

What treatment options are available?
The only treatment option for cataracts is surgical cataract extraction and placement of an intraocular lens (IOL) implant. Cataract surgery is a very safe and relatively quick procedure in which the patient can have a total visual recovery within days if there is no other pathology affecting the vision. With current cataract extraction techniques, this procedure can be done as soon as the person notices any change in visual acuity. Since there is no real visual acuity cutoff at which the surgery is performed, the patient must be told that this is an elective procedure and must also be informed of all possible risks of surgery.

Complications. Diabetes is not a contraindication for cataract surgery. However, cataract surgery can stimulate additional problems for persons with diabetes, specifically if the cataract surgery results in a capsulotomy (rupture in the bag that holds the lens). In this case, the angiogenic factors produced by the retina that can cause proliferative diabetic retinopathy flow from the posterior segment forward to reach the iris. This, in turn, may stimulate neovascular glaucoma, a recognized complication of cataract surgery in diabetic patients. [9] Proper stabilization of any diabetic retinopathy prior to cataract extraction can significantly reduce the risk of the development of these complications. In some cases, lens extraction may be needed to improve retinal surveillance.[11]

Glaucoma

Glaucoma is the second leading cause of blindness in the United States with more than 1.6 million people having significant visual impairment.[12] There are several categories of glaucoma, which are based on chronology or etiology. Those most commonly associated with diabetes are discussed here:

- Primary open-angle glaucoma
- Neovascular glaucoma

Primary Open-Angle Glaucoma

Primary open-angle glaucoma (POAG) is described as a multifactorial optic neuropathy (optic nerve disease) that is characterized by a chronic and progressive loss of optic nerve fibers (clinically, this can be evaluated according to a cup-to-disc ratio, which usually ranges from 0.1 to 0.4). Such loss develops in the presence of an open anterior chamber angle (the eyes' main drainage system), characteristic visual field abnormalities, and intraocular pressure that is too high for the continued health of the eye (normal intraocular pressure ranges from 8 to 22 mm Hg). Because of the silent nature of the disease, patients usually will not present with any visual complaints until late in the course. At this time, patients present with complaints of a constriction in the visual field (decrease in peripheral vision) or a decrease in visual acuity. Although there is still controversy, some epidemiologic studies show that primary open-angle glaucoma is found more often in type 2 diabetic patients when compared with age-matched nondiabetic populations.[13-15]

Treatment of POAG is limited to the reduction of intraocular pressure (IOP). This is mainly performed through topical medications (eye drops) and occasionally via laser or incisional surgery. The US Preventive Services Task Force (USPSTF) concluded in the March 2005 Recommendation Statement on Screening for Glaucoma that there is good evidence that screening can detect increased IOP and early POAG in adults.[16] The USPSTF also found good evidence that early treatment of adults with increased IOP detected by screening reduces the number of persons who develop small visual field defects and allows for early treatment to prevent progression. However, the Task Force did not find sufficient evidence to determine the extent to which screening, with earlier detection and treatment, would reduce impairment in vision-related function or quality of life. Harms associated with treatment of increased IOP and early POAG include local eye irritation and an increased risk for cataracts. Further research is needed to clarify the balance between the benefit from early treatment and the given known harm of early screening for glaucoma.

Glaucoma and diabetes:

The greatest visual threat to persons having both glaucoma and diabetes is development of neovascular glaucoma.

Neovascular Glaucoma

Neovascular glaucoma (NVG) is a secondary glaucoma. Retinal ischemia is the most common and important mechanism in NVG. Recently, it has been discovered that significantly higher vascular endothelial growth factor (VEGF)[17] levels occur in the ocular fluids of individuals with proliferative diabetic retinopathy than in persons with nonproliferative diabetic retinopathy. Extremely elevated levels of VEGF were found in the ocular fluids of patients with NVG. Currently, there are studies evaluating the use of anti-VEGF drugs in the management of these complications. Patients presenting with NVG may experience ocular pain or redness, multicolored halos, or headache, and some patients may be asymptomatic.

The management of this disorder is related to the stage of the disease, but panretinal photocoagulation (PRP) remains the primary treatment. PRP is a type of laser surgery delivered in a scatter pattern throughout the peripheral fundus; it is intended to lead to a regression of neovascularization. PRP reduces the areas of retinal ischemia; thus, angiogenic factors are reduced. In cases where PRP treatment does not lower the pressure, filtration surgery or the implantation of a drainage device may be necessary to control the pressure and salvage the optic nerve.[18]

Central Retinal Vein Occlusion

Central retinal vein occlusion (CRVO) is a retinal vascular disorder commonly seen in patients with a history of high blood pressure and/or diabetes mellitus.[19] The exact pathogenesis of the occlusion of the central retinal vein is not known. Various local and systemic factors play a role in the pathological closure of the central retinal vein. Clinically, CRVO presents with variable sudden visual loss. The fundus eye exam may show retinal hemorrhages, dilated tortuous retinal veins, cotton-wool spots (soft exudates that represent infarcts of the nerve fiber layer of the retina), macular edema (swelling, or thickening, in the central part of the retina), and swelling of the optic nerve. CRVO can be divided into 2 clinical types:

- Nonischemic CRVO
- Ischemic CRVO

Nonischemic CRVO is the milder form of the disease. It may present with good vision, a few retinal hemorrhages and cotton-wool spots, no relative afferent pupillary defect (abnormality in the pupils reaction to light), and good blood perfusion to the retina. Nonischemic CRVO may resolve fully with good visual prognosis, or it may progress to the ischemic type.

Ischemic CRVO is the severe form of the disease. Usually, ischemic CRVO presents with severe visual loss, extensive retinal hemorrhages and cotton-wool spots, presence of relative afferent pupillary defect, and/or poor blood perfusion to the retina. In addition, the disease may result in NVG and a painful blind eye.

No known effective medical treatment is available for either prevention or treatment of CRVO. If an underlying systemic medical condition is found, treatment may be indicated, but this rarely reverses the vein occlusion.[20] Treatment may, however, help prevent the opposite eye from developing a vascular occlusion. The exact pathogenesis of the CRVO is not known. Various medical modalities for the treatment of CRVO have been advocated by multiple authors with varying success in preventing complications and preserving vision. Laser photocoagulation is the treatment of choice in the management of various complications associated with retinal vascular diseases (diabetic retinopathy, branch retinal vein occlusion). That is why PRP has been used in the treatment of neovascular complications of CRVO such as neovascular glaucoma for numerous years. Guidelines on treatment modalities and follow-up care of patients with central retinal vein occlusion were provided by the Central Vein Occlusion Study (CVOS),[21] a multicenter prospective study sponsored by the National Eye Institute.

Neuropathies

Prolonged diabetes is a risk factor in the development of a number or neuropathies. The mechanism responsible for the observed neurological defects is believed to be an injury that damages the small vessels nourishing the nerves. Defects of this nature that affect the eye include the following:

- Ischemic optic neuropathy
- Ocular palsies
- Diabetic corneal neuropathy

Ischemic Optic Neuropathy

Ischemic optic neuropathy (ION) refers to irreversible optic nerve damage due to loss of blood flow to the nerve. Patients present with complaints of loss of central field and/or a characteristic altitudinal visual field defect. This ocular complication occurs more frequently in persons with diabetes and can lead to permanent visual loss.

Ocular Palsies

Ocular palsies result from ischemia to the third, fourth, and sixth cranial nerves. Impairment of extraocular muscle function leads to strabismus (crossing of the eyes) or diplopia (double vision). This condition is temporary, and normal function usually returns within a few months.

Diabetic Corneal Neuropathy

This disease can lead to severe dry eye and corneal ulcers. (The cornea is the transparent front part of the eye that covers the iris pupil and anterior chamber and provides most of the eyes' optical power.) In addition to these corneal epithelial problems, the corneal endothelium has an increased incidence of dysfunction in individuals with diabetes.[22,23] Usually, these patients will complain of tearing, occasional ocular pain, and blurry vision. This condition needs to be treated with topical lubricants to decrease the occurrence of further complications.

Other Visual Impairments

Blurring of Vision

Blurring of vision due to instability of blood glucose is related to osmotic changes in the lens of the eye. This problem occurs commonly at the onset of diabetes and during periods of fluctuating blood glucose control. The patient needs to be reassured that this condition is transient and instructed to delay testing for new refractive lenses until the blood glucose has been stabilized for 6 to 8 weeks.

Temporary Visual Changes

Temporary visual changes such as dimming of vision, bright flashing lights, or double vision may be experienced during periods of hypoglycemia (low blood glucose levels).[1,24,25]

Diabetic Retinopathy

Diabetic retinopathy is the leading cause of legal blindness in people with diabetes in the United States. It is the most common and most important eye disease affecting the diabetic patient.

Diabetic retinopathy[2,4,5,24,26] occurs when the microvasculature nerve layer that nourishes the retina is damaged. The damage permits leakage of blood components through the vessel walls. (The retina is a layer of nerve tissue at the back of the eye that is responsible for processing images and light.) These images are then relayed along the optic nerve to the brain. Any disturbance to the nerve layer can cause visual symptoms.

There are many theories regarding the pathogenic mechanisms that lead to the development of diabetic eye disorders. The most popular of these theories relate to abnormalities of (1) protein glycosylation, (2) aldose reductase activity, and (3) glycosylated hemoglobin. All of these mechanisms can result in a relative tissue hypoxia, which may be the final common pathway.[9]

The first clinical findings of diabetic retinopathy are abnormalities of the retinal blood vessels. For instance, the first identifiable lesion is a microaneurysm located within 30° of the center of the macula.[27] (The macula is the small central area of the retina surrounding the fovea; it is the area of acute central vision used for reading and discriminating fine detail and color. A microaneurysm is a minute bubble in the wall of a small blood vessel.) After these first abnormalities are detected, more will tend to occur.

> ***Preventing Blindness***
>
> Diabetic retinopathy, the most common and most important eye disease affecting persons with diabetes, is the nation's leading cause of legal blindness. Cataracts and glaucoma also are leading causes of blindness.

Intervention impedes the leading cause of blindness in those with diabetes:

Without appropriate intervention, diabetic retinopathy can progress from a mild asymptomatic form to a severe, rapidly progressing condition.

Retinopathy is staged from its mildest form, using the terms nonproliferative (mild, moderate, and severe), to its most-advanced form, called proliferative retinopathy.[28] Table 22.1 summarizes the stages. Retinopathy is often detectable within 5 years of the onset of diabetes.[1,2] Since type 2 diabetes may go undetected for well over 5 years after its onset, 21% of persons with type 2 diabetes already have retinopathy at the time of diagnosis.

Ninety percent of the people with diabetes who acquire the disease (either type 1 or type 2 diabetes) at less than 30 years of age will develop nonproliferative retinopathy within 20 years after the initial diagnosis, and 50% will progress to proliferative retinopathy.

Risk Factors

The development and progression of retinopathy correlates strongly with the degree of glycemic control and the duration of diabetes.[4,5,24]

Modifiable risk factors: hyperglycemia and blood pressure

The severity of hyperglycemia is the key alterable risk factor associated with the development and progression of diabetic retinopathy.[29-31] Blood pressure control is also important.

Glucose Control. The relationship of hyperglycemia severity to the development and progression of diabetic retinopathy was demonstrated in the Diabetes Control and Complications Trial (DCCT) for type 1 diabetes and in the UK Prospective Diabetes Study (UKPDS) for type 2 diabetes.[30,32] The data resulting from these studies

Case—Part 2: Poor Follow-Up Prevents Timely Intervention

Three years passed. MG had missed all his follow-up appointments with the retina service after the initial exam, but he saw the glaucoma specialist once. The glaucoma specialist had started him on eye drops to control the eye pressure, but MG stopped using the eye drops 2 years ago. He returned to the retina service approximately 3 years after his initial examination. By this time, he noticed his vision had decreased and he had started seeing several "cobwebs," especially in the right eye.

- On examination, he had a visual acuity of 20/200 in the right eye and 20/40 on the left.
- IOP was 22 and 21 mm Hg, respectively, in the right and left eyes.
- A 2+ posterior subcapsular cataract was noted (unchanged since last visit) on the right eye and mild cataract on the left eye.
- On the fundus exam, the cup-to-disc ratio was unchanged from last visit.
- The retinal evaluation revealed that MG had progressed to a more severe stage of diabetic retinopathy with neovascularization at the disc. Multiple intraretinal hemorrhages, microaneurysms, and cotton-wool spots along with hard exudates were noted within the macular area. There were several areas of retinal thickening (edema) on both eyes.
- Fluorescein angiography (FA), macular optical coherence tomography (OCT), and visual field tests were performed. They showed a large amount of dye leakage from both eyes, macular thickening, and visual field defects in both eyes.

Diagnosis

- Proliferative diabetic retinopathy
- Clinically significant macular edema
- Subcapsular cataract in right eye
- Primary open-angle glaucoma

Treatment

- MG was given laser treatment (panretinal photocoagulation and focal laser) in both eyes according to standards of care and scheduled for follow-up in 6 to 8 weeks.
- He was also referred to the glaucoma specialist to restart glaucoma treatment.

Follow-Up

Six weeks later, MG's visual acuity was 20/80 in the right eye and 20/30 in the left eye, and significant improvement was noted in the retinal exam. There was regression of the neovascularization and improvement of the macular edema. He saw the glaucoma specialist, who restarted him with glaucoma eye drops. His IOP was reduced to 14 mm Hg on both eyes. For 2 years, MG then continued his eye examinations as indicated and remained stable.

The progression of eye disease might have been prevented in this case or at least delayed through continued close treatment and ongoing observation of the patient's eye disease. Application of effective teaching strategies might have helped this man realize the implications of his self-care choices and motivated him to engage in successful comprehensive self-management.

emphasized the importance of achieving tight blood glucose control in all persons with diabetes in an attempt to decrease the severity of its complications. Once retinopathy is present, duration of diabetes appears to be less of a factor than hyperglycemia; therefore, it must be stressed to the patient and healthcare providers that controlled blood glucose levels will greatly determine progression to the later, more-advanced stages of diabetic retinopathy.[31] (See chapter 8 on hyperglycemia.)

Blood Pressure. Another important alterable factor is high blood pressure. Intensive management of hypertension has been demonstrated to slow retinopathy progression.[33,34]

Other Risk Factors. There is less agreement concerning the importance of other factors such as age, clotting factors, renal disease, and use of specific types of high blood pressure medication.[31,35-37]

TABLE 22.1 Diabetic Retinopathy—International Clinical Disease Severity Scale	
No apparent retinopathy:	No abnormalities
Mild nonproliferative diabetic retinopathy:	Microaneurysms only
Moderate nonproliferative diabetic retinopathy:	More than just microaneurysms, but less than severe nonproliferative diabetic retinopathy
Severe nonproliferative diabetic retinopathy:	Any of the following: • More than 20 intraretinal hemorrhages in each of 4 quadrants • Definite venous beading in 2 or more quadrants • Prominent intraretinal microvascular abnormalities in 1 or more quadrants • And no signs of proliferative diabetic retinopathy
Proliferative diabetic retinopathy:	One or both of the following: • Neovascularization • Vitreous or preretinal hemorrhage

Source: Wilkinson CP, Ferris FL 3rd, Klein RE, et al (Global Diabetic Retinopathy Project Group). Proposed international clinical diabetic retinopathy and diabetic macular edema disease severity scales (review). Ophthalmology. 2003 Sep;110(9):1677-82.

Evidence Base. Several large clinical studies have provided excellent information on the natural history and effective treatment strategies that can prevent severe vision loss. These studies include 5 major clinical trials: the Diabetes Control and Complications Trial (DCCT),[30,38,39] the Diabetic Retinopathy Study (DRS),[40,41] the Early Treatment Diabetic Retinopathy Study (ETDRS),[42,43] the Diabetic Retinopathy Vitrectomy Study (DRVS),[44,45] and the UK Prospective Diabetes Study (UKPDS).[32,33,46]

Natural History

In its earliest stages, diabetic retinopathy, termed nonproliferative diabetic retinopathy (NPDR), is characterized by retinal vascular abnormalities. These include microaneurysms (which are seen as sacular outpouchings along weakened vascular walls), intraretinal hemorrhages that may appear as dots or a flame shape, and cotton-wool spots. Increased retinal vascular permeability can occur in this or later stages of retinopathy and may result in retinal thickening (edema) and fluid deposits (hard exudates). Clinically significant macular edema (CSME) is a term used frequently for retinal thickening and/or hard exudates that either involve the center of the macula or threaten to infiltrate it.

As retinopathy progresses, there is a gradual closure of the retinal vessels, which results in decreased perfusion and ischemia. Signs of increased ischemia include vascular abnormalities (eg, beading, loops), intraretinal microvascular abnormalities (IRMA) that appear as dilated capillaries that arise around ischemic areas where there is capillary closure, and increased retinal hemorrhages and exudation.

The more advanced stage, proliferative diabetic retinopathy (PDR), is characterized by the growth of new blood vessels along the surface of the retina (neovascularization). These vessels may extend to the vitreous cavity using the posterior vitreous surface as a scaffold. (The vitreous is the transparent, colorless, gelatinous mass that fills the rear two-thirds of the eyeball, between the lens and the retina.) The blood vessels are fragile and rupture easily. For this reason, neovascularization in the optic disc (NVD) or neovascularization elsewhere (NVE) is prone to bleeding, which ultimately results in a vitreous hemorrhage. (The optic disc is the ocular end of the optic nerve; it denotes the exit of retinal nerve fibers from the eye and entrance of blood vessels to the eye.) This and other fibrous proliferation may result in epiretinal membrane formation, vitreoretinal traction bands, retinal tears, and retinal detachments.[47] See Tables 22.1 and 22.2 for specific classifications of diabetic retinopathy stages and findings, including macular edema.

Diabetic Macular Edema

The macula is the specialized portion of the retina responsible for central vision. Macular edema is leakage of fluid and exudate from the vessels into the macula. This is a serious consequence that affects the primary area of focus.[2,4] Macular edema may accompany nonproliferative or proliferative diabetic retinopathy. Table 22.2 outlines the progression and severity of macular edema.

Macular edema is defined as retinal thickening within 2 disc diameters (~3 mm) from the center of the macula. Focal edema is associated with hard exudate rings that result from leakage of the microaneurysms. Diffuse edema results from the breakdown of the blood-retinal barrier

TABLE 22.2 Diabetic Macular Edema—International Clinical Disease Severity Scale

Diabetic macular edema apparently absent:	No apparent retinal thickening or hard exudates in posterior pole
Diabetic macular edema apparently present:	Some retinal thickening or hard exudates in posterior pole
Mild diabetic macular edema:	Some retinal thickening or hard exudates in posterior pole, but distant from the center of the macula
Moderate diabetic macular edema:	Retinal thickening or hard exudates approaching the center of the macula, but not involving the center
Severe diabetic macular edema:	Retinal thickening or hard exudates involving the center of the macula

Source: Wilkinson CP, Ferris FL 3rd, Klein RE, et al (Global Diabetic Retinopathy Project Group). Proposed international clinical diabetic retinopathy and diabetic macular edema disease severity scales (review). Ophthalmology. 2003;110(9):1677-82.

with leakage from microaneurysms, retinal capillaries, and arterioles.

CSME results when retinal thickening and exudates are sufficient enough to threaten or impair the central vision. Visual loss may vary from mild blurring to a visual acuity of 20/200 or less (legal blindness). (The higher the bottom number, the more vision is decreased. Normal visual acuity is 20/20.) The risk for development of CSME is 10% to 15% for all persons having diabetes for 15 to 20 or more years. CSME, as defined by the ETDRS, exists with any of the following findings:

- Retinal thickening within 500 µm of the center of the fovea (the central pit in the macula that produces the sharpest vision)
- Hard exudates within 500 µm of the center of the fovea with adjacent retinal thickening
- At least 1 disc area (1.5 × 1.5 mm) of retinal thickening, any part of which is within 1 disc diameter (~1.5 mm) of the center of the fovea[48]

CSME is determined through a dilated pupil, by slitlamp biomicroscopy and/or stereoscopic fundus photography. Fluorescein angiography is a study used to evaluate the retinal vessels, and it helps to guide treatment and monitor progression and therapeutic results. Macular edema that is not clinically significant is observed and not usually treated with laser surgery. CSME is treated with laser surgery by using focal argon photocoagulation to seal the leaking blood vessels. Focal photocoagulation is a laser technique directed to abnormal blood vessels with specific areas of focal leakage to reduce chronic fluid leakage in patients with macular edema.

Timely treatment of macular edema reduces severe vision loss:

Although multiple laser surgeries are often necessary, results from the ETDRS trial demonstrated that timely treatment can reduce the risk of severe vision loss by 50% in the 3 years after diagnosis of clinically significant macular edema.[49]

Eye Examination

The initial diabetic eye examination should include the following components as a minimum. Other studies such as diagnostic imaging are performed when indicated.

- Best corrected visual acuity
- IOP
- Ocular motility
- Gonioscopy (a test to visualize the anterior chamber angle and help classify glaucoma), when indicated
- Slitlamp biomicroscopy
- Dilated funduscopy including stereoscopic examination of the posterior pole
- Examination of the peripheral retina and vitreous

Frequency of Examination

Recommended frequencies for diabetic eye exams, for both type 1 and type 2 diabetes, are listed in the sidebar on the following page. See chapter 11 for information on progression of retinopathy as a maternal complication in pregnancy; see also the first case study's discussion of preconception care in that chapter.

Recommended Frequency of Diabetic Eye Examination

Type 1 Diabetes

Individuals with type 1 diabetes should have a routine diabetic eye exam at puberty, if diabetes is diagnosed by then, and within 3 to 5 years of receiving a diagnosis of diabetes. Thereafter, exams are annual and when pregnant.

Type 2 Diabetes

All persons with type 2 diabetes should be referred for an ophthalmic evaluation at the time of diagnosis.[50] Routine diabetic eye exams should be scheduled yearly thereafter as well as when pregnant.

Type 1 Diabetes. Type 1 diabetes usually has an abrupt onset; therefore, one can usually determine how long a person has had diabetes. Diabetic retinopathy usually becomes apparent as early as 6 to 7 years after onset of the disease, but since the development of vision-threatening retinopathy is rare in children prior to puberty,[51,52] ophthalmic examination is recommended to begin 3 to 5 years after the diagnosis of type 1 diabetes and every year thereafter.[47,53] The eye-care provider may need to evaluate the patient more often if progression of retinopathy warrants it.

Type 2 Diabetes. At the time an individual is diagnosed with type 2 diabetes, the disease has usually been present for an undetermined period of time. For this reason, up to 3% of those diagnosed with diabetes at age 30 years or older have CSME at the time of the initial diagnosis.[53] Almost 30% of patients will have some manifestation of diabetic retinopathy at diagnosis.

Table 22.3 summarizes the recommended frequency of ophthalmologic examinations based on the stage of retinopathy.

Blood Pressure, Blood Glucose, and Eye Disease

To slow retinopathy progression, intensively manage hypertension. Blood glucose control also greatly influences disease progression.

Care Process

The primary purpose of evaluating and managing diabetic retinopathy is to prevent, retard, or reverse visual loss. Doing so maintains and/or improves vision-related quality of life (see sidebar for self-management and self-care strategies). Once diabetic retinopathy is established, treatment is divided according to its severity scale or retinopathy stage (see Tables 22.1 and 22.2).

Early treatment reduces visual loss by 50% after 3 years[49]

Within 1 year of diagnosis of eye disease, 5% to 10% of patients will progress to a more advanced stage.[7] These guidelines are, thus, imperative:

- Normal-to-mild nonproliferative retinopathy requires observation and should be reexamined annually[53]
- Moderate nonproliferative retinopathy without macular edema should be reexamined within 6 to 12 months, as disease progression is common[54]
- Mild-to-moderate nonproliferative retinopathy with clinically significant macular edema should be treated with focal argon photocoagulation to seal leaking blood vessels

Vision improves in only a minority of patients; for the majority, the goal of laser photocoagulation treatment is to stabilize visual acuity.

TABLE 22.3 Suggested Schedule for Ophthalmologic Examination

Stage of Retinopathy	*Frequency of Examination*
No retinopathy	Annually
Mild nonproliferative retinopathy	Annually
Moderate nonproliferative retinopathy	6 to 12 months
Clinically significant macular edema or proliferative retinopathy	3 to 4 months
Proliferative retinopathy with high-risk characteristics	Individualized to patient needs

Source: Bernbaum M, Stich T. Eye disease and adaptive diabetes education for visually impaired persons. In: A Core Curriculum for Diabetes Educators: Diabetes and Complications, 5th ed. Franz MJ, ed. Chicago, Ill: American Association of Diabetes Educators; 2003:131.

Importance of Self-Management Education and Self-Care

Treatment of retinopathy begins with preventive measures such as optimizing blood glucose, lipids, and blood pressure. Smoking cessation may also be of value. Routine annual screening and follow-up by an ophthalmologist are essential to assure that any intervention is appropriately timed.[2,4,24,26,48,49,57]

Patient education about the following topics is an important part of the care process:[47]

- Importance of maintaining near-normal glucose levels
- Importance of maintaining near-normal blood pressure
- Lowering serum lipid levels

See also the resource listing at this end of this chapter and chapter 20 for additional information on topics and strategies appropriate to diabetes education regarding eye disease.

Patients with CSME and excellent visual function should be considered for treatment before visual loss occurs. When treatment is deferred because the center of the macula is not involved or imminently threatened, the patient should be observed at least every 3 to 4 months for progression.[47]

Severe nonproliferative retinopathy and (non-high-risk) proliferative diabetic retinopathy have a similar clinical course. Consequently, subsequent recommendations and treatment are similar, as shown in the ETDRS.

Laser Surgery. In eyes with severe diabetic retinopathy, the risk of progression to proliferative disease is 50% to 75% within 1 year. The ETDRS also studied the value of laser surgery for these patients. Panretinal photocoagulation should be considered and should not be delayed if the eye has reached the high-risk proliferative stage (if neovascularization of the optic disc is extensive or vitreous/preretinal hemorrhage has occurred recently). Careful follow-up at 3 to 4 months is important. The goal of laser therapy is to reduce the risk of visual loss. The ETDRS protocol provides detailed guidelines for treatment.[55,56] The patient should be seen for a follow-up visit every 1 to 4 weeks until completion of panretinal photocoagulation and then every 2 to 4 months thereafter.

When panretinal photocoagulation is to be carried out in eyes with macular edema, it is preferable to perform focal photocoagulation before panretinal photocoagulation. There is evidence that panretinal photocoagulation may exacerbate macular edema and may cause moderate visual loss compared with untreated eyes.[42] Panretinal laser should not be delayed if the diabetic retinopathy is in the high-risk stage. In these cases, panretinal and focal photocoagulation may be performed concomitantly.[47]

Vitreous Surgery. In cases of high-risk proliferative diabetic retinopathy, photocoagulation may not be delivered due to cataracts or severe vitreous or preretinal hemorrhage. In other cases, active proliferative diabetic retinopathy may persist despite extensive panretinal photocoagulation. In these cases, it may be necessary to perform vitreous surgery. Vitreous surgery is frequently indicated in patients with tractional retinal detachment and in nonclearing vitreous hemorrhage precluding panretinal photocoagulation. Patients with vitreous hemorrhage and rubeosis iridis (neovascularization of the iris) also should be considered for prompt vitrectomy and intraoperative photocoagulation, as demonstrated in the DRVS.[44,45]

Other Treatments Being Investigated. Currently, there are different drugs being studied for the management of diabetic retinopathy. Some of these drugs include the administration of short- and long-acting corticosteroids for diabetic macular edema. Other drugs with anti-angiogenic activity (inhibitors of the vascular endothelial growth factor) are also being studied. Although good results have been reported, at this time there is insufficient evidence to guide treatment recommendations for these therapies.[47]

Ancillary Tests. If used appropriately, a number of tests ancillary to the clinical examination may enhance patient care. These include the following:

- *Color Fundus Photography.* This is a more reproducible technique than a clinical examination for detecting diabetic retinopathy in clinical research studies. However, clinical examination is superior for detecting retinal thickening and at identifying fine-caliber neovascularization (NVD or NVE).
- *Fluorescein Angiography.* This is a clinically valuable test for selected patients with diabetic retinopathy and can be used as a guide for treating diabetic macular edema.[48] It is also helpful as a means for evaluating areas of retinal ischemia or the cause of unexplained decreased visual acuity.

- *Ultrasonography (echography).* This is a valuable test for diabetic eyes with opaque media. The test should be considered when media opacities preclude exclusion of retinal detachment or retinal masses by indirect ophthalmoscopy.
- *Optical Coherence Tomography (OCT).* Provides high-resolution (10-µm) imaging of vitreoretinal interface, retina, and subretinal space. OCT can be useful for quantifying retinal thickness and macular edema and identifying vitreomacular traction.[58]

Counseling and Referral

While it is clearly the responsibility of the ophthalmologist to manage eye disease, the ophthalmologist also has the responsibility to ensure that people with diabetes are referred for appropriate management of their systemic condition.[24]

An important aspect of treatment is meeting the patient's needs in adapting to loss of vision.[44,59-62] An offer of psychosocial counseling should be made before there is actual deterioration of vision to help alleviate anxiety and depression. Chapter 4 can be of value in assessing and addressing anxiety and depression; chapter 34, on healthy coping, also has content of relevance.

Low-vision evaluation is indicated as soon as vision loss impacts normal daily activities. Referral to rehabilitation services as early as possible will allow the person to acquire adaptive skills and maintain participation and independence in work and recreational activities. Patients need information and instruction in adaptive diabetes self-care as soon as vision is compromised, preferably before adaptive equipment is required.

The extent of vision impairment and the individual's ability to adapt to the vision loss must be evaluated before undertaking adaptive education. The adaptive education and training needs of persons with preexisting eye disease due to other causes may differ from persons experiencing a new onset of diabetic retinopathy. The diabetes educator can play a key role in referring patients with visual impairment to the proper rehabilitative and psychosocial services.

Questions and Controversies

Effect of Laser Therapy on Vision

Panretinal laser photocoagulation (PRP) is the standard treatment for proliferative diabetic retinopathy. Vision will improve with PRP in only a minority of patients. For the majority, the goal is to stabilize the disease and help reduce the progression of vision loss. In some cases, PRP may be associated with a decrease in vision, a partial loss of peripheral vision, and/or some degree of night blindness. Still, PRP has been proven to prevent severe vision loss for years ahead.

Pharmacologic Therapies

Vascular endothelial growth factor (VEGF) has been shown to play a key role in retinal neovascularization. For this reason, anti-VEGF treatments have been hypothesized as an alternative adjunctive treatment for retinal neovascularization. Studies are being conducted to determine the safety and efficacy of different anti-VEGF medications as an adjunctive treatment to panretinal laser photocoagulation and also to determine if proliferative diabetic retinopathy can be controlled solely with intravitreal medications without applying laser photocoagulation.

The standard treatment for macular edema has been focal laser. Presently, there are several studies under investigation using different medications in their treatment, including intravitreal steroids and anti-VEGF medications. Although they have shown promising results, the pros and cons of these medications are still under investigation.

Smoking Cessation

The effect of tobacco use (smoking) on certain eye diseases is a subject of controversy. The 2004 Surgeon General's Report entitled The Health Consequences of Smoking: A Report of the Surgeon General indicated there is insufficient evidence regarding a causal relationship between smoking and the onset or progression of diabetic retinopathy.[63] The report further indicated there is suggestive but insufficient evidence for a causal relationship between smoking and nuclear cataract, or between smoking and age-related macular degeneration. There was inadequate evidence to infer either the presence or absence of a causal relationship between smoking and glaucoma.

Focus on Education: Pearls for Practice

Teaching Strategies

- **Provide hope, prevent vision loss.** Most diabetic eye diseases can be controlled without significant visual loss if they are diagnosed and managed in time. Blindness does not have to be part of diabetes. The primary purpose in managing retinopathy is to prevent, retard, or reverse vascular loss. In addition, consistent, frequent monitoring of blood pressure, blood glucose, and lipids is needed.

- **Prepare adequately for those with visual impairment.** Teaching methods need to include large print, magnifiers, and the option of recording instructor's information or directions or obtaining prerecorded instructions. Provide hands-on time and extra time for return demonstration when teaching people with varied levels of visual capacity.

- **Emphasize timely referrals.** Rehabilitative and psychosocial services are available and referral needs to be made promptly to prepare patients for vision loss as well as to help them adapt to vision already lost.

Messages for Patients

- **Emphasize maintaining good diabetes control.** Keeping blood sugars at target maintains strict control of diabetes and helps preserve vision.

- **Involve family.** Invite family or significant others to attend education sessions for support and to assist in "helping" roles. Ensure, however, that "helpers" do not take over, for example when vision is compromised.

- **Ask about vision changes.** Blurriness may be temporary due to elevated blood sugars. Wait until blood sugar resolves before considering eye glasses or changes in lenses.

- **Discuss eye care.** Be knowledgeable about both screening to protect vision and other reasons to consult an eye care specialist. Understand what the recommendations are for diabetic eye examinations, both for initial visits and follow-up. Identify the frequency of eye care visits that will best protect vision for the individual.

- **Protect vision through eye examinations.** Knowing the current status of eye disease and what symptoms to watch for is important. Schedule a retinal evaluation by an ophthalmologist to assess eye condition. This examination is not just a fitting for glasses; it is a dilated eye exam. Use the appointment to ask these kinds of questions: explain what condition my eyes are in, what can I do to keep my vision, is it okay to exercise, and what do I need to change?

- **Seek out specialists when help is needed.** To help alleviate anxiety, depression, and begin the process of adapting to loss of vision, psychosocial counseling is appropriate to include *before* deterioration of vision occurs.

Resources

Consumer and Service Organizations

American Council of the Blind
1155 Fifteenth Street, NW, Suite 1004
Washington, DC 20005
202-467-5081
800-424-8666
www.acb.org

American Foundation for the Blind
11 Penn Plaza, Suite 300
New York, NY 10001
212-504-7600/800-232-5463
www.afb.org

LIONS Club International
300 West Twenty-Second Street
Oakbrook, IL 60523
630-571-5466
www.lions.org

National Eye Institute
Information Officer
Building 31, Room 6A32
Bethesda, MD 20205
301-496-5248
www.nei.nih.gov

National Federation of the Blind*
1800 Johnson Street
Baltimore, MD 21230
410-659-9314
www.nfb.org

Prevent Blindness America
500 East Remington Road
Schaumburg, IL 60173
847-843-2020
800-331-2020
www.preventblindness.org

Sources for Audiotaped and Braille Reading Material

American Printing House for the Blind
1839 Frankfort Avenue
Louisville, KY 40206
502-895-2405
800-223-1839
www.aph.org

National Library Service for the Blind and Physically Handicapped
Library of Congress
1291 Taylor Street, NW
Washington, DC 20542
202-287-510
800-424-8567
www.lcweb.loc.gov/nls

Recording for the Blind and Dyslexic
20 Roszel Road
Princeton, NJ 08540
800-221-4792
www.rfbd.org

Correspondence Courses (including courses on diabetes and adjustment to vision loss)

Hadley School for the Blind
700 Elm Street
Winnetka, IL 60093
847-446-8111/800-323-4238
www.hadley/school.org

Diabetes-Related Products

*A Braille Exchange List (ADA Diet-1995) and a comprehensive listing of diabetes products for people with vision impairment are available from the National Federation of the Blind. (See above listing for contact information.)

References

1. Klein R, Klein BEK. Vision disorders in diabetes. In: Diabetes in America, 2nd ed. National Diabetes Data Group, eds. National Institutes of Health; 1995:293-337.
2. Ferris FL III, Davis MD, Aiello LM. Treatment of diabetic retinopathy (review). New Engl J Med. 1999;341:667-78.
3. Javitt JC, Aiello LP. Cost effectiveness of detecting and treating diabetic retinopathy. Ann Intern Med. 1996;124:164-9.
4. Aiello LP, Gardner TW, King GL, et al. Diabetic retinopathy (technical review). Diabetes Care. 1998;21(1):143-56.
5. Aiello LP, Cavallerano J, Bursell SE. Diabetic eye disease. Endocrinol Metab Clin North Am. 1996;25:271-91.
6. Harris MI. Summary. In: Diabetes in America, 2nd ed. National Diabetes Data Group, eds. National Institutes of Health; 1995:1-13.

7. Ferris FL III, Davis MD, Aiello LM. Treatment of diabetic retinopathy (review). New Engl J Med. 1999;341:667-78.

8. Ferris FL 3rd. How effective are treatments for diabetic retinopathy? JAMA. 1993;269:1290-1.

9. Feman SS. Diabetes and the eye. In: Duane's Clinical Ophthalmology on CD-ROM. Philadelphia, Pa: Lippincott Williams & Wilkins; 2004.

10. Ederer F, Hiller R, Taylor HR. Senile lens change in diabetes in two population studies. Am J Ophthalmol. 1981;91:381.

11. Flanagan DW. Current management of established diabetic eye disease. Eye. 1993;7:302.

12. Leske MC. The epidemiology of open-angle glaucoma: a review. Am J Epidemiol. 1983;118:66.

13. Becker B. Diabetes mellitus and primary open-angled glaucoma. Am J Ophthamol. 1971;71:1.

14. Klein BE, Klein R, Jensen SC. Open-angle glaucoma in older onset diabetes: The Beaver Dam Eye Study. Ophthalmology. 1994:101:1173.

15. Dielemans I, de Jong PTVM, Stolk R, et al. Primary open-angle glaucoma, intraocular pressure, and diabetes mellitus in the general elderly population. The Rotterdam Study. Ophthalmology. 1996;103:1271.

16. US Preventive Services Task Force. Screening for glaucoma (recommendation statement). Ann Fam Med. 2005;3:171-2.

17. Aiello LP, Avery RL, Arrig PG. Vascular endothelium growth factor in ocular fluid of patients with diabetic retinopathy and other retinal disorders. N Engl J Med. 1994;331:1480.

18. Molteno ACB, VanRooyen MNB, Bartholomew RS. Implants for draining neovascular glaucoma. Br J Ophthalmol. 1977:61:120.

19. The Eye Disease Case-Control Study Group. Risk factors for central retinal vein occlusion. Arch Ophthalmol. 1996;114:545.

20. Schwab PJ, Okun E, Fahey FJ. Reversal of retinopathy in Waldenstrom's macroglobulinemia by plasmapheresis: a report of two cases. Arch Ophthalmol. 1960;64:67.

21. Central Vein Occlusion Study Group. A randomized clinical trial of early panretinal photocoagulation for ischemic central vein occlusion. The Central Vein Occlusion Study Group N report. Ophthalmology. 1995;102(10):1434-44.

22. Schultz RO, Peters MA, Sobocinski K. Diabetic corneal neuropathy. Trans Am Ophthamol Soc. 1983;81:107.

23. Busted N, Olsen T, Schmitz O. Clinical observations on the corneal thickness and the corneal endothelium in diabetes mellitus. Br J Ophthalmol. 1982;65:687.

24. Frank KJ, Dieckert JP. Diabetic eye disease: a primary care perspective. South Med J. 1996;89:463-70.

25. Cox DJ, Kiernan BD, Schroeder DB, Cowley M. Psychosocial sequelae of visual loss in diabetes. Diabetes Educ. 1998;24:481-4.

26. Sanders R, Wilson M. Diabetes-related eye disorders. J Natl Med Assoc. 1993;85:104-8.

27. Feman SS. The natural history of the first clinically visible features of diabetic retinopathy. Trans Am Ophthalmol Soc. 1994;92:744.

28. Wilkinson CP, Ferris FL, 3rd, Klein RE, et al. Proposed international clinical diabetic retinopathy and diabetic macular edema disease severity scales. Ophthalmology. 2003;110:1677-82.

29. Klein R, Klein BE, Moss SE, et al. Glycosylated hemoglobin predicts the incidence and progression of diabetic retinopathy. JAMA. 1988;260:2864-71.

30. The Diabetes Control and Complications Trial (DCCT) Research Group. The effect of intensive treatment of diabetes on the development and progression of long-term complications in insulin-dependent diabetes mellitus. N Engl J Med. 1993;329:977-86.

31. Davis MD, Fisher MR, Gangnon RE, et al. Risk factors for high-risk proliferative diabetic retinopathy and severe visual loss: Early Treatment Diabetic Retinopathy Study Report #18. Invest Ophthalmol Vis Sci. 1998;39:233-52.

32. UK Prospective Diabetes Study (UKPDS) Group. Intensive blood-glucose control with sulphonylureas or insulin compared with conventional treatment and risk of complications in patients with type 2 diabetes (UKPDS 33). Lancet. 1998;352:837-53.

33. UK Prospective Diabetes Study Group. Tight blood pressure control and risk of macrovascular and microvascular complications in type 2 diabetes (UKPDS 38). BMJ. 1998;317:703-13.

34. Snow V, Weiss KB, Mottur-Pilson C. The evidence base for tight blood pressure control in the management of type 2 diabetes mellitus. Ann Intern Med. 2003;138:587-92.

35. Klein R, Klein BE, Moss SE, et al. The Wisconsin epidemiologic study of diabetic retinopathy: IX. four year incidence and progression of diabetic retinopathy when age at diagnosis is less than 30 years. Arch Ophthalmol. 1989;107:237-43.

36. Klein R, Klein BE, Moss SE, et al. The Wisconsin epidemiologic study of diabetic retinopathy: X. four year incidence and progression of diabetic retinopathy when age at diagnosis is 30 years or more. Arch Ophthalmol. 1989;107:244-9.

37. Klein R, Sharrett AR, Klein BE, et al. The association of atherosclerosis, vascular risk factors, and retinopathy in adults with diabetes: the atherosclerosis risk in communities study. Ophthalmology. 2002;109;1225-34.

38. The Diabetes Control and Complications Trial (DCCT). The relationship of glycemic exposures (HbA1c) to the risk of development and progression of retinopathy. Diabetes. 1995;44:968-83.

39. The Diabetes Control and Complications Trial (DCCT) Research Group. The effect of intensive diabetes treatment on the progression of diabetic retinopathy in insulin dependent diabetes mellitus. Arch Ophthalmol. 1995;113:36-51.

40. The Diabetic Retinopathy Study (DRS) Research Group Report No. 14. Indications for photocoagulation treatment of diabetic retinopathy. Int Ophthalmol Clin. 1987;27:239-53.

41. The Diabetic Retinopathy Study (DRS) Research Group. DRS report No. 3. Four risk factors for severe visual loss in diabetic retinopathy. Arch Ophthalmol. 1979;97:654-5.

42. Early Treatment Diabetic Retinopathy Study Research Group ETDRS Report No. 9. Early photocoagulation for diabetic retinopathy. Ophthalmology. 1991;98:766-85.

43. Early Treatment Diabetic Retinopathy Study Research Group ETDRS Report No. 19. Focal photocoagulation treatment of diabetic macular edema: relationship of treatment effect to fluorescein angiographic and other retinal characteristics at baseline. Arch Ophthalmol. 1995;113:1144-55.

44. The Diabetic Retinopathy Vitrectomy Study Research Group. Study report no. 2. Early vitrectomy for severe vitreous hemorrhage in diabetic retinopathy: two-year results of a randomized trial: Diabetic Retinopathy Vitrectomy. Arch Ophthalmol. 1985;103:1644-52.

45. The Diabetic Retinopathy Vitrectomy Study Research group. Study report no. 5. Early vitrectomy for severe vitreous hemorrhage in diabetic retinopathy: four-year results of a randomized trial. Arch Ophthalmol. 1990;108:958-64.

46. UK Prospective Diabetes Study (UKPDS) Group (UKPDS 34). Effect of intensive blood-glucose control with metformin on complications in overweight patients with type 2 diabetes. Lancet. 1998;352;854-65.

47. American Academy of Ophthalmology Quality of Care Committee Retina Panel. Preferred Practice Pattern for Diabetic Retinopathy. San Francisco, Calif: American Academy of Ophthalmology; 2003.

48. Early Treatment Diabetic Retinopathy Study Research Group. Early Treatment Diabetic Retinopathy Study report 1. photocoagulation for diabetic macular edema. Arch Ophthalmol. 1985;103:1796-1806.

49. The Diabetic Retinopathy Study Research Group. Preliminary report on effects of photocoagulation therapy. Am J Ophthalmol. 1976;81:383-96.

50. Klein R, Klein BE, Moss SE, et al. The Wisconsin epidemiologic study of diabetic retinopathy III. prevalence and risk of diabetic retinopathy when age of diagnosis is 30 or more years. Arch Ophthalmol. 1984;102:527-32.

51. Klein R, Klein BE, Moss SE, et al. Retinopathy in young-onset diabetic patients. Diabetes Care. 1985;8:311-5.

52. Krolewski AS, Warram JH, Rand LI, et al. Risk of proliferative diabetic retinopathy in juvenile onset type I diabetes: a 40-year follow-up study. Diabetes Care. 1986;9:443-52.

53. Klein R, Klein BE, Moss SE, et al. The Wisconsin epidemiologic study of diabetic retinopathy II. prevalence and risk of diabetic retinopathy when age at diagnosis is less than 30 years. Arch Ophthalmol. 1984;102:520-6.

54. Klein R, Klein BE, Moss SE, et al. The Wisconsin epidemiologic study of diabetic retinopathy: IX. four-year incidence and progression of diabetic retinopathy when age at diagnosis is 30 years or more. Arch Ophthalmol. 1989;107:237-43.

55. Early Treatment Diabetic Retinopathy Study Research Group. Early Treatment Diabetic Retinopathy Study report no. 2. Treatment techniques and clinical guide-

lines for photocoagulation of diabetic macular edema. Ophthalmology. 1987;94:761-74.

56. Early Treatment Diabetic Retinopathy Study Research Group. ETDRS report 3. Techniques for scatter and local photocoagulation treatment of diabetic retinopathy. Int Ophthalmol Clin. 1987;27:254-64.

57. Ferris F. Early photocoagulation in patients with either type I or type II diabetes. Trans Am Ophthamol Soc. 1996;94:505-37.

58. Strom C, Sander B, Larsen N, et al. Diabetic macular edema assessed with optical coherence tomography and stereo fundus photography. Invest Ophthalmol Vis Sci. 2002;43:241-5.

59. Bernbaum M, Albert SG. Referring patients with diabetes and vision loss for rehabilitation—who is responsible? Diabetes Care. 1996;19:175-7.

60. Bernbaum M, Albert SG, Duckro PN. Psychosocial profiles in patients with visual impairment due to diabetic retinopathy. Diabetes Care. 1988;11:551-7.

61. Jacobson AM. Current concepts: the psychological care of patients with insulin-dependent diabetes mellitus. N Engl J Med. 1996;334:1249-53.

62. Wulsin LR, Jacobson AM, Rand LI. Psychosocial adjustment to advanced proliferative diabetic retinopathy. Diabetes Care. 1993;16:1061-6.

63. US Department of Health and Human Services. The health consequences of smoking: a report of the Surgeon General. Atlanta, Ga: US Department of Health and Human Services, Centers for Disease Control and Prevention, National Center for Chronic Disease Prevention and Health Promotion, Office on Smoking and Health; 2004. On the Internet at: www.surgeongeneral.gov/library/smokingconsequences. Accessed 20 Feb 2006.

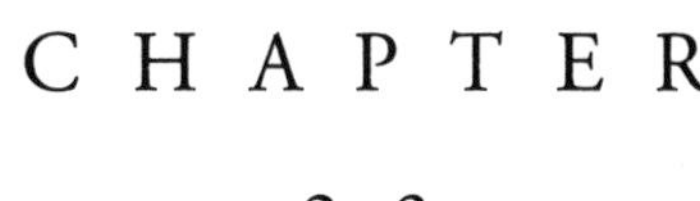

CHAPTER

23

Diabetic Kidney Disease

Author

Laura D. Byham-Gray, PhD, RD, CNSD

Key Concepts

- Early detection and diagnosis of chronic kidney disease is essential for preventing and/or delaying further disease progression.
- Laboratory parameters and diagnostic tests aid in classifying the stages of chronic kidney disease, the various types of kidney failure, and nephrotic syndrome.
- Other concomitant health considerations, such as hyperparathyroidism and anemia, require early treatment.
- Cardiovascular disease is a concern. The risk of cardiovascular disease in persons with chronic kidney disease is 30 times the norm.

Introduction

The spectrum of changes in the kidney that occur among individuals diagnosed with diabetes that cannot be ascribed to other causes has been called diabetic nephropathy; more recently, the term **diabetic kidney disease** is being used.[1] At the severe end of this spectrum is overt (or clinically apparent) diabetic kidney disease, which is characterized by persistent **proteinuria**, hypertension, and a progressive decline in kidney function that often leads to chronic kidney disease (CKD). CKD leads to renal replacement therapies (RRT) (ie, hemodialysis, peritoneal dialysis, or transplantation) and/or premature mortality from cardiovascular disease (CVD). Toward the milder end of the spectrum is **microalbuminuria**. Appropriate and timely clinical intervention may delay or prevent microalbuminuria from progressing to kidney failure.[2]

CKD is a growing public health problem in the United States. Twenty million US adults have CKD, and another 20 million are at increased risk for developing it.[3] Diabetes is the most common primary diagnosis in persons with kidney failure, accounting for approximately 45% of new cases.[4] The increased prevalence of diabetes in the CKD population is related to 2 major factors:[5] the increased incidence of type 2 diabetes in the general population and the innovative therapeutic approaches that have allowed persons diagnosed with diabetes to live longer. These factors likely influence the number of individuals eligible for conservative renal management and/or RRTs.

A glossary of terms related to pathophysiology appears at the end of this chapter.

As measured in the 5-year survival data by disease etiology (diabetes, hypertension, **glomerulonephritis**), one-half of all persons diagnosed with diabetic kidney disease who receive dialysis die within 2 years of initiation of dialysis; this is the highest mortality rate among the 3 leading causes for kidney failure.[6] Regardless of disease etiology, the primary cause of death among persons with CKD is CVD. Persons with CKD have an increased risk of CVD. Their risk is 30 times higher than that of the general population.[7] Thus, the need for a "proactive, comprehensive, integrated intervention and treatment approach to successfully manage diabetes, CKD, and CVD" is appropriate to emphasize.[5]

Early identification is essential:

Early identification of diabetic kidney disease facilitates appropriate treatment that may have the following desired effects:

- Prevent the onset of CKD
- Improve outcomes of people with diabetic kidney disease, and/or
- Slow the progression of kidney failure

Interventions are most effective when instituted early:

The onset and course of diabetic kidney disease can be ameliorated by several interventions, including the following:[8-12]

- Attaining and maintaining glycemic and blood pressure control
- Using antihypertensives
- Decreasing protein intake

These interventions are most effective when instituted early. Thus, detecting microalbuminuria and monitoring kidney function before diabetic nephropathy is clinically evident are important strategies.[2]

Ethnicity and Genetics

To deliver the highest quality care possible to all persons diagnosed with diabetes, the changing demographics among the CKD population must be recognized. Diabetes is the leading cause of kidney failure among all major races reported in the US Renal Data System (USRDS) (Whites, Blacks, Native Americans, Hispanics, or Asians), with dramatic increases occurring within the Native American, Hispanic, and Black cultures. By the mid-1990s, diabetes surpassed hypertension as the leading etiology for kidney failure among Black Americans.[4] Research evidence also supports that there is a strong genetic predisposition for diabetic nephropathy.[13-15]

Age

The median age of persons with kidney failure treated with RRTs over the past 25 years has risen to 58.2 years. This represents a 15% overall increase in age. The largest increase has been reported in persons over the age of 75 years, with the incidence rate doubling in the last decade.[4]

Treatment Approaches

Treatment approaches to CKD will be described in detail later in the chapter. Treatment consists of conservative management with emphasis on lifestyle modification as well as RRT.

A case study is woven throughout the chapter to show one method for applying the best research evidence to clinical practice. The chapter uses the case of a 55-year-old, African American woman with type 2 diabetes of 15 years' duration and at considerable risk for kidney disease as a tool to examine appropriate screening, assessment, and treatment options. Teachable moments are emphasized throughout the chapter as well, and strategies are provided for dealing with the challenges of this complicated condition. This chapter also identifies unanswered clinical questions related to diabetic kidney disease and offers insight into additional topics for scientific inquiry. At the end of the chapter, the reader will find clinical pearls for practice, featuring teaching strategies and messages for patients.

Kidney Function in Health and Disease

The kidney is an intricate organ. It maintains homeostatic control through regulation of fluid volume, sodium and potassium levels, acid-base ratios, and calcium-phosphorus balance.[16] The kidney is one of the main detoxifying organs of the body; it excretes waste products such as excess water, electrolytes, metabolites, drugs, and other potentially harmful toxins. Lastly, it supplies endocrine functions necessary for bone maintenance, blood pressure control, normal metabolism, and red blood cell production.

To fully appreciate all these diverse functions, one must first examine how the kidneys and the entire system work.[16] The urinary system is composed of the kidneys, ureters, bladder, and urethra. Each kidney weighs about 6 oz and is approximately the size of a human fist. The outer core of the kidneys is encapsulated by a fibrous, rigid sheath that forms the renal cortex. Directly underneath this cortex is the medulla. Between these 2 segments, the **nephrons** and collecting tubules are housed. The functional unit or "workhorse" of the kidney is the nephron. Each kidney has well over 1 million nephrons. Within each nephron are several components:[17]

- *Glomerulus and Bowman Capsule.* Fifty capillaries make up the branches of small arteries in the glomerulus. Through this tuft of afferent and efferent arterioles, blood flows into the kidney. The exchange of waste products occurs at the Bowman capsule. Approximately 180 L of filtrate pass through the kidneys at the glomerulus, and 1 to 2 L of urine are actually excreted.
- *Proximal Convoluted Tubule.* This section of the nephron, which is directly connected to the Bowman's capsule, is the main location where glucose, sodium, bicarbonate, potassium, chloride, calcium, phosphate, water, and other solutes are absorbed. The reabsorption of fluid through sodium pumps also occurs in the proximal convoluted tubule.
- *Loop of Henle.* This is the site where urine is concentrated or diluted. The process is largely dictated by the fluid requirements of the body.
- *Distal Tubule.* This tubule has 3 parts: the ascending limb of the Loop of Henle, the macula densa, and the distal convoluted tubule. Ninety-nine percent of the water filtered by the kidneys is reabsorbed here.
- *Collecting Duct.* Secretion of potassium is a major function of the collecting duct. As urine is produced in the nephrons, it flows from the collecting duct to the main cavity of the renal pelvis and then on to the ureter into the bladder, and finally it is expelled through the urethra.

Renal Physiology

Through glomerular filtration, tubular secretion, and reabsorption, the kidneys are able to regulate the chemical composition of the body fluids and eliminate metabolic wastes.[16] Homeostatic regulation of the urine osmolality is controlled by the distal convoluted tubules and collecting ducts. Reabsorption and transport of water greatly varies with cellular permeability and is largely affected by secretion of the **antidiuretic hormone** (ADH). As plasma osmolality increases in a dehydrated condition, ADH secretion increases so that water is conserved by the kidneys; the opposite is true in a hypervolemic state.

The kidneys are also the major site where calcium and phosphorus levels remain in balance. **Parathyroid hormone** (PTH), secreted by the parathyroid glands, is paramount to achieving this balance. The hormone maintains this balance by enhancing calcium and phosphorus absorption from the gastrointestinal tract and bone. During episodes of increased calcium intake, there is a transitory rise in circulating levels of calcium with a subsequent fall in PTH secretion. This results in more calcium filtered by the kidneys and excess amounts excreted. The inverse occurs during periods of low dietary calcium intake. PTH synthesis and release also responds to variations in circulating levels of serum phosphorus, irrespective of serum calcium or vitamin D levels.[18] The final step in the activation of vitamin D occurs within the kidneys. Vitamin D is essential for assisting with the absorption of calcium from the intestinal lumen as well as augmenting bone resorption. Vitamin D, in concert with **calcitonin** and PTH, maintains calcium-phosphorus homeostasis and protects overall bone health.

As already described, the kidneys are greatly affected by a number of hormones.[16] However, the kidneys are invaluable to the endocrine system as well. For instance, 2 other hormones that are produced by the kidneys are released to stimulate effects elsewhere in the body system. These substances are **renin** and **erythropoietin**. Renin is vital for maintaining normal blood pressure and is generated by the kidneys in response to decreased blood volume. Renin acts to form **angiotensin**, which serves as a powerful vasoconstrictor and triggers the release of **aldosterone**, which enhances sodium and water retention. Erythropoietin is also manufactured by the kidneys. This hormone stimulates the bone marrow to produce red blood cells, which in turn prevents severe **anemia** from developing. As evident, the kidneys are one of the most vital organs in the body in maintaining homoeostasis and optimal health. Achieving such balance is increasingly difficult during declining kidney function.

Renal Pathophysiology

Kidney failure may be either sudden, causing **acute renal failure** (ARF), or progressive in nature, as in CKD.[17]

Acute Renal Failure

Persons with ARF have a rapid onset of symptoms, including the following: elevation in **blood urea nitrogen** (BUN), **creatinine**, electrolytes, and minimal urinary output. ARF is typically caused by ischemic or nephrotoxic injury, multiorgan system failure, sepsis, obstructive uropathy, or acute glomerular nephritis.[17] Morbidity and mortality rates can be as high as 80%, depending on etiology. Usually with adequate dialytic support and nutritional intervention, the condition will reverse itself. Only when ARF is superimposed with other illnesses, such as diabetes, may additional medical and nutritional support be required.

Chronic Kidney Disease

In 2002, a standard for classifying the stages of CKD was outlined by the National Kidney Foundation–Kidney Disease Outcomes Quality Initiative (NKF-K/DOQI).[19] The K/DOQI presents evidence-based practice guidelines for the management and treatment of all phases of kidney disease. It was launched in 1995, with routine updates and reviews of the practice guidelines given as necessary. Additional guidelines continue to be developed. For example, the Clinical Practice Guidelines for Diabetes and Chronic Kidney Disease are scheduled for release in mid-year 2006.[1] The language associated with kidney disease has been standardized because synonymous terms were easily confused. The stages of CKD replace commonly used terms such as predialysis, pre-ESRD (end-stage renal disease), and chronic renal insufficiency. This system classifies CKD by an "at risk" stage and 5 progressive stages as defined by the **glomerular filtration rate** (GFR).

Stages of Chronic Kidney Disease. Table 23.1 summarizes the classification for CKD, according to K/ DOQI. Kidney function is dependent on the measurement of the GFR through a number of validated equations. Some decreases in kidney function may be secondary to the normal aging process.[17] If decline persists, kidney function should be monitored to enable appropriate and timely intervention.

Persons diagnosed with CKD experience a permanent loss of GFR that occurs over a period of months to years, such as in diabetic nephropathy. Eventually, CKD may lead to Stage 5, requiring RRT, such as dialysis or transplantation, to sustain life. Although RRTs are discussed, the focus of this chapter is on how to delay or prevent further disease progression.

TABLE 23.1 Stages of Chronic Kidney Disease (CKD)—A Clinical Action Plan

Shaded area identifies CKD; unshaded area designates increased risk for developing chronic kidney disease. Chronic kidney disease is defined as either kidney damage or GFR <60 mL/min/1.73 m^2 for ≥3 months. Kidney damage is defined as pathologic abnormalities or markers of damage, including abnormalities in blood or urine tests or imaging studies.

Stage	*Description*	*GFR (mL/min/1.73 m^2)*	*Action**
	At increased risk	≥60 (with chronic kidney disease risk factors)	Screen Reduce risks for chronic kidney disease
1	Kidney damage with normal or ↑ GFR	≥90	Diagnose and treat Treat comorbid conditions Slow progression Reduce risk for CVD
2	Kidney damage with mild ↓ GFR	60–89	Estimate progression
3	Moderate ↓ GFR	30–59	Evaluate and treat complications
4	Severe ↓ GFR	15–29	Prepare for kidney replacement therapy
5	Kidney failure	<15 (or dialysis)	Replacement (if uremia present)

*Includes actions from preceding stages

Key: CVD—cardiovascular disease; GFR—glomerular filtration rate

Source: Adapted with permission from National Kidney Foundation. Clinical practice guidelines for chronic kidney disease: evaluation, classification, and stratification. Am J Kidney Dis. 2002;39 2 suppl 1:S1-S266.

Nephrotic Syndrome

Nephrotic syndrome is considered "one of the most challenging conditions of nephrology."[17] Changes in the glomerular basement membrane occur, secondary to diabetes, glomerulonephritis, or amyloidosis, that lead to profound proteinuria. Clinical signs present as increased urinary losses of albumin (>3 g/day urinary albumin in adults, proportional in children), decreased circulating serum levels of albumin, high blood pressure, elevated serum lipids, and retained fluid.[17]

Medical Management. Proteinuria represents a significant risk factor for CVD and kidney failure. Thus, medical management is directed towards minimizing such losses, controlling blood pressure, and correcting hypervolemia through the use of corticosteroids, immunosuppressants, and angiotensin receptor blockers. To correct dyslipidemia, hydroxymethylglutaryl coenzyme A reductase inhibitors may be prescribed. See chapter 18 for more on pharmacologic therapies for dyslipidemia and hypertension.

Nutritional Management. Dietary manipulation may have minimal impact on serum lipids during episodes of nephrotic syndrome. A moderate protein restriction of 0.8 g per kilogram standard body weight may be assistive in reversing the proteinuria experienced as long as iatrogenic malnutrition does not result. The protein level may be changed to 1.0 g per kilogram standard body weight in the attempt to achieve adequate nutritional status. More research is needed to establish optimal nutritional management for proteinuria. Sodium restriction should be based on fluid status and the need to control edema. Other electrolytes and minerals should be monitored, with the meal plan individualized accordingly.

Pathogenesis of Diabetic Kidney Disease

Hyperglycemia plays a role in the pathogenesis of diabetic kidney disease. Alteration in tubuloglomerular feedback occurs, resulting in renal vasodilation, increased renal blood flow, and hyperfiltration.[2] Accelerated formation of nonenzymatic advanced glycosylation end-products (AGEs) in tissues is directly correlated with hyperglycemia. An increase in circulating AGE peptides parallels the severity of renal dysfunction in diabetic nephropathy. Glycosylation of proteins in the capillary basement membrane may stimulate mesangial expansion. Glycation of albumin can also contribute to its loss across the glomerular basement membrane.

Other hormonal imbalances, aside from insufficient insulin, have been implicated in the pathogenesis of diabetic kidney disease. Growth hormone and glucagon, which are both elevated in poorly controlled diabetes, have been shown to produce glomerular hyperfiltration.[2] Changes in circulating levels of angiotensin II, catecholamines, and prostaglandins, or altered responsiveness to these vasoactive hormones, may also result in hyperfiltration. Angiotensin II may promote cellular and glomerular hypertrophy as well as mesangial expansion.

Renal hemodynamic changes play a role in the pathogenesis of diabetic kidney disease. Glomerular hypertension contributes to increased pressure and flow across the glomerular membrane, resulting in hyperfiltration. Glomerular hypertension and the associated renal vasodilation and hyperfiltration increase glomerular protein filtration, leading to proteinuria and glomerulosclerosis with consequent destruction of nephrons.

Screening and Detection

Recommended frequency of screening for nephropathy:

- *Type 1 Diabetes:* 5 years after diagnosis; annually thereafter
- *Type 2 Diabetes:* At diagnosis and annually thereafter; also during pregnancy

In type 2 diabetes, screening should be initiated at the time of diagnosis because the disease (diabetes) may have gone unrecognized and been affecting the kidneys for several years. Those with type 1 diabetes have an even greater risk of overt nephropathy and kidney failure as the disease progresses. Annual screening facilitates early detection and slowing the progression of kidney disease.

The Dialysis Morbidity and Mortality Study (DMMS) found that 30% of all persons with Stage 5 CKD did not see a nephrologist until 3 months before initiating RRT, and 50% never consulted with a dietitian before starting such therapy.[20] In the 12 months before initiation of RRT, appropriate and timely medical care for those diagnosed with CKD greatly reduces morbidity and mortality.[21]

Screening Tests for Diabetic Kidney Disease

Urine Tests. The amount of microalbumin in the urine needs to be measured, and various tests are used for this with varying levels of reliability. A random or timed (4 hour or overnight) urine albumin-to-creatinine ratio (mg/g) can be used to screen for diabetic kidney disease; a 24-hour urine albumin (mg) can be used for confirmation. In the absence of infection, strenuous exercise, or hematuria, an elevated level should be confirmed prior to starting drug therapy.[22]

- Microalbuminuria is diagnosed at >30 mg
- Clinical albuminuria is described at >300 mg

Blood Tests. Regardless of the degree of urine albumin excretion, serum creatinine should be measured at least annually in all adults with diabetes to estimate the GFR. Serum creatinine alone should not be used as a measure of kidney function, but instead be used to estimate GFR and stage the level of CKD.

Estimating Glomerular Filtration Rate. A more accurate predictor of kidney function than serum creatinine alone is an estimation of the GFR. Serum creatinine may be affected by body shape, size, and dietary intake. A number of methods for estimating GFR (eGFR) may be used; 2 validated approaches include the abbreviated Modifications of Diet in Renal Disease (MDRD) Study equation or the Cockcroft-Gault equation. Both take into account a number of factors that may affect kidney function, such as sex, age, race, weight, and serum creatinine (SCr) levels.[23] A GFR calculator is available at the National Kidney Foundation website (www.kidney.org) so the practitioner is able to readily predict the level of kidney function.

Abbreviated MDRD Study Equation

$$\text{GFR (mL/min/1.73 m}^2\text{)} = 186.3 \times \text{SCr} - 1.154 \times \text{Age} - 0.203 \times 0.742 \text{ (if female)} \times 1.210 \text{ (if African American)}$$

Cockcroft-Gault Equation

$$\text{Ccr} = \text{(mL/min)} \quad \frac{(140 - \text{Age}) \times \text{Weight in kg}}{72 \times \text{SCr}} \times 0.85 \text{ if female}$$

Stages of Nephropathy

The stages of nephropathy, summarized in the sidebar, provide a developmental framework. Kidney failure will ensue if the nephropathy is left untreated or not controlled. Do not confuse the stages of nephropathy with the stages of CKD, which are described in Table 23.1.

Individuals may progress through the stages of nephropathy at differing rates. Progression varies according to age and comorbidities, such as atherosclerosis, hypertension, or autonomic neuropathy. The first sign of incipient nephropathy (stage 3) is microalbuminuria (>30 mg/day).[24]

Progression of Disease. In the absence of medical intervention, 80% of persons with type 1 diabetes will progress in 10 to 15 years to overt nephropathy (clinical albuminuria >300 mg/day) with hypertension. Recent literature has indicated that the incidence rate of persons

Stages of Nephropathy[2,24]

These are not to be confused with Stages of CKD, which are described in Table 23.1.

Stage 1 is characterized by hyperfiltration and renal hypertrophy. These changes frequently are seen at the time of diagnosis of diabetes. Hyperglycemia leads to increased kidney filtration.

Stage 2 involves structural changes, including glomerular basement membrane thickening and mesangial expansion. These structural changes appear to initiate the decline in renal function. This phase is clinically silent, but hyperfiltration continues.

Stage 3, incipient diabetic kidney disease, develops after 7 to 15 years of diabetes duration. Microalbuminuria first appears. Functional and structural renal alterations lead to abnormal filtration of microscopic amounts of protein into the urine. Blood pressure during this stage may be normal or slightly elevated; individuals at stage 3 are generally asymptomatic. The presence of microalbuminuria in type 1 diabetes appears to be a strong predictor of clinical or overt diabetic nephropathy.

Stage 4 is overt (clinical) diabetic kidney disease. Abnormal filtration of protein increases progressively and becomes persistent in this stage. Nephrotic syndrome and hypertension are usually present. Suboptimal blood pressure and glucose control are positively correlated with the rate of GFR decline.

Stage 5, end-stage renal disease, develops when GFR is less than 15 mL per minute and uremia is present.

diagnosed with type 1 diabetes and risk for ESRD is decreasing, in comparison to previous reports.[25] There are wide variations among the study samples cited in the research; however, the following can be generally said:

- *Type 1 Diabetes.* At present, the common conception is that kidney failure will develop in approximately 50% of persons diagnosed with type 1 diabetes in 10 to 20 years.[25,26]
- *Type 2 Diabetes.* Conversely, in persons diagnosed with type 2 diabetes, only 20% to 40% will develop incipient nephropathy that progresses to overt nephropathy, and, within 20 years only 20% will then progress to kidney failure.[24]

Prevention and Delay of Chronic Kidney Disease

The following are important parameters to monitor and control in preventing and delaying the progression of CKD. Each is discussed separately below, with targets summarized in a chart.

- Blood glucose control
- Blood pressure control
- Lipid levels, for CVD risk
- Hemoglobin, for anemia
- Serum markers of bone and mineral metabolism

Do not confuse stages of nephropathy with stages of chronic kidney disease.

Blood Glucose

Good glycemic control is the mainstay of therapy for preventing or delaying further disease progression. Maintaining the A1C level at less than 7% reduces risk for complications. The Diabetes Control and Complications Trial (DCCT) demonstrated that tight glycemic control lowered the risk for microalbuminuria in type 1 diabetes by 30%, and among persons with microalbuminuria, the risk for further disease progression was reduced by 50%.[8] The UK Prospective Diabetes Study (UKPDS) indicated that individuals with type 2 diabetes had a 25% risk reduction in nephropathy when intensive diabetes therapy was initiated.[9,10] Additionally, for every 1% drop in A1C, there was a 35% reduction in risk for complications. See chart at end of this section for targets.

Blood Pressure

Controlling blood pressure slows the decline of GFR in persons with diabetic kidney disease. In fact, the most recent release of USRDS data indicates that the ESRD rate has stabilized, perhaps indicating that adequate screening and preventive measures (eg, ACEi, ARBs, and/or diuretics) are decreasing the incidence of disease progression.[4] A number of studies have substantiated the inverse relationship between blood pressure and GFR; ie, as blood pressure rises, there is a drop in GFR.[27]

A target blood pressure of <130/80 mm Hg has been given; nonetheless, tighter control is necessary in the existence of nephropathy <120/70 mm Hg.[28] Blood pressure should be measured at every ambulatory care visit, and treatment, as will be discussed, should encompass a number of antihypertensive agents, namely angiotensin converting enzyme inhibitors (ACEi) and/or angiotensin receptor blockers (ARBs) in the presence of proteinuria. See chart at end of this section for targets.

Lipids

As suggested earlier, the presence of proteinuria is a significant risk factor for CVD.[7] The relationship between these factors may be related to genetic predisposition, endothelial dysfunction, associated hypertension, insulin resistance, atherogenic dyslipidemias, hyperglycemia, and anemia.[29] See summary chart at end of this section for targets.

Hemoglobin

In the RENAAL (Reduction of Endpoints in NIDDM with the Angiotensin II Antagonist Losartan) Trial, baseline hemoglobin predicted kidney failure in type 2 diabetes with nephropathy.[30] Early treatment of anemia is associated with improved outcomes.[1] Symptoms associated with anemia in CKD are decreased exercise tolerance, impaired cognitive function, sexual dysfunction, impaired functional status, anorexia, and decreased quality of life. Reversing the anemia experienced in CKD has been shown to decrease left ventricular hypertrophy and increase survival on dialysis as well as enhance quality of life and improve exercise capacity.

When GFR is <60 mL/min/1.73 m^2 (Stage 3 CKD), the hemoglobin should be evaluated. If hemoglobin is suboptimal, additional lab studies are recommended, inclusive of complete blood count (CBC), reticulocyte count, serum iron, total iron binding capacity (TIBC), serum ferritin, and transferrin saturation (TSAT). Depending on lab values, iron supplementation and possibly erthyropoietin administration may be necessary. See summary chart for targets.

Serum Markers of Bone and Mineral Metabolism

Abnormalities in bone and mineral metabolism are frequently seen in persons diagnosed with CKD.[3] Compromises in bone remodeling occur when the GFR drops below 60 mL/min/1.73 m^2 (ie, when 50% of kidney function is lost), suggesting that by the time an individual is diagnosed at Stage 5 CKD (eg, GFR <15 mL/min/1.73 m^2), severe osteodystrophy complications requiring treatment and management have developed.[3] During CKD, the activation of vitamin D to 1, 25-dihydroxycholecalciferol (ie, calcitriol) is disrupted, resulting in hyperphosphatemia, hypocalcemia, and secondary **hyperparathyroidism**

Summary of Target Values in Preventing and Delaying Progression of CKD

Blood Glucose Targets

Target ranges for fasting plasma glucose levels should be as follows:[39,40]

- <120 mg/dL in CKD
- <140 mg/dL in hemodialysis
- <160 mg/dL in peritoneal dialysis
- A1C checked twice a year, or quarterly in individuals with poor glycemic control

Blood Pressure

The goals for blood pressure control are similar to those for the general population as outlined by the Joint National Committee (JNC) for Prevention, Detection, Evaluation and Treatment of High Blood Pressure (Seventh Report):[41]

- Blood pressure <130/80 mm Hg, measured at each healthcare visit
- Blood pressure <120/70 mm Hg in the presence of nephropathy

Lipids

Since CVD is the leading cause of death in diabetic kidney disease, aggressive management of lipids is suggested. As per the K/DOQI Practice Guidelines on Managing Dyslipidemias, serum lipids need to be kept within target ranges similar to the Adult Treatment Panel (ATP) III Guidelines published by the National Cholesterol Education Program:[31]

- Total cholesterol < 200 mg/dL
- Low-density lipoprotein cholesterol <100 mg/dL
- Triglycerides <150 mg/dL
- High-density lipoprotein cholesterol >40 mg/dL
- Serum lipids monitored at least annually and checked more frequently when abnormalities are detected

Hemoglobin

- Hemoglobin between 11 to 12 g/dL, measured annually

Serum Markers

The K/DOQI Practice Guidelines for Bone Disease and Chronic Kidney Disease recommend the following:[33]

- PTH: in CKD Stage 3, target is 35 to 70 pg/mL; in CKD Stage 4, target is 70 to 110 pg/mL
- Phosphorus at or above 2.7 mg/dL and no higher than 4.6 mg/dL in CKD Stages 3 and 4
- Serum calcium within normal ranges, preferably 8.4 to 9.5 mg/dL
- PTH, serum calcium, and phosphorus measured annually in CKD stage 3, quarterly in CKD Stages 4 and 5

> ***Treat the Trio***
>
> Diabetes educators must seek to help individuals manage not only their diabetes, but also CKD and CVD. A proactive, integrated approach ensures the best outcome.

(SHPT). Besides the conditions often associated with renal osteodystrophy (such as muscle and bone pain, bone fractures, and pruritis), the systemic effects of such imbalances include soft tissue and vascular calcification as well as erythropoietin-resistant anemia.[33-35] A paucity of evidence currently exists that identifies the effect of such metabolic derangements on morbidity and mortality among this patient population.[31] Scientific efforts toward reversing these trends or outcomes have been and continue to be supported.[36-38] Calcium, phosphorus, and plasma parathyroid hormone (PTH) levels should be monitored closely. See summary chart (sidebar) for targets.

Treatment for Chronic Kidney Disease

Treatment options for those diagnosed with CKD are described below. The individual's right to self-determination is central to the decision to undergo treatment for CKD—whether to choose or not choose RRT. Proceeding without RRT should be presented as a treatment option to patients and their family or caregivers. If no treatment is administered, death is imminent in less than a year.[2] The patient and family should be encouraged to discuss this decision with clergy, a psychologist, a social worker, the healthcare team, and/or other family members. Plans for supportive care (eg, home care, hospice care) are necessary for the person who wishes to forgo treatment.

CKD Stages 1-4

Treatment options for individuals with diabetic kidney disease are dependent on the stage of CKD.

- For persons with diabetes in the early stages of CKD (Stages 1 through 3) or with preclinical nephropathy, intervention is geared toward glycemic control, hypertensive management with the use of medications that are active on the renin-angiotensin system, and protein restriction

To attain A1C goals without undesired hypoglycemia and weight gain, management of diabetic kidney disease must be appropriately balanced according to diet, insulin, and activity levels.[22] Irregular blood glucose levels may be partially explained by changes in oral intake and appetite. Nonetheless, episodes of hyperglycemia and/or hypoglycemia may also result secondary to alterations in insulin metabolism with changing kidney function. One-fourth to one-third of injected insulin is catabolized by the kidney.[2]

Case in Point: A Woman With Type 2 Diabetes of Long Duration

MG was a 55-year-old, widowed African American woman who had type 2 diabetes for approximately 15 years. She was referred to the diabetes clinic for intensive education and self-management training. Physical findings revealed some shortness of breath upon exertion, blood pressure elevated to 155/90 mm Hg, height 5 ft 3 in, weight 200 lb. MG's laboratory tests revealed the following:

Test	*Results*	*Target Range*
Hemoglobin (g/dL)	9.4	>11.0
Creatinine (mg/dL)	1.9	0.6–1.2
Serum albumin (g/dL)	3.3	$\geq$ 4.0
A1C (%)	8.5	<7.0
LDL-C (mg/dL)	130	<100
HDL-C (mg/dL)	45	>40
Glucose (casual) mg/dL	175	<140
Albumin (mg/g CR)	283	<30
Calcium (mg/dL)	8.9	8.4–9.5
Phosphorus (mg/dL)	4.0	2.7–4.6
PTH (pg/mL)	75	35–70

From the serum biomarker results, it was evident MG was currently at Stage 3 CKD, with an eGFR of 48 mL/min/1.73m^2, experiencing profound microalbuminuria (>30 mg). This diagnosis is substantiated by the noted elevation in the casual glucose level and A1C. MG was anemic (hemoglobin <11.0 g/dL) and showing early signs of osteodystrophy (secondary hyperparathyroidism). MG was also at considerable cardiovascular risk, not only due to the proteinuria, but also because she presented with classic dyslipidemia and uncontrolled hypertension.

Insulin. As kidney function declines, exogenous insulin acts longer and in an unpredictable manner, characterized by recurrent or severe hypoglycemia in some individuals. The use of multiple daily insulin injections and hypoglycemia awareness training may reduce the frequency and severity of hypoglycemic episodes.

Energy Requirements. Energy requirements should be established between 30 to 35 kcal per kilogram of standard body weight, with 50% to 60% originating from carbohydrates and 20 to 30 g of dietary fiber (Table 23.2).

Hypertension Medications. Systematic reviews of ACEi and ARBs on mortality and outcomes in diabetic kidney disease have indicated that these medications are preferable to other antihypertensives in reducing microalbuminuria and slowing decline.[27,42] The K/DOQI Practice Guidelines for Hypertension provide recommendations as to when to seek further treatment and the best way to manage hypertension in CKD.[27] In persons with advanced stages of CKD, potassium levels should be monitored, as both ACEi and ARBs may cause hyperkalemia. Conversely, if the patient is on a potassium-wasting diuretic, it may have an opposite effect. Sodium intakes should be decreased to less than 2400 mg per day in the presence of hypertension, and fluid restrictions are only necessary in progressive nephropathy (Stage 4 CKD) (Table 23.2).

Dietary Manipulation. A meta-analysis of several small studies demonstrated that a protein-controlled diet may be beneficial in some persons whose nephropathy appears to be progressing.[24,43] With the onset of overt nephropathy, a protein restriction of no more than 0.8 g per kilogram standard body weight (<15% total kcalories) should be implemented (Table 23.2). Further protein restriction (0.6 g per kilogram standard body weight) may be helpful in slowing the decline in individuals who are stable, but they must be monitored for clinical signs of malnutrition. Once the GFR drops below 60 mL/min/1.73 m^2, there is a spontaneous decline in appetite and oral intake.[44] Weight loss is an independent risk factor for mortality on dialysis, so an adequate, palatable, and realistic meal plan during the early stages of CKD is of first and foremost importance. High biologic value (HBV) protein sources, or foods that contain a high proportion of essential amino acids, will be helpful in minimizing the nitrogen load and consequent **azotemia** that may develop once advanced stages of CKD are experienced. Vegetarian meal plans can be used in early as well as later stages of CKD, but the practitioner must assure that the individual is following the principles of a healthy diet (eg, adequacy, balance, moderation, and variety). Plant proteins, such as soy, are excellent alternatives to animal proteins and may have a heart-protective effect of improving serum lipids if consumed with regularity.[24] When soy is used, the practitioner will need to monitor serum phosphorus and potassium levels; soy foods are rich sources of these minerals, and overconsumption may negatively impact homeostasis, especially in CKD Stages 4 and 5. To provide sufficient energy, fats can and should be used in the meal plan, but adjusted according to recommendations from the ATP III Guidelines (Table 23.2).

Other Lifestyle Changes. Dietary manipulation is a major factor in the therapeutic lifestyle changes (TLC) suggested, but other risk factors for CVD also need to be reduced, such as sedentary activity and cigarette smoking or tobacco use.

Pharmacologic Interventions. Pharmacologic agents may be used in CKD and should be tailored to the individual's lipid profile. For example, a person experiencing an elevation in LDL-C may benefit from TLC as well as a statin medication. A multiple of medical approaches may be used depending on laboratory results, and the K/DOQI Practice Guidelines on Dyslipidemias provide excellent examples and insight for the practitioner.[29]

As mentioned, treating the early signs of anemia and osteodystrophy has a significant effect on patient outcomes. Individuals with a low serum hemoglobin may benefit from iron supplementation (200 mg/day) if diagnosed as deficient. If the blood count does not improve, even with supplemental iron, synthetic erythropoietin may be administered. Evidence is strong that the use of calcitriol (activated vitamin D) is beneficial for retarding or preventing metabolic bone disease in early stages of CKD with minimal risk for the individual.[45] The challenge arises in correcting the imbalance of one serum value while not disturbing the balance of another biomarker. For example, suppressing PTH with activated vitamin D may lead to a concomitant rise in serum calcium level, with consequent effects and additional systemic complications. Finding and maintaining the right balance among the serum markers of bone disease (eg, serum calcium, serum phosphorus, and PTH level) is as much of an art form as it is a scientific intervention. The K/DOQI Clinical Practice Guidelines for Bone Metabolism and Disease in CKD strongly encourage the achievement of target values, supported by research evidence and clinical expertise/opinion, for calcium, phosphorus, and PTH levels in the attempt to minimize or reduce renal osteodystrophy complications.[31] Close monitoring of serum markers and responding to abnormalities in a timely fashion are required to achieve such target ranges. If the PTH level is above target, the person should be evaluated for serum levels of vitamin D,

TABLE 23.2 Recommended Dietary Modifications at Stages of Diabetic Nephropathy

Nutrient	*Preclinical Nephropathy Stages 1-3*	*Progressive Nephropathy Stage 4*	*Hemodialysis*	*Peritoneal Dialysis*	*Transplantation*
Energy (kcal/kg/d)	30–35; adequate to achieve and maintain healthy body weight	30–35; adequate to achieve and maintain healthy body weight	30–35; adequate to achieve and maintain healthy body weight	30–35; allows for dialysate kcalories	30–35; adequate to achieve and maintain healthy body weight
Protein	12%–15% of kcalories 0.8–1.0 g/kg/day	10% of kcalories; 50% HBV 0.6–1.0 g/kg/day*	12%–20% of kcalories 50% HBV 1.2 g/kg/day*	12%–20% of kcalories 50% HBV 1.2-1.3 g/kg/day*	1.3–2.0 g/kg after surgery 0.8–1.0 g/kg in stable patients
Carbohydrate	50%-60% of kcalories; ↑fiber to 20–30 g	50%-60% of kcalories; ↑fiber 20–30 g	50%-60% of kcalories; ↑fiber 20–30 g	50%-60% of kcalories (35% oral and 15% dialysate); ↑fiber 20–30 g	50%-60% of kcalories; ↑fiber 20–30 g
Fat	25%-35% kcalories <7% saturated fat Emphasis on MUFA <200 mg cholesterol/day	25%-35% kcalories <7% saturated fat Emphasis on MUFA <200 mg cholesterol/day	25%-35% kcalories <7% saturated fat Emphasis on MUFA <200 mg cholesterol/day	25%-35% kcalories <7% saturated fat Emphasis on MUFA <200 mg cholesterol/day	25%-35% kcalories <7% saturated fat Emphasis on MUFA <200 mg cholesterol/day
Sodium (mg/d)	No HTN: ≤3000 HTN: ≤2400	No HTN: ≤3000 HTN: ≤2400	2000–2400	No HTN: ≤2000-4000 Monitor fluid balance	No HTN: ≤3000 HTN: ≤2400
Potassium (g/d)	No restriction	Monitor labs: 2 if hyperkalemic	2-3; adjust to serum levels	Unrestricted if serum levels are normal	Unrestricted unless hyperkalemic
Phosphorus	Maintain serum value WNL; 800–1000 mg/d; adjust for protein	10-12 mg/g protein or 10 mg/kg/d; 800–1000 mg/d	0-12 mg/g protein or 800–1000 mg/d; adjust for protein	10-12 mg/g protein or 800–1000 mg/d; adjust for protein	DRI; supplement as needed
Calcium (g/d)	Maintain serum value WNL 1.0–1.5	1.0–1.5; daily limit including binder load: <2.0	Daily limit including binder load: <2.0	Daily limit including binder load: < 2.0	0.8–1.5
Fluid	No restriction	Output plus 1000 mL	Output plus 1000 mL	Maintain balance	Unrestricted unless overloaded

*1.2–1.5 g per kilogram per day during catabolic stress

Abbreviations: HBV = high biological value protein; HTN = hypertension; MUFA = monounsaturated fatty acids; DRI = dietary reference intakes; WNL = within normal limits

Source: Reprinted with permission from Pagenkemper JJ. Nutrition management of diabetes in chronic kidney disease. In: A Clinical Guide to Nutrition Care in Kidney Disease. Byham-Gray LD, Wiesen K, eds. Chicago, Ill: American Dietetic Association; 2004.

Case Wrap-Up

Use of a 24-hour food recall and diet history helped reveal that MG was following a high-protein diet 6 months ago and lost 10 lb, but was not able to comply with the low-carbohydrate plan. MG had regained over 15 lb. She generally skipped breakfast, ate salad for lunch at her desk, drank diet sodas throughout the day, and sometimes ordered food in or stopped at a local fast-food restaurant for dinner. MG rarely cooked since her husband died last year from cancer. MG remarked that she often ate a lot at night when she was feeling the most "out of sorts." Treatment goals were this:

- Tight glycemic control
- Regulation of blood pressure
- Lowered protein intake

Medical Nutrition Therapy

- The meal plan was geared toward weight loss (BMI 36), but without a high-protein diet approach, to prevent further damage to the kidneys.
- Meal planning was simplified and incorporated the use of quick meal ideas/recipes and alternatives to the typical fast-food menu options.
- Education was essential on the macronutrient components of the prescribed meal plan.
- The concerns with consuming a high-protein intake and the need for regular rather than erratic eating patterns were emphasized.

Psychosocial Aspects

- MG's feelings about the loss of her husband and the frequency of her night binges needed to be considered to determine if referrals to psychological services might be warranted to enable MG's successful management of her diabetes.
- The educator also helped MG examine familial and friends/peer support and available networking opportunities.
- MG needed to be active in her treatment plan, learn how to complete routine meter testing, and be empowered to take on the responsibility for how to adjust her diet, activity, and/or medications as necessary.

Physical Activity

To further assist with weight loss, the educator discussed the need for MG to be engaged in physical activity. MG was encouraged to use a pedometer as one safe way to monitor her activity level throughout the day, as long as it was medically advisable.

Pharmacologic Therapy

- *Diabetes.* Because of the poor glycemic control over the last several months, options to intensify treatment were reviewed and evaluated. Insulin therapy was discussed.
- *Hypertension.* The educator identified that MG required either an ACEi or ARB to assist with hypertensive control and to reduce proteinuria.
- *Anemia.* Further testing would determine whether she needed supplemental iron and/or erythropoietin administered to reverse the anemia and its effects on fatigue.
- *Bone Health.* Since her PTH was mildly elevated, further assessment of vitamin D status was warranted to determine if calcitriol should be initiated.
- *CVD.* Statin medication would not need to be started immediately. MG indicated she was able to make modifications in diet that would improve the serum lipids.

Follow-Ups and Referrals

Lastly, MG was told about the importance of maintaining regular check-ups with her diabetes team and how referral to a nephrologist was paramount. The nephrologist would seek to further retard disease progression and, if appropriate, prepare MG for further treatment options in kidney failure.

and activated vitamin D provided if suboptimal levels are identified. Serum phosphorus levels may be controlled with a low-phosphorus diet as well as phosphorus binder medications. The K/DOQI Clinical Practice Guidelines for Bone Metabolism have wonderful treatment algorithms concerning PTH, calcium, and phosphorus in the early stages of CKD.[3]

CKD Stage 5

Once kidney failure results (Stage 5 CKD), a number of options are available either as maintenance dialysis (hemodialysis and peritoneal dialysis) and/or transplantation:

- *Hemodialysis:* In center or at home
- *Peritoneal Dialysis:* Either continuous ambulatory, continuous cyclic, or intermittent
- *Transplantation:* Kidney or kidney-pancreas

The person diagnosed with kidney failure and family members need to be involved in treatment decisions. This part of the chapter reviews treatment options in Stage 5 CKD and the effects of such modalities on glycemic control. Since the individual diagnosed with kidney failure will likely be followed closely by a healthcare team (nephrologist, nurse, dietitian, social worker) associated with a dialysis treatment facility, it is important for the patient and family to discuss issues relating to RRT with the nephrology team, as appropriate.

Hemodialysis

Hemodialysis (HD) is a process of cleansing or filtering the blood of nitrogenous wastes. The blood of the person being treated is circulated and cleansed outside of the body.[2] With effective dialysis treatments, uremia can be treated and the person can achieve an improved level of health and well-being. The process is described below, with related factors for consideration noted after the description.

Process. The filter used for hemodialysis is a semi-permeable membrane. The membrane, a thin material with holes, permits passage of small particles, but retains larger particles. During dialysis, the patient's blood passes on one side of the membrane, while dialysate (prepared dialysis solution) passes on the other side of the membrane. The solution removes fluid and particles (waste products) from the blood by diffusive clearance. Blood is withdrawn through a needle inserted in a specially prepared blood vessel, usually a synthetic graft or an arteriovenous fistula (using the patient's own blood vessels) located in the patient's forearm. The needle is attached by plastic tubing to a hemodialysis machine. A pump keeps blood moving through the dialyzer as wastes and fluid are filtered out. The cleansed blood returns to the patient through another needle in the same or an adjacent blood vessel. Hemodialysis can be performed in an ambulatory setting or in the person's home.

Considerations. Treatments are usually 3 to 4 hours long, 3 times per week, on average. Because the blood is not being cleansed 24 hours a day, the person must still follow an individualized meal plan with fluid restriction. The meal plan is designed to minimize azotemia and the buildup of waste products and provide adequate protein, energy, electrolytes, and fluids (Table 23.2).

In comparison with individuals with other types of kidney disease, persons with diabetes, at the initiation of dialysis, generally have more comorbid conditions, have a higher incidence of complications, and are less well-nourished.[24]

Blood Glucose Control. Factors that can alter glucose levels for the person receiving hemodialysis treatment include the glucose concentration in the dialysate bath, appetite alteration on dialysis days and nondialysis days, decreased activity on dialysis days, and emotional stress.[2] Probing the individual about glucose patterns, eating habits, and activity level on dialysis and nondialysis days helps explain fluctuations in blood glucose levels. Because of the lack of glucosuria in diabetic kidney disease, these individuals may experience extreme fluctuations in blood glucose level.[24] Hyperglycemia causes polydipsia, which negatively influences fluid control. Serum potassium levels may also vacillate during hyperglycemic episodes as it creates cellular shifts of potassium.

Peritoneal Dialysis

Peritoneal dialysis (PD) takes place inside the body, employing the body's own capillary and serosal membranes.[2] Blood is filtered through the peritoneal membrane that lines the abdominal cavity. Surgery is required to place a catheter through an opening in the wall of the abdominal cavity. This opening allows the dialysis solution to be instilled into the peritoneal cavity and waste products to pass from the bloodstream into the dialysis solution. The used solution is drained and replaced with a new solution on a regular basis. Currently, 3 types of peritoneal dialysis are being used.

- *Continuous Ambulatory Peritoneal Dialysis (CAPD).* This is a manual method of performing peritoneal dialysis. The patient exchanges new fluid (dialysate) every 4 to 6 hours during a 24-hour period each day. The dialysate passes from a plastic bag through the catheter and stays in the patient's abdomen with the catheter sealed. The dialysate is drained after several hours, then the process begins again with fresh dialysate solution.

- *Continuous Cyclic Peritoneal Dialysis (CCPD).* This is like CAPD except a machine that is connected to the catheter automatically fills and drains the dialysate solution from the patient's abdomen.
- *Intermittent Peritoneal Dialysis (IPD).* This form of dialysis uses the same type of machine as CCPD to fill and drain the dialysate solution from the patient's abdomen. IPD treatments take longer than CCPD, and assistance from a family member, friend, or health professional is required.

Treatment Modality Considerations. PD is often a preferred treatment modality because of its ability to achieve steady state in terms of serum chemistries and fluid balance.[24] Persons receiving this treatment often report greater satisfaction with PD over HD because of the liberalization in diet that occurs. PD allows the removal of uremic toxins on a daily basis, and therefore generally does not require strict potassium or fluid restrictions (Table 23.2). Despite glucose absorption from dialysate, glycemic control can be achieved with intraperitoneal insulin added to the dialysate.[2] Such administration allows for continual delivery of insulin into the portal circulation. There may be some insulin loss due to difficulties with absorption or its adsorption to dialysate bag; hence, supplemental subcutaneous insulin may still be required. Intraperitoneal insulin can also be an additional source of bacterial contamination for the dialysate, resulting in a higher total insulin dose required.

Blood Glucose Control. Factors that can affect blood glucose regulation for persons on PD include the following:

- Concentration of the dialysate solution
- Method(s) of insulin delivery (eg, intraperitoneal, subcutaneous, or both)
- Infection (peritonitis)

To understand variability in blood glucose levels, the practitioner should assess the following:

- Glucose concentration used in the dialysate (eg, 1.5% 2.5%, or 4.25%)
- Type and amount of insulin, as well as the location of insulin injection
- Any clinical signs of infection

Kidney Transplantation

Kidney transplantation can be performed using a kidney from a living related donor, a living unrelated donor, or a suitable cadaveric donor.[2] Once transplantation has occurred, immunosuppressive medications are required throughout the recipient's life to prevent the body from rejecting the transplanted organ. Persons with diabetes must take additional insulin following transplantation because the newly functioning kidney catabolizes insulin once again, because posttransplant steroid therapy has a hyperglycemic effect, and because the person experiences a notable increase in appetite, which can lead to weight gain.

Blood Glucose Control. Following transplantation, blood glucose control may be altered by the following factors:[2]

- Degree of function of the transplanted kidney
- Treatment for transplant rejection
- Changes in steroid dose: Immunosuppressant agents (specifically, corticosteroids, cyclosporine, and tacrolimus) may contribute to posttransplant diabetes
- Patient's increased appetite and ability to consume a more liberal diet with subsequent weight gain
- Diuretic therapy
- Presence of infection: Transplant recipients are more susceptible to infection because of immunosuppression

Simultaneous Transplant: Kidney and Pancreas

Persons with type 1 diabetes may be considered for a simultaneous kidney-pancreas transplantation.[2] A kidney-pancreas transplantation restores both glucose metabolism and kidney function. Criteria for patient selection vary at each transplant center, but typically include the criteria listed in Table 23.3. Contraindications and complications are also summarized in the table.

TABLE 23.3 Kidney-Pancreas Transplantation: Criteria, Complications, and Contraindications

*Criteria (may include the following)**	*Contraindications (may include the following)*	*Complications (may include the following)*
• Diagnosis of type 1 diabetes • Evidence of secondary complications such as renal insufficiency or preproliferative retinopathy • Metabolic instability • Adequate financial resources/ insurance (insurance carriers review eligibility for payment case by case)	• Presence of HIV • Malignancy • Psychosis • Any active infection • Severe neuropathies • Inoperable cardiovascular disease	• Cardiac incompetence • Arterial or venous thrombosis • Anastomotic leaks, bleeding • Side effects of immunosuppression • Pancreatitis • Metabolic acidosis related to exocrine pancreatic function

*Criteria for patient selection vary at each transplant center; the above are typical.

Questions and Controversies

Despite medical advances in diabetic kidney disease, the morbidity and mortality of individuals with diabetes on RRTs are higher than among those who do not have diabetes. Early detection, referral, and treatment are essential to preserve residual kidney function. Although tight glycemic control and hypertensive management focused on minimizing proteinuria seem effective in slowing the disease progression, the evidence is not strong to suggest that severe protein restriction is required, even in the earliest stages of CKD (Stages 1 and 2). Malnutrition and weight loss may result from such restrictive diets and will have a significant impact on survival and treatment outcomes. Adequate energy coupled with a palatable diet, and perhaps the availability of ketoacid analogs, may improve the diets prescribed in CKD. The interrelated nature of diabetes, CVD, and CKD complicate treatment and management. Nonetheless, further research into how best to manage these conditions is warranted. Greater understanding into the role of anemia and secondary hyperparathyroidism on CKD and diabetes should not only elucidate the relationship of CKD to CVD, but also, perhaps, determine the variability in incidence rates of disease progression in type 1 and type 2 diabetes.

Focus on Education: Pearls for Practice

Teaching Strategies

Screening. Reinforce the need to determine kidney function regularly: in type 1, annually after 5 years' onset; in type 2, annually. Screen annually with a 24-hour urine; also for anemia and osteodystrophy. Blood tests are required periodically, as are tests for potassium and cholesterol. Discuss which tests measure what function, define expected and normal lab values, and provide a record-keeping tool to bring to each clinic/ education visit.

Referrals. Nephrology is necessary when loss of function is noted. Referral to a registered dietitian is necessary for a comprehensive nutrition evaluation. Educator is appropriate for assistance with changes and coping with chronic disease. Assist with scheduling these appointments. Include family and significant others for support and reinforcement.

Meals. Prescribe meal plans and diets that are adequate, palatable, and realistic. Protein restriction may be warranted in later stages of CKD to slow disease progression and when RRT is not initiated.

Treatment. Medical management minimizes function loss and complications; this includes control of blood pressure and blood glucose; correction of hypervolemia; and pharmacologic intervention to correct dyslipidemia, hypertension, and elevated glucose. Review the purposes for testing for these, demonstrate tools for home monitoring, and discuss signs for change.

Messages for Patients

Therapeutic lifestyle changes. Begin making lifestyle changes of value in minimizing complications, as tight control makes a difference. Actively participate in home monitoring (of weight, blood pressure, and blood glucose) and record-keeping to determine progress toward goal. Follow medication, activity, and meal plan suggestions; control diet as recommended (sodium or potassium, for example). Follow up with clinic visits and laboratory testing to monitor kidney function.

Care options. Select the best care by learning about the choices, particularly for RRTs. Invite involvement of family and appropriate others for support and clarity.

A Brief Glossary

Acute renal failure (ARF). Usually a sudden and rapid onset of kidney failure that is often reversed once the etiological factors are treated.

Albumin. The major plasma protein. Albumin is generally too large to be filtered out of the blood as it passes through the glomeruli; thus, it is normally found in only minute amounts in the urine. Increased amounts of albumin in the urine indicate glomerular damage.

Albumin excretion rate (AER). The amount of albumin that is excreted in the urine over a given period. AER is commonly expressed in mcg/min or mcg/24 h. An increase in the AER can indicate an abnormality at the glomerular filter that is allowing albumin to enter the filtrate in greater amounts.

Aldosterone. Hormone that causes the kidneys to retain water and sodium.

Anemia. A hemoglobin level less than 12 g/dL in postmenopausal women. Widely prevalent in CKD because of the consequent lack of erythropoietin and red blood cell production.

Angiotensin. A powerful vasoconstrictor that triggers the release of aldosterone.

Antidiuretic hormone. Maintains fluid homeostasis within the body.

Azotemia. An excess of nitrogenous bodies in the blood as a result of declining kidney function.

Bowman capsule. A cuplike structure that surrounds the glomerulus.

Blood urea nitrogen (BUN). The blood level of urea. Urea is the end product of protein metabolism and is formed in the liver. After synthesis, urea travels through the blood and is excreted in the urine. The normal plasma value of urea is 8 to 20 mg/dL (2.9 to 7.1 mmol/L), varying with the quantity and quality of protein intake, state of hydration, and kidney function. The blood level rises as kidney function deteriorates.

Calcitonin. Hormone secreted by the thyroid gland that also regulates calcium levels by increased calcium deposition in the bones.

Creatinine (Cr). A nitrogen compound formed mainly from the metabolism of muscle. An individual's daily production rate of creatinine is relatively constant. The normal plasma value is 0.5 to 1.4 mg/dL (44 to 124 µmol/L), varying with body size and gender; males have higher levels than females. Serum creatinine rises as kidney function deteriorates, but not indefinitely (ie, it will eventually stabilize despite continued deterioration of renal function).

Creatinine clearance (CrCl). CrCl measures the rate at which creatinine is removed from the blood by the kidney and is used as an estimate of the glomerular filtration rate (GFR) and an approximate measure of kidney function. CrCl compares the amount of creatinine in a serum or plasma sample with the amount found in a timed urine specimen, which approximates how much creatinine the kidneys filter out of the blood each minute. Most people clear about 100 to 125 mg/min. A fall in CrCl is a sign of declining renal function. However, as the true GFR decreases in renal disease, the estimation of GFR by CrCl becomes uncertain.

Diabetic kidney disease. A term describing the progressive nature of kidney disease among persons with type 1 or type 2 diabetes.

End-stage renal disease (ESRD). The term used to describe advanced kidney failure. Renal replacement therapy (eg, dialysis or transplantation) must be implemented for life to continue.

Erythropoietin. A hormone manufactured by the kidneys that is largely responsible for stimulating bone marrow to produce red blood cells.

Glomerulonephritis. Inflammation of the glomeruli that often develops after an infection, but may be related to other systemic diseases, such as lupus, Goodpasture syndrome, or diabetes.

Glomerulus. The filtering component of the nephron. It is a tuft of capillaries in which filtration of blood takes place. A kidney biopsy will show structural changes in the glomeruli of a person with diabetic nephropathy.

Glomerular basement membrane. A selectively permeable structure located between the glomerular capillaries and the Bowman capsule that serves as a dialyzing membrane to regulate the passage of water and solutes.

Glomerular filtration. A process that initiates the production of urine with the formation of an ultrafiltrate as blood passes through the glomerular capillaries. Glomerular filtration is governed by a number of factors, including the anatomy of the glomerulus and its Bowman capsule (eg, the size of the pores and the electrical charges within the glomerular filter and the relative diameters of the afferent and efferent arterioles).

Glomerular filtration rate (GFR). The rate at which the kidney produces glomerular filtrate. GFR represents the amount of fluid that passes from the blood into the capsular space over a given period of time. Normal GFR is approximately 100 to 125 mL/min. This rate is determined using a precise technique that measures the renal clearance of a marker substance; GFR values are used primarily in research. GFR decreases with aging, the presence of kidney or vascular diseases, sodium and water depletion, hemorrhage, and vigorous exercise. The rate increases with dietary protein intake, hyperglycemia, and pregnancy. Repeated measurements of GFR over time provide more useful information than a single value.

Mesangium. The central core tissue in the glomerulus, bounded by the capillary endothelium and the glomerular basement membrane. The mesangium may play a role in regulating glomerular blood flow.

Microalbuminuria. An increase in the urinary AER above normal but below the level of overt proteinuria. More specifically, microalbuminuria is defined as an AER >20 mcg/min but <200 mcg/min (which is approximated by 30 to 300 mg/24 h).[12] There is a large intra-individual day-to-day variation in AER in individuals with diabetes.[13-17] Therefore, the absence or presence of microalbuminuria should be determined based on more than a single urine collection.

Nephrons. The functional units of the kidneys that serve to clear the blood of waste materials and form urine. Each kidney contains about 1 million nephrons. Each nephron consists of a glomerulus that leads to a long tubule in which the filtrate is concentrated and modified before it is eliminated as urine.

Nephrotic syndrome. A state characterized by urinary protein excretion >3.5 g/24 h (which roughly corresponds to an AER >2400 mcg/min). Typically, the rate of protein excretion can increase from 4 to 30 g/24 h, resulting in low blood protein levels and massive fluid retention. Hypertension, weight gain, peripheral edema, hyperlipidemia, hyperfibrinogenemia, hypercoagulability, increased blood viscosity, congestive heart failure, and pulmonary edema are common clinical manifestations of the nephrotic syndrome. Although many people with diabetes manifest nephrotic-range proteinuria, true nephrotic syndrome occurs in only 10% to 20% of patients.

Parathyroid hormone. Regulates calcium and phosphorus levels by causing more to be excreted through the kidneys during periods of excess and retention at times of suboptimal intakes.

Proteinuria. The presence of protein in the urine. While the degree of proteinuria is often assessed by concentration, it is more precisely measured when quantified as the amount of protein excreted over a given period of time. The normal amount of protein excreted is approximately 0.1 g/24 h. Excess amounts of protein are pathologic, indicating either systemic disease or kidney disease. Overt proteinuria is indicated by the excretion of albumin at a rate >200 mcg/min (300 mg/24 h) or by the excretion of >0.5 g of total protein in 24 h.

Renin. A hormone vital in regulating blood pressure.

Uremia. A syndrome characteristic of ESRD that develops as renal function declines, causing an accumulation of urea, creatinine, and other metabolic waste products in the blood. This extra amount of urea results in anemia, osteodystrophy, neuropathy, and acidosis. Nausea, hypertension, susceptibility to infection, and generalized organ dysfunction frequently accompany this syndrome.

Urinary albumin/creatinine ratio (A/C ratio). The ratio of the urinary albumin concentration to the urinary creatinine concentration. Use of the A/C ratio can help reduce inaccuracies that can occur in assessing albumin excretion based on concentration alone—inaccuracies (particularly false negative results) that especially can occur in individuals with diabetes whose urinary volume, and possibly concentration, can vary depending on the degree of glucosuria and polyuria. A/C ratios, however, have been shown to have little or no less intraindividual day-to-day variation than AERs. The A/C ratio of a midmorning single-void urine sample collected after initial morning voiding has been shown to be both highly correlated with and highly predictive of an individual's AER measured from a 24-h urine collection. This test is often found to be the easiest to carry out in an office setting.

References

1. National Kidney Foundation. Clinical Practice Guidelines. On the Internet: www.kidney.org. Accessed 1 Dec 2005.
2. Coonrod B, Ernst KL. Nephropathy. A Core Curriculum for Diabetes Education: Diabetes and Complications, 5th ed. Chicago, Ill: American Association of Diabetes Educators; 2003.
3. National Kidney Foundation. Clinical practice guidelines for chronic kidney disease: evaluation, classification, and stratification. Amer J Kidney Dis. 2002;392 suppl 1:S1-266.
4. National Institutes of Health. US Renal Data System, USRDS 2005 Annual Data Report: Atlas of End-Stage Renal Disease in the United States. Bethesda, Md: National Institutes of Health, National Institute of Diabetes and Digestive and Kidney Diseases; 2005.
5. Goeddeke-Merickel C. The goals of comprehensive and integrated disease state management for diabetic kidney-disease patients. Adv Chronic Kidney Dis. 2005;12(2):236-42.
6. National Institutes of Health. USRDS 2004 Annual Report. Bethesda, Md: National Institutes of Health, National Institute of Digestive, Diabetes and Kidney Diseases; 2004.
7. Levey A, Beto JA, Coronado BE, et al. Controlling the epidemic of cardiovascular disease in chronic renal disease: what do we know? what do we learn? where do we go from here? National Kidney Foundation Task Force on Cardiovascular Disease. Am J Kidney Dis. 1998;32:853-906.
8. Diabetes Control and Complications Trial Group. The effect of intensive treatment of diabetes on the development and progression of long-term complications in insulin-dependent diabetes mellitus. N Engl J Med. 1993;329:977-86.
9. UK Prospective Diabetes Study Group. Intensive blood glucose control with sulphonylureas or insulin compared with conventional treatment and risk of complications in patients with type 2 diabetes (UKPDS 33). Lancet. 1998;352:837-53.
10. UK Prospective Diabetes Study Group. Effect of intensive blood glucose control with metformin on complications in overweight patients with type 2 diabetes (UKPDS 34). Lancet. 1998;352:854-62.
11. Gross J, DeAzevedo, MR, Silveiro, SP, et al. Diabetic nephropathy: diagnosis, prevention, and treatment. Diabetes Care. 2005;28:176-88.
12. Waugh N, Robertson AM. Protein restriction for diabetic renal disease. The Cochrane Library. 2005:4.
13. Seaquist E, Goetz FC, Rich S, Barbosa, J. Familial clustering of diabetic kidney disease: evidence for genetic susceptibility to diabetic nephropathy. N Engl J Med. 1989;320:1161-5.
14. Sedor J. Frontiers in diabetic nephropathy: can we predict who will get sick? J Am Soc Nephrol. 2006;17:336-8.
15. Rich S. Genetics of diabetes and its complications. J Am Soc Nephrol. 2006;17:353-60.
16. Byham-Gray L. Medical Nutrition Therapy for Renal Disease: Understanding the Implications, 2nd ed. Clarksville, Md: Wolf Rinke Associates, Inc; 2004.
17. Gonyea J, McCarthy M. Overview: pathophysiology of the kidney. In: A Clinical Guide to Nutrition Care in Kidney Disease. Byham-Gray LD, Wiesen K, eds. Chicago, Ill: American Dietetic Association; 2004.
18. Knapp S, Liftman, C. Renal osteodystrophy. In: A Clinical Guide to Nutrition Care in Kidney Disease. Byham-Gray LD, Wiesen K, eds. Chicago, Ill: The American Dietetic Association; 2004.
19. National Kidney Foundation. Clinical Practice Guidelines. Available at: www.kidney.org/professionals/KDOQI/. Accessed 1 Dec 2005.
20. National Institutes of Health, National Institute of Digestive, Diabetes and Kidney Diseases. USRDS 1997 Annual Data Report. On the Internet: www.usrds.org/adr_1997.htm. Accessed 29 Nov 2005.
21. Moore H, Reams SM, Wiesen K, Nolph KD, Khanna R, Laothong C. National Kidney Foundation Council on Renal Nutrition Survey: past-present clinical practices and future strategic planning. J Renal Nutr. 2003;13:233-40.

22. American Diabetes Association. Clinical practice recommendations. Diabetes Care. 2006;29 Suppl 1: S4-32.

23. Levey AS, Coresh J, Balk E, et al. National Kidney Foundation practice guidelines for chronic kidney disease: evaluation, classification, and stratification. Ann Intern Med. 2003;139(2):137-47.

24. Pagenkemper JJ. Nutrition management of diabetes in chronic kidney disease. In A Clinical Guide to Nutrition Care in Kidney Disease. Byham-Gray LD, Wiesen K, eds. Chicago, Ill: American Dietetic Association; 2004.

25. Finne P, Reunanen A, Stenman S, Groop PH, Gronhagen-Riska C. Incidence of end-stage renal disease in patients with type 1 diabetes. JAMA. 2005;294(14):1782-7.

26. DeFronzo R. Diabetic nephropathy. In: Therapy for Diabetes Mellitus and Related Disorders. Lebovitz H, ed. Alexandria, Va: The American Diabetes Association; 2004.

27. National Kidney Foundation. K/DOQI clinical practice guidelines on hypertension and antihypertensive agents in chronic kidney disease. Am J Kidney Dis. 2004;43:1-290.

28. American Diabetes Association. Standards of medical care in diabetes. Diabetes Care. 2005;28Suppl 1: S4-36.

29. National Kidney Foundation. K/DOQI Clinical practice guidelines for managing dyslipidemias in chronic kidney disease. Am J Kidney Dis. 2003;41suppl 3: S1-152.

30. Mohanram A, Zhang Z, Shahinfar S, Keane WF, Brenner BM, Toto RD. Anemia and end-stage renal disease in patients with type 2 diabetes and nephropathy. Kidney Int. 2004;66(3):1131-8.

31. NKF-KDOQI. K/DOQI clinical practice guidelines for bone metabolism and disease in chronic kidney disease. Am J Kidney Dis. 2003;42 suppl 3:S1-202.

32. Malluche H, Faugere MC. Effects of 1,25(OH)2D3 administration on bone in patients with renal failure. Kidney International. 1990;29suppl:S48-53.

33. de Francisco A. Secondary hyperparathyroidism: review of the disease and its treatment. Clin Ther. 2004;26:1976-93.

34. Goodman W. The consequences of uncontrolled secondary hyperparathyroidism and its treatment in chronic kidney disease. Sem in Dial. 2004;17:209-16.

35. Block G. Prevalence and clinical consequences of elevated Ca x P product in hemodialysis patients. Clin Nephrol. 2000;54:318-24.

36. Pisoni R, Greenwood RN. Selected lessons learned from the Dialysis Outcomes and Practice Patterns Study (DOPPS). Contrib Nephrol. 2005;149:58-68.

37. Young E, Akiba T, Albert JM, McCarthy JT, Kerr PG, Mendelssohn DC, Jadoul M. Magnitude and impact of abnormal mineral metabolism in hemodialysis patients in the Dialysis Outcomes and Practice Patterns Study (DOPPS). Am J Kidney Dis. 2004;44:34-8.

38. Young E, Albert JM, Satayathum S, et al. Predictors and consequences of altered mineral metabolism: the Dialysis Outcomes and Practice Patterns Study (DOPPS). Kidney Int. 2005;67:1179-87.

39. American Diabetes Association. Clinical practice recommendations. Diabetes Care. 2006;29suppl 1: S4-32.

40. McCann L. Pocket Guide to the Nutrition Assessment of the Patient with Chronic Kidney Disease, 3rd ed. New York: National Kidney Foundation; 2002.

41. Chobanian AV, Bakris GL, Black HR, et al. Seventh report of the Joint National Committee on Prevention, Detection, Evaluation, and Treatment of High Blood Pressure. Hypertension. 2003;42(6):1206-52

42. Strippoli G, Craig M, Deeks JJ, et al. Effects of angiotensin converting enzyme inhibitors and angiotensin II receptor antagonists on mortality and renal outcomes in diabetic nephropathy: systematic review. BMJ. 2004;329:828-939.

43. Yu H, Pedrini MT, Levey AS, et al. Progression of chronic renal failure. Arch Intern Med. 2003;163:1417-29.

44. National Kidney Foundation. Kidney Disease Dialysis Outcome Quality Initiative (K/DOQI) clinical practice guidelines for nutrition in chronic renal failure. Am J Kidney Dis. 2000;35suppl 2:S1-140.

45. McCann L. K/DOQI practice guidelines for bone metabolism and disease in CKD: another opportunity for renal dietitians to take a leadership role in improving outcomes for patients with CKD. J Renal Nutr. 2005;15:265-274.

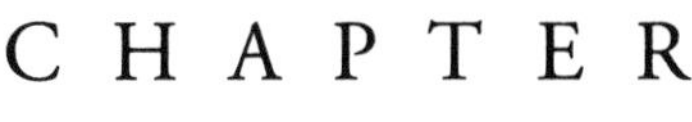

CHAPTER

24

Diabetic Neuropathies

Authors

Aaron I. Vinik, MD, PhD, FCP, MACP
Etta J. Vinik, MA (Ed)

Key Concepts

- The specific syndrome guides the treatment. Management of this multifaceted disease is complex, and the key to success depends on separating out the underlying pathological processes in each particular clinical presentation.
- A careful history and detailed physical examination are essential for the diagnosis, together with objective testing.
- Preventive strategies and patient education are key in reducing complication rates and mortality.
- Somatic and autonomic neuropathies are among the most common long-term complications of diabetes as well as its precursors—impaired glucose tolerance and the metabolic syndrome.
- Diabetic neuropathy, which includes somatic and autonomic neuropathies, is associated with considerable morbidity and mortality and significant impact on quality of life.
- Entrapments occur in one-third of patients and can be treated medically or surgically.
- Proximal neuropathy is an inflammatory condition that coexists with diabetic neuropathy and is amenable to anti-inflammatory therapy.
- Focal mononeuropathies occur involving single nerves and for the most part resolve spontaneously.
- Diabetic neuropathy is highly prevalent in diabetic populations, but often not recognized by physicians.
- Small-fiber neuropathy may lead to foot ulceration and subsequent gangrene and amputation.
- Large-fiber neuropathy produces numbness, ataxia, and impairment of quality of life and may lead to falls and fractures.
- A number of simple tests that can be done in the clinic are useful for detecting diabetic neuropathy and predicting complications, such as foot ulcers and gangrene.
- Standard and validated quantitative measures of disease progression are now available and allow better interpretation of responses to different treatments and study results.
- The pathogenesis of neuropathy is still poorly understood. Recent studies on new agents that target the pathophysiological mechanisms have led to a better understanding of the pathogenesis of diabetic neuropathy as well as the pain mechanisms for the different types of pain syndromes.
- These newer symptomatic treatment modalities, based on etiologic factors, have potential for significant impact on morbidity and mortality.

Introduction

Translation of the science of neuropathy into clinical care is a major challenge for diabetes care providers. It requires knowledge on the one hand and careful attention to patient histories, symptoms, and signs on the other. The emergence of the study of neuropathy as a science in its own right, enhanced by technological and biological advances, has resulted in more knowledge about neuropathy. However, we still await major research breakthroughs in understanding its pathophysiology and etiology.

Diabetic neuropathy (DN) is not a single entity, but rather a number of different syndromes, each with a range of clinical and subclinical manifestations. Effective management is based on recognizing the particular manifestation and underlying pathogenesis of the particular form of DN in each patient, and using this information to initiate therapy at a level that avoids undesirable side effects. Since different syndromes can now be distinguished by different affected nerve fibers, the artful physician, by mindful interaction with the patients and a carefully honed skill set, is able to separate out the different and often intertwined neuropathic entities and administer individualized treatment.

State of the Disease

Diabetic neuropathy is the most common form of neuropathy in developed countries and is responsible for 50% to 75% of nontraumatic amputations.[1] These disorders are among the most frequent complications of diabetes mellitus and a significant cause of morbidity and mortality. The major morbidity is foot ulceration, which can lead to gangrene and ultimately to limb loss. The true prevalence is not known and reports vary from 10% to 90%, depending on the criteria and methods used to define neuropathy.[1-5] Each year 86,000 amputations are performed on diabetic patients in the United States, yet up to 75% of them are preventable.[4] The national annual direct cost of foot ulcers in the United States has been estimated as approximately $5 billion.[6] DN is clearly a huge global economic burden; on an individual level, it also has a tremendous impact on a patient's quality of life.[7,8]

A Problem Diabetes Education Can Address

Educators have a large opportunity to assist in preventing the painful, devastating, and costly complications of DN.

- Although DN is highly prevalent in the diabetic population, physicians often do not recognize it.
- When DN is recognized, most physicians regard it as a single disease (rather than a heterogeneous group of disorders) and dismiss it with, "Nothing can be done; learn to live with it." At most, physicians will prescribe a palliative for pain or other symptoms.

This chapter suggests opportunities for dealing with these problems. Educators have the following opportunities to assist patients affected by these common, painful, and potentially devastating diabetic complications:

- Acquire more information about neuropathy
- Recognize the different components of the disease
- Elicit useful information from patients by asking the right questions
- Use the information to guide interventions
- Explain importance of controlled blood sugar in preventing and reversing certain neuropathies
- Emphasize meticulous foot care to prevent and reverse certain neuropathies

The diabetes educator can play a significant role in helping to prevent and reverse neuropathy (in some instances) by explaining the importance of controlled blood sugar and meticulous foot care. Blood glucose, blood pressure, lipids, and lifestyle modifications remain as essential measures to reduce the risk of macrovascular disease.

This chapter also provides information about new research on different treatment modalities that not only relieve symptoms, but also provide hope for actually changing the course of the disease.

Definition

A detailed definition of neuropathy was agreed upon at the San Antonio Consensus Conference in 1998:[10] "diabetic neuropathy is a descriptive term meaning a demonstrable disorder, either *clinically* evident or *subclinical*, that occurs in the setting of diabetes mellitus *without other causes* for peripheral neuropathy. The neuropathic disorder includes manifestations in the somatic (voluntary) and/or autonomic (involuntary) parts of the peripheral nervous system." A minimum of 2 abnormalities (symptoms, signs, nerve conduction abnormalities, quantitative sensory tests or quantitative autonomic tests) are required for diagnosis and for clinical studies, one of these 2 abnormalities should include quantitative tests or electrophysiology.[11-13]

Since asymptomatic (subclinical) neuropathy is common, a careful clinical examination is needed for the diagnosis.[11] In fact, absence of symptoms cannot be equated with absence of neuropathy. The importance of excluding nondiabetic causes was emphasized in the Rochester Diabetic Neuropathy Study, in which up to 10% of peripheral neuropathy in diabetic patients was found to be due to nondiabetic causes.[13]

Thus, the general consensus is that DN should not be diagnosed based on a single symptom, sign, or test: a minimum of 2 abnormalities (from symptoms, signs, nerve conduction abnormalities, quantitative autonomic tests) is recommended by Dyck.[13] However, neuropathy remains underdiagnosed by endocrinologists as well as non-endocrinologists, as shown in the Glycemic Optimization with Algorithms and Labs At Po1nt of Care (GOAL A1C) study.[14] Identification of neuropathy in 7000 patients in the presence of mild neuropathy was only accurate one-third of the time and reached 75% *only* if neuropathy was severe. Clearly, physician education is needed on criteria for neuropathy diagnosis.

Case in Point: Neuropathic Pain

A 48-year-old woman, CM, with an 18-year history of type 2 diabetes returned to see her primary care provider after a 2-year absence. Her complaint was numbness and pain in both feet. She had a past medical history of obesity, hypertension, hypertriglyceridemia, and background retinopathy.

Physical Signs

- BP 152/88 mm Hg; HR 80 beats/min; BMI 38.9
- Microaneurysms
- 2/6 Systolic ejection murmur
- Normal thyroid, carotids, heart, abdomen
- Dorsalis pedis pulses 2+ symmetrically
- *Calluses* over 5th metatarsal heads and lateral edge of great toes, bilaterally
- *Ankle jerks* absent
- *Vibratory sense* absent
- *Touch pressure* absent (5.07 Semmes-Weinstein monofilament)

Medications

- Metformin (Glucophage) 1 g bid
- Glipizide GITS (Glucotrol XL) 10 mg/d
- Trandolapril (Mavik) 4 mg/d
- Aspirin 81 mg/d, MVI

Questions to Consider

What is the significance of these physical findings (especially italicized ones)?

How common is this problem?

Is this a typical presentation?

What investigations should be conducted?

Diagnosis

Scoring Systems

Symptoms of neuropathy can vary markedly from one patient to another, making the correct assessment of these disorders difficult at times. For this reason, symptom questionnaires with similar scoring systems have been developed. These are useful to assess responses to treatment. The neurologic symptom score[15, 12]; has 38 items that capture symptoms of muscle weakness, sensory disturbances, and autonomic dysfunction.

Screening Recommendations

Table 24.1 contains DN screening recommendations from the American Diabetes Association (ADA).

Combinations of more than 1 test have more than 87% sensitivity in detecting chronic sensorimotor neuropathy.[16,17] Longitudinal studies have shown that these simple tests are good predictors of foot-ulcer risk.[18] Numerous composite scores to evaluate clinical signs of DN, such as the nerve impairment score (NIS), are useful in documenting and monitoring neuropathic deficits.[19]

Diagnostic Testing

Quantitative Sensory Testing. Quantitative sensory testing is of value in detecting subclinical neuropathy, assessing progression, and predicting risk for foot ulceration.[19,20] These standardized measures of vibration and thermal thresholds also play an important role in multicenter clinical trials as primary efficacy end-points, as do quality of life measures.[7]

TABLE 24.1 Diabetic Neuropathy: Screening Recommendations

Frequency

- All persons with type 2 diabetes be screened for DN at diagnosis and annually thereafter
- All persons with type 1 diabetes should be screened 5 years after diagnosis and annually thereafter

Method

Screening must include sensory examination of the feet and ankle reflexes.* One or more of the following can be used to assess sensory function:

- Pinprick
- Temperature
- Vibration perception (using 128-Hz tuning fork)
- 10-g monofilament pressure perception at the distal halluces

*Boulton AJ, Vinik AI, Arezzo JC, Bril V, Feldman EL, Freeman R et al. Diabetic neuropathies: a statement by the American Diabetes Association. Diabetes Care 2005; 28(4):956-962.

Case—Part 2: Neuropathic Discomfort

Diagnosis and Initial Treatment

CM's physician ordered the following investigations and obtained the results noted:

- Electrolytes: normal
- Thyroid function tests, $B_{12:}$ normal
- A1C: 9.5% (4.1-6.5%)
- Albumin/creatinine ratio: 98 (g/mg (>30)
- Triglycerides: 298 mg/dL
- Cholesterol: 187 mg/dL

CM had previously mentioned numbness and pain. What other questions were appropriate to ask about the discomfort in her feet?

When CM described her pain, she mentioned 3 kinds of pain:

- Constant diffuse, sharp burning
- Knife-life lightning episodes that occur episodically at night
- Dull, gnawing "bone" pain, similar to a toothache

Is there any significance to these descriptions? What do they reveal? Into which of the following categories does her pain fit: distal symmetric polyneuropathy? Acute or chronic (greater or less than 6 months?)? Small- or large-fiber? What initial approach to the management of her neuropathic discomfort would you have recommended?

- In an attempt to improve her glycemic control, NPH insulin at bedtime was added to her medications
- Topical capsaicin 0.025% (Zostrix) was suggested 4 times per day

Finding Acceptable Pain Relief

One Month Later

CM returned for follow-up. Her NPH insulin was then titrated upwards, and her overall glycemic control appeared improved. She demanded further pharmacologic help. In addition to improved glycemic control, what agents would you have suggested?

- Her trandolapril (Mavik) was doubled to 8 mg per day
- Amitriptyline (Elavil), 10 mg nightly, was added, with instructions to increase by 10 mg per week until side effects or relief was achieved

Three Months Later

CM returned for continued follow-up. Her A1C had declined to 7.4% (4.1-6.5%) with the addition of 70 units of NPH insulin nightly. With 80 mg per day of amitryptyline, she had acceptable relief from the superficial burning symptoms, but not the deep-seated gnawing symptoms. What recommendations would you have made?

- Clonidine (Catapres) 0.1 mg at bedtime was added

Subsequent Follow-Up

CM had acceptable relief from all of her symptoms. But 1 year later, she again complained of burning, superficial (just below the skin) discomfort. She could not tolerate more than 100 mg per day of amitryptyline (Elavil). What would you have suggested? Was what the physician suggested likely to be effective?

- Gabapentin (Neurontin) was added, titrated to 3200 mg per day, with cessation of amitryptyline (Elavil)
- Clonidine (Catapres) was continued.
- Evening primrose oil was added

Acceptable pain relief was achieved with a combination of Clonidine and tramadol (Ultram) as needed and daily morphine sulfate sustained release (MS Contin). Evening primrose oil did not help.

This chapter's section "treatment of diabetic neuropathy based on pathogenetic mechanisms" helps readers consider whether the therapies chosen were appropriate and if there were alternatives.

Nerve Conduction Velocity. The use of electrophysiologic measures (measures of nerve conduction velocity, or NCV) in both clinical practice and multicenter clinical trials is recommended.[10] In type 2 diabetes patients,[21] NCV abnormalities in the lower limbs increased from 8% at baseline to 42% after 10 years of disease. A slow progression of NCV abnormalities in type 1 diabetes was observed in the Diabetes Control and Complications Trial (DCCT).[22] NCV, nevertheless, plays a key role in ruling out other causes of neuropathy and is essential for the identification of focal and multifocal neuropathies.[11,23]

Skin Biopsy. The importance of the skin biopsy as a diagnostic tool for chronic sensorimotor neuropathy is increasingly being recognized.[24-26] This technique quantitates small epidermal nerve fibers through antibody staining of the pan-axonal marker protein gene product 9.5 (PGP 9.5). (An axon is the central core of nerve fiber.) Though minimally invasive (3-mm diameter punch biopsies), this technique enables a direct study of small fibers, which cannot be evaluated by NCV studies.

Quality of Life. The effect of neuropathy per se on the quality of life (QOL) of the person with diabetes is widely recognized. The Norfolk QOL questionnaire for DN is a validated tool addressing specific symptoms and impact of large, small, and autonomic nerve-fiber functions; the tool has been used in clinical trials and is available in several validated language versions.[7] The NeuroQol[8] measures patients' perceptions of the impact of neuropathy and foot ulcers.

The diagnosis of distal polyneuropathy is mainly clinical, aided by specific diagnostic tests according to the type and severity of the neuropathy; however, nondiabetic causes of neuropathy must always be excluded, depending on the clinical findings.

The spectrum of clinical neuropathic syndromes described in persons with diabetes includes dysfunction of almost every segment of the somatic peripheral and autonomic nervous system[27]—thus, the adage, "knowing neuropathy means to know the whole of medicine." Distinguishing each syndrome by its pathophysiologic, therapeutic, and prognostic features is feasible. This theme will be reiterated throughout the chapter.

Overview of Diabetic Neuropathies

This chapter describes different aspects of DN; explains the various nomenclatures; presents a clear, comprehensible classification of this complex disease state; and describes treatment options for specific neuropathic disorders.

As mentioned, DNs are a heterogeneous group of disorders that include a wide range of abnormalities, ranging from subclinical to clinical manifestations. Diabetes-related neuropathies have been classified based on their clinical manifestations as well as anatomical findings[28] (see Table 24.2). Most of the pathology of DN occurs in the peripheral (surrounding) nervous system, although there may be some central nerve involvement. The peripheral nerve system is comprised of the autonomic nervous system (ANS) (sympathetic and parasympathetic) and the sensorimotor nervous system. Autonomic nerves control *involuntary* functions (eg, breathing, heart beat), while sensory nerves send information from the skin and internal organs about sensory perception (eg, hot and cold sensation), and motor nerves send commands from the brain to the body (eg, remove your hand from the hot stove), thus controlling voluntary functions.[6]

TABLE 24.2 Clinical Diabetic Neuropathies: Classification

Rapidly Reversible Neuropathy
Hyperglycemic neuropathy

Generalized Symmetrical Polyneuropathy
Acute sensory neuropathy
Chronic sensorimotor neuropathy (distal diabetic polyneuropathy)

- Small-fiber neuropathy
- Large-fiber neuropathy

Autonomic Neuropathy
Cardiac Autonomic Neuropathy
GI Disorders Related to Autonomic Neuropathy
Sexual Dysfunction Related to Autonomic Neuropathy
Bladder Dysfunction Related to Autonomic Neuropathy
Sudomotor Dysfunction Related to Autonomic Neuropathy
Pupillomotor and Visceral (Metabolic) Response Related to Autonomic Neuropathy

Focal and Multifocal Neuropathies
Focal-limb
Cranial neuropathy
Proximal-motor neuropathy (amyotrophy)
Truncal radiculoneuropathy
Coexisting chronic inflammatory demyelinating neuropathy

Sources: Adapted from the following.

1. Boulton AJ, Vinik AI, Arezzo JC, et al. Diabetic neuropathies: a statement by the American Diabetes Association. Diabetes Care. 2005;28(4):956-62.
2. Thomas PK, Ward JD, Watkins PJ. Diabetic neuropathy. In: Complications of Diabetes. Keen H, Jarrett J, eds. London, UK: Edward Arnold Publishing Company; 1982: 109-36.

Subclinical Neuropathies

According to the San Antonio Convention,[10] the main neurological disturbances in diabetes include the following:

- Subclinical neuropathy
- Diffuse clinical neuropathy
- Focal syndromes

Since no obvious symptoms are present, characteristics of subclinical sensory neuropathy, small-fiber neuropathy, and autonomic neuropathy should be determined by abnormal results in the following tests:

- Electrodiagnostics (nerve conduction velocity and amplitudes)
- Quantitative sensory testing
- Abnormal quantitative autonomic function tests

Characteristics of Subclinical Neuropathy

- Early stages of sensory neuropathy may manifest as deterioration of nerve function and development of subtle sensory-motor deficits. At this stage, symptoms are minimal and barely clinically detectable.
- Neurological deficits may be found during a physical examination, such as injury to a foot with unrecognized loss of sensation.[29]
- Very mild neuropathy may not be detectable even by careful physical examination, but may become apparent with nerve physiology, sensory or autonomic testing, or skin or nerve biopsy.

Implications for Diabetes Education and Care Because of the prevalence of neuropathy stated above, and because it is an insidious and often silent disease, educators are advised to bring even the slightest suspicion of sensory and autonomic neuropathy to the physician's attention for nerve function testing.

Clinical Neuropathies

The natural history of clinical neuropathies separates them into 2 distinct entities:

- *Diffuse:* Those that progress gradually with increasing duration of diabetes
- *Focal:* Those that usually remit completely

Sensory and autonomic neuropathies generally progress gradually, while the focal mononeuropathies, and acute painful neuropathies, although symptoms are severe, are short-lived and tend to recover. Thus, each syndrome is characterized by either *diffuse* or *focal* damage to the peripheral somatic (voluntary) or autonomic (involuntary) nerve fibers.

Rapidly Reversible Hyperglycemic Neuropathy

Reversible abnormalities of nerve function with distal sensory symptoms may occur in patients with recently diagnosed or poorly controlled diabetes. Recovery soon follows restoration of euglycemia.[11]

Implications for Diabetes Education and Care. In patients recently diagnosed with diabetes or those with poorly controlled diabetes, the opportunity exists to reverse neuropathy. A concerted effort to encourage the patient to achieve this goal by tight blood sugar control is essential. The patient must be advised and understand that the pain may get worse with initiation of glycemic control before it gets better.

Generalized Symmetrical Polyneuropathy

Acute Sensory Neuropathy

Acute painful sensory neuropathy (ASN) is a variant of chronic sensorimotor neuropathy that is characterized by severe pain, wasting, weight loss, depression, and, in males, erectile dysfunction.[30] Patients report, especially in the feet, unremitting burning, deep pain, and hyperesthesia. Other symptoms include sharp stabbing or "electric shock-like" sensations in the lower limbs that appear more frequently during the night. Signs are usually absent with a relatively normal clinical examination, except for allodynia (interpretation of all stimuli as painful, even light touch). Occasionally, ankle reflexes are absent or reduced.[31] ASN is usually associated with poor glycemic control, but may also appear after rapid improvement of glycemia. It has been hypothesized that changes in blood glucose flux produce alterations in epineurial blood flow, leading to ischemia.[32] Other authors propose an immune-mediated mechanism.[33]

Implications for Diabetes Education and Care. The key to management of this syndrome is achieving blood glucose stability. Most patients also require medication for neuropathic pain. The natural history of this disease is resolution of symptoms within 1 year.[31]

Chronic Sensorimotor Neuropathy

Chronic sensorimotor neuropathy (also referred to as distal diabetic polyneuropathy or distal symmetric polyneuropathy) is the most common form of *diffuse* neuropathy in diabetes. Chronic sensorimotor neuropathy primarily involves the sensory nerves. Sensory deficits occur in the distal portions of the limbs, spreading over time from the toes to the legs and then from the fingers up the arms in a "stocking-glove" pattern, involving small nerve fibers, large nerve fibers, or both.

Small-Nerve-Fiber Neuropathy

Small-nerve-fiber neuropathy often presents with pain, but without objective signs or electrophysiologic evidence of nerve damage. Table 24.3 lists clinical manifestations of small-fiber neuropathies.

Ulceration, gangrene, and amputation are risks with small-fiber neuropathy:

With small-fiber neuropathy, the greatest risk is for foot ulceration and subsequent gangrene and amputation.

Diagnostic Testing. Small, unmyelinated nerve fibers are affected early in diabetes and are not reflected in NCV studies. Other methods that do not depend on conduction, such as quantitative sensory testing or skin biopsy with quantification of intraepidermal nerve fibers (IENF), are necessary to identify these cases.[33] However, NCV plays a key role in ruling out other causes of neuropathy and is essential for the identification of focal neuropathies and entrapments as well as multifocal neuropathies.[11, 23] Also, the importance of the skin biopsy as a diagnostic tool for chronic sensorimotor neuropathy is increasingly being recognized.[24-26] This technique quantitates small epidermal nerve fibers through antibody staining of the pan-axonal marker protein gene product 9.5 (PGP 9.5).

TABLE 24.3 Small-Fiber Neuropathies: Clinical Manifestations

- Symptoms are prominent. Pain is the C-fiber type, which is burning and superficial and associated with allodynia (interpretation of all stimuli—ie, touch—as painful)
- Late in the condition, there is hypoalgesia (lack of sensation)
- Defective warm thermal sensation
- Defective autonomic function with decreased sweating, dry skin, impaired vasomotion and blood flow, and a cold foot
- Reflexes and motor strength are remarkably intact
- NCV studies show no deficit
- Loss of cutaneous nerve fibers is shown using PGP 9.5 staining
- Diagnosed clinically by reduced sensitivity to 1.0 g Semmes Weinstein monofilament and pricking sensation using the Waardenberg wheel or similar instrument*
- Abnormalities in thresholds for warm thermal perception, neurovascular function, pain, quantitative sudorimetry and quantitative autonomic function tests
- Risk is foot ulceration and subsequent **gangrene**

*Vinik AI, Suwanwalaikorn S, Stansberry KB, Holland MT, McNitt PM, Colen LE. Quantitative measurement of cutaneous perception in diabetic neuropathy. Muscle Nerve. 1995; 18:574-584.

Pain Mechanism. The mechanism for pain in small-fiber neuropathy is not well understood.[34] Hyperglycemia may be a factor in lowering the pain threshold. A striking amelioration of symptoms with the intravenous administration of insulin can be achieved.[9] Disappearance of pain may not necessarily reflect nerve recovery but rather nerve death. When patients volunteer the loss of pain, progression of the neuropathy must be excluded by careful examination.

Implications for Diabetes Education and Care. A comprehensive clinical examination is key to the diagnosis of chronic sensorimotor neuropathy. Feet must be examined in detail to detect ulcers, calluses, and deformities, and footwear inspected at every visit. All persons with chronic sensorimotor neuropathy are at increased risk of foot ulceration and Charcot neuroarthropathy.

Large-Nerve-Fiber Neuropathies

Large-nerve-fiber neuropathies may involve sensory and/or motor nerves. These tend to be the neuropathies of *signs*, with a lesser degree of *symptoms*. Large fibers mediate motor function, vibration perception, position sense, and cold thermal perception. Unlike the small nerve fibers, these are the myelinated, rapidly conducting fibers that begin in the toes and have their first synapse in the medulla oblongata. (Myelin is a fat-like substance that forms a sheath around certain nerve fibers.) These fibers tend to be affected first because of their length and the tendency in diabetes for nerves to "die back." Because they are myelinated, they are the fibers represented in the electrophysiologic nerve conduction studies, and subclinical abnormalities in nerve function are readily detected.

The symptoms may be minimal: sensation of walking on cotton, floors feeling "strange," inability to turn the pages of a book, or inability to discriminate among coins.

Guard Against Amputation

Of the 86,000 amputations in the United States each year—1 every 10 minutes—50% are preventable

Large-nerve-fiber neuropathy produces numbness, ataxia and in-coordination, impairing activities of daily living and causing falls and factures.[35] See Table 24.4 for clinical manifestations of large-fiber neuropathies.

TABLE 24.4 Large-Fiber Neuropathies: Clinical Manifestations

- Impaired vibration perception and position sense are often the first objective evidence
- Depressed tendon reflexes
- Pain is described as deep-seated gnawing, dull, like a "toothache" in the bones of the feet, or crushing or cramp-like pain (called type A-δ nerve fibers)
- Sensory ataxia (waddling like a duck)
- Wasting of small muscles of feet with hammertoes or weakness of hands and feet
- Shortening of the Achilles tendon with pes equines (horses' foot)
- Increased blood flow (hot foot)

Combinations of Large- and Small-Fiber Damage

Most patients with chronic sensorimotor neuropathy have a "mixed" variety of neuropathy, with both large-nerve-fiber and small-nerve-fiber damages. Early in the course of the neuropathic process, multifocal sensory loss also might be found. In some individuals, severe distal muscle weakness can accompany the sensory loss, resulting in an inability to stand on the toes or heels. Some grading systems use this as a definition of severity.

Implications for Diabetes Education and Care. Severe weakness is rare and, if present, should raise the question of a possible nondiabetic neuropathy, such as Gullain-Barré syndrome, chronic inflammatory demyelinating polyneuropathy (CIDP), or monoclonal gammopathies (MGUS).[2,11,33] Another important point is that chronic sensorimotor neuropathy is frequently accompanied by diabetic autonomic neuropathy (DAN), which is easily determined by methods discussed below.

Case in Point: Complexities of Autonomic Neuropathy

RK was a 36-year-old white, nonobese male (height 5 ft 7 in, weight 142 lb) with a 15-year history of type 1 diabetes. His diabetes had been poorly controlled for many years on a regimen of a single dose of 35 units 70/30 insulin per day without regular blood glucose monitoring. He had repeated admissions to hospitals for diabetic ketoacidosis and resisted attempts at intensification of treatment or improved monitoring.

Over the past few weeks, RK had developed intractable burning pain in the feet, which he described as a "dog gnawing at the bones" or like somebody who has a "toothache in the feet." He found it unbearable to have his feet come in contact with the bed clothes, and putting on his shoes and socks in the morning was close to or near impossible. The pain was worse at night, and he was getting little sleep.

Symptoms:

- Constantly tired, felt weak, apathetic, lethargic, and incapable of carrying out his normal daily activities.
- Had become significantly *depressed* by the pain and was not eating well
- Felt *bloated* and full after eating only little bits of food, and occasionally *vomited* and could taste food on his breath that he had eaten maybe a day or two before.
- *Irregular bowels*; varied from marked constipation to explosive diarrhea, with episodes sometimes so sudden and forceful he would soil himself

Physical Signs:

- A lean individual, who displayed signs of weakness
- Resting BP: 80/64 mm Hg; HR: 96 beats/min
- *On standing,* BP fell to 50/40 mmHg; HR did not change
- Background retinopathy
- No renal disease or clinical evidence of cardiovascular disease

Question to Consider

What kind of neuropathy did RK have?

Case—Part 2: Complexities of Autonomic Neuropathy

Diagnosis

RK had clear evidence of mixed sensory motor polyneuropathy with autonomic neuropathy. What tests should be ordered?

The physician ordered the following tests, with results as noted:

- Gastroparesis: documented with a gastric emptying time of solid foods of 55 min (normal of <17 min)
- Cholesterol: 132 mg/dL; triglycerides: 101 mg/dL; A1C: 11.5% (normal <6.05%)
- Urine protein: 500 mg, creatinine: 1.7, BUN: 40 mg/dL
- Supine norepinephrine: 196 pg/mL, rising to 369 pg/mL after standing 15 min
- Resting cardiac ejection fraction: 61%, no increase with maximal exercise
- Resting heart rate: 100 beats/min
- Beat-to-beat heart rate variability: 12 beats/min between deep inspiration; expiration E:I ratio: 1.01 (normal >1.3)
- Valsalva ratio: 1.06 (normal >1.10)
- Heart rate response to standing (the 30:15 ratio): 1.0 (normal >1.0)
- Orthostatic systolic pressure drop: 36 mm Hg (normal < 30 mm Hg) and he became quite dizzy

Treatment

What would you suggest to help control his hyperglycemia?

- NPH insulin at bedtime was added to his medications

What about his painful neuropathy?

- Topical capsaicin 0.025% (Zostrix) was suggested, 4x/day

How would you address the autonomic neuropathy?

What can be done for the orthostasis?

Is there anything that would improve gastric emptying?

This chapter's section on autonomic neuropathy helps readers answer questions raised in this case.

Autonomic Neuropathy

Autonomic neuropathy (AN) is often referred to in the diabetic population as diabetic autonomic neuropathy (DAN).

Autonomic neuropathy significantly impacts survival and quality of life:

Although serious and common, AN (or DAN) is among the least recognized and poorly understood complications of diabetes.[17]

The reported prevalence of AN varies widely (7.7% to 90.0%), depending on the study population and methods used for diagnosis.[36,37]

The autonomic nervous system (ANS) supplies all organs in the body and consists of an afferent and an efferent system, involving both the parasympathetic and sympathetic nervous systems. AN may involve any system in the body. Involvement of the autonomic nervous system can occur as early as the first year after diagnosis and major manifestations are cardiovascular, gastrointestinal, and genitourinary system dysfunction.[27,38]

Disturbances in the ANS may be *functional* (eg, gastroparesis with hyperglycemia and ketoacidosis) or *organic*, wherein nerve fibers are actually lost. This creates great difficulty in diagnosing and treating as well as establishing true prevalence rates. Many conditions affect the ANS (AN is not unique to diabetes); thus, the diagnosis of diabetic autonomic neuropathy rests with excluding other causes. Subclinical involvement may be widespread, whereas clinical symptoms and signs may be focused within a single organ.

Symptoms. The following are some common symptoms of autonomic neuropathy:

- Reduced exercise tolerance
- Edema
- Paradoxical supine or nocturnal hypertension

- Intolerance to heat (due to defective thermo-regulation)
- Gastrointestinal and genitourinary dysfunction

Table 24.5 lists the most common clinical features, diagnostic methods, and treatment options for AN.

Cardiac Autonomic Neuropathy

Cardiovascular dysfunction is associated with abnormalities in heart rate control and vascular dynamics. The first sign of cardiac impairment is usually *resting tachycardia*. Parasympathetic nerves slow the heart rate, and sympathetic nerves increase the speed and force of heart contractions and stimulate the vascular tree to increase the blood pressure. Cardiovascular impairment is present in up to 40% of patients with diabetes. The 3 major associated syndromes are these:[6]

- Cardiac denervation syndrome
- Abnormal cardiovascular response to exercise
- Orthostatic (postural) hypotension

Cardiac Denervation Syndrome

Cardiac denervation is defined as a fixed heart rate that does not change in response to stress, exercise, breathing patterns, or sleep. This syndrome results from both parasympathetic and sympathetic system impairment. Initially, parasympathetic tone decreases, which causes a relative increase in sympathetic tone and an increase in heart rate. Progressive impairment of sympathetic tone causes a gradual slowing of the heart. Over time, both parasympathetic and sympathetic tone become impaired.[17]

Initially, a fixed heart rate of 100 to 120 beats per minute is common. In the later stages, the fixed heart rate will be in the range of 80 to 100 beats per minute. The heart rate is unresponsive to stress, exercise, or tilting.[39,40] In the later stages, the person may suffer myocardial ischemia or myocardial infarction without experiencing pain. The resulting delay or failure to seek treatment contributes to increasing mortality rates. These persons are also at risk for cardiac arrhythmias and sudden death.[17]

Diagnosis. Cardiac denervation is assessed using specific devices designed to test for autonomic neuropathy (eg, ANSAR by ANSAR). The device records the pulse or heart rate during deep breathing (6 breaths per minute) or before or after a Valsalva maneuver or exercise. No variation in heart rate is indicative of cardiac nerve damage.[17]

Implications for Diabetes Education and Care. Teach patients with cardiac denervation syndrome to avoid heavy exercise, aerobic exercise, and straining. Stress testing is a requirement before initiating any type of exercise program. In addition, these patients should to be carefully evaluated prior to initiation of intensive insulin therapy because of the risk of hypoglycemia, which can result in cardiac arrhythmias.[17]

Abnormal Cardiovascular Response to Exercise

Some people with diabetic autonomic neuropathy may lose their normal increased cardiac output and vascular tone response to exercise and become hypotensive with aerobic activity.[17]

Postural Hypotension

Blood pressure is normally maintained upon standing by a sympathetic reflex that increases the heart rate and by peripheral vascular resistance in association with an increase in norepinephrine levels. Orthostatic hypotension is defined as a drop in systolic blood pressure of more than 30 mm Hg or a diastolic drop of more than 10 mm Hg within 2 minutes of changing from a supine to standing position. This syndrome occurs late in diabetes and signals advanced autonomic impairment.

Orthostatic hypotension, which results from blood pooling in the feet, can occur without symptoms, but often is accompanied by dizziness, light-headedness, weakness, visual impairment, or syncope.[17] This places the patient at risk for injury from falls. All persons with diabetes must have their blood pressure and pulse rates assessed in the lying, sitting, and standing positions. Greater accuracy in the assessment can be achieved by having the patient rest in a supine position, then stand quietly while the blood pressure is measured at 1-minute intervals for 3 to 5 minutes.[17]

Treatment. Treatment of symptoms involves raising the head of the bed 30 degrees at night, increasing venous pressure with supportive elastic whole body stockings or at least to the waist that are applied while supine, and wearing an antigravity suit. Other therapies can include correcting hypovolemia, midodrine, β-blockers, clonidine (Catapres), octreotide (Sandostatin), and erythropoietin. (Refer to Table 24.5.)[17]

Implications for Diabetes Education and Care. Patients should receive education on the proper application and use of elastic body stockings, which need to be waist high. (Knee or thigh-high stockings that cut into the leg are hazardous as they may restrict the blood supply). Patients should also receive instruction on rising slowly from a recumbent position and graded supervised exercise to improve strength and balance is recommended, as well as nutritional counseling on salt intake. Silent

TABLE 24.5 Autonomic Neuropathy: Clinical Features, Diagnosis, and Treatment

Symptoms	*Tests*	*Treatments*
Cardiac		
Resting tachycardia, exercise intolerance	HRV, MUGA thallium scan, MIBG scan	Graded supervised exercise, ACE inhibitors, β-blockers
Postural hypotension, dizziness, weakness, fatigue, syncope	HRV, supine and standing BP, catecholamines	Mechanical measures, clonidine, midodrine, octreotide, erythropoietin
Gastrointestinal		
Gastroparesis, erratic glucose control	Gastric emptying study, barium study	Frequent small meals, prokinetic agents (metoclopramide, domperidone, erythromycin)
Abdominal pain, early satiety, nausea, vomiting, bloating, belching	Endoscopy, manometry, electrogastrogram	Antibiotics, antiemetics, bulking agents, tricyclic antidepressants, pyloric botox, gastric pacing
Constipation	Endoscopy	High-fiber diet and bulking agents, osmotic laxatives, lubricating agents
Diarrhea (often nocturnal, alternating with constipation)	None	Soluble dietary fiber, gluten and lactose restriction, anticholinergic agents, cholestyramine, antibiotics, somatostatin, pancreatic enzyme supplements
Sexual Dysfunction		
Erectile dysfunction	H&P, HRV, penile-brachial pressure index, nocturnal penile tumescence	Sex therapy; psychological counseling; 5'-phosphodiesterase inhibitors; PG E1 injections, devices, or prostheses
Vaginal dryness	None	Vaginal lubricants
Bladder Dysfunction		
Frequency, urgency, nocturia, urinary retention, incontinence	Cystometrogram, postvoiding sonography	Bethanechol, intermittent catheterization
Sudomotor Dysfunction		
Anhidrosis, heat intolerance, dry skin, hyperhidrosis	Quantitative sudomotor axon reflex, sweat test, skin blood flow	Emollients and skin lubricants, scopolamine, glycopyrrolate, botulinum toxin, vasodilators
Pupillomotor and Visceral Dysfunction		
Visual blurring, impaired adaptation to ambient light, Argyll-Robertson pupil	Pupillometry, HRV	Care with driving at night
Impaired visceral sensation: silent myocardial infarction, hypoglycemia unawareness		Recognition of unusual presentation of myocardial infarction, control of risk factors, control of plasma glucose levels

Key: ACE = angiotensin-converting enzyme; BP = blood pressure; H&P = history and physical examination; HRV = heart rate variability; MI = myocardial infarction; MIBG = metaiodobenzlyguanidine; MUGA = multigated angiography; PG = prostaglandin

Source: Copyright © 2005 American Diabetes Association. Modified with permission Boulton A J, Vinik A, Arezzo J, et al. Diabetic Neuropathies (position statement). Diabetes Care. 2005;28(4):956-62.

myocardial infarction, respiratory failure, amputations and sudden death are hazards for the diabetic patients with cardiac autonomic neuropathy.[41,42] Therefore, it is imperative to make this diagnosis early so that appropriate intervention can be instituted.[43]

Treatment for the Underlying Cause of Autonomic Neuropathy. Treatment of the underlying cause can include management of the following:

- Hyperglycemia
- Lipids
- Blood pressure
- Use of antioxidants[37,44]
- Angiotensin-converting enzyme (ACE) inhibitors[45,46]

Gastrointestinal Disorders Related to Autonomic Neuropathy

If the nerves are affected by autonomic neuropathy, gastric emptying of both liquids and solids may be delayed. Vagal nerve dysfunction is usually responsible for motility.

Upper Gastrointestinal Dysfunction

Most upper gastrointestinal dysfunction may involve the esophagus, stomach, and upper small intestine. Symptoms of gastroparesis (delayed gastric emptying) can include heartburn, reflux, anorexia, early satiety, nausea, abdominal bloating, erratic blood glucose levels due to delayed absorption of food, and vomiting undigested food eaten several hours or days earlier.[47,48] Signs associated with gastroparesis include weight loss and a succussion splash over the left quadrant of the abdomen, although delayed gastric emptying can also occur without symptoms.[47,48]

Diagnosis. A barium series of the upper gastrointestinal tract is useful to rule out obstruction. A solid-phase gastric emptying phase study is the most specific way to diagnose delayed gastric emptying.[48,49] Gastroscopy may be needed to exclude a bezoar. The blood glucose must be normal when the test is performed.

Implications for Diabetes Education and Care. Normalizing blood glucose levels may improve gastric emptying. The presence of gastroparesis complicates balancing insulin doses with food absorption. Frequent monitoring of pre- and postprandial blood glucose levels is a requirement to detect hypoglycemia and hyperglycemia and determine the insulin dose. Rapid-acting insulin is probably not appropriate for some patients with gastroparesis, although some find it useful if taken after the meal.

Treatment. Treatment includes the following:

- Referral to a dietitian for a low-fat, low-fiber diet
- Use of multiple, small, and mostly liquid meals eaten throughout the day
- Referral to a gastroenterologist
- Medications to decrease inhibition of gastric motility such as metoclopramide (Reglan), taken 30 minutes before all meals, snacks, and at bedtime
- Other medications that increase the motility of the stomach such as erythromycin, Zelnorm or bethanechol may be useful
- In the most severe stages jejunostomy tube feedings may be necessary
- New treatments include gastric pacing

Lower Intestinal Tract Dysfunction

Lower intestinal tract dysfunction is the result of damage to the efferent autonomic nerves and leads to hypotonia and poor contraction of the smooth muscles to the gut, which results in constipation.

Constipation. Constipation is fairly common and has been reported in up to 60% of all persons with diabetes. Treatment involves increasing fiber in the diet while avoiding excess fiber, judicious use of laxatives, adequate hydration, increased activity, stool softeners and bulk laxatives such as psyllium (Metamucil), and medications such as metoclopramide (Reglan) or neostigmine (Prostigmin) to increase intestinal motility.[47,50]

Diarrhea. Diarrhea can also occur as a result of both decreased small intestinal motility and hypermotility without bacterial overgrowth.[47,48] Although constipation is more common, diarrhea is usually more troublesome to patients. Diarrhea may be nocturnal, intermittent with constipation, and associated with fecal incontinence; it may occur without cramping or pain. Treatment involves the use of antibiotics (eg, tetracycline or metronidazole) to decrease the bacterial overgrowth. It is better to drive the bowel (eg, with metoclopramide or erythromycin) than to inhibit motility. Nonetheless medications that may be useful for slowing intestinal motility are loperamide, codeine, diphenoxylate hydrochloride, or atropine sulfate. However, care should be exercised because they may aggravate the situation. Fiber and psyllium may increase stool bulk and consistency. In addition, some patients may benefit from biofeedback, relaxation, and bowel training. Early treatment of diarrhea may help prevent the development of incontinence.[47,48]

Implications for Diabetes Education and Care. Include a discussion of how these symptoms are related to diabetes. Stress the need to inform providers of symptoms to allow for early detection and treatment. Explain with care diagnostic tests, test results, and therapies.

Sexual Dysfunction Related to Autonomic Neuropathy

Sexual dysfunction is common among people with diabetes. As many as 75% of men and 35% of women experience sexual problems due to DN.[51] Male sexual dysfunction involves erectile dysfunction and retrograde ejaculation. Retrograde ejaculation is unusual and may respond to use of an antihistamine, desipramine, or phenylephrine.[52]

Male Sexual Dysfunction

Erectile dysfunction (ED) occurs in men with diabetes at an earlier age than in the general population. The incidence of ED in men with diabetes aged 20 to 29 years is 9% and increases to 95% by 70 years of age. ED may be the presenting symptom of diabetes. More than 50% notice the onset of ED within 10 years of the diagnosis, but it may precede the other complications of diabetes. The etiology of ED in diabetes is multifactorial. Neuropathy, vascular disease, diabetes control, nutrition, endocrine disorders, and psychogenic factors as well as drugs used in the treatment of diabetes and its complications play a role.[52,53] Diagnosis of the cause of ED is made by a logical step-wise progression.[53,54]

Diagnostic Assessments. Assessments should include a careful medical and sexual history; physical and psychological evaluations; blood test for diabetes and levels of testosterone, prolactin, and thyroid hormones; a test for nocturnal erections; tests to assess penile, pelvic, and spinal nerve function, penile blood supply and blood pressure. A simple test of autonomic function using heart rate variability will exclude a neurologic cause of ED. A flow chart can assist in defining the problem.[52,53]

The healthcare provider must ask questions to help distinguish the various forms of organic erectile dysfunction from those that are psychogenic in origin. Physical examination must include an evaluation of the autonomic nervous system, vascular supply, and hypothalamic-pituitary-gonadal axis.

AN causing ED is almost always accompanied by loss of ankle jerks and absence or reduction of vibration sense over the large toes. More direct evidence of impairment of penile autonomic function can be obtained by demonstrating normal perianal sensation, assessing the tone of the anal sphincter during a rectal exam, and ascertaining the presence of an anal wink. These measurements are easily and quickly done at the bedside and reflect the integrity of sacral parasympathetic divisions.

Test for nocturnal penile tumescence (NPT) distinguish psychogenic from organic dysfunction. Normal NPT defines psychogenic ED, and a negative response to vasodilators implies vascular insufficiency. However, the NPT test is not so simple. It is much like having a sphygmomanometer cuff inflate over the penis many times during the night while the patient is trying to sleep.

Treatment of Erectile Dysfunction. A number of treatment modalities are available, and each treatment has positive and negative effects. Therefore, patients must be made aware of both aspects before a therapeutic decision is made. Before considering any form of treatment, every effort should be made to have the person withdraw from alcohol and eliminate smoking. If possible, the patient should be removed from drugs that are known to cause erectile dysfunction and metabolic control should be optimized.

Recent research has revealed the ability to have and maintain an erection depends on nitric oxide (NO) and cGMP. Agents such as sildenafil (Viagra), vardenafil (Levitra),and tadalafil (Cialis) exert their effect by increasing NO and cGMP levels that may be low in men with diabetes. Before any of these agents are prescribed, ischemic heart disease must be excluded. These medications are absolutely contraindicated in persons being treated with nitroglycerine or other nitrate-containing drugs. Severe hypotension and fatal cardiac events can occur.[49]

Direct injection of prostacylin into the corpus cavernosum will induce satisfactory erections in a significant number of men. Also, surgical implantation of a penile prosthesis may be appropriate. The less expensive type of prosthesis is a semi-rigid, permanently erect type that may be embarrassing and uncomfortable for some men. The inflatable type is three times more expensive and subject to mechanical failure, but it avoids the embarrassment caused by other devices.

Implications for Diabetes Education and Care. The advent of therapies such as sildenafil, vardenafil, and tadalafil have created a new era of openness regarding sexual issues. However, many patients may still be reticent about their sexual function. The diabetes educator should be aware that a problem may exist and alert the physician. When appropriate, including both sexual partners in selecting therapy is extremely important. Review all therapeutic options as well as their costs and benefits.

Female Sexual Dysfunction

Women with diabetes mellitus may experience decreased sexual desire, difficulties in arousal, and more pain during sexual intercourse, but they are at risk of decreased sexual arousal. They also have decreased vaginal lubrication even if stimulated.[55] However, female sexual dysfunction, decreased vaginal lubrication, vaginal flushing, and delayed or absent orgasmic response need further assessment.

Sexual difficulties not related to autonomic neuropathy include loss of libido related to depression as a result of diabetes and its complications as well as the frequent occurrence of yeast and other vaginal infections in women with diabetes.

Implications for Diabetes Education and Care. Diabetes educators need to address sexual concerns because these issues may be difficult for patients to discuss. Discuss sexual function, the potential for diabetes-related problems, and the need to bring problems to the attention of providers. Offer to include patients' partners in the discussion and point out the importance of their inclusion in treatment decisions. Management includes application of estrogen or lubricating vaginal creams and referral to a gynecologist. Offer the patient and her partner referral for counseling with a sex therapist.

Bladder Dysfunction Related to Autonomic Neuropathy

In AN, the motor function of the bladder is unimpaired, but afferent fiber damage results in diminished bladder sensation. Symptoms of a neurogenic bladder are usually insidious and progressive. In the early stages, the sensation of the need to void may be blunted. This infrequent urination may be misinterpreted as decreased polyuria due to improved blood glucose control. In later stages, difficulty in emptying the bladder, dribbling, and overflow incontinence may occur.[17] The urinary bladder can be enlarged to more than three times its normal size. Patients are seen with bladders filled to their umbilicus, yet they feel no discomfort. Loss of bladder sensation occurs with diminished voiding frequency, and the person is no longer able to void completely. An untreated neurogenic bladder often leads to urinary tract infections as a result of urinary stasis. These frequent infections may accelerate deterioration of renal function. More than 2 urinary tract infections per year among men and 3 among women indicate of the need for further evaluation of bladder function.

Diagnosis. Bladder insensitivity is diagnosed by a cystometrogram. A post-voiding residual of greater than 150 cc confirms bladder dysfunction or cystopathy, which may put the patient at risk for urinary infections.

Treatment of Cystopathy. A patient with cystopathy should be instructed to palpate his or her bladder and, if unable to initiate micturition with a full bladder, use Crede's maneuver (massage or pressure on the lower portion of abdomen just above the pubic bone) to start the flow of urine. The principal aim of the treatment should be to improve bladder emptying and to reduce the risk of urinary tract infection. Parasympathomimetics such as bethanechol are sometimes helpful, although frequently they do not help to completely empty the bladder. Extended sphincter relaxation can be achieved with an α_1-blocker, such as doxazosin (Cardura). Self-catheterization can be particularly useful, with the risk of infection generally being low.

Implications for Diabetes Education and Care. Stress the need for frequent, complete urination; the signs and symptoms of urinary tract infections; and the importance of early treatment for infections. Teach patients to palpate for bladder fullness.

Sudomotor Dysfunction (Sweating Disturbances) Related to Autonomic Neuropathy

Excessive perspiration (hyperhidrosis) of the upper body, often related to eating (gustatory sweating) and deficiency of sweat (anhidrosis) of the lower body, are characteristic features of AN. Gustatory sweating accompanies the ingestion of certain foods, particularly spicy foods and cheeses. Application of glycopyrrolate (antimuscarinic compound) has been suggested for persons with diabetes who experience with gustatory sweating.[32] Symptomatic relief can be obtained by avoiding the specific food irritant.

Emphasize foot care:

Loss of lower body sweating can cause dry, brittle skin that cracks easily, predisposing one to ulcer formation that can lead to limb loss. Special attention must be paid to foot care as many individuals do not recognize the sweating or other problems.

Implications for Diabetes Education and Care. Patients rarely think to report abnormal sweating. However, this symptom is a red flag for the potential for heat stroke and foot ulcers. A careful history and examination of the feet for dryness and fissures are important to conduct at each visit.[17] Patient education should include inspection for fissures and lubrication for dry feet; avoidance of hot, spicy or other offending foods; and prevention of hyperthermia and heat stroke.

Research studies have shown defective blood flow in the small capillary circulation.[56-58] The clinical counterpart is dry cold skin, loss of sweating, development of fissures and cracks that are portals of entry for organisms leading to infectious ulcers and gangrenes. This is an example of the value of research translating into clinical care. Awareness of the consequences of defective blood flow and education towards behaviors for preventing fissures and cracks can protect against the ravages of foot ulcers and gangrene.

Pupillomotor and Visceral (Metabolic) Response Related to Autonomic Neuropathy

Abnormal Pupillary Response

The iris is innervated by both parasympathetic and sympathetic nerve fibers. Sympathetic nerve fibers cause the pupils to dilate and are generally more severely affected. Abnormal pupillary responses are related to duration of diabetes.[17] Slow dilation of pupils in response to darkness may be observed during clinical examination. Patients may report slow adaptation when entering a dark room.

Implications for Diabetes Education and Care. Stress using caution during night driving, the importance of turning on lights when entering a dark room, and using nightlights in darkened hallways and bathrooms to help prevent injuries.

Hypoglycemia Unawareness

Blood glucose concentration is normally maintained during starvation or increased insulin action by an asymptomatic parasympathetic response with bradycardia and mild hypotension, followed by a sympathetic response with glucagon and epinephrine secretion for short-term glucose counter-regulation and growth hormone and cortisol in long-term regulation. The release of catecholamine alerts the person to take the required measures to prevent coma due to low blood glucose. The absence of warning signs of impending neuroglycopenia is known as "hypoglycemic unawareness." Failure of glucose counterregulation can be confirmed by the absence of glucagon and epinephrine responses to hypoglycemia that is induced by a standard, controlled dose of insulin.[59]

In persons with type 1 diabetes mellitus, the glucagon response is impaired with diabetes duration of 1 to 5 years, and after 14 to 31 years of diabetes, the glucagon response is almost undetectable. The glucagon response is not present in those with AN. However, a syndrome of hypoglycemic autonomic failure occurs with intensification of diabetes control and repeated episodes of hypoglycemia. The exact mechanism is not understood, but it does represent a real barrier to physiologic glycemic control. In the absence of severe autonomic dysfunction, hypoglycemic awareness associated with hypoglycemia is at least partly reversible.

Patients with hypoglycemia unawareness and unresponsiveness pose a significant management problem for the healthcare team. Although autonomic neuropathy may improve with intensive therapy and normalization of blood glucose, there is a risk to the patient, who may become hypoglycemic (without being aware of it) and be unable to mount a counterregulatory response. These are some recommendations:

- In pump therapy, use boluses of smaller than calculated amounts and in intensive conventional therapy use long-acting insulin with very small boluses
- In general, modify goals for glucose and A1C levels in these patients to avoid the possibility of hypoglycemia[60]

Further complicating management for some patients is the development of a functional autonomic insufficiency associated with intensive insulin treatment, which resembles AN in all relevant aspects. In these instances, relaxing therapy, as for the patient with *bona fide* AN, is prudent. If hypoglycemia occurs in these patients at a certain glucose level, it will take a lower glucose level to trigger the same symptoms in the next 24 to 48 hours. Avoidance of hypoglycemia for a few days will result in recovery of the adrenergic response.

Implications for Diabetes Education and Care. Include prevention of hypoglycemia, appropriate treatment, the value of frequent home blood glucose monitoring, caution while driving, and wearing appropriate diabetes identification. Teach family members the signs and treatment of hypoglycemia, including glucagon administration. Blood glucose awareness training may improve functional capacity.[37,61]

Focal and Multifocal Neuropathies

The various focal neuropathies are acute and unpredictable. They are not specific to diabetes and are not related to the duration of diabetes. There are no strategies for prevention or early detection. Focal neuropathies are generally classified into the following types:

- Mononeuropathies
- Entrapment syndromes

The primary symptom of focal neuropathies is acute local pain.

Focal Limb Neuropathies

Focal limb neuropathies are usually due to entrapments. Entrapment syndromes start slowly and progress and persist unless intervention is prescribed. Carpal tunnel syndrome (compression or entrapment of the median nerve of the wrist) occurs 3 times as frequently in diabetics compared with healthy populations[23,62] and is found in up to one-third of patients with diabetes.[23] The diagnosis can be made by a careful history and physical and confirmed by electrophysiological studies.

Treatment consists of resting, aided by placement of wrist splint in a neutral position to avoid repetitive trauma. Anti-inflammatory medications and steroid injections are sometimes useful. Surgery should be considered if weakness appears and medical treatment fails.[11,63]

Mononeuropathies

Mononeuropathies occur primarily in older people; the onset is acute, associated with pain, and their course is self-limiting, resolving within 6 to 8 weeks. They are due to vascular obstruction.[64] Mononeuropathies, characterized by their acute onset, should be distinguished from entrapment syndromes. (See Table 24.6)

Cranial Neuropathies

Cranial neuropathies in diabetic patients are extremely rare (0.05%) and occur in older individuals with a long duration of diabetes.[65] The third cranial nerve is most often affected. The onset is generally abrupt with headache, eye pain, or dysesthesias of the upper lip preceding palsy. The patient is unable to move the eye. After a few weeks the pain subsides and the ocular function improves, with full recovery in 3 to 5 months.

Implications for Diabetes Education and Care. Assure the patient that this is a temporary situation that will soon resolve. Suggest the use of an eye patch for affected eye.

TABLE 24.6 Mononeuropathies Versus Entrapment Syndrome

Feature	*Mononeuropathy*	*Entrapment Syndrome*
Onset	Sudden	Gradual
Pattern	Single nerve, but may be multiple	Single nerve exposed to trauma
Nerves involved	Cranial nerves III, VI, VII; ulnar; median; peroneal	Median, ulnar, peroneal, medial and lateral plantar
Natural history	Resolves spontaneously	Progressive
Treatment	Symptomatic	Rest, splints, local steroids, diuretics, surgery

Source: Adapted with permission from Elsevier from Vinik A, Mehrabyan A. Diabetic neuropathies. Med Clin North Am. 2004;88(4):954.

Proximal-Motor Neuropathy (Amyotrophy)

Proximal-motor neuropathy typically occurs in older patients (50 to 60 years of age) with type 2 diabetes and presents with severe pain and unilateral or bilateral muscle weakness and atrophy in proximal thighs. Pathogenesis is still unclear, although immune-mediated epineurial microvasculitis is the culprit in some cases. Immunosuppressive therapy is recommended using high-dose steroids or intravenous immunoglobulin.[66]

Implications for Diabetes Education and Care. Treatment of proximal neuropathies can be very rewarding, as 91% are due to coexistence of CIDP and respond to intravenous immunoglobulin therapy. For those who fail to respond, immunosuppressive agents may be effective.[67]

Chronic Inflammatory Demyelinating Polyneuropathy

When an unusually severe, predominantly motor and progressive polyneuropathy develops in diabetic patients, chronic inflammatory demyelinating polyneuropathy (CIDP) should be considered. Progressive motor deficit and progressive sensory neuropathy in spite of optimal glycemic control together with typical NCV findings and an unusually high cerebrospinal-fluid protein level suggest the possibility of an underlying demyelinating neuropathy. This neuropathy occurs 11 times more frequently in people with diabetes than in those without diabetes.[67-70]

Implications for Diabetes Education and Care. The diagnosis is often overlooked, but it is very important to recognize the condition, because it is treatable. Immunomodulatory therapy with intravenous immunoglobulin or immunotherapy can produce a relatively rapid and substantial improvement.[70]

Diabetic Truncal Radiculoneuropathy

Diabetic truncal radiculoneuropathy affects middle-aged to elderly persons, especially males. (Radiculopathy is the disease condition of the nerve roots in spinal nerves.) Pain is the most important symptom, occurring in a girdle-like distribution over the lower thoracic or abdominal wall, unilaterally or bilaterally distributed. Pain and/or loss of sensation is usually worse at night. Motor weakness is rare. Resolution generally occurs within 4 to 6 months.

Implications for Diabetes Education and Care. Nonnarcotics or simple analgesics may help control the pain, which generally subsides in 6 to 24 months.

Treatment of Diabetic Neuropathy Based on Pathogenetic Mechanisms

Glycemic and Metabolic Control

Studies have shown a relationship between hyperglycemia and the development and severity of DN. The DCCT research group reported that clinical and electrophysiological evidence of neuropathy was reduced by 50% in type 1 patients treated intensively with insulin.[71] In the UK Prospective Diabetes Study (UKPDS), control of blood glucose was associated with improvement in vibration perception.[72,73]

Vascular Risk Factors and Diabetic Neuropathy

The Steno trial, using multifactorial intervention, reported a reduction in the development of AN in patients with type 2 diabetes.[46] The EURODIAB, a prospective study that included 3250 patients across Europe, has shown that the incidence of neuropathy is also associated with potentially modifiable cardiovascular risk factors, including a raised triglyceride level, body mass index, smoking, and hypertension.[74]

Treatment and Prevention. Treatment and prevention of neuropathy should, therefore, include measures to reduce both microvascular and macrovascular risk factors: hyperglycemia, blood pressure, lipid control, and lifestyle modifications including exercise and weight reduction, smoking cessation, a diet rich in omega-3 fatty acids, and avoidance of excess alcohol consumption.[46]

Oxidative Stress

A number of studies have shown that hyperglycemia causes oxidative stress in tissues, including peripheral nerves that are susceptible to complications of diabetes. Studies show that hyperglycemia induces an increased presence of markers of oxidative stress, such as superoxide and peroxynitrite ions, which are now measurable in tissues and in body fluids. Persons with diabetic peripheral neuropathy have a reduced internal antioxidant defense mechanism against free radicals.[75]

Treatment. Therapies known to reduce oxidative stress are recommended.[76] Therapies under investigation include aldose reductase inhibitors (ARIs), α-lipoic acid, γ-linolenic acid, benfotiamine, and protein kinase C (PKC) inhibitors.

- ARIs reduce the flux of glucose through the polyol pathway, inhibiting tissue accumulation of sorbitol and fructose. (Sorbitol is a crystalline alcohol that is the intermediate product in the metabolism of glucose in the nerve and other tissues.) Newer ARIs are currently being explored,[77] but it is becoming clear that these agents may be insufficient per se and combinations of treatments may be needed.[63]
- *γ-Linolenic acid* can cause significant improvement in clinical and electrophysiological tests for neuropathy.[78]
- *α-Lipoic acid*, or thioctic acid, has been used for its antioxidant properties and for its thiol-replenishing redox-modulating properties. A number of studies show its favorable influence on microcirculation and reversal of some symptoms of neuropathy.[79] Ongoing studies will examine its long-term effects on electrophysiology and clinical assessments.

Inhibition of the enzyme PKC B has been shown in a phase 2 study to reduce symptoms due to DN[80] in those patients who had mild neuropathy detectable by the presence of a sural nerve amplitude on nerve electrophysiology.[81] Although the phase 3 study did not meet the endpoint of symptom relief, ongoing studies of the effects of ruboxistaurin on more objective measures of nerve function are carried out.

Some of the research studies mentioned above could provide models for the translation of the results of clinical trials involving neuropathy into preventive medicine and optimal clinical care. However, the art of a skilled physician will still be required to interact fully with the patient and maximize the outcomes of translational research.

Controversies in Neuropathy Management

Mechanical Measures

Transcutaneous Nerve Stimulation

Transcutaneous electrical nerve stimulation (TENS or electrotherapy) may be helpful and is one of the more benign therapies for painful neuropathy.[82,83] Caveat: It is important to move the electrodes around to identify sensitive areas and obtain maximal relief.

Static Magnetic Field Therapy

Static magnetic field therapy has been reported to be of benefit, but blinding in these studies was difficult.[84]

Frequency-Modulated Electromagnetic Neural Stimulation

Frequency-modulated electromagnetic neural stimulation (FREMS) has been shown to induce a significant reduction in daytime and nighttime pain. In addition, a significant increase in tactile threshold was detected using Semmes Weinstein Monofilament (SMW), lowering of the vibration detection threshold (VDT), and improved motor nerve conduction velocity using a biosthesiometer. There was an extra benefit shown in measures of quality of life using the SF-36 Health Survey, a short-form, 36-question health survey, in terms of general health, physical, and social functioning.[85] This finding suggests that FREMS may be an active, safe method to improve *symptoms* of neuropathy with the possibility of enhancing *neurological function.*

Infrared Light

Infrared light had benefits in a study of 27 patients whose extremities were treated for 2 weeks with sham or active infrared. There was reportedly a reduction in the number of insensate sites in patients with mild neuropathy, but not in those with greater sensory loss. Improved balance was also reported, but was not quantified objectively. Clearly, these observations need to be extended for longer periods, and more objective measures need to be applied to evaluating responsiveness to treatment.[86]

Implanted Spinal Cord Stimulation

An implanted spinal cord stimulator was used in a series of patients with severe painful neuropathy unresponsive to conventional therapy.[87] However, this cannot be generally recommended except in very resistant cases, as it is invasive, expensive, and unproven in controlled studies.

Vibration

Vibration on the sole of the foot below the individual's threshold for 30 to 60 seconds has been shown to enhance sensitivity, neurotransmission, and vibration detection threshold.[88] Although monofilament application to the sole of the foot after vibration resulted in enhanced detection, this enhancement did not apply to the big toe. The ability to amplify signals from the neuropathic foot may have relevance to protecting feet from injury and possibly even enhancing postural stability. These studies need to be expanded to longer term to determine the durability of their effects.

Surgical Treatment of Neuropathy

Tarsal Tunnel Release

The role of tarsal tunnel release in the management of the person with diabetes who has a painful foot syndrome remains controversial.[23] The major problem is the application of tarsal tunnel release in patients with diabetic peripheral neuropathy *in general* and not *specifically* for those patients with tarsal tunnel entrapment syndrome (TTS). TTS is not difficult to diagnose clinically when DSPN is not severe and NCV is moderately abnormal. Mild symmetric peroneal and tibial NCV abnormality with intact ankle jerks and sensation of the dorsal aspect of the foot with the above-mentioned clinical signs are the most important diagnostic features of TTS. When the neuropathy is severe, diagnosis may be impossible. A positive Tinel sign, tapping just below the medial malleolus, may be helpful, but may also simply reflect nerve damage in peripheral neuropathy, a negative sign suggesting that nerve damage predicts a poor outcome of surgery. Caveat: *If patients are carefully selected,* release of the tibial nerve through the tarsal tunnel in the diabetic may improve plantar sensibility and help prevent plantar ulceration and ultimate lower extremity amputation. Several recent studies lend credence to this notion, though some are subject to design flaws.[89,90]

Summary

The following are key issues in diabetic retinopathy.

- Diabetic neuropathies are among the most common long-term complications of diabetes although they often are not recognized by physicians
- Management of the disease is complex
- A thorough history and detailed physical examination, together with the aid of simple tests (performed in the clinic), are essential for the diagnosis
- In each particular clinical situation, decision of the best treatment option should be made based on the underlying pathological process, the clinical presentation, and cost in relation to effectiveness
- There has been increasing understanding of the pathogenesis of DN over the last decades and new therapies are currently being studied that hold promise for the treatment of this disease

This chapter has addressed the challenges facing diabetes educators and suggested opportunities for dealing with DN. The message is powerful: DN is not a single entity, but rather a number of different syndromes, each with a range of clinical and subclinical manifestations. Effective management is based on recognizing the particular manifestation and underlying pathogenesis of the particular form of DN in each patient and using this information to initiate therapy at a level that improves quality of life for the person with diabetes.

Focus on Education: Pearls for Practice

Teaching Strategies

- **Theory.** Offer assurance that treatment of many of the neuropathies can be rewarding. Some conditions are due to coexistence of other problems and respond to therapy.

- **Diagnosis.** Often, neuropathies are overlooked or "tolerated" as a natural progression of a disease. The key is screening, early detection, and treatment. Emphasis needs to be placed on routine annual and semi-annual exams. Detection can be difficult; thus, clinicians are to inspect feet and skin at every visit to detect change or symptoms.

- **Control.** Neuropathies can be controlled by treatment. Pain associated can be helped with nonnarcotics or simple analgesics.

Education

- **Pain.** Read about the condition and its treatment, openly describe and talk about pain associated with neuropathies, and use the medications (prescription and over-the-counter) appropriately. Relieving pain improves the quality of life and allows for clearer problem solving.

- **Checkups.** Schedule appointments in advance and note them on the calendar. Make this a priority. Identification and early treatment increase good response and reduction in symptoms. Insist that the healthcare provider "look at skin and feet" at every visit. Insist that the healthcare provider talk about the pain and problems to look for with neuropathies.

- **Medication and treatment regimens.** Pay attention to timing of medicines. Use only the supplements advised by the healthcare team. Obtain a routine review of medicines with a pharmacist and the healthcare team: this is advisable to offer the best combination of treatments.

References

1. Holzer SE, Camerota A, Martens L, Cuerdon T, Crystal-Peters J, Zagari M. Costs and duration of care for lower extremity ulcers in patients with diabetes. Clin Ther. 1998; 20:169-81.
2. Dyck PJ, Kratz KM, Karnes JL, et al. The prevalence by staged severity of various types of diabetic neuropathy, retinopathy, and nephropathy in a population-based cohort: The Rochester Diabetic Neuropathy Study. Neurology. 1993;43:817-24.
3. Vinik AI, Mitchell BD, Leichter SB, Wagner AL, O'Brian JT, Georges LP. Epidemiology of the complications of diabetes. In: Diabetes: Clinical Science in Practice. Leslie RDG, Robbins DC, eds. Cambridge, UK: Cambridge University Press; 1995:221-87.
4. Caputo GM, Cavanagh PR, Ulbrecht JS, Gibbons GW, Karchmer AW. Assessment and management of foot disease in patients with diabetes. N Engl J Med. 1994;331(13):854-60.
5. Young MJ, Boulton AJM, MacLeod AF, Williams DRR, Sonksen PH. A multicenter study of the prevalence of diabetic peripheral neuropathy in the United Kingdom hospital clinic population. Diabetologia. 1993;36:1-5.
6. Vinik A, Erbas T, Pfeifer MA. Diabetic autonomic neuropathy. In: Ellenberg & Rifkin's Diabetes Mellitus. Porte D Jr, Sherwin RS, Baron A, eds. New York: McGraw Hill; 2003;789-804.
7. Vinik E, Hayes R, Oglesby A, et al. The development and validation of the Norfolk QOL-DN: a new measure of patients' perception of the effects of diabetes and diabetic neuropathy. Diabetes Technol Ther. 2005;7(3):497-508.
8. Vileikyte L, Peyrot M, Bundy C, et al. The development and validation of a neuropathy- and foot ulcer-specific quality of life instrument. Diabetes Care. 2003;26(9):2549-55.
9. Vinik A, Mehrabyan A. Understanding diabetic neuropathies. Emerg Med. 2004;36(5):39-44.
10. Consensus Statement. Report and recommendations of the San Antonio conference on diabetic neuropathy. American Diabetes Association and American Academy of Neurology. Diabetes Care. 1988;11:592-7.
11. Boulton A, Malik T, Arezzo JC, Sosenko J. Diabetic somatic neuropathies (technical review). Diabetes Care. 2004;27:1458-86.
12. Dyck PJ. Severity and staging of diabetic polyneuropathy. In: Textbook of Diabetic Neuropathy. Gries, FA, Arnold F. Stuttgart, eds. New York, Thieme: 2003; 170-175.
13. Dyck PJ, Karnes JL, O'Brien PC, Litchy WJ, Low PA, Melton III LJ. The Rochester Diabetic Neuropathy Study: reassessment of tests and criteria for diagnosis and staged severity. Neurology. 1992;42:1164-70.
14. Herman WH, Kennedy L. Underdiagnosis of peripheral neuropathy in type 2 diabetes. Diabetes Care. 2005;28(6):1480-1.
15. Dyck PJ. Detection, characterization and staging of polyneuropathy: assessed in diabetes. Muscle Nerve. 1988;11:21-32.
16. Vinik AI, Suwanwalaikorn S, Stansberry KB, Holland MT, McNitt PM, Colen LE. Quantitative measurement of cutaneous perception in diabetic neuropathy. Muscle Nerve. 1995;18:574-84.
17. Boulton AJ, Vinik A, Arezzo J, et al. Diabetic neuropathies (position statement). Diabetes Care. 2005;28(4):956-62.
18. Abbott CA, Carrington AL, Ashe H, et al. The North-West Diabetes Foot Care Study: incidence of, and risk factors for, new diabetic foot ulceration in a community-based patient cohort. Diabet Med. 2002;19(5):377-84.
19. Dyck PJ, Davies JL, Litchy WJ, O'Brien PC. Longitudinal assessment of diabetic polyneuropathy using a composite score in the Rochester Diabetic Neuropathy Study cohort. Neurology. 1997;49(1):229-39.
20. Yarnitsky D, Sprecher E. Thermal testing: normative data and repeatability for various test algorithms. J Neurol Sci. 1994;125:39-45.
21. Partanen J, Niskanen L, Lehtinen J, Mervaala E, Siitonen O, Uusitupa M. Natural history of peripheral neuropathy in patients with non-insulin-dependent diabetes mellitus. N Engl J Med. 1995;333:89-94.
22. DCCT Research Group. The effect of intensive diabetes therapy on the development and progression of neuropathy. Ann Intern Med. 1995;122:561-68.
23. Vinik A, Mehrabyan A, Colen L, Boulton A. Focal entrapment neuropathies in diabetes. Diabetes Care. 2004;27(7);1783-8.
24. Kennedy WR, Wendelschafer-Crabb G, Johnson T. Quantitation of epidermal nerves in diabetic neuropathy. Neurology. 1996;47:1042-8.

25. Polydefkis M, Hauer P, Griffin JW, McArthur JC. Skin biopsy as a tool to assess distal small fiber innervation in diabetic neuropathy. Diabetes Technol Ther. 2001;3(1):23-8.

26. Pittenger GL, Ray M, Burcus NI, McNulty P, Basta B, Vinik AI. Intraepidermal nerve fibers are indicators of small-fiber neuropathy in both diabetic and nondiabetic patients. Diabetes Care. 2004;27(8):1974-9.

27. Vinik AI, Holland MT, Le Beau JM, Liuzzi FJ, Stansberry KB, Colen LB. Diabetic neuropathies. Diabetes Care. 1992;15(12):1926-75.

28. Thomas PK, Ward JD, Watkins PJ. Diabetic neuropathy. In: Complications of Diabetes. Keen H, Jarrett J, eds. London, UK: Edward Arnold Publishing Company; 1982:109-36.

29. Vinik A. Management of neuropathy and foot problems in diabetic patients. Clinical Cornerstone. 2003;5(2):38-52.

30. Thomas PK. Classification, differential diagnosis and staging of diabetic peripheral neuropathy. Diabetes. 1997;46 suppl 2:S54-7.

31. Oyibo SO, Prasad YD, Jackson NJ, Jude EB, Boulton AJ. The relationship between blood glucose excursions and painful diabetic peripheral neuropathy: a pilot study. Diabet Med. 2002;19(10):870-3.

32. Tesfaye S, Malik R, Harris N, et al. Arterio-venous shunting and proliferating new vessels in acute painful neuropathy of rapid glycaemic control (insulin neuritis). Diabetologia. 1996;39:329-35.

33. Sinnreich M, Taylor BV, Dyck PJ. Diabetic neuropathies: classification, clinical features, and pathophysiological basis. Neurologist. 2005;11(2):63-79.

34. Vinik A, Pittenger G, Barlow P, Mehrabyan A. Diabetic neuropathies: an overview of clinical aspects, pathogenesis, and treatment. In: LeRoith D, Taylor S, Olefsky J, ed. Diabetes Mellitus, 3rd ed. Philadelphia, Pa: Lippincott Williams and Wilkins; 2004: 1343-4.

35. Resnick HE, Vinik AI, Schwartz AV, et al. Independent effects of peripheral nerve dysfunction on lower-extremity physical function in old age: the Women's Health and Aging Study. Diabetes Care. 2000;23(11):1642-7.

36. Ziegler D, Dannehl K, Muhlen H, Spuler M, Gries FA. Prevalence of cardiovascular autonomic dysfunction assessed by spectral analysis, vector analysis, and standard tests of heart rate variation and blood pressure responses at various stages of diabetic neuropathy. Diabet Med. 1992;9(9):806-14.

37. Vinik AI, Maser RE, Mitchell BD, Freeman R. Diabetic autonomic neuropathy. Diabetes Care. 2003;26(5):1553-79.

38. Zola BE, Vinik AI. Effects of autonomic neuropathy associated with diabetes mellitus on cardiovascular function. Coron Artery Dis. 1992;3:33-41.

39. Vinik AI, Erbas T. Diabetic Autonomic Neuropathy. Germany, Academy Germany: Aventis, Inc.; 2001:100-39.

40. Vinik A, Erbas T. Neurological disease and diabetes, autonomic. In: Encyclopedia of Endocrine Disease 3. 2004;334-9.

41. Ziegler D. Diabetic cardiovascular autonomic neuropathy: prognosis, diagnosis and treatment. Diabetes Metabolism Rev. 1994;10:339-83.

42. Valensi P. Diabetic autonomic neuropathy: what are the risks? Diabets Metab. 1998;24:66-72.

43. Mancia G, Paleari F, Parati G. Early diagnosis of diabetic autonomic neuropathy: present and future approaches. Diabetologia. 1997;40:482-4.

44. Ziegler D, Gries FA. Alpha-lipoic acid in the treatment of diabetic peripheral and cardiac autonomic neuropathy. Diabetes. 1997;46 suppl 2:S62-6.

45. Athyros VG, Didangelos TP, Karamitsos DT, Papageorgiou AA, Boudoulas H, Kontopoulos AG. Long-term effect of converting enzyme inhibition on circadian sympathetic and parasympathetic modulation in patients with diabetic autonomic neuropathy. Acta Cardiol. 1998;53:201-9.

46. Gaede P, Vedel P, Larsen N, Jensen G, Parving H, Pedersen O. Multifactorial intervention and cardiovascular disease in patients with type 2 diabetes. N Engl J Med. 2003;383-93.

47. Vinik A, Mehrabyan A, Johnson D. Gastrointestinal disturbances. In: Lebovitz H, ed. Therapy for Diabetes Mellitus and Related Disorders, 4th ed. Alexandria, Va: American Diabetes Association; 2004: 426-429.

48. Jones KL, Russo A, Stevens JE, Wishart JM, Berry MK, Horowitz M. Predictors of delayed gastric emptying in diabetes. Diabetes Care. 2001;24(7):1264-9.

49. Vinik A, Mehrabyan A. Diagnosis and management of diabetic autonomic neuropathy. Compr Ther. 2003;29(2/3):130-45.

50. Horowitz SH, Ginsberg-Fellner F. Ischemia and sensory nerve conduction in diabetes mellitus. Neurology. 1979;29:695-704.

51. Vinik AI, Richardson D. Erectile dysfunction in diabetes. Diabetes Reviews. 1998;6:16-33.

52. Richardson D, Vinik A. Etiology and treatment of erectile failure in diabetes mellitus. Curr Diab Rep. 2002;2(6):501-9.

53. Vinik AI, Richardson D. Erectile dysfunction in diabetes: pills for penile failure. Clinica Diabetes. 1998;16:108-19.

54. Vinik A, Richardson D. Erectile dysfunction. In: Diabetes in Old Age, 2nd ed. New York: Wiley; 2001;89-102.

55. Enzlin P, Mathieu C, Vanderschueren D, Demyttenaere K. Diabetes mellitus and female sexuality: a review of 25 years' research. Diabet Med. 1998;15(10):809-15.

56. Stansberry KB, Hill MA, Shapiro SA, McNitt PM, Bhatt BA, Vinik AI. Impairment of peripheral blood flow responses in diabetes resembles an enhanced aging effect. Diabetes Care. 1997;20:1711-6.

57. Stansberry KB, Peppard HR, Babyak LM, Popp G, McNitt PM, Vinik AI. Primary nociceptive afferents mediate the blood flow dysfunction in non-glabrous (hairy) skin of type 2 diabetes. Diabetes Care. 1999;22(9):1549-54.

58. Haak ES, Usadel KH, Kohleisen M, Yilmaz A, Kusterer K, Haak T. The effect of alpha-lipoic on the neurovascular reflex arc in patients with diabetic neuropathy assessed by capillary microscopy. Microvasc Res. 1999;58:28-34.

59. Meyer C, Hering BJ, Grossmann R, et al. Improved glucose counterregulation and autonomic symptoms after intraportal islet transplants alone in patients with long-standing type I diabetes mellitus. Transplantation. 1998;66(2):233-40.

60. Vinik A. Diagnosis and management of diabetic neuropathy. Clinics in Geriatr Med. 1999;15(2):293-319.

61. Cox DJ, Gonder-Frederick L, Julian DM, Clarke W. Long-term follow-up evaluation of blood glucose awareness training. Diabetes Care. 1994;17(1):1-5.

62. Perkins B, Olaleye D, Bril V. Carpal tunnel syndrome in patients with diabetic polyneuropathy. Diabetes Care. 2002;25:565-9.

63. Vinik A, Mehrabyan A. Diabetic neuropathies. Med Clin North Am. 2004;88(4):947-99.

64. Vinik A, Mehrabyan A. Diabetic monoradiculopathy/amyoradiculopathy. In: Therapy for Diabetes Mellitus and Related Disorders, 4th ed. Lebovitz H, ed. Alexandria, Va: American Diabetes Association; 2004: 416-23.

65. Watanabe K, Hagura R, Akanuma Y, et al. Characteristics of cranial nerve palsies in diabetic patients. Diabetes Res Clin Pract. 1990;10(1):19-27.

66. James P, Dyck B, Windenbank A. Diabetic and non-diabetic lumbosacral radiculoplexus neuropathy: new insights into pathophysiology. Muscle Nerve. 2002;25:477-91.

67. Vinik AI, Anandacoomaraswamy D, Ullal J. Antibodies to neuronal structures: innocent bystanders or neurotoxins? Diabetes Care. 2005;28(8):2067-72.

68. Sharma K, Cross J, Farronay O, Ayyar D, Sheber R, Bradley W. Demyelinating neuropathy in diabetes mellitus. Arch Neurol. 2002;59:758-65.

69. Krendel DA, Zacharias A, Younger DS. Autoimmune diabetic neuropathy. Neurol Clin. 1997;15:959-71.

70. Ayyar DR, Sharma KR. Chronic inflammatory demyelinating polyradiculoneuropathy in diabetes mellitus. Curr Diab Rep. 2004;4(6):409-12.

71. DCCT Research Group. The effect of intensive treatment of diabetes on the development and progression of long-term complications in insulin dependent diabetes mellitus. N Engl J Med. 1993;329:977-86.

72. UK Prospective Diabetes Study (UKPDS) Group. Effect of intensive blood-glucose control with metformin on complications in overweight patients with type 2 diabetes (UKPDS 34). Lancet. 1998;352:854-65.

73. UK Prospective Diabetes Study Group. Tight blood pressure control and risk of macrovascular and microvascular complications in type 2 diabetes: UKPDS 38. BMJ. 1998;317:703-13.

74. Tesfaye S, Chaturvedi N, Eaton SE, et al. Vascular risk factors and diabetic neuropathy. N Engl J Med. 2005; 352(4):341-50.

75. Ziegler D, Sohr CG, Nourooz-Zadeh J. Oxidative stress and antioxidant defense in relation to the severity of diabetic polyneuropathy and cardiovascular autonomic neuropathy. Diabetes Care. 2004; 27(9):2178-83.

76. Vincent AM, Russell JW, Low P, Feldman EL. Oxidative stress in the pathogenesis of diabetic neuropathy. Endocr Rev. 2004;25(4):612-28.

77. Bril V, Buchanan RA. Aldose reductase inhibition by AS-3201 in sural nerve from patients with diabetic

sensorimotor polyneuropathy. Diabetes Care. 2004; 27(10):2369-75.

78. Keen H, Payan J, Allawi J, et al. Treatment of diabetic neuropathy with g-linolenic acid. Diabetes Care. 1993;16:8-15.

79. Ziegler D, Nowak H, Kempler P, Vargha P, Low PA. Treatment of symptomatic diabetic polyneuropathy with the antioxidant alpha-lipoic acid: a meta-analysis. Diabet Med. 2004;21(2):114-21.

80. Vinik A. The protein kinase C-beta inhibitor, ruboxistaurin, for the treatment of diabetic microvascular complications. Expert Opin Investig Drugs. 2005;14(12):1547-59.

81. Vinik AI, Bril V, Litchy WJ, Price KL, Bastyr EJ, III (MBBQ Study Group). Sural sensory action potential identifies diabetic peripheral neuropathy responders to therapy. Muscle Nerve. 2005;32(5):619-25.

82. Somers DL, Somers MF. Treatment of neuropathic pain in a patient with DN using transcutaneous electrical nerve stimulation applied to the skin of the lumbar region. Phys Ther. 1999;79(8):767-75.

83. Hamza MA, White PF, Craig WF, et al. Percutaneous electrical nerve stimulation: a novel analgesic therapy for diabetic neuropathic pain. Diabetes Care. 2000;23(3):365-70.

84. Weintraub MI, Wolfe GI, Barohn RA, et al. Static magnetic field therapy for symptomatic diabetic neuropathy: a randomized, double-blind, placebo-controlled trial. Arch Phys Med Rehabil. 2003;84(5):736-46.

85. Bosi E, Conti M, Vermigli C, et al. Effectiveness of frequency-modulated electromagnetic neural stimulation in the treatment of painful diabetic neuropathy. Diabetologia 2005;48(5):817-23.

86. Leonard DR, Farooqi MH, Myers S. Restoration of sensation, reduced pain, and improved balance in subjects with diabetic peripheral neuropathy: a double-blind, randomized, placebo-controlled study with monochromatic near-infrared treatment. Diabetes Care. 2004;27(1):168-72.

87. Tesfaye S, Watt J, Benbow SJ, Pang KA, Miles J, MacFarlane IA. Electrical spinal-cord stimulation for painful diabetic peripheral neuropathy. Lancet. 1996; 348:1698-1701.

88. Khaodhiar L, Niemi JB, Earnest R, Lima C, Harry JD, Veves A. Enhancing sensation in diabetic neuropathic foot with mechanical noise. Diabetes Care. 2003;26(12):3280-3.

89. Wieman TJ, Patel VG. Treatment of hyperesthetic neuropathic pain in diabetics: decompression of the tarsal tunnel. Ann Surg 1995;221:660-5.

90. Dellon A. Treatment of symptomatic diabetic neuropathy by surgical decompression of multiple peripheral nerves. Plast Reconstr Surg. 1992;89(4):689-97.

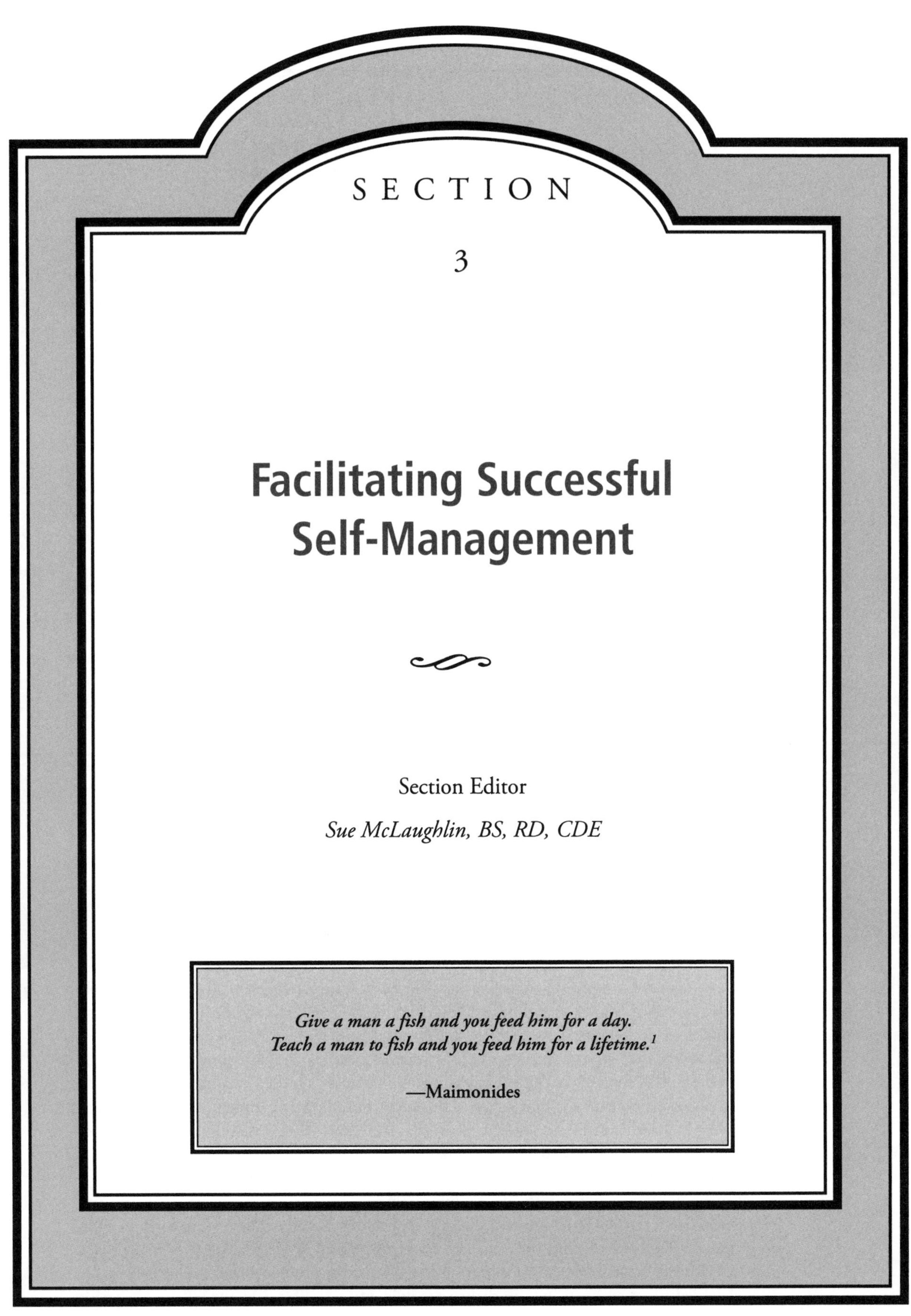

SECTION

3

Facilitating Successful Self-Management

Section Editor

Sue McLaughlin, BS, RD, CDE

Give a man a fish and you feed him for a day.
Teach a man to fish and you feed him for a lifetime.[1]

—Maimonides

SECTION 3 OVERVIEW

Sue McLaughlin, BS, RD, CDE

Give a man a fish and you feed him for a day.
Teach a man to fish and you feed him for a lifetime.[1]

—Maimonides

Simple yet provocative, these words of wisdom speak to the essence of education. Following the emergence of the team approach in the late 1970s to early 1980s, diabetes education has been increasingly recognized as being more than just the teaching of concepts about the disease. The diabetes care team has learned through experience that individuals with diabetes and their families must have more than a basic understanding of the physical effect that the disease process has on the body. Those whose lives are affected by diabetes must learn and be able to internalize behaviors that promote, over the long term, a healthy lifestyle and higher quality of life.

The material presented in Section 1 of the *Desk Reference* makes the following clear: to be effective, diabetes education must take into consideration the needs of the individual. Chapters in Section 2 show how medical knowledge related to diabetes and its complications needs not only to be well understood by the diabetes educator, but also must be translated and transformed by the educator into meaningful information and skills of value to those living with the disease. This final section of the book focuses on what all educators strive for, yet are not always successful in achieving—the *art* of our profession, which is the delivery of truly effective diabetes education, education whose outcome is positive behavior change. Section 3 of the book lays out the critical components of the education effort, elucidating how, through a behavior change curriculum, diabetes educators can help individuals develop and refine important self-management skills. Chapters in this section answer questions such as these:

- What are the keys to building a relationship of trust with the person affected by diabetes so that the individual is successful in achieving desired outcomes?
- How does the educator convey medical information in such a way that it makes an understandable and compelling argument for the learner? What can the educator do to guide individuals toward internalizing the components of diabetes management into their lives and viewing this as an achievement?
- What teaching strategies have been shown to be most effective in helping individuals across the spectrums of age, culture, and literacy levels?
- How does the diabetes educator assist the individual in determining short-, intermediate-, and long-term goals that translate into successful outcomes?

Material in Section 3 is organized around 2 areas of concentration: process and content. First, the fundamental approach to delivering diabetes education—assessment, planning, implementation, and evaluation—is delineated and discussed. Described in the literature as basic competencies in the Standards of Practice and Standards of Professional Performance for Diabetes Educators,[2] each step of this approach is dealt with separately in chapters 25 through 28. Then, in the final 7 chapters of the book, chapters 29 through 35, the overriding message of the book—that behavior change is best achieved by understanding what influences the individual's health behaviors and choices—is applied to the diabetes education curriculum. Specific content for diabetes education is outlined and articulated.

Approaches to teaching vitally important self-care behaviors are detailed at length in separate chapters, with an emphasis on identifying teaching strategies, pearls for practice, and proactive messages for patients at the end of each chapter. In addition, case studies or scenarios are included. They serve to illustrate chapter concepts, identify potential barriers that persons with diabetes may encounter, and facilitate discussion about problem-solving alternatives that the diabetes educator and person with diabetes may identify. Collectively, the self-care behaviors detailed in this section have been presented in the literature as the AADE 7 Self-Care Behaviors™ and identified in the National Standards for Outcomes Measurement.[3] They are dealt with more comprehensively here than in any other publication and made more powerful by the content that surrounds them in Sections 1 and 2. Chapters provide information on how self-care behaviors and outcomes measures can be applied to the practice of diabetes education in a practical and meaningful way.

Evident throughout this section is the paradigm shift that has occurred in diabetes education. The skilled diabetes educator of today does far more than deliver education and skills training. The educator's work is no longer primarily evaluated based on the learner's receipt or attainment of content and knowledge. Behavior change is the unique and expected outcome of diabetes self-management education; it is the measure of effective intervention by the diabetes educator as part of the diabetes care team.

The material in Section 3 is, in essence, the practical application or "how to" part of the *Desk Reference*. Within these chapters, readers find valuable information and examples that show how individuals with diabetes as well as diabetes educators and their colleagues may achieve successful outcomes by focusing on self-care behaviors, within a behavior change curriculum. This holistic approach recognizes that at the center of the diabetes team is the individual who has been diagnosed with diabetes. This person has all the wants, desires, fears, temptations and, at a minimum, as many challenges as the next person. He or she deserves to be given the same respect, appreciation, and nonjudgmental attitude as any other human being.

Finally, the material this section's authors have provided also serves to inspire and challenge readers to reexamine their teaching approaches and practices. Positive and meaningful experiences await those who incorporate these strategies and concepts into their work. Indeed, work is anticipated to become more personally fulfilling as a result. Lastly, success in implementing these lessons helps fulfill the broader mission and calling of those in the healthcare profession—to improve the lives of those afflicted by disease, to shape healthy and supportive communities, and to foster a culture that strengthens a society's health and quality of life.

Teach them to fish . . .

References

1. Rabbi Moshe ben Maimon (1135-1204), Jewish rabbi, physician, and philosopher (known also as Maimonides). Maimonides. Wikipedia Wikiquote. Available on the Internet at: http://en.wikiquote.org/wiki/Maimonides. Accessed 11 April 2006.
2. Martin C, Daly A, McWhorter LS, Shwide-Slavin C, Kushion W. The scope of practice, standards of practice, and standards of professional performance for diabetes educators. Diabetes Educ. 2005;31(4):487-511.
3. American Association of Diabetes Educators. Standards for outcomes measurement of diabetes self-management education (position statement). Diabetes Educ. 2003;29(5):804-16.

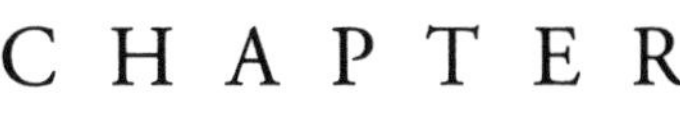

CHAPTER

25

Assessment: Gathering Information and Facilitating Engagement

Authors

James W. Pichert, PhD
David G. Schlundt, PhD

Key Concepts

- Understand the goals of assessments and effective strategies for conducting them
- Focus on recognizing and improving individual assessment skills in practice
- Use the opening part of the assessment to build trust and rapport, set expectations, and elicit priorities
- Learn alternatives regarding what and how to ask for needed information so that management plans and interventions best address the person's needs
- Appreciate the importance of skillfully eliciting concerns, values, misunderstandings, and priorities
- Identify alternatives to interviewing, such as questionnaires, surveys, and self-monitoring diaries for conducting assessments

Introduction

Diabetes educators are problem solvers. Their best solutions address persons' pressing problems. But real problem solving cannot begin until those real problems are revealed and understood. This chapter is the first of 4 in this section of the *Desk Reference* that focuses on the 4-step process of providing diabetes education. Assessment is first in the process:

Assessment → Planning →
Implementation → Evaluation and outcomes

By understanding what the interests, needs, and problems of the person with diabetes are, the diabetes educator is more likely to provide appropriate and useful information that will assist in meeting desired outcomes. This is the focus of the assessment.

This chapter contains a variety of practical tips and strategies about how to best obtain the information needed to facilitate productive problem solving. The method for achieving good assessments involves consistently creating environments in which persons with diabetes will honestly discuss their behaviors, outcomes, goals, motivation, resources, obstacles, assumptions, perceptions, and values. Because the educator cannot read another's mind, the educator must determine the appropriate scope and level of detail for each assessment interview, and then guide the interaction. Readers of this chapter will be challenged to practice any contents they believe may help them open their assessments, gain the trust of the persons they serve, ask appropriate questions, use various information-gathering strategies, and thereby set the stage for effective problem solving.

Overview of an Assessment

Fundamentally, diabetes educators are problem solvers.[1,2] The importance of the assessment cannot be stressed enough as the groundwork for their service in helping persons with diabetes learn to live well and cope effectively with the disease and its complications.

No one expects to learn all there is to know about a person in a single interview, let alone in the few minutes of time usually available. The objective of the assessment is to gather enough information to know the person sufficiently well so that the patient and the educator, as well as the care team, can collaborate on mutually satisfactory outcomes. Evidence from both research and clinical experience supports a 2-part method that is challenging but useful for accomplishing a successful patient-centered assessment.[3-12]

Two steps to successful, patient-centered assessment:

- Create an environment in which people feel comfortable talking about their needs, motivations, goals, problems, and feelings
- Artfully employ a range of assessment strategies and interviewing skills to develop an understanding of clients and their specific problems

The educator's very challenging task is to determine both the *scope* and *content* of individual and family assessments. If assessments are focused too narrowly, diabetes educators can miss important contextual information. Allowing assessments to range too broadly, however, can

Case in Point: A Man With Type 1 Diabetes of Long Duration

CT, a 39-year-old man with longstanding type 1 diabetes, has arrived for his appointment with a diabetes educator. He is sitting in the waiting area feeling discouraged about his diabetes care, in general, and his seeming inability to avoid hypoglycemia, in particular. CT has experienced several episodes of severe hypoglycemia in the past year, and he is concerned that he has lost some symptom awareness. He is very worried about acting stuporous or losing consciousness while driving, at work, and in social situations.

Meanwhile, the diabetes educator is reviewing CT's medical record. The diabetes education checklist reveals that most contents have been addressed over the past 24 months, with the exception of foot care education, despite the presence of an apparent slow-healing lower extremity wound, noted 6 months earlier. When the two meet a few minutes later, discussion confirms the following:

- History of a slow-healing, lower extremity lesion
- No prior foot care education, but willingness to spend time talking about foot care now
- Blood glucoses that have been running high

The educator delivers a carefully prepared, well-rehearsed lesson on foot care, designed to help any person with diabetes understand and remember. And CT does.

- Have this man's needs been met?
- While the educator had good intentions by evaluating the medical record and completing the checklist, was foot care education the most urgent concern of this person with diabetes?
- Might the educator have done anything differently?
- How and to what extent might the person's other needs for education and support have been taken into consideration?

As suggested above, the lack of an adequate assessment may cause an educator to miss the most pressing needs felt by persons with diabetes, their important health and life goals, and the problems posing obstacles to attaining desired goals. Effective assessments—the topic of this chapter—allow educators to spend more of their precious clinical time solving the highest-priority problems and promoting health and quality of life.

consume so much time that the educator is unable to accomplish anything specific and helpful.

Above all, diabetes professionals need to maintain some control of the direction and flow of the assessment portion of a clinical encounter if they are to have sufficient time to engage in problem solving. How, then, can diabetes educators learn the stories of the persons they treat while simultaneously—and reasonably efficiently—arriving at a specific plan for problem solving?

Conducting an Effective Assessment

The American Association of Diabetes Educators has defined the Scope of Practice, Standards of Practice, and Standards of Professional Performance for Diabetes Educators. The Standard for Assessment[13-14] is the first on the list. According to the Standards, "The diabetes educator conducts a thorough, individualized assessment of the person with or at risk for diabetes." The assessment process requires ongoing collection and interpretation of relevant data. As shown in Table 25.1, the Assessment Standard outlines both the information appropriate to obtain and an approach to obtaining it.

Characteristics of Effective Assessments

Effective assessments succeed in obtaining the information that is important in solving the pressing problems of the individual (or family) being served. The following are characteristic of an effective assessment:

- Effective assessments reveal lifestyle issues and factors
- They are patient-centered, elicit sufficient participation, and facilitate honest self-disclosure; they also involve family members and caregivers as appropriate
- They identify the needs of those in special populations and factors that interfere with an individual's activities of daily living; they effectively cross cultures to garner cooperation, information, and trust

TABLE 25.1 Data Needed for Effective Assessment

Approach to Gathering Information
A systematic and organized approach is called for, with data collected from the following sources: • From the person with diabetes • From family members and members of the client's social support network, as appropriate • From existing medical records • From referring healthcare providers
Data To Be Collected
Information on the following topics is appropriate to gather: • Health and medical history • Nutrition history and practices • Physical activity and exercise behaviors • Prescription and over-the-counter medications; complementary and alternative therapies uses and practices • Factors that influence learning, such as education and literacy levels, health beliefs, perceived learning needs, motivation to learn, and learning style (eg, audio, visual, kinesthetic) • Diabetes self-management behaviors, including experience self-adjusting the treatment plan • Previous diabetes self-management training, actual knowledge, and skills • Physical factors, including age, mobility, visual acuity, hearing, manual dexterity, alertness, attention span, and ability to concentrate; special needs or limitations requiring accommodations or adaptive support and use of alternative skills • Psychosocial concerns, factors, or issues, including family and social supports • Current mental health status, including history and treatment of eating disorders • History of substance use including alcohol, tobacco, and recreational drugs • Occupation; vocation; financial status; and social, cultural, and religious practices • Access to and use of healthcare resources
Data for Prediabetes Assessment
For an individual with prediabetes, the following information must be gathered in addition to the above information: • *Knowledge of Prediabetes and Risks:* Evaluate person's understanding of prediabetes and the risks associated with it • *Weight Loss and Weight Management:* Evaluate the person's understanding of the role of weight loss and weight management through nutrition modification and healthy eating in the management of prediabetes • *Physical Activity:* Determine the individual's habits and behaviors associated with physical activity and the individual's understanding of the role of physical activity in management of prediabetes • *Motivation:* Assess the individual's motivation skills for maintaining positive behavioral change

- Effective assessments find the high-priority problems to be solved

In the paragraphs that follow, these characteristics are discussed more fully.

Lifestyle Issues:

Effective assessments address lifestyle as well as diabetes-specific content

Most diabetes educators are aware of and very knowledgeable about the diabetes-specific elements of an assessment, as listed above. However, even this lengthy list presents only a portion of thorough assessments. It is important that diabetes educators employ strategies to learn about both the diabetes- and lifestyle-related components of assessments. The following are lifestyle-related aspects to be addressed:[15-16]

- Current behaviors
- Current outcomes and desired outcomes and goals
- Motivations
- Resources
- Obstacles
- Psychosocial and cultural contexts
- Assumptions
- Perceptions, cognitions, emotions, values

Patient-Centered:

Effective assessments are patient-centered

Diabetes management involves assessing the person's current eating habits, medication use, patterns of exercise and physical activity, acute and chronic complications, and other diabetes-specific contents captured in the Assessment

Standard. As suggested above, effective assessments must also evaluate and achieve an accurate understanding of a person's current lifestyle.[1-17] Together, the findings provide the clues needed to negotiate the sort of patient-centered management plans that will achieve the desired level of glycemic control with acceptable degrees of lifestyle change.

Effective assessments also reveal a person's existing or potential obstacles to self-management. Knowing these obstacles allows the educator to share realistic expectations concerning the difficulty of meeting glucose targets in everyday situations. Discussing obstacles and expectations sets the stage for subsequent assessments, during which the educator aims to help the person sustain those lifelong self-management practices that minimize complications while they maximize quality of life. Such assessments also help identify which behavioral strategies might best help an individual achieve and sustain successes in daily life.

Family and Caregivers:

Involvement creates challenges and opportunities

Every diabetes educator has had the experience of conducting assessments in the presence of family members. In general, directing questions to the person with diabetes is best, to learn his or her responses first. Asking the individual if there are any family members who assist them with diabetes care is helpful; if the answer is yes, the educator can suggest inviting them to the education session.

Family members may agree, disagree, elaborate on, or interrupt the person with diabetes' responses or try to provide all the answers themselves. Every one of these actions provides important assessment information and insights into family dynamics. Therefore, it is wise to have a strategy for anticipating and dealing with the potential problems (confusion, tangents, conflicting information) that undesired family responses can create. Many educators find it works best if they set the stage by explaining that they want to hear directly from the person with diabetes and that the family members will have a chance to add their insights afterward. Sometimes, clinicians choose to interview the person with diabetes and the family member separately. What is important is reassuring each party that their input is valued, but in the order most helpful in conducting the assessment.

Special Populations:

Special needs and challenges are brought to light

Assessments should attend to the special challenges frequently faced by members of particular population segments. For example, the population of older adults includes persons who possess the entire gamut of knowledge, skills and abilities; yet, compared to their younger counterparts, older adults suffer more physical limitations (eg, visual, auditory, olfactory, activity-limiting joint pain).

Importantly, 2 individuals who seem to have the same disease status may be assessed as quite different from one another. Each individual's functional ability reflects not only measures of metabolism and complications, but also one's capacity for adaptation (eg, the blind person with longstanding diabetes who has had substantial time to adapt plus successful rehabilitation training). Therefore, it is appropriate to address such factors during assessments. Similarly, an assessment of language preferences, literacy, and numeracy skills often needs to be conducted.

Practice Setting:

Setting affects the goals of the assessment

Assessments must be appropriate to the demands of the practice setting and the patient's previous history in that setting. For example:

- *Initial Inpatient.* Assessments conducted on inpatient units for immediate "survival" skills training and/or discharge planning must focus on those elements germane to those immediate needs.
- *Repeat Hospitalization:* A patient repeatedly hospitalized for DKA, on the other hand, will require a more specific, targeted assessment.
- *Outpatient:* Assessments conducted in outpatient clinics with high probability of continuous follow-up visits may be more comprehensive, at least over time.
- *Consultant:* Assessments conducted by consultants who refer persons with diabetes back to other professionals in "shared care" arrangements may focus on previously negotiated elements of the assessment standards.

Educators must understand and clearly explain the purpose of their assessments to the persons they are trying to serve. The educator's questions must be reasonably focused, yet allow enough flexibility so the person with diabetes can elaborate on his or her answers and provide information that assists in guiding and refining the educational process.

Activities of Daily Living:

Determines individual's ability to perform as desired

The questions that follow may help the educator understand how to help persons with diabetes with the activities of daily living that they value and wish to perform.

- Does the person have adequate skills to perform necessary self-care tasks and use standard instruction materials?

- Can the person read the lines on a syringe or medication container?
- Can the person see, read, and interpret the display on a blood glucose meter and the spot on which to apply a blood drop?
- Does the person need assistance in any of the following areas: shopping and preparing food appropriate to the meal plan, walking about the home, personal hygiene, transportation to medical appointments, social activities, and other important activities?
- What, if any, assistance is available from family, friends, colleagues, community, and social groups?
- Does the person want (or has the person had) any education in daily living skills?
- Does the person have adequate cognitive ability to learn new skills?
- Is the person so anxious, disoriented, or depressed by the diagnosis of diabetes or the onset of a new complication that learning a new skill would be extremely difficult? If so, more time may be needed for learning or teaching diabetes skills.
- Has the individual experienced short-term memory loss? If so, does he or she have adequate memory to learn new ways of performing reliable diabetes self-care?

Cultural Sensitivity:

Assessments of individuals from other cultures can be challenging

In addition to all the other strategies outlined in this chapter, sociologist Arthur Kleinman[18] recommends the following 8 questions for gaining insights into the health-and-disease-related understandings of individuals from other cultures:

- What do you call the problem?
- What do you think has caused the problem?
- Why do you think it started when it did?
- What do you think the sickness does? How does it work?
- How severe is the sickness? Will it have a short or long course?
- What kind of treatment do you think you (or the person) should receive? What are the most important results you hope will be achieved from this treatment?
- What are the chief problems the sickness has caused?
- What do you fear most about the sickness?

Eating behavior, food preferences, leisure time activities, and physical activities are all affected by ethnicity and culture.[19] A full discussion of this issue is beyond the scope of this chapter. Direct questioning about eating behaviors for both routine times and special celebrations may be required. Honesty is the best policy. For example, admitting, "I may not be as familiar with the foods you choose to eat day in and day out, so I would like to ask you some questions about them." Also, "My knowledge about the foods included in your holiday celebrations may not be correct. I would like to ask you some questions about them so that your diabetes care plan includes the traditional foods that you enjoy."

The diabetes educator should never assume that persons from other cultures share the educator's perspective about the world, their behavior, their relationships, or their health.

Pressing Needs:

High-priority problems are identified

The educator can remain task-focused by seeing the immediate objective as finding and defining the most pressing problems to be solved.[17,20] At the end of the assessment, the educator should be able to share with the person a brief summary of whatever problem(s) have been identified. For example, in the opening scenario, the educator might have identified both fear of severe hypoglycemia *and* need for foot care instruction as high priorities, even if time permitted only one to be fully addressed during that session. Understand and define the problem. Look beyond merely identifying the problem that needs to be solved and seek to understand the details surrounding it.

- How did the problem come about?
- What impact does it have on health, well-being, or quality of life?
- What has the person done previously to try to solve this problem?
- What coping strategies have worked and which have not?
- Do certain situations or conditions make the problem better or worse?
- How does this problem impact other aspects of the person's life, diabetes control, or ability to adhere to elements of the recommended health care regimen?
- How does this problem affect the family or status in the community?

These are just a few examples of questions that will help the educator develop a better understanding of a person's problems. There are many others. Table 25.2 presents many common influences that affect regimen adherence. Each entry in the table represents a type of everyday situation that makes adherence difficult and suggests interview questions to confirm the educator's hypothesis. These questions may be adapted to assess the influence of other lifestyle-related factors on the diabetes regimen and diabetes outcomes.[12]

TABLE 25.2 Assessing Lifestyle Effects on the Diabetes Regimen

Hypothesized Problem	*Description of Problem*	*Sample Interview Questions*
Negative emotions	You overeat, change frequency of exercise/glucose monitoring to cope with stress and negative feelings	Are there any situations in your life that are currently causing you a lot of stress? How does your regimen change when you feel upset, depressed, or stressed?
Resisting temptation	Foods, cues, and cravings tempt you to eat extra amounts of food; fatigue tempts you to do less exercise	What foods or situations trigger cravings? What foods or situations tempt you to eat inappropriately? What situations make it tempting to forego planned activity?
Being away from home and routines	Being away from home makes it hard to control what and how much you eat (eg, in restaurants) and when and how much you exercise or test glucose	How do exercise and testing differ when you are away from home? How do the amounts or kinds of foods you eat differ when you eat away from home or at a restaurant?
Feeling deprived	You feel deprived because you feel you cannot eat foods or do activities you enjoy, so you are tempted to give up and give in	How often do you feel like giving up on taking good care of your diabetes because it keeps you from eating the way you enjoy? What foods do you feel like you should give up eating?
Time pressure	Having many demands on your time makes regimen demands difficult	What kinds of social, family, or job pressures make it hard for you to find the time to take care of your diabetes the way you want to?
Tempted to relapse	When you feel discouraged or feel like a failure, you consider no longer trying to follow your diabetes care plan	How often do you feel so discouraged about your care plan that you want to just give up? Do you see your current plan as rigid or flexible?
Planning	A hectic schedule makes it hard for you to plan what and when to eat, how and when to exercise and test, even when to take medications	How difficult is it for you to plan when, where, and what you will do to follow your diabetes care regimen?
Competing priorities	Many responsibilities and obligations (eg, family and job) interfere with your ability to make healthy choices	What important priorities in your life get in the way of making healthy choices? Do you sometimes feel like you have to choose between good diabetes care and other important life goals?
Social events	Your care plan goes out the window at parties, holidays, special occasions, and other social events, especially those that involve food	How do the amounts or kinds of food you eat differ when you eat at parties or social events? How do parties and social events affect the other elements of your diabetes care plan?
Family support	Your family's behaviors do not support healthy choices	Describe the things your family does to support or hinder your efforts to manage your diabetes the way you want to?
Refusals	Someone offers choices of food or activity that you find hard to refuse	How hard is it for you to refuse tempting options for food or activity when someone offers them to you?
Friend's support	Friend's behaviors do not support healthy choices	Describe the things your friends do to support or hinder your efforts to care for your diabetes the way you want to.
All-or-nothing thinking	Seeing yourself and the world in black-and-white terms; alternating between being in control and out of control of self-care	How do you react when you are unable to achieve an important goal or if you are unable to stick to a plan? Are there times when you alternate between being in control and out of control?

(continued)

TABLE 25.2 Assessing Lifestyle Effects on the Diabetes Regimen

Hypothesized Problem	*Description of Problem*	*Sample Interview Questions*
Regimen complexity	Self-management plan has too many parts or is too difficult	How easy or hard is it for you to do each part of your care plan?
Fatalism	Nothing you do can change the outcome: "It's all in the hands of my Higher Power"	Do you believe that your efforts to follow this self-care plan will help keep you healthy?
Lack of confidence in regimen	You don't believe the self-management plan will work	Do you believe that following this self-care plan will help keep you healthy?
Other hypotheses		

Interaction: Alternative methods are used to elicit participation

Assessment is very much an interactive process. Unless the educator can engage persons in assessment interactions, little information will be obtained. The educator has to spend brief, but sufficient time building rapport.[21] Strategies to draw out reluctant participants include the following:

- Begin with easy questions
- Encourage each individual to feel free to speak
- Reassure each individual that discussions are confidential
- Show interest in what each person has to say
- Be accepting and nonjudgmental
- Be very slow to interrupt

Simply counting slowly (and silently) to 5 will create the kind of silence that (1) shows the educator to be patient and (2) helps the person become the one to break the awkward silence.

Trust and Rapport: Environment is created that supports honest self-disclosure

Honest self-disclosure occurs only when people trust each other. The educator's tasks are to develop an atmosphere of trust and to do so quickly. Therefore, the educator must avoid saying or doing things that will destroy a person's trust. Specifically, the most important thing an educator can do is to maintain an attitude of nonjudgmental acceptance.[1,22] This means listening, repeating, and asking more questions while avoiding criticism, sarcasm, horror, stereotyping, or disgust. Remaining nonjudgmental is especially important when working with persons from other economic, racial, and ethnic backgrounds. The educator's job is to learn of peoples' problems, progress, and successes—not to pass judgment on them.

Assessing problems and situations efficiently:

- Take charge of the interaction
- Ask appropriately direct questions
- Be willing to bring the interaction back on task

Educators no doubt feel there is always more information that could be obtained, but because their time is limited, they must limit the information sought to what is actually needed.[20]

Assessment Skills

In effective assessments, the diabetes educator uses 4 critical skills:[12]

- Gathers information
- Facilitates engagement
- Tests hypotheses
- Analyzes problems

Information Gathering

Information-gathering skills are the behaviors and strategies the educator uses to obtain data from individuals. These include skills related to the management of an interview session; for example:

- Opening and closing the assessment
- Using summaries and transitions
- Formulating appropriate questions
- Using various strategies to gather data about health and behavior

Facilitating Engagement

These are skills the diabetes educator uses to create a safe, trusting atmosphere in which the individual feels comfortable divulging details about personal health, self-management, and lifestyle. These include the following:[23]

- Listening skills
- Social skills
- Nonverbal behaviors

Hypothesis Testing

The process of identifying and understanding a person's problems is best accomplished via hypothesis testing. The most effective and efficient interviewers develop hypotheses—educated guesses—about problems that are specific to a particular person. As suggested in Table 25.2, the interviewer then asks questions designed specifically to elicit information that will eliminate some hypotheses and confirm others. Using a hypothesis testing approach, the educator can zero in on a problem and develop a sophisticated understanding of the issues in a relatively short period of time.

Problem Analysis

Problem analysis refers to developing an understanding of the "what's and why's" of a person's medical and self-management problems. Understanding the kinds of problems typically faced and the most common obstacles to behavior change helps the educator develop reasonable hypotheses. These can then be tested by asking pertinent questions, analyzing the answers, and thereby increasing the understanding of the issues for subsequent problem solving.

Opening the Assessment:

The time to create expectations, build trust, and signal transitions

Creating Expectations

It happens all too often: a person with a chronic disease enters the examination or teaching area, sits down, and the health-care provider begins asking a series of increasingly detailed and personal questions. The person answers, but wonders the entire time: "Why is this person asking me all these questions?" This approach generates suspicion and mistrust.

Effective Openings. Situations such as the one described above may be avoided by including an opening in every assessment. The most effective openings have 4 phases:

1. **Provide Brief Orientation.** Begin by introducing yourself, saying who you are, explaining why you have come, and stating in broad terms what you will be doing.
2. **Share the Objectives.** Tell the person what you hope to learn from him or her.
3. **Explain Rationale.** Provide a rationale that helps the person understand why you need this information and the benefits of disclosing this information.
4. **Assess Receptivity.** Invite the person's agreement to move on. Listen to and observe the response. Does the person find this proposal acceptable, or do they express reluctance, dissatisfaction, or discomfort? Be sure to listen to what the person says and observe nonverbal behaviors. Decide whether or not the person is ready to engage in assessment or whether more discussion and negotiation are necessary.

This 4-part process may appear time consuming, but the straightforward example given in the sidebar suggests how quickly these elements may be conveyed.

Opening the Assessment:

The chance to build trust and support

Orientation:	Briefly introduce yourself and what you will be doing
Objectives:	Describe the areas of information you need to address
Rationale:	Explain why you need this information
Receptivity:	Invite assent or comment so you can observe the reaction and what it tells you about the person you are assessing

Example

Clinician:	*I'm Bob and I'm one of the exercise specialists here. To help you choose the physical activities that will help you feel better, we need to start by asking some questions about your past experiences with exercise. The reason for this is to make sure that the kinds of exercises we recommend fit your interests and preferences. How does that sound to you?*
Client:	*Sounds good, but I hope we'll have time for you to address a couple of questions I've had . . .*

Building Trust and Rapport

Remember the Golden Rule, "Treat others as you would like to be treated"? Consider this a strategy for building trust and rapport in diabetes education and problem-solving sessions. Trust and honesty are integral to creating an atmosphere that promotes the educator's ability to obtain the needed information. The paragraphs below highlight a number of "do's and don'ts" that can help build a relationship of trust and good rapport.

Trust and Honesty:

Treat others as you would like to be treated

Do

- Build trust
- Encourage honesty
- Express empathy
- Accept unconditionally
- Listen

Do Not

- Use fear to motivate
- Be judgmental
- Interrupt too quickly
- Ignore feelings and emotions

Strategies that Develop Good Rapport

Build Trust

People trust other people and form collaborative relationships when they feel safe with them. Much of the work involved in building trust is nonverbal. Through both voice and body, express that the client can share information and feelings in this relationship without fear of judgment or criticism. All professional educators must strive to be culturally appropriate in provider-client interactions, but few in the profession are universally culturally competent. Therefore, one goal is to *avoid the most culturally inappropriate actions*—those that erode trust and interfere with collaborative relationships. Sometimes the healthcare professional must frankly admit that he or she does not understand everything the person would like them to with respect to someone's culture; the educator must follow-up, though, and express sincere interest in learning more about that culture with the client's help.

Similarly with families, one goal is to form and maintain to the greatest extent possible a bond of trust with all those involved in diabetes care, and especially the person with diabetes. When that is not possible due to significant cognitive, emotional, or physical disabilities, the bond of trust must be formed with the principal caretaker(s).

Encourage Honesty

Educators must tell people directly that they can be most helpful to the individual if the person agrees to be completely honest in this relationship. Reiterating the educator's commitment to confidentiality also helps.

Communicate Empathy

Empathy is being able to see things from the other person's point of view. *Experiencing* empathy is good, but, even better, educators need to *communicate* that they have seen things from the client's point of view.

Accept Unconditionally

This facet is essential if the assessment is to be useful. During an assessment, the educator needs to suspend judgment and refrain from criticizing or correcting the person being served. Showing disgust or revulsion at something a person has revealed serves only to inhibit the quality of further assessment information. Controlling personal reactions can be difficult because the tendency is to apply personal standards and values. There will be times when the educator is tempted to allow personal values to influence his or her response to another person. However, the health professional's goal is to be a helper and a facilitator. The way to help is by learning the truth about people's lives. Being judgmental during assessments—or any time—creates significant and sometimes insurmountable obstacles to achieving understanding. Even during subsequent problem solving, discussing the pros and cons of alternative behavior choices will likely be far more effective and persuasive than pronouncing judgments.

Listen Well

Virtually all health professionals have had the experience of missing things said during interviews because they were busy thinking about the next question, deciding the best way to address the person's emerging issues, or even daydreaming. The educator must not only ask good questions, but listen carefully to the answers. Listening includes attending to the words, to the meanings behind the words, and to the nonverbal behaviors that clarify or belie the words people say. Sometimes, more can be learned about persons and how they really feel about an issue by observing their nonverbal behaviors, rather than by accepting their words alone. When working with families or caretakers, observe and listen carefully to all parties, noting any discrepancies worthy of follow-up.

Strategies That Should Not Be Used

Do Not Use Fear to Motivate

Many health professionals believe they can motivate persons to change behavior via scare tactics. Saying things like, "do you realize that lung cancer is an agonizing way to die?" does little to motivate most persons to quit smoking. There is a difference between helping people see and understand the consequences of their choices and trying to scare them into doing something. In many cases, scare tactics are actually counterproductive, leading people to withdraw from the interaction, stop listening, and abandon the relationship and other relationships like it. Trying to frighten people clouds the atmosphere of trust that is so essential for building a working rapport.

Do Not Be Judgmental

This is important enough to emphasize again. There are many ways to be judgmental. Some are explicit, like responding to a description of a person's binge eating with, "that is disgusting." Others are less pointed (largely nonverbal), but felt nevertheless: such as shaking your head, rolling your eyes, averting your gaze, shaking or pointing your finger, or changing tone of voice. Guard against both the obvious and the subtle expressions of judgment.

Do Not Interrupt

When asking a client a question, give the person plenty of time to answer. If the person is talking, allow the person to come to some closure before asking another question. While it is important for the educator to be able to guide and direct the flow of an interaction, the educator must refrain from interrupting, or at least be very slow to interrupt when an interruption is needed to keep the assessment from straying too far afield.

Do Not Ignore Feelings and Emotions

Persons with diabetes often have very strong feelings, both positive and negative, about their health and their efforts to take care of their health. In doing a general assessment, topics will often come up that are permeated with strong emotional content. Part of being a good listener involves picking up on the client's emotional experience and acknowledging awareness of their feelings. Mostly, this involves summary comments like, "that must make you feel sad," or "you seem to be unsure of your ability to accomplish the goals you just set." Attending to emotion builds trust because the person is aware you are interested and listening carefully. Ignoring emotion makes the educator seem either insensitive or uncaring.[24,25] Some studies suggest that rates of depression are significantly higher among persons with chronic diseases, including diabetes, making it very important to attend to depression-related verbal and nonverbal cues.

Signaling transitions:

Transitions indicate movement from one content area to another during the course of the interview. For example:

> "Now that you've told me about your recent glucose values and we've established that they've been running high in the mornings, I'd like to ask you a few questions about your experiences lately with hypoglycemia, low glucose values."

Transition statements serve as signposts to mark progress through the interview. They serve to keep the interview, the interviewer, and the interviewee on track. As in the example, in many cases transition statements follow a summary of what was learned or decided during the previous interview segment. In effect, transitions provide the opening for each domain the educator has chosen to assess in the interview.

Knowing What to Ask:

You get what you ask for,
so ask for what you want

Interviewing skills usually take many years to master. In fact, most good interviewers will admit they still have much to learn and are improving all the time. One way an educator can improve his or her interviewing skills is to take the time, just a small amount, to identify how well the following techniques are employed.

Knowing What to Ask:

You get what you ask for,
so ask for what you want

Skills:

- Pause and think
- Be direct
- Ask for specifics
- Be persistent
- Ask follow-up questions
- Make mental notes
- Ask for examples

Strategies:

- Use direct questions
- Review regimen
- Review deviations from routine
- Propose hypothetical situations
- Inquire about common obstacles
- Recall a specific example

Pause and Think

One mistake health professionals can make is hurrying through an interview. When unsure what question to ask, the best strategy is to pause and think. The pause may seem long, but when most professionals see a videotape or listen to an audiotape of their interviews, they discover that these pauses are not long at all. Pausing for a moment to formulate a good question is far better than moving prematurely to another topic.

Be Direct

Some in the profession so strongly emphasize the use of open-ended questions during assessment interviews that they may leave an impression that close-ended questions have no place.

The authors of this chapter respectfully disagree. Every question asked by the educator should simply be the type that will provide the kind of answer needed:

- *To Elicit A Description:* Ask an open-ended question. For example: "Please tell me about your weekly exercise routine."
- *To Eliminate or Confirm A Hypothesis:* "Yes or no" questions may be more helpful. For example: "It sounds like other priorities get in the way with exercising. Do these include family responsibilities? Work?"

Ask for Specifics

The authors of this chapter have conducted research that has involved systematic observation and analysis of many videotaped conversations between individuals and their healthcare providers.[25-30] The findings show that many healthcare providers appear to take a great deal for granted. They ask a question, get a very general answer, and then move on to the next question. Those watching the video wonder what the professional really learned.

Very often, the educator must follow-up after initial questions, asking for more specific information. Such requests might be as straightforward as, "Can you please be more specific?" The response may reveal that the assumptions the educator made about the general answer were not correct and that a great deal more is learned by asking for specifics.

Be Persistent

Interviewers sometimes make the mistake of thinking they have only one opportunity to ask particular questions. The best interviewers know how to be persistent and to keep asking questions, even the same questions over and over again, until the necessary information has been obtained. A simple approach is to follow up with, "Please tell me more about that." Often asking the same question phrased in a slightly different way will allow the person to open up a little more and communicate useful information on the second or even third try.

Ask Follow-Up Questions

An important interviewing skill is to evaluate information right after it is given. This enables the interviewer to determine when a follow-up question may help to either clarify or provide more detail. Again, there is no rule that says once an educator has asked about a topic, the topic cannot be brought up again. The educator must listen carefully and ask good follow-up questions.

Make Mental Notes (or Jot Ideas Down)

Sometimes while individuals are talking about one topic, they reveal important pieces of information that stimulate a new or different hypothesis. Rather than jumping abruptly to a new topic before an assessment in one area has been completed, make a mental note, or, if need be, jot down a key word. This reminds the educator to move to the new subject once work on the current topic has been completed.

Ask for Examples

A simple way to obtain increasingly detailed and specific information from an individual is to ask for examples. When someone is providing a general description or speaking abstractly about a problem, have the person think about a recent incident and ask the person to describe the situation as one example of the general problem.

Knowing What to Ask:

Strategies for getting information

A variety of strategies may be used to systematically gather information.[3-17] Sometimes, especially when the educator does not have strong hypotheses about what the problem or problems might be, the following information-gathering strategies can help.

- Direct questions
- Regimen review
- Deviation review
- Specific examples
- Hypothetical situations
- Common obstacles

Direct Questions

Sometimes the best way to get information is to ask for it directly. Decide what information is needed, then formulate a question that will get at that information directly.

Regimen Review

A regimen review asks individuals to summarize or describe what they typically do to take care of themselves. For example: "Please tell me what you do to care for your diabetes in the morning when you get up."

Deviation Review

When asking people to describe their typical routines, ask them also to describe times when they deviate from their routines. The educator benefits from knowing both about usual routines and exceptions to them.

Specific Examples

People will often find it easier to provide details about a general problem or a behavior if asked to describe a specific example. Ask the person to recall a recent incident or day, and have them describe each episode in detail.

Hypothetical Situations

The educator can sometimes learn a great deal and have hypotheses confirmed or negated by posing a hypothetical situation. Hypothetical situations ask the person to consider what they would say, think, or do if a certain situation were to occur. For example, the educator might ask the person to describe what he or she would do at a restaurant after suddenly realizing that blood glucose testing supplies or insulin were left at home. Many times these hypothetical situations can provide a great deal of useful assessment information.

Common Obstacles

Hypothesis testing offers diabetes educators opportunities to evaluate whether any common obstacles to regimen adherence may be interfering with a person's self care.[1,2,12,17,26] When the person's diabetes control is not consistently in the target range, what might be preventing better self-care? Thoughtful educators will ask questions designed to reveal problems in areas such as these:

- Lack of knowledge or skill
- Competing priorities (lack of time)
- Treatment costs (money, social sacrifices)
- Habit patterns
- Family or social support
- Stress
- Unhelpful cognitions
- Language-learning difficulties
- Other aspects

The obstacles to adherence that are present (or may arise) can often be anticipated. When the educator sees potential trouble, assessing for its presence can relieve and help the person heading toward it. The assessment sets the stage for the educator and client to develop both a plan for overcoming existing obstacles and plans for dealing with potential ones. The focus is on helping the person devise new and more effective ways of responding to situations that present adherence obstacles. The person may be encouraged to practice or rehearse the plan to ensure success.

Hypothesis Testing:

Generating predictions and testing them during assessments

Areas for healthcare professional "hypothesizing":

- Assess readiness to change
- Assess knowledge and skill
- Assess adherence
- Assess obstacles to adherence

How to test hypotheses:

- Ask questions
- Listen to verbal cues and look for nonverbal cues
- Pose hypothetical scenarios and "what ifs"
- Provide hands-on tasks
- Ask patient to review the regimen, ie "day in their life"
- Request counter-examples and exceptions
- Request specific examples

Assessing obstacles to adherence:

- Lack of important knowledge or skill
- Costs and competing priorities
- Habitual behaviors
- Social support
- Stress and emotions
- Unrealistic expectations

Encouraging Participation:

If you do all the talking, how can it be an assessment?

Diabetes educators are accustomed to talking. Sometimes they find they have done most of the talking while, for most of the session, the person being assessed has been sitting quietly. When this occurs, the educator is unlikely to have obtained sufficient assessment information. Several strategies may be employed to encourage the client's active participation.

- Use active listening skills: clarify, paraphrase, reflect feelings, use minimal encouragers
- Give time to answer
- Summarize
- Give feedback

Give Time to Answer

Conducting an assessment can be difficult when the client is slow to respond or reticent. People have different response times, information processing rates, and social interaction styles. Not only that, these factors vary widely from one culture to another. Trying to rush the discussion along may be perceived as disrespectful. Especially in these cases, before moving on, be patient and provide enough time for inquiries to be answered.

Use Active Listening Skills

Most diabetes educators are aware of and employ 1 or more of 4 verbal and nonverbal behaviors generally referred to as active listening skills: clarifying, paraphrasing, reflecting feelings, and using minimal encouragers.

Clarification. Asking for clarification helps the interviewer ensure understanding of what has been said by the person. What the interviewer is doing is checking his or her understanding of a particular word, phrase, or idea used by the person. To ask for clarification, the interviewer can simply tell the person the word or words that are vague, ambiguous, or otherwise unclear, then ask for elaboration.

- For example: "Please tell me what you mean when you say you went on a diet?" If the person with diabetes has trouble responding and is accompanied by a family member or caretaker, the educator can consider whether it is "safe" to ask those persons to offer their insights as well.

Paraphrasing. Paraphrasing tells the other party that he or she has been heard and understood. The interviewer simply restates what the person has said in slightly different words that have the same meaning. A paraphrase need not be long. Paraphrasing responds to the factual or informational content of what the person is saying. Unlike clarification, paraphrasing does not involve asking a question. Instead, the interviewer confirms what was heard by restating it to the person.

- For example, a person may be describing difficulties with social support around meals in their family. The educator then says, "It sounds like your family is not very supportive when it comes to fixing healthy meals."

Reflecting Feelings. Reflecting feelings involves giving feedback to the person on the affective tone of what is being said. Thus, the emotion or feeling that is expressed in the person's verbal or nonverbal behavior is made explicit by reflecting feeling. Paraphrasing, in contrast, involves giving feedback on factual information. When a person is expressing an emotional reaction, reflect this emotion back to the person is often helpful. Sometimes, people are not aware of their emotional reactions, so by reflecting feelings, the interviewer is able to help them become more aware of how they appear to be reacting emotionally to a particular situation. Reflecting feelings can also be useful as a way for interviewers to check whether they are getting an accurate reading of the person's feelings about a particular event or situation.

- For example, a person might grimace and then ask, "My spouse told me I was looking a bit plump, so I wondered whether I needed to go on a diet?" The educator might reflect feelings by saying, "The comment about looking plump seems to be upsetting to you."

Minimal Encouragers. Minimal encouragers are the verbal and nonverbal behaviors people use to signal to another person that they are listening and the person speaking should continue. The best way for educators to learn how well they use minimal encouragers is to watch one of their interviews on videotape.

- Examples: eye contact while listening; nodding the head; saying little phrases like "yes," "continue," "uh-huh," and "ok"

One caveat: Avoid minimal encouragers if and when individuals engage in any kind of "jousting," such as blaming other professionals or family members for their poor control, for creating barriers to regimen adherence, or for their complications. People may interpret minimal encouragers as agreement with their negative evaluations of others. In such cases, the educator must be especially attentive to listening carefully, but studiously avoid any appearance of agreeing. Otherwise, the educator may become an enabler or encourager of such behavior. The educator may also one day hear from colleagues or family members who were surprised to hear the educator had "accused" them of some wrongful behavior.

Techniques important in closing:

Two techniques are important to employ during closure:

- Summarizing
- Giving feedback

Summarize

Summarizing is similar to paraphrasing, in that the interviewer restates what the person just said. However, a summary covers a greater amount of information and serves a more integrative function than paraphrasing. A summary allows the interviewer to see if he or she has learned the gist of what the person has been talking about. Summaries are appropriately used when the interviewer has gathered all the information he or she needs on a particular topic and is ready to move on to the next topic. A summary gives the person an opportunity to correct the interviewer's perception or to add information that has been omitted and also serves to create a smooth transition between topics.

Give Feedback

At the end of an assessment or when a portion of the assessment has been completed, the educator should give feedback to the individual. Feedback involves not just a summary, but an interpretation of what the educator learned in the interview. People generally appreciate feedback, especially when their particular problems are put into context. A man who is experiencing impotence may appreciate feedback that while this problem occurs in more than half of all men with diabetes, the educator really appreciates his willingness to share his problems and feelings.

Other Ways to Assess:

Alternatives to interviewing

While interviewing is the most important tool for gathering assessment information, several other techniques are worth using in certain situations.[1,2,13,14]

- Paper and pencil measures
- Biological data

- Self-monitoring
- Observation

Paper and Pencil Measures

The educator may use formal assessment tools such as inventories, forms, and questionnaires. A variety have been devised by experts to evaluate the behaviors of persons with diabetes. The chosen tool (whether selected from existing questionnaires or devised personally) should be designed with the following ideals in mind:

- The items are written in clear and easily understood language
- The way the person should respond is clearly defined
- Each item asks only 1 question
- Each item addresses a specific event or behavior
- If the questionnaire employs multiple choice responses, the alternatives cover the range of possible responses

Biological Data

There are many different biological tests and data that can be collected to help the educator answer assessment questions. For example, to know if a weight-loss program is working, collect body weight data. To assess blood glucose control, obtain an A1C or review the person's blood glucose log book or memory meter.

Self-Monitoring

Self-monitoring involves asking people to keep records of their behavior. For example, the person can be asked to self-monitor—count—the number of cigarettes smoked each day. A diary's purpose is twofold:

- *Provides the person* with immediate feedback on his or her success at meeting the treatment goal
- *Provides the healthcare professional* with an ongoing record of behavior that can be used to identify specific problems

Tips on diaries:

The following are some tips for obtaining high-quality self-monitoring data.

- *Definition.* The target behaviors to be monitored must be clearly defined.
- *Entries.* The person must be shown what kind of record to make when a behavior occurs. Ideally, the educator provides a clear, simple form for keeping records.
- *Use.* The person should be told where to keep the record and when to complete it.
- *Rationale.* Give a clear rationale for keeping records. Explain how the data will be used, and why a diary will be helpful. People who understand the importance of keeping good records are more likely to comply.
- *Willingness.* Make sure the person is willing to keep a diary.
- *Simplicity.* Make the record-keeping task as simple as possible.
- *Understanding.* Ask the person to reiterate the instructions. For example: "Tell me in your own words what I have asked you to record." Educators should not assume the person understands; in fact, they are often surprised that an assignment they thought was clear confused the client.
- *Receipt.* Make a note in the medical record to be sure to ask for the diary at the next meeting. When given a completed diary, give ample praise. Use the information in the teaching/counseling session. Help the person feel the effort was worthwhile.

Observe Behavior

Sometimes the educator has questions about a person's skills and abilities to do certain things. Arranging to observe the person performing the skill is often more preferable than simply asking about self-perceived capabilities. For example, to assess someone's skill in using a particular blood glucose meter, give them the meter and ask them to perform a blood glucose test. Use role-playing techniques, too. For example, give the person a restaurant menu and say, "please pretend I am the waiter and order a meal that fits the meal plan you just agreed to."

Summary

This chapter has discussed a variety of practical strategies and skills that are used to conduct assessments of persons with diabetes. A summary appears in Table 25.3. The major goal of the assessment is to come to understand the person and the problems that need to be addressed. The assessment process is a matter of generating and testing hypotheses. Skills that can be used to improve the educator's ability to conduct a good assessment include listening skills, questioning skills, and information-gathering strategies. For more information on developing cultural competence, see chapter 5, on social support; also, for information on learning styles, see chapter 3, on self-management of health.

TABLE 25.3 Effective Assessments at a Glance

Set the tone
- Decrease background sounds, especially for those who may have hearing or attention deficits
- Avoid interruptions
- Include family members, caregivers
- When addressing an elderly adult, speak clearly and face-to-face
- Avoid patronizing titles ("dear," "hon"); use formal salutations ("Ms. Jackson," "Dr. Jones")

Open and close effectively

Opening
- Orientation
- Objectives
- Rationale
- Receptivity

Closing
- Summary
- Transitions

Build trust and encouraging honest communication

Do:
- Build trust
- Encourage openness and honesty
- Form a collaborative relationship, including caregivers as appropriate
- Accept the person unconditionally
- Express empathy
- Be an active listener

Don't:
- Don't use fear or scare tactics
- Don't be judgmental
- Don't interrupt or hurry
- Don't ignore feelings and emotion
- Don't use jargon or unfamiliar terms
- Don't underestimate people's desire and ability to learn

Improve skill in information gathering
- Use this checklist while reviewing videotaped assessments
- Watch and emulate expert colleagues
- Offer to teach these skills to others

Ask good questions
- Pause and think
- Be direct
- Ask for specifics
- Be persistent
- Ask follow-up questions
- Make mental notes
- Ask for examples

Identify sensory and cognitive deficits
- Assess for hearing deficits
- Assess for visual impairment
- Assess for literacy and language problems
- Assess for cognitive impairment

Know what type of questions to ask
- Direct questioning (what you want to know)
- Regimen review: *What do you usually do?*
- Deviation review: *Tell me about exceptions or special circumstances*
- Specific examples: *Give me an example of when that happened*
- Hypothetical situations: *What would you do if...*

Encourage patient participation
- Allow time to answer, recognizing individual and cultural differences
- Use active listening skills
- Summarize
- Give feedback

Gather information using a variety of strategies
- Paper and pencil measures
- Biological data
- Self-monitoring
- Observe behavior
- Solicit information from client, family, caregivers

Acknowledge client's feelings and frustrations
- Listen to how it is said
- Watch body language
- Give feedback
- Be sympathetic

Focus on Education: Pearls for Practice

Teaching Strategies

- **View assessment as critical to problem solving.** An accurate and comprehensive assessment of current skills, knowledge base, and coping is the first step toward helping the individual with diabetes effectively create a plan. Spend more time listening than talking.

- **View the whole person.** Learn about the person—his or her joys, challenges, and expectations. This will assist you in identifying information to be taught and behavioral strategies to plan. When given permission to do so, include family members and significant others as a part of the assessment process.

- **Foster an atmosphere conducive to problem solving.** Build trust by maintaining a nonjudgmental attitude. Create an atmosphere that promotes honesty and trust. Learn the truth. The right atmosphere helps clients feel comfortable sharing details about their health, self-management, and lifestyle.

- **Identify special challenges.** Determine what may impact the individual's ability to manage diabetes. For example, visual or auditory problems will influence the methods of presenting educational information; joint-related problems will affect the type of physical activity the person is able to do; financial concerns may result in inability to get to clinic visits, fill medication prescriptions, or buy food. Family support or lack thereof has been shown to have a significant effect on successes in managing diabetes.

- **Incorporate new techniques.** Try new strategies for conducting assessments. Some options to consider are hypothesis testing, problem analysis, paraphrasing, and reflecting feelings. Videotape and review sessions to develop and refine these techniques. Teach a class to peers or a general in-service on assessment and interviewing skills.

- **Shadow a colleague.** Shadow diabetes educators with reputations for excellent skills (ask their permission). Identify the interviewing strategies and skills they use and resolve to emulate what is helpful.

- **Tune in to culture.** Be sensitive to differences in cultural and ethnic backgrounds during assessment. Appropriate voice tone, rate of questioning, and nonverbal cues are critical in establishing rapport and the success of future educational encounters.

Messages for Patients

- **Recognize your opportunities.** View the assessment process as one of many opportunities to share the successes, challenges, and concerns you have about diabetes management. Realize that assessment-type questions help the healthcare professional assist you by correctly targeting your personal goals.

- **Ask as well as answer.** No question or answer is silly or dumb. Clarify what each person on the care team is expecting and ask for help so you have a clear path to progress.

References

1. Anderson BJ, Rubin RR, eds. Practical Psychology for Diabetes Clinicians: How to Deal with the Key Behavioral Issues Faced by Patients and Health Care Teams. Alexandria, Va: American Diabetes Association; 1996.
2. Schlundt DG, Pichert JW. A behavioral approach to dietary intervention in IDDM. Diabetes Spectrum. 1995;8(1):60-3.
3. Lipkin M Jr, Putnam SM, Lazare A. The Medical Interview, Clinical Care, Education and Research. New York: Springer-Verlag; 1995:71-2.
4. Tresolini CP and the Pew-Fetzer Task Force. Health Professions Education and Relationship-Centered Care. San Francisco, Calif: Pew Health Professions Commission; 1994.
5. Lewin SA, Skea ZC, Entwistle V, Zwarenstein M, Dick J. Interventions for providers to promote a patient-centered approach in clinical consultations. Cochrane Database of Systematic Reviews. 2001;(4): CD003267
6. Greenfield S, Kaplan S, Ware JE. Expanding patient involvement in care—effects on patient outcomes. Ann Intern Med. 1985;102:520-8.
7. Orth JE, Stiles WB, Scherwitz L, et al. Interviews and hypertensive patients' blood pressure control. Health Psychol. 1987;6:29-42.
8. Smith RC. Patient-Centered Interviewing: An Evidence-Based Method, 2nd ed. Philadelphia, Pa: Lippincott Williams & Wilkins; 2002.
9. Lipkin M Jr, Frankel RM, Beckman HB, Charon R, Fein O. Performing the interview. In: Lipkin M Jr, Putnam SM, Lazare A, eds. The Medical Interview: Clinical Care, Education, and Research. New York: Springer-Verlag; 1995:75-6.
10. Stewart M, Brown JB, Donner A, et al. The impact of patient-centered care on outcomes. J Fam Pract. 2000;49:796-804.
11. Swenson SL, Buell S, Zettler P, White M, Ruston DC, Lo B. Patient-centered communication: do patients really prefer it? J Gen Intern Med. 2004;19:1069–79.
12. Schlundt DG, Pichert JW, Gregory B, Davis D. Eating and diabetes: a patient-centered approach. In: Practical Psychology for Diabetes Clinicians: How to Deal with the Key Behavioral Issues Faced by Patients and Health Care Teams. Anderson BJ, Rubin RR, eds. Alexandria, Va: American Diabetes Association; 1996.
13. Funnell MM, Hunt C, Kulkarni K, Rubin R, eds. A Core Curriculum for Diabetes Education, 3rd ed. Chicago, Ill: American Association of Diabetes Educators; 1998.
14. Franz MJ, ed. A Core Curriculum for Diabetes Education: Diabetes Education and Program Management, 4th ed. Chicago, Ill: American Association of Diabetes Educators; 2001.
15. Roter D, Hall JA, Kern DE, Barker LR, Cole KA, Roca RP. Improving physicians' interviewing skills and reducing patients' emotional distress: a randomized clinical trial. Arch Intern Med. 1995;155:1877-84.
16. Roter DL, Hall JA. Physicians' interviewing style and medical information obtained from patients. J Gen Intern Med. 1987;2:325-9.
17. Schlundt DG, Rea MR, Kline SS, Pichert JW. Situational obstacles to dietary adherence for adults with diabetes. J Am Diet Assoc. 1994;94:874-6.
18. Kleinman A. The Illness Narratives: Suffering, Healing, and the Human Condition. New York: Basic Books; 1988.
19. Lipson JG, Dibble SL, Minarik PA, eds. Culture and Nursing Care: A Pocket Guide. San Francisco, Calif: UCSF Nursing Press; 1996.
20. Branch WT, Malik TK. Using 'windows of opportunities' in brief interviews to understand patients' concerns. JAMA.1993;269:1667-8.
21. Cohen-Cole SA, Bird J. Function 2: building rapport and responding to patient's emotions (relationship skills). In: The Medical Interview: The Three-Function Approach. Cohen-Cole SA, ed. St. Louis, Mo: Mosby Year Book;199:21-6.
22. Suchman AL, Markakis K, Beckman HB, Frankel R. A model of empathic communication in the medical interview. JAMA.1997;277:678-82.
23. Nardone DA, Johnson GK, Faryna A, Coulehan JL, Parrino TA. A model for the diagnostic medical interview: nonverbal, verbal, and cognitive assessments. J Gen Intern Med. 1992;7:437-42.
24. Robinson JW, Roter DL. Psychosocial problem disclosure by primary care patients. Soc Sci Med. 1999;48:1353-62.
25. Lang F, Floyd MR, Beine KL. Clues to patients' explanations and concerns about illnesses. Arch Fam Med. 2000;9:222-7.

26. Pichert JW, Lorenz RA, Schlundt DG, Stetson BA. Adherence-related questioning by fourth year medical students interviewing ambulatory diabetic patients. Teach Learn Med. 1989;1(3):146-50.

27. Stetson BA, Pichert JW, Roach RR, Lorenz RA, Boswell EJ, Schlundt DG. Registered dietitians' teaching and adherence promotion skills during routine patient education. Patient Educ Couns. 1992;19(3):273-80.

28. Pichert JW, Roach RR, Lorenz RA, Boswell EJ, Schlundt DG. Translating the "Effective Patient Teaching" course to a second university setting. J Nutr Educ. 1994;26(3):149-52.

29. Gregory RP, Pichert JW, Lorenz RA, Antony M. Interviewing skills of dietetic interns and experienced dietitians. J Nutr Educ. 1995;27(4):204-8.

30. King EB, Schlundt DG, Pichert JW, Kinzer CK, Backer BA. Improving the skills of health professionals in engaging patients in diabetes-related problem-solving. J Cont Educ Health Prof. 2002;22:94-102.

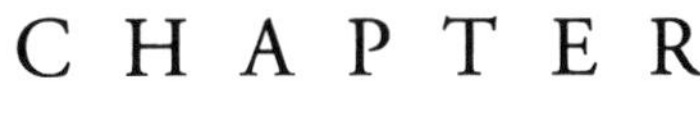

CHAPTER 26

Developing the Plan for Education

Author

Melinda D. Maryniuk, MEd, RD, CDE, FADA

Key Concepts

- Successful management of diabetes requires collaboration between the person with diabetes, the healthcare providers, and others in the support system.
- Planning is the second step in the diabetes self-management education and training process. Planning is included in the AADE Standards of Professional Practice for Diabetes Educators. The plan for education must be individualized and appropriately paced and address not only the objectives outlined in the medical plan, but equally or more importantly, the needs and capabilities of the person with diabetes.
- Key components of the planning process include the following. (*1*) Specific, desired outcomes are addressed. (*2*) Specific instructional strategies to be used are identified; these reflect the needs, skills, learning styles, and preferences of the person seeking assistance. (*3*) Respect for the individual's cultural, lifestyle, and health beliefs is demonstrated. (*4*) A dynamic plan for diabetes self-management education (DSME) is included that reflects inevitable changes in the individual's needs and goals. (*5*) A description of the process to be used for evaluating effectiveness is included. (*6*) DSME is recognized as a lifelong process.
- Effective education plans differentiate between learning objectives and behavioral objectives and recognize that both are essential and should not be substituted for each other.
- To meet the American Diabetes Association's Education Recognition Program (ERP) criteria, documentation of the education provided must be included in the medical record of all individuals who have received diabetes education.
- Group education is the method recognized for Medicare reimbursement; however, the diabetes educator must determine if the individual would be better served by a one-on-one session. If so, this must be communicated immediately to the physician.
- Skill sets that promote effective learning in groups include consideration of the teaching environment, including space, room arrangement, sound, lighting, and teaching materials (handouts and audiovisuals).
- The empowerment model of diabetes education provides information to enable people with, or at risk for, diabetes to make informed decisions about their behaviors, rather than providing information so the person knows why behaviors need to change.
- According to the Chronic Care Model, optimal chronic care is achieved when a prepared, proactive healthcare team interacts with an informed, activated patient.

Introduction

Planning and goal setting is a critical component in successful diabetes self-management education (DSME). This chapter discusses the components of the planning process listed below:

- Overview of planning
- Considerations
- Skills for developing the education plan
- Writing objectives
- Implementing the plan
- Adapting quickly to change
- Personal improvement for professional development

Case in Point: An Education Plan

DS, a 72-year-old widow, had patiently answered all the questions asked of her by the diabetes educator. Six months prior, she had learned she had type 2 diabetes. She had been taking metformin (Glucophage) since then. The objectives from the referring physician that were communicated to the diabetes educator were to teach DS insulin injection skills, since DS would be starting on glargine (Lantus), and record keeping for self-monitoring of blood glucose (SMBG). The physician also recommended that DS attend the "Balance and Control" comprehensive education series that took place on 5 consecutive Wednesday afternoons.

The diabetes educator had learned about DS's medical history, including that her blood pressure had been controlled on medication for the past 10 years. DS demonstrated correct skills for monitoring, but did not know target glucose goals, when to monitor, and what to do with the results. DS took care of her grandchildren most afternoons while her daughter was at work. She loved to play piano, but complained that the frequent blood glucose (BG) checks made her fingers sore.

After the assessment discussion, the diabetes educator proceeded to demonstrate proper insulin injection technique and discuss the importance of writing the results of SMBG in a logbook. The educator instructed DS to bring the logbook to her next visit and told her how to register for the afternoon diabetes class series.

In the medical record at the end of the visit, the diabetes educator wrote the following:

The patient was instructed to

- Inject insulin and rotate sites
- Record BG results in a record book
- Attend diabetes education classes

Is the plan based on the assessment? Is the plan personalized and patient centered? Does it focus on key priorities? Does the plan that was documented illustrate learning objectives or behavioral objectives? As the chapter progresses, readers gain insight to answer these questions.

Overview of Planning

He who fails to plan, plans to fail.
—A proverb

Planning is the part of the DSME process that involves the selection of specific interventions and goals based on a multifaceted assessment. Planning requires collaboration between the diabetes educator, the person seeking assistance (and family members as appropriate), the referring provider, and other members of the healthcare team to ensure a mutually agreeable, individualized, realistic, and effective approach to DSME.

As described in the chapter on assessment, the major goal of the assessment is to understand the person seeking assistance and the problems that need to be addressed. The next step is to take that assessment information and develop a plan that is personalized and appropriately paced and that prioritizes both the needs of the medical plan and the wants and desires of the person seeking assistance.

A therapeutic plan based on the assessment is essential to individualize the intervention and to select and prioritize the knowledge, skills, and behaviors that may be addressed by the diabetes educators. In this way, the intervention becomes tailored to the individual's specific needs. Also, the likelihood that suggested behavior changes will be adopted, resulting in improved clinical indicators and quality of life, is increased. During the planning phase, the diabetes educator identifies the outcomes to be monitored and measured throughout the DSME process. Understanding the variables that may affect the plan assists the diabetes educator in defining plans that are flexible and realistic.

At its most basic level, the education plan is an outline of the participant's individual objectives for the education program. The plan can be documented simply and succinctly using a checklist of common behavioral objectives. In Figure 26.1, the education documented indicates that although this person is competent in monitoring skills, additional teaching is needed to ensure that monitoring is actually done according to the recommended plan and that the results are used.

Diabetes, or the management of any chronic illness, requires collaborative management. Collaborative management is care that strengthens and supports self-care in chronic illness while assuring that effective medical, preventive, and health maintenance interventions take place. Goal setting and planning are essential elements of health care that can enhance collaborative management.[1] This

Assessment Summary Date: 2/3/06	*Basic Diabetes Self-Management Skills*	*Instruction Given*					*Goal reached*
		Insert total time spent with patient below.					
		60 min					
		Date: 2/3/06	*Date:*	*Date:*	*Date:*	*Date:*	*Date/initial*
	Monitoring						
(1) 2 3 0	Demonstrates monitoring skill						✔ 2/3/06 MM
1 (2) 3 0	Monitors BG according to plan						
1 2 3 (0)	Uses results of monitoring						
3	Identifies meter and locations for alternate site BG monitoring	✔					

1=competent, 2 = review needed, 3 = full education needed, 0 = not applicable

Source: Education record (sample section) from Joslin Diabetes Center, Boston, Mass.

FIGURE 26.1 Sample Education Record

occurs after the person seeking assistance and the person providing diabetes education mutually agree on the specific problem(s) to be addressed. Action planning has the following steps:

- Identify options for achieving a goal
- Choose 1 option
- Develop specific implementation plans, foreseeing obstacles and making a commitment to put the plan into effect

What You Must Think About

Organizing is what you do before you do something, so that when you do it, it is not all mixed up.

—A.A. Milne

The AADE lists planning as a Standard of Professional Performance for Diabetes Educators. As defined by the AADE, the diabetes educator develops the DSME plan to attain the mutually defined outcomes. The plan integrates current diabetes care practices and established principles of teaching and learning. The plan is coordinated among the diabetes healthcare team members, the person with, or at risk for, diabetes, his or her family and other relevant support systems, and the referring provider.[2]

This standard further defines measurement criteria that the planning process should include, as follows:

- Addresses specific desired outcomes
- Identifies and describes specific instructional strategies to be used—these must reflect the needs, skills, learning style, and preference of the person with diabetes
- Demonstrates respect for the individual's cultural, lifestyle, and health beliefs
- Uses measurable, behaviorally focused terms
- Recognizes the DSME plan as dynamic, and the plan reflects inevitable changes in an individual's needs and goals
- Describes the process to be used for evaluation of effectiveness
- Recognizes DSME as a lifelong process—because of the chronic nature of the disease, the evolving knowledge related to management of diabetes, and the changing needs, desires, and abilities of the person living with the disease

In addition, the Education Recognition Program (ERP) of the American Diabetes Association (ADA) requires that an education plan be documented in every patient's medical record.[3] Auditors are instructed to review a selection of diabetes education records to ensure there is documentation of an education plan. This is defined to include both measurable learning objectives and patient-selected behavioral objectives that are based on the assessment.

Case—Part 2: Recognizing Priorities

If the educator had been listening more carefully during the assessment and not focusing primarily on meeting the requests of the referring provider, the educator's teaching priorities would have been reorganized.

A more collaborative approach might have led the diabetes educator to recognize that DS could not attend afternoon education classes until childcare options for her grandchildren were addressed. Also, DS was not recording BG results because she was not doing any checks (due to the discomfort in her fingers). Despite the fact that she listened respectfully to the educator as the insulin injection process was described, DS had no intention of following through with this therapy because she had heard insulin can make your diabetes worse and leads to blindness.

A better plan for DS would have been to explore a bit more about the sore fingers and the reasons that results were not recorded. The diabetes educator might have discovered that DS had virtually stopped checking (therefore, no results to write down) due to the discomfort in her fingers. When the diabetes educator presented the options of alternate sites for checking blood glucose, DS was most interested. Thus, the priority goal for teaching was to address DS's concerns first.

Based on this standard, there are several things to think about in developing an effective education plan:

- The education plan has to be mutually determined
- The plan must have buy-in from the person for whom it is developed
- Teaching strategies used must match learning styles
- The plan must differentiate between learning objectives and behavioral objectives
- The plan should use checklists as a guide, not a crutch
- The person for whom the plan is developed must be understood and respected as an individual

Each of these topics is discussed in the paragraphs that follow.

Mutually Determine Education Plans

An important part of assessment is understanding the individual's expectations and desired outcomes as well as those of the referring provider. They may not be the same. In addition, while conducting the assessment, the diabetes educator may identify additional needs that should be addressed in the education plan, including the needs and objectives that may be described by family members who are part of the visit. The skilled educator will identify all the areas that need to be covered for comprehensive education and then carefully outline the options for how this can be accomplished over time.

Obtain Buy-In

Successful diabetes management involves lifelong learning. The best education plan is of very little value if the person with diabetes never returns for follow-up visits or additional classes. Establishing an ongoing relationship with a diabetes educator, similar to that established with the primary care provider, can be discussed during the initial education encounter.

Discuss commitment to attend follow-up visits

Perhaps the most important objective of the education plan is to have the person with diabetes state the importance of keeping appointments and commit to a follow-up visit. This may raise a discussion of possible barriers to coming to class.

Match Teaching Strategies to Learning Styles

Each individual has character traits, personality styles, and learning preferences that can affect the overall education intervention. Acknowledging that these differences exist is an important first step by the diabetes educator toward adapting and adjusting teaching styles.

Each individual comes into a DSME encounter with personal preferences for learning new information. Some people prefer to watch a video. Others prefer to read. However, experts agree that most participants benefit from sessions that are as interactive as possible, rather than a lecture format in which the educator tells people what to do. Although Medicare regulations dictate that most patients receive their education in a group setting in order to qualify for reimbursement, the following are exceptions:[4]

- No group session is available within 2 months of the date the education is ordered
- The individual has severe vision, language, or hearing limitations
- Other conditions are identified by the treating physician or nonphysician practitioner

Match educational materials to health literacy skills

Since so much of what is typically delivered in traditional diabetes education relies on a considerable amount of written material, health literacy skills must be assessed and addressed in the planning process.

When interventions are tailored according to an individual's literacy needs, patient outcomes will improve, as demonstrated in a diabetes disease management program.[5] A validated knowledge scale has been developed for use with patients with type 2 diabetes and poor literacy, entitled Spoken Knowledge in Low Literacy Patients with Diabetes (SKILLD). It is administered orally and takes less than 10 minutes to complete.[6] Chapter 27, on implementation, provides more information on meeting literacy needs.

If the education assessment indicates that individual instruction would better meet a person's needs, then the diabetes educator should let the referring physician know this promptly, so the referring provider can document this request.

Differentiate Between Learning and Behavioral Objectives

There are 2 kinds of education plans that may be set at a single educational encounter. As part of the initial interview and assessment process, the diabetes educator determines the purpose of the visit (as requested by the referring provider) as well as the needs described by the individual. From that assessment and with the individual's agreement, an education plan with learning objectives for the visit is established. At the end of the session, behavioral objectives are determined, specifying what the individual will do at home and before the next visit.

Use Checklists as a Guide, Not a Crutch

Most diabetes educators rely on forms and checklists to streamline the documentation process and to help ensure compliance in documenting an education plan. Of course, no checklist is ever perfect for every individual. The diabetes educator must recognize when modifications need to be made to a checklist so that specific issues unique to an individual may be addressed. For example, in Figure 26.1, which outlines monitoring skills, the diabetes educator may add another learning objective, such as this: "Identifies meter and locations for alternate site BG monitoring."

Understand and Respect Each Person as an Individual

Each individual comes for DSME with a unique set of experiences. These experiences affect the individual's ability to learn and level of readiness to change behaviors. The individual's cultural, lifestyle, and health beliefs may be very different than those familiar to the health educator, and this needs to be acknowledged, honored, and respected. A large body of research underscores the existence of disparities in health care. The literature shows that US racial and ethnic minorities are less likely to receive routine medical procedures and more likely to experience a lower quality of health services compared to their counterparts in the white population. This research is summarized in a report published by the Institute of Medicine titled *Unequal Treatment: Confronting Racial and Ethnic Disparities in Health Care.*[7] The Web site of the Office of Minority Health of the US Department of Health and Human Services (www.omhrc.gov/templates/browse.aspx?lvl=1&lvlIID-13) offers resources on cultural competence for healthcare professionals as well as links to patient education materials in different languages.

An analysis of data from the 2001 Behavioral Risk Factor Surveillance System demonstrated that frequency distributions of selected diabetes management variables were widely variant across levels of race/ethnicity. Overall, those in the Hispanic population were significantly less likely to have positive self-management behaviors.[8] When the provider understands the cultural factors and beliefs that can contribute to these differences, more tailored and effective interventions can be designed.

Case—Part 3: Defining Learning and Behavioral Objectives

The documentation by the diabetes educator in DS's medical record did not list objectives of either kind: learning or behavioral. The educator only documented what she did, not what DS's learning objectives were, nor what DS would aim to do behaviorally once at home.

The objectives listed in Figure 26.1 are a better example of learning objectives. A particular advantage of this type of education record is the opportunity to set up a plan over time and then note (in the far right column) when the objective has finally been met.

The differences between learning objectives and behavioral objectives are described in more detail later in this chapter. Recognizing that both are essential and one does not replace the other is important.

A Word About Children. The examples and scenarios in this chapter deal primarily with the adult learner. Readiness to learn in childhood changes considerably with age and maturation.[9] A wide array of caregivers, including parents, siblings, grandparents and other family members, the primary care provider, school personnel, coaches, and babysitters are included as part of the healthcare team and considerable planning must occur for all to be included in the education process at relevant times. In addition to imparting facts and teaching practical skills, diabetes education should promote desirable health beliefs and attitudes in the young person. This is often best accomplished in a setting where age-appropriate peer education can occur, such as in summer camps or moderated Web site discussion boards.[10]

Skills for Developing an Education Plan

Proper preparation prevents poor performance
—Charlie Batch

The development of a successful education plan requires the diabetes educator to use a number of important skills:

- Synthesis of information
- Maintaining engagement
- Prioritizing interventions
- Developing objectives
- Targeting outcomes

Synthesizing Information

During the assessment phase, a considerable amount of information is gathered from a variety of sources including the person, family, referring provider, and medical record. The challenge of the diabetes educator is to analyze all available information and propose a realistic plan within the time constraints of the visit.

Maintaining Engagement

Just as with the assessment process, in which an essential skill is facilitating engagement, the educator needs to maintain that connection. Thoughtful communication on the part of the educator includes not only the words, but paying careful attention to the tone of voice, body language, and pace of language so the person seeking assistance does not feel rushed and thus feels comfortable in dialogue.

Cultural Considerations

Since studies confirm that culture influences the effectiveness of health care, diabetes educators are encouraged to become familiar with the health-related cultural influences of the populations they are most likely to encounter. Ensure that educational materials are not only available to meet the language needs of your patients, but that they are culturally appropriate as well. A list of traditional American foods translated into Spanish will not work for most individuals of Hispanic background! Consider incorporating community health workers into the healthcare team. Generally, these lay health workers are trusted and respected members of the community who act as a link between the healthcare system and the community.[8]

Prioritizing Interventions

In most cases, the assessment will reveal more that should be taught or reviewed than can possibly be covered in a single class or individual appointment. The educator must prioritize the learning objectives into those that must be handled immediately (for patient safety, such as hypoglycemia teaching, if starting on insulin) and those that can wait. Principles of adult learning theory (discussed in chapter 27, on implementation) should be kept in mind when setting priorities; this increases the likelihood for success. For example, adults learn best when they feel the need to know, when it relates to what is already known, when it is made personally relevant, and when it is active and not passive.[11]

One technique to help engage an individual in setting priorities is to show a comprehensive list of all the possible topics that can be covered over time through diabetes education. This serves to illustrate that everything cannot possibly be done in a single session (as some individuals think!). A tool such as this also helps in the collaborative selection of goals. The educator might ask that individual, "As you look over this list, is there something you see that is of particular interest to you to discuss right now?" As the person thinks about the banquet she has been invited to attend this weekend, she might reply, "Yes, I would like to talk about eating out when there is lots of food around."

Targeting Outcomes

The desired outcomes must be clearly specified and mutually agreed upon. To do this, ideally, the educator must obtain as much information as possible from the referring provider regarding his or her desired outcomes of the education session. These outcomes may be knowledge based, behavior based, or clinical. For example, the educator and person with diabetes both need to know the provider's targets for A1C and blood glucose levels in order to set up realistic action steps and expectations.

As described by the AADE position statement on Standards for Outcome Measurement, behavior change is the unique outcome measurement for DSME.[12] So although an A1C of 7% is a goal to aim for, the diabetes educator will be able to more effectively plan counseling strategies and measure success if behavioral interventions are selected to drive toward outcomes that would lead to this goal. For example, goals of taking medications as prescribed, eating according to the meal plan, and following the exercise recommendations are behaviors that will target this outcome.

Variations in outcomes desired by the person with diabetes, versus those desired by the diabetes clinicians, must be discussed and rectified. For example, if the person defines losing 100 lb and staying off insulin as the desired goal, the educator will need to discuss a more realistic set of outcomes.

Developing Objectives

An important aspect of designing the education plan is developing objectives that are mutually agreeable—to the person with diabetes, the referring provider, and the diabetes educator—that will result in improved outcomes. Emphasis should be placed on behaviorally focused outcomes. The initial assessment should include documentation of activities for each self-care behavior, as in the AADE 7 Self-Care Behaviors™. The documentation must be quantifiable and objective so that subsequent assessment of these same targets can easily demonstrate if changes have been made. For example, if the learning objective is to increase physical activity and the person's selected behavioral goal is to record 8000 steps per day on a pedometer, then it is good idea to record a baseline pedometer measurement so progress can be measured. The following section provides more detail on writing objectives.

Writing Objectives

A goal properly set is halfway reached.
—Zig Ziglar

"Diabetes self-care behaviors should be evaluated at baseline and then at regular intervals during and after the education program." This is 1 of the 5 AADE Standards for Outcomes Measurement of Diabetes Self-Management Education.[13] A required component of a diabetes education program recognized by the ADA is for each patient to have a specific action plan including at least 1 self-selected behavior change goal that is monitored over time.[3]

Action Planning

Action planning has been found to be an effective component of health education programs.[14] Polonsky (written communication, January 2006) describes the critical elements of action planning to include the following:

- *Specificity:* The patient clearly understands exactly what he or she needs to do
- *Reasonableness:* The patient believes the plan for action is achievable
- *Patient Centered:* The patient perceives some sense of personal ownership of the plan and its development; it is not merely a set of instructions delivered by the educator
- *Meaningfulness:* The patient perceives that accomplishing the plan will be of personal value

An excellent example of how behavioral objectives that meet these criteria can produce positive outcomes is illustrated in a study assessing implementation intentions. Sheeran and Orbell[15] asked a sample of 114 women to make appointments for cervical cancer screening. Half of the sample served as controls (ie, they were given no further instructions), while the remaining half were asked to specify in writing their intention to implement this recommendation. They were asked to write down when, where, and how they would make the appointment. Of this latter group, 92% attended screenings. In contrast, only 69% of the control group attended screenings. These data lend further support to the importance of personalized, specific behavioral objectives or action planning. When people have detailed their own "implementable" plan for action, they are equipped with a plan that is likely to be specific, reasonable, and, of course, patient centered. This enhances their intent to take action; therefore, behavior change is more likely to happen.

The National Standards for Diabetes Self-Management Education address the importance of having a written curriculum with measurable learning objectives or outcomes.[16] The standards also describe the importance of the periodic reassessment of participant behaviors, the inclusion of a continuous quality improvement (CQI) process to evaluate the effectiveness of the education experience provided, and the role of an established system (advisory board) to annually review outcomes. The ADA's application and instructions for ERP more specifically interpret these standards and delineate the following elements related to writing objectives, which must be part of a complete program:

- An education plan that includes measurable learning objectives and patient-selected behavioral objectives
- Evaluation of progress towards or achievement of learning and behavioral objectives and related outcomes
- Tracking of behavioral outcomes in at least 1 of the following areas: nutrition, physical activity, medications, monitoring, acute complications, risk reduction, or psychosocial adjustment

Learning Objectives Versus Behavioral Objectives

Although there are a variety of definitions, for purposes of consistency with ERP terminology, this text defines and distinguishes between learning and behavioral objectives as follows:

- **Learning Objective** (also known as an educational objective): What the participant is expected to meet at the completion of a teaching session
- **Behavioral Objective** (also known as a behavior change goal or behavioral outcome): A planned change in behavior that is expected to result in improved health or quality of life; a behavior under the participant's direct control that is selected by and/or written by the participant

Both learning objectives and behavioral objectives are written as measurable, observable statements so the participant and educator can clearly determine if objectives have been met.[17] Table 26.1 gives examples of each type of objective. Table 26.2 is an aid, based on Bloom's Taxonomy, for writing both types of objectives.[17]

Since learning cannot be witnessed directly, objectives provide a basis for making the best possible inferences about whether learning has occurred. Objectives clarify the purposes and intent of instruction. Objectives enable the person with diabetes to know what is expected, which helps improve communications.

Behavioral Objectives: Characteristics

A behavioral objective should have the following characteristics:

The participant:

- Values the goal and perceives a need for it
- Understands the steps needed to change the behavior
- Believes that changing the behavior will improve his or her health or quality of life
- Believes he or she is likely to be successful in changing the behavior

A simple acronym to guide educators in assessing the completeness of their objectives is to determine if they are SMART: specific, measurable, achievable, realistic, and time bound (that is, stated in terms of a specific time when they will happen).

Common Mistakes. The following 3 examples represent behavioral objectives that are not well written. As you read each, consider why it is not a good example.

Example 1: *"I will eat healthier foods."*

- Rationale: This is not a specific objective. What is a "healthier food"? Guide the patient in making this more specific and measurable, such as, "I will eat 5 servings of fruits and vegetables each day for the next month and reevaluate the goal at my next clinic visit."

Example 2: *"I will lose 5 pounds."*

- Rationale: This is not an objective, but an outcome of practicing healthy behaviors (such as eating less or exercising more). An objective is something the person can actually do that will result in weight loss, such as "I will limit my meat servings at lunch and dinner to 4 oz at least 5 evenings per week."

Example 3: *"I will join a gym and go for one hour every day."*

- Rationale: You would want to double check with the person to learn if this is really achievable. A daily, hour-long visit to the gym may be tough for even the most avid exercise enthusiast to meet. It is important to guide the person in setting small goals to ensure they can be met and evaluate them after a short period to reward success.

TABLE 26.1 Differentiating Between Learning and Behavioral Objectives

Sample Learning Objectives
• Identify carbohydrate foods • List 4 treatments for hypoglycemia • Discuss differences between saturated and unsaturated fats
Sample Behavioral Objectives
• Record food intake and activity in a logbook 4 days per week for 1 month • Eat 4 carbohydrate servings at lunch and dinner and one 1-carbohydrate snack for 2 weeks and reevaluate with registered dietitian • Drink noncaloric beverages instead of sweetened ones until follow-up class

Source: Hill JVC. Writing behavioral objectives: tips from an educator and auditor. On the Cutting Edge. Maryniuk MD, theme ed. 2005; 26:2, 25-29.

TABLE 26.2 Guide for Writing Learning and Behavioral Objectives

Sample Verbs	*Learning Objective*	*Behavioral Objective*
1) KNOWLEDGE Student recalls or recognizes information, ideas, and principles in the approximate form in which they were learned.		
• List • Identify • Record • State	List 3 treatments for hypoglycemia.	Record how I treat hypoglycemia in my log for the next 2 weeks and evaluate with registered dietitian next visit.
2) COMPREHENSION Student translates, comprehends, or interprets information based on prior learning.		
• Describe • Discuss • Differentiate • Compare	Describe rationale for the 15-15 rule in hypoglycemia treatment.	Describe treatment for hypoglycemia to my husband and coworker within the next week.
3) APPLICATION Student selects, transfers, and uses data and principles to complete a problem or task with a minimum of direction.		
• Demonstrate • Choose • Examine • Complete	Choose food models of 15-g carbohydrate portion sizes.	Choose foods that match meal plan during the next month and discuss with registered dietitian at follow-up class.
4) ANALYSIS Student distinguishes, classifies, and relates the assumptions, hypotheses, evidence, or structure of a statement or question.		
• Analyze • Determine • Summarize • Use	Determine carbohydrate foods that have a higher glycemic index based on case example information.	Analyze effect of different carbohydrate foods on blood glucose by keeping records for 1 month.
5) SYNTHESIS Student originates, integrates, and combines ideas into a product, plan, or proposal that is new to him or her.		
• Design • Order • Prepare • Produce	Prepare a sample meal incorporating carbohydrate allowance and principles of healthy eating.	Prepare a set of sample menus for 1 week incorporating carbohydrate allowances and principles of healthy eating.
6) EVALUATION Student appraises, assesses, or critiques on a basis of specific standards and criteria.		
• Assess • Critique • Evaluate • Rank	Evaluate relationship between different meals and activity by reviewing blood glucose records in case examples.	Evaluate relationship between food and BG by reviewing records for 2 weeks and discussing with registered dietitian in scheduled phone call.

Source: Developed by Melinda Maryniuk, based on Bloom's taxonomy. Hill JVC. Writing behavioral objectives: tips from an educator and auditor. On the Cutting Edge. Maryniuk MD, theme ed. 2005; 26:2;25-29.

Implementing the Plan

Without goals, and plans to reach them,
you are like a ship that has set sail without a destination.
—Fitzhugh Dodson

DSME may be conducted in either group or individual counseling settings. Not only is group education the method recommended for Medicare reimbursement, the group setting has been found to be effective both from a clinical and cost perspective.[18-20] Nonetheless, the educator must efficiently ascertain if each individual is appropriate for the group or if that person would be better served in a one-on-one counseling session.

Mensing and Norris describe how the process of group education has evolved over time.[21] Not long ago, diabetes group education might have been described as a set of didactic "classes," presented lecture style, where the "teacher" would impart knowledge. Now, group education meetings are more interactive "sessions" or "gatherings" where the "facilitator" elicits discussion based on the participants' interests and needs.

These authors also describe several crucial skill sets that diabetes educators must have to effectively lead groups, the first being "preparation." This includes careful consideration of the teaching environment (space, room arrangement, sound, light), teaching materials (handouts, chalkboard, markers), and audiovisuals. Whenever possible, a room arrangement that encourages interaction and discussion is recommended instead of rows of chairs set up in a traditional classroom style. Will the educator be sitting in a circle with the class, standing in the front, moving around, or a blend of all 3? Generally, a combination works best for most kinds of groups. Plan ahead so that handouts and materials to be distributed are well organized for easy referencing and accessibility and to minimize excessive paper shuffling. Practice delivering a mini-presentation to colleagues to confirm that the use of audiovisual aids, the light, sound, your voice projection, and other elements all work well in a particular room.

Despite the fact that an assessment should be the basis of the education plan, the diabetes educator is quite likely to encounter an individual for the first time in a group class environment with no prior access to medical records or referral information. A basic needs assessment of all participants can be conducted efficiently by having each individual complete a very short, written assessment tool and answer questions during group introductions. In addition to asking participants to share some basic diabetes information such as type of diabetes medication being taken, current A1C, target goal, and previous diabetes education, the educator might also ask, "what one question do you hope to have answered in this next hour?"

When conducting a brief, group assessment, the educator must also focus on anything that may be a risk for the class. Pay close attention to physical signs and symptoms that a person may be exhibiting. Make sure there is easy access to a phone, emergency phone numbers, hypoglycemia treatment, and a blood glucose meter. Discuss with colleagues what to do in the event of different emergency situations that may arise so you can react promptly and appropriately.

Last but not least, the educator must think about the order in which topics are to be presented. Are you planning to teach about diabetes the way you, as a healthcare professional, were taught, beginning with definitions, basics of diagnosis, pathophysiology, treatment, and so on? Are psychosocial issues pushed to the very end? It should be the opposite way around! In general, individuals are not interested in diabetes as an academic subject, but in how it affects them in their day-to-day life. Funnell and Anderson have long been describing an empowerment model, making the experiences of the person with diabetes as the basis for the curriculum.[22] Discussing the nature of a self-managed disease such as diabetes at the beginning of an education program helps participants understand why the interaction with the group and information presented is so important. Participants also then see that the role of the healthcare professional is to be a source of expertise, support, and inspiration rather than a teacher or caregiver. This approach recognizes that the person living with diabetes has as important a contribution to make to the session as the diabetes educator. This view redefines the purpose of diabetes education, taking it from providing information so individuals will know why their behaviors need to change to providing information so individuals can make informed decisions about their behaviors.

Plan "B": Adapting Quickly to Change

Bad planning on your part does not
constitute an emergency on my part.
—A proverb

As important as it is to have a plan, having a backup plan is also important. Diabetes educators need to be able to be flexible, spontaneous, and maintain an even course even

> Diabetes education today helps individuals make informed decisions about their care behaviors. Simply providing information so individuals know why their behaviors need to change is inconsistent with the Chronic Care Model.

through what may feel like stormy seas. Listed below are a couple of scenarios that diabetes educators may face from time to time, with suggestions for how to quickly make the best of the situation.

A Group of One?

You have spent time preparing for class. You have PowerPoint slides and handouts and are ready for a 1-hour session, but when you arrive at the classroom, there is only one person there. You are tempted to deliver the class you are accustomed to giving each week, but do not! Instead of delivering the class you had planned, treat the session as one-to-one counseling. Determine exactly what the person's needs are and individualize your messages to meet those needs directly. Although the person will not have the benefit of the group interaction, he or she will benefit from much more personal attention.

The More the Merrier?

If you enter the classroom expecting to encounter 8 individuals and instead you find 15, think about what you might do to appear calm, cool, and collected. After all, this is a good thing! Acknowledging your surprise with the bigger group is fine, but avoid showing that you feel hassled or annoyed. Ask the group to assist you in making a few adjustments so that everyone with diabetes can be best accommodated. For example, guests who have accompanied class participants can be asked to sit in the outer circle behind their partners to give them priority at the table or inner circle. Ask if participants would share materials and say that you will promptly arrange to get everyone a set by the next class. Smile. Show a sense of humor and all will be fine.

Technical Difficulties?

Access to technologies means more chance for equipment failures! Are you prepared if your PowerPoint projector does not work or your handouts do not get delivered from the copy center? Unless you have unlimited financial resources, you do not need 2 of everything "just in case." Instead, think about how you might get by on your own. If you are accustomed to using overheads or slides, have a handout set for yourself so you can at least use them as prompts to know what topic comes next. Use a flipchart or a white board on which to write key points that may need emphasis. In fact, teach some classes without any audiovisual aids from time to time. Avoid overreliance on technology and ensure room for individualization and flexibility based on group needs.

Personal Improvement for Professional Development

When planning for a year, plant corn.
When planning for a decade,
plant trees. When planning for life,
train and educate people.

—Chinese Proverb

Planning and preparation to ensure positive patient encounters is critically important. One aspect often overlooked is a review of one's own counseling and teaching skills. There is often room for improvement. Following a CQI model, diabetes educators are encouraged to specify their own Personal Improvement Plan. Figure 26.2, at the end of chapter, outlines the 4 steps of this plan and references 2 checklists (also at the end of the chapter) by which educators can evaluate their own counseling skills and group teaching techniques.[23]

Questions and Controversies

According to the Chronic Care Model, optimal chronic care is achieved when a prepared, proactive healthcare team interacts with an informed, activated patient.[24] This collaborative approach, or patient-provider partnership, requires much planning, but results in improved outcomes for self-managed chronic conditions such as diabetes.[25] Looking ahead and facing the realities of the business of health care and the ever-tightening fiscal environment, practitioners are seeking ways to build on these opportunities while maintaining efficiencies. Questions such as the following deserve further exploration:

Can a patient's time before the actual encounter with the provider be used more effectively to be truly prepared for the visit?

Research shows that "preactivated" patients—those who are prepared to interact and ask questions during the medical visit—have better outcomes than those who have not been similarly prepared.[26]

Does the planned visit, or group visit model, make sense for people with diabetes?

The planned or group visit model has been recommended as an excellent mechanism for helping patients become more involved in their care. A planned visit involves the time of at least 2 healthcare providers (physician and educator) and could involve a group meeting of 8 to 10 patients for a 2-hour block of time. Results published thus far for diabetes group visits demonstrate significantly improved outcomes and both patient and provider satisfaction.

Are there opportunities to increase the role of community health workers—particularly in preactivating or in planned group visits—to provide more personal connections with patients of differing ethnic and cultural backgrounds?

One provider cannot possibly speak all the languages spoken by patients or be expected to fully understand all the customs and traditions that may influence health behaviors. A variety of programs around the country are training community members to work as liaisons between patients and providers to best insure that information is understood and realistic goals are agreed upon.

With proper planning, the diabetes educator is able to guide patients through self-management education experiences that result in improved behavioral outcomes, yet are delivered in an efficient manner that makes the best use of resources.

The art of learning how to get the most out of life under all circumstances must be cultivated by any patient. It takes time, thought and practice to accommodate one's method of living to changed conditions, but it pays to study the problem.

—E.P. Joslin, MD, 1935[26]

Personal Improvement Plan for Diabetes Educators

As a diabetes educator, in addition to all the continuous quality improvement (CQI) you do for your diabetes program, you should perform CQI on your own diabetes education and counseling skills. The following steps are especially recommended for new diabetes educators.

Assess

Establish Baseline Within 3 Months. Complete a baseline skills assessment documentation tool within 3 months of starting to teach classes. How this is done (self-evaluation, peer-to-peer review, or completed by a supervisor) does not matter, as long as it is done! Use the 2 accompanying forms to document baseline skills: the 2-page Group Education Skills Checklist and the 1-page Clinical Techniques of Diabetes Education Evaluation, which assesses one-on-one counseling skills.

Plan

Identify 2 to 3 Goals. Based on a review of the baseline skills assessment, develop a written Personal Improvement Plan. Identify 2 to 3 specific areas for improvement. Determine if additional education is needed to help support your improvement plan.

Implement

Strengthen Individual Components. Practice your new skills. Establish incremental steps to attain measurable goals that promote development of the skills and areas being targeted. Include both learning and behavioral objectives, as appropriate. Identify barriers and appropriate feedback mechanisms. Review progress toward goals at a predefined frequency.

Reevaluate

Measure in 1 to 2 Years. Complete another skills assessment tool and measure improvement in the targeted areas. Determine if new areas of focus, adjustment, and improvement will be targeted. Develop strategies to maintain or extend progress toward goals. Repeat a self-evaluation every 1 to 2 years.

Group Education Skills Checklist

Use this checklist as a guide when conducting an assessment of group teaching skills.

Rating key: 1= met all noted elements; 2 = needs some improvement (specify)			
Objective: Demonstrates skills essential to effective class communications			
Skill	*Specific elements to observe*	*Rating/comments*	
Preparation	• Arranges room conducive to interaction (if able) • Gathers materials; organizes for logical flow • Reviews available info on participants • Name of class, educator, and contact info visible	1	2
Vocal and listening	• Demonstrates a relaxed, friendly, confident style	1	2
	• Minimizes reliance on notes, slides, etc.	1	2
	• Uses humor when appropriate; smiles	1	2
	• Effective voice volume and tone	1	2
	• Listens well; summarizes and applies	1	2
	• Connects with audience using eye contact; saying names	1	2
	• Uses techniques to manage diverse audience styles, from the quiet listener to the avid talker	1	2
	• Avoids distracting motions or phrases (pacing, wringing hands or too many “ums” or “ahs”)	1	2

FIGURE 26.2 (part 1 of 3) Enhancing Your Skills: Personal Improvement Plan for Educators

Rating key: 1= met all noted elements; 2 = needs some improvement (specify)		
Objective: Demonstrates skills essential to effective class communications (continued)		
Skill	***Specific elements to observe***	***Rating/comments***
Audiovisual aids and handouts	Audiovisual aids • Uses aids appropriately to reinforce material • Clear, simple messages • Design encourages interaction Handouts • Handouts are referred to during class • Activities to personalize content • Clear, simple messages	1 2 1 2
Class flow	• Maintains appropriate pace of class • Uses evaluations from class to make improvements • Starts and ends on time • Mindful of class dynamics; adjusts as needed	1 2
Documentation	• Completes documentation clearly and efficiently • Documents measurable goals and behavioral objectives • Documents follow-up recommendations	1 2
Comments:		

Objective: Leads the group through the 4 parts of an effective class		
Part	***Specific elements to observe***	***Rating/comments***
Engages and personalizes	• Introductions: self and group (as appropriate) • Asks for participant expectations and goals • Assesses knowledge, interest, need for class • Reviews objectives of class (with emphasis on what participant will be able to DO, not just know, and incorporates participant needs) • Reviews "ground rules" (time, structure)	1 2
Informs	• Delivers accurate information • Ensures both learner objectives and class objectives are met (with priority to learner)	1 2
Interacts	• Incorporates 1 or more activities into class for the purpose of practicing a behavior and applying it to home/real-world setting	1 2
Evaluates and sets goals	• Evaluates group understanding of topic/ competence with objectives • Discusses application of learning to home setting • Guides learner to define own action plan/goals (clear, measurable, achievable) • Summarizes key points and action steps (including follow-up plans)	1 2
Comments:		

FIGURE 26.2 (part 2 of 3) Enhancing Your Skills

Clinical Techniques of Diabetes Education: Evaluation Form

Use this checklist as a guide when observing and evaluating an educator's counseling skills. Each diabetes educator should be observed by a peer at least once per year. Circle a rating (1 = poor, 3 = fair, 5 = excellent).

Skill	*Specific elements to observe*	*Rating*
Establishes a trust level (rapport)	• Is organized and prepared • Introduces self to participant • Explains purpose, length of visit, fees • Asks participant's goals and purpose	1 2 3 4 5
Communication skills	• Listens attentively • Asks for clarification • Questions effectively • Speaks succinctly • Uses voices, tone, body language well • Communicates with other team members when needed	1 2 3 4 5
Data-gathering skills	• Obtains accurate information • Asks for clarification when needed	1 2 3 4 5
Intervention and guiding skills	• Controls direction of the session • Gets participant back on track • Handles outside distractions well • Helps participant set realistic goals	1 2 3 4 5
Teaching skills	• Provides accurate information • Uses common words and phrases • Teaches essentials; not too much detail • Uses teaching tools appropriately • Uses interactive format	1 2 3 4 5
Client-centered skills	• Assesses participant's emotional and intellectual position accurately and continually throughout the interview	1 2 3 4 5
Closing session	• Signals end of session • Summarizes session • Makes agreement about follow-up • Makes referral as appropriate	1 2 3 4 5
Documentation	• Completes documentation clearly and efficiently • Documents measurable goals and behavioral objectives • Documents follow-up recommendations	1 2 3 4 5
Comments:		

FIGURE 26.2 (part 3 of 3) Enhancing Your Skills

Focus on Education: Pearls for Practice

Teaching Strategies

- **Plan ahead.** Flexibility is the key. Plan to deliver information in several ways, adjusting the teaching plan based on patient needs or what the day or moment requires.

- **Prioritize.** A person's goals, interests, and needs guide how much and what to cover. There will always be more information and topics to discuss than there is time available. Keep the focus on making safe and informed decisions and not overwhelming the patient.

- **Keep the pace.** There is plenty of time to wrap up and discuss goals, application, and next steps. Covering fewer topics than intended, but ensuring there is a behavioral action plan is always better than covering many topics with no discussion of implementation intentions.

- **Plan some problem solving.** Provide tools and resources to discover answers and solve day-to-day dilemmas. Diabetes requires daily decision making, and problem-solving experience develops confidence. Have patients write action plans, "experiment" when implementing a new behavior, try something for a few weeks until the next class or visit, and then be prepared to discuss the effects.

- **Be practical.** Use teaching models and examples that are culturally appropriate and related to what activity might be done at home. In this way, you can assess skills and offer a chance to give something new a try. Typically, this approach is used for insulin injection and monitoring skills, but it can be effective for so much more—including foot inspection, portion size, label reading, basic stretching exercises, and reviewing the practicalities of hypoglycemia treatments.

- **Personal improvement plan.** Videotape yourself conducting a teaching event. Review the tape and consider discussing it with a peer. Look for alternative ways to set up a plan. Identify behaviors that enhance the visit and those that set up barriers.

Patient Education

- **Avoid information overload.** Recognize that although being a diabetes educator may be a full-time job, having diabetes is just a tiny piece of the patient's universe. Mutually agreeing on actionable expectations increases the likelihood of improved outcomes.

- **Ability to adjust.** Full involvement, commitment to each step, and willingness to look to next steps is helpful. If a plan does not seem to work, problem solving and making a new plan is appropriate. Expect that there will always be some problem solving and new choices to make. Power comes from the process of planning.

References

1. Von Korff M, Gruman J, Schaefer J, Curry S, Wagner E. Collaborative management of chronic illness. Ann Intern Med. 1997;127:1097-102.

2. Martin C, Daly A, McWorter LS, Shwide-Slavin C, Kushion W. The scope of practice, standards of practice, and standards of professional performance for diabetes educators. Diabetes Educ. 2005;31(4):487-512.

3. American Diabetes Association. Education Recognition Program. On the Internet at: www.diabetes.org/recognition. Accessed 18 Feb 2006.

4. Centers for Medicare and Medicaid Services. Medicare Benefit Policy Pub. 100-2, transmittal B, change request 3185. US Department of Health and Human Services. On the Internet at: http://new.cms.hhs.gov/transmittals/Downloads/R13BP.pdf. 28 May 2004. Accessed 6 April 2006.

5. Rothman RL, Dewalt DA, Malone R, et al. Influence of patient literacy on the effectiveness of a primary-care based disease management program. JAMA. 2004;292:1711-6.

6. Rothman RL, Malone R, Bryant B, et al. The Spoken Knowledge In Low Literacy In Diabetes Scale: a diabetes knowledge scale for vulnerable patients. Diabetes Educ. 2005;31:215-24.

7. Smedley BD, Stith AY, Nelson AR, eds. (Committee on Understanding and Eliminating Racial and Ethnic Disparities in Health Care). Unequal Treatment: Confronting Racial and Ethnic Disparities in Health Care. Washington, DC: National Academies Press; 2002.

8. Thackeray R, Merrill RM, Neiger BL. Disparities in diabetes management practice between racial and ethnic groups in the United States. Diabetes Educ. 2004;30:665-75.

9. Redman BK. The Practice of Patient Education, 9th ed. St Louis, Mo: Mosby; 2001;27.

10. Laffel L, Pasquarello C, Lawlor M. Treatment of the child and adolescent with diabetes. In: Joslin's Diabetes Mellitus. 14th ed. Kahn CR, Weir G, King GL, et al, eds. Philadelphia, Pa: Lippincott Williams & Wilkins; 2005.

11. Knowles, MS. The Adult Learner: A Neglected Species, 4th ed. Houston, Tex: Gulf Publishing; 1990.

12. American Association of Diabetes Educators. Standards for outcomes measurement of diabetes self-management education (position statement). Diabetes Educ. 2003;29(5):804-16.

13. Mulcahy K, Maryniuk M, Peeples M, et al. Diabetes self-care management education core outcomes measures. Diabetes Educ. 2003;29(5):768-803.

14. Gibson PG, Powell H, Coughlan J, et al. Self management education and regular practitioner review for adults with asthma. Cochrane Database Syst Rev. 2003;(1):CD001117.

15. Sheeran P, Orbell S. Using implementation intentions to increase attendance for cervical cancer screening. Health Psychol. 2000;19(3):283-9.

16. Mensing C, Boucher J, Cypress M, et al. National standards for diabetes self-management education. Diabetes Care. 2000;23:682-9.

17. Hill JVC. Writing behavioral objectives: tips from an educator and auditor. On the Cutting Edge. Maryniuk MD, theme ed. 2005; 26:2, 25-29.

18. Rickheim PL, Weaver TW, Flader JL, Kendall DM. Assessment of group versus individual diabetes education: a randomized study. Diabetes Care. 2002;25:269-74.

19. Heller SR, Clarke P, Daly H, et al. Group education for obese patients with type 2 diabetes: greater success at less cost. Diabetes Med. 1988;5:552-6.

20. Campbell EM, Redman S, Moffitt PS, Sanson-Fisher RW. The relative effectiveness of educational and behavioral instruction programs for patients with NIDDM: a randomized trial. Diabetes Educ. 1996;22:379-86.

21. Mensing CR, Norris SL. Group education in diabetes: effectiveness and implementation. Diabetes Spectrum. 2003;16:96-103.

22. Funnell MM, Anderson RM. Empowerment and self-management of diabetes. Clinical Diabetes. 2004;22:123-7.

23. Joslin Diabetes Center. Diabetes Educator Orientation Manual—Affiliated Programs. Boston, Mass: Joslin Diabetes Center; 2005:section C.

24. Bodenheimer T, Lorig K, Holman H, Grumbach K. Patient self-management of chronic disease in primary care. JAMA. 2002;2469-75.

25. Bodenheimer T. Helping patients improve their health related behaviors: what system changes do we need? Dis Manage. 2005;319-30.

26. Joslin EP. The Treatment of Diabetes Mellitus. Philadelphia, Pa: Lea & Febiger; 1935.

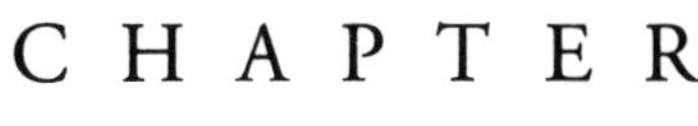

CHAPTER

27

Implementation of Diabetes Education

Author

Gayle M. Lorenzi, RN, CDE

Key Concepts

- To effectively implement the diabetes education process, educational content and delivery must be tailored to the learner. This may require adaptation of one's usual teaching styles and methods so they are sensitive to learning styles, learner readiness, and the special needs of persons with diabetes and their family and support network.
- When working with adult learners, recognize these characteristics: adults prefer information they can apply and that meets their needs. Problem-oriented learning helps facilitate problem solving. Most adults prefer to learn by participating in discussions and sharing personal experiences.
- Children often learn best by example and simple explanations. Involvement by their parents, families, and support at school are critical to the education process.
- The compliance and empowerment approaches may both be used during the education process, depending on where the person is in the learning process.
- Healthcare education processes need to consider the cultural and ethnic backgrounds of participants if they are to be effective in providing culturally appropriate and responsive care.
- Literacy level must be assessed so learning deficits can be identified and appropriate teaching methods and written materials tailored to the person's needs.
- The Americans with Disabilities Act (1990) defines the rights of those with disabilities. People with diabetes should receive appropriate adaptive devices, diabetes self-management education, tools, and techniques to help them manage their diabetes.

Introduction

For many decades, personal healthcare decision-making rested largely on the shoulders of the healthcare provider, generally the physician. As the authority figure, the healthcare provider was given the power by the person with diabetes to make all the decisions and to respond in a parental fashion when instructions were not followed as prescribed. Those who were unable or unwilling to comply were labeled "noncompliant" and, over time, were often dismissed by the healthcare provider as being unmotivated, lazy, rebellious, or even stupid. After all, how could anyone with intelligence not understand the importance of "doing as told" by someone who was educated to know more than they about their health condition? In that era, collaborative care, individualized approaches to treatment, multidisciplinary team management, and patient empowerment were relatively unheard of concepts. Diabetes was managed as a "white coat" disease. This approach worked relatively well during the era when treatment choices were few, care focused on preserving life, and outcomes short of death were considered a success.

Over the past 2 to 3 decades, scientific discoveries have fostered the development of innovative pharmacologic therapies, drug delivery devices, and glucose monitoring systems. The availability of these tools, in conjunction with the data that substantiated the importance of striving for optimal glycemic control from the Diabetes Control and Complications Trial (DCCT)[1] and UK Prospective Study (UKPDS),[2] changed the face of diabetes management. Despite all these innovations, individuals with diabetes nonetheless continue to struggle to achieve optimal levels of glycemic control.

Managing diabetes involves more than scientific knowledge and innovations; it requires translating this knowledge into daily self-care practices. The AADE 7 Self-Care Behaviors™ (discussed individually in subsequent chapters) are based on scientific knowledge and represent desired education outcomes for individuals with diabetes. These outcomes include Healthy Eating, Being Active, Taking Medication, Monitoring, Problem Solving, Healthy Coping, and Reducing Risks.

Educating involves imparting information and assisting the individual to make informed decisions about how to best integrate diabetes management strategies into daily life. The accessibility and effectiveness of this education influence future acquisition of knowledge and skills, the person's attitude about diabetes, his or her motivation to actively participate in self-management as well as the person's ability and/or willingness to make recommended changes.

The education process has 4 basic components: assessment, planning, implementation, and evaluation. This chapter highlights issues to consider when implementing the education process and illustrates several concepts pertinent to this phase of diabetes education. It discusses various education strategies, reviews teaching and learning principles pertinent to diabetes management, and identifies factors to consider when assessing individual needs and readiness to learn. Additionally, factors that interfere with educator effectiveness and patient readiness to learn are identified, and techniques to improve learning and decision-making are discussed.

Keys to Effectively Implementing Diabetes Education

- Education content and delivery must be appropriate
- Effective implementation requires adaptation of teaching styles and methods that are sensitive to learning styles, learner readiness, and special needs
- Teaching does not always result in learning or behavior change
- Learning is a dynamic and ongoing process

Case in Point: Developing An Effective Plan of Care

SS is a 48 year-old male who was diagnosed with type 1 diabetes at the age of 17. Prior to diagnosis, he was an accomplished baseball player with the demonstrated skill and motivation needed to pursue a professional athletic career. The months preceding diagnosis were characterized by progressive hyperglycemic symptoms, increasing lethargy, and weakness. At the time of diagnosis, he presented in severe ketoacidosis and remained in the hospital for 2 weeks. When discharged, he was instructed to take a single mixed injection of regular and NPH insulin each morning and test his urine twice daily. He was also told that his dreams of a baseball career should be forgotten. Determined to overcome the skepticism, he worked to regain strength, speed, and skill and subsequently obtained a baseball scholarship to the state university.

During the subsequent 20 years, his diabetes treatment regimen was progressively intensified to keep step with therapeutic advances. However, despite using multiple daily insulin injections combined with careful attention to dietary choices, consistent physical activity, and frequent blood glucose monitoring, glycemic control as measured by A1C continued above 9%. In 1995, he began using continuous subcutaneous insulin infusion (CSII) and increased his blood glucose monitoring to 3 to 4 times per day, which enabled him to achieve consistent A1C values in the 8.0% to 8.5% range. However, by age 47, the complications associated with diabetes were well established, and he presented with aggressively progressing retinopathy and significant visual impairment, bilateral carpal tunnel syndrome, peripheral neuropathy, hypertension, and albuminuria.

His new clinical care team was challenged to assist SS with ongoing glycemic management in the face of physical disabilities and progressive complications associated with long-standing diabetes. In developing the plan of care, the following needed to be considered.

What are the medical goals for treatment?

- Improve level of glycemic control
- Prevent further physical deterioration via appropriate pharmacologic intervention

How does the person with diabetes perceive the treatment goals?

- Do his or her goals align with the medical goals for treatment? If not, discuss the differences and prioritize. Keep in mind that medical recommendations that are not perceived as important to the individual will be difficult to implement regardless of the value of the intervention.
- Is the person's reluctance to follow through with recommendations related to a real or perceived fear? Previous negative experience? Lack of knowledge? Lack of resources? Avoid jumping to the conclusion that the individual is noncompliant and unmotivated.

(continued)

Case in Point: Developing An Effective Plan of Care (continued)

Are there physical limitations that must be considered?

- How significant is the visual impairment?
  —Does this individual need a sight-assisted blood glucose monitoring device?
  —Is the individual able to accurately program and deliver insulin using the insulin pump?
  —What are the limitations for reading text? Do materials need to be in larger, bolder type?
- How significant is the pain and limitation?
  —How much is the pain interrupting daily life? How effectively is the pain being managed?
  —Is manual dexterity compromised? If so, are the devices currently being used to manage the diabetes still a realistic option for him? Are there other devices that may be easier to use?
  —How much is pain or decreased dexterity interfering with diabetes self-care behaviors?
  —How is this person coping with the pain and limitations?

Is mobility affected by the peripheral neuropathy?

- Has neuropathy interfered with his ability to continue an athletic lifestyle?
- Has he integrated other physical activities that take this into consideration? Has he withdrawn from all activity due to fear? Pain? Lack of knowledge? Depression?

Does the person have a support network to support self-management efforts?

- Is there a significant other that can provide support for this person?
- What is their level of understanding of the issues facing this man?
- Is their relationship with this individual a source of positive or negative support?
- Will including this support person in the education and intervention planning be an asset to the person?
- Are there community resources that could assist the individual and family in dealing with the physical and/or emotional challenges?

Are there emotional or psychological issues that are interfering with this person's ability to effectively care for himself?

- Is the individual frightened, depressed, or thinking fatalistically?
- What is or has contributed to the current psychological state?
- Are the emotions related to lack of knowledge?
- Would psychological intervention be helpful? Would this person be open to this intervention?

Careful assessment is critical to developing an effective plan of care for the person with diabetes. An individual's response to physical or emotional challenges is influenced by past experiences as well as current status. Successful intervention requires attention to the physical, educational, and emotional issues that may influence the individual's ability to self-manage the disease.

Are there other issues that may influence this person's ability to implement treatment recommendations?

- Is he particularly concerned about specific aspects of his current health status?
- What is of concern and what is most important to this person?
- What is he capable of hearing and learning?
- What are his current physical limitations?

Standards of Practice for Diabetes Education

Diabetes is a lifelong disease that requires daily management. As such, opportunities for education are needed throughout the disease process and throughout the life span of those affected. As the primary managers of their disease, persons with diabetes require sufficient, appropriate education to enable informed decision-making and effective self-care. This is best achieved when the education is a collaborative effort between the healthcare team and the person with diabetes.[3] Standard 4 of the AADE Standards of Practice for Diabetes Educators[4] is titled "Implementation" and follows after the standards for Assessment, Outcome Identification, and Planning.

Note that the Standards consider the terms diabetes self-management training (DSMT) and diabetes self-management education (DSME) to be interchangeable; however, this book uses the term DSMT to refer only to training of practitioners. This chapter discusses DSME (education), not DSMT (practitioner training).

Implementation of the education plan as defined in Standard 4 lists the following requirements:

- Identify an accessible, safe, and appropriate setting for the conduct of DSME
- Use teaching materials appropriate to the learner's age, culture, learning style, and abilities
- Provide sequential education, progressing from basic safety and survival skills to advanced information for daily self-management and improved outcomes
- Include basic diabetes self-management content, namely, safe medication use, meal planning, self-monitoring of blood glucose, and recognizing when and how to access professional services
- Provide increasingly advanced DSME that is goal-directed and based on the person's needs; this includes preventing and managing chronic complications, psychosocial adjustment, developing problem-solving skills, managing physical activity, adjusting medication treatment regimens, pattern management, and coping with travel and stress
- Incorporate opportunities for peer support
- Integrate the DSME plan into the overall plan of care
- Communicate the diabetes education plan and the individual's progress to the referring healthcare providers
- Establish means for follow-up and continuity of DSME, including referrals to other healthcare professionals
- May provide a forum for group education to foster support, encouragement and empowerment of persons with diabetes[4]

As described, Standard 4 emphasizes the chronic and dynamic nature of diabetes, reinforces the need for sequential learning (from survival learning to empowered, advanced self-management) and ongoing learning, and recognizes the importance of peer and professional education and support. While the Standards of Practice for Diabetes Educators provide guidance for educating people with diabetes, providing education is not owned by diabetes educators. Any healthcare professional who interacts with the person with diabetes has the opportunity and obligation to support efforts toward successful self-management. In order for this educational opportunity to be successful, an appreciation of basic teaching and learning principles is helpful.

Understanding Basic Teaching and Learning Principles

Have you ever tried to convince a teenager to do something that was important to you—such as meet a curfew, clean his or her room, or curtail use of the phone? The attempt generally results in a struggle, largely because the outcome is something you want or need, not something the teen wants or needs at the time. However, attempting to teach a teenage male how to change the oil in the family car, so that he may use the car, can be a very different experience. Why? Because, the teen sees the need to learn this skill in order to get something important to him. So it is with adult learners: *the information must be salient and aligned with the individual's need.*[5,6]

Now let's consider the science class. While it is important to learn the basic principles behind the scientific process, without the lab portion of the course, how many students would know how to conduct an experiment? The same applies to learning about a disease that must be managed. The scientific explanations and rationale represent important learning, but given alone, are insufficient in helping the person cope with daily situations. So it is with adult learners: *problem-oriented learning provides information that is critical to solving problems and making appropriate decisions.*[5,6]

What about teaching someone about the importance of making appropriate adjustments to medication and/or food intake when physical activity is unexpectedly increased? If the person has recently experienced a significant hypoglycemic event, his or her ability to hear alternate suggestions may be better. So it is with adult learners: *learning that incorporates sharing of personal experiences has more relevance and encourages the development of improved problem-solving skills.*[5,6]

Have you ever attended a program for continuing medical education where the speaker spoke nonstop, did not engage the audience, and the program ended without the moderator or audience asking a single question? How much did you learn? How satisfied were you with the experience, and how relevant was the education to you? So it is with most adult learners: *participatory learning that encourages questions, promotes a problem-solving approach, and actively engages the participants is more likely to result in effective learning.*[5,6]

Improving the Effectiveness of Diabetes Education

To summarize, the effectiveness of diabetes education (individual or group) will be influenced by incorporating the following principles into the education process:

- Information presented must be perceived as important to the recipient
- Problem-oriented learning provides information that is critical to solving problems and making appropriate decisions
- Learning that incorporates sharing of personal experiences has more relevance and promotes the development of improved problem-solving skills
- Participatory learning that encourages questions, promotes a problem-solving approach and actively engages the participants is more likely to result in effective learning

The above principles apply, in varying degrees, across the spectrum of ages. The effectiveness of education depends on modifications in the methods and delivery of information that are appropriate for the different age groups and learning capabilities.

Children and Their Families. Children often learn best by example and simple explanation. The explanations need to use words they are familiar with, incorporating play whenever possible. Assuming responsibility for daily tasks (for example, blood glucose testing, injections, pump programming, or food choices) is a gradual process that should be guided by the child's developmental phase, intellect, ability, and willingness to assume responsibility. Understanding what the child is managing in his or her routine life can serve as a guide for encouraging increasing independence in diabetes management.[6,7]

Educating the child with diabetes requires educating the family about diabetes. While the teaching and learning principles discussed above apply to the parents, their learning will be challenged by the fear of diagnosis, the sense of responsibility for their child's diagnosis and the turmoil of the emotional and financial burdens attributable to diabetes. Ideally, the child and parents receive the same education messages, but the detail, depth, focus, and delivery vary.

Older Adults. The older adult also requires modifications to the education style and approach. While age-related changes can affect the processing and recall of new information, the capacity to learn and integrate new information remains intact throughout the life cycle.[8] Older adults may require more time to assimilate the information and benefit from slower-paced education sessions. In some instances, inclusion of appropriate significant others and/or caretakers in the education sessions may be helpful or necessary to ensure appropriate and safe home care practices.

Whether planning for group education or individual education sessions, consider age as well as the individual's stage of life. The needs, capabilities, issues, and treatment strategies will vary across time, with children or adolescents and their parents, young adults, working adults, active retirees, and the elderly in dependent care each having unique issues and needs. Regardless of age or stage of life, the education process must accomplish the following:

- Include information that is viewed as important to the individual
- Recognize and integrate the individual's experiences into the learning process
- Foster the development of problem-solving skills
- Promote active participation in one's personal care

Implementing Education: Considering the Options

A frequently asked question when the DCCT ended was "How was it done?" Specifically, healthcare professionals and people with diabetes were curious: what strategy was used to treat the intensive treatment group that resulted in achievement of the desired outcome? The DCCT illustrated the need for patient education, the importance of multidisciplinary team care, the value of incorporating regimens that were most consistent with the individual's lifestyle, and the importance of ongoing support. Various education strategies and tactics that recognized and capitalized on the individual's needs, attributes, and limitations were used. However, no universal strategy or education approach could be identified.

So, what does this tell us about how to best educate people with diabetes? If there is no "right" way to do it, what factors should be considered to improve effectiveness?

Compliance and Empowerment: Two Approaches to Education

Two education approaches have particular relevance to diabetes education: the compliance-based approach and the empowerment approach. The compliance-based approach has been the basis for the delivery of diabetes care for many years. This approach focuses on the healthcare professional as the expert, while those with the disease are passive learners who are instructed on what to do, told why it is important, and expected to follow recommendations given.[9] Contrast that approach to the empowerment approach. Using this approach, persons with diabetes are expected to be active in the management of their diabetes, provided with information needed to make informed daily care decisions, and responsible for making these decisions.[9-12] The empowerment approach to education is discussed in greater detail in chapter 3, on self-management of health. However, Table 27.1 lists 12 strategies for facilitating patient empowerment.

TABLE 27.1 Facilitating Patient Empowerment

- Ask questions
- Begin with the individual's agenda
- Individualize the treatment plan
- Specifically define the problem(s)
- Use a stepped approach
- Develop problem-solving skills
- Focus on behaviors, not outcomes
- Use contracts, as needed
- Involve the individual's support network
- Maintain contact between in-person visits
- Help develop effective coping skills
- Ask for help from colleagues, refer to specialists when needed

Source: Adapted from Rubin RR, Napora JP. Behavior change. In: A Core Curriculum for Diabetes Education: Diabetes Education and Program Management, 4th ed. Franz MF, ed. Chicago, Ill: American Association of Diabetes Educators; 2001:75.

While the compliance and empowerment approaches to education have specific attributes and limitations, they are not mutually exclusive, nor is one approach ideal for all individuals throughout the learning process. Consider the person recently diagnosed with diabetes. He requires basic information and instruction to prevent hospitalization and ensure safety. Adjusting insulin doses for eating out may not be relevant to him at this time. However, learning how and why he got diabetes, what has gone wrong in his body, how and when to take medication or give an injection, and why medication is needed everyday are all vital pieces of information during these early weeks. Conversely, the individual who has had diabetes for several years may gain little from a didactic lecture about carbohydrate counting that does not include opportunities to ask about adjustments that would be needed to cover their favorite foods or how to make healthy choices at their favorite restaurant. Table 27.2 highlights distinct characteristics of the compliance and empowerment approaches to patient education.

TABLE 27.2 Approaches to Patient Education

	Compliance Approach	*Empowerment Approach*
Assumptions	• Healthcare professionals are the experts • Patients comply with recommendations • Following instructions is criteria for success	• Patients are capable of making complex decisions • Patients have the right and responsibility to manage their diabetes • Healthcare professionals provide guidance and support
Strategies	• Healthcare professional identifies important aspects of care and provides education • Instructions are directive and approach is often uniform over time	• Basic understanding of disease and management tools needed • Healthcare professional provides guidance regarding specific aspects of management, directed by the patient • Recommendations often replace standardized instructions • Education focuses on self-care, self-management, and coping skills
Goal	• Patient complies with treatment recommendations	• Patient assumes primary responsibility for daily decision-making
Usefulness of Approach to Patient	• Early in disease process, beyond survival skills • If unable to assume greater responsibility for personal healthcare decisions • If unable to focus on specifics of self-care due to other life issues	• After individual has a good understanding of diabetes survival skills • If willing to actively participate in care decisions • If able to make informed decisions and recognize when to seek assistance

Assessing Need and Readiness to Learn

While the education approach may be well matched to the person or population being served, if those on the receiving end are not ready to receive information or if the information is unimportant to them at the time, learning will likely be compromised.

Consider the following: An individual with type 2 diabetes has just been given a prescription for insulin. You are responsible for educating her. The information you have to share is important. Does the person agree—or is she angry and resistant to learning about insulin today? You are adamant that the information you have to share is important for the person to know and understand. However, the person you are trying to help may not agree with your assessment. You know that her history of glycemic control has been suboptimal for years; however, she reports feeling "just fine." What are the chances that the information you have to offer her will be heard today? Will this one-time education session achieve your goals or meet the patient's need(s)?

The situation described above is neither unusual nor rare. There are general questions that the healthcare professional should ask when developing an individual or group education plan. Is the information something that needs to be known? To whom is it important? Why is this information important? What can interfere with the information being heard? Without an awareness of these issues, the education plan risks failure.

Method and message must match learner readiness

In situations where the education method and message are not aligned with learner readiness, the outcome will likely be less than desired.[9-12] Issues to consider when assessing educational needs and readiness to learn are summarized in Table 27.3.

Teaching Strategies and the Learning Experience

For learning to occur, the individual must be open and ready to learn. However, issues that interfere with learning are not confined to the learner. The outcome of the education is also influenced by the methods used and effectiveness of delivery of the information. Choosing the appropriate method of instruction is a critical determinant to effective education. While teaching and learning can occur informally, in person or remotely via phone or computer, more formal education requires planning to maximize success. Identification of content and skills to be learned, access to audiovisual materials, class size and composition, time, and available resources all should be considered when developing a teaching plan.

Several teaching strategies can be considered, individually or collectively, to deliver information depending on the education needed and expected outcome. (See Table 27.4). No single format is conducive for teaching all components of diabetes self-management to all persons with diabetes. Using a combination of various media, tools, and materials can enhance integration of the information and skills needed to effectively self-manage diabetes. Creativity and ongoing assessment of the methods used to impart information to the learner will prevent monotonous delivery of outdated or irrelevant content—and make the education experience more rewarding for teacher and learner.

Beyond the Initial Education Interaction

Understanding what has gone awry in the body in the presence of diabetes is *important.* However, understanding how to manage the disease on a daily basis is *critical* to the individual's short- and long-term health and quality of life. Beyond the "what" and "why," adequate attention must be paid to the "how."

For example, a person who is newly diagnosed with diabetes is told that his blood glucose is high and must be controlled in order to avoid the complications of diabetes. He may be told to get a glucose meter, check his blood glucoses values, and return for a follow-up appointment in 2 weeks. He has been told he has diabetes (*what*), has been told that testing blood glucose is important (*why*), but no instruction was received about *how*—which meter to purchase, how and when to check blood glucose, and what to do with the results, for example. The brief education he received has limited his ability to carry out the prescribed action, and integration of the diabetes into his daily life was not even discussed.

The challenge for healthcare educators is to effectively provide the individual with sufficient information to facilitate translation of new information into positive behavior change. An individual's management of diabetes requires integration of several skill sets: specific self-care skills, self-management skills, and coping skills.

Self-Care Skills. Essential self-care skills include making food choices, monitoring blood glucose, taking medications (orally or by injection or inhalation), adjusting for food or activity variations, and managing

TABLE 27.3 Assessing Education Needs and Readiness to Change

Assessment	*Issues to Consider*	*Negative Impact if...*
Knowledge, psychomotor skills, and attitudinal learning	• Attitude and health beliefs about diabetes • Attitude toward participating in education program • Individual goals of treatment: A1C, BP, weight, etc • Experience with diabetes to date • Presence of other confounding health conditions • Presence or absence of a support network	• Diabetes is viewed as unimportant, education is not desired, goals are different, diabetes is not a priority, or support is lacking
Current level of self-care	• Individual ability to perform complex tasks • Willingness to devote more time to management	• Individual not interested in being actively involved in self-management
Learning style	• Preferred method: read, listen, discuss • Usual method of acquiring new information: media, internet, friends/family, etc • Preference for group vs. individual instruction	• Ability to learn depends on a method that is not available • Individual instruction is required but not available
Level of stress	• Acute vs. chronic • Influence on ability to learn or make changes	• Stress is high enough to interfere with learning or prioritization of diabetes
Social, cultural, religious preferences	• Influence on willingness to learn new behaviors • Potential for conflict between treatment recommendations and cultural beliefs	• Education message or methods or treatment recommendations conflict with belief system
Literacy	• Years of formal education • Learning style and ability to tolerate complexity • Directive teaching may be beneficial	• Assumptions are made solely on years of education • Literacy level of education method and materials is not appropriate
Readiness for change	• Extent that need for change is recognized • Create conditions that stimulate desire to change or capitalize on readiness to change	• Expressed desire to change does not reflect willingness to change • Readiness for change is not aligned with education goals • Assumptions are made that the individual will never change

Source: Adapted from Anderson RM. Applied principles of teaching and learning. In: A Core Curriculum for Diabetes Education: Diabetes Education and Program Management, 4th ed. Franz MJ, ed. Chicago, Ill: American Association of Diabetes Educators; 2001:7-8.

TABLE 27.4 Teaching Strategies and the Learning Experience

Teaching Format	*Goal*	*Learning Experience*	*Attributes*	*Limitations*	*Example*
Lecture	Present information	Passive—listens	Easier to implement and control content	Limited applicability of information to the individual	Present physiology of diabetes
Discussion	Seek and acquire information	Active—asks questions, shares information and experiences	Active participation and learning; ability to learn from others	Less control over content and time; agenda may be influenced by outspoken few	Review of factors that influence blood glucose response
Demonstration	Teach psycho-motor or social skills	Active—if return demonstration included	Allows learner to observe, perform, and be evaluated	Takes more time; easier to do in small groups or one to one	Self-monitoring of blood glucose; instruction in insulin administration
Print Materials	Provide and/or reinforce information	Passive—self-initiated	Augments in-person education and provides enduring resource	Does not replace in-person education; effectiveness influenced by congruence between materials and individual characteristics (literacy, language, etc)	Sick day management; insulin-to-carbohydrate ratio
Audiovisual Aids	Enhance presentation of information	Passive and active learning	Provides variety in presentation of information; assists those who are visual learners; adaptable to audience size and composition	Can decrease integration of information if used alone; complexity vs simplicity need to be balanced and targeted to audience	Physiology presentation
Computers	Enhance self-directed education	Active learning—information resource with interactive potential	Provides opportunity for self-directed learning and problem-solving; 24-hour accessibility	Comfort with technology varies by age, socioeconomic status, and prior comfort and/or experience	Simulated daily management: ability to make decisions and observe outcome
Role-Playing	Practice, express, explore, discuss. share	Active learning—facilitates sharing of information	Useful in individual or group setting	Requires cohesiveness of participants and instructor with good interpersonal skills; facilitates exploration of "what if" situations	Dealing with alienation from peers or over- or under-involved significant other(s)
Games	Enhance learning	Active learning—interactive	Can make learning more enjoyable or comfortable	Can detract from learning if not well planned or executed	Adaptable to various topics and settings

Source: Adapted from Anderson RM. Applied principles of teaching and learning. In: A Core Curriculum for Diabetes Education: Diabetes Education and Program Management, 4th ed. Franz MJ, ed. Chicago, Ill: American Association of Diabetes Educators; 2001:9-11.

hyperglycemia and hypoglycemia. These are commonly referred to as "survival skills"; many people with diabetes have, however, "survived" knowing less than this amount of information.

Self-Management Skills. Mastery of the essential self-care management skills requires incremental learning that incorporates information and personal experience. Diabetes education is an ongoing process, not a once in a lifetime experience. Development of self-management skills requires that learning be pushed to the next level. For this to happen, an individual must incorporate previously acquired information into situational decision-making. Utilization of anticipatory planning and problem-solving promote the development of self-management skills. For example, adjusting the insulin dose to compensate for pizza and beer involves anticipatory planning. Evaluating the outcome of this adjustment using postmeal blood glucose data allows the individual to assess the effectiveness of his decision.

Coping Skills. Equally important to self-care is the identification and cultivation of appropriate coping skills. The presence of diabetes adds multiple stressors to the individual's life. The ability to manage the usual stresses (job, family, etc) will directly influence the individual's ability to manage the stressors associated with diabetes (inconvenience of daily care, potential for hypoglycemia, evolving complications, etc). Thus, helping the individual to recognize and evaluate his or her usual coping strategies assists in the development of diabetes-specific coping behaviors. For example, if an individual typically responds to unplanned situations with frustration and agitation, helping him or her to anticipate and problem solve about delayed meals or unexpected schedule changes may decrease the frustration and agitation felt during these unplanned times. In this way, the event may be viewed as a learning opportunity, rather than a threat.

Finally, the person with diabetes needs to understand the goals and limitations of diabetes management. Maintenance of daily glycemic control is a potential challenge. If the learner has access to self-management information and that information is presented in an effective manner, diabetes can be managed.

Cultural Competency

The education process is further challenged by the presence of multiple languages and cultural beliefs and practices. The globalization of society has had a significant impact on the healthcare community, necessitating attention to the materials and methods used to educate people about how to care for themselves. This has particular relevance for diabetes management in the United States, where the incidence of diabetes is disproportionately higher in the races of color.[14,15] Healthcare and education programs must consider the cultural and ethnic backgrounds of the participants during program development and implementation. The National Center for Cultural Competence provides rationale for the development of cultural competence: (*1*) to improve quality of services and outcomes; (*2*) to meet legislative, regulatory, and accreditation mandates; (*3*) to gain a competitive edge in the marketplace; and (*4*) to decrease the likelihood of liability and malpractice claims.[16]

> Our challenge as healthcare educators is to effectively provide individuals with information sufficient to help them translate new information into positive behavior change.

Campinha-Bacote describes a practice model of cultural competence that is guided by 4 basic assumptions:[16]

- Cultural competency is a dynamic process, not an end-point
- The process of achieving cultural competence incorporates 5 interrelated constructs: cultural desire, cultural awareness, cultural knowledge, cultural skill, and cultural encounters (see Table 27.5)
- Cultural competence is needed to ensure effective and culturally responsive care
- All encounters are cultural encounters

Culturally competent healthcare and education recognize differences in the interpretation and relevance of wellness versus illness, present versus future, self-care versus directed care, and preventable versus inevitable outcomes. Providing essential information and self-care skills education using terms, descriptions, and situations that are meaningful to the specific population enhances one's learning experience and increases the possibility that the information provided will translate to the desired behavior change.[15,16,17]

A common misconception is that translation of education materials from English to another language is sufficient for educating non–English-speaking individuals. Specifically, how often have you witnessed patients being given non-English pamphlets and told to read them and, with that, their education is considered "complete"? Is this an effective means of providing education? Direct translation of words without an appreciation of the context or interpretation can result in confusion and misconceptions. A culturally sensitive and informed healthcare professional understands and addresses the cultural beliefs and myths that may influence their patient's ability and willingness to follow directions, ask questions, or seek additional information.

TABLE 27.5 Cultural Competence in the Delivery of Healthcare Services: Foundation of the Practice Model

Cultural Awareness	• Recognize personal prejudices and biases toward other cultures • Understand personal cultural/ethnic background
Cultural Humility	• Commit to ongoing self-evaluation and self-critique • Be willing to address power imbalances in patient-provider relationship • Develop mutually beneficial partnerships with communities/organizations on behalf of defined populations
Cultural Knowledge	• Develop an education foundation that incorporates various worldviews of different cultures • Identify and integrate knowledge regarding biological variations, disease and health conditions, and variations in drug metabolism
Cultural Skill	• Collect culturally relevant data regarding the individual's presenting problem and health history • Conduct culturally based physical assessments in a culturally sensitive manner
Cultural Desire	• Commit to engage in the process of cultural competence • Demonstrate compassion, authenticity, humility, openness, availability, and flexibility • Provide care, regardless of conflict

Source: Adapted from Campinha-Bacote J. The process of cultural competence in the delivery of healthcare services: a model of care. J Transcult Nurs. 2002;13:181-4.

Understanding the usual practices, myths, and beliefs of particular cultures provides important context to the education process. However, labeling and making broad assumptions based on cultural background interferes with effective learning. Asking questions, listening to the responses, and adjusting the education intervention based on what is said, observed, and/or heard enhances learning and promotes a sense of trust between the patient and healthcare professional. This type of interchange also helps the educator uncover what is important to the individuals they serve regarding their life and healthcare.

Literacy

Developing a level of cultural awareness and competency improves the communication and increases the possibility that the educator's message will be heard. While new information must fit within the construct of the learner's cultural context, the information must also be presented at an appropriate level. Thus, identifying and incorporating the literacy level of the patient population into program development and implementation increases the possibility of influencing the person's actions and decisions.[18,19]

Consider the following example: You are covering the inpatient diabetes service and are scheduled to meet with a 45-year-old plumber to provide basic diabetes education before discharge. You go armed with all of the pamphlets and handouts you can find, knowing that your time with him is limited to 45 minutes. Early in the conversation, he shares that he "doesn't read much." However, his medical record indicated he has a very successful business, and thus you expect he will be able to understand the new information in the written materials with minimal difficulty. He must be literate; after all, he is successful. Is your assumption accurate? See the sidebar for common fallacies about literacy.

Common Fallacies About Literacy

There are several common *fallacies* about literacy:[20]

- People will tell you if they cannot read
- Most illiterates are poor, immigrants, or minorities
- Years of schooling is a good measure of literacy level
- Illiterates are dumb and learn slowly, if at all

The National Literacy Act of 1991 defines literacy as an individual's ability to read, write, and speak in English and to compute and solve problems at levels of proficiency necessary to function on the job and in society to achieve one's goals and to develop one's knowledge and potential.[20] The ability to use reading, writing, and computational skills at levels adequate to deal with everyday circumstances is called functional literacy or functional competency.[19] In the above example, the plumber likely falls into the functionally literate category. He is clearly a functioning and successful member of society. However, will he be able to read the pamphlets, let alone understand the medical jargon? Health literacy pertains to the presence of skills adequate to participate in self-care and achievement of health

> ***Low Literacy is Not Uncommon***
>
> About 50% of adults in America function at the 2 lowest literacy levels. Less than 20% function at the 2 highest levels.

goals. While this man's reading skills may be inadequate, using discussion, demonstration, audiovisual materials, and/or role-playing will provide information the plumber needs in a more understandable format. Written materials that use illustrations and graphics to "tell the story" will also help this individual. See Table 27.4 to review 8 teaching formats and their uses and limitations.

Word recognition and understanding are components of literacy. Can the individual read *and* interpret the words before them? Literacy can be assessed by asking the person to read text and subsequently explain what the text said. Many people with low literacy skills have underdeveloped skills in reading and limited ability to analyze and synthesize the written word. Understanding the differences between skilled and unskilled readers can provide valuable insight into the education strategies used for an individual or group. Unskilled readers tend to do the following:[19]

- Take instructions literally and not be able to apply the instructions to different situations
- Read one word at a time and not be able to link the words together to provide meaning
- Skip over uncommon words and often not able to think in terms of categories or classes of information
- Miss the context of the information and/or not be able to make inferences based on facts or additional information

Literacy does not equate to a particular grade level in school, and low literacy does not uniformly mean low intelligence or functioning. Additionally, physical appearance, speech, and race/ethnicity are not accurate predictors of literacy.

Think in terms of the 5 levels of proficiency in literacy

The National Adult Literacy Survey (1992) defined 5 levels of proficiency.[20] Using this scale, level 1 is at the low end and level 5 is at the high end of the literacy scale. To understand the potential impact of literacy on the delivery of healthcare education, consider the following facts based on a cross-section of the average US adult population:

- Average reading level is at 8th to 9th grade level (between literacy levels 2 and 3)
- Approximately 1 in 5 people read at or below the 5th grade level (literacy level 1)
- For adults 65 years of age and older and inner city minorities, approximately 2 in 5 read below the 5th grade level (literacy level 1)
- Most adults are successful in hiding their literacy deficit[19]

More specifically, approximately 50% of the US adult population fall into literacy levels 1 and 2, with only approximately 18% of the population at levels 4 or 5. Most individuals are capable of learning despite their literacy level, so long as the method of instruction is designed to recognize and compensate for the literacy deficits.[19] Within health care, there is a mismatch between the general literacy level and the literacy demands of healthcare instructions, with readability of most healthcare instructions being 9th grade or above.[19] The lack of agreement between the general literacy level and the complexity of healthcare instructions also impacts healthcare costs. Those with lower levels of literacy are more apt to put off preventive care measures or delay seeking medical assistance than those at high literacy levels, contributing to higher healthcare costs.[21]

Healthcare professionals have a professional responsibility to educate persons with diabetes about issues that influence their health and to ensure that the instructions they give are understandable. The challenge to create instructions that are simpler and more tailored to the learning capabilities of a major portion of the population remains. For those with the lowest literacy skills, methods of instruction that focus on nonprint media are more effective. Table 27.6 describes skills and offers suggested interventions specific to different levels of literacy. The sidebar offers guidelines for creating education materials effective at lower literacy levels.

Education Materials Effective at Lower Literacy Levels

The following are practical guidelines to consider when creating education materials, especially for lower literacy levels:[19]

- Use active voice; write the way you talk
- Use short, simple sentences and common words
- Give examples to explain difficult words or concepts
- Include the opportunity for interaction and information review

Physical Disabilities

All too often, persons with physical disabilities are assumed to be less capable than others of learning the complexities of managing life, let alone managing their diabetes. Imagine being a corporate financial executive who has had

TABLE 27.6 Literacy Level Attributes and Education Considerations

Literacy Level	*Capabilities*	*Limitations*	*Education Considerations*
1, 2	• Single-word recognition • Short, simple text • Simple addition	• Difficulty reading • Unable to interpret information • Difficulty following written instructions • May be embarrassed by or not admit to reading or comprehension difficulties	• Demonstration and repeat demonstration • Discussion • Audiovisual aids • Allow adequate time to learn • Involve support persons • Ensure mastery of simple concepts before advancing to complex
3	• More complex text • Able to identify cause and effect • Able to read and explain basic information • Low-level inferences and integration of information • Guided problem solving	• Comprehension may lag behind word recognition • Familiar with written instructions, but may be reluctant to admit to decreased understanding	• Lecture with associated written materials • Discussion • Role-playing • Interactive computer programs
4, 5	• Self-education • Use of more complex materials and concepts • High-level inferences and integration of information • Independent problem solving		• Additional reading or education materials • Theoretical or advanced discussions • May challenge the healthcare professional for additional information

Sources: Doak CC, Doak LG, Root JH. Teaching patients with low literacy skills. Philadelphia, Pa: JB Lippincott Co; 1996:1-9, 73-89; Kirsch IS, Jungeblut A, Jenkins L, Kolstad A. Adult literacy in America: a first look at the results of the national adult literacy survey. Washington, DC: National Center for Education Statistics, US Department of Education; 1993.

type 1 diabetes since he was a teen who is now experiencing aggressive advancement of retinopathy resulting in severe visual impairment. As a sighted person, this man was an ideal candidate for the latest technological advances available to care for his diabetes. Historically, he received both solicited and unsolicited information at levels appropriate for his cognitive abilities. Now significantly impaired, he is no longer able to continue working and must go to an alternate facility for his diabetes care. At this facility, he asked about a new medication that he had heard about for the treatment of diabetes. He thought the medication might be helpful in controlling some of the wide swings in blood glucose levels that had been characteristic of his diabetes for many years. However, asking his new healthcare provider about using this medication, he was met by a response that insulted his intellect, limited his access to the same resources that were available to him as a sighted individual, and undermined his confidence in his ability to self-manage his diabetes. So, what is wrong with this picture?

While disabilities related to accidents, genetic, or environmental influences occur across the population, those with diabetes are more apt to be challenged by disabilities than the general population. In 1990, the Americans with Disabilities Act was enacted to offer protection to those with disabilities in the workplace, healthcare setting, and general community.[22] Specifically, the act prohibits discrimination against those with disabilities and ensures they are afforded the same opportunities related to employment, services, commercial and public facilities, and transportation as those without disabilities. This act further defines the rights of those with disabilities:

- A right to reasonable accommodations to make goods, services, and facilities available
- Access to the goods, services, facilities, accommodations, privileges, and advantages available to those without disabilities, provided this is appropriate for the individual

The AADE offers guidance to healthcare providers caring for those with diabetes and physical disabilities. The AADE position statement, Diabetes Education for People with Diabetes, states the following:

- Disabilities do not necessarily preclude effective diabetes self-management. People who have disabilities and diabetes are usually capable of caring for themselves when they are provided with appropriate adaptive diabetes self-management education, tools, and techniques.
- People who have disabilities should receive diabetes education equivalent to that received by people without current disabilities. Disability per se should not be a barrier to the pursuit of desirable levels of glucose control.
- As new diabetes self-management tools and technologies are developed, durable medical equipment manufacturers, government and private third party payors, and diabetes care professionals are urged to make reasonable accommodations to ensure that these resources are available to people with visual and physical disabilities.[23]

Disabilities encompass any medical, physical, or emotional condition that affects the ability to learn. Thus, the presence of a disability must be incorporated into the entire education process. Assessment of individual capability, planning that incorporates accommodations specific to the person, implementation of the plan that includes ongoing evaluation, and subsequent modification as needed are key components of an education intervention designed for success. Additionally, including others that assist in the care of the disabled person can provide helpful insight about the disabled person's capabilities and challenges, while also educating them about appropriate diabetes management. Community and professional organizations that support the needs of those with disabilities can be excellent resources for education programs and materials, adaptive devices, and general information about the issues to be considered in dealing with a particular disability. In addition, several of these organizations offer support resources for both the person with diabetes and their support network. (Table 27.7)

TABLE 27.7 Resources for Information Related to Disabilities

Disability	*Organization*	*Web Site*
Amputation	Amputee Coalition of America Amputee Information Network	www.amputee-coalition.org www.amp-info.net
Hearing Impairment	Hearing Exchange National Association of the Deaf	www.hearingexchange.com www.nad.org
Kidney Diseases	National Institute of Diabetes, Digestive, and Kidney Diseases National Kidney Foundation Kidney Foundation of Canada	www.niddk.nih.gov www.kidney.org www.kidney.ca
Learning/Attention	Children and Adults with Attention Deficit Disorders (CHADD) Learning Disabilities Association of America National Center for Learning Disabilities	www.chadd.org www.ldanatl.org www.ncld.org
Macrovascular Disease	American Heart Association American Stroke Association National Stroke Association	www.americanheart.org www.strokeassociation.org www.stroke.org
Mental Illness	Center for Mental Health Services Knowledge Exchange Network Mental Help Net National Alliance for the Mentally Ill National Depressive and Manic-Depressive Association National Institute of Mental Health PsyCom.net Substance Abuse and Mental Health Services Administration	www.mentalhealth.org www.mentalhelp.net www.nami.org www.mdmda.org www.nimh.nih.gov www.psycom.net www.samhsa.gov
Mental Retardation	American Association on Mental Retardation	www.aamr.org
Visual Impairment	American Council of the Blind American Foundation for the Blind Lighthouse International National Federation of the Blind	www.acb.org www.afb.org www.lighthouse.org www.hfb.org

Source: Adapted from American Association of Diabetes Educators. Diabetes education for people with disabilities (position statement). Diabetes Educ. 2002;28(6):916-21.

Conclusion

Teaching is not a singular event and, even when repeated, does not always result in the desired learning or behavior change. Learning is a dynamic and ongoing process. As healthcare professionals, we are responsible for implementing appropriate healthcare education that promotes longevity and productivity for the people we serve. Appropriate education incorporates information that is tailored to the individual and delivered in a manner that facilitates learning. Those providing diabetes education must, therefore, adapt teaching styles, methods, and materials to be sensitive to the learning capability, readiness, needs, and cultural influences of the learner.

Standard 4 of the AADE Standards of Practice for Diabetes Educators addresses implementation of diabetes self-management education. Components and issues to consider when implementing an education plan have been addressed in this chapter. In summary, to implement diabetes education successfully, confirm the individual's readiness to learn, identify teaching methods appropriate for the person's literacy level, recognize the importance of cultural influences, and integrate these factors into the education process. Additionally, strive to motivate the people with diabetes you serve. Understand what is important to them (and why), help them identify barriers they may encounter, and work with them to address these barriers. Keep in mind that you cannot "make" someone learn, and inability or unwillingness to learn is not a permanent state. If the individual is not ready, try another time, listen a little differently, or try another method perhaps, but do not give up. Teaching can be done in many ways, at many times. By asking a question or answering one, you have likely succeeded in providing some "education."[24]

Focus on Education: Pearls for Practice

Teaching Strategies

- **Educational content.** Consider learning styles, learner readiness, and special needs of the learner (vision, concentration, physical health, etc) when determining educational content and delivery.

- **Learning Principles.** Become familiar with the principles that enhance learning: The information must be perceived as important and applicable to the person immediately or in the near future. Problem oriented learning develops problem-solving and decision-making skills. Sharing personal experiences provides more relevance. Participatory, interactive teaching is encouraged and preferred. Gather information to understand the individual and maximize the effectiveness of education; this applies to determining literacy goals as well.

- **Educational content.** Ensure that materials and methods are at the appropriate literacy level. Move in sequence from simple to more complex information. Practice sensitivity and awareness of cultural differences, and adjust teaching options to fit the person's style.

- **Individualized services.** Provide special services, when indicated, to meet a person's needs. Learners may require modifications: a deaf interpreter, large-print materials, or recorded sessions, for example.

- **Teacher skills.** Be aware of your teaching style and comfort level in teaching. Be flexible regarding content delivery and presentation; for example, avoid being bound to teaching only the information outlined in the teaching plan or too much of it. Communicate by speaking and listening well! Recognize that your accessibility and effectiveness will influence the learners' attitudes, motivation, and willingness to self-manage diabetes and make appropriate choices. Recognize that managing diabetes requires the individual with the disease to translate the science into daily self-care practices.

Patient Education

- **Education is ongoing.** Diabetes education is not just a one-time event. Take as much time as you need to understand and make choices.

- **Your rights.** You have the right and responsibility to ask questions, seek clarification, and make decisions and changes in managing your diabetes and overall health. You have a right to know all the choices, alternatives, and potential outcomes of your choices. You have the right to a second opinion, to ask your family or others for advice, and to take as much time as is needed.

References

1. Diabetes Control and Complications Trial Research Group. The effect of intensive treatment of diabetes on the development and progression of long-term complications in insulin-dependent diabetes mellitus. N Engl J Med. 1993;329:977-86.
2. UK Prospective Diabetes Study (UKPDS) Group. Intensive blood glucose control with sulfonylureas or insulin compared with conventional treatment and risk of complications in patients with type 2 diabetes (UKPDS 33). Lancet. 1998;345:837-53.
3. Funnell MM, Mensing CR. Diabetes education in the management of diabetes. In Complete Nurse's Guide to Diabetes Care. Childs B, Cypress M, Spollet G, eds. Alexandria, Va: American Diabetes Association; 2005:188-98.
4. Martin C, Daly A, McWhorter LS, Shwide-Slavin C, Kushion W; for the American Association of Diabetes Educators. The scope of practice, standards of practice, and standards of professional performance for diabetes educators. Diabetes Educ. 2005;31(4):487-512.
5. Walker EA. Characteristics of the adult learner. Diabetes Educ. 1999;25(6):16-24.
6. Redman BK. The Practice of Patient Education. St Louis, Mo: Mosby; 2001:7-79.
7. Grey M, Boland ED, Davidson M, Li J, Tamborlane WV. Coping skills training for youth with diabetes mellitus has long-lasting effects on metabolic control and quality of life. J Pediatr. 2000;137:107-13.
8. American Association of Diabetes Educators. Special considerations for the education and management of older adults with diabetes (position statement). Diabetes Educ. 2002.
9. Anderson RM. Applied principles of teaching and learning. In: A Core Curriculum for Diabetes Education: Diabetes Education and Program Management, 4th ed. Franz MF, ed. Chicago, Ill: American Association of Diabetes Educators, 2001:3-18.
10. Rubin RR, Napora JP. Behavior change. In: A Core Curriculum for Diabetes Education: Diabetes Education and Program Management, 4th ed. Franz MJ, ed. Chicago, Ill: American Association of Diabetes Educators, 2001:72-92.
11. Weinger K, McMurrich SJ. Behavioral strategies for improving self-management. In: Complete Nurse's Guide to Diabetes Care. Childs B, Cypress M, Spollet G, eds. Alexandria, Va: American Diabetes Association, 2005:199-206.
12. American Association of Diabetes Educators. Standards for outcome measurement of diabetes self-management education (position statement). Diabetes Educ. 2003;29(5)804-15.
13. Kirsch IS, Jungeblut A, Jenkins L, Kolstad A. Adult Literacy in America. Washington, DC: National Center for Education Statistics, US Department of Education; 1993:xvi.
14. Melkus GD, Newlin K. Cultural context of diabetes education and care. In: Complete Nurse's Guide to Diabetes Care. Chicago, Ill and Alexandria, Va: American Diabetes Association; 2005:207-19.
15. Campinha-Bacote J. A culturally conscious approach to holistic nursing. Program and abstracts of the American Holistic Nurses Association 2005 Conference; June 2005; King of Prussia, Pa.
16. Campinha-Bacote J. The process of cultural competence in the delivery of healthcare services: a model of care. J Transcult Nurs. 2002;13:181-4.
17. Robins LS. Cultural competence in diabetes education and care. In: A Core Curriculum for Diabetes Education: Diabetes Education and Program Management, 4th ed. Franz MJ, ed. Chicago, Ill: American Association of Diabetes Educators; 2001:99-114.
18. Pichert JW, Anderst JD, Miller S. Teaching persons with low literacy skills. In: A Core Curriculum for Diabetes Education: Diabetes Education and Program Management, 4th ed. Franz MJ, ed. Chicago, Ill: American Association of Diabetes Educators; 2001:123-38.
19. Doak CC, Doak LG, Root JH. Teaching patients with low literacy skills. Philadelphia, Pa: JB Lippincott Co; 1996:1-9, 73-89.
20. Kirsch IS, Jungeblut A, Jenkins L, Kolstad A. Adult literacy in America: a first look at the results of the national adult literacy survey. Washington, DC: National Center for Education Statistics, US Department of Education; 1993.
21. Weiss BD, Blanchard JS. McGee DL, et al. Illiteracy among Medicaid recipients and its relationship to health care costs. J Health Care Poor Underserved. 1994;5(20):99-111.
22. Americans with Disabilities Act of 1990: Public Law 101-336, 101st Congress. Washington, DC: US Government Printing Office; 1990.
23. American Association of Diabetes Educators. Diabetes education for people with disabilities (position statement). Diabetes Educ. 2002;28(6):916-21.
24. Kanzer-Lewis G. Patient education: You can do it! Alexandria, Va: American Diabetes Association; 2003.

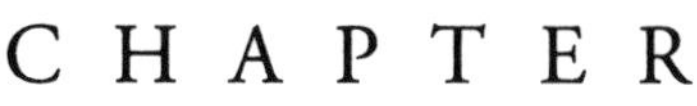

CHAPTER

28

Evaluating and Documenting Outcomes

Authors

Jackie L. Boucher, MS, RD, BC-ADM, CDE
Jeffrey J. VanWormer, MS

Key Concepts

- Documentation and evaluation of education and patient care should include immediate, intermediate, post-intermediate, and long-term outcomes.
- Documentation at the aggregate level provides data for future educational planning; program outcome evaluation can be used to determine how well a program of diabetes self-management education is meeting the needs of individuals with diabetes.
- Data can be analyzed to determine if the needs of the greater community are being met (eg, populations at risk or the underserved).
- Implementation of a continuous quality improvement process is critical to problem solving and identifying whether individuals are achieving their personalized goals and if program goals have been met or are in need of improvement.
- The AADE 7 Self-Care Behaviors™ are one system upon which outcomes can be evaluated. Use of the AADE 7 Self-Care Behaviors™ Goal Sheet facilitates documentation while reinforcing important behavior changes.
- A framework can be of value in evaluating an education program's impact. Two models to consider are the RE-AIM model (organized around the dimensions of reach, effectiveness, adoption, implementation, and maintenance) and the PIPE model (organized around 4 coefficients: penetration, implementation, participation, and effectiveness).

Introduction

This chapter discusses documentation and evaluation of individual participant outcomes and aggregate data of value in improving diabetes education. The fundamental steps preceding documentation and evaluation—assessment, planning, and implementation—are discussed in chapters 25 through 27.

Documentation, the focus of the first part of this chapter, is critical to the process of diabetes self-management education (DSME). The information is needed both to evaluate outcomes related to the individual and to evaluate a DSME program's achievement of its goals. Without such documentation, providing ongoing education that evolves to match the changing needs of the person with diabetes is virtually impossible.

Evaluation is the focus in the second part of the chapter. As with documentation, the chapter looks at the role of evaluation in helping both the individual with diabetes who is seeking care as well as the DSME program, which can enhance individual outcomes by examining aggregated data. Tools of value in evaluating outcomes are also discussed.

Guidelines for documentation and evaluation are outlined in Standard 9 of the National Standards for Diabetes Self-Management Education (NSDSME).[1] This chapter provides information to help diabetes educators meet this standard.

Documentation

Documentation for the Individual

Standard 9 of the NSDSME states that, "there shall be documentation of the individual's assessment, education plan, intervention, evaluation, and follow-up in the permanent confidential education record."[1] This documentation must occur at every step in the DSME process. DSME is defined as an interactive, collaborative, ongoing process involving the person with diabetes and the educator(s).[2] The process includes the following steps:[2,3]

Case in Point: Diabetes Education With an Outcomes Focus

Two months ago, TM was referred to a diabetes education program for assistance. She had been recently diagnosed with type 2 diabetes and started on metformin. During her first visit, an in-depth assessment was completed. TM was 50 years old and had a body mass index of 30, a blood pressure of 120/80 mm Hg, and a fasting blood glucose of 200 mg/dL. She also had 3 children, worked full-time and as a result, had limited time to lead an active lifestyle. She was interested in eating healthier so that both she and her family might benefit.

During her initial visit, TM was taught how to self-monitor blood glucose, given basic information on carbohydrate counting, and provided with a pedometer to promote a walking program and help assess her activity level. When she left the visit, her identified goals were to self-monitor her blood glucose at least twice a day, wear the pedometer for at least 3 days before she returned to assess her baseline activity level, and eat 3 meals per day with 3 to 4 carbohydrate choices per meal. When TM returned for follow-up 2 months later, she had met her goals and was ready to learn more to manage her diabetes.

TM achieved her goals, but will these changes last and ultimately lead to improved health and quality of life? Do your patients return for follow-up? Can you determine if they achieve their goals? Most of these questions can be answered if key elements of care are documented and an evaluation plan is in place.

Step 1: Assessment
The individual's specific education needs should be assessed
↓
Step 2: Outcomes Identification
The individual's specific diabetes self-management goals should be identified
↓
Step 3: Planning
A plan is mutually developed to achieve the outcomes identified
↓
Step 4: Implementation
Education and behavioral interventions directed toward helping the individual achieve identified self-management goals as planned are provided
↓
Step 5: Evaluation of Outcomes
Attainment of identified self-management goals for each individual are evaluated

Developing the documentation is an ongoing process, not a one-time event. Its purpose is to support each step of DSME and result in the final product, a program evaluation. Quality documentation should be relevant, accurate, and timely.[4] Table 28.1 describes the information to be included at each step to ensure accurate, high-quality documentation throughout the DSME process.

Deciding exactly what should be documented can be difficult. Individual patient outcomes are perhaps the most important. For an individual patient to be successful, the following written elements are required:[5]

- *Outcomes Measurement:* Consistent measurement of specific indicators
- *Outcomes Monitoring:* Measurement of these indicators at specified intervals
- *Outcomes Management:* Use of these outcomes to drive educational and clinical decision-making

Standards for measurement of diabetes education outcomes:

The AADE has developed standards for outcomes measurement.[5] These standards, which complement the NSDSME, are listed below.

1. Behavior change is the unique outcome measurement for DSME.
2. Seven diabetes self-care behavior measures—known as the AADE 7 Self-Care Behaviors™—can be used to determine the effectiveness of DSME at the individual, participant, and population level:
    - Being Active
    - Healthy Eating
    - Taking Medication
    - Monitoring
    - Problem Solving
    - Reducing Risks
    - Healthy Coping

    (See chapters 29 to 35 for more information on each of these behaviors.)
3. Diabetes self-care behaviors should be evaluated at baseline and then at regular intervals following the initial education program.

TABLE 28.1 Documentation of the Process of Diabetes Self-Management Education

Process	*What to Document*
Step 1: Assessment	• Date and time of assessment • Pertinent data collected from medical records, referring providers, person with diabetes, and family members/support persons • Comparison of data collected with standards • Patient's readiness to change, values, and perceptions • Changes in level of understanding, self-care behaviors, and pertinent clinical or functional outcomes
Step 2: Outcomes Identification	• Date and time • Specific treatment and behavioral goals and expected outcomes as identified by the assessment process
Step 3: Planning	• Date and time • Recommended interventions and instructional strategies to be used and who on the care team will be providing those interventions • Plans for follow-up and frequency of care and how the care will be evaluated
Step 4: Implementation	• Date and time interventions provided • Description of interventions provided, including educational materials used, and patient receptivity/understanding • Referrals made, resources used, and communication with referring provider (if appropriate) • Rationale for discharge/discontinuation of care, if appropriate
Step 5: Evaluation	• Date and time • Specific outcomes measured (ie, learning, behavioral, clinical, and health status) and results • Progress toward goals and/or barriers to achieving goals

Sources: American Association of Diabetes Educators. The Scope of Practice, Standards of Practice, and Standards of Professional Performance for Diabetes Educators. Diabetes Educ. 2005;31:487-513; Lacey K, Pritchett E. Nutrition care process and model: ADA adopts road map to quality care and outcomes management. J Am Diet Assoc. 2003;103(8):1061-72.

4. The continuum of outcomes, including learning, behavioral, clinical, satisfaction, and health status, should be assessed to demonstrate the interrelationship between DSME and behavior change in the care of individuals with diabetes (see Figure 28.1).
5. Individual patient outcomes are used to guide the intervention and improve care for that individual. Aggregate population outcomes are used to guide programmatic services and for continuous quality improvement (CQI) activities for the DSME program and the population it serves.

Desired outcomes should be measured before and after the educational intervention for each individual receiving care.[5] Additional follow-up measurements are ideal and should be applied as appropriate to the practice setting. Short hospital stays and lack of return for follow-up do not preclude evaluation.[4]

Innovative methods of contacting patients help monitor progress:

Mailings, telephone, and Internet follow-up are some of the innovative methods that can be used to contact patients to monitor their progress[4] and improve outcomes.

Documenting what the diabetes educator has done (the interventions provided) and what goals the educator and the individual with diabetes have collaboratively established is one component of the educational process. This documentation is then in place to assess and evaluate progress. Having this documentation also assists in meeting the criteria established by the American Diabetes Association (ADA) for recognition of the diabetes education program and in evaluating a program's achievements.

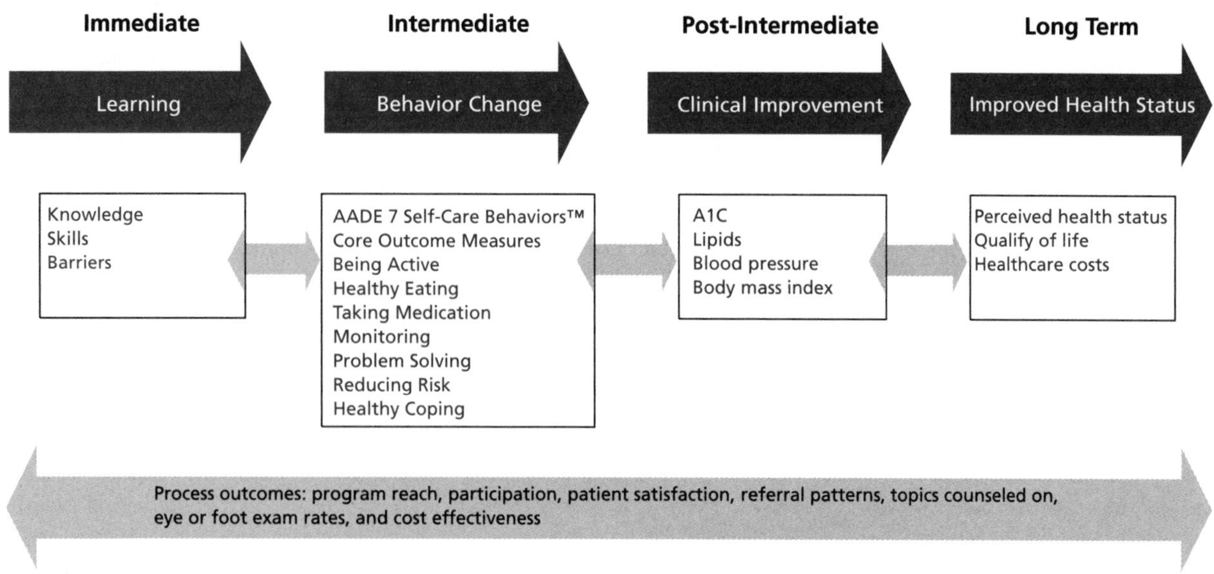

FIGURE 28.1 Diabetes Self-Management Education Outcomes Continuum

Sources: Adapted from the following: Lacey K, Pritchett E. Nutrition care process and model: ADA adopts road map to quality care and outcomes management. J Am Diet Assoc. 2003;103(8):1061-72; American Association of Diabetes Educators. Standards for outcomes measurement of diabetes self-management education. Diabetes Educ. 2003;29:804-16.

Determining the Desired Outcome

The first step in this phase is to determine the outcome that is being sought. Ultimately, the long-term goal is to help the individual with diabetes improve his or her health through more effective management—in large part by identifying potential behavior reinforcement or changes that will help the person accomplish his or her goals. The diabetes educator will want to work collaboratively with each patient to identify and monitor individual goals. In addition, the educator needs to assess how an individual's achievements, or lack thereof, have affected outcomes. This is a step toward addressing barriers, acknowledging successes, and revising goals as appropriate.

Collaboratively Establishing Goals

In collaboration with each patient, the diabetes educator should establish and document specific goals and objectives. The aim is to set goals and write specific behavioral objectives that are important to the individual and that the individual feels confident about achieving.

Additionally, those working in an ADA-Recognized Education Program must establish goals, learning objectives, and behavioral objectives (for more information see www.diabetes.org/for-health-professionals-and-scientists/recognition/edrecognition.jsp). These 2 distinct types of objectives are defined as follows:

- *Goal.* This serves as a big-picture, directional guide; it is the focal point for the objectives and end result of meeting the objectives
- *Learning Objective.* This is the objective the individual with diabetes is expected to meet at the end of the educational intervention. Examples of learning objectives are "identify 3 foods with carbohydrate" and "discuss sick day treatment guidelines."
- *Behavioral Objective.* Also called a behavioral goal, this is a planned, measurable change in behavior that is expected to achieve a positive health outcome over a period of time once the initial intervention is completed. Examples of behavioral objectives are "eat 3 to 4 carbohydrate choices per meal" and "monitor blood glucose 4 times per day."

Using Tools to Track Progress

Documenting goals, objectives, and outcomes of those goals is important to assess impact and refocus treatment. When the documentation is in the patient's chart and the goals and outcomes are tracked in various notes, tracking and identifying progress or opportunities for improvement is not always easy. Use of forms or checklists can help the educator and the patient track different behaviors, assess progress toward goals, and see how achievement or lack of achievement of those goals impacts treatment outcomes.

Forms can be used for both individual-level interventions and group classes.

One example of a tool for tracking progress is the AADE 7 Self-Care Behaviors™ Goal Sheet (part of the AADE 7 IMPACT™ product) (see Figure 28.2). This tool allows the educator to not only introduce the concept of 7 critical self-care behaviors to patients, but to also allow the educator, care team, colleagues, and patients to track goals and goal achievement in a consistent manner.

Evaluating Goals and Objectives

The following are some key areas to consider when evaluating the goal.

What is the patient's assessment of the goal?

- Did the patient feel he or she achieved the goal?
- How would the patient rate his or her progress?
- Both open-ended questions and scales can be of value. For example, the person can be asked to rate his or her progress on a Likert scale of 1 to 10 (1= did not meet goal; 10 = achieved goal) or given word choices (eg, met goal most of the time, some of the time, did not meet goal, or changed goal).

What is your collaborative assessment of the goal?

- Was the goal appropriate for the patient?
- Did the patient have adequate time to achieve the goal?
- Did the goal achieve the expected outcome?
- Did that outcome impact the diabetes treatment plan?
- If so, does therapy need to change?

What should the next steps be?

- Should the goal be changed or continued?
- Should additional goals be added or other goals changed?
- When will new goals be evaluated?
- What other changes in the diabetes treatment plan need to occur to support the goal(s)?

Once evaluation of the information has taken place, the educator should summarize this information and send a summary of results to the referring provider. This information can also be reviewed by the educational team, summarized (blinded), and presented to the advising group, who may offer suggestions, interpretation, and ideas for possible improvements to the educational process.

Using Protocols With Time Frames

The DSME practice should establish standardized time frames (protocols) for following up on individual outcomes. Standardized protocols are useful for tracking how many classes a patient attends, the number of one-to-one visits a patient keeps, and the combination of group and individual follow-up visits. As part of the educational process, the educator must think about time frames when documenting the education provided and the outcomes achieved.

Outcomes related to the AADE 7 Self-Care Behaviors™ can, for example, be documented at baseline (ie, first visit or class) and then at specified time points, such as months 1, 3, 6, and 12. As part of the protocol, the practice should determine if the most effective way to obtain this information (based on the practice's patient population) is via face-to-face visits, group classes, mail, e-mail, or phone. The key is to document the information with a standardized method. If the information is to be used as part of an overall diabetes program evaluation strategy, this will enable the practice to track the same information at these specified time points so data can be aggregated and reviewed with the instructional staff and advising group. The purpose is to determine if the best possible methods and educational strategies are being used to gain the best health outcomes with each patient. One approach to doing this is to identify one team member to be in charge of this process, then shepherd that person to see that follow-up and evaluation actually occur (ie, patients are contacted, feedback is collected, and so on).

Documentation for the Aggregate

Aggregate-level activities start with high-quality documentation at the individual level (see Mulcahy and colleagues[6]). As described, documentation should take place at least before and after the intervention.[5] Ideally, documentation should take place more frequently to identify aggregate-level trends in a program evaluation.

- Program performance can be assessed and compared against standards and/or other benchmarks
- Data can be used to improve the quality of care and/or identify subpopulations of patients who may benefit from additional care

Many relevant data points at the aggregate level, however, are not captured in the individual-level charting of standard DSME outcomes. Because of this, important process and logistical variables are easy to overlook. Capturing data that answers aggregate-level questions such as the following can be exceptionally challenging:

- How many patients received care in the program?
- What were the most common interventions?
- How much did treatment cost?

As outlined in Standard 2 of the NSDSME, program managers should identify all needed data points a priori so that proper investments can be made in the technical systems and/or staff processes that can realistically capture the needed information.[1] If resources permit, managers should consider automating or outsourcing difficult methods of process data collection. For example, the number of

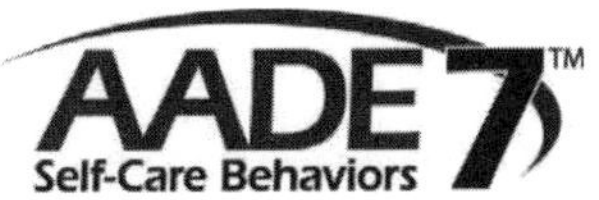

Patient name: ______________________

Addressograph/Stamp Area

Goal Setting		Follow Up		Goal Review
Date	Goal	Date	Achievement	Documentation
Date:	☐ **Healthy eating**	Date:		☐ Achieved ☐ Continued ☐ Modified
	☐ Make better food choices ☐ Reduce portion size ☐ Follow meal plan Goal individualization: ______	☐ 1 mo. ☐ 3 mo. ☐ 6 mo. ☐ 12 mo.	Rate 0-10 _____	
Date:	☐ **Being active**	Date:		☐ Achieved ☐ Continued ☐ Modified
	☐ Exercise longer ☐ Exercise more often ☐ Follow exercise plan Goal individualization: ______	☐ 1 mo. ☐ 3 mo. ☐ 6 mo. ☐ 12 mo.	Rate 0-10 _____	
Date:	☐ **Monitoring**	Date:		☐ Achieved ☐ Continued ☐ Modified
	☐ Follow monitoring schedule ☐ Monitor more often ☐ Monitor health status Goal individualization: ______	☐ 1 mo. ☐ 3 mo. ☐ 6 mo. ☐ 12 mo.	Rate 0-10 _____	
Date:	☐ **Taking medication**	Date:		☐ Achieved ☐ Continued ☐ Modified
	☐ Increase taking medications on time ☐ Miss fewer medications ☐ Take medications as prescribed Goal individualization: ______	☐ 1 mo. ☐ 3 mo. ☐ 6 mo. ☐ 12 mo.	Rate 0-10 _____	
Date:	☐ **Problem solving**	Date:		☐ Achieved ☐ Continued ☐ Modified
	☐ Identify potential problems ☐ Plan problem situation treatment ☐ Prevent problem situations Goal individualization: ______	☐ 1 mo. ☐ 3 mo. ☐ 6 mo. ☐ 12 mo.	Rate 0-10 _____	
Date:	☐ **Healthy coping**	Date:		☐ Achieved ☐ Continued ☐ Modified
	☐ Cope with diagnosis of disease ☐ Adapt to lifestyle changes ☐ Get support from family/friends Goal individualization: ______	☐ 1 mo. ☐ 3 mo. ☐ 6 mo. ☐ 12 mo.	Rate 0-10 _____	
Date:	☐ **Reducing risks**	Date:		☐ Achieved ☐ Continued ☐ Modified
	☐ Stop smoking ☐ Get health checkups ☐ Perform daily self-care activities Goal individualization: ______	☐ 1 mo. ☐ 3 mo. ☐ 6 mo. ☐ 12 mo.	Rate 0-10 _____	

Diabetes Educator Name and Initial Index:

Name: ______ Initial: ____	Name: ______ Initial: ____
Name: ______ Initial: ____	Name: ______ Initial: ____

FIGURE 28.2 AADE 7 Self-Care Behaviors™ Goal Sheet (part of the AADE 7 IMPACT™ product)

participants seen by diabetes educators, as well as the type of interventions used, could be automatically "pulled" from electronic medical records into convenient reports. Likewise, cost data could be ascertained from records of insurance claims. It is important to note, however, that all levels of documentation are protected under the Health Insurance Portability and Accountability Act.[7] Personal health information must always be stored, analyzed, and reported in a manner that protects the identification of individuals.

Documentation should ultimately capture immediate, intermediate and post-intermediate, and long-term outcomes.[6]

- *Immediate outcomes* are those that can be measured at the time the intervention is delivered—Learning, for example, is an immediate outcome
- *Intermediate and post-intermediate outcomes* result over time—behavior changes and clinical improvements are examples
- *Long-term outcomes* result from multiple variables over an extended period of time—reduction in healthcare costs and improvements in quality of life are possible long-term outcomes

These types of outcomes can be measured using a variety of tools (see Table 28.2),[8] leading to the eventual product of high-quality documentation and program evaluation. Table 28.3 provides examples of outcomes specific to the AADE 7 Self-Care Behaviors™ measures.[6] For specific examples of diabetes-related surveys, see the Michigan Diabetes Research and Training Center Web site at www.med.umich.edu/mdrtc/survey/index.html.

Key Terms

Aggregate-level outcomes are pooled data that is routinely assessed, summarized, and reported.

Continuous quality improvement (CQI) is a management approach that attempts to correct program shortcomings via the timely use of program evaluations. Steps often used in CQI include the following: identify the opportunity for improvement, collect data, analyze data, choose an approach, develop the concepts and processes, implement, evaluate, and improve.

Evaluation is the act of examining processes and outcomes to determine whether the desired goals and objectives (individual or program) were achieved.

Immediate outcomes are those that can be measured at the time of the intervention (eg, learning as assessed by testing or direct observation).

Intermediate and post-intermediate outcomes are those that result over time, require more than a single measurement, are sensitive to change, and may show a statistical change (eg, behavior change or clinical improvements).

Long-term outcomes result from multiple variables over an extended time (eg, improved health or quality of life).

Outcomes management is how outcomes are used for educational and clinical decision making.

Outcomes measurement is the process of consistently measuring specific indicators.

Outcomes monitoring is the frequency and interval of measuring specific indicators.

Program evaluation is the systematic collection of information about the activities, characteristics, and outcomes of programs to make judgments about the program, improve program effectiveness, and/or inform decisions about future program development.

TABLE 28.2 Data Collection Tools

Method	*Examples of Outcomes Collected*	*Easy to Use?*	*Yields Reliable Data?*	*High Response Rate?*
Survey Method used to question individuals in writing, face-to-face, by phone, or by mail	Learning; behavior change; quality of life; satisfaction	Yes; can be designed to be simple and easy to use	Yes; although respondents' interpretation of survey questions can vary	Depends; telephone or face-to-face surveys can have a high response rate
Chart/File Audit Review of closed, open, or computerized medical records to retrieve information	Lab data (AlC, lipids); process data (eye or foot exam)	Depends; paper chart review can be labor-intensive and time-intensive	Depends on skill of individuals doing the review	Yes
Checklist Data collection sheet for gathering concurrent information during a study	Behavior change; process and implementation tasks	Yes; can be designed to be simple and easy to use	Depends; all people who will be completing the checklist during the data collection must be trained on how to use the data collection instrument	Depends on the cooperation and availability of the personnel completing the forms
Time Study Concurrent information about time to complete a process such as turnaround time	Cycle time to schedule a patient for a visit	Usually very time-intensive and labor-intensive	Depends; all people who will be completing the time study during the data collection must be trained on how to use the instrument	Depends on the cooperation and availability of the personnel completing the study

Source: Adapted from Mulcahy K. Management of diabetes education programs. In: A Core Curriculum for Diabetes Educators, 5th ed. Franz MJ, ed. Chicago, Ill: American Association of Diabetes Educators; 2003:203.

TABLE 28.3 Outcomes for the AADE 7 Self-Care Behaviors™

	Immediate Outcome*			Intermediate Outcome†	
	Knowledge	*Skill*	*Barriers*	*Measures*	*Methods of Measurement*
Being Active physical activity, exercise	Type; duration; intensity; safety precautions.	Develops appropriate activity plan; balances food and medication with activity.	Physical limitations; time; environment; fear.	Type; frequency; duration; intensity.	Patient self-report; observation; use of tools such as a pedometer.
Healthy Eating	Effect of food on blood glucose; sources of carbohydrate; meal plan (what to eat, when to eat, how much to eat); resources to assist in food choices.	Meal-planning; weighing and measuring food; carbohydrate counting; label reading.	Environmental triggers; emotional eating; cultural influences; financial issues.	Type of food choices; amount of food eaten; timing of meals; alcohol intake; effect of food on glucose; special situations and problem solving.	Patient self-report; observation; records of food and blood glucose; food recall (eg, 24-hour recall or food frequency questionnaires).
Taking Medication	Name, dose, frequency; medication action; action for missed dose; side effects, toxicity; action for side effect; storage, travel, safety; recognition of efficacy.	Preparation, technique, administration; safe handling, disposal of equipment; dose adjustment; recognition, treatment, prevention of low blood glucose.	Vision or dexterity; financial; fear of needles; cognitive, math skills; embarrassment.	Adherence to medication; dose accuracy.	Pill count; review of pharmacy refill; demonstration, patient self-report; records of blood glucose and medication; observation and role playing.
Monitoring of blood glucose	Testing schedule; target values; proper disposal of sharps; interpretation, use of results.	Self-blood glucose monitoring techniques; records of blood glucose values; equipment use, care.	Physical; financial; cognitive; time; inconvenient; emotional.	Frequency of missed tests; frequency and schedule of monitoring (eg, times/day, days/week); planned, unplanned testing; review of pharmacy refill record.	Review of log book; meter memory review or printout; patient self-report; demonstration of technique.
Problem Solving especially for blood glucose: high and low levels and sick days	Signs, symptoms, causes; treatment, guidelines, prevention strategies; sick day rules; safety concerns (eg, driving, operation equipment).	Hypoglycemia treatment; glucagon administration (if applicable); use of blood glucose data to determine appropriate actions related to food, exercise, medication.	Cognitive; financial; coping strategies; emotional; physical.	Blood glucose testing; adjusting food, medication, activity; contact with healthcare provider for problem resolution; checking meter and strips for function; number of blood glucose tests per month that require assistance; number of times ketones are tested (when appropriate); missed days from work, school, or related activities.	Patient self-report; review of log book; meter memory review or printout; medical chart review; frequency of medication adjustment.

TABLE 28.3 Outcomes for the AADE 7 Self-Care Behaviors™

	*Immediate Outcome**			*Intermediate Outcome†*	
	Knowledge	*Skill*	*Barriers*	*Measures*	*Methods of Measurement*
Reducing Risks of diabetes complications	Standards of care; therapeutic goals; how to decrease risks (through preventive services).	Foot exam; blood pressure (self); self-monitoring of blood glucose; maintaining personal care record.	Financial; time; unaware of disease process or seriousness; lacking rapport with provider; travel; physical disabilities.	Smoking status; frequency of foot self-exam; aspirin therapy; eye exam; MD visit; diabetes educator visit; RD visit; lipids checked; blood pressure checked; flu vaccine, pneumonia vaccine; urine check for protein; prepregnancy counseling.	Patient self-report; chart or exam code audit for demonstration of self-care activities.
Healthy Coping living with diabetes (psychosocial adaptation)	Recognizing that everyone has problems; benefits of treatment and self-care; motivation is internal function.	Goal setting; problem solving; coping strategies; self-efficacy.	Lack of awareness; financial; lack of support; physical; psychosocial distress.	Depression score; stress; quality of life; functional measurement; treatment self-efficacy; patient empowerment; self-report.	SF-36/SF-12; PAID; Zung/Beck Depression Scale; D-SMART.

*Immediate outcomes are those that can be measured at the time of the intervention (eg, learning).

†Intermediate outcomes result over time (eg, behavior change) and require more than a single measurement.

Source: Adapted from Mulcahy K, Maryniuk M, Peeples M, et al. Diabetes self-management education core outcomes measures. Diabetes Educ. 2003;29:768-88.

Evaluation

Individual Evaluation

Evaluation is the final step in DSME, before the process cycles again into reassessment, planning, and implementation. At the individual level, evaluation helps examine processes and outcomes to determine whether an individual achieved the agreed-upon goals.[9]

- Patients get measurable feedback on how they are doing (eg, when comparisons are made against standards) and it helps drive the interventions selected to help them achieve their goals.
- The effectiveness of specific interventions can be determined which helps make decisions on what interventions to continue in practice.

Setting goals and monitoring/evaluating progress provide both the educator and the person with diabetes with information on what is working and what is not. Evaluation is based on individual variables, but allows others to see the bigger picture. With systematic collection of information about the activities, characteristics, and outcomes of programs, judgments can be made about the program to improve its effectiveness and/or enable informed decision making for future program development.[10]

Examples of evaluation as they relate to patient outcomes include the following:

- *Knowledge:* Based on pre- and post-tests to determine what information presented was retained
- *Skill Mastery:* By return demonstration
- *Satisfaction Level:* Regarding the DSME training provided

One method of determining satisfaction is to provide the patient and the referring provider with a brief satisfaction survey. This can be completed and returned to the educational team. Content includes items related to education and may use a Likert scale (in which information is ranked from 1 to 10) or word choices. Statements such as, "Patient was able to identify targets for blood glucose (eg, 70 to 140 mg/dL) and blood lipid levels (eg, LDL-C under

100 g/dL)" and "Patient is able to demonstrate types of food and their portions that would equal a meal with 60 g of carbohydrate" are examples of the latter.

Program Evaluation

Program evaluation has at least 4 general purposes:[11]

1. *To Gain Insight:* For example, documenting or assessing an innovative approach to practice
2. *To Change Practice:* For example, improving operations, refining program strategy, or improving quality or efficiency
3. *To Assess Effects:* For example, documenting program outcomes, both intended and unintended
4. *To Affect Participants:* For example, serving as a catalyst for self-directed change among stakeholders, spurring staff development, contributing to organizational change

As outlined in Figure 28.1, evaluations basically reveal how well the program works. Such information empowers the care team to improve their performance in a manner that is consistent with evidence-based medicine.[12] Conducting a program evaluation, however, is more complicated than merely summing up and reporting each of the outcomes. Traditionally, program evaluations have been overly focused on efficacy.[13,14] A simple literature search of published randomized, controlled trials that employ counseling by diabetes educators illustrates the fact that most interventions are nearly exclusively concerned with answering the question, "Does the treatment reduce A1C level?" Although the answer to this research question likely represents the bottom line in the minds of most consumers and healthcare purchasers, it ignores other key elements that portray a program's true impact.

Impact is essentially the ability of a program to improve the health of a targeted community. Several evaluation frameworks have been developed that expand on efficacy and attempt to illustrate program impact,[15,16] but most are complicated and difficult to use. In addition to the CQI process, which has been promoted for some time, at least 2 other models have been developed recently to help managers evaluate their health education programs more meaningfully, including diabetes education.

> ***CQI Resource***
>
> *CQI: A Step-by-Step Guide for Quality Improvement in Diabetes Education* is an AADE publication that can help improve patient care and program management.

Evaluation Tools and Frameworks

This section discusses 3 widely used tools that can be of value in evaluating a DSME program:

- The CQI process
- The RE-AIM model
- The PIPE framework

Using What You Know: Continuous Quality Improvement

As implied in Standard 10 of the NSDSME,[1] documentation and evaluation are not particularly useful activities if the information is not put into action in making real performance improvements. To ensure program managers are using the information gathered, the NSDSME recommend implementing a CQI process. CQI is a management approach that attempts to correct program shortcomings via the timely use of program evaluations.[17,18] It is essentially a program-level approach to problem solving.

CQI is as much a management philosophy, however, as it is a set of techniques.[19] To implement a CQI program effectively, program managers must adopt a plan that meets its customers' needs.

The first step is to identify exactly who the customers are. The obvious selection is individuals with diabetes, but third party payors and regulatory agencies may also need to be considered.

The next step is to determine what outcomes will be assessed to gauge performance. Again, the obvious selection may be the AADE 7 Self-Care Behaviors™ identified by Mulcahy and colleagues,[6] but managers should consider programmatic challenges as well. For example, if a program has low enrollment, managers should strive to capture accurate participation rates. Technical process issues (eg, equipment functioning, computer systems utilization) may also be of interest.

Once the customers and outcomes of interest are identified, a formal plan can be developed by recording the goals and who is responsible for what.

Program managers can appoint a team to lead the CQI effort and decide on a schedule of regular meetings to receive updates on the process. During such meetings, a simple cycle of Plan, Do, Check, Act (PDCA) can be used to carry out attempts at improving performance.[20]

The PDCA cycle can be illustrated using the weight management program implemented by HealthPartners. During the regular CQI meetings conducted by HealthPartners management, penetration was quickly identified as a potential deficit in the program (the goal of penetrating a community will be discussed more fully in the discussion of the PIPE model). As a result of these CQI discussions, the team *planned* to report on penetration in the upcoming final analysis. A critical action identified to *do* was to contact the HealthPartners clinics to obtain an estimate of the total overweight population (so penetration could be calculated from participation data). Penetration was then formally *checked* in a review of the final data analysis. Based on this, several solutions for improving penetration were identified (eg, offering the weight management program for a longer amount of time, marketing the program more intensely, expanding the referral capacity to ancillary staff, limiting the scope of the target population) to *act* on in future program roll-outs.

The RE-AIM Framework

Perhaps the model most widely used in evaluating the overall impact of health intervention programs is the RE-AIM framework.[13] RE-AIM is an acronym for the program dimensions to be evaluated: reach, effectiveness, adoption, implementation, and maintenance. Each dimension, or element, is summarized in the adjacent sidebar.

The essential purpose of the RE-AIM framework is to help managers determine the characteristics of their program that can reach large volumes of people, be adopted across many different settings, be easily and consistently implemented by staff, and produce long-term benefits (at a reasonable cost).[21] Eakin, Bull, Glasgow, and Mason recently used the RE-AIM framework to evaluate studies that employed DSME with underserved (eg, low-income, minority) populations.[22] About half of the studies reported on the percentage of patients who participated, but data on adoption and implementation were almost never reported. The investigators concluded that studies of modalities that explicitly address the issues within a community are needed to increase the reach (and improve the long-term effectiveness) of DSME across underserved populations.

When starting a program or evaluating an existing program, program management may want to review each of the RE-AIM dimensions. By asking key questions related to each dimension of RE-AIM, program management can gather important information on all aspects of the programs and services delivered, thereby improving not only the quality of the program, but engaging staff, referring providers, and the diabetes care team in the process. The RE-AIM Web site, at www.re-aim.org, provides more questions and information, including interactive calculators and checklists.

The PIPE Model

The PIPE model (an acronym for penetration, implementation, participation, and effectiveness) is perhaps the most straightforward evaluation framework,[14] although it

Dimensions of the RE-AIM Framework

Reach is the participation rate of eligible individuals and representativeness of patients treated. Evaluations of reach consider issues such as the following:

- How many patients comprise our target population?
- How many participated (ie, were reached)?
- How many completed the program?

Effectiveness is the results in terms of the primary outcomes, quality of life, and negative outcomes. Evaluations of effectiveness consider issues such as the following:

- What outcomes (ie, health, behavior, satisfaction, cost of program, quality of life) were measured on our patients over the past year?
- What were the actual outcomes for the specified time period?

Adoption is the participation of the potential settings and representativeness of the setting(s) that actually delivered treatment. Evaluations of adoption consider issues such as the following:

- Did we get referrals from organizations we targeted?
- Did we get the patients we targeted into the program?
- What were the barriers?
- Can we address these barriers?

Implementation is the time and cost of the intervention as well as the extent to which it was delivered as intended. Evaluations of implementation consider issues such as the following:

- Did we deliver the program as planned?
- How many classes planned were delivered?
- Did we follow up with providers who referred patients as planned?
- Did we follow up with patients as planned?

Maintenance is the program sustainability, participant attrition, and long-term effects on individual outcomes after 6 months or more. Evaluations of maintenance consider issues such as the following:

- Have we communicated with referring providers and gathered input on the referral process and/or patient expectations and outcomes?
- Are we maintaining long-term contact with patients and providers?

is similar to RE-AIM in some ways. As outlined in Figure 28.3, the PIPE model generates an overall "impact score" based on the degree to which a program does the following:

- Penetrates the community
- Is implemented according to its design
- Is participated in
- Is effective

The actual metric is simply the product of these 4 coefficients:

penetration × implementation ×
participation × effectiveness

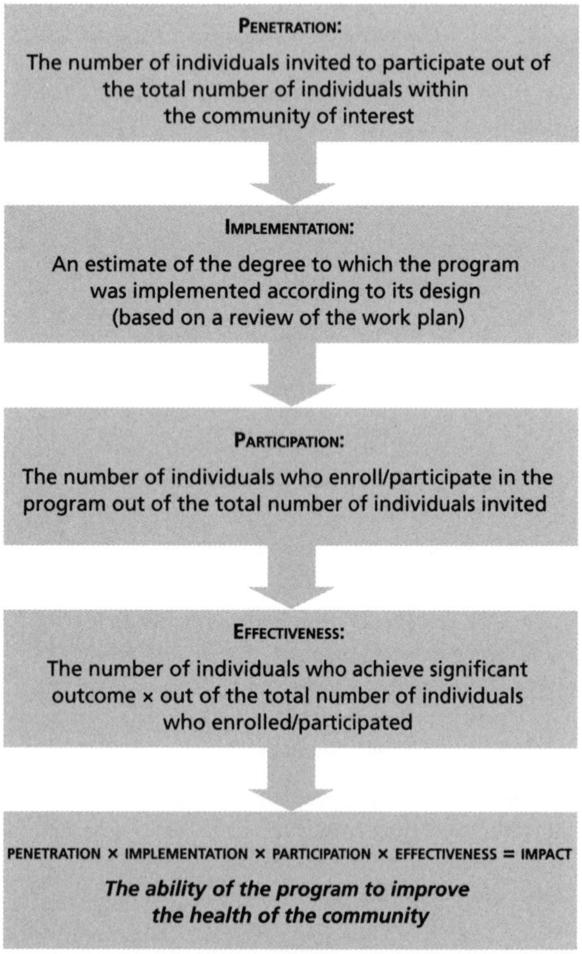

PENETRATION:
The number of individuals invited to participate out of the total number of individuals within the community of interest

↓

IMPLEMENTATION:
An estimate of the degree to which the program was implemented according to its design (based on a review of the work plan)

↓

PARTICIPATION:
The number of individuals who enroll/participate in the program out of the total number of individuals invited

↓

EFFECTIVENESS:
The number of individuals who achieve significant outcome x out of the total number of individuals who enrolled/participated

↓

PENETRATION × IMPLEMENTATION × PARTICIPATION × EFFECTIVENESS = IMPACT
The ability of the program to improve the health of the community

FIGURE 28.3 The PIPE Model for Improving Health Outcomes

This metric provides a global estimate of impact, or the investment (ie, work) and influence (ie, effectiveness) that a program has.

As an illustration, the PIPE model was recently used by HealthPartners to evaluate a provider referral–based weight management program. This program was piloted over 6 months and involved medical providers referring their overweight patients to a HealthPartners phone-based weight management program. The population of interest was an estimated 3000 overweight patients receiving care at a HealthPartners clinic. Of this patient pool, 115 (4%) were referred to the weight management program. Based on a review of the work plan, an estimated 90% of the implementation procedures (eg, marketing, data entry, referral follow-up contact) were carried out as planned. Sixty-two (54%) patients enrolled in the program and, of these, 19 (31%) lost at least 5% of their baseline body weight. The overall PIPE impact metric, then, was 1% (0.04 × 0.90 × 0.54 × 0.31).

The impact of this program on the target community was small, but the individual coefficients were quite useful in highlighting the areas in greatest need for improvement. For this program, the subscore from the users' perspective (participation × effectiveness = 17%) was much higher than the total impact metric (1%). This indicated that the program was relatively effective, but had a very limited outreach across the population of overweight patients. Clearly, penetration represented the greatest opportunity for program improvement.

Conclusion

Documentation and evaluation are critical components of the DSME process. Both are considered "standards" of diabetes care. Knowing what to document about the individual at the educational program level is often a difficult decision; patient outcomes are perhaps the most important elements. For individuals and programs to be successful, the following elements are required:[5]

- *Outcomes Measurement:* Consistent measurement of specific indicators
- *Outcomes Monitoring:* Measurement of these indicators at specified intervals
- *Outcomes Management:* Use of these outcomes to drive educational and clinical decision making

Standardized tools and methods to track and report outcomes can help the educational process and improve the health of individuals and the quality of programs when the documentation is reviewed on a regular basis.

Case Wrap-Up

TM had been referred to the diabetes education program. The following Learning Objectives were identified as Immediate Outcomes, to be mastered by the end of the education program: (*1*) Patient will be able to correctly demonstrate how to use the blood glucose meter provided, (*2*) Patient will be able to state the food items she would include in a meal with 3 to 4 carbohydrate choices, and (*3*) Patient will be able to demonstrate how to reset the step counter on her pedometer. In addition, TM, in collaboration with the diabetes educator, had set these initial Behavioral Goals: to self-monitor her blood glucose twice a day, wear the pedometer for at least 3 days before she returned to assess her baseline activity level, and eat 3 meals per day with 3 to 4 carbohydrate choices per meal.

To document these goals and track progress, the diabetes educator working with TM began using the AADE 7 Self-Care Behaviors™ Goal Sheet. When TM returned for the second visit, her goals were reviewed. TM scored her achievement of these goals on a scale of 0 to 10, with 10 being 100% achieved. Regarding her goal for meal planning, TM rated her achievement at 8, stating "I have done well most of the time, but still need to work on keeping carbohydrate choices at 3 to 4 per meal."

By exploring goals and success toward achieving them, the diabetes educator had the opportunity to discuss barriers that TM may have encountered. This allowed discussion about problem solving and how TM might change her environment or behavior to aid her in achieving her goals.

For example, further discussion might reveal that one of TM's older children was usually responsible for helping prepare the evening meal and that she often made several meal items that were high in carbohydrate. Because she did not want to hurt her daughter's feelings, TM found it hard to turn down the various food items, which resulted in a combined carbohydrate intake that was above her goals. The educator might have suggested that TM purchase a cookbook that included the use of nonnutritive sweeteners in cooking and that she work with her daughter to prepare some of these food items, which would be healthier for the whole family.

At the end of her educational visits, TM and her diabetes educator had agreed upon 3 behavioral objectives/goals:

1. Continue to self-monitor her blood glucose twice daily: before breakfast and 2 hours after eating her big meal of the day
2. Wear her pedometer and aim for 5000 steps per day (her baseline step measurement averaged 4000 steps per day)
3. Eat 3 to 4 carbohydrate choices per meal

The diabetes educator assisted TM in recording these goals on the AADE 7 Self-Care Behaviors™ Goal Sheet.

Follow-Up

TM was scheduled to return to the clinic 1 month later. The time and date were noted on the scheduling card that TM received. TM was advised to check in by phone before the appointment.

By following up with TM in 1 month, the diabetes educator could assist TM in monitoring her progress toward identified goals, resolving barriers, and reevaluating treatment strategies based on outcomes of the goals. Additionally, by using the AADE 7 Self-Care Behaviors™ Goal Sheet, information could be documented in TM's medical record. Eventually, the information obtained could also be used at the aggregate level as part of the DSME program evaluation.

In addition, the educator could remind TM of the importance of following up with her physician at 3- and 6-month intervals so that post-intermediate and long-term outcomes, such as trends in body mass index, A1C, blood pressure, and lipid levels could be monitored. This was valuable information, not only for TM, but for DSME program evaluation and planning.

Questions and Controversies

More research is needed on the outcomes of DSME as it relates to improved health and quality of life for individuals with diabetes. Most published research focuses on the question, "does the treatment reduce AlC level?" While this is important, there are other key elements that portray a program's true impact. The RE-AIM framework and PIPE model are 2 methods that can be used to assess program impact; however, more research is also needed to assess these tools' value for DSME programs.

Focus on Education: Pearls for Practice

Teaching Strategies

- **Documentation is critical.** Written information includes assessment of the individual's immediate concerns, interventions that are included in the planning, short- and long-term goals, and expected outcomes. Interdisciplinary forms and documents are needed that capture this information and remind educators to make comments on topic areas, promoting complete teaching.

- **Documentation is an ongoing process.** Create a form or format that allows for multiple team use, offers opportunity for accumulation of information and measurement between visits, captures information that should be retained, and fosters reinforcement.

- **Behavior change.** Behavior change is the unique outcome measurement of DSME. Behavioral outcome measurements are to be reviewed at intervals, reinforcing the need to check if goals remain appropriate or have changed with the changing needs of the individual. Using the AADE 7 Self-Care Behaviors™ Goal Sheet can help standardize and streamline this process.

- **Evaluation.** Data can be captured, reviewed, and evaluated more easily and consistently when forms and formats are provided to the educator. CQI, RE-AIM, and PIPE frameworks are useful methodologies. Patient educational outcome data as well as program data can be used to update curriculum, educational delivery, and instructor styles or content and enhance care as well as program goals.

Patient Education

- **Documenting goals and objectives.** Though sometimes difficult to determine, identifying areas where behavior change is needed and writing this information down is often the first step toward establishing new behaviors. Discussing your goals with the healthcare team and documenting them will help to objectively determine if goals and objectives are appropriate, if plans are useful to achieve the goals, and if care has been, or can be, improved upon. The key is to be involved! Make certain your preferences and confidence in being able to achieve a goal are acknowledged. You want to "own" both the process and the plan.

- **Tracking progress.** Working with the education team, use the personal goals you have identified as a discussion tool at each of the next follow-up visits. This type of written tool helps to track progress and identify barriers and challenges and goals and objectives that need to be revised as situations change. The written tool can be as simple as a sheet of paper or as formal as a printed, typed document.

- **Not about failure.** Deciding that the plan is not working, the goal or objective is not right, or the steps to accomplish changes are too hard does not equate to a failure to achieve on your part. Evaluation is really about recognizing differences, taking charge of making changes, and looking for success! Developing a better path—in effect, identifying different behaviors, objectives or goals—serves as a way to take care of oneself.

References

1. Mensing C, Boucher J, Cypress M, et al. National standards for diabetes self-management education. Task Force to Review and Revise the National Standards for Diabetes Self-Management Education Programs. Diabetes Care. 2000;23:682-9.
2. Report of the Task Force on the Delivery of Diabetes Self-Management Education and Medical Nutrition Therapy. Diabetes Spectrum. 1999;12:44-7.
3. American Association of Diabetes Educators. The Scope of Practice, Standards of Practice, and Standards of Professional Performance for Diabetes Educators. Diabetes Educ. 2005;31:487-513.
4. Lacey K, Pritchett E. Nutrition care process and model: ADA adopts road map to quality care and outcomes management. J Am Diet Assoc. 2003;103(8):1061-72.
5. American Association of Diabetes Educators. Standards for outcomes measurement of diabetes self-management education. Diabetes Educ. 2003;29:804-16.
6. Mulcahy K, Maryniuk M, Peeples M, et al. Diabetes self-management education core outcomes measures. Diabetes Educ. 2003;29:768-88.
7. US Department of Health and Human Services. Summary of the HIPAA privacy rule. Last revised 2003 May (cited Dec 2005). Available on the Internet at: www.hhs.gov/ocr/privacysummary.pdf
8. Mulcahy K. Management of diabetes education programs. In: A Core Curriculum for Diabetes Educators: Diabetes Education and Program Management, 5th ed. Franz MJ, ed. Chicago, Ill: American Association of Diabetes Educators; 2003:181-218.
9. Johnson EQ. Measuring and monitoring behaviors in medical nutrition therapy—how do you know it worked? On the Cutting Edge. 2005;26(2):13-5.
10. Patton MQ. Utilization-Focused Evaluation: The New Century Text, 3rd ed. Thousand Oaks, Calif: Sage Publications; 1997.
11. Centers for Disease Control and Prevention. Framework for program evaluation in public health practice. MMWR 1999;48(no. RR-11): 1-40. Available on the Internet at: www.phppo.cdc.gov/phtn/Pract-Eval/workbook.asp. Accessed 4 Apr 2006.
12. Davidson KW, Goldstein M, Kaplan RM, et al. Evidence-based behavioral medicine: what is it and how do we achieve it? Ann Behav Med. 2003;26:161-71.
13. Glasgow RE, Vogt TM, Boles SM. Evaluating the public health impact of health promotion interventions: the RE-AIM framework. Am J Public Health. 1999;89:1322-7.
14. Pronk NP. Designing and evaluating health promotion programs: simple rules for a complex issue. Dis Manag Health Outcomes. 2003;11:149-57.
15. Green LW. Kreuter MW. Health Promotion Planning: An Educational and Environmental Approach. Mountain View, Calif: Mayfield; 1991.
16. Rohrer JE. Planning for Community-oriented Health Systems. Baltimore, Md: APHA United Book Press; 1996.
17. American Association of Diabetes Educators Research Committee. CQI: A Step-by-Step Guide for Quality Improvement in Diabetes Education. Chicago, Ill: American Association of Diabetes Educators; 2005.
18. Garvin DA. The process of organization and management. Sloan Manage Rev. 1998(summer);30-50.
19. Lowrie EG. A continuous quality improvement paradigm for health care networks. In: Quality Assurance in Dialysis, 2nd ed. Henderson LW, Thuma RS, eds. Kluwer, England: Academic Publishers: 1999:7-26.
20. Walton M. Deming Management Method. New York, NY: Dodd, Mead; 1986.
21. re-aim.org [home page]. Frequently Asked Questions about RE-AIM: The Basics. Last revised 2004 July (cited Dec 2005). Available on the Internet at: www.re-aim.org/2003/FAQs_basic.html.
22. Eakin EG, Bull SS, Glasgow RE, Mason M. Reaching those most in need: a review of diabetes self-management interventions in disadvantaged populations. Diabetes Metab Res Rev. 2002;18:26-35.

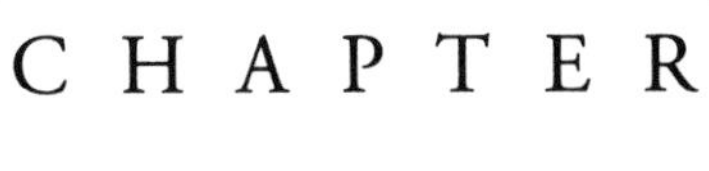

CHAPTER

29

Healthy Eating

Author

Patti B. Geil, MS, RD, FADA, CDE

Key Concepts

- Healthy eating is an effective, but challenging self-care behavior that improves glycemic control.
- To achieve the outcome of successful behavior change for healthy eating, the diabetes educator must assist the person with diabetes, and those being treated to prevent diabetes, in acquiring specific knowledge and skills.
- Healthy eating behaviors can be supported by well-designed diabetes nutrition self-management education that uses the Nutrition Care Process and Nutrition Practice Guidelines.
- While the goals of medical nutrition therapy apply to everyone with or at risk for diabetes, the individual's circumstances must always be considered. The nutrition issues are different depending on if the goal is diabetes prevention or treatment and if the disease is type 1 or type 2 diabetes. Also, special populations—pregnant women, children and adolescents, older individuals, and ethnically and culturally diverse populations—have distinct nutrition issues.
- Matching the appropriate meal planning resources to the needs of the person with diabetes results from an individualized and comprehensive nutrition assessment.
- A variety of meal planning resources are available for use. These help in educating and promoting behavior changes directed at making healthier food choices.
- Educators must stay abreast of the controversies and trends in healthy eating for diabetes. Currently, these include use of the glycemic index, complementary therapies for diabetes, new methods of delivering diabetes self-management education, and the expanded role of diabetes educators in addressing healthy eating not only for diabetes itself, but also for its comorbidities.

Introduction

Healthy eating has a significant effect on the metabolic control of diabetes. Many diabetes educators and clinicians consider healthy eating to be the most challenging of the AADE 7 Self-Care Behaviors™ to implement with success. Healthy eating involves basic behaviors and decisions such as when to eat, what to eat, and how much to eat. Influencing these decisions are complex individual factors such as habits, emotions, food preferences, food availability, and family and cultural eating patterns. To help individuals achieve effective behavior change related to healthy eating, the educator's role encompasses the following:

- Providing the person with or at risk for diabetes with knowledge and skills training
- Helping the person identify barriers
- Facilitating problem solving and coping skills

Successful self-management of healthy eating leads to improved metabolic control, a reduced risk for diabetic complications, and improved overall health and quality of life. In addition, for individuals who are at risk for type 2 diabetes, healthy eating strategies which promote weight loss have been shown, along with physical activity, to delay or prevent the progression to type 2 diabetes, as shown in the Diabetes Prevention Program (DPP), which is discussed elsewhere.

Promoting Healthy Eating: Role of Medical Nutrition Therapy

Diabetes medical nutrition therapy (MNT) is the term for the specific nutrition services provided to treat diabetes and promote healthy eating habits.[1] Successful MNT can be provided in a variety of settings, including these:

- Inpatient and outpatient settings[2,3]
- Individual sessions and group sessions[4,5]
- Newly evolving options of online or telemedicine care[6,7]

Comprehensive assessment is essential to successful treatment

In-depth, comprehensive assessment of the nutritional status of the individual is an essential first step. Treatment—nutrition therapy and counseling—for diabetes and prediabetes is based on the assessment.

Although every educator involved in diabetes treatment and management must be able to apply the principles of MNT and use the same core set of behaviors to measure outcomes, the registered dietitian (RD) is the

Case in Point: Healthy Eating Via Self-Management Education

SM is a 35-year-old Caucasian female who has had type 1 diabetes since age 17. She is interested in preconception planning for her first pregnancy.

Assessment Data

- Height: 65 in
- Weight: 130 lb
- BMI: 21
- Blood pressure: 128/77 mm Hg

Most Recent Lab Values

- A1C: 8.5%
- Fasting blood glucose: 145 mg/dL
- Total cholesterol: 226 mg/dL
- Triglycerides: 128 mg/dL
- HDL-C: 42 mg/dL
- LDL-C: 113 mg/dL

SM lived with her husband and traveled frequently for her pharmaceutical sales job. She had previously been instructed on an 1800-calorie Exchange Diet, but she was not consistent with her intake. She often ate sporadically due to her hectic travel schedule. Breakfast during the work week was typically a large bagel with low-fat cream cheese, a piece of fruit, and black coffee; on weekends at home she slept late and enjoyed making a brunch of bacon, eggs, and fruit salad. Lunch was generally a chef's salad with low-fat ranch salad dressing, 2 packages of crackers, and a diet drink. SM often went out for a late dinner with friends, choosing items such as pasta with tomato sauce or grilled chicken, salad, bread, and an occasional alcoholic beverage.

SM currently took 10 units of a rapid-acting insulin analog with meals and 20 units of glargine (Lantus) at bedtime. She was not adjusting her mealtime insulin doses. She was interested in using an insulin pump. SM checked her fasting blood glucose daily and tried to check her blood glucose at least 1 more time each day. SM was taking St John's Wort because she occasionally felt "overwhelmed." She denied other medications.

Her physical activity program consisted of running 3 miles per day on the weekends. Her activity level during the week was much less, although she tried to attend a step aerobics class twice a week. Otherwise, her activity was rather sedentary, as she spent much of her day in the car, driving between physicians' clinics in rural Kentucky.

Questions to Consider

1. What are the key issues the educator might address at the initial visit?
2. What is SM's nutrition diagnosis?
3. What behavior changes would you encourage that focus on healthy eating?
4. Which nutrition intervention and meal planning resources would you choose for SM?
5. List 1 clinical goal that would be appropriate for SM.
6. List 2 behavioral goals that would be appropriate for SM.
7. How would you document the initial encounter with SM?
8. What would you evaluate on a 6-week return visit?

health professional with the greatest expertise in providing MNT. The RD's effectiveness has been demonstrated in the research studies that have achieved positive outcomes. Pastors et al have published a comprehensive review of the evidence for the effectiveness of MNT and healthy eating in diabetes management.[8] The authors cite randomized, controlled trials in which MNT was either implemented independently or delivered as part of an overall diabetes self-management training program. The studies demonstrated the following:

- *Decreases in A1C*: Approximately 1% in subjects with newly diagnosed type 1 diabetes, 2% in subjects with newly diagnosed type 2 diabetes, and 1% in subjects with type 2 diabetes with an average duration of 4 years
- Reductions in use of health services and costs: Suggesting MNT is also cost-effective

Strong evidence also suggests that interventions such as intensive lifestyle modifications based on healthy eating habits and physical activity are effective in delaying or preventing the onset of type 2 diabetes by 58% to 71%.[9]

Care Planning

MNT should be part of the care plan of every individual with diabetes, regardless of his or her medication regimen. MNT is also part of diabetes prevention. Chapter 2, on lifestyle intervention for diabetes prevention, discusses the possibility that Medicare and private insurance may soon cover MNT for prediabetes and obesity.

For Diabetes. For individuals with diabetes, the goal is to prevent and treat the chronic complications of diabetes. The main tactic is this:

- Attain and maintain optimal metabolic outcomes in blood glucose level, A1C level, low-density lipoprotein cholesterol (LDL-C) and high-density lipoprotein cholesterol (HDL-C) and triglyceride levels, blood pressure, and body weight

For Prediabetes. For individuals with prediabetes, the goal is to decrease the risk of diabetes and cardiovascular disease. The main tactic is this:

- Promote physical activity and healthy food choices that result in moderate weight loss that is maintained or, at a minimum, prevents weight gain

A summary of the current recommendations[10] for metabolic outcomes for adults with diabetes is outlined in Table 29.1.

Registered Dietitian

The team member with the most expertise and demonstrated effectiveness in fostering healthy eating for diabetes is the RD.

Outcomes Focus

For the individual who participates in self-management education focused on healthy eating, for either diabetes management or prevention, the goal is a positive outcome. Measuring outcomes demonstrates the effectiveness and unique contribution that can be made by the diabetes educator. For each of the AADE 7 Self-Care Behaviors™, a continuum of outcomes related to diabetes education are expected:[11]

- *Immediate Outcome:* Goal is learning
- *Intermediate Outcome:* Goal is behavior change
- *Post-Intermediate Outcome:* Goal is clinical improvement
- *Long-Term Outcome:* Goals include improvement in health status and cost savings

Immediate Outcome. Learning is the immediate outcome sought. After teaching a healthy eating behavior such as label reading, the diabetes educator can immediately ask the learner to demonstrate the new skill. The

TABLE 29.1 Summary of Recommended Metabolic Outcomes for Adults With Diabetes

Glycemic Control	
A1C	<7.0%
Preprandial Capillary Plasma Glucose	90–130 mg/dL (5.0–7.2 mmol/L)
Peak Postprandial Capillary Plasma Glucose	<180 mg/dL (<10.0 mmol/L)
Lipids	
LDL-C	<100 mg/dL (2.60 mmol/L)
Triglycerides	<150 mg/dL (1.7 mmol/L)
HDL-C	Men: >40 mg/dL (1.15 mmol/L) Women: >50 mg/dL (1.44 mmol/L)
Blood Pressure	<130/80 mm Hg

Source: Adapted with permission from American Diabetes Association. Standards of medical care in diabetes, 2006. Diabetes Care. 2006;29:S4-42.

educator asks the learner, for example, to read a sample label for critical information, such as portion size or carbohydrate content; this enables the educator to determine if the person learned the material that was taught.

Intermediate Outcome. Behavior change, the intermediate outcome sought, is the unique outcome measurement for diabetes self-management education. Although the learner may have acquired important information regarding label reading, the desired outcome is that this person use the information to change his or her behavior and make healthier food choices. Behaviors such as choosing the proper type and amount of food or dealing with special situations such as illness or travel can be measured by observation, self-report of food intake, and review of records of blood glucose readings.

Post-Intermediate Outcome. Clinical improvement, the desired post-intermediate outcome, can be measured via laboratory tests and clinical measurements.

Long-Term Outcomes. At the end of the continuum of outcomes are long-term outcomes such as health status improvement. Long-term outcomes can be measured as improvement in quality of life, economic benefits from reduced healthcare costs, and increased productivity.

Expected outcomes from MNT[8] are listed in Table 29.2. Achieving successful self-care behaviors that are focused on making healthy food choices requires knowledge and skill on the part of the learner. This chapter focuses on the art of diabetes education as it relates to healthy eating; its contents highlight the areas that are important to teach, support, and promote to guide behavior change in the individual at risk for or with diabetes.

Supporting Healthy Eating Behaviors: Well-Designed Nutrition Self-Management Education

Two recommended tools are the Nutrition Care Process (NCP) and the Nutrition Practice Guidelines (NPG), both developed by the American Dietetic Association. Each is discussed separately below.

Nutrition Care Process

The American Dietetic Association has developed the NCP,[12] which outlines the consistent and specific steps to be used when delivering MNT. Although the NCP is primarily intended for dietetics professionals, other healthcare professionals may find the process useful in providing quality care. Central to effective provision of MNT is the relationship between the individual seeking care and the dietetic professional.

Four Steps in the Nutrition Care Process:
Assessment → Diagnosis →
Intervention → Monitoring and Evaluation

Step 1: Nutrition Assessment

An RD who provides MNT and education on healthy eating should follow a systematic process that begins with a nutrition assessment. Other team members often provide information valuable in making the assessment.

TABLE 29.2 Expected Outcomes from Medical Nutrition Therapy

Glycemic Control	
Evaluate at 6 weeks and 3 months:	
A1C:	Decrease of 1%–2% unit (15%–22% overall)
Plasma Glucose (Fasting):	Decrease of 50-100 mg/dL (2.77–5.55 mmol/L)
Lipids	
Evaluate at 6 weeks; if goals not achieved, intensify MNT and evaluate again in 6 weeks:	
LDL-C:	Decrease of 19–25 mg/dL (1.05–1.38 mmol/L) (12%–16%)
Total Cholesterol:	Decrease of 24–32 mg/dL (1.33–1.77 mmol/L) (10%–13%)
Triglycerides:	Decrease of 15–17 mg/dL (0.83–0.94 mmol/L) (8%)
HDL-C:	• With no exercise, decrease of 3 mg/dL (0.16 mmol/L) (7%) • With exercise, no decrease
Blood Pressure	
Measure in hypertensive patients at every medical visit:	
BP	5 mm Hg decrease in systolic, 2 mm Hg decrease in diastolic

Source: Adapted with permission from Pastors JG, Franz MJ, Warshaw H, Daly A, Arnold M. How effective is medical nutrition therapy in diabetes care? J Am Diet Assoc. 2003;103: 827-31.

Gathering Relevant Data. To specifically assess nutrition status, the following data are essential:

- *Referral Data:* Medical history, medications, laboratory data, information from the individual and any family members
- *Anthropometric Measures:* Weight, height, waist-to-hip ratio, body mass index (BMI)
- *Food and Nutrition History:* These can be obtained based on a 24-hour recall or a typical day's food intake with specific details on eating times, alcohol intake, and the use of vitamins, minerals, and herbal supplements
- *Physical Activity Patterns:* Type(s), frequency, duration, intensity; whether activity is aerobic or strengthening type, or both

Learning About the Individual. A complete nutrition assessment includes all past nutrition education, or lack there of, as well as the individual's perception of that experience. Conducting the assessment establishes rapport, which is particularly helpful as the process of diabetes self-management education continues. The educator must learn the following about the individual:

- Individual's diabetes management goals
- Level of knowledge and skills
- Attitude and motivation
- Readiness to learn new behaviors and interest in changing old ones, if appropriate
- Preferred ways of learning

During the assessment phase, the educator can determine the way in which an individual prefers to learn. This enables the educator to present information in a style tailored to promote success. Osterman identified several characteristics that differentiate 4 styles of learning that may be useful:[13]

- *Thinkers:* Look for facts and may best gain knowledge by lecture
- *Sensors:* Learn by problem solving and may benefit by demonstration
- *Feelers:* Learn by listening and may respond to discussion
- *Intuitors:* Learn by trial and error and may learn better through self-discovery

Process of Behavior Change: Precontemplation → Contemplation → Preparation → Action → Maintenance

In the Transtheoretical Model of behavior change, Prochaska et al outlined 5 stages an individual progresses through toward behavior change: precontemplation, contemplation, preparation, action, and maintenance. The stages are useful to consider when planning and implementing nutrition care. (See chapter 3 on self-management of health.) In making changes, people progress through these 5 stages, yet they also move through the stages unsystematically. Aware of the nature of this process, the educator can better understand and help the individual progress toward behavior changes that result in healthy eating.[14] Recognizing that behavior change is a multistep process helps minimize unrealistic expectations.

Recognizing Barriers. Health beliefs need to be considered. Food choices and why a person eats as he or she does are deeply embedded in the psyche and may be a result of strong cultural or ethnic traditions. The supportiveness or family members may not be obvious; further probing may be required. Visual status, disabilities, and socioeconomic status are all important factors to determine in the assessment. Barriers to learning, literacy level, and the way in which the person learns best are also key points.

A comprehensive assessment is the crucial step in providing individualized diabetes nutrition therapy. The assessment requires adequate time to perform thoroughly, but provides a wealth of information that allows the professional to tailor the intervention and the diabetes nutrition therapy to the individual. The RD cannot begin to develop a nutrition diagnosis or design a nutrition intervention without the sound basis of an assessment. A high-level assessment involves obtaining appropriate data as well as analyzing and interpreting the data in light of evidence-based standards.

Step 2: Nutrition Diagnosis

The nutrition diagnosis determines the specific healthy eating behaviors that need to be modified. The nutrition diagnosis is not the same as the medical diagnosis, which is diabetes mellitus. While the patient may have a medical diagnosis of type 1 diabetes, after completing a nutrition assessment the RD establishes the nutrition diagnosis. The following are examples:

- "Inconsistent carbohydrate intake"
- "Overly large portion sizes"
- "High fat intake"

Determining a nutrition diagnosis will guide the person with or at risk for diabetes and the educator toward the appropriate selection of goals for behavior change and their desired outcomes.

Step 3: Nutrition Intervention

The third step of the NCP, nutrition intervention, involves planning and implementing the activities that specifically

> ### *Expecting Changes*
>
> Promote flexible thinking and adaptability. As diabetes progresses, goals change. As learners develop skills, more advanced concepts can be added to better support the individual.

facilitate or support the individual's healthy eating behavior. Education, the process of providing accurate and timely information to the individual who has or is at risk for diabetes, is key at this step. However, the role of the educator goes beyond merely supplying facts. The educator is a counselor and a coach, whose role is to help the person understand the disease and cope with its implications. The educator is a partner in disease management, assisting individuals in making their own decisions about self-care and helping them discover how they may be motivated to change their behavior.

At this stage, the person seeking assistance and the educator work together to formulate goals and determine a plan of action. When establishing goals, the RD should distinguish not only between short-term goals for behavior change and long-term goals, but also behavior change outcomes that are the goals of the person seeking assistance and those that are the goals of the healthcare provider. Goals for both parties should be specific, reasonable, attainable, and measurable.[15] Examples of behavior change goals for healthy eating are shown in Table 29.3. If the professional has established a good rapport with the person, negotiating attainable goals is easier. Healthy eating goals evolve over time and need to be evaluated and renegotiated as circumstances change.

After the nutrition diagnosis is made and behavior goals and desired outcomes are established, the nutrition intervention begins and healthy eating skills can be taught. A number of healthy eating resources are available; quite a few are summarized below. No single meal planning approach works for every individual. The initial meal planning approach is chosen with the understanding that it may change as the person's understanding of the disease and motivation to self-manage evolves

Outline for a well-designed diabetes nutrition education encounter

1. *Focus on the Individual.* The encounter begins with the educator asking the individual what questions and concerns he or she has regarding healthy eating.
2. *Assess, Diagnose, Plan.* The educator then completes the nutrition assessment, establishes a nutrition diagnosis, and works with the individual to set behavior change goals and plan a nutrition intervention using an individualized healthy eating approach.
3. *Wrap Up for the Individual's Benefit.* The session ends with the educator answering remaining questions, summarizing key points, and making a follow-up plan for future appointments.

TABLE 29.3 Sample Behavior Change Goals for Healthy Eating

- I will measure my food and beverage intake for 3 days, record the amounts, and bring the records to my next clinic appointment
- I will substitute diet soda or water for sweetened soda at lunchtime at least 3 days per week
- I will check and record my blood glucose levels 2 hours after each meal every day
- I will modify 3 favorite recipes into lower-fat and lower-carbohydrate versions before my next clinic appointment
- I will limit my carbohydrate intake to 60 g of carbohydrate at each of my 3 meals and 15 g of carbohydrate at each of my 2 snacks at least 5 days per week

Source: Leontos C, Geil P. Individualized Approaches to Diabetes Nutrition Therapy: Case Studies. Alexandria, Va: American Diabetes Association; 2002.

Step 4: Nutrition Monitoring and Evaluation

Successful MNT involves the process of problem solving, adjustment, and readjustment. Food and records, such as blood glucose readings, are reviewed, evaluated, and reassessed. Measurable goals help make evaluation a simple task. Helping the person with diabetes think in terms of a course correction, rather than a goal evaluation, helps make this discussion less threatening. If initial goals are not met, they may need to be changed or renegotiated. If they have been met, new reasonable, attainable, and measurable goals should be designed.

Documentation. At each stage of the Nutrition Care Process, documentation should be recorded. Documentation in the medical record aids in communication with other members of the healthcare team.

- *After the First Visit:* Document both clinical and behavioral goals, including nutrition recommendations, chosen meal planning approach, and educational topics covered.

- *After Subsequent Visits*: Document and communicate acceptance and understanding, behavior changes made, and plans for ongoing care to the person's primary caregiver (usually the referral source) and other team members. Written documentation can be shared with the individual to demonstrate his or her progress and encourage further efforts.

Nutrition Practice Guidelines

Nutrition practice guidelines (NPGs) for type 1, type 2, and gestational diabetes[16] have been developed to delineate the process or system by which optimal care is provided. The NPGs are evidence-based protocols that when used to deliver MNT result in positive health outcomes.[17-19] These guidelines outline clinical outcomes as well as necessary lifestyle changes and suggest the frequency and length of contact with the RD as well as the amount of time between encounters, based on the specific situation of the person. For example, due to the time-sensitive nature of gestational diabetes, more frequent contacts in a shorter period of time are generally required as compared to routine follow-up for an individual with long-standing type 2 diabetes. Together, the Nutrition Care Process and NPGs form the framework for well-designed self-management education regarding healthy eating.

Evaluation is Ongoing:
Solve Problems → Adjust → Readjust

Healthy Eating for Specific Medical Conditions and Special Populations

Successful self-management for healthy eating requires diabetes education that focuses on concerns that are specific to the person's medical condition. The general goals of diabetes MNT are to prevent and treat the chronic complications of diabetes by attaining and maintaining optimal metabolic outcomes. Although these apply to everyone with or at risk for the disease, one size does not fit all when educating an individual. Focus areas for healthy eating for type 1 diabetes are quite different than those for gestational diabetes, for example. Below are specialized issues that must be considered.

Diabetes Prevention

Results from the DPP confirm that lifestyle modification was nearly twice as effective as medication in preventing diabetes (58% versus 31% relative reductions, respectively).[9]

Lifestyle intervention should be the first choice for diabetes prevention

The greater benefit of weight loss and physical activity strongly suggests that lifestyle modification should be the first choice to prevent or delay diabetes. The following are recommended goals:

- *Modest weight loss:* 5% to 10% of body weight
- *Modest physical activity:* 30 minutes daily

Because this intervention not only has been shown to prevent or delay diabetes, but also has a variety of other benefits, healthcare providers should urge all overweight, obese, and sedentary individuals to adopt these changes, and such recommendations should be made at every opportunity.[10] Chapter 2 on prevention offers these guidelines from the National Institutes of Health (NIH) and World Health Organization (WHO):

- The NIH defines overweight as a BMI of 25.0 to 29.9 kg/m^2 and obesity as a BMI ≥30 kg/m^2
- For Asian populations, the WHO defines the observed risk cut-off point for BMI as varying from 22 kg/m^2 to 25 kg/m^2 and the high-risk cut-off point as a BMI varying from 26 kg/m^2 to 31 kg/m^2

Chapter 2 also discusses diabetes prevention and the importance of lifestyle intervention more thoroughly.

Type 1 Diabetes

Individuals with type 1 diabetes require exogenous insulin, so their primary nutrition goal is to establish an insulin regimen that fits into their preferred eating routine and lifestyle. The total and type of carbohydrate in meals and snacks directly affects blood glucose levels, so this is a main area of focus. Those individuals on a fixed insulin regimen should strive for consistency of carbohydrate intake. Those on a flexible insulin regimen or insulin pump should adjust their insulin and food intake based on their carbohydrate-to-insulin ratio. Because hypoglycemia occurs more frequently in individuals with type 1 diabetes, reviewing the basics of hypoglycemia prevention and treatment is important. Finally, the blood glucose–lowering effect of physical activity means that the educator should share strategies such as adjusting insulin dosage for planned exercise or having a carbohydrate snack prior to exercise.[20] More information on this can be found in chapter 19, which deals with physical activity. Nutrition issues pertinent to children and teens with type 1 diabetes are described in a subsequent section.

Type 2 Diabetes

Because most individuals with type 2 diabetes are overweight and insulin-resistant, the educator should emphasize therapeutic lifestyle change, which includes a reduction in energy intake and an increase in physical activity.

- *Weight Loss.* A moderate decrease in caloric balance (500 to 1000 kcal per day) will result in a slow, but progressive weight loss (1 to 2 lb per week). For most patients, weight-loss diets should supply at least 1000 to 1200 kcal per day for women and 1200 to 1600 kcal per day for men.
- *Physical Activity.* Initial physical activity recommendations should be modest and based on the person's willingness and ability to change. Physical activity should gradually increase in duration and frequency to 30 to 45 min of moderate aerobic activity, 3 to 5 days per week (the goal is at least 150 min per week). Greater activity levels of at least 1 hour per day of moderate (walking) or 30 min per day of vigorous (jogging) activity may be needed to achieve successful long-term weight loss.[10]

Information about the types of foods that contain carbohydrate as well as the importance of reasonable portion sizes and timing of meals and snacks are also key considerations when educating a person with type 2 diabetes. Nutrition issues pertinent to children and teens with type 2 diabetes are described in a subsequent section.

Pregnancy

MNT for pregnancy with diabetes should focus on providing adequate calories and nutrients to meet the needs of pregnancy while maintaining optimal blood glucose control.[20]

Breastfeeding is encouraged in all women with diabetes, with an emphasis on education for the prevention and treatment of hypoglycemia for women who require insulin.[21-23] Specific nutrition issues with preexisting diabetes and gestational diabetes mellitus are noted below.

Preexisting Diabetes

Whether type 1 or type 2, the goal is "control before conception" since the risk of fetal anomalies is greater when blood glucose control is poor during fetal organogenesis, which occurs early in pregnancy.

Pregnancy for a woman with type 1 diabetes is often a time for intensive diabetes management involving an insulin pump or multiple daily injections of insulin. Thus, concepts such as insulin-to-carbohydrate ratio must be mastered. The educator should also emphasize issues relating to food and the response of blood glucose during pregnancy. Hypoglycemia occurs more commonly in the first trimester because insulin requirements decrease and morning sickness leads to decreased food intake. As the pregnancy progresses, insulin resistance increases due to weight gain and increased placental hormones, necessitating increased insulin dosages to maintain optimal blood glucose control.

Women with type 2 diabetes who become pregnant require much of the same information as women with type 1 diabetes. If the women were overweight or obese when they became pregnant, the educator should discuss the need for modest calorie restriction (25 cal/kg of actual weight per day) to reduce hyperglycemia.

Additional information can be found in chapter 11, on pregnancy with preexisting diabetes.

Gestational Diabetes

Emphasis should be placed on maintaining normal blood glucose while consuming enough calories and carbohydrate to promote appropriate weight gain yet avoid maternal starvation ketosis. Women who develop gestational diabetes should also be made aware of the lifestyle changes they need to adopt to delay or prevent their increased risk for developing type 2 diabetes later in life. Additional information can be found in chapter 12, on gestational diabetes.

Children and Adolescents With Diabetes

Nutrition education to promote healthy eating for children and adolescents with or without diabetes, should involve the entire family and caretakers and be geared toward the appropriate developmental stage of the child. Food plans must be developed with consideration of both treatment goals and realistic lifestyle choices in mind. Consider these points for all children, with diabetes or at-risk for type 2 diabetes, when creating the nutrition plan:

- Adjust the food plan to meet energy requirements for growth and activity
- Focus on an intake of nutrient-dense foods (ie, fruits, vegetables, whole grains, and calcium-rich foods) versus nutrient-sparse foods (ie, excessive amounts of sweets or large amounts of juice and fruit drinks)
- Use the term "food plan" or "meal plan," rather than "diet," to avoid furthering negative connotations regarding the same
- Engage the child or adolescent in development of the food plan as well as shopping for and preparing healthy foods for the entire family

Type 1 Diabetes

In addition to that mentioned above, nutrition education for children with type 1 diabetes revolves around achieving blood glucose goals without excessive hypoglycemia while promoting normal growth and development. The key concepts mentioned earlier about type 1 diabetes in adults also apply to children with type 1 diabetes. MNT discussions should also address the following:[24]

- Nutrition issues for school and day care, irregular schedules, sports activities, and peer influences and level of acceptance
- Effects of growth and hormonal changes on blood glucose
- Additional adjustments to be made in insulin administered at mealtime, due to picky eaters

Type 2 Diabetes

According to statistics from the US Centers for Disease Control and Prevention, an estimated 1 out of 3 children born in the United States in the year 2000 will have diabetes in their lifetime. This is due, in part, to the increasing number of children who may be medically classified as "pediatric overweight." In addition to that mentioned above, nutrition education for children at risk for or diagnosed with type 2 diabetes should include the following:

- Controlling portions by encouraging children to "eat to appetite," rather than "cleaning their plates" filled with adult-sized portions
- Slowing their rate of eating
- Striving for regular mealtimes and limiting distractions, such as eating while watching TV
- Promoting physical activity of a minimum of 60 minutes per day
- Decreasing the number of hours of sedentary activity, such as TV watching or time spent playing video games or Internet surfing

Because of the strong genetic component of type 2 diabetes, the entire family will often benefit by being involved in the lifestyle change program.[25] Successful lifestyle change outcomes for children with type 2 diabetes are defined as follows:[26]

- Cessation of excessive weight gain with near normal linear growth
- Near-normal fasting blood glucose and A1C values

Older Adults

Recommendations for making healthy food choices should be individualized, regardless of a person's age, but the need for this is even more apparent when the numerous factors affecting the older adult are considered.

> *Older Adults*
>
> One-on-one sessions often eliminate visual and auditory barriers to learning. Family and caregivers can easily attend.

Older adults with diabetes vary widely in their physical and cognitive status; in the presence or absence of underlying chronic conditions and comorbidities; and in their cultural backgrounds, traditions, and beliefs. An older individual who is able and willing to undertake the responsibility for diabetes self-management should be encouraged to do so and be treated using the previously stated metabolic goals for adults.[10] The educator should provide meal planning guidelines that incorporate cultural food favorites and also meet calorie and nutrient needs while promoting glycemic control. Physical activity should also be encouraged as a regular part of the individual's daily routine. With the individual's permission, family and caregivers should be encouraged to attend the teaching sessions; one-to-one sessions may be preferable to group classes in which visual and auditory barriers could arise. Healthy eating issues such as taste preferences and lifelong eating habits, finances, and food preparation ability are also important.[27]

Ethnic and Cultural Appropriateness

Because ethnic diversity continues to increase and the prevalence of diabetes in minority groups throughout the United States is extremely high, the diabetes educator must be prepared to tailor MNT and education for healthy eating to fit a variety of cultural practices. Chapter 27, on implementation, can help educators and other clinicians improve their effectiveness in cross-cultural encounters. Cultural competency is the ability to work effectively with people of different cultural backgrounds. Successful diabetes prevention and treatment in diverse ethnic populations requires sensitivity to cultural differences in health beliefs and eating habits.

> ***Educators can use a 4-step process to improve cross-cultural counseling:***

Eating is a personal matter that may carry great cultural significance. Health professionals can use a 4-step process to improve cross-cultural counseling:[28]

1. Self-evaluation of the educator's own cultural heritage
2. Preinterview research on the cultural background of each individual

3. In-depth, cross-cultural interview to establish individual's personal preferences and cultural background and eating habit adaptations made in the United States
4. Unbiased analysis of the data

In cross-cultural counseling, as in other situations, the person who came for assistance should be involved in problem solving and in developing strategies for behavior change. Include family members who are involved in food preparation. Establish respect and trust by keeping a nonjudgmental attitude and accepting cultural differences. Include as many familiar foods as possible in the healthy eating plan and explore the person's uses of special foods or beverages as folk remedies.[29,30] (Refer to chapter 19, on biological complementary therapies, for more information and a list of resources.)

A variety of resources are available for learning more about a specific culture and are useful when providing MNT.[31] Existing educational materials may also be adapted to be culturally specific. Invite the individual with diabetes to teach the educator about the ingredients in and preparation of cultural and ethnic foods. Combining an individual's cultural expertise with the diabetes and nutrition knowledge of the educator allows for a true exchange of information that benefits both parties.

Meal Planning Resources for Healthy Eating

No single meal planning approach works for every individual, and no single approach has been proven to be more effective than another. Attaining behavior change for healthy eating depends greatly on readiness to learn and the individualized needs of the person with diabetes. For each phase of education, different educational resources may be needed.

Initial Education. Basic nutrition interventions are needed for beginning or "survival" education, while more in-depth tools may be needed as the counseling process continues. Basic or initial education provides the information needed at the time of diagnosis, when the treatment plan or person's lifestyle changes, or at the time of initial contact with an RD. Initial skill topics include the following:

- Information about basic nutrition guidelines
- Instruction on sources of carbohydrate, amount of carbohydrate to consume, portion sizes, and the need to space carbohydrates throughout the day to control blood glucose
- Symptoms and treatment of hypoglycemia, if appropriate

More Advanced Topics. Continuing self-management training provides more advanced education and includes both management and lifestyle skills. Topics to cover are chosen based on the individual's situation; level of nutrition knowledge; and experience in planning, purchasing, and preparing food. People with diabetes can be taught more in-depth topics such as these:

- Making adjustments in food and medication for sick days, physical activity, travel, and eating away from home

Meal Planning Resources

Preplanned, printed diet sheets are ineffective and should not be used.[32] A number of meal planning approaches are available to teach basic diabetes nutrition guidelines as well as more in-depth nutrition interventions. The person with diabetes and the educator may begin with one meal planning approach and then try other resources as the counseling process continues.

Dietary Guidelines for Americans[33] and *MyPyramid*[34] can be used as an introduction to basic nutrition and to begin the process of changing eating behaviors. However, these resources do not address issues specific to diabetes; therefore, a diabetes-related resource might prove more effective.

The First Step in Diabetes Meal Planning (English and Spanish)[35] is a basic, self-contained nutrition pamphlet based on the Food Guide Pyramid. This pamphlet is designed to be given to persons with diabetes for use until a dietitian can develop an individualized meal plan. General guidelines are provided for the recommended number of servings from each food group, and space is provided for the person using it to identify health goals and steps for reaching goals and to write in an individualized food/meal plan. Foods containing carbohydrate are grouped to facilitate the introduction of this concept, and guidelines for increasing physical activity are included. Servings must be measured and food intake can be tracked in a diary that indicates the number of servings eaten from each group daily.

Healthy Food Choices (English and Spanish)[36] is a pamphlet that illustrates the basics of good nutrition and the exchange lists. It opens into a small poster that provides a general overview of what to eat and when. Space is provided to write in a detailed meal plan in any "meal planning language" (ie, carbohydrate servings, exchange groups, or actual menu items).

The Plate Method[37,38] uses a simple graphic of a dinner plate to teach general portion control, consistency, and basic food categories. Using this meal planning method, a plate is "divided" into 4 sections:

- *At Breakfast:* 1/2 is for starches and 1/2 is for meat
- *At Lunch:* 1/4 is for starches, 1/4 is for meat, and 1/2 is for vegetables
- *At Dinner:* 1/4 is for starches, 1/4 is for meat, and 1/2 is for vegetables
- *At Each Meal:* A piece of fruit and a glass of milk are added

This meal planning approach is especially useful for visual learners, those who do not speak English, persons with poor reading or math skills, and individuals with cognitive limitations.

Menus. Individualized menus can be developed by the RD to provide a written description of exactly what and when to eat. Individualized, preplanned menus help people with diabetes achieve healthy eating by specifying the foods and amounts to be consumed for meals and snacks each day. Preplanned menu resources often include simple recipes to help people with diabetes prepare their foods. Menus are useful for initial or simplified diabetes meal planning; for those who have little experience or interest in meal planning; and for individuals with poor reading and math skills, cognitive limitations, or difficulty using more structured approaches. The American Diabetes Association has developed healthy menus available as the Month of Meals series.[39]

Eating Healthy with Diabetes: Easy Reading Guide[40] is intended for persons with diabetes who have limited reading skills or impaired vision. The guide offers larger print, more photos, and very little text. Food lists are presented in the context of breakfast, lunch, dinner, and snack choices.

Exchange Lists for Meal Planning (English and Spanish)[41] lists groups of measured foods of approximately the same nutritional value; foods in each list can be substituted or exchanged for other foods in the same list. This continues to be the most complete set of food lists on which all other diabetes nutrition resources are based. The exchange lists are used with an individualized meal plan that specifies when and how many exchanges from each group are to be eaten for meals and/or snacks.

Carbohydrate Counting

Carbohydrate affects blood glucose more directly than protein and fat, the other 2 sources of energy. Both the amount (grams) and type of carbohydrate in a food influence the blood glucose level.[42] Low-carbohydrate diets are not recommended in the management of diabetes. Monitoring total grams of carbohydrate remains a key strategy in achieving glycemic control. Using the carbohydrate counting method, the person with diabetes counts the exact number of grams of carbohydrate in the foods eaten. Alternatively, each serving of starch, fruit, or milk can be counted as 1 carbohydrate serving. Each carbohydrate serving has about 15 g of carbohydrate. A registered dietitian can help the person with diabetes determine the optimal number of carbohydrate servings or grams of carbohydrate to eat per day; the individual then follows this recommendation in planning meals. Food records and self-monitoring of blood glucose can be used to determine if the amount of carbohydrate prescribed is appropriate. Carbohydrate counting can be effective for individuals with all types of diabetes. Meal planning resources for carbohydrate counting are divided into 2 levels of instruction.

Basic Carbohydrate Counting[43] is a foldout pamphlet that introduces basic concepts of carbohydrate counting and blood glucose management. This pamphlet encourages consistency of carbohydrate intake and portion control using abbreviated food lists.

Advanced Carbohydrate Counting[44] is a booklet that is designed to teach blood glucose and pattern management and how to use insulin-to-carbohydrate ratios. An advanced carbohydrate-counting vocabulary list, a list of needed skills, practice exercises, and questions and answers are included. This booklet is intended to be used in conjunction with the Exchange Lists for Meal Planning or other carbohydrate-counting nutrition references, as food lists are not included.

For more information on carbohydrate counting, see chapter 16 on pattern management, and chapter 17, on insulin pump therapy.

Case Wrap-Up

What are the key issues the educator might address at the initial visit?

- Improve glycemic control prior to conception
- Match insulin to carbohydrate intake
- Improve consistency of carbohydrate intake
- Improve consistency of physical activity
- Address use of complementary therapy

What is SM's nutrition diagnosis?

- Needs to intensify glycemic control prior to pregnancy

What behavior changes should the educator encourage that focus on healthy eating?

- More consistency in meal times and carbohydrate intake
- Begin taking a multivitamin with folic acid daily
- More frequent blood glucose monitoring with occasional postprandial monitoring
- Design physical activity program to achieve consistent level of physical activity most days of the week, perhaps include use of pedometer
- Review implications of using St John's Wort during pregnancy

Which nutrition intervention and meal planning resources could the educator choose for SM?

- Initially, Basic Carbohydrate Counting, until consistent carbohydrate intake and improved glycemic control is achieved
- Move to Advanced Carbohydrate Counting to learn insulin-to-carbohydrate ratio technique

List 1 clinical goal that would be appropriate for SM.

- "I will achieve an A1C as close to normal as possible prior to conception"

List 2 behavioral goals that would be appropriate for SM.

- "I will use an insulin-to-carbohydrate ratio of 1:15 to calculate my insulin lispro injection (Humalog) dosage at mealtime"
- "I will check my blood glucose 4 times daily on a rotating basis and occasionally postprandially for 2 weeks"

How should the educator document the initial encounter with SM?

- Note clinical and behavioral goals, including nutrition recommendations, suggested meal planning approach, and educational topics covered. Share with referring physician and diabetes care team.

What should the educator evaluate on a 6-week return visit?

- Progress toward behavioral goals
- Progress toward clinical goals

Progress Toward Behavioral Goal 1. If during her follow-up visit, SM voices having a problem with hypoglycemic episodes several times a week after lunch and subsequent fear of driving to appointments (barrier identification), the diabetes educator may suggest that recording carbohydrate at this meal and doing premeal and postmeal lunch checks for a week to determine if (a) the carbohydrate intake is being counted accurately, (b) the carbohydrate-to-insulin ratio needs adjustment, and/or (c) other adjustments in insulin or activity are needed (possible barrier resolutions). It also might be suggested that SM fax the record of her food and blood glucose logs to the diabetes educator in 1 week for further review and evaluation.

Progress Toward Behavioral Goal 2. If during her follow-up visit, SM voices difficulty with remembering to test her blood glucose 4 times per day (barrier identification), the diabetes educator might suggest that she write "test BG" in her appointment book at appropriate times and highlight it, to help her remember to check blood glucose (possible barrier resolution).

Progress Toward Clinical Goals. Clinical goals such as A1C, blood pressure levels, and serum lipids should be evaluated at the 3-month follow-up and quarterly appointments. In addition, reviewing kidney function status and the results of an ophthalmologic exam are important. Based on this data, SM may be advised to postpone pregnancy a bit longer, until blood glucose or blood pressure levels are more tightly controlled.

Controversies and Trends

Two controversial topics in diabetes nutrition are use of the glycemic index and complementary therapies. Each is discussed briefly below. As the chapter concludes, trends and fascinating opportunities in the field are also noted. Those on the diabetes care team can expect continued emphasis on prevention of diabetes and prevention and delay of chronic complications, use of computer technologies for educational delivery, and interest in community-based programs.

Controversies in Healthy Eating for Diabetes

Nutrition is an evolving science; new information is discovered daily. Persons with diabetes and prediabetes can access the latest information via the media or Internet and may have questions about controversial areas and nutrition trends that the educator should be prepared to discuss.

Glycemic Index

Glycemic index (GI) is a method of measuring the acute postprandial glycemic impact of a carbohydrate-containing food. Foods that break down quickly during digestion cause a rapid rise in blood glucose, followed by a rapid fall, while those that break down slowly produce a steady, less-steep rise coupled with a slower, extended decline. Over 800 foods have been tested for the glycemic index. Test subjects are given 50 g of carbohydrate from a test food, and the food is ranked on a scale of 0 to 100, according to the blood glucose response it produces. Pure glucose has a GI of 100. Factors that influence the GI include the physical form of the food; type of sugar or starch it contains; protein, fat, and fiber content; acidity of the food; and the method by which the food is cooked and processed.[45] Below are examples of GI values:

- *Breads:* Whole grain pumpernickel (GI of 41), white bread (GI of 70)
- *Cereals:* Oat bran (GI of 55), corn flakes (GI of 92)
- *Starches:* Baked beans (GI of 38), baked potato (GI of 85)
- *Fruits:* Cherries (GI of 22), bananas (GI of 52)
- *Cookies:* Oatmeal cookies (GI of 54), vanilla wafers (GI of 77)

Research studies examining the effectiveness of GI have had mixed results. However, this method of classifying carbohydrate may be useful to those who wish to establish an individual-specific glycemic index of foods. This may provide an additional benefit for controlling glycemic excursions over that observed when total carbohydrate alone is the focus of meal planning.[42,46] Further information on this topic can be found in the chapter on medical nutrition therapy, chapter 13.

Complementary Therapies for Diabetes

Many persons with diabetes use dietary supplements to lower blood glucose or treat diabetes-related comorbidities or diabetes-related complications. These products may cause serious side effects or potential drug interactions. In addition, they are not required to undergo the same stringent approval process that is required for drugs and are not required by the US Food and Drug Administration (FDA) to prove safety and effectiveness prior to being marketed. While many products have no proof of effectiveness in diabetes, some are more promising. For example, randomized, controlled trials in persons with type 2 diabetes taking sulfonylureas found that cinnamon (1/2 teaspoon daily) improved glucose and blood lipids.[47] On the other hand, the FDA has determined that chromium, a popular product used by individuals for diabetes and weight loss, has insufficient evidence of effectiveness to support health claims.[10] Patients should be encouraged to discuss their use of complementary therapies with the diabetes care team, which should act as a knowledgeable resource in this controversial area. More information and a resource list can be found in chapter 19, on biological complementary therapies.

Trends in Diabetes Self-Management Education for Healthy Eating

The epidemic of diabetes will to continue to affect diabetes self-management education for healthy eating in a variety of ways. In the future, there will be a continued emphasis on prevention of diabetes and its complications on a primary, secondary, and tertiary level. Methods of delivering education will rely more on electronic, online, and telemedicine approaches. Community-based programs will be used to deliver education alongside the traditional clinic-based programs.

Diabetes educators must be prepared to address healthy eating not only for diabetes itself, but also for the many comorbidities, such as cardiovascular disease and hypertension, that are experienced by individuals with diabetes. Behavior change, rather than content mastery, will be the gold standard for outcomes of effective diabetes self-management education for healthy eating.[48]

Focus on Education: Pearls for Practice

Teaching Strategies

Be a team coordinator. Achieving healthy eating goals requires a coordinated team effort that centers around the active involvement of the person with prediabetes or diabetes. Because of the complexity of nutrition issues, the RD is the team member with the most skill and expertise in implementing MNT into diabetes management and education. However, all team members must be knowledgeable about nutrition therapy and support and model lifestyle changes.

Encourage topic selection. Start MNT sessions by asking the individual an open-ended question such as "What would you like to work on today?" or display a list of nutrition-related topics and let the individual choose what seems most beneficial to learn. This technique encourages patient empowerment and relieves the educator of the unrealistic burden of trying to teach everything in a single session. Use colorful waiting room displays of charts or test tubes showing the amounts of sucrose or fat in common foods to stimulate discussions of healthy eating.

Make teaching creative and fun! Ask for food labels from home to teach carbohydrate awareness. Use the Nutrition Facts to point out the grams of carbohydrate, protein, fat, and number of calories per serving. Use the label to illustrate that the serving size may differ from the exchange value; for example, a label for brown rice lists a serving size of 1 cup while its serving size from the starch list is 1/3 cup.

Visualize portion sizes. Knowing portion sizes is crucial to successful diabetes control. Use plastic food models to demonstrate portion sizes and foods that contain carbohydrate. Compare small portions of common foods such as a cookie, frozen yogurt, or ice milk with the sucrose in a 12-oz can of regular soft drink, gelatin, fruited yogurt, and other foods. Have the individual weigh and measure foods at home occasionally to improve portion-estimating abilities when eating away from home. Teach convenient guides to portion sizes:

- Thumb tip = 1 teaspoon
- Thumb = 2 tablespoons or 1 ounce
- Fist = 1 cup
- Palm = 3 ounces of meat
- Handful = 1 to 2 ounces of snack food

Engage the learner. Use menus from local restaurants or fast-food chains to help individuals plan a meal according to their healthy eating plan. Role-play so individuals can practice assertiveness skills by asking their "waiter" partner questions about ingredients, preparation, and presentation of food.[49]

Recognize cultural, ethnic, and familial traditions. Work to incorporate preferences or adapt recipes to include favorite foods and family traditions into meal planning to promote good health for their family.

Foster acceptance of natural progressions. Changing medications or adjusting dosages is a natural progression in the management of diabetes. Discourage people from thinking that they have failed. A change in therapy may be needed to meet blood glucose goals.

Stay current. Nutrition is ever-evolving. The knowledge that "sugar is not a poison" is just one example of how evidence-based research on dietary carbohydrate has guided the remarkable changes that have occurred in clinical practice recommendations in recent years.

Messages for Patients

Be open to new information. Recognize that learning about making healthier food choices takes time, but the extra effort will help achieve goals for improved diabetes management and overall health. Also, remember that recommendations for diabetes nutrition change and evolve as more is learned. Learning about the most current guidelines is worthwhile.

Meal planning is individualized. What works for your friend or neighbor may not be appropriate for you. For example, whether a person with diabetes includes snacks in his or her meal plan depends on that person's medication, activity level, blood glucose levels, and nutrient needs. Children with type 1 diabetes may require frequent snacks to maintain normal blood glucose levels, but adults with type 2 diabetes who are controlled by lifestyle changes alone may not need the extra calories that snacks provide. A meal plan can be designed to meet needs and work as a part of a management plan.

References

1. Identifying patients at risk: ADA's definitions for nutrition screening and nutrition assessment. J Am Diet Assoc. 1994;94:838-9.
2. Nettles AT. Patient education in the hospital. Diabetes Spectrum. 2005;18:44-8.
3. Tang TS, Gillard ML, Funnell MM, et al. Developing a new generation of ongoing diabetes self-management support interventions. Diabetes Educ. 2005;31:91-7.
4. Rickheim PL, Weaver TW, Flader JL, Kendall DM. Assessment of group versus individual diabetes education: a randomized study. Diabetes Care. 2002;25:269-74.
5. Rizzotto JA. Meal planning in groups. Diabetes Spectrum. 2005;18:132-4.
6. Heidgerken AD, Lewin AB, Geffken GR, Gelfand KM, Storch EA, Malasanos T. Online diabetes education: design and evaluation with prospective diabetes camp counselors. J Telemed Telecare. 2005;11:93-6.
7. Izquierdo RE, Knudson PE, Meyer S, Kearns J, Ploutz-Snyder R, Weinstock RS. A comparison of diabetes education administered through telemedicine versus in person. Diabetes Care. 2003;26:1002-7.
8. Pastors JG, Franz MJ, Warshaw H, Daly A, Arnold M. How effective is medical nutrition therapy in diabetes care? J Am Diet Assoc. 2003;103:827-31.
9. Diabetes Prevention Program Research Group. Reduction in the incidence of type 2 diabetes with lifestyle intervention or metformin. N Engl J Med. 2002;346:393-403.
10. American Diabetes Association. Standards of medical care in diabetes, 2006. Diabetes Care. 2006;29: S4-42.
11. Mulcahy K, Maryniuk M, Peeples M, et al. Diabetes self-management education core outcomes measures: technical review. Diabetes Educ. 2003;29:768-803.
12. Lacey K, Pritchett E. Nutrition care process and model: ADA adopts road map to quality care and outcomes management. J Am Diet Assoc. 2003;103:1061-72.
13. Osterman DN. The feedback lecture; matching teach and learning styles. J Am Diet Assoc. 1984;84:1221-2.
14. Prochaska J, Redding C, Evers K. The Transtheoretical Model and Stages of Change, 2nd ed. San Francisco, Calif: Jossey-Bass, Inc; 1997:60–84.
15. Leontos C, Geil P. Individualized Approaches to Diabetes Nutrition Therapy: Case Studies. Alexandria, Va: American Diabetes Association; 2002.
16. American Dietetic Association Medical Nutrition Therapy Evidence-Based Guides for Practice: Guidelines for Type 1, Type 2 and Gestational Diabetes Mellitus. Chicago, Ill: American Dietetic Association; 2001.
17. Kulkarni K, Castle G, Gregory R, et al, for the Diabetes Care and Education Dietetic Practice Group. Nutrition practice guidelines for type 1 diabetes mellitus positively affect dietitian practices and patient outcomes. J Am Diet Assoc. 1998; 98:62-70.
18. Monk S, Barry B, McClain K, Weaver T, Cooper N, Franz M. Practice guidelines for medical nutrition therapy provided by dietitians for persons with non-insulin-dependent diabetes mellitus. J Am Diet Assoc. 1995;95:999-1006.
19. Reader D, Sipe M. Key components of care for women with gestational diabetes. Diabetes Spectrum. 2001;14:188-91.

20. Franz MJ, Bantle JP, Brunzell JD, et al. Evidence-based nutrition principles and recommendations for the treatment and prevention of diabetes and related complications (technical review). Diabetes Care. 2002;25:148-98.

21. Reader D. Diabetes in pregnancy and lactation. In: American Dietetic Association Guide to Diabetes Medical Nutrition Therapy and Education. Ross TA, Boucher JL, O'Connell, eds. Chicago, Ill: American Dietetic Association; 2005:189-97.

22. American Diabetes Association. Gestational diabetes mellitus (position statement). Diabetes Care. 2004;27suppl 1:S88-S90.

23. American Diabetes Association. Preconception care of women with diabetes (position statement). Diabetes Care. 2004; 27suppl 1:S76–8.

24. American Diabetes Association. ADA Statement: care of children and adolescents with Type 1 diabetes. Diabetes Care. 2005;28:186-212.

25. Evert E, Gerken S. Birth through adolescence. In: American Dietetic Association Guide to Diabetes Medical Nutrition Therapy and Education. Ross TA, Boucher JL, O'Connell, eds. Chicago, Ill: American Dietetic Association; 2005:161-78.

26. American Diabetes Association. ADA Consensus Statement: type 2 diabetes in children and adolescents. Diabetes Care. 2000;23:381-89.

27. McLaughlin S. Diabetes in older adults. In: American Dietetic Association Guide to Diabetes Medical Nutrition Therapy and Education. Ross TA, Boucher JL, O'Connell, eds. Chicago, Ill: American Dietetic Association; 2005:179-88.

28. Kittler PG, Sucher KP. Diet counseling in a multicultural society. Diabetes Educ. 1990;16:127-34.

29. Brown TL. Ethnic populations. In: American Dietetic Association Guide to Diabetes Medical Nutrition Therapy and Education. Ross TA, Boucher JL, O'Connell, eds. Chicago, Ill: American Dietetic Association; 2005:227-38.

30. Brown TL. Meal-planning strategies: ethnic populations. Diabetes Spectrum. 2003;16:190-2.

31. American Dietetic Association. Ethnic and Regional Food Practices Series. Chicago, Ill: American Dietetic Association; 1994-2000.

32. Maryniuk MD. Counseling and education strategies for improved adherence to nutrition therapy. In: American Diabetes Association Guide to Medical Nutrition Therapy for Diabetes. Franz MJ, Bantle JP, eds. Alexandria, Va: American Diabetes Association; 1999:369-86.

33. Dietary Guidelines for Americans 2005. US Department of Health and Human Services. On the Internet: www.healthierus.gov/dietaryguidelines. Accessed 31 Dec 2005.

34. MyPyramid. US Department of Agriculture. On the Internet: www.mypyramid.gov. Accessed 31 Dec 2005.

35. American Diabetes Association and American Dietetic Association. The First Step in Diabetes Meal Planning. Alexandria, Va and Chicago, Ill: American Diabetes Association and American Dietetic Association; 2003.

36. American Diabetes Association and American Dietetic Association. Healthy Food Choices. Alexandria, Va and Chicago, Ill: American Diabetes Association and American Dietetic Association; 2003.

37. Rizor HM, Richards S. All our patients need to know about intensified diabetes management they learned in fourth grade. Diabetes Educ. 2000;26:392-404.

38. Idaho Plate Method. On the Internet at: www.platemethod.com. Accessed 31 Dec 2005.

39. American Diabetes Association. The Month of Meals Series. Alexandria, Va: American Diabetes Association; 1998-2004.

40. American Diabetes Association and American Dietetic Association. Eating Healthy with Diabetes: Easy Reading Guide. Alexandria, Va and Chicago, Ill: American Diabetes Association and American Dietetic Association; 2003.

41. American Diabetes Association and American Dietetic Association. Exchange Lists for Meal Planning. Alexandria, Va and Chicago, Ill: American Diabetes Association and American Dietetic Association; 2003.

42. Sheard NF, Clark NG, Brand-Miller JC, et al. ADA Statement: dietary carbohydrate (amount and type) in the prevention and management of diabetes. Diabetes Care. 2004;27:2266–71.

43. American Diabetes Association and American Dietetic Association. Basic Carbohydrate Counting. Alexandria, Va and Chicago, Ill: American Diabetes Association and American Dietetic Association; 2003.

44. American Diabetes Association and American Dietetic Association. Advanced Carbohydrate Counting. Alexandria, Va and Chicago, Ill: American Diabetes Association and American Dietetic Association; 2003.

45. Brand-Miller J, Wolever TMS, Foster-Powell K, Colagiuri S. The New Glucose Revolution: The Authoritative Guide to the Glycemic Index. New York, NY. Marlowe & Co; 2003.

46. Geil PB. Glycemic index: measuring the impact of carbohydrate on postprandial blood glucose. In: Pediatric Diabetes: Health Care Reference and Client Education Handouts. Evert AB, Hess-Fischel A, eds. Chicago, Ill: American Dietetic Association; 2005:12-4.

47. Khan A, Safdar M, Ali Khan MM, et al. Cinnamon improves glucose and lipids of people with type 2 diabetes. Diabetes Care. 2003;26:3215-8.

48. Austin MM. Learning from the past: setting the course for the future. Diabetes Educ. 2005;31:305-6.

49. Franz MJ. Medical nutrition therapy for diabetes. In: A Core Curriculum for Diabetes Education: Diabetes Management Therapies, 5th ed. Franz MJ, ed. Chicago, Ill: American Association of Diabetes Educators; 2003.

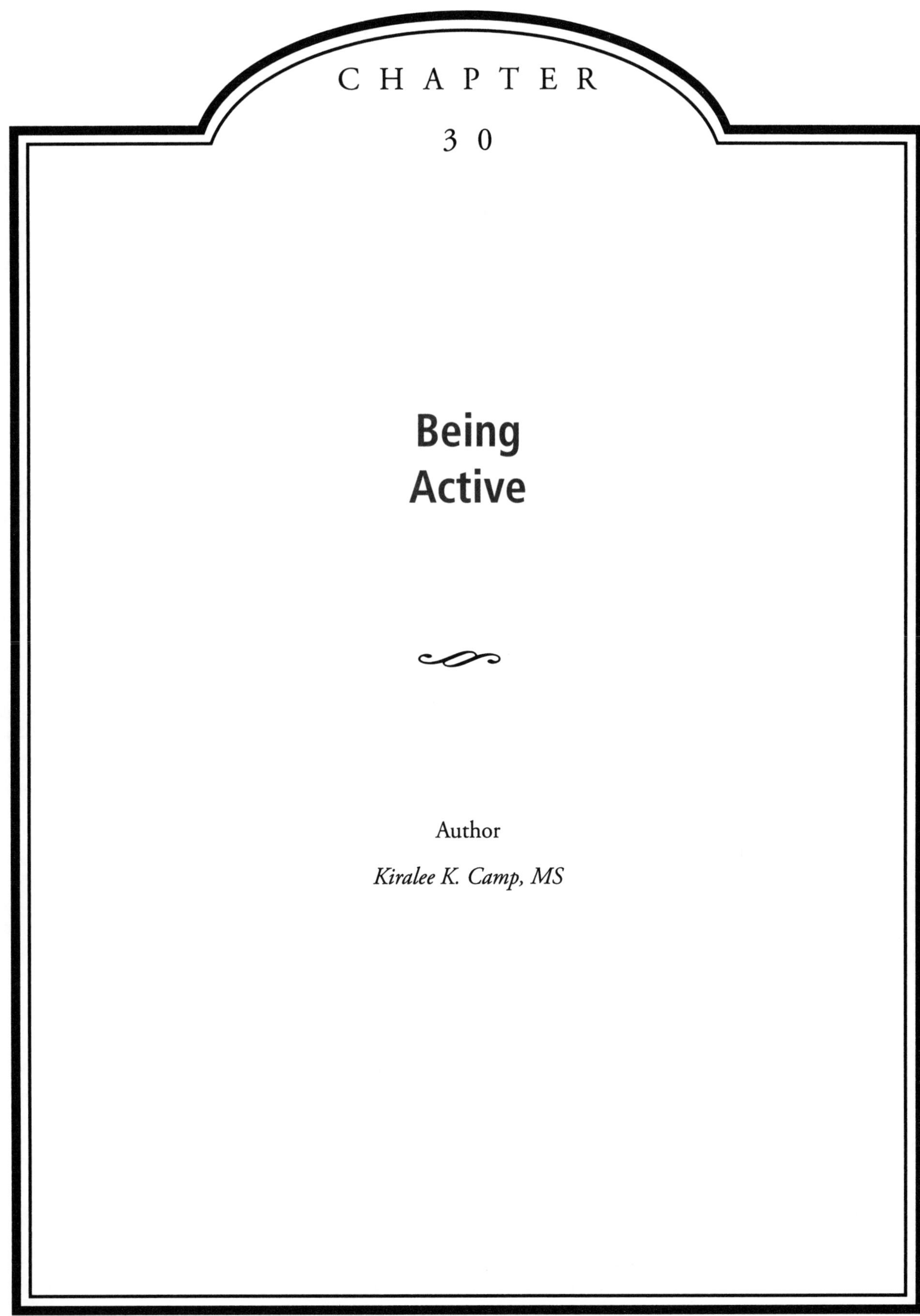

CHAPTER

30

Being Active

Author

Kiralee K. Camp, MS

Key Concepts

- Support public health recommendations for physical activity and exercise by identifying lifestyle interventions.
- Define physical activity and exercise.
- Understand behavior change strategies that are effective in promoting self-care behaviors related to being active.
- Use evidence-based strategies for goal setting: staged-matched "readiness" and the SMART acronym for goal setting, for example.
- Use motivational interviewing to foster the individual's readiness to make positive behavior changes in physical activity.

Introduction

Most Americans, with or without diabetes, do not meet recommended guidelines for physical activity.[1,2] Diabetes educators, therefore, have an important and challenging role in helping individuals with diabetes and prediabetes be more physically active. Effective behavior change strategies, coupled with a solid understanding of current recommendations for physical activity and exercise, can be powerful tools for helping individuals incorporate physical activity into their diabetes management program.

Physical activity and exercise are important in both the prevention and treatment of diabetes. Regular physical activity can prevent and delay the onset of type 2 diabetes and its complications: this is well established.[3-9] The Diabetes Prevention Program (DPP)[4,5] was a landmark randomized clinical trial of 3234 overweight individuals with impaired glucose tolerance. The DPP found lifestyle intervention to be more effective than metformin in preventing type 2 diabetes. The trial reported that intensive lifestyle intervention decreased the incidence of type 2 diabetes by 58%, compared with 31% in the group using metformin.[4] The lifestyle intervention included 150 minutes per week of moderate-intensity physical activity such as brisk walking and a healthy low-calorie, low-fat diet. The goal for participants in this group was to decrease and maintain a 7% reduction in their initial body weight. This lifestyle intervention is similar to current public health recommendations for physical activity and exercise.

The mechanisms by which physical activity helps prevent type 2 diabetes continue to be investigated. However, current evidence suggests physical activity improves insulin action, lowers blood glucose levels, improves body mass index, and reduces several risk factors for cardiovascular disease.[3,8] These important findings demonstrate the significant role physical activity and exercise have in the prevention and management of diabetes.

Physical activity and exercise can be defined separately; however, these terms will be used interchangeably throughout this chapter. Physical activity is defined as any bodily movement produced by skeletal muscle that requires energy expenditure in excess of resting energy expenditure.[10,11] Exercise is defined as planned, structured, and repetitive bodily movement done to improve or maintain one or more components of physical fitness.[10,11] Recommended exercise programs for individuals with diabetes typically include activities to enhance cardiorespiratory endurance, muscular fitness, and flexibility.

This chapter provides diabetes educators with tools and strategies to be used when helping individuals with and at risk for diabetes make positive and lasting changes in physical activity and exercise habits.

Preparing Individuals for Being Active

Medical Evaluation

Physical activity assessments are useful when an individual plans to begin a physical activity or exercise program. A thorough medical evaluation is recommended for individuals with diabetes to screen for the presence of macrovascular and microvascular complications that may be worsened by exercise. The medical history and physical examination should focus on the signs and symptoms affecting the heart, blood vessels, eyes, kidneys, feet, and nervous system.[12,13]

The American Diabetes Association (ADA) recognizes the value of a graded exercise test with electrocardiogram (ECG) for individuals at high risk for underlying cardiovascular disease and who are planning to participate in a moderate- to high-intensity exercise program based on the following criteria:[12]

- Age >35 years
- Age >25 years and
  —Type 2 diabetes of >10 years' duration
  —Type 1 diabetes of >15 years' duration
- Presence of any additional risk factor for coronary artery disease
- Presence of microvascular disease (proliferative retinopathy or nephropathy, including microalbuminuria)
- Peripheral vascular disease
- Autonomic neuropathy

Individuals who exhibit nonspecific ECG changes in response to exercise or who have nonspecific ST and T wave changes on resting ECG may need alternative tests such as radionuclide stress testing to rule out atherosclerotic heart disease.[12,13]

Other Program Design Considerations

A thorough screening for underlying diabetes-related complications is the first step in preparing an individual with diabetes for a safe and enjoyable activity program. Clinical status and health needs as well as the individual's personal interests and past and present activity patterns should be considered in program planning. In all cases, specific goals identified by the individual are the ultimate target. All exercise programs need to be designed in terms of intensity (how difficult), duration (how long), frequency (how often), and mode (type of activity). The appropriate rate of progression must also be considered. This depends on an individual's functional capacity, medical and health status, age, individual activity preferences and goals, and tolerance to the current level of activity.[13]

- *Type 1 Diabetes:* For individuals with type 1 diabetes without complications, exercise recommendations are similar to those for individuals with no known health problems
- *Type 2 Diabetes:* Recommendations for individuals with type 2 diabetes more closely align with obesity and hypertension guidelines and focus on calorie expenditure[10]

Case in Point: Weight, Blood Pressure, and Type 2 Diabetes

MT, a 48-year-old woman diagnosed with type 2 diabetes 7 years earlier, was having trouble controlling her weight and blood pressure. She was referred to a diabetes educator by her physician to discuss safe and appropriate ways to be more physically active so that she might address these issues and improve her overall health.

She had received medical clearance to start increasing her activity level with no specific restrictions. Her medications included a sulfonylurea and an antihypertensive agent. MT reported testing her blood glucose fairly regularly. She was not currently doing any structured physical activity and had not regularly participated in the past. She stated that she was motivated to be more active, mainly because of her physician's recommendation and her unhappiness with the weight gain she had experienced.

Vitals

- Height: 64 in
- Weight: 190 lb
- BMI: 33
- Heart rate: 65 beats per minute
- Blood pressure: 138/86 mm Hg

Lab Data

- Fasting plasma glucose: 158 mg/dL
- A1C: 7.2%
- Total cholesterol: 190 mg/dL
- Triglycerides: 200 mg/dL
- HDL-C: 38 mg/dL
- LDL-C: 132 mg/dL

Questions to Consider

1. What recommendations would you give to this individual for increasing her activity level?
2. What precautions would you suggest?
3. Most importantly, what strategies might you suggest to help motivate and support her efforts to establish regular physical activity as a lifelong habit?

In general, young individuals in good metabolic control can participate in most of the same activities as other healthy individuals. Middle-aged and older individuals are to be encouraged to be physically active, but advised of the need to be screened first for complications that may be worsened by physical activity.[8,12]

Developing a Physical Activity Program

Exercise Session Format

Exercise sessions should generally have 3 parts:

- Proper warm-up
- Conditioning
- Cool-down

Warm-Up. The warm-up phase includes 5 to 10 minutes of low-intensity aerobic activity. This helps to safely prepare the skeletal muscles, heart, and lungs for progressive increases in exercise intensity.[12,13] The warm-up may also help reduce muscle injury and facilitates a safe transition from rest to exercise by stretching postural muscles, increasing blood flow, elevating body temperature, increasing oxygen availability, and increasing metabolic rate.[13]

Conditioning. The conditioning phase includes activities to enhance cardiorespiratory fitness, muscle strength and endurance, or flexibility.

Cool-Down. The cool-down includes low-intensity activity to help the body gradually recover from the conditioning phase and safely transition back to a resting state. The cool-down helps prevent blood pooling in the arms and legs, removes metabolic by-products, and may reduce risks for cardiovascular complications immediately after exercise.

Flexibility and Stretching Exercises

Flexibility exercises can be included as part of the warm-up or cool-down.[12,13] According to the American College of Sports Medicine (ACSM),[13] flexibility is defined as the ability to move a joint though its complete range of motion. Stretching exercises help improve and maintain joint and muscle range of motion if performed properly. Current ACSM guidelines[10,13] for achieving and maintaining flexibility include the following:

- Complete a warm-up to increase muscle temperature before stretching
- Focus on muscle groups and joints with reduced range of motion
- Use static stretching, which involves slowly stretching a muscle to the end of its range of motion, without causing discomfort, and holding the position
- Hold each stretch for 15 to 30 seconds
- Complete 2 to 4 repetitions for each stretch
- Do stretching exercises at least 2 to 3 days per week and up to 5 to 7 days per week

Flexibility training summary:

- *Activity:* Stretch all major muscle groups; focus on joints with reduced range of motion
- *Frequency:* 2 to 3 days per week, up to 5 days per week
- *Duration:* 2 to 4 repetitions for each stretch; hold each stretch 15 to 30 seconds
- *Intensity:* Stretch to the muscle's end range of motion without causing discomfort

The ADA's current position on flexibility exercises notes that there is insufficient evidence to recommend for or against it as a routine part of the exercise prescription.[11] Therefore, flexibility exercise recommendations should be based primarily on the individual's specific needs and interests.

Aerobic Exercise

Cardiorespiratory or aerobic exercise is defined as continuous, dynamic exercise that uses large muscle groups and requires aerobic metabolic pathways to sustain the activity.[10,13] Examples include walking, jogging, biking, swimming, water aerobics, rollerblading, and cross-country skiing. Aerobic, compared to anaerobic, exercise provides the greatest benefits for people with diabetes in terms of blood glucose control and cardiovascular status. Table 30.1 summarizes recommendations for aerobic exercise for individuals with diabetes.

Mode of Activity

The recommended *types* or *modes* of aerobic activity for individuals with diabetes are highly dependent on the individual's preferences and skill level. Health-related benefits of improved physical fitness do not appear to depend on the type of aerobic exercise. Identifying activities that can safely and effectively improve cardiovascular endurance and maximize caloric expenditure is important.[14] Walking is the most common type of physical activity done by individuals with diabetes and often the most convenient. However, other low-impact or non-weight-bearing types of activity, such as bicycling, swimming, or aquatic exercises, may be more appropriate for those with complications or coexisting conditions such as peripheral neuropathy or degenerative arthritis.[14,15]

TABLE 30.1 Summary of Aerobic Exercise Recommendations for Individuals with Diabetes

Screening For patients intending on participating in moderate- to high-intensity physical activity, a graded exercise test (GXT) may be helpful based on the following criteria:* • Age >35 years • Age >25 years and —Type 2 diabetes of >10 years' duration —Type 1 diabetes of >15 years' duration • Presence of any additional risk factor for coronary artery disease • Presence of microvascular disease (proliferative retinopathy or nephropathy, including microalbuminuria) • Peripheral vascular disease • Autonomic neuropathy
Exercise Prescription, Type 2 Diabetes** Aerobic preferred; anaerobic allowed if no secondary limitations (twice weekly) • *Intensity:* 55% to 90% of age-adjusted maximal heart rate (equal to 40% to 85% of maximum oxygen uptake or heart rate reserve) † • *Duration:* 20 to 60 min (can be divided into three 10-minute sessions) ** • *Frequency:* 3 to 4 nonconsecutive days and up to 5 times per week
Exercise Prescription, Type 1 Diabetes* All levels of exercise can be performed by those who do not have complications and are in good blood glucose control
Safety Precautions • Warm-up and cool down • Careful selection and progression of exercise program • Patient education • Monitor blood glucose pre- and post-exercise • Adjust guidelines to prevent hypoglycemia • Management by healthcare personnel

*Brownell KD, Wadden TA. Etiology and treatment of obesity: understanding a serious, prevalent, and refractory disorder. J Consult Clin Psychol. 1992;60:505-17.

**Williams KV, Erbey JR, Becker D, Orchard TJ. Improved glycemic control reduces the impact of weight gain on cardiovascular risk factors in type 1 diabetes. Diabetes Care.1999;22:1084-91.

†Whaley MH, Brubaker PH, Otto RM, eds. American College of Sports Medicine: Guidelines for Exercise Testing and Prescription, 7th ed. Baltimore, Md: Williams & Wilkins; 2006.

Source: Adapted from SH, Ruderman NB. Exercise and NIDDM (technical review). Diabetes Care. 1990;13:785-9.

Intensity of Activity

Low-to-moderate intensity physical activity is generally recommended to achieve aerobic and metabolic improvements.[10,12,13]

Estimating Intensity. Intensity of aerobic activity is based on measured or estimated maximal oxygen uptake ($\dot{V}O_2$max) or heart rate.[10] The ACSM recommends the following:[10,13]

- Exercise intensity of 40% to 85% of oxygen uptake reserve ($\dot{V}O_2R$) or *heart rate reserve* (HHR)

This corresponds to 55% to 90% of *maximum heart rate* (HRmax). The recommended intensity range is intended to be broad to reflect that deconditioned individuals can gain improvements in cardiorespiratory fitness at lower intensities, while individuals with greater fitness typically require a higher minimal threshold, at least 45% $\dot{V}O_2R$.[13] The prescribed intensity range should be based on one's fitness level, duration of diabetes, degree of complications, and individual goals. The ACSM also recommends, based on recommendations from the ADA, that a more conservative intensity range of 50% to 80% $\dot{V}O_2R$ or HRR be considered for individuals with diabetes.[12,13]

Exercise performed at low levels (<50% HRmax) has less effect on glucose disposal than exercise performed at higher intensities. The effect on glucose disposal during high-intensity exercise is roughly proportional to the total work performed (time × intensity). However, high-intensity exercise may result in transient hyperglycemia and cause an excessive rise in blood pressure.

Formulas for Estimating Exercise Intensity

- $\dot{V}O_2R$ = $\dot{V}O_2max$ – Resting $\dot{V}O_2$
- HHR = Maximum heart rate – Resting heart rate
- Percent HHR = HHR × Percent intensity
- Percent HRmax = Maximum heart rate × Percent intensity

Determining Heart Rate. Exercise intensity can be calculated accurately using the results of an exercise stress test. Based on the individual's maximum heart rate response to the exercise stress test, the following HRR formula, also known as the Karvonen formula, is commonly used to calculate target heart rate range in beats per minute (bpm):[13]

Target heart rate range = [(HRmax – HRrest)%] + HRrest

Using HHR Formula to Determine Target Heart Rate Range

Example: Calculate the target heart rate range for a 50-year-old man with a resting heart rate of 70 bpm and a maximum heart rate of 170 bpm.

Lower estimated range = [(170 – 70) × 0.40] + 70
= [100 × 0.40] + 70
= 40 + 70
= 110 bpm

Higher estimated range = [(170 – 70) × 0.85] + 70
= [100 × 0.85] + 70
= 85 + 70
= 155 bpm

Target heart rate range = 110 to 155 bpm

If the actual maximal heart rate is not known, target heart rate range can be estimated using the following equation, although caution is required:

Estimated HRmax = 220 – Age

This equation should be used with caution due to the large standard deviation, which can cause the heart rate estimation to be off by 12 to 15 bpm.[13] This procedure may also overestimate the maximal heart rate of some individuals with type 2 diabetes, particularly those with autonomic neuropathy.[8,13] Due to the high prevalence of occult cardiovascular disease, use caution when applying standard heart rate formulas to the diabetes population.

Rating of Perceived Exertion (RPE). The RPE is another useful guide for estimating exercise intensity (Table 30.2). This is a subjective rating based on general fatigue and can be used along with target heart rate estimations or as a substitute to guide the intensity of activity.[13] There are 2 RPE scales appropriate to use with individuals with diabetes:

- Original RPE scale, which rates intensity from 6 to 20
- Revised RPE scale, which rates intensity from 0 to 10

TABLE 30.2 Rating of Perceived Exertion (RPE)

Category Scale	*Category-Ration Scale*	
6	0 Nothing at all	No intensity
7 Very, very light	0.3	
8	0.5 Extremely weak	Just noticeable
9 Very light	0.7	
10	1 Very weak	
11 Fairly light	1.5	
12	2 Weak	Light
13 Somewhat hard	2.5	
14 Hard	4	
16	5 Strong	Heavy
17 Very hard	6	
18	7 Very strong	
19 Very, very hard	8	
20	9	
	10 Extremely strong	Strongest intensity
	Absolute maximum	Highest possible

Source: Adapted with permission from Gunnar Borg. Borg's Perceived Exertion and Pain Scales. Champaign, Ill: Human Kinetics; 1998.

When RPE scales are used, the individual is instructed to focus on feelings of exertion and general fatigue. While performing the activity within his or her target exercise intensity, the individual is asked to identify feelings of exertion and fatigue. This elicits the recommended RPE range. Generally, an exercise intensity that corresponds to an RPE range of 12 to 16 (using the 6 to 20 scale) or 2 to 5 (using the 0 to 10 scale) is recommended.[12,13]

Duration of Activity

The duration of exercise is directly related to caloric expenditure requirements and inversely related to the intensity of exercise required to achieve the same results. To gain maximum benefit, lower intensity exercise needs to be performed for longer periods of time compared to higher intensity exercise. The exercise duration required to meet the recommended weekly energy expenditure is 20 to 60 minutes per session.[13,16]

Physical activity can be broken down into three 10-minute sessions throughout the day. Studies have shown that similar cardiorespiratory gains occur when physical activity is accumulated throughout the day in shorter bouts (~10 minutes) compared to a single prolonged activity session of similar duration and intensity (~30 minutes).[13,17] However, 30 to 60 minutes of continuous exercise seems to have a greater impact on weight loss.[14] Severely deconditioned individuals may need to exercise in multiple sessions of short duration (~10 minutes), begin at low levels (50% $\dot{V}O_2R$) with brief rest intervals, and progress weekly to higher intensity, continual exercise.[13] Initially, sessions can be done in 10 to 15 minutes, increasing progressively over time to 30 to 60 minutes.[13]

Frequency of Activity

Recommendations for frequency ought be given in sessions per day and in days per week. Individuals with diabetes are generally advised to participate in at least 3 to 4 nonconsecutive days and up to 5 sessions per week to improve glycemic control and cardiorespiratory endurance and achieve target caloric expenditure.[8,13,14] Exercise that is limited to 2 days per week generally does not result in significant improvements in cardiorespiratory endurance. Since the duration of glycemic improvement after an exercise session is usually greater than 12 hours but less than 72 hours, regular physical activity is needed to lower blood glucose.[14,18] For individuals taking insulin, being active on a daily basis may help to balance caloric needs with insulin dosages.[14] Obese individuals may need to be active more frequently (5 to 7 days per week) at lower intensities to optimize weight loss and maintenance.[13,14] To achieve sustained major weight loss, the optimal volume of activity needed is typically greater than the volume needed to achieve improved glycemic control.[11]

Energy expenditure can also be used to guide exercise programming. The ACSM recommends a target range of 150 to 400 calories per day of energy expenditure in physical activity.[10,13] This represents a minimum threshold of 1000 calories a week, which is associated with reduction in all-cause mortality risk. For previously sedentary individuals, recommend the minimum threshold as the initial goal. Encourage progress toward the upper target range of expending 300 to 400 calories per day in physical activity to achieve maximal health benefits and weight loss. Energy expenditure in excess of 2000 calories per week in physical activity has been associated with successful short- and long-term weight loss.[10]

Progressing Toward Goals

Recommend appropriate rates of progression to help individuals effectively and safely achieve aerobic exercise goals. Initially, suggest a focus on increasing frequency and duration of the exercise, rather than its intensity. This provides a safe level of activity that can be done with little effort and increases the likelihood of sustaining the activity habit.[14] See also the discussion that follows on putting the activity program into action and chapter 14, on physical activity and exercise, for more information on maintaining a program of physical activity.

Aerobic exercise summary:

- *Frequency:* 3 to 5 days per week
- *Duration:* 20 to 60 minutes
- *Intensity:* 40% to 85% of $\dot{V}O_2R$ or HHR (55% to 90% of HRmax)

Anaerobic Exercise

Anaerobic exercise is defined as an activity that does not require sustained oxygen to meet energy demands and generally does not induce the same health benefits as an aerobic exercise program. Anaerobic exercise and vigorous or high-intensity aerobic exercise may cause excessive rises in blood pressure, cardiac workload, and intraocular pressure. These reactions could be potential problems for those with diabetes and vascular disease or complications. Therefore, aerobic exercise is the preferred form of activity for these individuals.

Resistance (Strength) Training

Resistance exercise or strength training, along with aerobic activity, has been shown to improve musculoskeletal health, maintain independence in performing daily activities, and reduce the possibility of injury.[17,19] Studies suggest that properly designed resistance programs may improve indices of cardiovascular function, glucose tolerance, strength, and body composition, provided the person with diabetes does not have contraindications to strength training.[20,21]

The term "muscular fitness" refers to both muscular strength and endurance. Muscle strength is the ability of the muscle to exert force, while muscle endurance is the ability of the muscle to continue to perform without fatigue.[11,13] Resistance exercises, such as the types listed below, are used to improve muscular fitness:

- Weight lifting
- Weight machines
- Resistance bands
- Isometric exercises

Guidelines

Consider the following guidelines when helping individuals develop a resistance training program.

Exercise Selection. Select approximately 8 to 10 exercises that train each of the major muscle groups, which include the back, chest, shoulders, arms, legs, and abdomen.[22] Base exercise selection on individual goals, preferences, and skill. Specific muscle groups may also be targeted to enhance other components of the activity program, such as biking or swimming.

Sequence. Exercise large muscle groups before small muscle groups, such as doing chest and back exercises before arm exercises. In addition, recommend performing exercises involving multiple joints before those for single joints, such as doing leg presses before leg extensions. Doing exercises in this sequence helps ensure that adequate energy is available to effectively perform all exercises within a training session.[23]

Amount of Resistance. Recommend using lower resistance loads. The resistance used is determined by the individual's repetition maximum (RM), which is defined as the amount of weight that allows for successful completion of a specified number of repetitions (no more, no less).[23] The ACSM recommends 40% to 60% of RM for individuals with diabetes.[10,13] This involves working the muscle to near fatigue (RPE of 16). Advise the individual to avoid maximal muscle fatigue.

Frequency. Recommend strength training exercises 2 to 3 times a week with 48 hours of rest between sessions.

Progression. One set of 10 to 15 repetitions, 2 to 3 times a week is sufficient for strength gains and is recommended for those in the initial stages.[11,13] When individuals are comfortable with the exercise and have demonstrated good technique (typically after several weeks), advise them to increase to 2 sets. For further strength gains and greater metabolic benefit, advise individuals to progress to 3 sets of 8 to 10 repetitions.[11]

Modifications. For individuals who need to maintain a lower resistance program, the ACSM recommends 1 set of exercises for all major muscle groups, starting with 10 to 15 repetitions and progressing to 15 to 20 repetitions.[13]

Rest. Adequate rest periods between sets are needed to successfully complete all sets. Typically, lower intensity training requires 15 seconds to 1 minute of rest, while higher intensity training may require up to 2 minutes of rest between sets.[22]

Resistance training summary:

- *Activity:* 8 to 10 exercises for all major muscle groups
- *Frequency:* 2 to 3 days per week
- *Duration:* 1 to 3 sets of 8 to 20 repetitions (eg, 1 set of 10 to 15 repetitions, 2 sets 10 to 15 repetitions, 3 sets 8 to 10 repetitions)
- *Intensity:* Lower resistance; 40% to 60% RM; RPE of 16

Considerations With Cardiovascular Disease

When working with individuals with cardiac disease, focus particular attention on blood pressure and heart-rate response to resistance training. Advise these individuals to start with lighter resistance and choose exercises that use a smaller amount of muscle mass. This helps decrease the myocardial oxygen demand on the heart.[23] The heart rate and blood pressure need to remain within the limits established by the exercise stress test and, therefore, need to be monitored throughout the training session.

Instruction and Supervision

Before starting a resistance exercise program, individuals must be instructed on proper weight lifting techniques to ensure all exercises are performed safely and correctly. Recommend that a qualified professional supervise the initial stages of the training program. Instruct individuals on the following guidelines:[13]

- Breathe continually and avoid breath-holding. Exhale during the exertion or lifting phase, and inhale while returning to starting position.
- Avoid sustained, tight gripping and static lifts that may cause hypertensive responses.
- Lift weights with slow, controlled movements.

- Emphasize using complete range of motion.
- Maintain good form and keep the body properly aligned throughout the lift.
- Adjust the equipment to fit the body frame.
- Stop exercising if warning signs or symptoms occur such as dizziness, unusual shortness of breath, or chest pain.

Resistance Training Precautions

- Individuals with long-term microvascular or macrovascular complications require program modifications to decrease strain on their cardiovascular systems.
- Advise those with proliferative retinopathy or nephropathy against doing resistive training due to increased risk for an excessive systolic pressure response.[23]
- Before starting resistance training, individuals with diabetes and cardiovascular disease need to have an ejection fraction >45% and a cardiorespiratory fitness level of 7 metabolic equivalents, without ischemic ST segment depression on their ECG, hypotensive or hypertensive responses, serious ventricular arrhythmias, or symptoms of cardiovascular disease.[24]
- Individuals with any complications that may be worsened by resistance training need to receive approval from their physician before starting a resistance program.

Safety Considerations

- Teach all individuals with diabetes who are treated with insulin, sulfonylureas, or meglitinides to carry some type of carbohydrate with them while performing physical activity
- Teach the individual to monitor blood glucose, both before and after activity, to promote safety and understanding
- Advise individuals to wear some form of diabetes and personal identification
- Advise individuals to avoid vigorous physical activity in extremely hot, humid, smoggy, or cold environments
- Since seasonal changes in A1C have been related to environmental temperature,[25] encourage individuals to find safe and available places to be active indoors when the weather is colder
- Encourage the individual to wear clothing and shoes appropriate for the activity to reduce chance of injury
- Be aware that certain medications can impair exercise tolerance; for example, β-adrenergic blocking agents alter the heart-rate response to physical activity and mask hypoglycemia and the body's counterregulatory response
- Advise individuals to stop the activity if pain, lightheadedness, or shortness of breath occurs

Modifications for Diabetes Complications

Individuals with chronic complications of diabetes often do not take part in regular physical activity. Yet, increasing the physical activity level is especially useful for this group to improve or maintain functional capacity, strength, and flexibility.[26]

Cardiovascular Disease

Since individuals with diabetes have an increased risk of cardiovascular disease, a comprehensive assessment is recommended to determine the most appropriate physical activity options.

- Individuals with established cardiovascular disease usually require supervision in a cardiac rehabilitation program
- Advise individuals to avoid activities that cause a hypertensive response (systolic blood pressure >260 mm Hg, diastolic blood pressure >125 mm Hg)[13]
- Advise individuals to avoid activities that involve heavy lifting, straining, and Valsalva-like maneuvers
- Recommend activities that use lower extremities such as walking, light jogging, and cycling; activities that primarily use the upper body and arms generally cause larger increases in systolic blood pressure
- Recommend using low resistance with high repetitions for resistance exercises[13]

Peripheral Vascular Disease

Individuals with peripheral vascular disease will experience ischemic pain during physical activity as a result of insufficient oxygen supply and demand for the active muscles. A walking program for intermittent claudication may improve collateral circulation and muscle metabolism and, in turn, decrease pain.[27] A training program using intervals of walk and rest periods may result in improved tolerance for exercise, which was previously limited due to pain.

- Help individuals determine the distance and duration for walking by a pain-limited threshold
- Advise individuals to keep the intensity low because higher intensity demands a greater blood supply and causes claudication pain[28]

- Encourage individuals to use conversation, music, and other elements to divert attention from the discomfort and pain
- Stop activity when the discomfort or pain increases from moderate to intense discomfort and attention cannot be diverted from the pain[13]
- Recommend weight-bearing activities, although non-weight-bearing activities may be used if longer duration and higher intensity workouts are the goal
- Advise individual that pain at rest and during the night are signs of severe peripheral vascular disease, which is an absolute contraindication for a walking program[29]
- Daily activity sessions will maximize tolerable pain[13]

Retinopathy

Individuals with advanced retinopathy will have significant restrictions regarding the level of physical exertion and activity options. The level of retinopathy determines which activities are appropriate and which activities are to be avoided (see Table 14.13 in chapter 14, on physical activity).[30] Provide physical activity recommendations based on the severity and stage of diabetic retinopathy. Individuals with proliferative diabetic retinopathy must receive clearance for exercise from their ophthalmologist due to risk of vitreous hemorrhage or traction retinal detachment.

Visual Impairment

Recommend appropriate options for physical activity such as swimming using lane guides, stationary cycling, treadmill walking, tandem cycling and dancing, using a sighted person as a guide.[26]

End-Stage Renal Disease

Individuals with end-stage renal disease usually have low functional and aerobic capacity. Aerobic activities are preferred, but the individual's degree of kidney impairment dictates his or her ability to perform aerobic activity.

- Recommend individuals begin aerobic activity at a low level, perhaps using interval work, followed by a gradual, progressive activity plan[31]
- Recommend brisk walking, swimming, and cycling activities

Peripheral Neuropathy

Physical activity cannot reverse the symptoms of neuropathy, but it can prevent further loss of muscle strength and flexibility. Such losses are commonly seen in individuals with sensory polyneuropathy.

- Recommend daily range-of-motion exercises to help minimize shortening of connective tissue. Extra care is needed to avoid injury and overstretching by sensory-impaired individuals.[26]
- In most cases, advise individuals to avoid weight-bearing activities because of an increased chance of soft tissue and joint injury.
- Recommend low-impact activities such as cycling and swimming to avoid orthopedic stress; brisk walking may be another alternative if balance is not impaired.[10]
- Advise individuals to avoid jogging because it places a threefold increase on the foot compared with walking.
- Encourage individuals to wear proper footwear and inspect their feet after physical activity to prevent blisters and detect injuries.
- Suggest chair exercises for individuals with limited mobility to improve flexibility and strength.

Autonomic Neuropathy

Advise individuals with autonomic neuropathy that increases in physical activity levels must be approached with caution because of the role of the autonomic nervous system in hormonal and cardiovascular regulation during exercise.

- Advise individuals to avoid high-intensity physical activities
- Advise individuals to avoid physical exertion in hot or cold environments since dehydration may be a risk for those who have difficulty with hemoregulation
- Caution individuals that hypotension and hypertension may occur after vigorous activities
- Recommend recumbent cycling or water aerobics for individuals with orthostatic hypotension
- Recommend frequent blood glucose monitoring during physical activity for people with defective counterregulatory mechanisms[26]

Modifications for Obesity

Combined programs of physical activity, meal planning, and behavior change are effective for obese individuals. Physical activity combined with meal planning has been shown to be more effective for long-term weight loss than either done alone. Approaches that emphasize physical activity offer enhanced calorie expenditure and provide the benefits of improved fitness in terms of influencing blood lipids, blood glucose control, blood pressure, mood, and attitude.[10] Regular physical activity also helps maintain muscle mass while promoting fat loss during weight loss. When working with individuals who are obese, consider the following guidelines to increase their physical activity level:

- Recommend initial goals of simply increasing the amount of activity from an inactive level
- Recommend continuous aerobic exercise that uses large muscle groups since it has the greatest impact on weight loss
- Recommend lower intensity, non-weight-bearing activities to reduce the risk of orthopedic injury; higher intensity, weight-bearing activities such as running are not recommended
- Recommend walking as an effective choice for continuous aerobic exercise; alternative types of exercise also include cycling and water exercise
- Advise individuals that swimming is less likely to induce weight loss
- Recommend moderate-intensity (40% to 60% $\dot{V}O_2R$ or HRR) activities with emphasis on increasing duration and frequency
- Advise individuals that intensity can progressively increase to 50% to 75% $\dot{V}O_2R$ or HRR to improve aerobic capacity; however, this is not necessary if the individual prefers lower intensity
- Recommend 45 to 60 minutes of activity 5 to 7 days per week
- Recommend a target range of 300 to 400 calories per day of energy expenditure or 2000 calories per week in physical activity

Modifications for Older Adults

When working with older adults, give special consideration to changes in body composition that may have occurred over the years (eg, declines in muscle mass and muscle strength, with resultant decreases in basal metabolic rate, activity level, and energy expenditure). Encourage older adults to identify an activity they enjoy and guide them in a stepped approach toward meeting the Surgeon General's recommendation of 30 minutes of moderate-intensity activity on most and preferably all days of the week.[13,32] Brisk walking, gardening, yard work, and housework are good examples of moderate-intensity activities.

Results from the DPP demonstrate that it is never too late to begin an exercise program. In that study, older adults who met the activity goal of 150 minutes per week were found to derive the greatest benefit from exercise in warding off type 2 diabetes, when compared to their younger counterparts.[4] Table 30.3 summarizes the guidelines for aerobic exercise in older adults. In general, population-based guidelines for aerobic exercise, resistance training, and flexibility also apply to them; however, the ACSM[10,13] recommends that special consideration be given to the following areas.

Aerobic Activity: Older Adults

- A thorough medical exam is needed before starting an exercise program
- Recommend aquatic exercises and stationary cycling for individuals with less tolerance for weight-bearing activities, such as those with degenerative joint disease or osteoarthritis
- Instruct individuals to increase exercise duration before intensity
- Recommend a conservative approach when increasing exercise intensity
- Since sedentary individuals have an increased risk for cardiac arrest and cerebral vascular accidents if the physical exertion is too vigorous, advise starting at lower levels, progressing more slowly, and gradually increasing the duration and frequency to reach the desired fitness level
- Advise individuals to consult their physician before doing vigorous exercise
- Advise individuals to limit vigorous aerobic exercise to 2 to 3 days per week (rather than 3 to 5)

Resistance Training: Older Adults

- Recommend 1 set of 8 to 10 exercises for each major muscle group 2 to 3 times a week
- Recommend 10 to 15 repetitions that are "somewhat hard" on the RPE scale (12 to 15)
- Advise individuals that the first several sessions should be supervised by a trained professional
- Recommend minimal resistance be used for the first 8 weeks to accommodate changes in connective tissue
- Suggest machines, rather than free weights, since machines are typically easier to use, help stabilize the body, and allow for more control over exercise range of motion
- Advise individuals with degenerative joint disease or osteoarthritis to avoid participation in resistance training during active periods of joint inflammation or pain

Flexibility Exercises: Older Adults

- Recommend a well-rounded stretching program to counteract decreases in flexibility and improve balance and agility
- For deconditioned individuals who are just beginning to be more active, recommend devoting the entire exercise session to improving flexibility

TABLE 30.3 Guideline Summary for Aerobic Exercise in Older Adults	
Activity Type	Cycling, brisk walking, swimming, dancing, rowing
Duration	30 to 40 minutes Intersperse initial activity sessions with brief rest periods until a continuous bout of activity can be achieved. Add 2 to 5 minutes per week until desired goal is met.
Frequency	5 to 6 days per week
Intensity	Typically 60% to 75% of maximal heart rate Base training intensity on the individual's graded exercise test (GXT), risk factors, and medical history
Assess progress and reevaluate the individual's fitness plan in approximately 4 to 6 weeks.	

*Graham C. Exercise and aging: implications for persons with diabetes. Diabetes Educ. 1991;17:189-95.

Considerations With Children and Adolescents

Type 2 diabetes is being diagnosed in children at an ever-increasing and alarming rate. While the causes for this looming epidemic are multiple, the decline in physical activity levels for children in the United States is partially responsible. The *Dietary Guidelines for Americans, 2005* recommend children and adolescents participate in at least 60 minutes of moderate intensity physical activity most days of the week, preferably daily.[33] When working with children and adolescents, focus activity recommendations on enjoyable playtime activities, rather than structured exercise bouts. Encourage participation in school physical education classes, recreation leagues, school sports, and active family outings. Encourage parental involvement in the planning and development of physical activity programs for children and adolescents. For a listing of Web sites with information on how to help children establish good activity habits and ongoing advocacy efforts in this area, see the list of Internet resources at the end of this chapter.

For children with type 1 diabetes, careful review of insulin dosages, insulin peaks and durations of action, injection sites, and timing of meals and snacks is critical if problems with widely variant blood glucose levels, related to physical activity, are to be avoided. Frequent self-monitoring of blood glucose (ie, before, during, and after the exercise period) will assist in guiding adjustments in insulin dosing that will help to avoid the extremes of glycemic control. Due to an increased uptake of glucose into skeletal muscle during exercise, children who have not had a regular pattern of activity or conditioning may be particularly susceptible to hypoglycemic episodes, near the time of the exercise or hours later. To avoid problems, a decrease in "insulin on board" during active periods, avoidance of injecting near the primary muscle areas to be used in the activity, and modifications in food intake may be needed.

Cultural Considerations

When assisting individuals in planning and preparing for physical activity, consideration must be given to their cultural practices and beliefs and how these may influence the adoption of physical activity behaviors. Understanding and being sensitive to beliefs and perceptions regarding physical activity is crucial for successful planning of physical activity goals. Promote physical activities that do not offend or ignore the cultural beliefs of the individual. Elicit information from individuals and provide culturally appropriate suggestions to help tailor suitable physical activity recommendations for their particular group.

Dance and music are a vital part of tradition and celebration for many ethnically diverse groups, including Native, Hispanic, and African Americans. The commitment and promise to pass traditions on to future generations is very strong. By reinforcing the regular inclusion of dance as a healthy lifestyle choice, the diabetes educator can help individuals with diabetes (and their family members who are at high risk to develop the disease) make physical activity a regular part of the family routine. The activity helps strengthen families as well.

Putting the Activity Program into Action

Most diabetes educators are adept in interpreting and promoting recommendations for physical activity and exercise to individuals with diabetes. Educators who are skilled in behavior change strategies and able to effectively tailor exercise programs to individual goals, needs, and interests are better equipped to help individuals be more active. Physical activity programs that are designed primarily by the individual are more likely to be sustained. When an individual chooses activities that are personally enjoyable and convenient, he or she is more likely to participate in the activity on a regular basis.

Using Stage-Matched Interventions

The Transtheoretical Model of behavior change, which uses progressive stages of readiness for behavior change, can be used to tailor exercise interventions.[34,35] Stage-matched interventions are widely accepted by healthcare practitioners in helping individuals make permanent lifestyle changes, including regular exercise.[2,9,10,13,36-38] The following stage-matched strategies can be used to help individuals overcome physical activity and exercise barriers.[5,9,10,39]

Stages of Change for Exercise Behavior[1,10,13,38]

1. *Precontemplation:* Not regularly active and has no intention to be active in the next 6 months
2. *Contemplation:* Not regularly active but thinking about starting in the next 6 months
3. *Preparation:* Doing some activity but not enough to meet current guidelines for regular physical activity
4. *Action:* Has become regularly physically active within the last 6 months
5. *Maintenance:* Has maintained regular physical activity for 6 months or more

Precontemplation

The goal at the precontemplation stage is for individuals to begin thinking about physical activity.

- Build trust with the individual and provide information as needed
- Emphasize the individual's autonomy in decisions to be more active
- Discuss pros and cons of physical activity
- Encourage the individual to think about personally relevant benefits
- Address individual's specific barriers and encourage the individual to come up with possible solutions to these barriers
- Use appropriate goal-setting activities focused on getting the individual to think about being more active, such as reading a pamphlet on the benefits of exercise
- Suggest that the individual write down benefits, barriers, reasons to be active, and reasons not to be active

Contemplation

The goal at the contemplation stage is for individuals to begin taking steps to be more active and think about setting physical activity goals.

- Continue to use strategies from the precontemplation stage
- Provide support and validation to the individual
- Offer information on physical activity and exercise, emphasizing social, psychological, and general health benefits
- Discuss the individual's personal preferences for physical activity
- Encourage the individual to think about what has been personally successful in the past regarding physical activity or examples of family and friends who have been successful
- Suggest that the individual use a reinforcement program that provides positive rewards when goals are achieved
- Suggest that the individual identify other people to use for support

Preparation

The goal at the preparation stage is for individuals to increase physical activity to recommended levels.

- Praise preparation
- Continue to use strategies from precontemplation and contemplation stages
- Assist the individual in setting goals to gradually increase physical activity levels
- Encourage individuals to track progress with a physical activity log that details activity type, amount, duration, and frequency
- Suggest the individual join an exercise class or club, as this is often helpful to individuals in this stage

Action

The goal at the action stage is for individuals to begin making physical activity a regular part of their life.

- Praise all efforts of the individual
- Work with the individual to develop a specific plan for tracking progress and setting short-term physical activity goals
- Suggest the individual try new activities or train for an upcoming exercise event (such as walking or a bicycle race)
- Limit suggestions for additional changes to 1 or 2
- Encourage the individual to begin to anticipate barriers

Maintenance

The goal at the maintenance stage is for individuals to prepare for possible setbacks and find ways to continue to increase enjoyment with the personalized physical activity program.

- Praise all efforts of the individual
- Use strategies from the action stage
- Help the individual find ways to avoid boredom
- Promote relapse prevention strategies—distinguish between a lapse (slight slip) and a relapse (return to former behavior patterns) by having the individual identify potential high-risk situations and develop a plan to deal with them
- Encourage the individual to reflect on the benefits personally achieved with regular physical activity

Keep in mind that most people are not successful with their first attempt at increasing physical activity. Some individuals may need 3 or 4 attempts before physical activity becomes a long-term habit. Individuals will progress through the stages as they learn from past attempts and try different methods for increasing activity. The more an individual takes action to become more physically active, the better his or her chances of progressing forward. The role of the diabetes educator is to support the individual in all stages and apply appropriate intervention strategies as needed.

Promoting Lifestyle Physical Activity

Consider lifestyle physical activity as a method to help individuals be more physically active. For individuals with diabetes, who may be deconditioned and sedentary, the first major challenge is to help them incorporate physical activity into daily living.[8]

According to the Surgeon General's Report *Physical Activity and Health*,[32] significant health benefits, such as reduction in coronary risk factors, can be obtained by incorporating frequent bouts of moderate-intensity activities on most, if not all days of the week. While lifestyle physical activity does not take the place of a traditional structured exercise program, it can be highly effective in helping individuals increase their daily activity level. In addition, those who have successfully implemented more physical activity into their daily lifestyle may feel more confident and ready to initiate more structured forms of activity.

Activity Pyramid. The Activity Pyramid is a useful tool to help individuals be more active (see Figure 30.1). It shows a variety of ways that physical activity, both structured and unstructured, can be included in daily life. Diabetes educators can use the Activity Pyramid to help individuals identify, plan, and progressively increase regular physical activity.

- Suggest individuals begin by focusing on daily activities from the base of the pyramid
- Once the individual has established a solid base, encourage the person to consider activities from other areas of the pyramid
- Specific fitness areas can be enhanced by doing activities from a specific level of the pyramid:
  - —Activities from the base enhance overall health
  - —Activities from the second level focus on improving aerobic fitness
  - —Activities from the third level focus on improving muscle strength and flexibility
  - —The tip of the pyramid suggests ways to decrease sedentary activities
- Encourage individuals to move more and sit less by eventually incorporating activities from all areas of the pyramid

Pedometers. Pedometers (small monitors that record the number of steps taken) can be useful tools for increasing lifestyle physical activity. Pedometers may be helpful to individuals in self-monitoring physical activity by providing immediate feedback, building confidence, and enhancing enjoyment.[40] However, pedometers only detect walking-based activities and cannot detect changes in type, intensity, or pattern of activity.[10] Assist individuals to effectively use a pedometer:

- Wear the pedometer correctly (usually attaches to waistband of pants and is centered above knee cap)
- Log steps each day
- Establish a baseline by tracking steps for a few days without intentionally increasing physical activity level
- Set appropriate step goals by progressively increasing steps from baseline

What determines if people are active?

According to the Surgeon General's Report *Physical Activity and Health*,[32] the following are central determining factors influencing activity across the life span:

- Self-efficacy—having confidence in one's ability to be active
- Enjoyment of physical activity
- Support from others to continue exercising
- Positive beliefs concerning the benefits of physical activity
- Lack of perceived barriers to being physically active

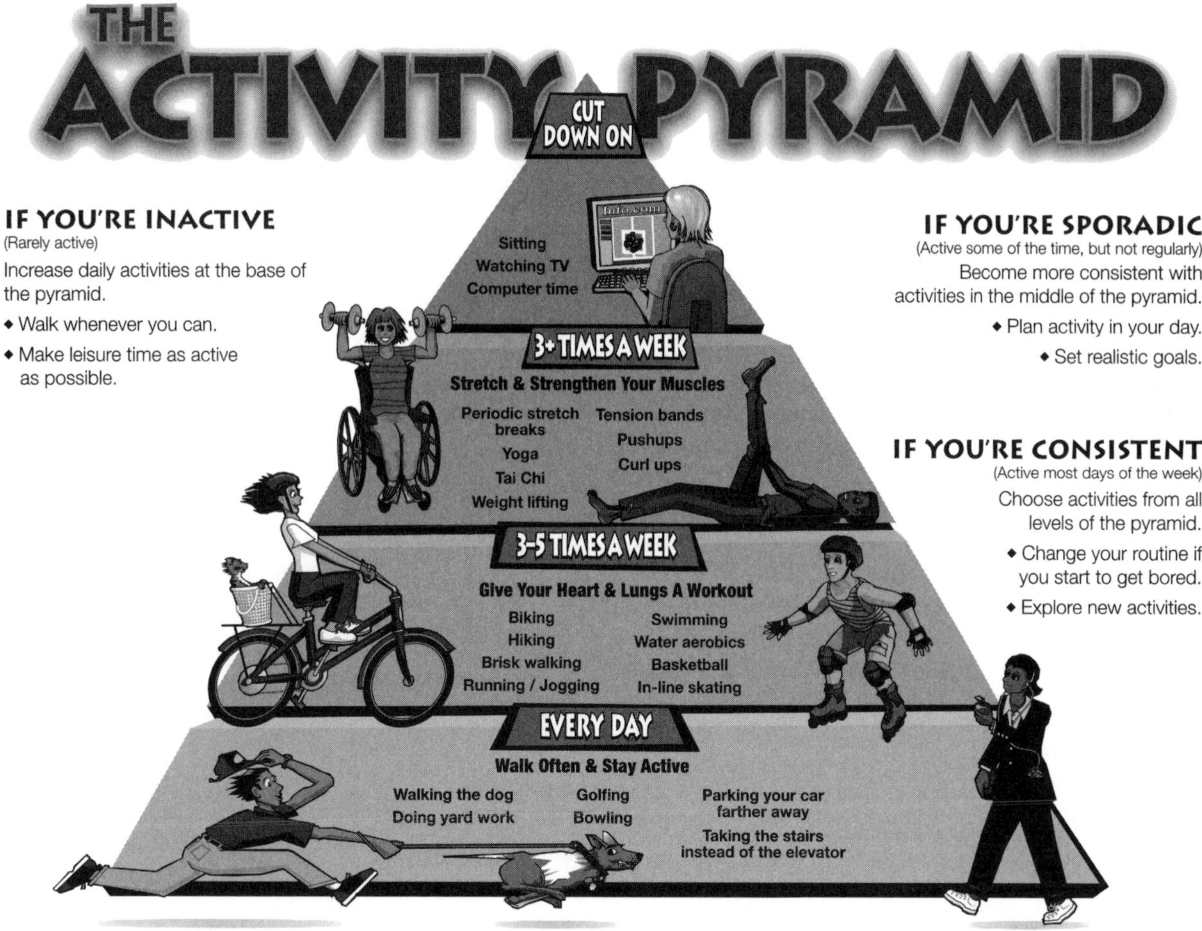

FIGURE 30.1 The Activity Pyramid

Source: From Type 2 Diabetes BASICS © 2004 International Diabetes Center. Adapted with permission from The Activity Pyramid © 2003 Park Nicollet HealthSource, Minneapolis, Minn.

Enhancing Self-Efficacy

Beliefs about self-efficacy influence health behaviors. Individuals tend to pursue tasks they feel competent to perform and avoid those in which they feel incompetent to perform.[10] Diabetes educators can help individuals enhance self-efficacy in the following ways:

- Help the individual develop realistic activity goals[41]
- Plan a gradual program with the individual, using small, incremental steps[9,41,42]
- Encourage setting goals that the individual is likely to attain, to promote feelings of mastery[10]
- Provide suggestions or opportunities to observe others succeeding at being physically active, such as watching a video or exercise class[10]
- Rehearse or practice the intended exercise behavior with the individual[41]
- Provide regular, supportive feedback

Goal Setting

When planning to increase physical activity levels, an important skill for individuals is to develop realistic and practical goals. Goals that are too vague, too ambitious, or too distant do not provide enough self-motivation to maintain long-term interest. Encourage individuals to write down and track their goals to help see their progress and identify barriers. The acronym SMART may be used to help individuals set appropriate physical activity goals. SMART stands for Specific, Measurable, Attainable, Realistic, and Time-frame specific, as explained below:[10]

- *Specific:* Encourage the individual to be specific and identify details of frequency, duration, intensity, and type of activity
- *Measurable:* Teach the person how to make goals measurable so he or she can accurately track and identify progress

- *Attainable:* Help the individual set goals that are challenging but attainable, to increase confidence and the likelihood of setting even more challenging goals in the future
- *Realistic:* Help the individual evaluate how realistic chosen goals are in a given situation
- *Timeframe-Specific:* Encourage the individual to set short-term goals that provide more immediate feedback, such as setting goals for just the next week

Using Motivational Interviewing

Motivational interviewing is an individual-centered directive method of communication for enhancing intrinsic motivation to change by exploring and resolving ambivalence.[43,44] This technique can be used with individuals to help increase motivational readiness to make positive behavior changes in physical activity.[10] (See also chapter 3.) Key strategies that diabetes educators can use with individuals experiencing ambivalence with physical activity participation include the following:[10,43,44]

- Emphasize the individual's autonomy and freedom to choose not to be physically active
- Encourage the individual's acceptance of responsibility for change and consequences of not changing activity habits
- Use strategic feedback, reflections, and questions to help the individual develop internal discrepancies for remaining inactive
- Use decisional balance scales to help the individual weigh the pros and cons of being more active to remaining inactive or less active
- Obtain permission from the individual before providing information or offering advice (the individual may give permission by asking for advice, and the educator can both ask permission to give advice and preface advice with permission to disagree or disregard)

A key tool of motivational interviewing is the use of rulers to explore importance and raise confidence regarding the individual's exercise behaviors.[10,43,44] Start by asking the individual to rate, on a 10-point scale, how important it is and how confident they are about a particular activity behavior, such as walking 3 times a week for 15 minutes. After the individual chooses a number, ask why that specific number was chosen, versus a lower number. See the sidebar for an example of how this technique is implemented.

Using Behavior Change Rules

Importance Rulers

1. On a scale of 0 to 10, how *important* is it for you to begin walking 3 times a week for 15 minutes?
   The answer given helps determine the individual's readiness to change physical activity patterns
2. And why are you a 6 and not a 2?
   The individual's answer elicits conversation regarding behavior change

Confidence Rulers

1. On a scale of 0 to 10, how *confident* are you that you could walk 3 times a week for 15 minutes?
   The answer given helps determine the individual's confidence regarding increasing physical activity
2. And why are you a 7 and not a 4?
   The answer given elicits conversation regarding the individual's ability to be more active

Readers are also referred to chapter 14, on physical activity. Whereas this chapter focuses on strategies for promoting self-care behaviors relevant to being active, chapter 14 provides a good deal of fundamental information about physical activity and exercise prescriptions for those with diabetes and prediabetes. Readers learn about current fitness terminology, the physiological responses to physical activity related to blood glucose levels, and the effects of the various modes of physical activity on diabetes management and chronic complications, including prevention. Medical considerations regarding chronic complications are reviewed. Hypoglycemia and hyperglycemia are discussed in detail as they relate to physical activity. Readers also find more information on the exercise prescription and considerations for children and older adults.

Summary

This chapter reviewed current physical activity and exercise guidelines for individuals with diabetes and discussed a variety of strategies to assist individuals, both those with and at risk for diabetes, in becoming more active. The basic elements of the exercise prescription serve as a guide to creating safe and effective physical activity programs. However, the true art of program planning lies in the effective use of behavior change strategies to tailor programs to each individual's health status, personal preferences, abilities, goals, and stage of readiness.

Case Wrap-Up

A thorough interview with MT to discuss her personal beliefs, past experiences, preferences, and concerns about being more active helped the diabetes educator gain a better understanding of MT's view of physical activity.

Education Goals

Education focused on the importance of monitoring blood glucose before and after exercise and carrying a form of carbohydrate during activity.

Exercise Program Goals

- *Activity:* The initial focus was on lifestyle physical activity using low- to moderate-intensity forms of physical activity
- *Frequency and Duration:* The educator encouraged use of short activity bouts, perhaps 10-minute sessions, that could be incorporated into MT's daily routine
- *Progression:* Long-term exercise goals focused on progressively increasing amounts and frequency of activity to minimum recommended levels (30 minutes most days of the week)

Tools and Strategies

- *Activity Pyramid:* The Activity Pyramid helped MT identify activities from the base of the pyramid that she might be interested in trying
- *Pedometer:* A pedometer was suggested as a way for MT to obtain feedback about her activity levels
- *Stages of Change:* Behavior change strategies appropriate for the contemplation and preparation stages were used, including offering information on the benefits of physical activity, discussing the pros and cons of increasing physical activity, helping to identify and build a support system, and identifying barriers to physical activity and brainstorming possible solutions
- *Self-Efficacy Through SMART Goals:* Self-efficacy was built by helping MT set "SMART" goals she was likely to be successful with, such as making a list of 5 ways to be more active throughout the day and trying 1 of them for the next week
- *Motivational Interviewing:* MT was encouraged to ask questions and come up with ideas and suggestions for becoming more active to promote autonomy and build confidence

Focus on Education: Pearls for Practice

Teaching Strategies

Use theory to guide interventions. Be familiar with theories to tailor and individualize interventions (for example, stage-matched strategies, goal setting, and motivational interviewing techniques).

Set goals using the SMART approach. Goals are set to achieve positive outcomes. Using the SMART approach (goals that are Specific, Measurable, Attainable, Realistic, and Time-specific), encourage positive outcomes and help establish lifelong habits. Encourage a plan for activity that is enjoyable, safe, and effective. Role model your own activity plan, and wear and encourage use of a pedometer. Plan a group program such as a walking club or exercise class; track activity and outcomes.

Identify protocols and professional exercise resources. Contact exercise physiologists or clinical specialists for advice, consultation, and/or participation in your program. Shadow them during a work session for an exercise prescription and testing. With permission, videotape your session with the exercise physiologist and have this professional review and offer recommendations.

Preexercise evaluation. Individuals at risk for or for whom vascular or cardiac complications have been documented need a preexercise evaluation. Once the evaluation is completed, a tailored program can be developed. Aerobic activities provide the greatest benefit and are recommended over other forms of exercise, but individuals must be evaluated for enrollment.

Patient Education

A routine is best. Establish a routine for physical activity. Physical activity is a vital part of improved or continued diabetes control, and it has a positive effect on blood pressure and blood cholesterol. It also aids in helping prevent type 2 diabetes. Choose an activity you enjoy! Involve family or friends in a swim class, biking or hiking trip, or neighborhood street dance.

Health issues. Contact your healthcare provider for approval of an exercise plan if you have high blood pressure or any other complications (such as neuropathy or arthritis).

Safety first. Wear identification. Test blood sugars before and after activity. Wear clothing that fits well to prevent injury. Wear layers so that if you get warm you can adjust what you are wearing. Stop the activity if you are light-headed or short of breath. If you are on medications for diabetes, be prepared: carry a carbohydrate product.

Internet Resources

The following Web sites are recommended as resources regarding physical activity in children.

10 Tips to Eating Healthy and Physical Activity for You, from the President's Council on Physical Fitness and Sports
www.fitness.gov/funfit/10tips.htm

99 Tips to Family Fitness and Fun
www.shapeup.org/publications/99.tips.for.family.fitness.fun/

Action for Healthy Kids
www.actionforhealthykids.org

After School Physical Activity
www.afterschoolpa.com

America on the Move
www.americaonthemove.org

Family Health & Fitness Day USA
www.fitnessday.com/family/

VERB: It's What You Do
www.verbnow.com

American Heart Association's online curriculum HeartPower! For teaching about the heart and how to keep it healthy
www.americanheart.org/heartpower

Outdoor Games
www.indianchild.com/outdoorgames.htm

Making Physical Activity Part of Your Life
www.cdc.gov/nccdphp/dnpa/physical/life/index.htm

Kids Walk to School
www.walktoschool.org

The National Association for Sport and Physical Education
www.aahperd.org/naspe/template.cfm

Suggested Readings

Albright A, Franz M, Hornsby G, et al, for American College of Sports Medicine. Exercise and type 2 diabetes: position stand. Med Sci Sports Exerc. 2000; 32:1345-60.

American College of Sports Medicine. ACSM's Exercise Management for Persons with Chronic Diseases and Disabilities, 2nd ed. Champaign, Ill: Human Kinetics; 2003.

American Diabetes Association. Physical activity/exercise and diabetes mellitus. Diabetes Care. 2003; 26 suppl 1: S73-77.

Barnes DE. American College of Sports Medicine. Action Plan for Diabetes: Your Guide to Controlling Blood Sugar. Champaign, Ill: Human Kinetics; 2004.

Kaminsky LA, Bonzheim KA, Garber CE, et al, eds. American College of Sports Medicine. Resource Manual for Exercise Testing and Prescription, 5th ed. Baltimore, Md: Williams & Wilkins; 2006.

Marcus BH, Selby VC, Niaura RS, Rossi JS. Self-efficacy and the stages of exercise behavior change. Res Q Exerc Sport. 1992;63:60-6.

Marcus BH, Simkin LR. The transtheoretical model: applications to exercise behavior. Med Sci Sports Exerc. 1994;26:1400-4.

Miller WR, Rollnick S. Motivational Interviewing: Preparing People for Change, 2nd ed. New York: Guilford Press; 2002.

Rollnick S, Mason P, Butler C. Health Behavior Change: A Guide for Practitioners. London, England/New York: Churchill Livingstone; 1999.

Sigal RJ, Kenny GP, Wasserman DH, Castaneda-Sceppa C. Physical activity/exercise and type 2 diabetes. Diabetes Care. 2004;27(10):2518-39.

Whaley MH, Brubaker PH, Otto RM, eds. American College of Sports Medicine. Guidelines for Exercise Testing and Prescription, 7th ed. Baltimore, Md: Williams & Wilkins; 2006.

References

1. Kirk AF, Mutrie N, Macintyre PD, Fisher MB. Promoting and maintaining physical activity in people with type 2 diabetes. Am J Prev Med. 2004;27(4):289-96.
2. Krug, LM, Haire-Joshu D, Heady SA. Exercise habits and exercise relapse in persons with non-insulin-dependent diabetes mellitus. Diabetes Educ. 1991;17:185-8.
3. Kriska A. Can a physically active lifestyle prevent type 2 diabetes? Exerc Sports Sci Rev. 2003; 31(3):132-7.
4. Diabetes Prevention Program (DPP) Research Group. Reduction in the incidence of type 2 diabetes with lifestyle intervention or metformin. N Engl J Med. 2002;346(6):393-403.
5. Diabetes Prevention Program (DPP) Research Group. The Diabetes Prevention Program (DPP): description of lifestyle intervention. Diabetes Care. 2002;25(12):2165-71.
6. Diabetes Prevention Program (DPP) Research Group. Achieving weight and physical activity goals among diabetes prevention program lifestyle participants. Obes Res. 2004;12(9):1426-34.
7. Ryan DH, Diabetes Prevention Program (DPP) Research Group. Diet and exercise in the prevention of diabetes. Int J Clin Pract Suppl. 2003;134:28-35.
8. Castaneda C. Diabetes control with physical activity and exercise. Nutr Clin Care. 2003;6(2):89-96.
9. Koenigsberg MR, Bartlett D, Cramer JS. Facilitating treatment adherence with lifestyle changes in diabetes. Am Fam Physician. 2004;69(2):309-16.
10. Kaminsky LA, Bonzheim KA, Garber CE, et al, eds. American College of Sports Medicine. Resource Manual for Exercise Testing and Prescription, 5th ed. Baltimore, Md: Williams & Wilkins; 2006.
11. Sigal RJ, Kenny GP, Wasserman DH, Castaneda-Sceppa C. Physical activity/exercise and type 2 diabetes. Diabetes Care. 2004;27(10):2518-39.
12. American Diabetes Association. Physical activity/exercise and diabetes mellitus. Diabetes Care. 2003; 26 suppl 1:S73-7.
13. Whaley MH, Brubaker PH, Otto RM, eds. American College of Sports Medicine. Guidelines for Exercise Testing and Prescription, 7th ed. Baltimore, Md: Williams & Wilkins; 2006.
14. Albright A, Franz M, Hornsby G, et al, for American College of Sports Medicine. Exercise and type 2 diabetes (position stand). Med Sci Sports Exerc. 2000; 32:1345-60.
15. Stewart KJ. Role of exercise training on cardiovascular disease in persons who have type 2diabetes and hypertension. Cardiol Clin. 2004;22(4):569-86.
16. Schneider SH, Amorosa LF, Khachadurian AK, Ruderman NB. Studies on the mechanism of improved glycemic control during regular exercise in type II diabetes. Diabetologia. 1984;26:355-60.
17. Castaneda C, Layne JE, Munoz-Orians L, et al. A randomized controlled trial of resistance exercise training to improve glycemic control in older adults with type 2 diabetes. Diabetes Care. 2002;25:2335-41.
18. Schneider SH, Khachadurian AK, Amorosa LF, Clemow L, Ruderman NB. Ten-year experience with an exercise-based outpatient lifestyle modification program in the treatment of diabetes mellitus. Diabetes Care. 1992;15(11):1800-10.
19. National Institutes of Health. NIH Consensus Statement: Physical Activity and Cardiovascular Health. Bethesda, Md: US Department of Health and Human Services, Public Health Service; 1995:13(3).
20. Durak EP, Jovanovic-Peterson L, Peterson CM. Randomized crossover study of effect of resistance training on glycemic control, muscular strength and cholesterol in type I diabetic men. Diabetes Care. 1990;13:1039-43.

21. Goldberg AP. Aerobic and resistive exercise modify risk factors for coronary heart disease. Med Sci Sports Exer. 1989;21:669-74.

22. Kraemer WJ, Fleck SJ. Resistance training: exercise prescription. Physician Sport Med. 1988;16:69-81.

23. Soukup JT, Maynard TS, Kovaleski JE. Resistance training guidelines for individuals with diabetes mellitus. Diabetes Educ. 1994;20:129-37.

24. Franklin B, Bonzheim K, Gordon S, Timmis G. Resistance training in cardiac rehabilitation. J Cardiopulm Rehabil. 1991;11:99-107.

25. Tseng CL, Brimacombe M, Xie M, et al. Seasonal patterns in monthly hemoglobin A1c values. Am J Epidemiol. 2005;161(6):565-74.

26. Graham C, Lasko-McCarthey P. Exercise options for persons with diabetic complications. Diabetes Educ. 1990;16:212-20.

27. Hiatt WR, Regensteiner JG, Hargarten ME, Wolfel EE, Brass EP. Benefit of exercise conditioning for patients with peripheral arterial disease. Circulation. 1990;81:602-9.

28. Schwartz RS. Exercise training in treatment of diabetes mellitus in elderly patients. Diabetes Care. 1990;13 suppl 2:77-85.

29. Levin ME. The diabetic foot. In: Ruderman NB, Devlin JT, eds. The Health Professional's Guide to Diabetes and Exercise. Alexandria, Va: American Diabetes Association; 1995.

30. Aiello LM, Cavallerano J, Aiello LP, Bursell SE. Retinopathy. In: Ruderman NB, Devlin JT, eds. The Health Professional's Guide to Diabetes and Exercise. Alexandria, Va: American Diabetes Association; 1995.

31. Painter P. Exercise in end-stage renal disease. In: Terjung RL, ed. Exercise and Sport Sciences Reviews. New York, NY: Macmillan; 1988:305-40.

32. Centers for Disease Control and Prevention. Physical Activity and Health: A Report of the Surgeon General. Atlanta, Ga: US Department of Health and Human Services; 1996.

33. US Department of Health and Human Services and US Department of Agricuture. Dietary Guidelines for Americans, 2005, 6th ed. Washington, DC: US Government Printing Office; 2005.

34. Marcus BH, Simkin LR. The transtheoretical model: applications to exercise behavior. Med Sci Sports Exerc. 1994;26:1400-4.

35. Marcus BH, Selby VC, Niaura RS, Rossi JS. Self-efficacy and the stages of exercise behavior change. Res Q Exerc Sport. 1992:63:60-6.

36. Kim CJ, Hwang AR, Yoo JS. The impact of a stage-matched intervention to promote exercise behavior in participants with type 2 diabetes. Int J Nurs Stud. 2004;41(8):833-41.

37. Clark M, Hampson SE, Avery L, Simpson R. Effects of a tailored lifestyle self-management intervention in patients with type 2 diabetes. Br J Health Psychol. 2004;9pt 3:365-79.

38. Kirk AF, Higgins LA, Hughes AR, et al. A randomized, controlled trial to study the effect of exercise consultation on the promotion of physical activity in people with type 2 diabetes: a pilot study. Diabet Med. 2001;18(11):877-82.

39. Koch J. The role of exercise in the African-American woman with type 2 diabetes mellitus: application of the health belief model. J Am Acad Nurse Pract. 2002;14(3):126-9.

40. Sidman CL. Count your steps to health and fitness. ACSM Health Fit J. 2002;6:1:13-7.

41. Allen NA. Social cognitive theory in diabetes exercise research: an integrative literature review. Diabetes Educ. 2004;30(5):805-19.

42. Di Loreto C, Fanelli C, Lucidi P, et al. Validation of a counseling strategy to promote the adoption and the maintenance of physical activity by type 2 diabetic subjects. Diabetes Care. 2003;26(2):404-8.

43. Rollnick S, Mason P, Butler C. Health Behavior Change: A Guide for Practitioners. New York, NY: Churchill Livingstone; 1999.

44. Miller WR, Rollnick S. Motivational Interviewing: Preparing People for Change, 2nd ed. New York, NY: Guilford Press; 2002.

CHAPTER

31

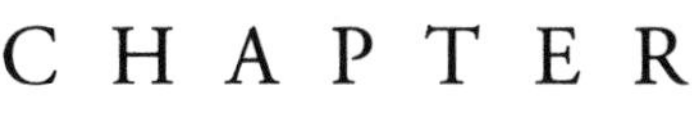

Taking Medications

Authors

Tommy Johnson, PharmD, CDE
Devra K. Dang, PharmD, BCPS

Key Concepts

- Self-care behaviors related to taking medications are important to develop, evaluate, and enhance. The diabetes educator plays an important role in this.
- The diabetes educator needs the ability to recognize potential barriers that interfere with an individual's appropriate taking of medications. An important part of the educator's job is to assist the person with diabetes in identifying and addressing these barriers.
- In particular, the diabetes educator must be familiar with special medication-taking considerations for people with diabetes.
- The educator must also be familiar with medications (both prescription and nonprescription) that can adversely affect diabetes control.
- Greater awareness of the unique medication-taking needs of special populations helps ensure that the person with diabetes benefits from the prescribed medications.

Introduction

Envision yourself in this situation. You are a diabetes educator, and today you have 2 individuals scheduled for their initial assessment.

The first is a 56-year-old female who has been recently diagnosed with type 2 diabetes mellitus. When you meet her, she is eager to learn how to manage her diabetes as long as she does not have to use insulin. You determine that she has a fear that insulin causes blindness and kidney failure because this is what happened to her mother. You also find out that she has hypertension, which is currently controlled with medications. During your initial assessment, one thing the woman asks about is use of over-the-counter products in treating occasional coughs, constipation, and headaches. She wants to know if there are any products that she should not take.

Your second patient is an 11-year-old male who was diagnosed with type 1 diabetes mellitus a week ago after being admitted to the hospital. His parents are noticeably upset and worried that their son will not be able to continue to play sports. They are overwhelmed with having to calculate different doses of insulin for different days of the week based on their son's activity level and are confused about the decision of whether to use an insulin pump or vial and syringe.

These are realistic scenarios, typical of many people with diabetes whom educators see and seek to help. In this chapter, issues relating to medication use in persons living with diabetes are discussed. The chapter especially focuses on the diabetes educator's role and opportunities in reinforcing individuals' self-care behaviors related to taking their diabetes medications. The chapter begins by examining what enhances the individual's ability to follow the regimen and what enhances the actual administration of the medication. Risk factors and warning signs for the diabetes educator to recognize are summarized. This section describes the following:

- Promoting use of medication administration aids that enhance the individual's ability to follow the medication plan
- Choosing medication delivery methods and treatment regimens appropriate to the individual
- Addressing issues of cost (affordability)

Strategies to improve individuals' ability to follow their medication regimens and derive the intended benefit of the medications are also discussed.

Next, the chapter describes clinical considerations relevant to specific medications used in diabetes control, with an emphasis on patient education strategies (instructional tips). In regard to this, each of the following are discussed separately:

- Sulfonylureas, meglitinides, metformin, thiazolidinediones, alpha-glucosidase inhibitors, insulin, exenatide, and pramlintide

The discussion of insulin includes consideration of delivery method options and regimen choices. An outline of basic and advanced education topics is presented plus a summary of teaching topics regarding insulin use.

Strategies to overcome issues of visual impairment, manual dexterity, and fears related to taking medication are presented to promote better self-care behaviors.

Other drugs that the individual with diabetes may be taking are considered next. Drug interactions and use of the following nonprescription medications and products are addressed:

- Alcohol- and sugar-free products
- Cough and cold products
- Pain and fever products
- Products for gastrointestinal ailments
- Dietary supplements
- Topical and dermatologic products
- Products for oral hygiene and dental care
- Ophthalmologic products

Before closing, the chapter attends to the unique needs of special populations with regard to medication taking. Special considerations are discussed individually for each of the following:

- Children and adolescents
- The elderly and those in long-term care facilities
- Women of reproductive age

The Medication Plan

Enhancing Follow-Through

Following a prescribed medication program is integral to the success of most medical treatment plans, but in the management of a chronic disease such as diabetes, following the medication regimen is crucial self-care behavior.

Following the medication plan includes not only taking prescribed medications, but also taking them on time and at the correct frequency. Long-term adherence to oral glucose-lowering agents has been reported as ranging from 36% to 93%, and insulin adherence in persons with type 2 diabetes ranges from 62% to 80%.[1,2] Poor follow-through has been shown to correlate with worse glycemic and lipid control.[1,3]

A multidisciplinary approach is important to determine if medications are being taken properly. The entire team of nurses, pharmacists, dietitians, physician assistants, social workers, and others can share information to increase the likelihood for positive clinical outcomes.

The pharmacist can identify if medications are being refilled at appropriate intervals. For example, if an individual is coming in to the pharmacy too early, the person may be taking more medication than prescribed due to elevations in blood glucose. The following are some reasons why a person may be late in picking up prescribed medications:

- May be experiencing adverse drug reactions
- May not have obtained expected beneficial clinical responses
- May just choose not to take medications
- May not have the financial resources to pay for the medication
- May have just forgotten

If the healthcare provider and diabetes education team are aware of this information, it will enable them to discuss it with the individual with diabetes at the next visit and identify potential barriers and solutions. Everyone involved in the care of the individual needs to share as much information about prescribed regimens as possible, and the individual's success in following the medication plan, if the desired outcomes are to be achieved.

Risk Factors and Warning Signs

Awareness of the risk factors for and warning signs of poor follow-through is the first step in resolving this issue. Risk factors include the following:[1,2,4,5]

- Age—the elderly and adolescents show poorer follow-through of the plan
- Medication dosing frequency and complexity of the regimen
- Presence of other concurrent medical conditions
- Presence of depression or other psychiatric disorders
- The individual's understanding of the treatment regimen and its potential side effects
- Socioeconomic status
- Health insurance status
- Cost of medications
- Poor family dynamics
- Poor patient-provider relationship

In addition to lapses in medication refills as described above, other warning signs of an individual's poor follow-through with the medication and treatment plans include the following:[4]

- Uncontrolled diabetes
- Erratic fluctuations in blood glucose
- Lack of follow-through with office visits and/or recommended clinical testing
- Lack of follow-through with self-monitoring of blood glucose or with reporting these results

Strategies to Improve Medication Plan Use

Relationship and Communication. Establishment of a trusting relationship between the healthcare professional and the person with diabetes is an important component in enhancing the individual's follow-through with medications and the treatment plan. The diabetes educator is in a unique position to explain to the person with diabetes the expected benefits and rationale of the medication and treatment plans. The diabetes educator should also acknowledge the potential for adverse drug reactions and discuss the expected likelihood that these may occur, ways that the individual can minimize or avoid these reactions, what the healthcare team is doing to monitor for these reactions, and how the individual can actively participate in this via self-monitoring. Cultural and religious beliefs and socioeconomic factors should also be taken into consideration when communicating about the treatment plans.

Regimen Changes and Adjustments. Medication-focused strategies to improve an individual's ability to follow the medication plan include the following:

- Decreasing the frequency of medication administration—by using once-daily medications whenever possible
- Decreasing pill burden—by using combination tablets

Combination tablets are available for glucose-lowering drugs (see Table 31.1) and many antihypertensive drugs, including various combinations of an angiotensin-converting enzyme (ACE) inhibitor or angiotensin II receptor blocker (ARB) plus the diuretic hydrochlorothiazide. Combinations of some calcium channel blockers and ACE inhibitors, such as amlodipine plus benazepril (Lotrel) or a calcium channel blocker and a HMG-CoA reductase inhibitor, such as amlodipine plus atorvastatin (Caduet), are also available.

Enhancing Medication Administration

Product Aids

A variety of medication administration aids are available from pharmacies, via online Web sites, and directly through manufacturers. Administration aids may help the individual follow the medication plan and include the following:

- Insulin injection aids
- Pill boxes
- Medication reminders, including alarms
- Medication calendars
- Blister packaging

TABLE 31.1 Cost of Oral Glucose-Lowering Agents

Name of Oral Agent		*Approximate Monthly Cost* of Generic (Branded) Product*
Generic Name	*Trade Name*	
Single-Ingredient Medications		
Glimepiride	Amaryl	$29.98 ($69.98)
Glyburide	Glynase	$23.99 ($94.52)
Glipizide	Glucotrol	$10.99 ($58.25)
Glipizide XL	Glucotrol XL	$39.98 ($59.98)
Metformin	Glucophage	$55.99 ($109.91)
Metformin XR	Glucophage XR	$79.98 ($95.98)
Pioglitazone	Actos	$179.99
Rosiglitazone	Avandia	$181.91
Acarbose	Precose	$87.45
Miglitol	Glyset	$81.20
Repaglinide	Prandin	$296.26
Nateglinide	Starlix	$99.97
Combination Medications		
Glyburide-Metformin	Glucovance	$95.99 ($119.98)
Glipizide-Metformin	Metaglip	$205.73
Rosiglitazone-Metformin	Avandamet	$227.39
Rosiglitazone-Glimepiride	Avandaryl	$229.97
Pioglitazone-Metformin	ACTO*plus* met	$219.96

*Prices (from www.drugstore.com, accessed 5 April 2006) are based on maximum daily doses for a 30-day supply.

One study found that 80% of adults with diabetes use at least one form of adherence aid, including use of a pill box in 50% of patients.[6] The diabetes educator should be aware of the different types of administration aids available in order to help persons with diabetes select the most appropriate product.

Delivery Methods Appropriate to Individual

As with other aspects of diabetes management, matching the insulin delivery device to the unique needs of the individual with diabetes is important. Any mismatch will increase the likelihood that the device or equipment will not be used as prescribed and the individual will be placed at increased risk for hypoglycemia or hyperglycemia. Chapter 15 describes insulin delivery devices: syringes, insulin pumps, jet injectors, pen devices, an inhalation device, and potential new modalities, including implantable pumps.

Addressing Issues of Medication Cost

Table 31.1 shows the average monthly cost of the oral agents currently available. No matter how effective a medication's glucose-lowering effect may be, those who can not afford to have the prescription filled cannot benefit from it. In 1 study in adults with diabetes, 19% of those surveyed reported decreasing medication use due to cost and 28% reported going without food or other essentials in order to afford medications.[7]

Resources

For individuals who are uninsured, this barrier of cost can be overcome by using manufacturer-sponsored medication assistance programs. Good sources of available programs are the Partnership for Prescription Assistance, a national program sponsored by pharmaceutical research companies via the Web site www.pparx.org, and the nonprofit NeedyMeds, whose Web site is www.needymeds.com. Other resources include health departments, which carry a limited formulary of medications for lower income individuals, and free clinics, where medical care and medications are provided free or at a minimal cost. For those who have health insurance, checking with the insurer to see what medications are on its formulary should be done.

Strategies to Reduce Cost

Occasionally, the use of more expensive medications is necessary to obtain clinical benefit and less expensive medications may be less desirable. However, this rarely occurs today with the choices of medications that are available. Tablet-splitting may be another option to save on medication cost since some medications are priced equally regardless of strengths. Consultation with a pharmacist should be performed prior to recommending this strategy as some medications should not be cut in half due to their physical, chemical, and/or therapeutic properties.

Clinical Considerations and Patient Education Strategies

Sulfonylureas and Meglitinides

Because most first-generation sulfonylureas have lower potency and higher risk for hypoglycemia, only second-generation sulfonylureas should be used. The second-generation sulfonylureas are glipizide (Glucotrol, Glucotrol XL), glyburide (Diabeta, Micronase, Glynase), and glimepiride (Amaryl). All of the second-generation sulfonylureas are dosed once or twice daily. The XL version of glipizide should not be cut in half because doing so may cause the medication to be released faster than intended and increase the risk of hypoglycemia. Meglitinides, repaglinide (Prandin) and nateglinide (Starlix), are given with meals to specifically lower postmeal glucose elevations. Persons taking these medications should be told to skip the dose if the meal is not eaten or delay the dose if the meal is delayed. Discussion of the risks of hypoglycemia and weight gain should be provided to persons taking either drug class. Sulfonylureas achieve their maximum glucose-lowering effect at half the maximum daily dose.[8] See also the more detailed discussion of each of these drug classes in chapter 15, on pharmacologic therapies for glucose management.

Metformin

Metformin (Glucophage) should be started at the lowest dose and titrated slowly, by 500 mg per week, to decrease the risk of gastrointestinal side effects such as cramping, bloating, and diarrhea. Taking metformin with meals also minimizes the risk of these side effects. Those taking this medication should be advised to report the use of metformin to all of their healthcare providers as its use is contraindicated during surgery, acute illness, and administration of intravenous contrast media. See also the more detailed discussion of biguanides (metformin) in chapter 15, on pharmacologic therapies for glucose management.

Thiazolidinediones

Persons taking a thiazolidinedione (TZD) should understand that the maximum glucose-lowering effect of these medications may not be apparent until after 8 to 12 weeks of use. Products available are pioglitazone (Actos) and rosiglitazone (Avandia). Those starting one of these medications need to be encouraged to keep taking it until a full effect can be determined. Persons taking TZDs should be educated about the risk of fluid retention and weight gain and how to self-monitor for these adverse events. See also the more detailed discussion of TZDs in chapter 15, on pharmacologic therapies for glucose management.

Alpha-Glucosidase Inhibitors

Alpha-glucosidase inhibitors work by delaying the absorption of carbohydrates from the intestinal tract, which reduces the rise of postprandial blood glucose. Products available are acarbose (Precose) and miglitol (Glyset). Normally, hypoglycemia is not a risk with monotherapy of these medications. However, in case hypoglycemia occurs due to taking acarbose or miglitol with other glucose-lowering drugs, the person needs to understand that only glucose tablets can be used for treatment, due to the mechanism of action of these drugs. See also the more detailed discussion of alpha-glucosidase inhibitors in chapter 15, on pharmacologic therapies for glucose management.

Insulin

Insulin is essential for treatment of type 1 diabetes and also is used in persons with type 2 diabetes with glucose toxicity or ineffective beta-cell functioning. Insulin is available in formulations that differ in their onset, peak and length of action, and source.

Delivery Method Options

The choice of administering insulin with a pump, pen device, syringe, needle-free jet injector, or inhaler (for mealtime doses only, adults only) may be determined by the individual's personal choice, physical limitations, and/or financial resources.

Regimen Choices

The choice of which insulin regimen to use should also be individualized based on the person's daily schedule, willingness to check blood glucose levels, and the number of daily insulin injections the individual is willing to receive or administer.

The most physiologic insulin regimen is the so-called "basal-bolus" regimen that uses a long-acting insulin as the basal dose and a rapid-acting insulin as the bolus dose given at meals. Additional advantages of this regimen include a lower risk of hypoglycemia and the ability to adjust the dose of the rapid-acting insulin according to meal content and timing.

Premixed insulins may be chosen over a basal-bolus regimen due to financial constraints, the individual's inability to calculate mixed doses and/or changing doses of insulin, or the person's preference for no more than twice-daily insulin injections.

The timing of meals and activity and adjustments in insulin are important to discuss. To minimize potential adverse events, the individual's understanding of and ability to perform these skills should be assessed before the medication is prescribed.

Education Topics

Minimal skills to be taught are these:

- Proper storage
- Preparation of dose
- Correct administration, including injection sites rotation and rolling the vials or inverting the pens for suspended insulin formulations prior to administration
- Safe disposal of syringes or needles
- Recognition of hypoglycemia symptoms and corrective actions to be taken

See the sections on hypoglycemia and insulin in chapter 15, on pharmacotherapy for glucose management.

The following are more advanced skills that are also important to teach; however, not all persons with diabetes will be able to learn and manage all of these skills:

- Mixing 2 insulins in the same syringe
- Pattern management
- Hypoglycemia prevention
- Insulin adjustments for physical activity, sick days, and differing amounts of carbohydrate intake

The diabetes educator must individualize the educational strategies and message to each person's educational and coping level. A number of chapters in this book address these topics individually (see index).

Overcoming Visual Impairment and Dexterity Issues

Individuals with dexterity problems or visual impairment may have difficulty in drawing up a dose of insulin. The use of different *injection aids* (eg, syringe magnifying guide) or easy-to-use devices such as an insulin pen device, needle-free jet injection device, or inhaled insulin for mealtime doses may be helpful for some. Individuals may be pleasantly surprised to learn that needle length and diameter are much smaller than they have anticipated. The *length of needles* for insulin injection varies from 3/16 in to 1/2 in. The *gauge of the needles* is also important for comfort. Most insulin syringes are available in the smaller 30 or 31 gauge, which may make the injection less painful. The *unit markings* on the side of the syringes also differ, depending on if the syringe holds 30 units (3/10 cc), 50 units (1/2 cc), or 100 units (1 cc). Individual markings may be in 1/2-unit, 1-unit, or 2-unit increments. If a person is injecting less than 30 units for a dose, using a syringe that closely matches the dose, in this case a 3/10 cc syringe, will allow the person to be able to see the units easier than using a 1-cc syringe. However, the risk for error in administration may be increased if the insulin dose is increased and the person is prescribed a different syringe size with a different unit increment, but not given education regarding this.

Overcoming Fears

Some people are resistant, or nonadherent, to insulin treatment due to fear of hypoglycemia and/or the development of diabetic complications. The fear of hypoglycemia because of past experiences with insulin may be engrained in a person's mind. The educator should make such persons aware of the availability of newer insulins that more closely mimic the body's natural release of insulin and which have been shown to decrease the incidence and severity of hypoglycemia. Detailed education regarding steps to avoid hypoglycemia, recognition of symptoms of hypoglycemia, and corrective actions to take should it occur should be provided. Some people also associate insulin initiation with the development of long-term complications of diabetes, such as nephropathy and dialysis. The diabetes educator should explain that the complication was mostly likely present before the insulin was initiated and most likely could have been avoided if insulin initiation had not been delayed.

Fear of injections is a significant barrier to treatment of diabetes, and educators need to be supportive of those who express this. Fear of injections extends to exenatide (Byetta) and pramlintide (Symlin) as well. Explanations of the benefits of the medication need to be carefully communicated. Use of these medications needs to be described as crucial for glycemic control and hence potential prevention of long-term complications of diabetes. Showing the person the different options for administration (which may, as appropriate, include short needles or an insulin pen device, needle-free jet injector, or insulin inhaler) may help alleviate some of the fears and allow the person to make some choices in how to improve individual outcomes. Some

Key Points on Insulin Use:

What to Review With Patients

- Determine what barriers to injection there may be. These may include fear of injection, cost, fear of complications, fear of hypoglycemia, social concerns, and weight gain.
- Discuss and show the person when and how the insulin is working to lower blood glucose levels and the proven clinical benefits of insulin therapy. Printed educational materials and information from the insulin manufacturer's Web site may be beneficial. Another commercially available product that is useful in teaching about insulin therapy is *Insulin Therapy Graphics* CD-ROM by Draheim Dimensional Presentations.
- Explain how to properly administer the insulin, including proper mixing and resuspension (if appropriate), appropriate injection sites, site rotation, and storage.
- Educate the person about the potential for hypoglycemia, recognition of hypoglycemic symptoms, and specific corrective actions that can be taken if this occurs. Discuss risk factors for hypoglycemia, including missed or irregular meals and hypoglycemia after exercise or physical activity. Discuss how to minimize the occurrence of hypoglycemic episodes. Educate the individual and family members and any caregivers about hypoglycemia unawareness and the use of glucagon emergency kits for treating severe hypoglycemia. Educate family members/caregivers about how to recognize signs and symptoms of hypoglycemia (see section in chapter 15).
- Properly matching the amount and timing of food to the type and dose of insulin should minimize hypoglycemic events. If the person is able to perform carbohydrate counting, carbohydrate-to-insulin ratios should be developed with persons using basal-bolus regimens. (See chapter 16, on pattern management, and chapter 17, on intensive insulin regimens.)
- Educate the person about what to do when eating out or traveling.
- Discuss the disposal of syringes and testing supplies. This varies by city, county, and state. One practice that is universal is to teach people to not recap syringes after use.
- Discuss reusing syringes and whether this is recommended. Some educators may think this is acceptable, except when contraindicated such as with insulin glargine and pramlintide acetate. Discuss that refrigerating the syringes if they want to reuse them and wiping the needle off with alcohol is not recommended.
- Discuss sick day management and the development of a sick day plan (see chapter 7).
- To avoid potential medication prescribing and dispensing errors, all persons taking these medications should know both the brand and generic names for their insulins; those taking insulin mixes should know the generic names of both insulin components.

people associate injections with drug abuse and do not want to be associated with this. Again, education about insulin administration and its crucial role in diabetes management can help to overcome this belief.

The fact that pramlintide (Symlin) may actually cause weight loss may be especially appealing for those with type 2 diabetes who are overweight and insulin resistant. Persons using exenatide (Byetta) or pramlintide (Symlin) should understand that these medications are not a substitute for insulin in those who require insulin for glycemic control, as they may mistakenly think they are trading one type of injectable medication for another.

See also the detailed section on insulin in chapter 15, on pharmacologic therapies for glucose management.

Exenatide and Pramlintide

When exenatide (Byetta) or pramlintide (Symlin) has been prescribed, the diabetes educator should explain the difference between the medication and insulin. Those who are prescribed these injectable therapies should be carefully taught regarding how to administer them, including differences in dosing units compared to insulin. Pramlintide (Symlin) is taken before meals and snacks that contain at least 250 calories or at least 30 g of carbohydrates and should be skipped if a meal is skipped or if the person is experiencing hypoglycemia. Persons taking pramlintide should also know that the mealtime insulin doses will need to be decreased by 50% initially. With both medications, education about the potential for hypoglycemia, recognition of hypoglycemic symptoms, and specific corrective actions that can be taken if this occurs should be provided. In addition, the potential for drug-induced nausea and vomiting should also be acknowledged. See also the discussions on these medications in chapter 15, on pharmacologic therapies for glucose management.

Drug Interactions

Persons living with diabetes often take a number of medications concurrently for comorbid conditions such as hypertension, hyperlipidemia, coronary artery disease, and heart failure. They may also be taking medications to treat long-term complications of diabetes such as peripheral neuropathy. Thus, the diabetes educator should be aware of the potential for drug interactions and increased adverse drug reactions. A complete discussion of the many potential drug interactions and medication-related problems that may occur is beyond the scope of this chapter. A brief discussion of medications that can adversely affect glycemic control is included in the paragraphs that follow. Chapter 15 also briefly discusses drug-drug, drug-disease, and drug-food interactions of concern when using medications for diabetes control. Consultation with a pharmacist and/or inclusion of a pharmacist into the healthcare team helps reduce the potential for medication misadventures.

Many medications have the potential to induce hyperglycemia and worsen glycemic control. Commonly used medications in this category include glucocorticoids, protease inhibitors, atypical antipsychotics, and niacin. Worsening of preexisting diabetes, new-onset diabetes, impaired fasting glucose, and impaired glucose tolerance have all been reported with these medications. Proposed mechanisms for hyperglycemia vary by drug class, but include decreased peripheral insulin sensitivity and insulin secretion and increased gluconeogenesis and insulin resistance. Atypical antipsychotics can also cause weight gain and dyslipidemia. Protease inhibitors can cause dyslipidemia and lipodystrophy. The risk of hyperglycemia may vary among drugs within a class. For example, clozapine (Clozaril) and olanzapine (Zyprexa) appear to have the highest association with hyperglycemia, although any of the atypical antipsychotics may adversely affect blood glucose levels. The risk of hyperglycemia is also dependent on other factors such as the dose used (as with glucocorticoids and niacin) and the route of administration (eg, lower risk with inhaled and topical, compared to oral, formulations of glucocorticoids).[9]

Recently, use of the oral fluoroquinolone antibiotic gatifloxacin (Tequin) has been associated with both hyperglycemia and hypoglycemia, including severe symptomatic cases. The use of gatifloxacin is now contraindicated in persons with diabetes. Risk factors for gatifloxacin-induced hypoglycemia and hyperglycemia include older age, renal impairment, and concomitant use of drugs affecting glucose regulation. Hypoglycemia typically occurred within 3 days of starting therapy, while hyperglycemia typically occurred after the third day of treatment. These disturbances in glucose levels have occurred in persons without diabetes.[10] Careful monitoring is required. Although the incidence is highest with gatifloxacin, other fluoroquinolones also have the potential to affect glucose and insulin regulation.[9]

Use of Nonprescription Medications

Approximately 1000 active ingredients comprise the more than 100,000 nonprescription medications (also commonly referred to as over-the-counter, or OTC, products) available in the United States.[11] According to the Consumer Products Healthcare Association, some of the more frequent ailments that are treated with nonprescription products include cough, cold and flu, pain and fever, allergy and sinus complaints, dermatologic conditions, gastrointestinal distress, and musculoskeletal pain.[12] People with diabetes may want to treat a common ailment, but may take something that may adversely affect their blood glucose or blood pressure. The labeling of the product should always be checked prior to administration as nonprescription products are frequently reformulated and ingredients may change. Educators need to be knowledgeable about the ingredients in these products to assist in selecting appropriate self-care therapies. Due to the complexity involved (eg, multitude of drug ingredients and formulations, adverse drug reactions, contraindications to self-care, potential for drug-drug, drug-disease, and drug-food interactions), consultation with a pharmacist prior to commencing use is especially important.

Alcohol-Free and Sugar-Free Products

Is it necessary for a person with diabetes to purchase alcohol-free and sugar-free products? This depends on the person's glycemic control, medications, and medical conditions. If a product contains carbohydrates, the carbohydrate count needs to be added into the number of grams of carbohydrates the person consumes. The dosage of these products varies by product so, just as with foods, labels have to be read carefully to prevent hyperglycemia or hypoglycemia. The amount of carbohydrate in some products may be so small that the potential increase in blood glucose may be minimal. The illness itself also may increase blood glucose levels, so this needs to be considered. Examples of the carbohydrate content of products can be found at each product's Web site or by calling the consumer toll-free phone number listed on the package. The alcohol content of many nonprescription products can also be found this way. The *Red Book* (formerly the *Drug Topics Red Book*), a product of Thomson Scientific and Healthcare (www.thomson.com), contains a list of sugar- and alcohol-free products.

Cough and Cold Products

One common mistake people make is taking a multi-symptom remedy when only a single symptom needs to be treated, for example with an antihistamine or cough suppressant. Nonprescription products marketed to treat cough and cold symptoms may contain ingredients that adversely affect blood glucose and blood pressure. This effect varies by product and formulation. Selecting a product that treats only the symptom(s) present, and being cognizant of the carbohydrates and alcohol content (especially with liquid formulations), allows people with diabetes to better select products for their care.

In most cases, tablet and gel-cap formulations to treat cough and cold symptoms do not contain any or only contain a limited amount of carbohydrate and alcohol. Nasal sprays used to treat nasal congestion and allergies should have limited systemic effects if used according to directions on the label. Oral decongestants such as pseudoephedrine or phenylephrine should be used with caution mainly due to their effects on increasing blood pressure and heart rate. They should be given only to persons with well-controlled hypertension and at the lowest dose possible for the shortest duration. They should not be used by persons with coronary artery disease. The labeling for oral and nasal decongestant products includes a warning against use in persons with diabetes, unless with medical supervision, since these sympathomimetic agents may increase blood glucose.

Pain and Fever Products

Pain and fever are commonly treated with nonprescription medications. Examples include aspirin, acetaminophen, and nonsteroidal anti-inflammatory drugs (NSAIDs) such as ibuprofen and naproxen. The person with diabetes should be aware that, unless directed by a healthcare professional, NSAID use should be avoided in those with renal impairment, hypertension, or heart failure. Aspirin may increase the risk of hypoglycemia when taken with sulfonylureas due to displacement of the sulfonylurea from plasma protein-binding sites. Aspirin also appears to possess hypoglycemic actions (proposed mechanisms include increasing pancreatic insulin secretion and insulin sensitivity and decreasing gluconeogenesis). However, these effects are usually only clinically relevant at higher (anti-inflammatory) doses.[9]

Products for Gastrointestinal Ailments

The diabetes educator should inquire about use of nonprescription products for gastrointestinal ailments as this may be a sign that the person with diabetes is experiencing gastrointestinal autonomic neuropathy. Most nonprescription products for the treatment of gas, heartburn, constipation, and diarrhea do not contain noticeable amounts of carbohydrate or alcohol and do not have any mechanisms of action that would adversely affect blood glucose levels. Most antacids contain magnesium, aluminum, a combination of the two, or calcium carbonate.

Products containing aluminum should be avoided in persons with impaired renal function or those at risk for constipation. Calcium antacids (and supplements), as well as products containing iron, may also induce constipation. Nonprescription agents for treating constipation include bulk-forming laxatives (eg, psyllium), osmotic agents (eg, magnesium citrate or hydroxide, glycerin), stimulant laxatives (eg, bisacodyl, senna, cascara, aloe), and stool softeners (docusate). Differences in these products include the onset of action and potential adverse drug reactions. These products do not affect blood glucose, but the stimulant laxatives and osmotic agents may lead to electrolyte imbalances. Senna, cascara, aloe, and mineral oil should not be recommended due to the potential for many adverse drug reactions.

The nonprescription agents approved by the US Food and Drug Administration (FDA) for the treatment of diarrhea include loperamide (eg, Imodium, Maalox

Anti-Diarrheal), bismuth subsalicylate (eg, Pepto-Bismol, KaoPectate Anti-Diarrheal), and kaolin. These do not adversely affect blood glucose levels. Products containing bismuth subsalicylate may interact with other medications that people with diabetes take such as aspirin and other antiplatelet drugs, NSAIDs, and anticoagulants, but generally do not adversely affect blood glucose levels in recommended nonprescription doses.

Dietary Supplements

When asked about dietary supplements and their effectiveness in lowering blood glucose or blood pressure, how should the diabetes educator respond? As noted by Cypress in the overview to Section 2 of this book, "Whether health professionals use or recommend these therapies is not as relevant in diabetes education as being aware of the alternative remedies people may be using and how those therapies interact with recommended or prescribed treatments."

Dietary supplements may include herbs, vitamins, minerals, and nutritional supplements. Unlike prescription products, dietary supplements are not regulated by the FDA and product quality may vary among manufacturers or even among lots of the same product. Some manufacturers of these products have voluntarily submitted to testing and verification by the US Pharmacopeia (USP), the organization responsible for setting standards and quality control for all FDA-approved prescription and nonprescription medications. If the diabetes educator recommends a dietary supplement, product recommendations should come from the list of USP-verified dietary supplements, available at www.usp.org/USPVerified/dietarySupplements/supplements.html. Evidence-based information about dietary supplements can be found via the Natural Medicine Comprehensive Database (www.naturaldatabase.com) and the National Center for Complementary and Alternative Medicine (http://nccam.nih.gov).

Cinnamon (*Cinnamomum cassia*), bitter melon (*Momordica charantia*), ginseng (both *Panax ginseng* CA *Meyer,* which is the Asian or Korean ginseng, and *Panax quinquefolius,* which is the American ginseng), ivy gourd (*Coccinia indica*), and chromium picolinate are a few examples of supplements that have been claimed to lower blood glucose levels. The agents with the most promising evidence-based data for efficacy are ivy gourd, ginseng, and cinnamon.[9,13] Persons with diabetes who wish to use an herbal product to help with glycemic control should be educated that the scientific evidence for effectiveness of these agents is equivocal and that these products cannot substitute for FDA-approved glucose-lowering medications. If a person still wishes to use these products, a careful check for potential drug interactions and adverse drug reactions should be completed. The diabetes educator should advise the person to use only USP-verified products, as noted above. Chapter 19 on biological complementary therapies provides more information to assist educators and those with diabetes in evaluating all complementary products. Specific products described above are also discussed in detail in that chapter.

Niacin, an ingredient in many nonprescription cholesterol-lowering products, may increase blood glucose levels when taken at therapeutic doses of 1 to 4.5 g per day (dose varies depending on the formulation used). Nonprescription niacin products include immediate-release (eg, crystalline niacin), long-acting (also known as sustained-release, controlled-release, or timed-release), and "no-flush" formulations. No-flush niacin products actually contain inositol hexanicotinate or a combination with inositol hexanicotinate and niacin. The diabetes educator should advise all persons with diabetes to avoid self-treatment with nonprescription niacin products as medical supervision and monitoring are required due to the potential for adverse drug reactions (eg, hyperglycemia, hepatotoxicity, and others). Nonprescription niacin products advertised as "no-flush" should be avoided as their efficacy is questionable.[14] Also see the section on niacin in chapter 21, on macrovascular disease.

Topical and Dermatologic Products

Persons with uncontrolled diabetes are at risk for fungal infections, dry skin, and possible skin ulcerations. Trauma to the skin from wearing ill-fitting shoes can lead to blisters. Education regarding proper foot care, discussed in chapters 20 and 35 (on chronic complications and reducing risks), should always be provided.

Tinea pedis or "athlete's foot" is common in many persons with diabetes. Nonprescription antifungal products may take 2 to 4 weeks of continuous treatment to resolve the problem. Many people do not use these products long enough, which leads to recurrent problems. If there is not significant improvement, systemic prescription medications may be needed.

Yeast infections may also occur in the folds of skin and vaginally. Antifungal products for treating vaginal yeast infection are available as creams, ointments, and suppositories and vary by the number of days required for treatment (1 to 7 days). Self-treatment for vaginal yeast infections can be recommended only if the person has symptoms consistent with those of an episode previously diagnosed by a healthcare professional and when less than 4 infections occur per year.[15]

Autonomic neuropathy and polyuria caused by hyperglycemia may lead to dry skin. Various moisturizers containing glycerin, mineral oil, and lanolin are available to prevent and treat dry skin. Those containing alcohol should be avoided, as the alcohol promotes drying of the skin.

Nonprescription products marketed for the removal of corns and calluses should not be used because excessive damage to the skin may occur due to the high salicylic acid content (12% to 40%).[16]

Products for Oral Hygiene and Dental Care

Gum disease and dental caries may occur more frequently in people with inadequately controlled blood glucose. Proper brushing and flossing and regular dental appointments will minimize this in most people. Many mouth rinses contain large amounts of alcohol, but can be used since they are not swallowed. Many people have problems with ill-fitting dentures if they have gingivitis. Candidiasis may occur in persons with poorly controlled blood glucose and may be prevented with adequate blood glucose control and removal of dentures at bedtime. Dentures should be cleaned once daily and rinsed thoroughly to prevent contact irritation. See also the discussion on oral care in chapter 20, on chronic complications.

Ophthalmologic Products

The use of moisturizing nonprescription eye drops containing lubricants only is usually safe. As with all nonprescription medications, labels should be read carefully as some products may contain more than one drug. Ophthalmic decongestants such as phenylephrine, naphazoline, oxymetazoline, or tetrahydrozoline are vasoconstrictors and are contraindicated in persons with angle-closure glaucoma. Medical supervision is advised when using these products, as incorrect administration or overuse may lead to appreciable systemic absorption and subsequent increases in blood pressure, heart rate, or blood glucose. Some ophthalmic decongestants are coformulated with ophthalmic antihistamines (eg, pheniramine) for the treatment of allergic conjunctivitis. Ophthalmic antihistamines are also contraindicated in angle-closure glaucoma.[17]

Considerations in Special Populations

Children and Adolescents

Medication administration for children can be challenging. Certain issues are of particular concern at different ages—when children are young, of school age, or adolescent. The issue of medication administration away from home can affect young children in day care as well as school-age children and sometimes still be a factor in the teen years. Psychosocial issues related to medication taking must also be considered.

Appropriate Medication

For young children, the availability of rapid-acting insulin analogs has allowed parents of fussy eaters to be able to give insulin after the child decides to eat as well as to adjust the dose based on the amount of carbohydrates the child actually ate. Prior to the availability of these insulins, a dose of short-acting insulin was prepared based on the child's blood glucose and the amount of carbohydrate for the meal. Since this type of insulin had to be administered 30 minutes before the meal, the risk of hypoglycemia was present if the child decided not to eat or consume the entire meal.

Medication Administration by Others

Some medications, including some regimens of insulin, may require administration of insulin doses at school and in care settings away from home. Education of school, day care, and camp staff is key to successful management. Another issue is that different insulin schedules may be used on different days, depending on the level of physical activity typical for that day. Children who usually take a mixed dose of NPH and a rapid-acting analog insulin may, on occasion, be advised to use a premixed insulin, such as 75/25, to allow for simpler administration (not requiring mixing) away from home. Some children may use premixed insulin to allow for administration to occur only at home. This may not provide the child with optimal blood glucose control, but may be a way to ensure that the insulin is given and given correctly. In all children taking glucose-lowering medication(s), both the child and personnel at school, day care, and camps need to be able to recognize the signs and symptoms of hypoglycemia and the necessary corrective actions. Parents and personnel at school, daycare, and camps also need to be educated on when to use glucagon to treat hypoglycemia. Too often teachers try to administer this to conscious children, causing unnecessary fear and anxiety. Chapter 9, on type 1 diabetes, contains a great deal of information relevant to issues that children with diabetes face when they are at school, away from home at other care settings, and physically active, such as when participating in sports.

Adolescent Issues

The combination of having diabetes and managing it well during adolescence can be challenging for a child with diabetes, the family, and others involved in their care and well being. This period of growth, with its hormonal changes, poses a challenge to even those teens and parents who are firmly committed to managing diabetes well. Unfortunately, adolescents with chronic medical conditions, including diabetes, have been reported to exhibit poor follow-through of treatment plans.[1,18] Teenagers need to be educated about the dangers of omitting their insulin doses. Some teenagers may feel that their parents are too protective and may become rebellious and seek attention through hospitalization. A teenager trying to lose weight may purposely omit his or her insulin to improve self-image. Teenagers also need to be educated on the detrimental effects of alcohol or illicit drug use on their medical condition and medications. Severe hypoglycemia may occur if they binge drink and pass out from intoxication. Referral to a psychologist or family counselor may be necessary for some families. Healthcare providers should be aware that insulin requirements will increase during puberty. See chapter 9 for more information on issues in adolescence relevant to taking medication and chapter 4 for psychological and mental health issues, such as eating disorders and depression, that may also have a bearing on medication-taking behavior.

Overcoming Fears

Insulin syringes have been improved to provide for "painless injections." The advent of the short needle, which is 31 gauge and 5/16-in long instead of 1/2-in long, allows most children to inject their insulin at a 90-degree angle and is less intimidating. In spite of the availability of this shorter needle, some pediatric endocrinologists will continue to recommend syringes with the 1/2-long needle to ensure an adequate injection into the subcutaneous fat. Advances in insulin pens have also allowed for more discrete insulin delivery. For children using an insulin pump, a variety of insertion sets with variable lengths of needles and cannulas are available to match individual preference for comfort and to promote best insulin absorption. Children may also use insulin pumps. Parents, the child, caregivers, and school/daycare/camp personnel need to be educated on how to address problems that may occur with pump use.

Type 2 Diabetes

For many years, the assumption was that the only type of diabetes children could develop was type 1 and terminology such as juvenile-onset diabetes was used. What we now know is that children may develop both type 1 and type 2 diabetes. In children older than 10 years of age with type 2 diabetes who require an oral glucose-lowering agent, the medication used is immediate-release metformin (Glucophage). These children may not need to have medication administered at school, since this medication can be given twice daily. In teenagers with type 2 diabetes treated with metformin, the risk of lactic acidosis and binge drinking needs to be discussed. Insulin is required for some children with type 2 diabetes and issues with medication taking and administration discussed earlier should be taken into consideration.

Coping Skills

Social support and education about coping skills should be provided to the child and his or her family members. The diabetes educator should also recognize psychosocial risk factors for poor diabetes control. According to the American Diabetes Association, these include the presence of other medical conditions, poor school attendance, learning disabilities, and emotional and behavioral disorders in the child. Family-related risk factors include a single-parent home, chronic physical or mental health problems in close relatives, a recent major life change for the parent, lack of adequate health insurance, complex childcare arrangements, health/cultural/religious beliefs affecting follow-through with treatment plans, and having a parent with diabetes.[19]

Healthcare professionals should understand the effect of these factors on self-management of diabetes and help children with diabetes and their families overcome these barriers. Community resources such as support groups and summer camps are available in some communities, but finding one that is age-appropriate, meets the needs of the family, and is within an acceptable geographic location may be a barrier. Resources such as the local chapter of the American Diabetes Association, the Internet (such as the American Diabetes Association resources at www.diabetes.org and others), and magazines can provide information for families.

The Elderly and Residents of Long-Term Care Facilities

Older individuals with diabetes who are living at home are at increased risk for medication-related adverse events (as described below), due to multiple factors, including polypharmacy issues, psychosocial issues, and the *possibility* that they will not be able to care for themselves. Medication planners and schedulers (such as pill boxes) and administration aids (such as insulin pens and injection guides) can help people remember to take their medications and to administer them correctly and at the right time. However, medication administration may prove to be difficult due to decreased manual dexterity and/or decreased vision and mobility. In addition, if inadequately or improperly trained, family members and other caregivers may give medication at the wrong time or in the wrong dosage. Involving them in the education session or discussing by phone can be critical in preventing errors from occurring.

Community-dwelling older persons with diabetes are more likely to be admitted to a long-term care facility than their counterparts without diabetes. Although this may present a difficult situation for the person with diabetes to accept, it provides an opportunity for members of the healthcare team to collaborate and work closely with the resident, family, and long-term care staff, while providing education and guidance, so problems with medication taking can be avoided.

The elderly and people living in assisted-living facilities may also have impaired liver and kidney function. They may be taking multiple medications that increase the risk of drug-drug interactions. Defects in the metabolism and excretion of medications can lead to episodes of hypoglycemia and hyperglycemia. Sulfonylureas and meglitinides are metabolized in the liver and excreted in the urine. In people with hepatic or renal impairment, the risk of hypoglycemia increases, especially if the individual does not eat at regular times or at all. If a sulfonylurea is chosen, glimepiride (Amaryl) or glipizide (Glucotrol and Glucotrol XL) are the drugs of choice due to minimally active or inactive metabolites, respectively. Metformin is excreted by the kidneys, and renal function should be monitored before therapy is started and at least annually, especially in the elderly and those with known renal impairment. In persons with renal insufficiency using insulin, the insulin dose will usually need to be adjusted downward as renal function worsens. TZDs can precipitate new-onset heart failure or worsen existing heart failure and may also precipitate or worsen diabetic macular edema (thus far reported with rosiglitazone only). Sudden weight gain, edema, and difficulty in breathing should be brought to the healthcare provider's attention. Body weight should be monitored in those receiving these agents. Liver function monitoring should be performed at baseline and then periodically to ensure safety. The recommendation for monitoring liver function has been relaxed due to the low incidence of this adverse effect in these agents. Finally, decreased thirst and hunger mechanisms in the elderly increase the risk for dehydration, malnutrition, and swings in blood glucose levels, including the risk for a hyperglycemic hyperosmolar state. (Chapter 8, on hyperglycemia, describes a case study with an elderly adult in rehabilitative care and provides more information.)

Women of Reproductive Age

Appropriate Medication

Diabetes. Insulin should be used in women with gestational diabetes when blood glucose levels are not adequately maintained at target levels. Only human insulin should be used for treating gestational diabetes to prevent the transfer of anti-insulin antibodies. Although there have been studies (mostly with insulin lispro), neither insulin glargine (Lantus) nor the rapid-acting insulin analogs aspart (Novolog), lispro (Humalog), or glulisine (Apidra) have been approved for use during pregnancy. The use of some sulfonylureas and metformin during pregnancy has been studied, and in clinical practice, some providers are using these medications; however, at this time, they are not widely accepted for use in the United States.[20]

Concurrent Medical Conditions. Women with prepregnancy hypertension and dyslipidemia should have their medications reevaluated at conception. ACE inhibitors, ARBs, and HMG-CoA reductase inhibitors (statins) are contraindicated in pregnancy and for women who are breastfeeding.

Also see the discussions on medications in pregnancy with preexisting diabetes in chapter 11 and in gestational diabetes, chapter 12.

Contraception. Table 11.3 on contraceptive use in chapter 11, on pregnancy with preexisting diabetes, describes methods and their efficacy and safety. Metformin and the TZDs have been used successfully in treating polycystic ovary syndrome (PCOS), including effecting a return in menstrual cycle regularity and ovulation.[21] Thus, women of childbearing age who are diagnosed with PCOS should be educated regarding pregnancy and contraception if they are taking metformin or a TZD. Pioglitazone has been shown to slightly decrease the concentration of ethinyl estradiol, the estrogen found in most combination oral contraceptives. Whether this is clinically significant is unknown.[22]

Overcoming Fears

Some women fear that injecting insulin into the abdomen will adversely affect their babies. These women need to be assured that this is untrue and that in contrast, the risks to the fetus caused by uncontrolled blood glucose, related to a refusal to take insulin, are much greater. Even in the third trimester, most pregnant women are able to give insulin injections in the abdominal area, using injection sites that are higher up near the midsection of the rib cage. In addition, other sites typically used for injection are options. Education about the risks to the fetus if blood glucose is inadequately controlled needs to be stressed.

Frequent contact with the mother and having her see her obstetrician are key in the delivery of a healthy baby.

Summary

There are many ways to ensure that optimal clinical outcomes are achieved without significant adverse effects when people who have diabetes and other conditions take prescription and nonprescription products. The person with diabetes, family members, caregivers, and healthcare professionals all need to contribute to the process. The diabetes educator should review all nonprescription and prescription medications taken with the person, and family and caregivers as appropriate, to prevent problems in following the medication plan and/or adverse reactions. Using an interprofessional approach to identify and correct barriers to therapy can also increase the likelihood for optimal clinical success. Most importantly, the persons living with diabetes should be active participants in their own care and be included in all healthcare decisions.

Focus on Education: Pearls for Practice

Teaching Strategies

Variety of diabetes medicines. Present information on all the options (prescription and nonprescription) for medicines on the market that may be considered by the person with diabetes. This would include over-the-counter products, weight-reduction products, "systems," "powders," nutrient supplements, and others the person may be considering.

Show and tell/demonstrate and discuss. Construct the information/presentation by function/categories of drugs, relating the information to how it affects the body and blood glucose (sensitizers, secretagogues, and so on). Pictures of how the medications are used in the body and what the medicine looks like are useful. A poster board display of actual pills helps identify actual dosing and aids in recognition. Involve family and others to assist with learning correct information, dosing, side effects, and other important information.

Assess medicines prescribed and ones actually taken. Ask to have all medicines brought in to clinic to determine date of prescription, dose, prescriber, pharmacy used, and other pertinent details. This will help create a more accurate accounting. Have the person describe how the medications are taken. Check for trade and generic duplication, outdated medicines, contraindicated medications, and other medication issues. Pharmacists may create a pharmacy care plan for this reason.

Patient Education

Safety. Establish one pharmacy or mail order house for consistency in medication refills. Keep an up-to-date listing of medicines including over-the-counter vitamins, supplements, and minerals. Bring to the physician, hospital, or procedure for review by the healthcare provider at each visit. Ask if there is any lab work to be done once you have started taking the medicine (to make certain the medicine is not causing any harm to your body).

Side effects. All medicines have the potential for a side effect. Follow the prescription. Do not add medicine on your own. Remind the healthcare provider of current medications. When new medicine is ordered, ask about side effects, how the medicine will work with the others taken, and exact information on how to take the medicine (such as before or after meals, with milk, at bedtime). Ask also what happens if illness occurs or if a procedure is scheduled requiring fasting overnight; ask if under those circumstances, you take the medicine or skip the dose and when to restart the medicine. When in doubt, contact your healthcare provider for instructions.

Plan ahead for family and caregiver involvement and education. Have a key member of your family, significant other, roommate, or close friend attend healthcare visits or classes with you to learn about the medicines you take. Give this person a list of medicines, side effects, treatment, and healthcare phone numbers in case of emergency situations. Have the person demonstrate use of blood testing equipment, discuss use of glucagon, or describe the number of glucose tablets used in case of low blood glucose.

References

1. Cramer JA. A systematic review of adherence with medications for diabetes. Diabetes Care. 2004;27:1218-24.
2. Rubin RR. Adherence to pharmacologic therapy in patients with type 2 diabetes mellitus. Am J Med. 2005;118suppl 5A:27S-34.
3. Pladevall M, Williams LK, Potts LA, Divine G, Xi H, Lafata JE. Clinical outcomes and adherence to medications measured by claims data in patients with diabetes. Diabetes Care. 2004;27:2800-5.
4. Leichter SB. Making outpatient care of diabetes more efficient: analyzing noncompliance. Clin Diabetes. 2005;23:187-90.
5. Lin EH, Katon W, Von Korff M, et al. Relationship of depression and diabetes self-care, medication adherence, and preventive care. Diabetes Care. 2004;27:2154-60.
6. Littenberg B, MacLean CD, Hurowitz L. The use of adherence aids by adults with diabetes: a cross-sectional survey. BMC Fam Pract. 2006;7.
7. Piette JD, Heisler M, Wagner TH. Problems paying out-of-pocket medication costs among older adults with diabetes. Diabetes Care. 2004;27:384-91.
8. Inzucchi SE. Oral antihyperglycemic therapy for type 2 diabetes. JAMA. 2002;287:360-72.
9. Dang DK, Haines S, Ponte CD, Calis KA. Drug-induced glucose and insulin dysregulation. In: Drug-Induced Diseases: Prevention, Detection, and Management. Tisdale JE, Miller DA, eds. Bethesda, Md: American Society of Health Systems Pharmacists; 2004:365-78.
10. Product Information. Tequin®, gatifloxacin. Princeton, NJ: Bristol-Myers Squibb Co; January 2006.
11. Consumer Products Healthcare Association. OTC facts and figures. Updated Feb 2006 (cited 5 Apr 2006). On the Internet at: www.chpa-info.org/web/press_room/statistics/otc_facts_figures.aspx.
12. Consumer Products Healthcare Association. Cited April 5, 2006. On the Internet at: www.chpa-info.org.
13. Yeh GY, Eisenberg DM, Kaptchuk TJ, Phillips RS. Systematic review of herbs and dietary supplements for glycemic control in diabetes. Diabetes Care. 2003;26:1277-94.
14. Niacin use: an update. Pharmacist Letter. 2005;21:211207.
15. Shimp LA. Vaginal and vulvovaginal disorders. In: Handbook of Nonprescription Drugs. Berardi RR, McDermott JH, Newton GD, et al, eds. Washington, DC: American Pharmacists Association; 2004:159-80.
16. Newton GD, Popovich NG. Minor foot disorders. In: Handbook of Nonprescription Drugs. Berardi RR, McDermott JH, Newton GD, et al, eds. Washington, DC: American Pharmacists Association; 2004:1037-60.
17. Fiscella RG, Jensen MK. Ophthalmic disorders. In: Handbook of Nonprescription Drugs. Berardi RR, McDermott JH, Newton GD, et al, eds. Washington, DC: American Pharmacists Association; 2004:659-89.
18. Kyngas H. Compliance of adolescents with chronic disease. J Clin Nursing. 2002; 9:249-56.
19. Silverstein J, Klingensmith G, Copeland K, et al. Care of children and adolescents with type 1 diabetes: a statement by the American Diabetes Association. Diabetes Care. 2005; 28:186-212.
20. American Diabetes Association. Gestational diabetes mellitus. Diabetes Care 2004; 27 suppl 1:S88-90.
21. Sharpless, JL. Polycystic ovary syndrome and the metabolic syndrome. Clin Diabetes. 2003;21:1564-61.
22. Product Information. Actos®, pioglitazone. Osaka, Japan: Takeda Pharmaceutical Company Ltd; August 2004.

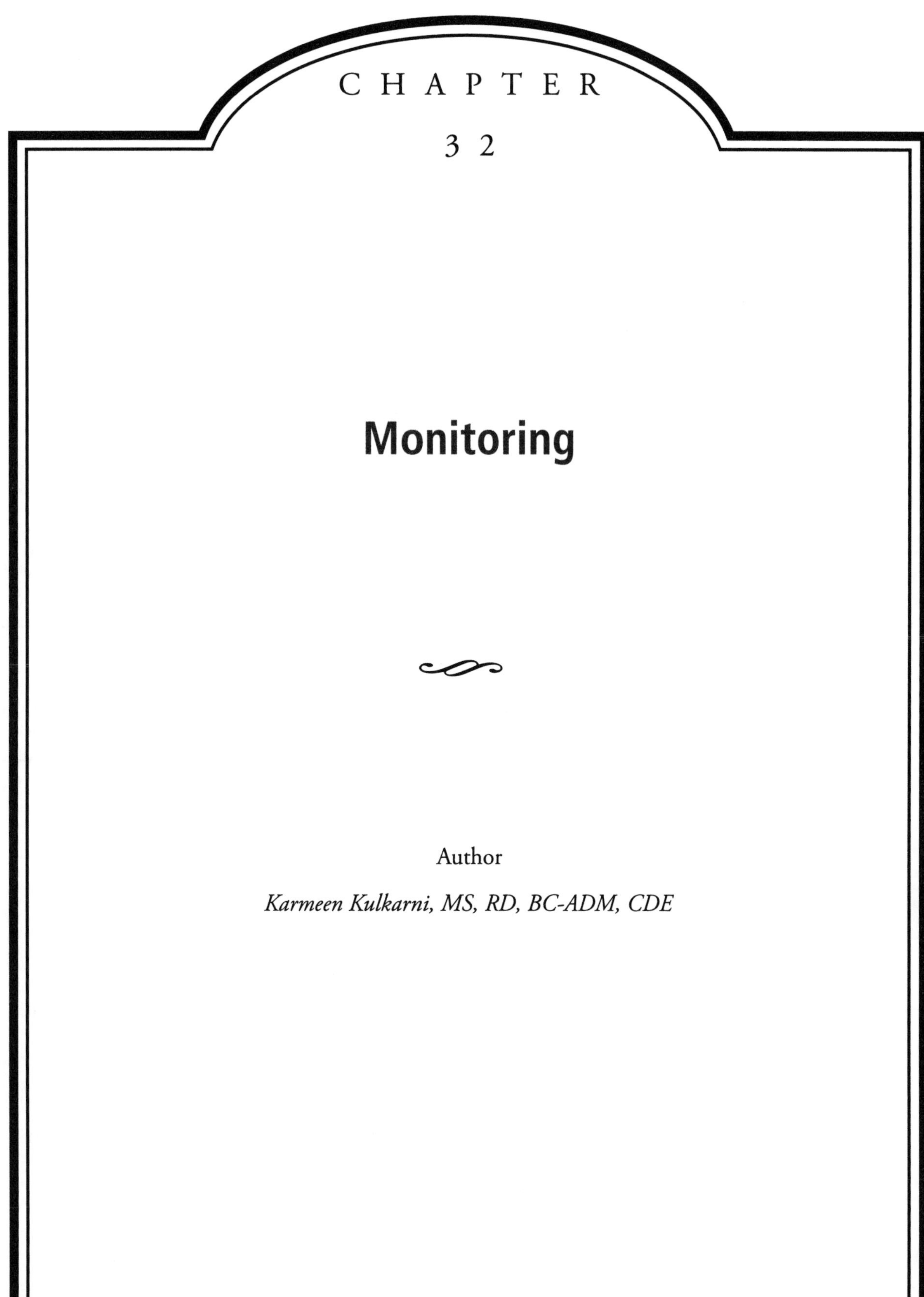

CHAPTER

32

Monitoring

Author

Karmeen Kulkarni, MS, RD, BC-ADM, CDE

Key Concepts

- Be familiar with recommendations for accurate self-monitoring of blood glucose
- Describe how the results of self-monitoring of blood glucose, ketone testing, and other laboratory data are useful in appropriate disease management
- Review the important role of routine, accurate testing in achieving target blood glucose levels for prevention of complications
- Identify the monitoring needs, adjustments, and alterations for special populations
- Review the benefits of new monitoring technology
- Identify the role self-monitoring plays in supporting self-care behaviors and decision making

Introduction

Monitoring is an all-too-familiar practice for many individuals with diabetes and for those who assist them in their care and management. Indeed, at times, life may seem to be one huge, never-ending, and overwhelming monitoring project. Questions such as these may become commonplace:

- When and how often do I check my blood glucose (BG)?
- Do I need to check for urine ketones?
- When and how much should I eat?
- How much insulin do I take to cover what I eat?
- Is adjustment needed in food intake or medication when I exercise?
- When am I at risk for hypoglycemia, and how do I prevent and treat it?
- Am I losing weight?
- When did I have my last eye or dental exam?
- When was my last A1C or cholesterol level drawn?

As Polonsky describes in Anderson and Rubin's book *Practical Psychology for Diabetes Clinicians*, some individuals with diabetes develop "diabetes burnout," wherein the multiple aspects of monitoring and managing diabetes seem much too overwhelming and people find themselves in a state of chronic emotional exhaustion.[1]

As healthcare professionals, we recognize and focus on gathering and monitoring various sets of data to help people with diabetes improve their metabolic control and maintain safety, while they also achieve the highest possible quality of life and well-being. Self-monitoring of blood glucose (SMBG) is not the only monitoring behavior that may be required of the person with diabetes. Monitoring of metabolic control by the healthcare team also encompasses the following:

- Reviewing blood glucose patterns and control over the longer term, as with measurements of A1C
- Monitoring the development and progression of long-term complications, including urinary protein measurements
- Blood pressure measurements and lipid levels
- Assessing growth for children and patterns of weight change in both children and adults

Although monitoring of all these parameters is valuable, this chapter focuses primarily on blood glucose monitoring that is performed by the person with diabetes. SMBG provides people with diabetes the information they need to assess how food, physical activity, and medications affect their blood glucose levels.

Other aspects of diabetes management that require monitoring, in a more global sense of the term, are outlined at the end of this chapter and more fully discussed in appropriate chapters throughout this book. Assisting persons with diabetes in behaviors and issues related to appropriate and useful monitoring is an area of diabetes care that clearly combines the diabetes educator's skills of management and education.[2]

Monitoring Blood Glucose

Monitoring has been identified as one of the AADE 7 Self-Care Behaviors™ and thereby is recognized as an important component of the treatment plan for persons with diabetes. This self-care behavior provides immediate feedback and data, enabling the person with diabetes to make changes in his or her management plan and reinforcing or challenging current lifestyle behaviors. Obtaining this data may help in the following ways:[3]

- In achieving and maintaining target goals for blood glucose
- In preventing and detecting hypoglycemia and avoiding episodes of severe hypoglycemia and hypoglycemia unawareness
- In preventing and detecting hyperglycemia and avoiding diabetic ketoacidosis
- In evaluating the glycemic response to types and amounts of food and physical activity
- In determining appropriate insulin-to-carbohydrate ratios, correction factors, and basal insulin rates for intensive management (multiple daily injections and insulin pumps)
- In adjusting treatment in response to changes in lifestyle and the need to add, subtract, increase, or decrease dosages or types of pharmacologic therapies
- In determining the need for adjustment in insulin dosages during illness
- In determining the need for insulin therapy in gestational diabetes

Integration and Facilitation Into Diabetes Education Practice

Immediate Outcomes:
The goal is a learning baseline

Acquiring Knowledge and Skills

As with other self-care behaviors, if individuals with diabetes are to integrate and embrace SMBG as part of their diabetes management, they must first learn the technical skills, understand their value, and be able to replicate the skill sets, as applicable. These are considered part of the Learning Baseline or Immediate Outcomes and include the following knowledge and skill sets:[4]

- Learning to use and care for the BG meter and test strips
- Performing quality control tests
- Proper disposal of lancets
- Identifying target BG values and knowing when to test BG
- Recording and interpreting data (pattern management)
- Knowing how to respond to it
- When and how to test for serum or urinary ketones (in type 1 diabetes)

Including Others Who Will Assist

It is also important to recognize that due to age limitations, physical or cognitive disabilities, and other factors, some individuals may need to rely on family members or caretakers to help them with or to perform these tasks. The diabetes educator must ask, prior to the initial teaching session, who may be involved with facilitating diabetes management so the appropriate individuals may be invited to be present in that and subsequent sessions. These individuals must be a part of the teaching and skills process. Also, as life's circumstances change, so does the level of involvement by others. For example, as the young child with type 1 diabetes grows and matures, the parents and other caregivers release increasingly greater amounts of the diabetes management skills to the child; conversely, as older adults age, physical limitations such as a decline in visual acuity or manual dexterity may result in the need for more assistance by others.

Identifying Barriers

Potential barriers to implementation of SMBG are important to identify up front so discussion of how to resolve these barriers may ensue. The following are examples of potential barriers:[4]

- *Physical:* Lack of manual dexterity; visual deficits
- *Financial:* Inadequate or lack of insurance coverage for testing supplies
- *Cognitive:* Too young or presence of physical or cognitive deficits that make it impossible to carry out the testing procedure without assistance
- *Time Constraints:* Choosing not to make time to perform BG checks; work or school situation that does not recognize need or allow time for BG checks
- *Inconvenience:* Choosing not to stop current activity to check BG, limited access to hand-washing facilities, working in climate extremes that make access to BG meter challenging
- *Emotional:* Fear of performing BG checks due to anticipated pain, fear of being noticed as being different, denial of diabetes, lack of support from family or caregivers

Intermediate Outcomes:
The goal is behavior change

Just learning the facts about diabetes management or the skills for monitoring is not enough. For what good is BG monitoring or the data obtained if it is not used to promote positive changes in behavior? Data used wisely enables the person with diabetes to make well-informed decisions. These decisions ultimately result in the long-term outcomes of improved glycemic control and may include the following desirable outcomes, to name just a few.

- Fewer admissions to the hospital for diabetic ketoacidosis
- Fewer days missed from work or school due to diabetes and illness
- Avoidance of dangerous or embarrassing situations related to hypoglycemia
- Avoidance of unwanted weight gain that can result from frequent treatment of hypoglycemia and ingestion of associated calories
- A more enhanced athletic performance
- Avoidance of diabetes complications
- Improved and desired quality of life

Successful behavior change results from the education interchange between the diabetes educator and the person with diabetes and the self-management efforts implemented by the person with diabetes.

Measures

To determine whether desired behavior changes have occurred, a status check needs to be done at follow-up visits after the initial teaching session(s). The Standards for Outcomes Measurement for Diabetes Self-Management Education (DSME) recommend that the person with diabetes return for this follow-up within 2 to 4 weeks after the initial teaching session as well as at 3-month intervals.[4,5] To determine the individual's success in implementing the monitoring behavior, the following measures can be used:

- *The Act and Frequency of Monitoring.* Is it being done and how often; for example, is it done the week prior to the follow-up clinic visit only, thus just to please the diabetes educator or other healthcare provider?
- *Schedule of Monitoring and Usefulness of the Data.* For someone using a carbohydrate-to-insulin ratio and correction factor before meals, is monitoring being done prior to meals? In addition, are postmeal checks done on occasion to evaluate whether either of these need adjustment?
- *Planned and Unplanned Testing.* Is the person only checking BG when he or she is in a crisis situation—for example, when there are signs of hypoglycemia or the meter reads "HI"?
- *Level of Data Documentation.* Is BG data being written down or downloaded and printed off the computer or insulin pump so it may be reviewed and patterns identified for use in making adjustments to the management plan?

Methods of Measurement. Tools available for measurement include the following:

- Logbooks
- Computer printouts of BG data
- Continuous glucose monitoring systems
- Manual retrieval of BG meter or insulin pump memory data
- Self-reports and demonstration of testing technique

Post-Intermediate Outcomes:
The goal is clinical improvement

Post-intermediate outcomes result over time and require a series of measurements at appropriate intervals. Clinical improvements reflect a combination of the following:

- Healthcare provider(s) clinical judgment and management
- DSME provided
- Efforts of the person with diabetes to self-manage his or her diabetes

Measures

Measures of clinical improvement include the following:

- Improved BG control, as evidenced by the A1C
- Fewer episodes of severe hypoglycemia or diabetic ketoacidosis
- Increased ability by the person with diabetes and caregivers to make informed decisions about management, independent of the diabetes educator
- Increased level of self-assurance by the person with diabetes and the family/caregivers, as evidenced by a resumed interest in taking part in activities that may have been put on hold while learning how to manage diabetes

For example, as a result of more frequent and timely BG monitoring, the person with diabetes may resume an activity that he or she had been fearful of doing, due to problems with severe episodes of hypoglycemia. Parents who had been hesitant to let their child stay overnight with friends may feel comfortable loosening up a bit, once they know that another parent has a good grasp of the monitoring procedure and understands adjustments to be made in insulin dosages or food intake to compensate for variations in blood glucose levels.

Case in Point: Native American Youth With Type 2 Diabetes

KB was a 14-year-old male. He was a member of the Winnebago Indian Tribe. He had been recently diagnosed with type 2 diabetes. This was found after the Community Health Educator conducted a routine screening at his high school for acanthosis nigricans. A follow-up fasting blood glucose was elevated and confirmed on a second occasion. Values were 165 and 149 mg/dL, respectively.

The diagnosis of diabetes did not surprise KB because many members of his family had diabetes. Several members had undergone dialysis, one member was in a wheelchair with bilateral below-the-knee amputations, and one aunt could no longer drive because she had lost her eyesight.

KB was angry about the diagnosis of diabetes, even though he had figured it would eventually happen to him. At the insistence of one of his uncles, KB had an appointment with one of the Indian Health Service physicians at the Reservation's hospital outpatient clinic. The physician drew an A1C, wrote a prescription for metformin 500 mg twice daily (before breakfast and the evening meal), and told KB that he wanted him to see the diabetes educator to learn about what to eat, exercise, and testing his blood glucose 2 to 3 times a day. He was also to set up an appointment to see the doctor in clinic in about 1 month.

Assessment Data

- Height: 68 in
- Weight: 200 lb
- BMI: 30.5
- BMI percentile: >97th percentile
- Acanthosis nigricans grading: 3+
- Blood pressure: 126/78 mm Hg
- A1C: 7.8%
- Lipid panel: pending

Other Data

Nutrition History. KB generally ate 2 meals per day. Lunch was eaten at school on weekdays, at a fast-food restaurant on Saturday, and often at a large family gathering on Sunday. The evening meal often included a soup of some type, several large pieces of fry bread, potato salad, fruited gelatin, and a sweetened soft drink. His afternoon snack was often a grabbed bag of chips and a 32-oz regular soda from the local store.

Physical Activity History. KB did not currently have a plan for regular physical activity. He had not been involved in team sports in the past, but would play basketball after school at the community Wellness Center with friends for an hour or so, once or twice a week.

Psychosocial History. KB enjoyed spending time with friends and family. He was living with an aunt and uncle and felt especially close to his uncle. He was a good student and had a good relationship with his teachers. His goals were to finish high school, go to a technical school or 4-year college, and then return to the Reservation to help improve life for others in his community.

At the meeting with the diabetes educator, KB voiced these concerns:

- Fear of the diagnosis of diabetes, as he viewed it as a death sentence. He had been hopeful about his future before, but now felt depressed and wondered if he could truly do anything to make a difference for his long-term health outlook.
- Hesitancy to take any of the information to heart, as he would "probably lose his eyesight or a leg anyway."
- Hesitancy to self-monitor his blood glucose (BG), as he did not want his friends to know that he had diabetes and did not know how he would make time to test at school anyway.

(continued)

Case in Point: Native American Youth With Type 2 Diabetes (continued)

Questions to Consider

What were the key issues for the diabetes educator to address with KB regarding the following:

- Self-monitoring of blood glucose (SMBG)
- Behavior changes that should be suggested for KB to focus on
- Two behavioral goals for KB
- A clinical goal for KB
- Documentation that should be included for the initial visit with KB
- Factors that should be evaluated during return visits with KB
- Potential barriers that might prevent KB from making desired behavior changes

Interventions and strategies for use by the diabetes educator in facilitating behavior changes such as those represented in this case can be found throughout the chapter.

Long-Term Outcomes:
Goals include improvement in health status and cost savings

Long-term outcomes include improvement in health status and can be measured in a number of ways:

- Perceived improvements in quality of life
- Economic benefits, such as fewer visits to the emergency room for treatment injuries caused by accidents related to hypoglycemia
- Fewer hospitalizations related to diabetic ketoacidosis
- Prevention of a myocardial infarction that might have occurred after years of uncontrolled hyperglycemia
- Improved pregnancy outcomes

These are all examples of long-term outcomes that may be achieved, in part, by monitoring blood glucose and making intelligent use of the data to improve glycemic control.

Knowledge Content Areas for SMBG

To assist persons in SMBG, diabetes educators need to understand issues in a number of areas. The following topics are discussed in the ensuing paragraphs:

- Ensuring meter accuracy
- Overcoming fears
- Using alternative sites appropriately
- Using the data obtained
- Selecting a meter

Ensuring Meter Accuracy

The data obtained from the BG meter must be accurate. This is critical. Anything less is an effort in futility by the person with diabetes and his or her healthcare provider. If the BG data obtained are erroneous due to an inadequate blood sample, outdated test strips, soiled fingertips, improper timing or testing procedure, or other factor, then the treatment decisions based on this data will be in error as well.

Blood glucose meters designed for home use are not completely accurate, but they are the best that technology has to offer at this point in time.

Recommended Accuracy. The American Diabetes Association (ADA) recommends the following performance goal for blood glucose meters:

- Total error of less than 10% at blood glucose levels of 30 mg/dL to 400 mg/dL (1.7 mmol/L to 22.2 mmol/L), 100% of the time[3]

Many products do not meet this performance goal. Table 32.1 lists guidelines that can be used by the diabetes educator to evaluate BG meter accuracy.

Other factors that may influence the results of SMBG systems include variations in the hematocrit (some systems are accurate with hematocrit ranges of 0% to 60%), altitude, environmental temperature and humidity, hypotension, hypoxia, and triglyceride concentrations.[2]

TABLE 32.1 Guidelines for Determining Accuracy of a Blood Glucose Meter

- *Against Lab Values.* Blood glucose meter results should be compared against the laboratory values, not against another meter.
- *Fasting Readings.* Compare fasting blood glucose levels only. After-meal levels will differ between capillary blood (as measured on the meter) and venous blood (as measured in the laboratory).
- *Simultaneous Testing.* To compare meter and laboratory results, the 2 tests must be done at the same time. Measuring blood glucose at home either before or after the venipuncture allows too much time between the readings for a valid comparison.
- *Timing.* The venous blood must be spun by a centrifuge to separate the plasma from the erythrocytes within 30 minutes after the time the blood sample was taken. If it is not spun, the glucose in the blood will begin to break down and the results will not accurately reflect the blood glucose levels at the time the sample was collected.
- *Sample.* Comparing meter readings to laboratory values involves a fingertip or alternative-site puncture and a venipuncture. Applying a drop of blood from the venipuncture needle is not acceptable. Some strips are designed for capillary blood only and will give false readings if venous blood is used.
- *Whole Blood Meter Reading.* A meter that reports whole blood glucose levels will have a reading 11% to 15% lower than the laboratory.

Source: Peragallo-Dittko V. How accurate is your meter? Diabetes Self-Manage. 2000;17(5):78-85.

User error is the most common reason for inaccurate SMBG results

Potential sources of user error include the following:

- Improperly stored, expired, or defective strips
- Uncalibrated meter
- Soiled meter
- Inadequate blood sample

Table 32.2 provides guidelines for teaching individuals how to use their blood glucose meters. Details on use of test strips, control solution, and meters as well as correct technique for obtaining the blood sample are given in the paragraphs that follow.

Test Strips. To yield accurate results, the strips must be stored according to the manufacturer's guidelines. These guidelines also refer to avoiding exposure to heat, cold, and humidity during shipping.

TABLE 32.2 Guidelines for Teaching Individuals How to Use a Blood Glucose Meter

- Use universal precautions: change lancets, end-caps, and gloves for each person seen*
- Encourage the individual to lance the finger or alternative site at the beginning of the session to minimize anxiety about the discomfort involved
- Demonstrate how to check blood glucose using control solution first and then using the individual's blood
- After demonstrating this technique, ask the individual to provide a return demonstration before teaching about control solution, calibration, cleaning, and using the logbook
- Explain how to dispose of lancets in an appropriate sharps container
- Evaluate the individual's technique at every opportunity

*American Association of Diabetes Educators. Educating providers and persons with diabetes to prevent the transmission of bloodborne infections and avoid injuries from sharps (position statement). Diabetes Educ. 1997;23:401-3.

Teach the individual to check the expiration date of the strips, especially when a mail-order shipment could include strips that expire within a few months—these should be used before all others. Because strips are costly, people are commonly tempted to use expired strips. This may lead to inaccurate readings. The strips and meter should be stored appropriately. Users should be instructed to store the strips in a dry place and always make sure the strip bottle has the lid on so strips are not exposed to light and temperature variations. Suggest that the meter and test strips not be stored in the bathroom, due to moisture variations. In addition, discourage leaving the meter in the car, as extremes of temperature in the car interior may damage the meter or cause a delay in its readiness to function (requiring several hours for the meter to "warm up" in very cold weather). Each meter and set of strips have their own storage requirements and these should be reviewed with the individual.

Control Solution. Control solution is a product provided by manufacturers to verify the integrity of the test strips. This is an underused method of verifying accuracy. A drop of control solution is placed on the test strip, or enters the test strip, in the same manner as when a drop of blood is used. Every manufacturer provides at least 1 control solution, and some have low-, normal-, and high-level control solutions to test the meter at extremes.

Follow-up discussions or initial visits with a person newly referred for education may reveal that an individual has not been using control solution for a variety of reasons: its use or importance had not been explained to them; they do not want to "waste" a strip (because strips are costly) that could have been used to test their own blood; and/or many insurance plans do not cover the cost of control solution. Therefore, when the bottle of control solution that came with their meter was emptied, they did not choose to pay for another as an out-of-pocket expense. The diabetes educator can discuss these issues with the person and problem solve regarding this procedural step.

Meter. The BG meter should be stored, used, and calibrated appropriately.

- *Meter Calibration.* Calibrating the meter is another way to ensure the most accurate results. Some meters automatically calibrate the strips with the meter, whereas other meters require setting a code or inserting a chip or strip to calibrate the meter.
- *Soiled Meter.* With some meters, the blood sample intended for the strip may come in contact with the meter and soil the optic window. This will yield inaccurate results. Manufacturers provide instructions for cleaning the meter.

Inadequate Sample. Some meters reject an inadequate sample, whereas other meters have a feature (usually an error message) that signals the user when the blood sample is not large enough to provide an accurate reading. Unfortunately, this feature creates a false sense of security because users assume that if they do not get the signal, they have given an adequate sample. The meter will only signal the user about a blood sample it cannot process; any other sample—even an inadequate one—registers a reading, but the reading can be inaccurate. At every opportunity, the educator should ask the individual to demonstrate his or her meter techniques. This demonstration gives the educator an opportunity to verify technique, provide advice, or clean a soiled unit.

An inadequate blood sample is the most frequent cause of inaccurate results and errors in subsequent treatment decisions

Some individuals have difficulty securing a drop of blood and may require guidance in choosing a lancing device or meter. Providing individualized guidance for each person's needs minimizes waste of strips and eases the person's frustration with blood glucose monitoring.

Securing an Adequate Blood Sample

Each person should be taught to follow specific directions for securing an adequate blood sample.[6] For example, when using the fingertips as a puncture site, the person should be aware of the following procedures:

- Vigorously wash hands with warm water to increase circulation to fingertips.
- Try hanging the hand at your side for 30 seconds so blood pools in that hand.
- Shake the hand to be pricked as though you were shaking down a thermometer.
- Use a lancing device or end-cap that will allow a deeper puncture or a larger gauge lancet.
- After your finger is punctured, gently milk the blood from the bottom to the tip of the finger until the blood drop is the correct size. Milking the finger works better than just squeezing the fingertips.

Overcoming Fears

Healthcare professionals, including some diabetes educators, may be surprised to find that many individuals, especially those newly diagnosed with diabetes, harbor considerable fear of the BG monitoring procedure. These fears may be described as "needle panic" and rise from previous negative experiences during childhood. For children, the activity may present a real and present danger as they are exposed to multiple probes and other invasive procedures associated with being newly diagnosed with diabetes. Although new technologies continue to become available (as presented later in this text), the majority of persons with diabetes will most likely continue to use fingerstick punctures to obtain a blood sample for BG testing.

Blood glucose monitoring is a must-do, if the person with diabetes strives to achieve good glycemic control. However, a skilled diabetes educator will learn to match and individualize the presentation of BG monitoring so that the fears of the person with diabetes may be alleviated. For example, when there are several components of diabetes management to be taught during a teaching session, explaining to the person what these components are and letting the person choose which to receive instruction in first is often advisable. Some people may share their fears related to monitoring and request to "just get it out of the way first," so they can absorb and participate in discussion of subsequent information more effectively. Very young children, although scared of the testing procedure to begin with, can be encouraged to take on increasing responsibility for doing their "finger pokes" and be rewarded with verbal praise for doing so when they return for clinic visits. In addition, an appropriate option for some individuals may be to consider using alternative-site testing. Due to the presence of fewer nerve endings in these sites, the testing procedure is often less painful than on the fingertips.

Using Alternative Sites Appropriately

Meters and strips have been designed to use alternative sites such as the forearm, palm of the hand, upper arm, or thigh for puncture. However, the following precautions are important for users to understand.

There is wide discordance between fingertip and alternative-site samples when blood glucose levels are changing rapidly due to circulatory physiology. Blood circulation in the skin of the fingers and palm of the hand is distinctly different from that in the arms and legs. The blood flow through the arteriovenous shunts in the fingertips proceeds at a higher velocity than the flow through other capillaries of the skin. Therefore, the transient difference between alternative site and fingertip during rapid blood glucose changes is a result of this decreased velocity of blood flow to sites such as the forearm.[7] When blood glucose concentration is falling rapidly, this lag between alternative site and fingertip could cause a delay in detection of hypoglycemia if an alternative site is being used for measuring glucose levels. In preprandial monitoring, glucose levels are in a steady state, so the difference between alternative-site and fingertip samples is small and not clinically significant, but for up to 2 hours postprandially the blood glucose is in flux.[7]

Alternative-site BG monitoring carries a level of risk. The individual must understand when it is not safe to use an alternative site.

- Alternative sites may be used before a meal and 2 hours after a meal
- Alternative sites should not be used when the person is hypoglycemic, prone to hypoglycemia (during peak activity of an injected basal insulin or up to 2 hours after injecting rapid-acting insulin), after exercise, during illness, when blood glucose levels are rapidly increasing or decreasing (such as any time less than 2 hours after a meal), or before driving
- Persons with a history of hypoglycemic unawareness should not use alternative sites

Because between-site differences of up to 100 mg/dL (5.6 mmol/L) have been reported,[8] the person performing the BG must document not only the result, time, medication, and relevant comments, but also the sampling site used. In addition, the diabetes educator should determine if there are sites the physician would prefer the person not use. For example, some pediatric endocrinologists prefer that children and adolescents use only the fingertips as puncture sites, due to the rapid changes in blood glucose levels often seen in these age groups due to spontaneous activity and glucose uptake into the muscle.

Samples taken from alternative sites less than 2 hours after a meal may reflect the wide discordance between fingertip and alternative-site samples. Teach pregnant women who check blood glucose levels 1 hour after a meal this difference between fingertip and alternative-site samples.

Using the Data

Many persons with diabetes are trained in the mechanics of using a meter, and how to record BG results, but not on how to use the data or why it is of value. This inadequacy may be related to patient education. Harris and associates[9] found that the frequency of monitoring was related to having attended a diabetes patient education class. Diabetes patient education was associated with an almost threefold greater probability that subjects monitored their blood glucose at least once per day. The critical uses of SMBG data by persons with diabetes are shown in Table 32.3.

Even when the case for SMBG has been presented to the person with diabetes by the diabetes educator, this is not sufficient, nor is it any assurance that a person will consistently monitor blood glucose. Indeed, it is the job of the diabetes educator to explain not only "why" and "how" to perform SMBG, but also to help individuals identify barriers that may prevent them from continuing this activity and making it a habit. A person may understand the value of SMBG, but perceive multiple challenges to actually performing the monitoring. Barriers to SMBG were mentioned previously in this chapter. Use of the AADE 7 Self-Care Behaviors™ Goal Sheet (part of the AADE 7 IMPACT™ product) combines data in a format that the person with diabetes and diabetes educator can use for problem solving and decision making.

While some decisions (eg, treating hypoglycemia or determining the need for a snack) require instant feedback for decision making, most decisions require reviewing

TABLE 32.3 How the Person With Diabetes Can Use SMBG Data

- To identify and treat hypoglycemia
- To make decisions concerning food intake or medication adjustment when exercising
- To determine the effect of food choices or portions on blood glucose levels
- For pattern management
- To manage intercurrent illness
- To manage hypoglycemia unawareness

numerous readings to identify a pattern (eg, adjusting medication dosages, changing the meal plan, or recognizing the impact of exercise). The memory feature of many meters is not intended to replace the logbook, but rather to provide the option of recording readings at a later date. Although a written record and graph of blood glucose readings yields important information, jotting down comments or explanations can be more helpful for teaching the impact of certain decisions related to medication, exercise, or food.

Educators and clinicians rely on SMBG to teach problem-solving skills, which are the essence of diabetes self-management, and complex management skills such as blood glucose pattern awareness and insulin dose adjustment. Diabetes educators use SMBG as the tool that links abstract principles of management with daily decision making. Educators can use blood glucose results to teach the concept of postexercise, late-onset hypoglycemia, and the behaviors necessary to prevent this condition. Behavior change concerning food choices or portions is facilitated by relating the food or portion to the postprandial blood glucose result.[10,11] For persons with type 2 diabetes who may be asymptomatic for hyperglycemia, the need for behavior change becomes personally relevant when they monitor and record blood glucose levels.

SMBG is used by educators to identify and influence psychosocial adaptations. SMBG can influence self-efficacy.[12] For example, persons with diabetes report increased confidence in their problem-solving abilities as a result of using SMBG. The act of monitoring can also have emotional consequences when an individual is confronted with an unacceptable number. This phenomenon, called "monitor talk," can help identify psychosocial needs and direct future learning.[13] Educators can discourage value judgment and replace the notion of good and bad readings with the terms "in range" or "out of range." Reference to blood glucose tests can be replaced with the terms "checks" or "measurements."

SMBG can be used to allay anxiety about hypoglycemia, especially parental anxiety, and is a critical tool for treating fear of hypoglycemia.[14] Although the influence of stress and stress management techniques on glycemic control is controversial, individuals may benefit from identifying a physical marker for their psychological distress.

The frequency and timing of SMBG are determined by how the data will be used. More frequent monitoring is beneficial during insulin dose adjustment, illness, pregnancy (to control outcomes), and heavy periods of exercise or physical activity and when an oral medication and/or injectable medication—pramlintide (Symlin), exenatide (Byetta), or a rapid-acting insulin analog—is prescribed that has a primary effect on postprandial glucose levels. Periodic postprandial checks may benefit someone who is learning about the glycemic effect of food portions.

Plasma and Whole Blood Glucose Levels. Another aspect of using the data appropriately is understanding what data the meter is gathering. While all meters use a drop of whole blood on the test strip, the majority of the meters read the plasma glucose level or have been programmed to calculate the plasma glucose level. A meter that provides plasma glucose levels will have results that are closer to the laboratory's results. Because a meter that reports whole blood values and a meter that reports plasma values will have different results for the same blood sample, there are different preprandial blood glucose treatment goals for whole blood or plasma.

Frequency of Monitoring

The following checklist is helpful to review when determining a realistic frequency for blood glucose checks:[15]

- What type of diabetes does the person have?
- What does the person with diabetes want to do?
- What is the current status of the diabetes control?
- What is the medication regimen?
- What is important about lifestyle/daily schedule with regard to activity, food, work?
- Physical ability to check blood glucose
- Does the individual have the ability to use the information and make management decisions?
- What is the attitude of the person toward BG testing?
- Are there financial limitations that may pose a barrier to BG testing?
- Are there other medical conditions?

Selecting A Meter

Meters for Home Use. The diabetes educator can assist individuals with meter selection by reviewing the following factors that affect choice:

- Overall size and shape of the meter
- Number of steps to check blood glucose
- Size of the readout
- Size of the drop of blood
- Time of the blood glucose check
- Memory capacity
- Computer download feature
- Cost of strips and meter
- Calibration and maintenance of the equipment
- Optional features for those with special needs (ie, visual deficits)

Meters for Healthcare Settings. Educators are frequently asked to provide consultation regarding the choice of a meter for a hospital or other facility. Although the scientific literature contains numerous reports of the statistical accuracy of systems for SMBG, most determine accuracy in ways that may not be clinically useful for these settings. The Error Grid Analysis[16] provides a useful methodological contribution for evaluating accuracy of glucose meters and clinical relevancy of statistical data related to SMBG.

Postprandial Monitoring

Postprandial monitoring is an essential part of diabetes self-management. Research has demonstrated that any therapy targeted at lowering postprandial blood glucose will also lower A1C level.[17] In individuals with type 1 and type 2 diabetes, abnormalities in insulin and glucagon secretion, hepatic glucose uptake, suppression of hepatic glucose production, and peripheral glucose uptake contribute to higher and more prolonged postprandial blood glucose excursions than in nondiabetic individuals.[18] In general, a measurement of plasma glucose 2 hours after the start of the meal provides a reasonable assessment of postprandial hyperglycemia. Specific clinical conditions such as gestational diabetes or pregnancy complicated by diabetes may benefit from the measurement of blood glucose 1 hour after a meal.[18]

Postprandial plasma glucose targets have been defined (see Table 32.4). There is controversy about the contributions of postprandial and fasting glucose increments to overall hyperglycemia. Monnier and colleagues tested the effect of overall glycemic control itself. They analyzed the diurnal glycemic profiles of patients with type 2 diabetes and investigated different levels of A1C. The conclusions from the study showed that in patients with fair control of their diabetes, the relative contribution of postprandial glucose excursions is predominant. As the diabetes worsens, the contribution of fasting hyperglycemia increases gradually.[19]

One of the most common barriers to postprandial monitoring is that people frequently forget to check after a meal because there is no trigger to remind them. With so many types of technology available today, the diabetes educator may suggest that people use it—by setting the alarm feature on their insulin pumps to sound or vibrate; programming an alert message into their desktop computers, cell phones, or Personal Data Assistants (PDAs)—or simply by writing and highlighting a reminder in their appointment books. Postprandial testing provides the person with diabetes information on the effect of the meal, the efficacy of the medication, and the impact of physical activity.

TABLE 32.4 Therapeutic Goals for Glycemia

	American Diabetes Association	*American College of Endocrinology*
A1C	<7.0%	<6.5%
Preprandial Capillary Plasma Glucose	90 to 130 mg/dL (5.0 mmol/L to 7.2 mol/L)	<110 mg/dL (6.1 mmol/L)
Peak Postprandial Capillary Plasma Glucose	<180 mg/dL (<10.0 mmol/L)	<140 mg/dL (<7.8 mmol/L)

Sources: American Diabetes Association. Standards of medical care in diabetes, 2006. Diabetes Care. 2006;29suppl:S4-42; American College of Endocrinology. Guidelines for glycemic control (consensus statement). Endo Pract. 2002;8suppl 1:6-11.

Frequency of Postprandial Monitoring

There are no set guidelines regarding the frequency of testing for type 1 and type 2 diabetes. Monitoring schedules are based on the person's needs, desires, and use of the data. Although some clinicians have not yet been convinced of the merit of SMBG for those not treated with insulin, the value of SMBG cannot be overemphasized as a teaching tool, motivator, and reinforcement and as an aid in prescribing appropriate dosages of the various combinations of oral glucose-lowering medications. Chapter 15, on pharmacologic therapy for glucose management, emphasizes SMBG with use of sulfonylureas, meglitinides, metformin, thiazolidinediones, and alpha-glucosidase inhibitors as well as with insulin.

Data Management Systems

Data management systems allow for downloading the memory stored in the BG meter to a computer (either directly or by modem) for record keeping or plotting the results on a graph. These systems can be accessed via personal computer or the Internet. Data summarization alone, however, does not identify the relationship that leads to the observed outcomes (eg, the 4 carbohydrate servings at breakfast that led to postprandial hyperglycemia). Data management systems can store hundreds of results and other information entered by the user, such as insulin or medication type and dose, meals, and exercise. Blood glucose monitor manufacturers provide information about compatible computer software on their Web sites. PDAs are also used as electronic logbooks. Combining the meter with the PDA allows automatic storage of the blood glucose result, and the user can log other helpful data.

Ensuring Quality

The Joint Commission for the Accreditation of Health Care Organizations and the Centers for Medicare and Medicaid Services require hospitals and other facilities to have quality assurance programs for bedside blood glucose monitoring.[20] Proficiency testing, use of control solutions, staff training, and correlation studies comparing bedside results with hospital laboratory values are essential elements of the quality assurance process.

The Clinical Laboratory Improvement Amendments of 1988 (CLIA '88)[21] require all laboratories that examine materials derived from the human body to be certified. This includes physician offices. Glucose tests performed on a meter approved by the US Food and Drug Administration (FDA) for home use are waived under CLIA and can be done at any site by any person. BG meters must have verified accuracy, and the provider's office must enroll in the CLIA program, follow the manufacturers' test recommendations, and submit fees for a waived test.

Meeting Unique Needs

Certain populations of people with diabetes have unique needs relating to SMBG. Issues specific to elderly adults, children, the visually impaired, and those hospitalized are discussed in the paragraphs that follow.

Elderly

Elderly adults with diabetes remain an underserved population despite the prevalence of diabetes in this population and the validity of SMBG as a management tool. Age should not be the sole criterion for decisions concerning SMBG. Indeed, research has shown that many older individuals perform equally as well, and in some cases better, than younger individuals in their follow-through with SMBG. The elderly are a heterogeneous population requiring personalized therapy and monitoring schedules. Educators need to consider the unique needs of some of the elderly that may influence the choice of products, such as potential limitations in manual dexterity, slowed reaction time, or fluctuating vision.[22]

Children

Children also have unique needs that influence product choice. Children especially benefit from strips that require a small sample of blood and lancing devices that hide the lancet and minimize discomfort. Parents often prefer meters that yield results quickly, have a back light (for testing in the middle of the night), and store multiple values in memory. This latter feature is particularly important because after a skin puncture, parents are focused on comforting their child and the meter may turn off before the parent can write down the results. At a very young age, many children begin to take responsibility for doing their BG "pokes" or "checks" (when speaking with children, these terms are preferred over "tests," which often has a pass/fail, negative connotation). It is important that they be verbally praised for participating in this critical part of their diabetes management. However, even after children have mastered the technique, it is important for parents and other caregivers to provide supervision of the testing procedure, so that data is recorded for use in treatment and pattern management.

Visually Impaired

Visually impaired persons with diabetes, including those with fluctuating vision to nonfunctional vision, need products that are fully accessible for them; limited products are currently available. Two meters for the visually impaired are the ACCU-CHEK Voicemate (Roche Diagnostics, www.accu-chek.com) and the Digi-Voice Mini and Deluxe modules (Captek/Science Products, Southeastern, Pa), which plug into the data port of certain BG monitors (www.captek.net). Equipment features that would be of benefit include tactile markings on the strip; clear speech output on a small, portable meter; and a method of consistent placement of the blood sample.[23]

Hospitalization

The case for monitoring blood glucose in the hospital is well established. As noted in the ADA Clinical Practice Recommendations, all patients with diabetes admitted to the hospital should have an order for blood glucose monitoring, with results available to all members of the healthcare team.[24] Observational studies suggest an association between hyperglycemia and increased mortality. When admissions on general medicine and surgery units were studied, patients with new hyperglycemia (ie, previously undiagnosed glucose intolerance) had a significantly increased in-hospital mortality, as did patients with known diabetes. In addition, length of stay was higher for the new hyperglycemic group, and both the patients with new hyperglycemia and those with known diabetes were more likely to require intensive care unit (ICU) care and transitional or nursing home care.

Conversely, better outcomes were demonstrated in patients with fasting and admission blood glucose <126 mg/dL (7mmol/L) and all random blood glucose levels <200 mg/dL (11.1 mmol/L). For these reasons, the ADA has suggested the following goals for blood glucose levels.[24]

- *Critically Ill:* Blood glucose levels should be kept as close to 110 mg/dL (6.1 mmol/L) as possible and generally <180 mg/dL (10 mmol/L). Intravenous insulin is usually required to meet these targets.
- *Not Critically Ill:* Premeal blood glucose levels should be kept as close to 90 to 130 mg/dL (5.0 to 7.2 mmol/L; midpoint of range 110 mg/dL) as possible given the clinical situation and postprandial blood glucose levels <180 mg/dL. Insulin should be used as necessary.

In addition, the ADA recommends the following guidelines for care of hospitalized patients with diabetes.[24]

- Scheduled prandial insulin doses should be given in relation to meals and should be adjusted according to point-of-care glucose levels. Traditional sliding-scale insulin regimens are ineffective and not recommended.
- A plan for treating hypoglycemia should be established for each patient. Episodes of hypoglycemia in the hospital should be tracked.
- All patients with diabetes admitted to the hospital should have an A1C obtained for discharge planning if the result of testing in the previous 2 to 3 months is not available.
- A diabetes education plan including "survival skills education" and follow-up should be developed for each patient. It has been suggested that hospitals develop standing orders for persons with diabetes to receive diabetes education as appropriate, including referrals for follow-up care when necessary.[25]
- As well, patients with hyperglycemia in the hospital who do not have a diagnosis of diabetes should have appropriate plans for follow-up testing and care documented at discharge.

From a realistic perspective, with regard to the skill and training of SMBG, all that may be accomplished before hospital discharge is checking to see that a patient has a BG meter and has been instructed in its use and understands BG targets, when to test, and the importance of following up with BG reporting by phone, fax, or email and follow-up visits with the physician and diabetes educators, as appropriate.

Continuous Glucose Monitoring

Continuous glucose monitoring (CGM) systems monitor glucose from interstitial fluid that is converted to an electronic signal. A sensor-type device transmits the signal to a monitor that acquires the data continuously. The typical measurement period is up to 72 hours.

CGM is intended for diagnostic and prescriptive use and can help identify glycemic effects of food, exercise, and insulin; previously unrecognized hypoglycemia; proper insulin doses to match food absorption in gastroparesis; and effects of dialysis on glucose levels.

The newer generation of CGM systems for home use will provide information for the person with diabetes to see the effect of lifestyle modification on glycemic control.[26] CGM assists in mealtime insulin delivery by determining the most effective way to use the dual-wave bolus feature on insulin pumps. By evaluating glucose trends, insulin adjustments can decrease fear of nighttime hypoglycemia and increase comfort with intensive plans.

Currently, a few CGM systems have been approved by the FDA, and many more are under development. Most of these measure glucose in the interstitial fluid. They need to be calibrated with a conventional blood glucose meter and provide a reliable estimate of glucose concentrations. The continuous monitoring systems currently available include these:[26]

- CGMS Gold—from Medtronic Diabetes, Northridge, California
- Glucowatch G2 Biographer—from Cygnus, Inc., Redwood City, California
- Freestyle Navigator CGMS—from Abbott Laboratories, Alameda, California

Clinical Observations

A study using a CGM system in children with type 1 diabetes who were in optimal glucose control (A1C <7.7%) found that 70% of the patients had prolonged asymptomatic hypoglycemia.[27] This study and others support the role of CGM in detecting and preventing hypoglycemia. CGM has also provided insight into postmeal glucose rises. When used in children under 6 years of age, CGM detected elevated postprandial values after meals 92% to 98% of the time.[28] These studies support the role of CGM for providing information on glucose patterns and trends. The postprandial information obtained from a CGM system can change how insulin is delivered for meals in the future. CGM could provide valuable information on how different macronutrients and micronutrients affect glucose levels.[26]

Future of Continual Monitoring

Continual glucose monitoring devices are, for the most part, simple to use and well tolerated by people with diabetes. Data from these devices have proved useful in projecting trends in glucose profiles and guiding therapy adjustments to enable people to better manage their diabetes.[26]The new generation of CGM technology offers not only the data, but also alarms for high and low blood glucose and has the potential to fulfill the promise of improved glycemic control.[26]

Other Glucose Monitoring Methods

Noninvasive Monitoring

Noninvasive monitoring involves measuring the concentration of glucose in the blood without puncturing the skin to obtain a drop of blood.[29] The system detects trends and tracks patterns in blood glucose levels. It is not intended to replace the immediate feedback provided by fingertip or alternative-site BG monitoring.

Urine Glucose Testing

Urine glucose testing was the original method of monitoring glycemic control. However, since the advent of BG monitoring, urine testing is no longer recommended. This is because urine glucose testing provides retrospective information and does not reflect current blood glucose. Some individuals may, however, still be using urine glucose testing due to very limited financial resources or because they are adamant in their refusal to do an invasive testing procedure. The results of urine glucose testing should be reported in percent values, not plus (+) values, for continuity of results among methods.

Urine testing for glucose has several distinct disadvantages:

- Elevated renal thresholds—that is, blood glucose >180 mg/dL (>10 mmol/L)—that occur with age will give false negative results
- Renal thresholds may be low in pregnancy
- Since urine testing gives a delayed picture of what is happening in the blood, it is not indicated in flexible insulin therapy
- False results (negative or positive) may occur with ingestion of certain medications (cephalosporins, large amounts of ascorbic acid)
- Urine testing can be awkward to do, especially when away from home
- Urine testing is limited to testing for elevated glucose levels

Ketone Tests

Monitoring for the presence of ketones remains an essential component of diabetes care. Individuals with type 1 diabetes are prone to ketosis, whereas those with type 2 diabetes are generally ketosis resistant. Either blood or urinary ketones can be measured. Blood ketones can be measured using a special meter designed for home use, and urinary ketones can be measured using a dipstick and matching the results to a color chart.

Situations When Ketone Testing is Appropriate

- Illness
- Consistently elevated BG with type 1 diabetes
- Pregnancy
- Weight-loss plan

Ketones should be tested routinely during illness by all individuals with diabetes. Individuals with type 2 diabetes can become ketotic during severe stress precipitated by infections or trauma.[30]

The ADA recommends that individuals with type 1 diabetes test for ketones when their blood glucose is consistently elevated: >300 mg/dL (>16.7 mmol/L).[31] For those using an insulin pump, ketonuria or ketonemia in the presence of hyperglycemia may indicate failure of the insulin delivery system. Patient teaching regarding ketone testing should include the reason why ketone spillage would occur, due to lack of adequate insulin and the body burning its own fat, of which ketones are a by-product. Teaching must also make clear that during ketone spillage fluid replacement—as well as carbohydrate replacement—is very important. Insulin users must be taught to continue to take their insulin and that additional insulin is often required to treat the accompanying hyperglycemia.

Pregnant women with diabetes (including gestational diabetes) are often advised to monitor urinary ketones every morning. These measurements are useful for detecting inadequate food intake (starvation ketosis) and providing warning of impending metabolic decompensation.[32]

What is Tested

Urinary ketones also may be measured on a regular schedule in individuals with diabetes who are actively trying to lose weight by calorie restriction. Because ketones are a waste product of fat metabolism, ketonuria in the presence of euglycemia can indicate weight loss, not metabolic decompensation. Individuals with type 1 diabetes who are restricting calories to lose weight require decreased dosages of insulin to prevent hypoglycemia. Too much of a reduction of insulin will result in hyperglycemia, ketonuria, and, if not corrected, metabolic decompensation to ketoacidosis.

Three ketone bodies are formed from the conversion of free fatty acids in the liver: acetoacetate, 3-13-hydroxybutyrate, and acetone. Urinary ketones are detected by the nitroprusside reaction in the treatment of acute diabetic ketoacidosis. The nitroprusside reagent predominantly reacts with acetoacetate and does not react with 13-hydroxybutyrate. Following the institution of insulin therapy, the concentration of acetoacetate increases and 13-hydroxybutyrate decreases. This shift accounts for the clinical observation that urine ketone test results may become more positive during the early phase of therapy and indicate clinical improvement rather than deterioration.

Rapid enzymatic methods have been developed to quantify 3-13-hydroxybutyrate levels in small-volume blood samples. These systems are designed for use at home and can measure 3-13-hydroxybutyrate levels on fingerstick blood samples.[33]

See also the section on ketone testing in chapter 9, on type 1 diabetes.

Long-Term Monitoring of Metabolic Control

A1C Measurement

A1C, the most abundant minor hemoglobin component in the red blood cell, increases in proportion to the blood glucose level over the preceding 3 to 4 months. Because the red blood cell has a life span of 90 to 120 days, the measurement of A1C reflects the blood glucose concentration over that period of time. The A1C test is an accurate, objective measure of chronic glycemia in persons with diabetes. A1C is the current preferred term, evolving from hemoglobin A1C and HbA1c.

Glycosylation occurs as glucose in the plasma attaches itself to the hemoglobin component of the red blood cell; this process is irreversible. The more glycosylation, the higher the values. The glycosylated hemoglobin (GHb) does not reflect the simple mean, but reflects the weighted mean over a long period of time.[26] The traditional idea that GHb reflects the simple mean and is referred to as the average of the blood glucose is inaccurate. For example, in an A1C measured on May 1, 50% of the A1C level is determined by the plasma glucose level during the preceding 1-month period (April), 25% of its level is determined by the plasma glucose level during the 1-month period before that (March), and the remaining 25% is determined by the plasma glucose level during the 2-month period before the past 2 months (February and January).

Measurement Methods

GHb can be measured by many different methods. Accurate interpretation requires knowledge of the method used to determine the GHb level, the component measured, and the normal range for the particular assay.

- *Affinity chromatography and colorimetric assay* methods measure total GHb, including all fractions of the hemoglobin molecule: HbA1a, HbA1b, and HbA1c.[20] Upper normal values of GHb may be in the range of 8% to 9%.
- *Ion-exchange chromatography, high-performance liquid chromatography (HPLC), and immunoassay* methods are used to measure A1C. The normal value is usually in the range of 4% to 6%.

Some laboratories measure total GHb, but report the ADA treatment goal of <7% in the reference range column, instead of listing the actual reference range of up to 9%. This may have clinical relevance if healthcare providers compare values from different laboratories. A result of 7.8% would be considered out of range if the reference range is 4.0% to 6.0% and within range if the reference range was 5.0% to 8.0%. The National Glycohemoglobin Standardization Program is an effort designed to encourage laboratories to standardized and report all glycosylated hemoglobin assays in values equivalent to the A1C as measured in the Diabetes Control and Complications Trial (DCCT).[34,35]

Interfering factors (sickle-cell hemoglobin and other hemoglobinopathies) may affect measurement of A1C level, depending on the method.[36]

A1C measurement is not a diagnostic test

A1C measurement is not currently recommended for diagnosis of diabetes, as it is an average of blood glucose levels for 3 to 4 months and not considered diagnostic. It is important to discuss with patients that both fingerstick checks and A1C testing are important to give both the day-to-day and longer term pictures of glycemic control.

Frequency of A1C Testing

Regular measurements of A1C permit timely detection of departures from the target range. In the absence of well-controlled studies that suggest a definite testing protocol, both the ADA[3] and ACE[37] suggest GHb testing at least once or twice a year for persons with a history of stable glycemic control and at least quarterly in those whose therapy has changed or who are in poor control.

Glycemic targets should be individualized for each individual. The DCCT[27] conclusively demonstrated, however, that the risk of retinopathy, nephropathy, and neuropathy in individuals with type 1 diabetes is reduced by intensive treatment regimens, as compared with conventional treatment regimens. These benefits were observed with an average A1C of 7.2% (normal range being 4.0%

to 6.0%) in the intensively treated group. The reduction in risk of these complications correlated continuously with the reduction in A1C produced by intensive therapy.[3] In the epidemiologic analysis of the UK Prospective Diabetes Study (UKPDS) data, the risk for occurrence of microvascular and macrovascular complications was shown to increase at A1C values of 6.5% or more.[38]

Hyperglycemia-induced oxidative stress is the chief underlying mechanism of glucose-mediated vascular damage. The hypothesis by Hirsch and Brownlee was that glycemic excursions were of greater frequency and magnitude among conventionally treated patients, who received fewer insulin injections. Subsequent studies correlating the magnitude of oxidative stress with fluctuating levels of glycemia support the hypothesis that glucose variability, considered in combination with A1C, may be a more reliable indicator of BG control and the risk for long-term complications than mean A1C alone.[39]

Glycemic Targets

Table 32.1, appearing earlier in the chapter, lists the glycemic goals established by the ADA and American College of Endocrinology (ACE); the reference range is 4.0% to 6.0%. A GHb result within the nondiabetic reference range may reflect frequent hypoglycemia and requires further evaluation. The GHb is a strong indicator of blood glucose control when compared with SMBG results.

GHb is a teaching tool as well as a marker of metabolic control. If an individual monitors only fasting blood glucose levels and finds values in the normal range but has an A1C result of 9.8% (normal range being 4.0% to 6.0%), the educator can encourage this individual to monitor at other times of the day (especially postprandial readings) to uncover periods of elevated blood glucose and identify the factors that may be associated with the elevated results.

Table 32.5 lists the correlation between A1C levels and mean plasma blood glucose levels based on data from the DCCT. Although this information may be helpful to clinicians in defining the relationship between plasma glucose and A1C, it is not appropriate for diabetes self-management education (DSME). For DSME, the educator would focus on helping the individual with diabetes develop an action plan designed to bring the A1C closer to goal.

Home A1C Testing

At-home A1C testing is available. Most products are certified by the National Glycohemoglobin Standardization Program. Insurance reimbursement varies with the insurance plan and the type of product.

TABLE 32.5 Correlation Between A1C Level and Mean Plasma Glucose Levels on Multiple Testing Over 2 to 3 Months

	Mean Plasma Glucose	
A1C (%)	*mg/dL*	*mmol/L*
6	135	7.5
7	170	9.5
8	205	11.5
9	240	13.5
10	275	15.5
11	310	17.5
12	345	19.5

Source: Modified with permission from the American Diabetes Association. Copyright © 2006 American Diabetes Association. Standards of medical care in diabetes, 2006. Diabetes Care. 2006;26suppl 1:S4-42.

Fructosamine Measurement

Fructosamine: glycosylated serum (fructosamine), a glycated serum protein test, measures glycemic control over 2 to 3 weeks. Normal ranges vary among the different methods of measurements. Fructosamine values are used in short-term follow-up of interventions that have been recently implemented to lower blood glucose or when there is a discrepancy between A1C level and the individual's reported blood glucose readings.[2] Fructosamine values may be useful in evaluation of recent glycemic control in gestational diabetes.

Monitoring for the Prevention and Management of Complications

Preventing and delaying the onset of the chronic complications of diabetes is an important part of patient care and education. These complications are discussed in detail in a number of other chapters in this book. Chapter 20 provides an overview of the topics and chapters 21 through 24 provide detail on specific conditions—namely, macrovascular disease, eye disease, diabetic kidney disease, and neuropathy (chapter 20 also covers foot and dental care). Within these chapters, guidance can be found on monitoring for the prevention and management of complications. More on hypertension and dyslipidemia in persons with diabetes can also be found in chapter 18. Standards of care regarding the complications of diabetes are also discussed at length in chapter 35, where the focus is on reducing risks. Below are highlights.

Cardiovascular Disease

Cardiovascular disease (CVD) is the major cause of mortality for persons with diabetes. Studies have shown the efficacy of reducing cardiovascular risk factors in preventing or slowing CVD. Monitoring blood pressure and blood lipids for the prevention and management of cardiovascular risk is considered part of the management of diabetes. Appropriate monitoring for each is briefly summarized in the paragraphs below. The presence of microalbuminuria is also a well-established marker of cardiovascular risk.[40] See monitoring information in the discussion of kidney disease that follows.

Target Blood Pressure Goals[24]

- Adults with diabetes: 130/80 mm Hg

Target Lipid Goals[24]

- *LDL-C:* <100 mg/dL (<2.6 mmol/L)*
- *HDL-C (men):* >40 mg/dL (>1.1 mmol/L)
- *HDL-C (women):* >50 mg/dL (>1.3 mmol/L)
- *Triglycerides:* <150 mg/dL (<1.7 mmol/L)

*Following the recommendations of the National Cholesterol Education Program's Report of the Expert Panel of Blood Cholesterol Levels in Children and Adolescents, LDL-C should be lowered to <110 mg/dL (<2.8 mmol/L) in children with cardiovascular risk factors in addition to diabetes.[41]

Hypertension

Hypertension is likely to be present in type 2 diabetes as part of the metabolic syndrome that is accompanied by high rates of CVD. In type 1 diabetes, hypertension is often the result of underlying nephropathy. See the sidebar for goals. See also the relevant material on both children and adults in chapter 20, on reducing risks, and chapter 21, on macrovascular disease, including the classification of hypertension in adults in Table 21.5

Dyslipidemia

Persons with type 2 diabetes have an increased prevalence of lipid abnormalities that contributes to higher rates of CVD. Lipid management aimed at lowering low-density lipoprotein cholesterol (LDL-C), raising high-density lipoprotein cholesterol (HDL-C), and lowering triglycerides has been shown to reduce macrovascular disease and mortality in persons with type 2 diabetes, especially those who have had prior cardiovascular events. See the sidebar for goals relevant material on both adults and children in chapter 35, on reducing risks, and the many pertinent tables in chapter 21, on macrovascular disease.

Liver Disease

Persons taking thiazolidinediones (Avandia and Actos) and HMG-CoA reductase inhibitors require periodic monitoring of liver function.

Kidney Disease

The ability to detect low levels of albumin in the urine (microalbuminuria) represents an important advancement in the diagnosis and treatment of diabetic kidney disease. The presence of microalbuminuria represents an early phase of nephropathy as well as a well-established marker of cardiovascular risk.[40]

In healthy individuals, small amounts of albumin can be found in the urine with a mean albumin excretion rate of 10 ± 3 mg per day (7 ± 2 mcg per minute).[42]

Frequency of Screening

The ADA Clinical Practice Recommendations state that an annual screening for the presence of urine microalbumin should be done in individuals with type 1 diabetes when they have had diabetes for 5 years' duration. Because of the difficulty in precise dating of type 2 diabetes, urinary microalbumin screening should begin at the time of diagnosis and also occur during pregnancy.[24]

Screening Methods

Screening for microalbuminuria can be performed by 3 methods: measurement of the albumin-to-creatinine ratio in a random spot collection, a 24-hour collection with creatinine, allowing the simultaneous measurement of creatinine clearance, or a timed (eg, 4-hour or overnight) collection. However, the analysis of a spot sample for the albumin-to-creatinine ratio is strongly recommended by authorities. The alternatives (24-hour collection and a timed specimen) are rarely necessary. See Table 32.6 for definitions of abnormalities in albumin excretion.

The reagent used in urinalysis test strips (Albustix) does not screen for microalbuminuria because it does not become positive until the albumin excretion rate (AER) exceeds 300 mg in 24 hours (200 mcg per minute).

TABLE 32.6 Definitions of Abnormalities in Albumin Excretion

Category	*Spot collection (mcg/mg creatinine)*
Normal	<30
Microalbuminuria	30 to 299
Macro- (clinical) albuminuria	≥300

Because of variability in urinary albumin excretion, 2 of 3 specimens collected within a 3- to 6-month period should be abnormal before considering a patient to have crossed one of these diagnostic thresholds. Exercise within 24 hours, infection, fever, congestive heart failure, marked hyperglycemia, and marked hypertension may elevate urinary albumin excretion over baseline values.

Source: Modified with permission from the American Diabetes Association. Copyright © 2006 American Diabetes Association. Standards of medical care in diabetes, 2006. Diabetes Care. 2006;26suppl 1:S4-42.

Contraindications

Screening for microalbuminuria should be avoided if the individual has a urinary tract infection, hematuria, fever, congestive heart failure, marked hyperglycemia, or marked hypertension or is menstruating or has exercised within 24 hours.[43]

See chapter 22, on diabetic kidney disease, and chapter 35, on reducing risks, for more complete information.

Assessment of Growth and Weight

Monitoring also involves assessment and tracking of growth in children, using height and weight charts, and weight gain in pregnancy. Obesity and central obesity are also factors to monitor. Brief information is given on each of these topics. More detail can be found in the specific chapters that discuss them: see especially chapter 9 for type 1 diabetes, chapter 10 for type 2 diabetes, and chapters 11 and 12 for pregnancy with preexisting diabetes and gestational diabetes mellitus.

Children With Type 1 Diabetes

For children with type 1 diabetes, adequate calories and insulinization are essential to promote euglycemia and optimal growth.

Children With Type 2 Diabetes

For children with type 2 diabetes, body mass index (BMI) is charted, as it is a more appropriate calculation for them. With the increased incidence of type 2 in children, a 4-year-old with a BMI plotted between the 85th and 95th percentiles for BMI-for-age and BMI-for-gender (also defined as at risk for overweight or overweight) has a 20% chance that overweight and obesity will continue into adulthood.[44] This information should be shared with the parents, and a lifestyle type of family plan can be emphasized in a nonjudgmental manner.

Pregnant Women

Tracking weight gain during pregnancy is also important. A weight chart is helpful for tracking.

Obesity and Central Obesity

Waist circumference measurement taken after inspiration and expiration at the midpoint between the lowest rib and iliac crest is helpful in identifying individuals with the metabolic syndrome. A waist circumference of greater than 40 in (102 cm) in men and 35 in (88 cm) in women has been identified as a risk factor for the metabolic syndrome.[45]

More information, including weight guidelines from the National Institutes of Health and World Health Organization, can be found in chapter 2, which focuses on disease prevention.

Documentation of weight is considered another indicator for diabetes management. Weight gain may reflect improvement in glycemic control, increased caloric consumption, frequent episodes of hypoglycemia, fluid retention, and eating disorders, among other conditions. Similarly, weight loss may reflect elevated blood glucose levels, decreased caloric consumption, or eating disorders. Fluctuations in weight can occur depending on the scale used and time of day.

Recap of Educational Considerations

There are a variety of meters available for monitoring blood glucose, and one meter that can also test for the presence of blood ketones. While the basic procedure used for testing BG is comparable between all meters (ie, turn on the meter, wait for signal/icon on screen to indicate that a blood drop may be applied, apply blood sample, and wait for results), each meter is unique. Differences were discussed earlier in this chapter, in the section on selecting a meter.

Diabetes educators are pivotal in guiding individuals to select the meter most appropriate for them and one for which they can easily obtain supplies. An individual's visual acuity and dexterity skills and insurance coverage need to be considered before recommending a specific meter.

Some insurers only cover the costs of certain meters and test strips, so having persons check on what is covered by their insurance plan (prior to their diabetes education

Case Wrap-Up

What are the key issues for the diabetes educator to address at this visit, related to SMBG?
KB had voiced a concern that he did not want his friends to know he had diabetes. It was thus important to talk with KB about what he foresaw as the consequences if he shared that he had diabetes with his friends. Once these concerns were identified, KB and the diabetes educator could then discuss the potential benefits and potentially negative consequences of a person not letting friends and family know about a medical condition and its treatment. The educator might suggest that KB first talk with relatives and other members of his tribe who have diabetes and associated complications. This would enable him to learn about what they might have done differently with their management if they had been diagnosed with type 2 diabetes at an early age and received diabetes self-management education. In addition, providing education about what it means to manage diabetes *well* and the value of SMBG as an important component of management were critical points to be discussed with KB.

What behaviors, related to SMBG, should be discussed with KB?
Since KB was a young person and newly diagnosed, the core components of treatment (ie, healthy eating and being active) needed to be discussed. The value of SMBG testing and using these results to help evaluate effectiveness of changes in the meal plan, exercise, and the effect of medication were to be emphasized. Table 32.3 lists the aspects of BG monitoring that needed to be reviewed with KB and his uncle.

List 1 behavioral goal, related to SMBG, that KB might identify to work on before the next appointment.
"I will test my BG twice daily, before breakfast and 2 hours after a meal (meals on a rotating basis) and record in my logbook."

As discussed in chapter 26, on DSME planning, the diabetes educator needed to help KB to establish goals that were SMART (specific, measurable, achievable, realistic, and time-bound).

List 1 clinical goal for KB.
At the end of the 3-month period, KB's A1C value will be 1% lower than at the present time (goal of 6.8%).

What should be included in the documentation for the initial visit?
Regarding monitoring, documentation regarding the initial visit with KB should include the following:

- Educational topics discussed
- Level of support by family members or friends (eg, who accompanied KB to the visit and what were their comments, positive or negative?)
- What type of BG meter was provided; whether he was able to master the skills of testing and return the demonstration
- KB's stated or suggested receptiveness to SMBG
- Identification of fears or hesitations related to carrying out the identified goals
- Plan for follow-up

What would you evaluate on a return visit with KB, specific to BG monitoring?

- Progress toward previously identified behavioral goals for frequency of monitoring
- Review of BG testing results (supplied by written records or BG meter memory)
- Use of BG testing results in the decision-making process for diabetes management
- Identification of barriers and potential solutions

At his return visit, KB related the following progress toward previously identified goals:

- He had switched from drinking regular to diet soda.
- He had begun to play basketball on an intramural tribal league 2 or 3 times a week.
- He said he had been testing BG in the morning before breakfast, but he had not been writing the data down. He forgot to bring his meter to the return visit; however, he said that he had been testing BG at fasting only, up until about 1 week ago. Values had been running between 130 to 140mg/dl at that time. When asked why he had quit testing, he said that he had run out of test strips and

(continued)

Case Wrap-Up (continued)

had not made time to pick more up from the pharmacy.

- He had been taking his metformin in the mornings only.
- His body weight had decreased by 2 lb.

What successes aided KB, and what barriers might potentially have prevented him from making desired behavior changes?

- First, recognize all the changes that KB had made and congratulate him on his accomplishments. Remember that BG monitoring is but *one* of several components of management that were suggested to KB. Ask to review his logbook with him, and ask him what things had enabled him to make positive changes in eating habits, increasing activity level, taking medication, testing once a day, and managing to lose 2 lb.
- Ask him to describe the challenges he was having with his management. What did he identify as barriers?
- KB's insecurity about how he would be accepted by peers with a diagnosis of diabetes might cause him to deny it and in turn, make him hesitant to check BG at a time of day when he was out with friends.
- The family had limited food dollars, so less access to healthier foods.
- KB had a sense of fatalism, related to poor health outcomes of other family members, and was indulging the position of "why does it matter anyway."

What barrier resolutions might impact his goals for BG monitoring?

- Suggest that KB consider alternative BG testing times, to help get a picture of his levels at times of the day other than just when fasting. Perhaps he would consider checking after breakfast or lunch on weekend days and after dinner in the evenings when he was home.
- Ask KB's permission to talk with school personnel about presenting an in-service to the student body on diabetes prevention and treatment, so that other students would understand the components of good management, which include BG monitoring. Since diabetes is so prevalent in Native American communities, the information presented on prevention would be beneficial for others as well. Community leaders who have had experiences with diabetes and could provide testament to the benefits of good control and detriments of poor control should also be invited to participate.
- Since KB and his uncle were said to have a close relationship, encourage them to problem solve how they could spend time together, participating in healthy lifestyle activities. Suggest to KB that he and his uncle talk with members of the Tribal Council about organizing a support group or talking circle in the community; healthcare professionals could be invited to talk about various health-related topics, such as prediabetes and diabetes. Incentives are used frequently in Native American communities to encourage people to attend various activities and programs. Perhaps these could also be incorporated into a Wellness program series that KB and his uncle could help organize.

visit) helps save time and prevent frustration. This also applies to individuals who obtain their meter and supplies through Veterans Affairs hospitals, county hospitals, or certain community programs..

Some insurance plans provide coverage for a variety of meters and supplies. If this is the case, a demonstration of several meters should be provided and the person with diabetes given the opportunity to "practice" using them. Many diabetes education centers, provider offices, and clinics are provided with free starter kits (meter, lancing device, and a small number of test strips and lancets) so that people can leave their appointments with their meter in hand.

Ask patients to bring their meters and all supplies to each visit. The meter can be cleaned, the strips and control solution can be tested, codes can be verified, and an actual blood glucose measurement can be performed.

Provide patients with the toll-free customer service number for the manufacturer of their meter. Experts are available at this number 24 hours a day to answer questions and provide assistance.

Careful and safe disposal of used lancets is critical. Teach people to dispose of used lancets in an appropriate sharps container (regulations vary from state to state). When monitoring blood glucose away from home, people can place their used lancets in an empty pill container or 35-mm film canister.

Consider the cost of supplies when the person decides on the frequency of monitoring. Be familiar with local suppliers who charge reasonable prices. Refer individuals to a social worker or community agency when appropriate.

Some individuals benefit from having a second meter that is compact, quick, and simple to use for easily checking their blood glucose level away from home or before driving. BG monitoring results will be most consistent if the same model of a meter is used all the time. If an individual chooses to use more than one type of meter, then the readings obtained from each should be identified as such in logbook.

Postprandial monitoring is effective for teaching the impact of food portions on blood glucose levels. For example, an individual may choose a meal high in carbohydrate content and have an elevated blood glucose reading 2 hours later, whereas after eating the same foods in smaller portions, the person may find the postprandial reading to be within goal range.

Teach the individual to record BG data in the logbook with the testing time and results recorded in linear and vertical fashion so the data can be more easily interpreted and patterns identified.

Recording BG levels on a graph, as well as having a numerical listing, provides a useful visual aid for teaching the concept of blood glucose patterns. Computer software marketed by meter manufacturers can be very helpful in providing graphs and other visual representations of the data.

If the person has stopped monitoring, investigate. Common causes are emotional reactions to elevated or fluctuating readings, consistent readings within range, discomfort related to lancing the skin, emotional response to blood letting or skin piercing, cost, inconvenience, and collection of meaningless data. As part of the assessment simply ask, "Is it helpful?"

Actual BG records of common patterns should be used when teaching self-management.

Provide the person with the opportunity to practice testing for urinary or serum ketones during the teaching appointment.

A supply sheet, signed by the healthcare provider, can be an effective organizational aid for the person with diabetes and the pharmacist and may serve as a prescription.

Teaching the concept of glycosylated hemoglobin can be challenging. This test can be referred to as the blood test with a memory that represents blood glucose levels over the last 3 months. A1C can be thought of as a long-term monitoring method as opposed to the day-to-day self-monitoring measurements that are performed with a home meter.

Avoid referring to A1C as an average of blood glucose levels. Besides being technically inaccurate, this language can lead persons to confuse A1C with the average in their meter memory.

The educator can use a picture of a pyramid or a thermometer to outline the various A1C levels and then demonstrate the goal range and the individual's most recent result. Ask individuals what they think about the results and what they would like to do about them, rather than offering judgments.

SMBG Basic Patient Education Components

- Focus the teaching session on the meaning of the BG results.
- Help the individual identify target ranges and review the dynamic nature of blood glucose so the person will expect fluctuations.
- Help the person choose a monitoring schedule that will provide meaningful data.
- Guide the individual in choosing a system for documentation of the readings, either using a written logbook, electronic logbook, or computer program. Documentation includes more than just the blood glucose reading; it also includes notes concerning food, activity, stress, and medication. Reinforce the importance of bringing this written documentation to clinic or diabetes education visits, so it can be reviewed with the other members of the healthcare team and informed decisions can be made about changes needed in the diabetes management plan.
- Choice of meter will depend on insurance reimbursement, an assessment of manual dexterity and visual acuity, plus the individual's unique needs or desires.
- Create the expectation that the person with diabetes will benefit from knowing the A1C results. Include the current A1C result, normal range, target range, and date for the next A1C test. Together, outline a plan for reaching that person's target range.
- Ketone testing is part of basic education for persons with type 1 diabetes, gestational diabetes, and pregnancy with preexisting diabetes.
- Advanced education components include benefits of monitoring urine for protein, ketone monitoring for persons with type 2 diabetes as part of sick day rules, and use of the data provided by SMBG.

See also Table 32.2 for guidelines for teaching how to use a BG meter and Table 32.3 for a summary of uses of BG data by those with diabetes.

Quick Summary on Monitoring in Pregnancy

- More frequent monitoring is beneficial during pregnancy to control and improve outcomes.
- As noted earlier, gestational diabetes or pregnancy complicated by diabetes may benefit from measuring blood glucose 1 hour after a meal.
- Teach pregnant women who check blood glucose levels 1 hour after a meal the difference between fingertip and alternative-site samples—differences of up to 100 mg/dL (5.6 mmol/L) have been reported, as explained earlier.
- A disadvantage of urine testing for glucose is that renal thresholds may be low in pregnancy.
- In gestational diabetes, fructosamine values may be useful in evaluation of recent glycemic control.
- Ketone testing is part of basic education for pregnant women with diabetes.
- Pregnant women with diabetes (including gestational diabetes) are often advised to monitor urinary ketones after an overnight fast. As noted earlier, these measurements are useful for detecting inadequate food intake (starvation ketosis) and warning of impending metabolic decompensation.
- Tracking weight gain during pregnancy is also important. A weight chart is helpful.

See also the section on monitoring in chapter 11, on pregnancy with preexisting diabetes, and the sections on glucose control and monitoring in chapter 12, on gestational diabetes mellitus.

Summary

Since SMBG is one of the essential tools of self-management, diabetes educators have the unique opportunity and responsibility to provide instruction concerning not only monitoring techniques, but also use of the data. Diabetes educators can teach individuals to approach monitoring as feedback (ie, helpful information) rather than evaluation (ie, punishment). Teach individuals that the results of monitoring metabolic control in the various ways provide more than feedback; they reinforce their active role in self-management and their position as the center of the healthcare team.

This chapter focused primarily on SMBG—the factors that affect the accuracy of SMBG results, the use of SMBG data by persons with diabetes, the current data systems available, and the SMBG needs of special populations. Monitoring of metabolic control by the healthcare team was also summarized—including assessing GHb, reviewing BG patterns, assessing growth and patterns of weight change, and monitoring the development and progression of long-term complications, including urinary protein measurements, blood pressure measurements, and lipid levels. This area of diabetes care—monitoring—clearly combines the diabetes educator's skills of management and education.[2] Readers are encouraged to consult the chapters specific to each topic for detail on these important topics.

Focus on Education: Pearls For Practice

Teaching Strategies

Appreciate a global definition of "monitoring." Monitoring activities in diabetes care include not only blood glucose, but also those activities related to metabolic control and the chronic complications associated with diabetes.

Demonstrate empathy for the additional work of patients embracing this tool. Monitoring the many aspects of diabetes management can be an overwhelming task, even for the most dedicated and goal-directed individuals with diabetes. At clinic appointments and outpatient visits, recognize and acknowledge the work that those you are serving have done in checking and recording BG levels.

Teach not just how, but why. The diabetes educator's job is not only to teach those with diabetes the "how" of using a BG meter, but also the "why" so individuals with the disease are empowered to use the knowledge gained to make healthy, informed choices in their food intake, exercise, medication adjustments, and sick day and stress management.

Setting realistic goals for monitoring. Consider what data will best serve the individual in making informed decisions about diabetes management and obtaining a specific, yet big-picture view of the individual's glycemic control.

Messages for Patients

Make the data work for you. BG monitoring is a tool that puts diabetes management in your hands, with some assistance by others. Take advantage of the technology available to make informed decisions and improve your BG control.

References

1. Polonsky WH. Understanding and treating patients with diabetes burnout. In: Practical Psychology for Diabetes Clinicians. Anderson BJ, Rubin RR, eds. Alexandria, Va: American Diabetes Association; 2002: 183-92.
2. Peragalla-Dittko V. Monitoring. In: A Core Curriculum for Diabetes Education: Diabetes Management Therapies, 5th ed. Franz MJ, ed. Chicago, Ill: American Association of Diabetes Educators; 2003: 189-212.
3. American Diabetes Association. Self monitoring of blood glucose (consensus statement). Diabetes Care. 1994;17:81-6.
4. Mulcahy K, Maryniuk M, Peeples M, et al. Diabetes self-management education core outcomes measures. Diabetes Educ. 2003;29:768-88.
5. Peeples M, Mulcahy K, Tomky D, Weaver T. National Diabetes Education Outcomes System (NDEOS). The conceptual framework of the National Diabetes Education Outcomes System (NDEOS). Diabetes Educ. 2001;27:547-62.
6. Peragallo-Dittko V. The lowdown on lancets and lancing devices. Diabetes Self-Manage. 1999;16(3): 64-71.
7. Peragallo-Dittko V. How accurate is your meter? Diabetes Self-Manage. 2000;17(5):78-85.
8. Jungheim K, Koschinsky T. Risky delay of hypoglycemia detection by glucose monitoring at the arm (letter). Diabetes Care. 2001;24:1303-6.
9. Harris MI, Crowe CC, Howie LJ. Self-monitoring of blood glucose by adults with diabetes in the United States population. Diabetes Care. 1993;16:1116-23.
10. Babione L. SMBG: the underused nutrition counseling tool in diabetes management. Diabetes Spectrum. 1994;7:196-7.
11. Ahern JA, Gatcomb PM, Held NA, Petit WA Jr, Tamborlane WV. Exaggerated hyperglycemia after a pizza meal in well-controlled diabetes. Diabetes Care. 1993;16:578-80.
12. Rubin RR, Peyrot M, Saudek CD. The effect of a diabetes education program incorporating coping skills training on emotional well-being and diabetes self-efficacy. Diabetes Educ. 1993;19:210-4.
13. Price MJ. Qualitative analysis of the patient-provider interactions: the patient's perspective. Diabetes Educ. 1989;15:144-8.
14. Cox DJ, Irvine A, Gonder-Frederick L, Nowacek G, Butterfield J. Fear of hypoglycemia: quantification, validation and utilization. Diabetes Care. 1987;10:617-21.
15. Austin MA, Kulkarni K, Powers MA. Blood Glucose Monitoring: Essential Skills for Health Care Professionals, 3rd ed. St. Paul, Minn: PT Publications; 2003.
16. Clarke WL, Cox D, Gonder-Frederick LA, Carter W, Pohl SL. Evaluating clinical accuracy of systems for self-monitoring of blood glucose. Diabetes Care. 1987;10:622-8.
17. Bastyr EJ III, Stuart CA, Broddows RG, et al. Therapy focused on lowering post-prandial glucose, not fasting

glucose, may be superior for lowering HbA1c. Diabetes Care. 2000;23:1236-41.

18. American Diabetes Association. Postprandial blood glucose (consensus statement). Diabetes Care. 2001;24:775-8.
19. Monnier L, Lapinski H, Colette C. Contributions of fasting and postprandial plasma glucose increments to the overall diurnal hyperglycemia of type 2 diabetic patients. Diabetes Care. 2003;26(3):991-5.
20. Walker EA. Quality assurance for blood glucose monitoring. Nurs Clin North Am. 1993;28:61-70.
21. American Diabetes Association. CLIA guidelines implemented. Diabetes Rev. 1993;1:30.
22. Peragallo-Dittko V. Clinical and educational usefulness of SMBG with the elderly. Diabetes Spectrum. 1995;8:17-9.
23. Bernbaum M, Albert SG, Brusca S, et al. Effectiveness of glucose monitoring systems modified for the visually impaired. Diabetes Care. 1993;16:1363-6.
24. American Diabetes Association. Standards of Medical Care in Diabetes-2006. Diabetes Care. 2006;29suppl 1:S4-42.
25. Clement S, Braithwaite SS, Magee MF, et al on behalf of the Diabetes in Hospitals Writing Committee. Management of diabetes and hyperglycemia in hospitals (technical review). Diabetes Care. 2004;27:553-91.
26. Block JM, Continuous glucose sensing technology: the latest in the evolution of glucose trend detection. On The Cutting Edge, DCE. Summer 2005:26(4).
27. Boland E, Monsod T, Delucia M, et al. Limitations of conventional methods of self monitoring of blood glucose. Diabetes Care .2001;24(11):858-62.
28. Jeha GS, Karaviti LP, Anderson B, et al. Continuous glucose monitoring and the reality of metabolic control in preschool children with type 1 diabetes. Diabetes Care. 2004;27(12):2,881-86.
29. Klonoff DC. Noninvasive blood glucose monitoring. Diabetes Care. 1997;20:433-7.
30. Fajans SS. Classification and diagnosis of diabetes. In: Ellenberg and Rifkin's Diabetes Mellitus: Theory and Practice, 5th ed. Porte D Jr, Sherwin RS, eds. Stamford, Conn: Appleton and Lang; 1997:357-72.
31. American Diabetes Association. Hyperglycemic crises in diabetes. Diabetes Care. 2004;27(Suppl 1): S94-S102.
32. Metzger BE, Phelps RL, Dooley SL. The mother in pregnancies complicated by diabetes mellitus. In: Ellenberg and Rifkin's Diabetes Mellitus: Theory and Practice, 5th ed. Porte D Jr, Sherwin RS, eds. Stamford, Ct: Appleton and Lange; 1997: 887-915.
33. Laffel L. Ketone bodies: a review of physiology, pathophysiology and application of monitoring to diabetes. Diabetes Metab Res Rev. 1999;15:412-26.
34. The Diabetes Control and Complications Trial Research Group. The effect of intensive treatment of diabetes on the development and progression of long-term complications of insulin-dependent diabetes. N Engl J Med. 1993;329:77-86.
35. American Diabetes Association. Tests of glycemia in diabetes (position statement). Diabetes Care. 2003;26(Suppl 1):S106-S108.
36. Goldstein DE, Little RR. More than you ever wanted to know (but need to know) about glycohemoglobin testing. Diabetes Care. 1994;17:938-9.
37. American College of Endocrinology. Guidelines for glycemic control (consensus statement). Endocrine Practice. 2002;8(Suppl 1):6-11.
38. Stratton IM, Adler AI, Neil HA, et al. Association of glycaemia with macrovascular and microvascular complications of type 2 diabetes (UKPDS 35): prospective observational study. BMJ. 2000;321:405-12
39. Hirsch I, Brownlee M. Should minimal blood glucose variability become the gold standard of glycemic control? J Diabetes Complicat. 2005;19:178-81.
40. Gall MA, Hougaard P, Borch-Johnsen K, et al. Risk factors for development of incipient and overt diabetic nephropathy in patients with non-insulin dependent diabetes mellitus: prospective, observational study. BMJ. 1997;314:783-8.
41. The Expert Panel of Blood Cholesterol Levels in Children and Adolescents. Treatment recommendations of the National Cholesterol Education Program Report of the Expert Panel on Blood Cholesterol Levels in Children and Adolescents. Pediatrics. 1992;89suppl:525-84.
42. DeFronzo RA. Diabetic nephropathy. In: Ellenberg and Rifkin's Diabetes Mellitus: Theory and Practice, 5th ed. Porte D Jr, Sherwin RS, eds. Stamford, Conn: Appleton and Lange; 1997:971-1008.
43. Morgensen CE, Vestbo E, Poulsen PL, et al. Microalbuminuria and potential con-founders. Diabetes Care. 1995;18:572-81.

44. US Department of Labor, Bureau of Labor Statistics. National Longitudinal Survey of Youth, 1986-1997. Available on the Internet at: www.bls.gov/nls/nlsy97.htm. Accessed 7 Sept 2004.

45. National Institutes of Health, National Heart, Lung, and Blood Institute. Clinical guidelines on the identification, evaluation, and treatment of overweight and obesity in adults—the evidence report. Obes Res. 1998;6:51S-209S.

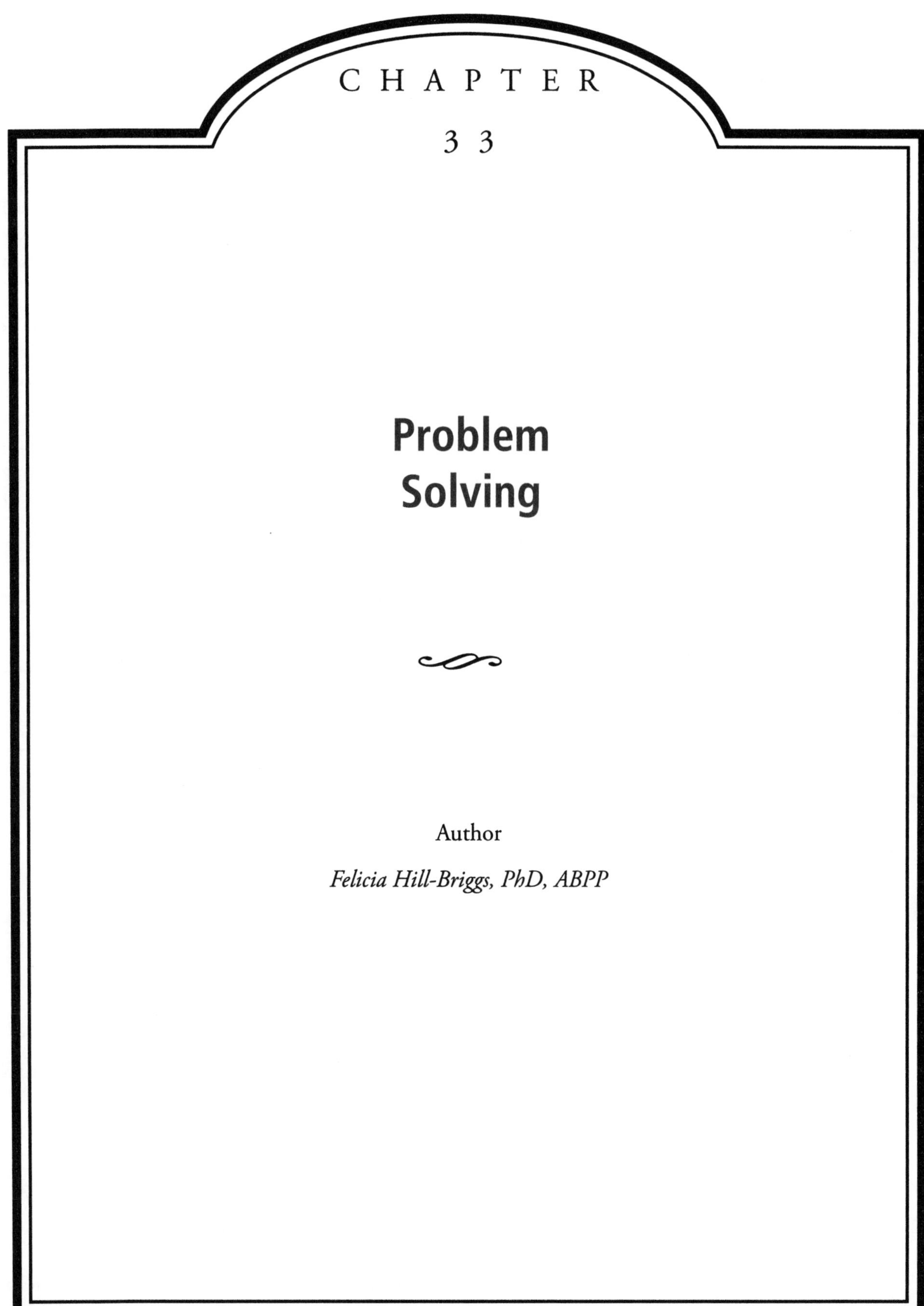

CHAPTER 33

Problem Solving

Author

Felicia Hill-Briggs, PhD, ABPP

Key Concepts

What is problem solving?

- Understanding what problem solving is (a definition) and using a theoretical model that identifies 5 components of problem solving

Using problem solving in diabetes self-management and education

- When to use direct instruction versus problem solving
- Identifying and assessing problems and barriers that impact diabetes self-management
- Recognizing that problems and barriers that affect diabetes self-management occur on 3 different levels: there are clinical markers and emergencies, problematic self-management behaviors, and problems impacting self-management
- Learning to drill down to identify the fundamental problem affecting the self-care behavior
- Applying problem-solving in diabetes education and counseling; choosing the right approach: when to be the problem solver, when to enlist the patient's contributions in problem solving, and when to further empower the individual in problem solving

Empowering the person with diabetes as a problem solver

- Assessing the individual's problem-solving ability and style when planning education and intervention, including interviewing and formal assessment tools
- Examining empirical research on diabetes problem-solving training
- Planning for problem-solving training and intervention, including strategies to use for individuals effective in problem solving as well as strategies appropriate when individuals are ineffective in problem solving due to specific reasons and situations

Recognizing special considerations and indications for problem-solving intervention:

- Recognizing cognitive impairment, age, education, ethnicity, and urgent situations

Introduction

Problem solving is an essential tool for diabetes self-management and for facilitating behavior change. As one of the AADE 7 Self-Care Behaviors™, Problem Solving can be viewed as cross-cutting in its application to Healthy Eating, Being Active, Taking Medication, Monitoring, Healthy Coping, and Reducing Risks. This chapter discusses application of problem-solving education and counseling by healthcare professionals and application of problem solving to self-management by the individual with diabetes.

> ***Problem-Solving Skills***
>
> These are not only the most difficult skill to teach; they are also the most difficult to learn.

What is Problem Solving?

> **Definition**
>
> As a core outcome of diabetes self-management education, problem solving is defined as follows:
>
> *A learned behavior that includes generating a set of potential strategies for problem resolution, selecting the most appropriate strategy, applying the strategy, and evaluating the effectiveness of the strategy.*[1(p. 788)]

Although problem solving is somewhat new to research and clinical practice as a method of training individuals in disease self-management, it has a long history in research and experimentation in the areas of psychology and behavior change. Historically, problem solving has been characterized as involving 3 components.[2,3]

- The individual is goal directed
- Reaching a solution or goal requires a sequence of mental processes
- The mental processes involved are cognitive rather than automatic

In applying this cognitive psychology definition to diabetes self-management, the goal-directed nature of diabetes self-management and regimen adherence is represented. Also represented are the effortful mental processes required to reach and maintain diabetes self-management goals. For persons with diabetes, these effortful mental processes generally evolve through education, training, and/or experiential learning rather than occurring spontaneously.[4]

Theoretical Model

Problem solving is often conceptualized as a process involving these steps:

- Identifying the problem
- Generating alternative solutions
- Selecting, implementing, and evaluating a solution

However, over time, research on problem solving has revealed problem solving to be complex and multidimensional, involving more than solely a process of logical thinking.[5] The complexity of problem solving from a theoretical perspective is consistent with the clinical observation that problem solving is the most difficult skill for diabetes educators to teach patients[6] and the most difficult skill for patients to learn.[7]

A multidimensional model of problem solving in diabetes self-management was developed as a tool to facilitate problem-solving assessment, training, and intervention in diabetes.[5] The model, which is depicted in Figure 33.1,

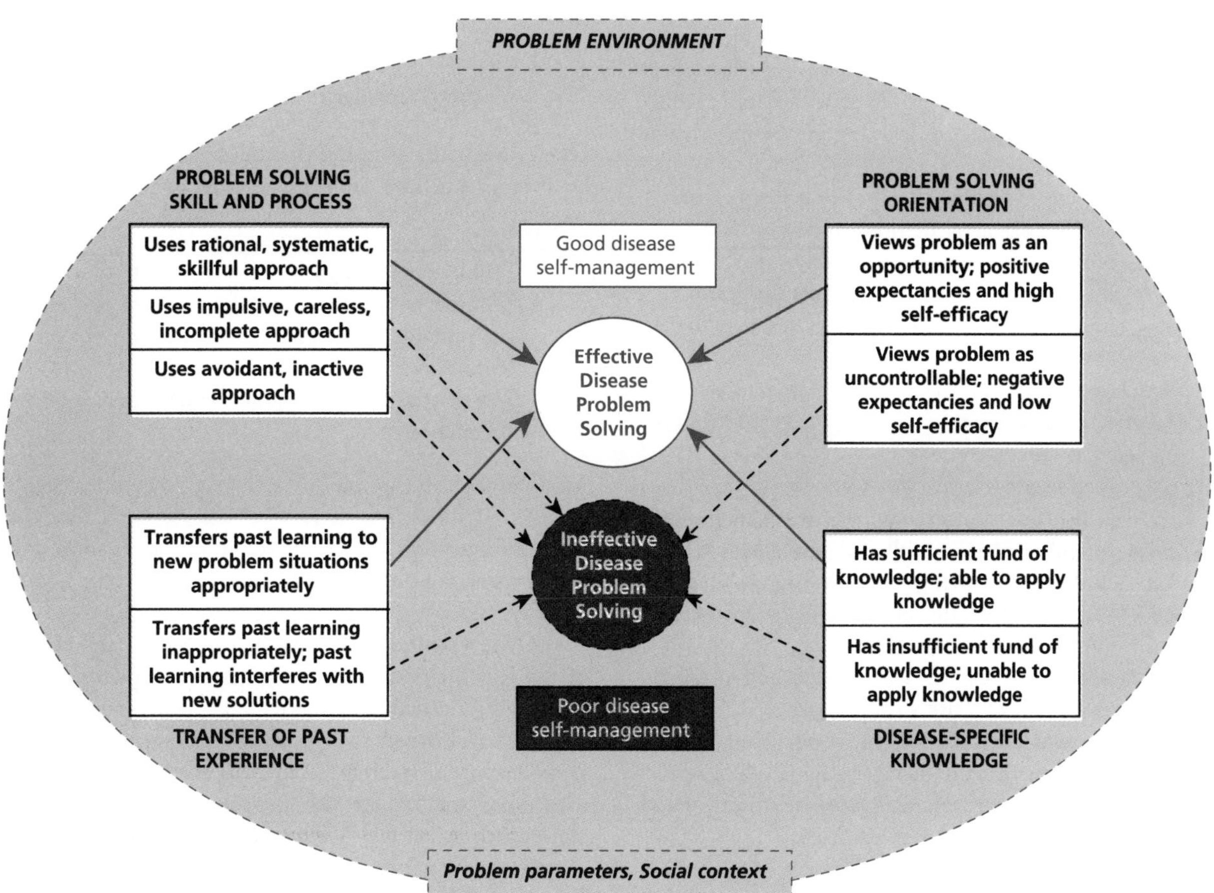

FIGURE 33.1 An Integrated Model of Problem Solving in Chronic Disease Self-Management

Source: Hill-Briggs F. Problem solving in diabetes self-management: a model of chronic illness self-management behavior. Ann Behav Med 2003;25:182-193. Reproduced by permission of Lawrence Erlbaum Associates.

integrates key components of problem solving from theories in cognitive psychology, education/learning, and social problem solving.

Components of Problem Solving

1. *Problem-Solving Skill.* Problem-solving skill represents approaches to dealing with problems and includes both effective and ineffective approaches.
   —Effective Approaches: Rational, logical
   —Ineffective Approaches: Impulsive, careless, avoidant
2. *Problem-Solving Orientation.* Problem-solving orientation or motivation reflects emotional and attitudinal cognitive sets toward dealing with diabetes-related problems and barriers. Orientation toward managing problems can be positive or negative.
   —Positive Orientation: Effective for promoting self-management
   —Negative Orientation: Ineffective for promoting self-management
3. *Transfer of Past Experience/Learning.* Problem solving leads to new learning because working through a problem creates potential for acquiring new knowledge or experience. Expert problem solvers are ones who can learn from prior experiences and apply that learning to new situations effectively. This transfer of learning can be effective or ineffective.
   —Effective Learning: Person learns from experiences and generalizes this learning to new problem situations appropriately
   —Ineffective Learning: Person does not learn from experiences or transfers experiences to new situations inappropriately
4. *Diabetes-Specific Knowledge.* A prerequisite for effective problem solving is knowledge in the problem domain.
   —Inadequate Knowledge: A knowledge base that is insufficient, inaccurate, or cannot be applied contributes to ineffective self-management
   —Adequate Knowledge: A knowledge base that is sufficient, accurate, and applicable contributes to effective self-management
5. *Problem Environment.* The above problem-solving components all exist within a problem environment, which represents the setting and context within which the problem occurs, including aspects of the person's social and physical environment and characteristics of the problem itself.

The components of this theoretical model, independently, are supported by a body of behavioral diabetes research demonstrating associations with diabetes self-management behaviors or diabetes control.[5]

Using Problem Solving in Diabetes Self-Management

Direct Instruction Versus Problem Solving

Knowledge is necessary but not sufficient for effective and maintained self-management, and problem solving requires more than knowledge or skill acquisition.[1] The healthcare professional must assess whether knowledge, through direct instruction and/or problem solving, is indicated for a given individual and presenting problem.

Situations in which direct instruction is recommended:

Direct instruction—rather than problem solving—would be recommended for problems meeting these criteria:

- Problem is well defined and straightforward[8]
- Problem has a single best strategy for resolution[8]
- Problem has a known, specific course of action that the individual with diabetes should take for problem resolution
- Use of trial and error could be detrimental or life threatening

Treating acute complications of hypoglycemia, hyperglycemia, and illness/sick days meet these criteria. See the sidebar discussing indications for direct instruction and problem-solving for hypoglycemia, hyperglycemia, and sick days.

Once the individual has mastered understanding of the specific courses of action to take and the technical skills needed to treat hyperglycemia, hypoglycemia, and sick days, then problem solving would serve as an important technique to help the individual plan to prevent and reduce risk associated with these acute complications.

Low Blood Glucose, High Blood Glucose, Sick Days: Direct Instruction or Problem Solving?

In the DSME Core Outcomes Measures, problem solving is listed as a diabetes self-care behavior to be used especially for low blood glucose, high blood glucose including ketones, and sick days.[1,72] The healthcare professional can assist* the person with diabetes through prevention, detection, and treatment in these areas.[63]

Decisions on which approach to use—direct instruction or problem solving—depend on the focus of the intervention. Is the goal prevention, detection, or treatment?

Treatment of Acute Complications of Hypoglycemia, Hyperglycemia, and Sick Days

Direct Instruction

Direct instruction is essential for educating the individual in specific courses of action to take in the treatment of these potentially life-threatening acute complications. The following are examples of types of instruction recommended for the healthcare professional's direct instruction to the person with diabetes:

- *Hypoglycemia.* Specific sources/forms of glucose for treating hypoglycemia, specific amounts of glucose for treating hypoglycemic episodes of different severities, guidelines regarding use of glucagon, and direction regarding when and whom to contact for emergency help.
- *Hyperglycemia.* Specific guidelines for treating hyperglycemia at different severities, including types and amounts of fluids for maintaining hydration, medication adjustment, and direction regarding when and whom to contact for emergency help.
- *Sick Days.* Specific guidelines for maintaining hydration, monitoring blood glucose and ketones, making adjustments to the medication regimen, and indications that signal need to contact the healthcare provider.

Detection of Hypoglycemia and Hyperglycemia

When the situation involves detection of hypoglycemia, hyperglycemia, or sick day management, a combination of direct instruction and problem solving is warranted.

Direct Instruction

This would include, for example, education about symptoms, blood glucose levels that indicate hypoglycemia or hyperglycemia requiring action, and technical skill in monitoring of blood glucose and ketones.

Problem Solving

This would include, for example, identifying specific and reliable symptoms the individual experiences during hypo- or hyperglycemia, identifying whether there are barriers to detection such as blood glucose unawareness or factors impeding sick day care, determining barriers to monitoring with appropriate frequency, and problem solving how monitoring data can be used fluidly to plan action or to adjust the regimen with regard to the individual's medication, eating, and activity.

Prevention of Hypoglycemia and Hyperglycemia

Problem Solving

For prevention, problem solving is a particularly important strategy to employ. There are many options for how preventive strategies can be incorporated. Selecting the most appropriate and effective strategies for a given individual to integrate and maintain in his/her lifestyle will result from problem solving. Problem solving can focus on identifying what unique situations tend to lead to these acute complications in the individual's life, devising tailored strategies for prevention, developing strategies to address both daily and long-term resolution of barriers to effective self-management, and planning for ongoing adjustment or maintenance of self-management behaviors for prevention.

Identifying and Assessing Problems and Barriers Impacting Diabetes Self-Management

Education or counseling that targets problem solving requires identification of the problems or barriers that are affecting diabetes self-management. Problem identification occurs on 3 different levels, listed below and elucidated in the sidebar:

- *Level 1:* Clinical markers and emergencies
- *Level 2:* Problematic self-management behaviors
- *Level 3:* Problems impacting self-management

When a person is referred for consultation due to difficulties with disease control (a Level 1 problem), assessment is needed to determine the individual's use of self-management behaviors (Level 2). (See chapter 25 for more on assessment.) To provide education and counseling to improve these behaviors, Level 3 factors must be determined. Once the Level 3 problems are identified, they become the target for problem-solving-oriented education or counseling.

Identification of Problems and Barriers

Level 1—Clinical Markers and Emergencies

- Suboptimal clinical control (eg, glycemia, blood pressure, lipids)
- Frequency and severity of acute complications (eg, hypoglycemia, hyperglycemia)
- Emergence and progression of diabetes complications
- Emergency room visits
- Preventable hospitalizations

Level 2—Problematic Self-Management Behaviors

- Unhealthy eating
- Being inactive
- Difficulties with taking medication
- Ineffective monitoring
- Difficulty coping
- Difficulty reducing risks

Level 3—Problems Impacting Self-Management

- Knowledge and understanding of self-management behaviors
- Technical skills to perform self-management behaviors
- Environmental barriers impeding implementation of self-management behaviors
- Psychosocial and emotional barriers impeding implementation of self-management behaviors

Common Problems in Diabetes Self-Management

Table 33.1 presents examples of Level 3 problems commonly documented in the literature regarding self-care behaviors:

- Taking Medication[9-13]
- Monitoring of blood glucose[12,14-16]
- Healthy Eating[12,17-22]
- Being Active[12,23-26]

Types of Barriers

Types of barriers that have been found to impact all self-management behaviors include the following:

- Emotional well-being and depression[27,28]
- Social pressures for children and adolescents[29]
- Financial barriers for middle and older adults[26,30]
- Among minority populations, socioeconomic, language, and knowledge barriers and the caregiver role[25,26,31]

For the healthcare educator, assessing and understanding these Level 3 problems is essential for comprehending the nature of the self-management problem and for ensuring that problem-solving interventions are appropriate for the unique barriers the individual is experiencing.

Measurement Tools

Formal or informal measures can be used to identify Level 3 problems.

- *Questionnaires:* Barriers can be assessed using formal measurement tools
- *Interviews:* The healthcare provider may use structured or unstructured interviewing to assess barriers

Formal measures provide the advantage of giving a broad view of problem areas and challenges across several self-management behaviors or regimen areas. For persons with diabetes who are unaware of what barriers are having an impact on their diabetes self-management, a list of several possibilities for them to consider and rate (on the extent to which they do or do not experience them) may be helpful. Formal measures can contribute to outcomes evaluation, as the healthcare professional can assess whether the number of barriers or impact of barriers has changed

TABLE 33.1 Evidence-Based Barriers to Diabetes Self-Management Behaviors (Level 3 Problems): Selected Examples

AADE 7 Self-Care Behaviors™	*Barriers*
Taking Medication	*Children and Adolescents* Technique accuracy and precision Diabetes knowledge Fear of needles/injecting *Adults* Medication knowledge Understanding of the medication regimen Perceived treatment benefits Medication side effects Medication costs Forgetting to take medications Running out of medications, forgetting to get prescriptions refilled Not using medications when out of the home or when around other people Having to take medications with food (not hungry) Number of medications Complexity of medication regimen Burden of injected insulin regimens Emotional factors
Monitoring Blood Glucose	*Children and Adolescents* Technique accuracy and precision Testing frequency Timing Diabetes knowledge Use of SMBG data Social supports Symptom beliefs Fear of hypoglycemia *Adults* Diabetes knowledge Painfulness Cost/expense Lifestyle interference Inconvenience Symptom beliefs Fear of hypoglycemia Fear of high blood glucose reading

(continued)

TABLE 33.1 Evidence-Based Barriers to Diabetes Self-Management Behaviors (Level 3 Problems): Selected Examples

AADE 7 Self-Care Behaviors™	*Barriers*
Healthy Eating	*Adolescents* Temptation to stop trying Negative emotional eating Facing forbidden foods Peer interpersonal conflict Competing priorities Eating at school Social events and holidays Food cravings Snacking when at home or when bored or alone Social pressure to eat *Adults* Negative emotions Resisting temptation to eat or to relapse Eating out Feeling deprived Time pressure Planning Competing priorities Social events, holidays, special occasions Family and friends Food refusal Expense/cost of healthy foods Difficulty with label reading Nutrition/meal planning knowledge deficit Portion size Quality of life/lifestyle Confusion or uncertainty about foods Food taste Rigid schedule or time constraints Communicating with health professionals about meal planning and constraints Hypoglycemia Not home for meals Lack of time to prepare foods Limitations of multiple aspects of diet (eg, carbohydrate, sodium, fat) Family functioning, level of support Having to eat when not hungry See sick day plan, chapter 7 (Hyperglycemia)

(continued)

TABLE 33.1 Evidence-Based Barriers to Diabetes Self-Management Behaviors (Level 3 Problems): Selected Examples

AADE 7 Self-Care Behaviors™	*Barriers*
Being Active	*Adults* Pain Time constraints Multiple responsibilities/competing demands Limited knowledge of exercises, variety Poor conditioning/functional status Unpleasant physical responses (shortness of breath, sweating, feeling ill, vertigo) Other medical conditions Hypoglycemia Distractions Lack of facilities/places to exercise Cost of facilities or equipment Vulnerability/safety concerns in environment Weather conditions (cold, rainy, windy) *Children and Adolescents* Vulnerability/safety concerns in environment Weather conditions Lack of local facilities/places to exercise (basketball courts, park, biking/walking trails, pool) Lack of parental or peer support Competing school or work activities Removal of physical education classes from school curriculum Poor conditioning Hypoglycemic episodes Cost of facilities or equipment Lack of neighborhood schools within safe walking distance

following intervention. Formal measures designed to assess problems and barriers include the following:

- *Barriers to Diabetes Self-Care Scale.*[32] This 31-item scale, originally designed for adults with type 2 diabetes, measures the frequency of environmental barriers (time, competing demands, social pressure) and cognitive barriers (eg, belief/attitude) in diabetes self-management.
- *Environmental Barriers to Adherence Scale* (EBAS).[33] EBAS subscales assess barriers in 4 regimen areas: medication, testing, exercise, and nutrition/meal planning.
- *Diabetes Distress Scale* (DDS).[34] The DDS is a measure of diabetes-related emotional distress developed from 3 former scales: the ATT39,[35] Questionnaire on Stress in Patients with Diabetes (QSD-R),[36] and Problem Areas in Diabetes (PAID).[37] The DDS assesses distress in 4 domains: emotional burden, physician-related distress, regimen-related distress, and diabetes-related interpersonal distress.

When working within a problem-solving training or education framework, one consideration for the healthcare educator is to ensure that use of a problem or barrier questionnaire does not negate the importance of problem identification as a part of the problem-solving process. When educating persons with diabetes in problem-solving techniques, this critical first step of identifying and defining the problem draws upon the person's ability to work backwards from a given problem situation to examine contributing factors. Use of a formal diabetes problem or barrier questionnaire can be viewed as a tool to assist the healthcare professional in understanding the scope of challenges faced by the individual with diabetes. Selecting the barriers to prioritize in education or counseling takes into account individual preference and goals that have been mutually agreed upon by the individual seeking assistance and the healthcare educator.

Applying Problem Solving in Diabetes Education and Counseling

There are different ways that problem solving might be used within an education or counseling session. Three applications in diabetes self-management are described below:

- Clinical problem solving by the healthcare professional
- Patient as observer or partial contributor to problem solving by the healthcare professional
- Patient as problem solver facilitated by the healthcare professional

Clinical Problem Solving by the Health Professional

Here, the healthcare professional is the problem solver.[38,39] Problem solving is used by the healthcare professional as a clinical skill to assist in identifying/diagnosing a problem, planning a course of action or treatment for the individual, and evaluating effectiveness. There are several contexts in which the healthcare educator is called upon to use clinical problem solving to teach the individual with diabetes self-management. Examples include core curriculum areas that require not only responsibility of the individual to carry out self-management, but responsibility of the healthcare professional to ensure proper medical management (eg, performing calculations for carbohydrate counting, medication adjustments, and managing the individual during illness, hospitalization, or surgery).

Patient as Observer or Partial Contributor to Problem Solving by the Health Professional

Here, although the person with diabetes may provide some input, the healthcare professional carries the active role as problem solver.[40] As a first step, the health professional identifies a problem or barrier. Next, the health professional generates solutions or options that the individual is encouraged to try or to select from, for implementation. This approach should be used carefully and only under special circumstances, such as when time or other constraints of the education session necessitate a more directive role by the healthcare professional[5,8,40] or when the person with diabetes is not able or does not prefer to assume an autonomous role in decision making (see the section on special considerations later in the chapter).

Problem Solving by Patient Facilitated by Health Professional

Here, the person with diabetes is the problem solver.[5,8,40] The healthcare professional, through skillful, patient-centered questions and responses, guides the person in using a problem-solving process to come up with his or her own solution(s)[41] or uses instructional methods to train the person in problem-solving as a method for resolving problems independently.[42]

Therapeutic Relationship. Maintaining a therapeutic rapport is essential throughout all stages of self-management education and counseling. The way in which problem solving is used can be a source of conflict between the individual and the healthcare professional. One study of such conflict described the perspectives of healthcare professionals and individuals regarding different uses of problem solving.[40] In this study, when the healthcare professional, rather than the individual, was in the role of problem solver, individuals viewed professionals as not understanding their difficulties and as unable to help them resolve problems. In contrast, when both the professional and the individual agreed that the individual ought to take the problem-solver role, mutuality and potential for supportive change by the individual was fostered. A model of the problem-solving conflict is shown in Table 33.2.

Use of communication methods from empowerment[43,44] and solution-focused therapy approaches[41] also facilitate maintaining a therapeutic relationship in which persons with diabetes feel valued and supported in their autonomy.

Empowering the Person With Diabetes as Problem Solver

Assessing Problem Solving for Planning Education and Intervention

Assessing problem solving in the context of self-management education provides useful information regarding the problem-solving skills or styles of the individual. This information helps guide the problem-solving training or education. In practice, interviewing (discussed in chapter 25, on assessment) is often used by the healthcare professional to determine an individual's intervention needs; however, formal measures are also valuable and have an advantage of standardizing the problem-solving assessment across individuals and settings, while quantifying the problem-solving ability in some manner. Moreover, problem-solving assessment allows for outcomes measurement to determine impact of education or intervention on an individual's problem-solving ability.[45]

Diabetes-Specific Measures. A majority of studies examining associations between problem solving and diabetes self-management behaviors or control have

TABLE 33.2 Conflict Between Patient and Healthcare Professional: Influence of Problem-Solving Approaches

Problem-Solving Approach	*Professional's View of Patient*	*Patient's View of Professionals*
Failure-Expecting Approach Conflict deadlocked	Patient is a problem	Professionals have had their chance
Compliance-Expecting Approach Conflict unchanged	Patient has a problem that we can solve	Professionals decide without knowing my difficulties in living with diabetes
Mutuality-Expecting Approach Conflict resolved; situational reflection takes advantage of a potential for change in different points of view	Patient is a problem solver	Professionals know my difficulties in living with diabetes and support me in solving them

Source: Adapted with permission from Sage Publications Inc. Zoffman V, Kirkevold M. Life versus disease in difficult diabetes care. Qualitative Health Research. 2005;15(6):758.

used diabetes-specific measures.[29,45-48,75] Problem-solving measures that have been developed for use in sample populations with diabetes are presented in Table 33.3. These measures represent different administration formats (interviews, questionnaires), response formats (multiple choice answer, open-ended response, Likert-scaled response), and content (diabetes knowledge-based problem solving, problem-solving style or ability).

Broader Measures. In addition to diabetes-specific measures, established generic measures have been used in diabetes studies. Generally, findings from these studies suggest that generic problem-solving measures may be somewhat less sensitive to diabetes outcomes than are problem-solving measures specific to diabetes content.[49-51]

Diabetes Problem-Solving Training: Examples from Empirical Research

Research studies have used varying methods for training individuals to problem solve for diabetes self-management, including use of visual media,[50,52,53] computer-based education,[54,55] and discussion group formats.[56,57] Interventions have been conducted in settings including routine classes for diabetes self-management education (DSME),[58] diabetes summer camps,[49,50] and the primary care office.[54,59] Some studies have incorporated problem solving as part of a more comprehensive intervention approach,[60,61] while others have focused on problem-solving skills training or specific problem resolution as the core intervention. Table 33.4 presents problem-solving intervention methods from selected studies.

Outcomes have been enhanced with problem solving as a component of intervention:

Among the interventions demonstrating strongest efficacy outcomes are those in which problem solving is included as a component with additional social learning, cognitive behavioral, and educational techniques.[45,60-62]

Planning for Problem-Solving Training and Intervention

The problem-solving ability and needs of an individual, as determined by assessment, can be used to tailor the focus of problem-solving training or intervention. A person may be an effective problem solver or an ineffective or inconsistent problem solver.

For persons with diabetes who are effective problem solvers, a problem-solving intervention may focus on reinforcing their use of problem solving for maintenance. For those whose problem-solving skills for diabetes self-management are ineffective or inconsistent (as determined by assessment), problem-solving training may be indicated. Problem-solving education and training can target any 1 or more of the components in the theoretical model of problem solving described at the beginning of this chapter. The following outlines basic intervention points based on individual problem-solving needs.

TABLE 33.3 Diabetes-Specific Problem-Solving Measures: Selected Examples

Measure	*Study Population*	*Description*
Test of Diabetes Knowledge: Problem Solving[*]	Children and adolescents with type 1 and parents (Caucasian)	A 36-item questionnaire describing situations patients might experience with their diabetes. Multiple-choice format for selecting best solution to the problem described.
Social Problem Solving for Diabetic Youth Interview (SPSDY)[†]	Children and adolescents with type 1 (Caucasian)	Structured interview with 10 vignettes of hypothetical social situations involving alcohol, diet-sweets, diet-timing, glucose testing, and hypoglycemia that require choice between regimen adherence or peer desires. Problem-solving ability factors including problem definition, number of solutions generated, chosen behavior, and anticipated consequences are scored.
Diabetes Problem-Solving Measure for Adolescents (DPSMA)[‡]	Adolescents with type 1 (predominantly Caucasian, 84%)	Structured interview with 17 vignettes of problem situations related to 5 areas: insulin adjustment, dietary management, glucose monitoring, recognizing and responding to glycemic deviation, psychosocial issues. Open-ended response format to each vignette.
Diabetes Problem-Solving Inventory (DPSI)[§]	Adult women with type 2 (predominantly Caucasian, 94%)	Survey format of previously validated interview procedure.[¶] Survey gives scenarios of a hypothetical problem in each of 3 diabetes self-management areas: healthful eating, physical activity, stress management. For each self-management area, respondents give their own personal example of a barrier or problem in the area, describe how they would respond to each depicted hypothetical scenario, and describe how they generally respond to each problem situation type.
Diabetes Problem-Solving Scale, Self-Report (DPSS-SR)[#] [**]	Adults with type 2 (African American, low socioeconomic status)	A 30-item questionnaire administered by interview. Items represent 6 subscales: effective problem-solving style, careless problem-solving style, avoidant problem-solving style, positive orientation/motivation, negative orientation/motivation, positive transfer of past experience, negative transfer past experience. Respondents reply to items describing problem-solving characteristics related to diabetes, using a 5-point Likert scale from "not at all true of me" to "extremely true of me."

[*] Johnson SB, Pollak RT, Silverstein JH, et al. Cognitive and behavioral knowledge about insulin-dependent diabetes among children and parents. Pediatrics. 1982;69(6):708-13.

[†] Thomas AM, Peterson L, Goldstein D. Problem solving and diabetes regimen adherence by children and adolescents with IDDM in social pressure situations: a reflection of normal development. J Pediatr Psychol. 1997;22(4):541-61.

[‡] Cook S, Aikens JE, Berry CA, McNabb WL. Development of the diabetes problem-solving measure for adolescents. Diabetes Educ. 2001;27(6):865-74.

[§] Glasgow RE, Toobert DJ, Barrera M, Jr, Strycker LA. Assessment of problem-solving: a key to successful diabetes self-management. J Behav Med. 2004;27(5):477-90.

[¶] Toobert DJ, Glasgow RE. Problem solving and diabetes self-care. J Behav Med. 1991;14:71-86.

[#] Hill-Briggs F, Yeh HC, Brancati FL. Development of the diabetes problem-solving scale. Ann Behav Med. 2005;30suppl:S-091.

[**] Hill-Briggs F, Gary TL, Yeh HC, Batts-Turner M, Brancati FL. Validity of a novel diabetes problem-solving scale. Diabetes. 2005; 54suppl 1:A471.

TABLE 33.4 Intervention Methods for Training Patients in Problem Solving: Selected Examples

Intervention Sample Age and Authors	*Setting/Format*	*Problem Solving Method*
Problem-Solving Training for Adolescents With Type 1 Diabetes		
Ages 11 to 14 Years Anderson, Wolf, Burkhard, Cornell, Bacon[*]	5 sessions, 90 minutes each. Sequential modules for adolescent group sessions and separate parent group sessions. Conducted at routine clinic visits.	Intervention targeted skills necessary for solving management problems using data from self-monitoring of blood glucose; included meal planning, physical activity, and intensive therapies.
Ages 13 to 19 years Schlundt et al[†]	8 sessions, 3 hours in duration each, conducted in a 2-week summer school setting.	Intervention targeted obstacles to dietary management, through a problem-based learning method using video scenarios of target problem situations involving a peer.[‡]
Ages 13 to 17 years Cook, Harold, Edidin, Briars[§]	The *Choices* program: 6 weekly problem-solving group sessions, each 2 hours long.	Content of the 6 sessions: (*1*) Making choices and keeping records, (*2*) Planning meals, (*3*) Timing your insulin, (*4*) Getting back on track, (*5*) Making adult decisions, (*6*) Dealing with the impact of diabetes. Used group discussion, individual goal setting, and workbooks for each session.
Problem-Solving Training for Adults With Diabetes		
Age ≥40 years, 77% with type 2 diabetes Glasgow et al[¶,#]	10-minute computer-based assessment and 20 minutes of individualized counseling, conducted in a medical office setting.	Touch-screen computer assessment to determine barriers to dietary self-management. Computerized personalized goal setting and 20-minute problem-solving counseling. Follow-up including interactive dietary education video and brief supportive phone calls.
Ages 19 to 53 years, type 1 diabetes Halford, Goodall, Nicholson[**]	6 group problem-solving sessions.	Content of the 6 sessions: Education on healthy diet (1 session); training in self-monitoring and identifying, coding, and graphing food intake (1 session); problem-solving training consisting of identifying high-risk situations, identifying solutions, skill training for implementing solutions, and implementing and evaluating solutions (4 sessions).

[*] Anderson BJ, Wolf FM, Burkhart MT, Cornell RG, Bacon GE. Effects of peer-group intervention on metabolic control of adolescents with IDDM. Randomized outpatient study. Diabetes Care. 1989;12(3):179-83.

[†] Schlundt DG, Flannery ME, Davis DL, Kinzer CK, Pichert JW. Evaluation of a multicomponent, behaviorally oriented, problem-based "summer school" program for adolescents with diabetes. Behav Modif. 1999;23(1):79-105.

[‡] See also (*1*) Pichert JW, Meek JM, Schlundt DG, et al. Impact of anchored instruction on problem-solving strategies of adolescents with diabetes. J Am Diet Assoc. 1994;94(9):1036-8 and (*2*) Schlundt DG, Rea M, Hodge M, et al. Assessing and overcoming situational obstacles to dietary adherence in adolescents with IDDM. J Adolesc Health. 1996;19(4):282-8.

[§] Cook S, Herold K, Edidin DV, Briars R. Increasing problem solving in adolescents with type 1 diabetes: the choices diabetes program. Diabetes Educ. 2002;28(1):115-24.

[¶] Glasgow RE, Toobert DJ, Hampson SE, Noell JW. A brief office-based intervention to facilitate diabetes dietary self-management. Health Educ Res. 1995;10(4):467-78.

[#] Glasgow RE, La Chance PA, Toobert DJ, Brown J, Hampson SE, Riddle MC. Long-term effects and costs of brief behavioural dietary intervention for patients with diabetes delivered from the medical office. Patient Educ Couns. 1997;32(3):175-84.

[**] Halford WK, Goodall TA, Nicholson JM. Diet and diabetes (II): A controlled trial of problem solving to improve dietary self-management in patients with insulin-dependent diabetes. Psychol and Health. 1997;12:231-8.

Individuals With Effective Problem Solving

- Give positive feedback about effective use of problem solving
- Facilitate discussion about how the individual is using problem solving
- Reinforce skills by making them explicit
- Encourage continued, independent, effective application of problem solving
- Ask whether the individual can anticipate any situations in which it may be difficult for the individual to problem solve effectively

Ineffective Problem Solving Due to a Diabetes Knowledge Deficit

- Remember that knowledge is a prerequisite for problem solving
- Give feedback about knowledge areas that are strong and areas where more education or information appears to be needed
- Provide diabetes education, as indicated, according to national standards[63]
- Check that the individual has gained understanding of the educational information presented, including ensuring that information presented met the language and literacy needs of the individual
- Determine whether correction of a knowledge deficit has resolved the self-management problem
- Determine any needs for problem-solving intervention
- If indicated, proceed with problem solving as needed

Ineffective Problem Solving Due to Problem-Solving Skill

- Discuss problem solving as a tool for self-management
- Give feedback regarding the person's problem-solving style, preferences, and ways to use problem solving more effectively
- Provide training in the rational problem-solving process
  —Identify problem
  —Generate alternative solutions (brainstorm)
  —Consider alternatives and weigh costs and benefits
  —Select an alternative to implement that maximizes benefits and reduces costs
  —Implement the solution
  —Evaluate the outcome (did it solve the problem?)
  —If the problem is solved, then the problem-solving process is complete
  —If the solution was not implemented effectively, then the problem-solving process examines barriers to implementation—these barriers may be addressed, or an alternative solution may be selected for implementation
  —If the solution was implemented effectively but the problem was not resolved, then the process begins again with reexamining and redefining the problem
- Use training tools such as modeling, rehearsal, and practice using hypothetical problem scenarios and actual problems
- Use worksheets or a diary approach to have the person practice identifying problems and thinking through the problem-solving process both during an educational/counseling session and at home
- Be consistent in reinforcing a problem-solving approach when new problems arise

Ineffective Problem Solving Due to Transfer of Past Experience/Learning

- Discuss self-management experiences as opportunities to learn for the future
- Discuss that diabetes self-management can be mastered by learning/gaining expertise about one's own diabetes with each experience
- Review, compare, analyze, and summarize effective and ineffective self-management experiences for use when new and similar types of problem situations are encountered
  —*After effective self-management experiences,* discuss what was done, how the individual made this decision, what made the outcome successful, and situations where this information might be useful in the future
  —*After ineffective self-management experiences,* discuss what was done, how the individual made this decision, and what made the outcome unsuccessful. Analyze what occurred in the problem situation that could cue the person toward a different solution in the future; anticipate similar problem situations and suggest problem-solving techniques to identify courses of action likely to be more effective

Ineffective Problem Solving Due to Emotional or Attitudinal Factors (Problem Orientation)

- Discuss the role of emotions and expectations in facilitating and hindering problem solving
- Clarify the nature and extent of emotional barriers and determine whether referral for professional counseling, psychotherapy, or pharmacotherapy evaluation is indicated
- To address negative emotions and expectancies (subclinical), recommend use of techniques to stop negative thinking and to replace negative thoughts

with more accurate/realistic expectations regarding self-management[42]

- Build in opportunities for success to build confidence
  - —Set very small goals that the individual can accomplish
  - —Build incrementally upon each success
  - —Provide positive feedback and reinforcement about strategies that are working
  - —Engage the individual in reflection and analysis about strategies that are working
  - —Empower the individual to use problem solving and analysis for barriers

Problematic Environmental Factors Impeding Self-Management and Problem Solving

- Clearly identify the source of environmental barriers
- Use problem solving to determine whether there are actions the person can take to overcome those barriers
- Be prepared to provide information regarding external resources/referrals to address barriers
- Use direct instruction and problem solving to assist the person in planning and taking action to access and use the resources successfully

Special Considerations and Indications for Problem-Solving Intervention

One reason that problem solving has been observed to be among the most difficult of skills to teach as well as to learn is that it relies on cognitive processes that can be influenced by a number of factors. Being aware of these factors is important when planning and implementing problem-solving based education or counseling.

Factors that Influence Problem Solving

- Cognitive impairment
- Age
- Education
- Ethnicity
- Urgent situations

Cognitive Impairment

Because problem solving is a cognitive skill, there are individuals who may not be able to participate fully in or benefit from interventions aimed at empowering them as an independent problem solver. Individuals who have severe cognitive impairment or dementia, for example, may not be able to engage the cognitive processes needed to carry out a complex analysis and decision-making process for resolving problems with their self-management. Individuals with uncontrolled psychiatric disorders that impair thinking may also be compromised in their capacity for independent, optimal problem solving. In such instances, a support person or caretaker would need to be enlisted to employ a problem-solving framework.

Age

In children, ability to problem solve has been observed as young as infancy; however, problem solving is initially rudimentary, and sophistication increases only with maturity.[2,64] Problem-solving approaches with children, therefore, must be aligned with early stages of cognitive development.

Early Childhood. During early childhood (2 to 6 years of age), while the child is in preoperational thought, decisions tend to be made based on immediacy, and the child has difficulty separating what seems apparent from what is real.[65] These young children would not be ready, from a cognitive development standpoint, to use fully independent problem solving to manage hyperglycemia, hypoglycemia, or anticipate and overcome barriers. Direct instruction, learned behavioral responses, and "rules" (eg, when your blood sugar is x, you do y) may be optimal.

Late Childhood. During late childhood (6 to 12 years of age), which is the cognitive stage of concrete operations, children begin to understand processes, to think more systematically, and to be able to make judgments based on quality versus quantity; however, thinking is not very flexible or abstract, and children at this age rely on concrete examples.[65] During this stage, the initial focus of problem solving with children with diabetes, therefore, might best target helping them see basic cause-and-effect processes with their diabetes (when this happens, then this happens). Children may accurately describe something that happened (an outcome), but without putting the pieces together with regard to the real cause(s). To help them put the pieces together, young children may benefit from such teaching methods as telling a story, enacting a situation through play, watching a video (animated or child peer), or demonstration/putting on an experiment. Generally, children benefit from repetition to facilitate learning. Research comparing such methods is needed to help identify techniques that may be optimal during different stages of child development.

Adolescence. Cognitive development during adolescence allows for more advanced problem-solving ability. During this cognitive development stage of formal operations, adolescents are able to manipulate ideas (not just concrete stimuli), use deductive logic, and approach problems systematically.[65] In addition, problem-solving skills such as capacity for planning to prevent obstacles, alternative thinking, and self-monitoring emerge.[2,64] The adolescent with diabetes, therefore, has more cognitive capability for learning a multiple-step problem-solving process that includes problem identification, generation of alternatives, selection of an alternative, solution implementation, and evaluation.

Competing social issues often affect teen problem solving:

Importantly, social developmental issues during adolescence must be considered.[65] *Having the ability* to use rational problem-solving skills does not necessarily result in *making good decisions*, particularly when competing social issues are present.

For adolescents, using groups for problem-solving training may be an effective method for reinforcing problem solving in a peer context.

Parental Support and Involvement. When children and adolescents are not able to perform independent problem solving (eg, due to their stage of cognitive development, individual differences in maturation of skills, preference, beliefs), assistance with problem solving is important. To address the need for supported problem solving, parents have been included in some studies of problem solving training with children[52,66] and adolescents,[59] and family therapy approaches have been used as well.[67]

Older Adults. Developmentally, during the transition from middle to older adulthood, while reasoning about familiar problems does not decline, both flexibility in thinking and reasoning for solving complex, unfamiliar problems show some decline.[68] As a result, older adults may have more difficulty with such problem-solving tasks as generating multiple and new alternatives. On a diabetes-specific problem-solving scale developed with a sample ranging in age from 39 to 75 years, with 15% over age 70 years, Glasgow and colleagues[69] found that older age was associated with reduced problem-solving scores prior to an intervention. Whether the improvements the researchers found in problem solving after intervention differed in the oldest participants was not reported in this study.

Education

In the neurocognitive literature, problem-solving skill is generally associated with education; that is, higher education is associated with higher problem-solving skill scores. Similarly, on one diabetes-specific scale, higher education was found to be associated with higher problem-solving scores, indicating better problem solving.[51,70] There is evidence that factors such as educational level or literacy may not automatically impede learning or use of problem solving, however. For example, in 1 study of problem-solving ability in everyday life (generic problem-solving ability), low-income African Americans with type 2 diabetes with a mean education of 11 years, but literacy near 6th grade level, demonstrated patterns in problem-solving scores similar to those of the scale's Caucasian normative samples, which were comprised of college students and professionals.[51] It may be that life experiences that require problem solving reinforce problem-solving skills, regardless of factors such as education.

Ethnicity

To date, neither the diabetes scale development nor intervention studies have examined whether diabetes-related problem-solving styles, abilities, and methods differ by ethnicity or culture. In the neurocognitive literature, problem-solving ability has not specifically been found to differ based on ethnicity or cultures, yet there is some evidence that level of acculturation to the majority culture may influence performance of some minorities on some tests.[70] Whether this occurs with regard to diabetes-related problem solving has yet to be examined. The educator must remember that factors including cultural appropriateness, education, and literacy must guide selection of educational strategies and materials for effective use.

Urgent Situations

Some individuals may not wish to assume the role of independent problem solver, based on personal preference, beliefs, or acculturation. Even so, problems may arise that call for immediate action when a healthcare professional or support person is not available. Therefore, it is important for the individual with diabetes to recognize that a degree of autonomy is needed to remedy the situation and prevent unwanted and often dangerous consequences. Having prepared guidelines available that outline the courses of action for treating hypoglycemia, hyperglycemia, and illness, for example, can reduce an individual's anxiety about assuming decision-making when managing acute complications. Family and caregivers are important to involve in the education and training process so they can assist with any problem solving needed in emergencies and other situations requiring independent problem solving.

Case in Point: New Job Disrupts Diabetes Control

MM was a 51-year-old man with a 2-year history of type 2 diabetes. On oral agents, he had been able to keep his A1C under good control, maintaining an A1C between 6.6% and 7.0% since starting treatment. Over the last 6 months, however, he had struggled with maintaining healthy eating and physical activity, leading to a weight gain of 9 lb and suboptimal control of blood glucoses, cholesterol, and blood pressure. He had been referred for diabetes education to work on improving his overall diabetes care to "get him back on track."

Physical Assessment Results:
Height: 68.4 in
Weight: 186 lb
BMI: 27.9
BP: 141/89 mm Hg

Lab Results:
A1C: 8.3%
Fasting blood glucose: 102 mg/dL
LDL-C: 145 mg/dL
HDL-C: 36 mg/dL

During his interview, MM revealed that he had not had time to give his diabetes care the attention he had in the past since being promoted to a managerial role at his work. Although he continued to take his medications, his nutrition and his physical activity had been disrupted significantly. In this new managerial role, he was involved in lunch meetings most days of the week. These meetings were catered by local restaurants. Prior to this, he usually bought something from the cafeteria that fit within his nutrition plan; he also had greater flexibility with the timing of his eating. Now, from 12 to 1 pm, he found himself presented with an array of foods that were generally high in fat, sodium, and/or sugars, including heavy sauces, creamed soups, and pastries, all of which he loved.

In addition, he had been working longer hours. With the longer hours, he tended to stop and "pick up something quick" so he would not have to eat his dinner late once he got home. He previously began his weekdays with a 1-hour exercise routine in his home. Over the past 6 months, he had missed his morning exercise more weekdays than not, largely because he had been going to bed later.

MM did not feel depressed, but he did feel overwhelmed. His endocrinologist was also frustrated because she had suggested several solutions both for his eating and his physical activity, such as bringing his own lunch and adhering to an earlier bedtime, so that he might return to doing his exercises in the morning. He had not followed up on any of these solutions. When asked about these suggestions, MM responded with, "Yeah, but. . ." or "that's not going to work." MM's endocrinologist had told him that if he did not stop the weight gain and improve his self-management, then he would likely need to start insulin as well as medication for his cholesterol and high blood pressure. MM did not want any changes in his medication regimen, as he felt any new changes would further complicate his life at that point. His endocrinologist knew MM was not open to changing his treatment at that time and hoped he would be able to resume his prior good self-management.

New Job—Case, Part 2

Questions for Consideration

1. MM was already somewhat disengaged from finding and trying solutions for his problem. He was overwhelmed, and he did not buy into the solutions given to him by his endocrinologist. Using components of the problem-solving model, how might you have reengaged him in a problem-solving process?

Problem-Solving Skill. Introduce problem solving as an important self-management tool. Help MM make explicit his current approach to solving his self-management problem (rational/logical, impulsive, careless, or avoidant?). Reinforce that taking a logical, step-by-step approach will make it less overwhelming and help him move forward.

Problem-Solving Motivation. Remind him that diabetes self-management is often about problem solving. Problems and barriers come up constantly, and how to care for diabetes in the midst of life is problem solving. Reinforce that what he was experiencing was not uncommon and that this was an opportunity for him to work on new tools for managing his diabetes—and his life.

Transfer of Past Experience/Learning. Find out what MM did in the past that worked for him. Reinforce that since he knew those things worked, it would be a good idea to work on making those possible again or modifying those to make them work now. Ask him what did not work (based on what he had been doing over the past 6 months). Reinforce that he discontinue doing those, or modifying those, since they did not work for him in the past.

Diabetes-Specific Knowledge. Check to see whether there was information he did not know or understand about the links between his self-management behaviors, his weight gain, and his metabolic control. Include information on the impact of stress on metabolic control and health behaviors. Make sure he was aware of the benefits of physical activity, not only for metabolic control but for stress as well.

2. Identifying the problem can be clarified by breaking his situation down into Level 1, Level 2, and Level 3 problems. What factors would be categorized in each level?

Level 1
- Suboptimal A1C, LDL-C, HDL-C, and blood pressure in the setting of progressive 9-lb weight gain

Level 2
- Not following his healthy eating plan
- Not getting regular physical activity

Level 3
- He was eating catered foods that were high in fat, sodium, and carbohydrate during lunchtime work meetings
- To avoid eating too late due to work schedule, he picked up fast food on the way home from work rather than eating prepared dinner food at home
- He was too tired to do his 1-hour routine weekday morning exercise

3. Setting goals becomes clearer when considering the 3 levels of problems. Level 1 goals were stated in the referral (stop weight gain and return to more optimal metabolic control). There are 2 areas for goals in Level 2 (healthy eating and physical activity). How might you have helped MM set Level 2 goals?
   - Have him choose which Level 2 problem he wants to work on first.
   - Help him set a goal for the problem that is specific, easily measured, and realistic. Give information, as needed, about specific clinical recommendations; relate the clinical recommendations to his particular situation to help with goal setting.

New Job—Case, Part 2

- Have him set a goal for the second problem, to be worked on after completing the first problem, and ensure that this goal is also specific, easily measured, and realistic. Give information, as needed, about specific clinical recommendations, to help with goal setting.

4. After setting Level 2 goals, decide which Level 3 areas will be targeted in order to reach set goals. How might you have helped MM identify the Level 3 areas he wanted to address first?
   - Look at the Level 3 problems and help him consider what was most doable
   - Help him consider what he felt most confident about being able to do
   - Help him consider what would give him the biggest payoff and motivate him to keep going
   - After selecting the first goal, suggest he line up the next goals to work on after goal 1 was met, to give a plan for ultimately reaching the Level 1 goal

5. How might you have helped MM generate alternative solutions?
   - Have him brainstorm as many ideas as possible, without worrying about whether they would work or not
   - Add additional ideas he might not have thought of
   - Ask him what worked before
   - Ask him what did not work before

6. How might you have helped MM select an alternative to try?
   - Have him consider what was most likely to work (have desired outcomes while minimizing undesired outcomes)
   - Have him consider what was most doable
   - Have him consider what he felt most confident about trying

7. How would you help MM evaluate the outcome and make further plans?
   - Ask him to anticipate what would be a sign that it was working and tell you what that would be
   - Ask him to anticipate what would be a sign that it was not working and tell you what that would be
   - Have him keep a record of what he was trying and the outcomes; use worksheets to help MM commit to his chosen action plan and then to evaluate whether it worked or did not, and why

8. How would you plan follow-up for MM?
   - See him for follow-up appointment(s) preferably through completion of all identified goals; follow up at least through completion of a successful first goal
   - Use time between follow-up with check-in phone calls for him to report on progress or reevaluation
   - If possible, have him fax worksheets that document what he was trying and the outcomes

Case in Point: Pharmacotherapy Nonadherence Due to Beliefs

RC was a 68-year-old African American man who was diagnosed with type 2 diabetes 3 years earlier. He was prescribed medications for diabetes and for hypertension at that time. RC stopped taking all the medications himself over 2 years ago because as he said, "they made me sick." He also had not returned to see the internist who was treating his diabetes since he stopped taking the medications. A cardiologist had referred RC for counseling and education due to poorly controlled diabetes and hypertension and refusal to take his diabetes and antihypertensive medications. RC was treated surgically by the cardiologist 6 years earlier for congestive heart failure stemming from a congenital heart defect. RC felt he had done a good job of controlling his health independently, by making wise food choices.

Physical Assessment Results:
Height: 68 in
Weight: 182 lb
BMI: 27.7
BP: 161/81 mm Hg

Lab Results:
A1C: 9.7%
Fasting blood glucose: 199 mg/dL
LDL-C: 102 mg/dL
HDL-C: 44 mg/dL

RC reported that when he was diagnosed with diabetes, his internist prescribed oral medications for him. He was not sure what the medications were, but "the names were long" and he had difficulty finding out information about them. He reported that the medications made him feel sick, and he therefore stopped taking them. When he told his internist of this concern, the internist reminded him of the importance of continuing to take the medications. RC then decided that he would not return for follow-up visits, since we was not planning to take the medications anyway.

He reported a family history of diabetes. Both parents had diabetes. RC's father suffered a stroke, and his mother suffered a heart attack. Both were now deceased. He described his father as always telling him to be careful about medications because they "do more harm than good." RC believed strongly, as his father taught him, that medications were designed to help pharmaceutical companies make a profit and that the properties of medication and the side effects were harmful and should be avoided. RC did not believe that medication had any place in the human body.

RC stated that he controlled his diabetes and blood pressure through healthy foods and natural supplements. He reported that he did not add salt to foods. He shopped for low-salt versions of foods like crackers and snacks. For breads, he relied on wheat and whole grain. RC did the cooking in his household. He would often cook large meals for his son and for neighbors, but he would not eat them "because I'm not supposed to have all that fried food." He often made himself his favorite meal, spaghetti and meat sauce. This he cooked with olive oil, prepared spaghetti sauce in a jar, and usually ground turkey instead of ground beef. He did not eat fresh fruits and vegetables, but bought canned vegetables, which he would cook without adding fat. He used seasoning salt for flavor. He ate canned fruits in light syrup. His weakness was candy bars, which he would crave in the evenings. He stated that he generally was able to resist his craving, but he kept a few bars in his nightstand drawer in case he needed extra energy.

RC quit smoking 6 years earlier when diagnosed with congestive heart failure. He had arthritis that limited his ability to do rigorous exercise, but got physical activity through routine walking. He did not own a car, so getting from one point to another always involved some walking—either to and from the bus or the destination itself. He felt confident that, with his healthy eating and the walking he did routinely, he could control his health without medication, and that, "What I can't do, I will turn over to God."

An adult son lived with RC in the home, and RC was divorced. RC had worked in a steel factory and was now retired. He completed education through the 10th grade. His reading level, assessed using the Wide Range Achievement Test (WRAT-3), was 6th grade. He had some vision problems that resulted in his needing very large print.

RC felt very confident that he was on the right track. He was hopeful about his ability to take control of his health. He stated that he planned to live to see his 100th birthday. The cardiologist wanted to see RC learn more about behavioral methods for controlling his blood glucose and blood pressure. He also hoped RC would return to seeing an internist who would resume medications if RC's metabolic control had not shown any improvement in 3 to 6 months' time.

Beliefs—Case, Part 2

Questions for Consideration

1. RC was disengaged from a problem-solving process because he felt he was already on the right track and doing a good job. Moreover, although his healthcare professionals considered his refusal to take medication a problem, he did not. Using components of the problem-solving model, how might you select ways to reengage him?

Diabetes-Specific Knowledge. RC's level of control did not match his stated understanding of diabetes and health behaviors—or his goal of seeing his 100th birthday. The discrepancy was an opportunity to establish that there was a problem to be worked on. What could be done? To help him evaluate whether he was fully on the right track and identify goals to work on, review target numbers for A1C, blood pressure, and BMI. Have him compare his current results with those targets. Ask if he knows why it is important for his numbers to be close to target. Share the connection between being in the target range and diabetes outcomes/complications; emphasize the importance of diabetes and blood pressure control for his heart. Provide information on how—and what—medications can help. Keep in mind that factors such as reduced literacy and difficulty seeing may have impeded his optimal understanding of health information he may have received previously. Make sure wording and materials are at or below a 6th grade reading level.

Problem-Solving Skill. Problem solving could be introduced as a self-management tool that would help him figure out what was going on and what he could change. What could be done? Help RC look at his current approach to dealing with his diabetes self-management (rational/logical, impulsive, careless, or avoidant?). Reinforce that taking a logical, step-by-step approach will help him make the best decisions regarding his health and self-management behaviors.

Problem-Solving Motivation. What could be done? Connect controlling his diabetes and blood pressure to his goal of living to see his 100th birthday. Reinforce that problem solving is an opportunity for him to work on new tools for managing his diabetes—ones that could help him have a better shot at reaching his goal.

Transfer of Past Experience/Learning. RC had learned a lot about diabetes and managing diabetes from his parents and from his experiences. Unfortunately, what he had learned was likely to maintain suboptimal self-management. This was an opportunity to help RC take a look at what he learned from his parents' situations and what happened to them. What could be done? Encourage him to learn from their experiences and from his own experiences so that his outcome would be different from theirs. Encourage him to think about modifying those things that have not been working as well as he thought they were.

2. Identifying the problem and where to begin to make changes can be clarified by breaking his situation down into Level 1, Level 2, and Level 3 problems. What would be the most immediate problems in each?

   Level 1
   - Blood glucose control, blood pressure control

   Level 2
   - Medication taking
   - Appointment keeping/medical follow-up
   - Healthy eating

   Level 3
   - He refused to take prescribed medications because he did not trust them; he believed that medications were unhealthy and that he would get sick if he used any
   - He would not see his internist because of communication issues and differences regarding the issue of medication taking
   - Although he had stopped adding table salt to foods, he continued to have a high sodium intake through canned and jarred foods and seasonings.
   - He was consuming more carbohydrate from canned fruit than he was aware of and kept candy bars readily available for when he had cravings.

3. Considering the 3 levels of problems can help clarify goals to be set. Level 1 goals were stated in the referral (improvement in control of blood

(continued)

Beliefs—Case, Part 2 (continued)

glucose and blood pressure in 3 to 6 months' time). There were 3 areas for goals in Level 2 (medication taking, appointment keeping, and healthy eating). How might you have helped RC set Level 2 goals?
- Have him choose which Level 2 problem he was willing to work on first.
- Help him set a goal for the problem that was specific, easily measured, and realistic. Give information, as needed, about specific clinical recommendations; relate the clinical recommendations to his own situation to help with goal setting.
- Have him set a goal for the second problem, to be worked on after completing the first problem, and ensure that this goal was also specific, easily measured, and realistic; give information, as needed, about specific clinical recommendations, to help with goal setting.

4. After setting Level 2 goals, specific Level 3 areas to address can be decided upon to reach the set goals. How might you have helped RC identify the Level 3 areas he wanted to address first?
   - Look at the Level 3 problems and help him consider what was most doable
   - Help him identify what would give him the biggest payoff and motivate him to keep going
   - Help him consider what he felt most confident about being able to do
   - After selecting the 1st goal, suggest he line up the next goals to work on after goal 1 is met (or a concurrent goal to work on), to give a plan for ultimately reaching the Level 1 goal
5. How might you have helped RC generate alternative solutions?
   - Have him brainstorm as many ideas as possible, without worrying about whether they would work or not
   - Add additional ideas he might not have thought of
   - Ask him what worked before
   - Ask him what did not work before
6. How might you have helped RC select an alternative to try?
   - Have him consider what was most likely to work (have desired outcomes while minimizing undesired outcomes) and to have the biggest payoff for his efforts; remind him that the goal was to see a change in his control numbers
   - Have him consider what was most doable
   - Have him consider what he felt most confident about trying
7. How would you help RC evaluate the outcome and make further plans?
   - Ask him to anticipate what would be a sign that it was working and tell you what that would be
   - Ask him to anticipate what would be a sign that it was not working and tell you what that would be
   - Have him keep a record of what he was trying and the outcomes; use worksheets to help RC commit to his chosen action plan and then to evaluate whether it worked or did not and why
8. How would you plan follow-up for RC?
   - See him for follow-up appointment(s) preferably through completion of all identified goals, but at least through completion of the first identified goal. Ideally, follow-up visits would extend over the 3- to 6-month time frame stated in the referral.
   - Use time between follow-up visits with check-in phone calls for him to report on progress or reevaluation.
   - If possible, between visits have him fax worksheets that document what he was trying and the outcomes.

Questions and Controversy

Effectiveness of Diabetes Problem-Solving Interventions

The effectiveness of problem-solving interventions in diabetes is an area that warrants continued research. Problem-solving intervention has demonstrated efficacy in treating other medical conditions,[42,71] but standard problem-solving interventions have not yet been widely applied in diabetes research. Because many of the diabetes studies that have demonstrated improved outcomes used several intervention components, including problem solving, it is difficult to isolate the extent to which problem solving was the active ingredient causing change. Diabetes studies examining problem-solving interventions specifically have had equivocal findings, largely due to methodological limitations.[5] In addition, because problem solving was not assessed in many of the studies of either problem solving individually or problem solving as a component of a larger, effective intervention, the impact of problem solving itself (eg, as indicated by change in problem solving after intervention) has been difficult to quantify across studies. Two studies incorporating problem solving as a component within larger interventions[45,62] have reported improvement in problem-solving ability along with diabetes outcomes.

Training Health Professionals to Facilitate Problem Solving

One area that deserves further research is methods of training healthcare professionals to facilitate problem solving in their work with individuals with diabetes; this is particularly important because problem solving has been identified as a difficult skill to teach.[6,7] Areas for study include what teaching strategies are effective, what method for systematic training of healthcare professionals would be effective for delivering problem-solving training, and what associations exist between healthcare professionals' problem-solving styles and experiences and their use of problem solving in education and counseling.

Models that Fit Practice Settings

Many of the current models for training patients in problem solving that have been considered in diabetes research generally use a series of sessions conducted over several days or weeks. While this is feasible in some settings in which ongoing behavioral or educational programs are offered, this model of problem-solving training does not lend itself to use in shorter, more time-limited programs, such as those common in many DSME and primary care practice settings. More research is needed on shorter problem-solving training methods and modalities that can be combined as part of a standard DSME or primary care setting.

Individual Versus Group Intervention

Finally, the majority of studies to date using healthcare professionals have generally focused on group interventions. Research is warranted to understand ways in which healthcare professionals routinely incorporate problem solving into individual education and counseling sessions. Those involved in diabetes education need to understand how effective these methods are with regard to timing, frequency, content, and outcomes. Problem solving is a tool that can be used to facilitate diabetes self-management across all AADE 7 Self-Care Behaviors™: Healthy Eating, Being Active, Taking Medication, Monitoring, Healthy Coping, and Reducing Risks.

Focus on Education: Pearls for Practice

Teaching Strategies

- **Assessment.** Use a variety of interviewing techniques and skills to identify problems and barriers that will be the focus of problem solving. Identify the problem-solving ability of the individual—for example, by role playing or discussing alternatives to real-life situations.

- **Direct instruction or problem solving?** Direct instruction is warranted when there is only a single best strategy to resolve a problem and when trial and error could be threatening—for example, in the case of severe hypoglycemia. Problem-solving is best used when there are a variety of options or courses of action from which to choose. In problem solving, behaviors chosen are not as structured and less focus is placed on choosing the one, right course of action; the patient has room for creative thinking and options that fit one's preferences, lifestyle, and goals.

- **Approaches to problem solving.** Approaches need to fit the capability and preference of the individual. For example, for a slower learner, pace the presentation of information, pausing long enough between topics to allow the learner to think and integrate the information. Educators often try to solve too many situations at once. Approach one topic at a time, one problem at a time. Keep in mind other special situations—such as religious preferences, culture, locus of control (internal, externally motivated), and learning style (audio, visual, kinesthetic)—that may alter the role the educator plays (collaborator, facilitator, confidant). Problem solving is not static; thus, practice and training matter. Individuals benefit from learning from experiences and generalizing to new situations.

Messages for Patients

- **Problem solving is a learned skill.** This skill can be learned and improved with practice. The level of skill may already be effective is some aspects of life situations, yet not as strong in new situations—for example, when learning to adjust to injections. Practice, discuss alternatives, and brainstorm potential situations to develop effective skill in problem solving.

- **Recognize the possibility of different approaches.** Take time to begin to identify potential problems and the variety of possible solutions. To broaden possible solutions, discuss, role play, and consider the experiences of others (caregivers, for example) and the different approaches they may offer. This adds choices and problem-solving skills when unusual situations are present, such as travel, rotating shifts, snow storms, illness, and other situations that alter the daily routine.

Suggested Readings

Funnell MM, Arnold MS, Barr PA, Lasichak AJ. Putting the pieces together. Life With Diabetes: A Series of Teaching Outlines by the Michigan Diabetes Research and Training Center, 2nd ed. Alexandria, Va: American Diabetes Association; 2000;347-89.

Patient handouts/worksheets with problem scenarios that can be used for training and practicing problem-solving skills

Touchette N. The Diabetes Problem Solver: Quick Answers to Your Questions About Treatment and Self-Care. Alexandria, Va: American Diabetes Association, 1999.

A guide on clinical problem solving for consumers (identifying medical symptoms and medical problems and answers for what to do)

Nezu AM, Nezu CM, Friedman SH, Faddis S, Houts PS. Helping Cancer Patients Cope: A Problem-Solving Approach. Washington, DC: American Psychological Association; 1998.

A guide on problem-solving training for patients, with handouts and worksheets for learning and implementing problem-solving

References

1. Mulcahy K, Maryniuk M, Peeples M, et al. Diabetes self-management education core outcomes measures. Diabetes Educ. 2003;29(5):768-70, 773-84, 787-8.
2. Mayer RE. Thinking, Problem Solving, Cognition, 2nd ed. New York, NY: Freeman; 1992.
3. Eysenck MW. Principles of Cognitive Psychology. Hillsdale, NJ: Lawrence Erlbaum Associates, Inc; 1993.
4. Paterson B, Thorne S. Expert decision making in relation to unanticipated blood glucose levels. Res Nurs Health. 2000;23(2):147-57.
5. Hill-Briggs F. Problem solving in diabetes self-management: a model of chronic illness self-management behavior. Ann Behav Med. 2003; 25(3):182-93.
6. Bonnet C, Gagnayre R, d'Ivernois JF. Learning difficulties of diabetic patients: a survey of educators. Patient Educ Couns. 1998;35(2):139-47.
7. Bonnet C, Gagnayre R, d'Ivernois JF. Difficulties of diabetic patients in learning about their illness. Patient Educ Couns. 2001;42(2):159-64.
8. King EB, Schlundt DG, Pichert JW, Kinzer CK, Backer BA. Improving the skills of health professionals in engaging patients in diabetes-related problem solving. J Contin Educ Health Prof. 2002;22(2):94-102.
9. Rubin RR. Adherence to pharmacologic therapy in patients with type 2 diabetes mellitus. Am J Med. 2005;118suppl 5A:S27S-34.
10. Vijan S, Hayward RA, Ronis DL, Hofer TP. Brief report: the burden of diabetes therapy: implications for the design of effective patient-centered treatment regimens. J Gen Intern Med. 2005;20(5):479-82.
11. Hill-Briggs F, Gary TL, Bone LR, Hill MN, Levine DM, Brancati FL. Medication adherence and diabetes control in urban African Americans with type 2 diabetes. Health Psychol. 2005;24(4):349-57.
12. Hill-Briggs F, Cooper DC, Loman K, Brancati FL, Cooper LA. A qualitative study of problem solving and diabetes control in type 2 diabetes self-management. Diabetes Educ. 2003;29(6):1018-28.
13. von Goeler DS, Rosal MC, Ockene JK, Scavron J, De TF. Self-management of type 2 diabetes: a survey of low-income urban Puerto Ricans. Diabetes Educ. 2003;29(4):663-72.
14. Wysocki T. Impact of blood glucose monitoring on diabetic control: obstacles and interventions. J Behav Med. 1989;12(2):183-205.
15. Vincze G, Barner JC, Lopez D. Factors associated with adherence to self-monitoring of blood glucose among persons with diabetes. Diabetes Educ. 2004;30(1):112-25.
16. Cox DJ, Irvine A, Gonder-Frederick L, Nowacek G, Butterfield J. Fear of hypoglycemia: quantification, validation, and utilization. Diabetes Care.1987;10(5):617-21.
17. Schlundt DG, Rea MR, Kline SS, Pichert JW. Situational obstacles to dietary adherence for adults with diabetes. J Am Diet Assoc. 1994;94(8):874-6, 879.
18. Schlundt DG, Pichert JW, Rea MR, Puryear W, Penha ML, Kline SS. Situational obstacles to adherence for adolescents with diabetes. Diabetes Educ. 1994;20(3):207-11.
19. Vijan S, Stuart NS, Fitzgerald JT, et al. Barriers to following dietary recommendations in type 2 diabetes. Diabet Med. 2005;22(1):32-8.
20. Wen LK, Parchman ML, Shepherd MD. Family support and diet barriers among older Hispanic adults with type 2 diabetes. Fam Med. 2004;36(6):423-30.

21. Galasso P, Amend A, Melkus GD, Nelson GT. Barriers to medical nutrition therapy in black women with type 2 diabetes mellitus. Diabetes Educ. 2005;31(5):719-25.

22. Wenzel J, Utz SW, Steeves R, Hinton I, Jones RA. "Plenty of sickness": descriptions by African Americans living in rural areas with type 2 diabetes. Diabetes Educ. 2005;31(1):98-107.

23. Wanko NS, Brazier CW, Young-Rogers D, et al. Exercise preferences and barriers in urban African Americans with type 2 diabetes. Diabetes Educ. 2004;30(3):502-13.

24. Thomas N, Alder E, Leese GP. Barriers to physical activity in patients with diabetes. Postgrad Med J. 2004;80(943):287-91.

25. Lawton J, Ahmad N, Hanna L, Douglas M, Hallowell N. 'I can't do any serious exercise': barriers to physical activity amongst people of Pakistani and Indian origin with type 2 diabetes. Health Educ Res. 2006;21(1):43-54.

26. Hill-Briggs F, Gary TL, Hill MN, Bone LR, Brancati FL. Health-related quality of life in urban African Americans with type 2 diabetes. J Gen Intern Med. 2002;17(6):412-9.

27. Peyrot M, Rubin RR, Lauritzen T, Snoek FJ, Matthews DR, Skovlund SE. Psychosocial problems and barriers to improved diabetes management: results of the Cross-National Diabetes Attitudes, Wishes and Needs (DAWN) Study. Diabet Med. 2005;22(10):1379-85.

28. Ciechanowski PS, Katon WJ, Russo JE. Depression and diabetes: impact of depressive symptoms on adherence, function, and costs. Arch Intern Med. 2000;160(21):3278-85.

29. Thomas AM, Peterson L, Goldstein D. Problem solving and diabetes regimen adherence by children and adolescents with IDDM in social pressure situations: a reflection of normal development. J Pediatr Psychol. 1997;22(4):541-61.

30. Schoenberg NE, Drungle SC. Barriers to non-insulin dependent diabetes mellitus (NIDDM) self-care practices among older women. J Aging Health. 2001;13(4):443-66.

31. Samuel-Hodge CD, Headen SW, Skelly AH, et al. Influences on day-to-day self-management of type 2 diabetes among African-American women: spirituality, the multi-caregiver role, and other social context factors. Diabetes Care. 2000;23(7):928-33.

32. Glasgow RE. Social-environmental factors in diabetes: barriers to diabetes care. In: Handbook of Psychology and Diabetes. Bradley CB, ed. United Kingdom: Harwood Academic Publishers; 1994:335-49.

33. Irvine AA, Saunders JT, Blank MB, Carter WR. Validation of scale measuring environmental barriers to diabetes-regimen adherence. Diabetes Care. 1990;13(7):705-11.

34. Polonsky WH, Fisher L, Earles J, et al. Assessing psychosocial distress in diabetes: development of the diabetes distress scale. Diabetes Care. 2005;28(3):626-31.

35. Dunn SM, Smartt HH, Beeney LJ, Turtle JR. Measurement of emotional adjustment in diabetic patients: validity and reliability of ATT39. Diabetes Care. 1986;9(5):480-9.

36. Herschbach P, Duran G, Waadt S, Zettler A, Amm C, Marten-Mittag B. Psychometric properties of the Questionnaire on Stress in Patients with Diabetes—Revised (QSD-R). Health Psychol. 1997;16(2):171-4.

37. Polonsky WH, Anderson BJ, Lohrer PA, et al. Assessment of diabetes-related distress. Diabetes Care. 1995;18(6):754-60.

38. Taylor C. Problem solving in clinical nursing practice. J Adv Nurs. 1997;26(2):329-36.

39. Taylor C. Clinical problem-solving in nursing: insights from the literature. J Adv Nurs. 2000;31(4):842-9.

40. Zoffmann V, Kirkevold M. Life versus disease in difficult diabetes care: conflicting perspectives disempower patients and professionals in problem solving. Qual Health Res. 2005;15(6):750-65.

41. Davis ED, Vander Meer JM, Yarborough PC, Roth SB. Using solution-focused therapy strategies in empowerment-based education. Diabetes Educ. 1999;25(2):249-7.

42. D'Zurilla TJ, Nezu AM. Problem-Solving Therapy: A Social Competence Approach to Clinical Intervention, 2nd ed. New York, NY: Springer Publishing Co; 1999.

43. Anderson RM, Funnell MM, Barr PA, Dedrick RF, Davis WK. Learning to empower patients: results of professional education program for diabetes educators. Diabetes Care. 1991;14(7):584-90.

44. Anderson B, Funnell MM. The Art of Empowerment: Stories and Strategies for Diabetes Educators. Alexandria, Va: American Diabetes Association; 2000.

45. Glasgow RE, Toobert DJ, Barrera M, Jr, Strycker LA. Assessment of problem-solving: a key to successful diabetes self-management. J Behav Med. 2004;27(5):477-90.

46. Johnson SB, Pollak RT, Silverstein JH, et al. Cognitive and behavioral knowledge about insulin-dependent diabetes among children and parents. Pediatrics. 1982;69(6):708-13.

47. Cook S, Aikens JE, Berry CA, McNabb WL. Development of the diabetes problem-solving measure for adolescents. Diabetes Educ. 2001;27(6):865-74.

48. Hill-Briggs F, Yeh HC, Brancati FL. Development of the diabetes problem-solving scale. Ann Behav Med. 2005;30suppl:S-091.

49. Kaplan RM, Chadwick MW, Schimmel LE. Social learning intervention to promote metabolic control in type I diabetes mellitus: pilot experiment results. Diabetes Care. 1985;8(2):152-5.

50. Schlundt DG, Flannery ME, Davis DL, Kinzer CK, Pichert JW. Evaluation of a multicomponent, behaviorally oriented, problem-based "summer school" program for adolescents with diabetes. Behav Modif. 1999;23(1):79-105.

51. Hill-Briggs F, Gary TL, Yeh HC, et al. Association of social problem solving with glycemic control in a sample of urban African Americans with type 2 diabetes. J Behav Med. 2006;29(1):69-78.

52. Lucey D, Wing E. A clinic based educational programme for children with diabetes. Diabet Med. 1985;2(4):292-5.

53. Pichert JW, Snyder GM, Kinzer CK, Boswell EJ. Sydney meets the ketone challenge—a videodisc for teaching diabetes sick-day management through problem solving. Diabetes Educ. 1992;18(6):476-7, 479.

54. Glasgow RE, Toobert DJ, Hampson SE, Noell JW. A brief office-based intervention to facilitate diabetes dietary self-management. Health Educ Res. 1995;10(4):467-78.

55. Glasgow RE, La Chance PA, Toobert DJ, Brown J, Hampson SE, Riddle MC. Long-term effects and costs of brief behavioural dietary intervention for patients with diabetes delivered from the medical office. Patient Educ Couns. 1997;32(3):175-84.

56. Cook S, Herold K, Edidin DV, Briars R. Increasing problem solving in adolescents with type 1 diabetes: the choices diabetes program. Diabetes Educ. 2002;28(1):115-24.

57. Halford WK, Goodall TA, Nicholson JM. Diet and diabetes (II): a controlled trial of problem solving to improve dietary self-management in patients with insulin-dependent diabetes. Psychol and Health. 1997;12:231-8.

58. Rubin RR, Peyrot M, Saudek CD. Effect of diabetes education on self-care, metabolic control, and emotional well-being. Diabetes Care. 1989;12(10):673-9.

59. Anderson BJ, Wolf FM, Burkhart MT, Cornell RG, Bacon GE. Effects of peer-group intervention on metabolic control of adolescents with IDDM: randomized outpatient study. Diabetes Care. 1989;12(3):179-83.

60. Wysocki T, Harris MA, Greco P, et al. Randomized, controlled trial of behavior therapy for families of adolescents with insulin-dependent diabetes mellitus. J Pediatr Psychol. 2000;25(1):23-33.

61. Grey M, Boland EA, Davidson M, Li J, Tamborlane WV. Coping skills training for youth with diabetes mellitus has long-lasting effects on metabolic control and quality of life. J Pediatr. 2000;137(1):107-13.

62. Trento M, Passera P, Borgo E, et al. A 5-year randomized controlled study of learning, problem solving ability, and quality of life modifications in people with type 2 diabetes managed by group care. Diabetes Care. 2004;27(3):670-5.

63. Mensing C, Boucher J, Cypress M, et al. National standards for diabetes self-management education. Diabetes Care. 2005;28 suppl 1:S72-9.

64. Ellis S, Siegler RS. Development of problem solving. In: Sternberg RJ, ed. Thinking and Problem Solving. San Diego, Calif: Academic Press; 1994:333-67.

65. Bee HL. The Developing Child, 9th ed. Boston, Mass: Allyn and Bacon; 2000.

66. Bloomfield S, Calder JE, Chisholm V, et al. A project in diabetes education for children. Diabet Med. 1990;7(2):137-42.

67. Wysocki T, Greco P, Harris MA, Bubb J, White NH. Behavior therapy for families of adolescents with diabetes: maintenance of treatment effects. Diabetes Care. 2001;24(3):441-6.

68. Lezak MD, Howieson DB, Loring DW. Neuropsychological Assessment, 4th ed. New York, NY: Oxford University Press; 2004.

69. Glasgow RE, Toobert DJ, Barrera M Jr, Strycker LA. Assessment of problem-solving: a key to successful diabetes self-management. J Behav Med. 2004;27(5):477-90.

70. Ferraro FR. Minority and Cross-Cultural Aspects of Neuropsychological Assessment. Exton, Pa: Swets & Zeitlinger Publishers; 2002.

71. Nezu AM, Nezu CM, Friedman SH, Faddis S, Houts PS. Helping Cancer Patients Cope: A Problem-Solving Approach. Washington, DC: American Psychological Association; 1998.

72. Peeples M, Mulcahy K, Tomky D, Weaver T. The conceptual framework of the National Diabetes Education Outcomes System (NDEOS). Diabetes Educ. 2001;27(4):547-62.

73. Pichert JW, Meek JM, Schlundt DG, et al. Impact of anchored instruction on problem-solving strategies of adolescents with diabetes. J Am Diet Assoc. 1994;94(9):1036-8.

74. Schlundt DG, Rea M, Hodge M, et al. Assessing and overcoming situational obstacles to dietary adherence in adolescents with IDDM. J Adolesc Health. 1996;19(4):282-8.

75. Hill-Briggs F, Gary TL, Yeh HC, Batts-Turner M, Brancati FL. Validity of a novel diabetes problem-solving scale. Diabetes. 2005;54suppl 1:A471.

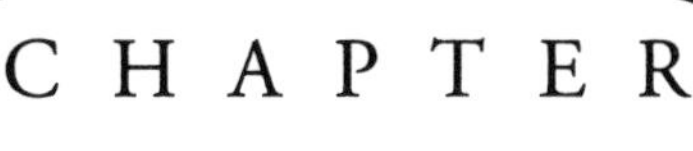

CHAPTER

34

Healthy Coping

Author

Gail D'Eramo Melkus, EdD, C-ANP, FAAN

Key Concepts

- Understanding healthy coping within the context of diabetes helps healthcare professionals on the diabetes care team guide individuals with diabetes, their families, and caregivers toward successful diabetes self-management and outcomes.
- Stress, illness adjustment, and coping are important to understand as well as related concepts of self-efficacy, perceived control, and coping styles.
- Understanding the various types of coping styles and strategies available guides the assessment process throughout the trajectory of diabetes and the continuum of related outcomes.
- Successful self-management depends on adaptation gained through mastery of the medical regimen as well as coping and adaptation to the emotional and social demands of living with diabetes.
- Coping strategies can be employed to identify, explore, and solve problems.

Introduction

The diagnosis of a chronic disease, such as diabetes mellitus, is often an unanticipated life event for an individual and family. Even when known risk factors exist, such as family history for type 2 diabetes or gestational diabetes, most individuals are caught off guard by the confirmation of a definitive diagnosis. The acute onset of symptoms and diagnosis of type 1 diabetes may be even more imposing because it occurs most frequently in youth. Thus, not surprisingly, the initial response is often one of disbelief or doubt regarding the accuracy of a diagnosis.

Individual responses to chronic disease are varied and depend on multiple personal and environmental factors. These factors may create conflict and emotional distress that distracts or discourages one from diabetes self-management, despite good intentions. Personal, familial and societal views, beliefs, and attitudes about the meaning of a chronic disease factor into the construction of a response. This begins the process of coping that is continuous and defined by appraisal and response.

The chronic phase of a disease or illness has been defined by the time span between initial diagnosis and a readjustment period made possible by the process of coping. In Rolland's *Psychosocial Typology of Chronic Illness*, this time span is characterized by periods of constancy, progression, or episodic change that require the individual and family to cope with psychological and organizational changes brought about by the nature of the condition.[1] Because diabetes requires daily self-management behaviors and decision-making, individuals and families need to be guided through the coping process at each period and stage in order to make necessary lifestyle adjustments. The core learning outcomes defined by the AADE for diabetes self-management education (DSME) identify as a goal of DSME the development of problem-solving and coping skills.[2] Implementing these skills helps the person with diabetes improve overall health status by overcoming barriers and implementing self-management behaviors.[2] This goal—to develop problem-solving and coping skills—recognizes the continual need to assess and intervene in the processes and outcomes of diabetes self-management so that individuals and families obtain and maintain healthy coping and psychosocial adaptation.

> ***Coping***
>
> Recognize that coping is a continuous process, one driven by appraisal and response.

Defining Terms and Processes

Stress is an observable or perceived circumstance that is exerted upon an individual. Such stress or stressors are unexpected or undesired events that upset the usual order of life. As stated earlier, the diagnosis of diabetes and resulting demands of disease self-management place numerous stressors on the individual and family.

The process of coping involves actions that are needed to restore order and a sense of well-being. **Illness adjustment** is necessary for healthy coping. Adjustment to a new or different self necessitates an integration of the chronic illness into one's way of being, in order for self-management to occur.

Frequently, however, such adjustment is difficult due to societal or self-imposed stigmas that are often associated with having a chronic condition. This gets at the core of an individual's **personal identity**, which, as the sidebar shows, is comprised of the following: the material self, psychological self, cognitive-affective self, social self, and ideal self.[3] Each of these components of the self is affected in coping with a chronic illness and is redefined by responses.

Personal Identity: Components of the Self

- *Material self* → The body itself
- *Psychological self* → Attitudes, beliefs, judgments
- *Cognitive-affective self* → Thinking, imagining, experiencing
- *Social self* → Roles and labels
- *Ideal self* → Aspirations

Further, one's cultural identity and affiliation often provide the foundation for personal identity and subsequent behaviors. This is because culture is comprised of the learned and shared beliefs, values, and lifestyle norms of a given group that have been passed down from one generation to another, thereby influencing the thinking and behaviors of its members.[4]

For instance, cultural spiritual and/or religious traditions often foster distinct healthcare practices and beliefs across and within ethnic groups affected by diabetes. Such beliefs may cause individuals to ask why they have been given the burden of being diagnosed with diabetes or a diabetes-related complication despite their adherence to beliefs and practices.[5] Many religions are based on belief in God or a higher power and, therefore, their members believe and accept that God or a higher power has ultimate control over their lives.[6] Such beliefs may result in passive coping, whereby perceived control over diabetes self-management outcomes is low and rests with external forces or a higher power.

Some cultural and ethnic groups among Asian, Hispanic, and Native American populations view illness as caused by an imbalance between the individual and the environment that may involve not only spiritual, but also emotional, social, and/or physical factors.[6,7] Such views and beliefs can be acknowledged by the diabetes healthcare professional and incorporated into motivational strategies for DSME that will assist with restoring balance between the individual and environment.

Stress, whether temporary or chronic, results in physiological and behavioral reactions that can affect diabetes self-management outcomes of glucose control, blood pressure, and psychosocial and emotional well-being. If unattended, such stressors or stressful life events have shown an association with increased frequency of both physiological and psychological illnesses.[8-10] The importance of coping with diabetes in a healthy optimal way, through the process of appraisal and response, is consistent with Maslow's Hierarchy of Needs.[11]

Basic needs must be met before other problems can be solved:

In Maslow's Hierarchy of Needs, individuals have a basic desire to maintain or attain the following:

1. Biological and physiological stability
2. Safety
3. Belonging to social networks
4. Self-esteem, personal identity
5. Self-actualization or potential

In the hierarchy, basic survival needs must be met before an individual can move toward self-actualization. Recognizing these basic human needs is important in understanding the role of motivation in diabetes self-management. The healthcare professional's assessment of an individual's motivation for self-management will reveal whether or not these basic human needs are being met and how they affect motivation.

The stress of diabetes and related self-management results in responses that begin the process and tasks of coping. This process takes place within the person and within the person's social networks and environment.[12] The impact and responses are often determined by the person's appraisal (primary appraisal) of the stressor or stressful life event, which in this case are the diabetes and self-management requirements, and the personal resources needed to respond to and manage the stressor (secondary appraisal).[13] Primary appraisal of diabetes and potentially serious complications may cause perceptions of severe risk and threat. This in turn may prompt coping efforts of problem management or ***problem-focused coping***, such as diabetes information seeking, and emotional regulation or ***emotion-focused coping***, such as verbalizing feelings and seeking support, that will eventually affect coping outcomes.

In some individuals, diabetes information seeking alone without emotional coping may result in a negative coping outcome of heightened emotional distress due to learning about the disease process and potential acute and chronic complications. In diabetes education or information seeking, the individual is attempting to find meaning through understanding what diabetes is and what caused it in order to perhaps answer the questions, "why me?" "what do I do?" and "how do I do it?"

The stages of denial, anger, bargaining, depression, and acceptance that Kubler-Ross[13] described for the process of grief in dying are similar to what an individual facing a new diagnosis of diabetes may feel. Table 34.1 describes how these stages may appear in an individual with a chronic disease. Basic to both of these demanding life situations—living with a chronic illness or living with dying—is the process of coping. A criticism of Kubler-Ross's theory and one that is important to keep in mind in understanding the concept and processes of coping is that there is no set order to when and how each task of coping is accomplished.

Numerous studies of the relationships of coping to psychosocial and treatment outcomes in populations with diabetes have been reported in the literature.

Some of these studies have found that despite age, duration of diabetes, presence of depressive symptoms, and quality of social support, depressive coping styles were used in persons who were not emotionally adjusting well to diabetes.[15] Further, psychological distress was related to avoidance, fatalistic, and emotional coping styles rather than optimistic, supportive, and self-reliant coping styles.[16]

Of the studies that have examined the relationship of coping styles to psychosocial and diabetes treatment outcomes in adults with type 2 diabetes and adolescents with type 1 diabetes, emotionally positive or problem-oriented coping styles and strategies have been shown to be significantly related to improved glycemic control.[17-20] Further, problem-solving strategies have been shown to be significantly related to the performance of self-management

TABLE 34.1 Adaptation to the Emotional Stages of a Chronic Disease: Therapeutic Approaches

Stage	*Presentation*	*Approach*
Denial	May question diagnosis and treatment especially if asymptomatic. Attempts to seek alternative diagnosis or may "doctor shop."	Don't agree but listen and acknowledge understanding. Limit teaching to survival skills and reinforcement of basic principles.
Anger	Resentment, anxiety, and guilt are common. Cognitive confusion results in need for repeated instructions. Children are especially susceptible to the "punishment" explanation. Family conflict may arise. "Why me?" "I can't do that."	Indicates that awareness is taking place. Learning begins at this stage. Provide clear, concise instructions, but do not focus on explanations of the "why."
Bargaining	May involve magical attempts to cure diabetes. Compulsive behavior to "make up" for prior nonadherence is common. "If I lose 20 pounds, can I come off of insulin?"	Identifies with others; group classes and support groups may be helpful. Education needs to focus on what the patient wants to know.
Depression and Frustration	Can occur at any time. Difficulty establishing or maintaining self-management. Feelings of anxiety, hopelessness, and loss of "control." "I can't handle this. No matter how hard I try, my blood sugar stays high."	Realization that diabetes treatment regimen and need for self-management is permanent; no vacation or breaks. Psychosocial support and referral as needed. Emphasize positive changes and accomplishments that have been made.
Acceptance and Adaptation	Becomes actively involved in management plan. Asks questions and seeks more information. "I never realized this." What do you mean by that? What should I do?	Indicates acknowledgement of condition and a sense of responsibility for care/self-management. This is not a permanent state, as new challenges always come along.

Adapted from readings and lectures by Kubler-Ross E, Peyrot M, Polansky WH, and Rubin RR.

activities and improved emotional outcomes and glycemic control compared to passive or emotionally-based action strategies.[21,22]

Lazarus and Folkman state that appraisal of possible options (secondary appraisal of what can be done) for dealing with the stressor(s) depends on the person's perceptions of control over the threat, the person's self-efficacy and confidence in dealing with the problem, and the person's response.[14] For example, if an individual has experienced a poor outcome related to a diabetes complication in a family member or friend, such as end-stage renal disease and hemodialysis, the person may then have a heightened perception of threat and a fatalistic view with regard to his or her own control over diabetes and being able to do anything that would prevent or minimize bad outcomes. Such perceptions may affect the level of self-efficacy or confidence in the ability to successfully self-manage diabetes in a way that complications may be avoided. Perceptions of ability to manage and emotionally cope with living with diabetes are then altered and daily self-management and lifestyle modifications perhaps avoided.

Given such a situation, the healthcare professional must remember that perceptions of personal control and self-efficacy for diabetes self-management may be further complicated by complex life demands such as financial concerns, employment demands, and other stressful life events. Diabetes is often perceived as a controllable disease in which problem-focused coping is a primary response. However, personal and environmental factors that affect daily self-management often require greater emotion-focused coping strategies. Although both forms of coping may be employed, the coping strategies used are based on an individual's appraisal of the stressor and his or her personal resources for dealing with it.

Assessment

Perceptions of how to "fit" daily diabetes self-management into an already busy or demanding life may cause emotional distress, anxiety, or depressive mood and symptoms. Perceptions of "fit" affect all aspects of personal identity and in particular the *social self*. Because stress responses and coping strategies are based on a complex set of health beliefs, perceptions, and practices that are culturally embedded, special considerations must also be given to the cultural context of coping.[23] A broad notion of culture is useful and should include, in addition to cultural and ethnic background and heritage, social, religious, employment, and other affiliations. With this as a basis for an assessment of stress responses and coping strategies, personal factors of health beliefs, attitudes, and practices, including cognitive factors of language, literacy, and learning styles, must be addressed. Assessment should also include attention to the following:

- Developmental age and stage
- Psychosocial factors of social support
- The family system and related roles and responsibilities
- Financial resources and insurance coverage
- Environmental factors of access to care and resources based on geographical location, transportation, and safety concerns

An understanding of the various types of coping styles and strategies will guide the assessment process throughout the trajectory of diabetes and the continuum of related outcomes. Coping styles, based on individual traits or dispositions, have been said to determine coping strategies and outcomes.[24] Individuals who adapt well despite serious stress or stressors, it has been suggested, possess the following:[25,26,27,28]

- Strong internal resources
- Sense of meaning and purpose
- Strong sense of confidence
- Overall hardiness
- An optimistic rather than pessimistic view

Of these coping styles, optimism has been studied most extensively and has been shown to affect behavior change outcomes.[28] In addition to optimism, information seeking or avoidance coping styles have also determined coping outcomes. Based on coping style, some individuals need to avoid, blunt, or minimize the extent of information seeking in order to cope with the stress confronting them. Initially, this is a healthy coping response that will ease an individual forward in the process. However, if continued for an extended period, such avoidance or minimizing can be maladaptive, thus affecting diabetes self-management and related outcomes.

In DSME, a thorough assessment of beliefs, attitudes, and readiness to engage reveals the extent of information exchange needed and the pace at which information exchange should take place. Identification of an individual's self-management goals, intentions, and barriers also contributes to shaping strategies for effective coping behaviors.

Assessment Tools. There are numerous scales to measure emotional distress, anxiety, depression, and generalized coping, such as the Problem Areas in Diabetes

> How much information to exchange and at what pace are strategic decisions the educator must make to assist the individual in healthy coping.

(PAID),[29] Crown Crisp Anxiety,[30] Beck Depression Scale,[31] and Center for Epidemiological Study of Depression (CESD),[32] Children's Depression Inventory (CDI),[33] Ways of Coping,[34] Adolescent Coping Orientation,[35] and Issues in Coping with Diabetes for Children.[36] More important than these formal tools, however, is the verbal history and report.

The most valuable assessment tool—the verbal history and report

Specifically asking the individual the following, as part of the verbal history, may be most beneficial in developing DSME for healthy coping outcomes:[37]

- How are you currently handling the concerns of diabetes self-management?
- How do you usually handle stressful situations?
- What strategies or behaviors have you found useful in dealing with stress?

Strategies for Intervention

Successful self-management depends on adaptation gained through mastery of the medical regimen as well as coping and adaptation to the emotional and social demands of living with diabetes.

Social Learning Theory

Social Learning Theory has provided the framework for much of the diabetes research related to self-management, adherence, and metabolic control. This theory is the foundation of diabetes education and behavioral interventions. The theory emphasizes learning that focuses on both personal and environmental variables that can be modified.[38] This consists of cognitive processes that lead to knowledge and skills acquisition through personal mastery and modeling, with consideration for efficacy and outcome expectations. Expectations of perceived control and self-efficacy with the diabetes care regimen determine whether coping behaviors will be initiated and maintained when the individual is faced with barriers to self-management. Given the multiple and complex challenges in managing diabetes, the affected individual's ability to generate solutions that enhance glycemic control, self-efficacy, and quality of life is critical to success. Personal and environmental factors that can be modified, including expectations of the effect and outcome of the desired self-management behavior, are found in the theories of behavior change.

Transtheoretical Model of Behavior Change

The Transtheoretical Model of Behavior Change incorporates the personal and environmental variables of Social Learning Theory that are modifiable, including expectancies of efficacy and outcome. The Transtheoretical Model has 2 main components, the experiential and behavioral processes of change.[39,40]

- *Experiential Processes:* These incorporate the cognitive, evaluative, and affective aspects of behavior change or problem-solving that are addressed in the AADE 7 Self-Care Behaviors™ and Standards for DSME.
- *Behavioral Processes:* These address more specific, observable change strategies.[41]

Ten processes of change are described in the sidebar on the following page: 5 are considered experiential and the other 5 are behavioral. Six of these processes, those in the top grouping of the sidebar, may be related to psychosocial behavioral interventions that address coping, such as cognitive behavioral therapy and coping skills training. As part of DSME, these 6 change processes help the individual transition from preparing or intending to participate and take action to taking action. In contrast, the 4 change processes grouped at the bottom appear to guide the individual's transition from action to maintenance. These transitions and processes are recognized and taught in cognitive behavior therapy and coping skills training and incorporated into DSME interventions.

Coping Strategies

Identify problem → Explore problem → Solve problem

Problem Identification

Coping strategies for *problem identification* or *stressor appraisal* can be initiated by having the participant first address the types of stressors that he or she may be facing.

- *Stressful Life Events:* Job change or loss, death in the family, marriage, or change of school, for example
- *Chronic Stressors:* Job, family, financial problems, or parents' divorce, for example
- *Internal Stressors:* Self-esteem issues or unrealistic expectation of self or others, for example

Problem Exploration

After the problem is identified, in a problem exploration exercise, the individual can be asked specific questions

Processes of Change (Transtheoretical Model)	
Experiential Processes	*Behavioral Processes*
Processes of value in transitioning from stages of preparing or intending to participate or take action to the stage of taking action:	
Consciousness Raising/Awareness What is diabetes and why is it important to know about it and to self-manage it?	Self-Liberation Making a choice—taking control as an active diabetes self-manager.
Self-Reevaluation What this means and how one can deal with it.	Counterconditioning Developing new ways to respond and resisting unproductive behaviors and thoughts.
Dramatic Relief, Understanding What diabetes is and that one can control it.	Stimulus Control Avoiding cues that initiate unproductive behaviors through self-talk, restructuring.
Processes of value in transitioning from action to maintenance:	
Environmental Reevaluation What will be needed to manage.	Reinforcement Management Self-reward, focus on positive aspects, progress, and outcomes.
Social Liberation Allowing one's self to make necessary behavior change.	Helping Relationships Allowing social support of others in a reciprocal, active manner.

such as those listed in Table 34.2. Strategies for problem exploration include techniques such as the following:

- Discuss with a friend or family member
- Think about the problem while alone
- Write about the problem
- Discuss the problem with a group
- Seek professional counseling

TABLE 34.2 Problem Exploration Coping Exercise

- Have I given myself time to consider all aspects of the problem?
- Who owns the problem? Does it really belong to me?
- Is there a new way to define the problem that might help manage it better?
- Do I need to gather more information?
- Can I break the problem down into smaller problems?
- Which problem is most important to address first?
- How do my values influence my thoughts about this problem and how it can be handled?

Problem Solving

Once the participant has identified the problem and chosen an exploration technique, the participant then determines if he or she has a new or different understanding of the problem that can be redefined. If successful in completing the tasks of identifying the problem and exploring it, the participant then moves on to problem solving. The problem-solving steps listed in Table 34.3 can be applied.

Finally, to prevent the problem from recurring or to help avoid a pattern, prevention strategies can be developed. Also at this point, other stressors can be addressed using the same processes. See Chapter 33 for more information on problem solving.

TABLE 34.3 Problem-Solving Coping Exercise

- Clarify the real or actual problem
- Envision possible outcomes, choose realistic goals
- Generate alternatives and examine possible coping strategies
- Weigh consequences, review advantages and disadvantages
- Select best approach to the problem
- Plan strategy, set objectives, and rehearse strategy
- Implement plan
- Evaluate plan

Prevention Strategies

- Acknowledge the behavior
- Take action against the behavior
- Substitute for the behavior
- Employ stress management techniques

One component of prevention is self-awareness. For behavior change to occur, one must be aware of and acknowledge the behavior, such as knowing that when stressed or anxious one eats more or smokes more. Another part of prevention, after self-awareness, is doing something about it—for example, saying no through use of assertiveness or refusal techniques in which negative thoughts and cues are reprogrammed. Substitution is also a useful prevention strategy that can be developed and maintained.

Using these strategies, individuals who are stressed or anxious can be taught to reprogram their response to avoid the unhealthy pattern—of eating or smoking, for example—by choosing a healthy substitute behavior, such as going for a walk or telephoning a friend. Stress management techniques such as deep breathing and relaxation exercises may also be useful in preventing recurrent stress.

Counterproductive Coping Strategies. Assessment for counterproductive coping strategies, such as the following, must be included:

- Antisocial behavior that is aggressive and destructive
- Health risk behaviors such as alcohol or drug use, eating disorders, and smoking
- Overcoping behavior such as excessive exercise or self-monitoring

If detected, these unhealthy coping strategies can be managed using the processes of problem identification, exploration, and solution.

Outcomes

As psychosocial behavioral interventions within DSME, coping strategies and processes of cognitive behavioral therapy and coping skills training may help individuals achieve, and more importantly, maintain disease self-management goals. These interventions may be particularly

Case in Point: A Maladaptive Coping Strategy

LP was a 56-year-old woman with a 10-year duration of diabetes who came in to the diabetes center because her blood glucose control had worsened over the past 6 months. She was accompanied by her daughter, who was a nurse. LP lived alone; however, her daughter lived nearby in the same city. LP admitted to poor dietary intake, with skipped meals and eating whatever was available when she did eat. During the report of dietary intake, the daughter encouraged LP to add more information about what she said she was eating and drinking. With some hesitation, LP reported that she was drinking alcohol and asked if that was causing the problem.

Assessment

The diabetes healthcare provider and educator could have begun responding to the question by providing knowledge about how alcohol can increase blood glucose and predispose one to hypoglycemia. However, an approach that would help the provider know best what knowledge to impart and to facilitate coping would be to first understand the drinking behavior.

- Was this something new or did LP drink in the past?
- When did it occur, daily or episodically?
- Did it occur with others or alone?
- Could LP recall when the drinking began to increase?
- Was there any reason that triggered the increase drinking?

Understanding the Behavior

One or many of these assessment questions might lead to an understanding of the issues LP was attempting to address.

LP responded to the questions, saying that in the past she only drank socially, but now she drank when she was alone, which was mostly the case currently. She stated that she began drinking in the afternoon and continued into the night, usually skipping lunch but having some supper. She stated that it began with, or was triggered by, mourning. When asked about the loss that resulted in mourning, LP reported that her husband, sister, and mother had all died within the past year.

LP was clearly trying to cope, but using a maladaptive strategy of alcohol abuse. A maladaptive strategy results in isolation and disengagement from others and also results in lack of motivation for diabetes self-management. Before LP could achieve better diabetes control, her losses had to be acknowledged as legitimate. The healthcare provider needed to ascertain if LP wanted to stop the maladaptive drinking behavior. If so, LP could be referred for alcohol treatment and also encouraged to join a grieving support group. Visits to the diabetes care provider should become more frequent until optimal glucose control could be achieved and LP demonstrated she was using positive strategies for coping with her losses and diabetes self-management.

valuable, given the multiple, and often stressful, competing demands of life.

Coping skills training for diabetes self-management has been tested in adolescents with type 1 diabetes[16,17,42] and in adults with type 2 diabetes.[18,43-45] In these studies, both adolescents and adults benefited from coping skills development using the strategies of problem identification, problem exploration, and problem solving. Significant improvements in glycemic control, quality of life, and self-efficacy and decreased diabetes-related emotional distress were demonstrated.

The Report of the Psychosocial Therapies in Diabetes Working Group provides further rationale and evidence for the importance of assessing psychosocial factors and providing interventions that will ensure optimal psychosocial functioning for optimal health and quality of life.[46] Positive outcomes of stress moderation or elimination and modified stress response can result in restoration and maintenance of physiological and psychosocial well-being. The coping appraisal and strategies used in psychosocial interventions such as coping skills training and cognitive behavioral therapy in the context of DSME are consistent with the AADE 7 Self-Care Behaviors™ and Core Outcomes and serve as a guide for the assessment, intervention, and evaluation of stress and coping in individuals and families with diabetes.

Focus on Education: Pearls for Practice

Teaching Strategies

- **Basic needs to be met.** Understand that basic survival needs must first be met before the process of identifying stressors and barriers can take place. This is key to problem solving and will affect motivation for higher order needs. For example, understand that the basic needs for physical comfort and safety must be met as well as the goal of stabilizing blood sugar before introducing higher level problems to solve.

- **Perceptions of risk and threat.** Cultural, spiritual, and/or religious and family traditions foster distinct beliefs and practices that shape future decision making. Before introducing problem solving and coping skills, assist individuals with identifying stressors and treatment plans for optimal coping and illness adjustment based on ethnic, cultural, and religious influences.

- **Different focuses.** *Problem-solving skills* focus on gathering information in self-management skill, technique, and judgment development. *Emotional problem solving* focuses on feelings, supports systems, emotional outcomes, and adjustments. Both types of problem solving are used jointly and facilitate change and coping with new challenges.

Messages for Patients

- **Medical regimens.** Begin to test the basic treatment plan, asking for assistance and clarification from the healthcare team. Frequent calls, emails, and clinic visits are expected in the first several weeks of a new plan, while comfort with the plan is mastered.

- **Coping skills develop.** Skills are developed through experience and information, trial and error. It is a process and can be guided by family, friends, and health professionals. An example of the process is this: Define one possible problem or concern and a potential solution; think about possible solutions and implement one plan; evaluate the plan, and decide to modify, change or adopt it.

References

1. Rolland JS. Toward a psychosocial typology of chronic and life-threatening illness. Family Systems Med. 1984;2(3):245-62.
2. Mulcahy K, Maryniuk M, Peeples M, Peyrot M, Tomky D, Weaver T, Yarborough P. Diabetes self-management education core outcomes. Diabetes Educ. 2003;29(5):1-25.
3. Dimond M, Jones S. Chronic Illness Across The Lifespan. Norwalk, Conn: Appleton-Century-Crofts; 1983:165-176.
4. Leininger M. What is transcultural nursing and culturally competent care? J Transcultural Nurs. 1999;10(1):9.
5. Melkus GD, Newlin, K. Cultural considerations in diabetes care. In: Nursing Care of Persons with Diabetes. Childs B, Cypress M, Spollett G, eds. Alexandria, Va: American Diabetes Association; 2005:207-19.
6. Minarik PA. Diversity among spiritual and religious beliefs. In: Culture & Nursing Care: A Pocket Guide. Lipson JG, Dibble SL, Minarik PA, eds. San Francisco, Calif: UCSF Nursing Press; 1996:11-22.
7. Still O, Hodgkins D. Navajo Indians. In: Transcultural Health Care, 2nd ed. Purnell LD, Paulanka, BJ, eds. Philadelphia, Pa: FA Davis; 2003:40-53.
8. Seyle H. The Stress of Life. New York, NY: McGraw-Hill; 1956.
9. Holmes TH, Rahe RH. The social readjustment scale. J Psychos Res. 1967;11:213-8.
10. Ciechanowski PS, Katon WJ, Russo JE. Depression and diabetes: impact of depressive symptoms on adherence, function, and costs. Arch Med. 2000;160(21):3278-85.
11. Maslow, AH. A theory of human motivation. Psychol Rev.1943;50:370-96.
12. Lazarus RS, Cohen JB. Environmental Stress. In: Human Behavior and Environment. Altman, I, Wohlwill JF, eds. New York, NY: Plenum; 1988.
13. Kubler-Ross E. On Death and Dying. New York, NY: Touchstone; 1969.
14. Lazarus RS, Folkman S. Stress, Appraisal, and Coping. New York, NY: Springer; 1984.
15. Enzlin P, Mathieu C, Vanderschueren K, Demytteraere K. Diabetes mellitus and female sexuality: a review of 25 years' research. Diabet Med. 1998;15:809-15.
16. Willoughby DF, Kee C, Demi, A. Women's psychosocial adjustment to diabetes. J Adv Nurs. 2000;32(6):1422-30.
17. Grey M, Boland EA, Davidson M, Chang Y, Sullivan-Bolyai S, Tamborlane W. Short term effects of coping skills training as an adjunct to intensive therapy in adolescents. Diabetes Care. 1998;21(6):902-8.
18. Grey M, Boland EA, Davidson M, Tamborlane W. Coping skills training for youths with diabetes on intensive therapy. Appl Nurs Res. 1999;12:3-12.
19. Peyrot M, McMurray J, Kruger D. A biopsychosocial model of glycemic control: stress, coping and compliance in early and late onset diabetes. J Health Soc Behav. 1999; 40(2):141-58.
20. Macrodimitris SD, Endler NS. Coping, control, and adjustment in Type 2 diabetes. Health Psychol. 2001;20(3):208-16.
21. Toobert DJ, Glasgow, RE. Problem solving and diabetes self-care. J Behav Med. 1990:14(1):71-85.
22. Lundman B, Norberg A. Coping strategies in people with insulin-dependent diabetes mellitus. Diabetes Educ. 1993;19(3):198-204.
23. Steffenson MS, Colker L. Intercultural misunderstandings about health care: recall of descriptions of illness and treatment. Soc Sci Med. 1982;16:1949-54.
24. Lazarus RS. Coping theory and research: past, present, and future. Psychosom Med. 1993;55:234-47.
25. Antonovsky A. Health, Stress and Coping. San Francisco, Calif: Jossey-Bass; 1979.
26. Kobasa SC. Stressful life events, personality and health: an inquiry into hardiness. J Personality Soc Psychol. 1979;42:168-77.
27. Pollack SE. The hardiness characteristic: a motivating factor in adaptation. Adv Nurs Sci. 1989;11(2):53-62.
28. Maciejewski PK, Prigerson HG, Mazure CM. Self-efficacy as a mediator between stressful life events and depressive symptoms: differences based on history of prior depression. Brit J Psychiatry. 2000;176:373-8.
29. Welch G, Weinger K, Anderson B, Polonsky WH. Responsiveness of the problem areas in diabetes (PAID) questionnaire. Diabet Med. 2003;20:69-72.
30. Crown S, Crisp AH. A short clinical diagnostic self-rating scale for psychoneurotic patients: the Middlesex Hospital questionnaire. Br J Psychiatry. 1966;112:917-23.

31. Beck AT, Rial WY, Ricket K. Short form of Depression Inventory: Cross-validation. Psychol Repo. 1974;34(3):1184-6.

32. Roberts RE, Vernon SW. The Center for Epidemiologic Studies Depression Scale: its use in a community sample. Am J Psychiatry. 1983;140:41-6.

33. Lang M, Tisher M. Childrens Depression Scale Manual, North American Edition. Palo Alto, Calif: Consulting Psychologists Press; 1987.

34. Folkman S, Lazarus R. Ways of Coping Manual. Redwood City, Calif: Mind Garden; 1988.

35. Patterson JM, McCubbin HI, A-COPE: Adolescent Coping Orientation for problem Experiences. In Family Assessment Resiliency, Coping and Adaptation. McCubbin, HI, Thompson AI, McCubbin MA, eds. Madison, Wis: University of Wisconsin Press; 1995:537-538.

36. Kovacs M, Brent D, Feinberg TF, Paulauskas S, Reid J. Children's self-reports of psychologic adjustment and coping strategies during the first year of insulin-dependent diabetes mellitus. Diabetes Care. 1986;9:472-9.

37. Grey M. Coping and diabetes. Diabetes Spectrum. 2000;13(3):167.

38. Bandura A. Social foundations of thought and action: a social cognitive theory. Englewood Cliffs, NJ: Prentice Hall; 1986.

39. Prochaska JO, DiClemente CC. The Transtheoretical Approach: Crossing Traditional Boundaries of Therapy. Pacific Grove, Calif: Brookes-Cole; 1984.

40. Prochaska, JO, DiClemente CC, Norcross JC. In search of how people change, applications to addictive behavior. Am Psychologist. 1992;47(9):1102-14.

41. Ruggiero L, Glasgow RE, Dryfoos, JM, et al. Diabetes self-management: self-reported recommendations and patterns in a large population. Diabetes Care.1997;20(4):568-76.

42. Grey M, Boland EA, Davidson M, Li J, Tamborlane WV. Coping skills training for youth with diabetes has long-lasting effects on metabolic control and quality of life. J Pediatr. 2000;137:107-3.

43. Rubin R, Peyrot M, Saudek C. The effect of a comprehensive diabetes education program incorporating coping skills training on emotional well being and diabetes self-efficacy. Diabetes Educ. 1993;19(3):210-4.

44. Peyrot M, McMurry J. Stress-buffering and glycemic control: the role of coping styles. Diabetes Care. 1992;15(7):842-6.

45. Surwit RS, van Tilburg MAL, McCaskill CC, et al. Stress management improves long-term glycemic control in type 2 diabetes. Diabetes Care. 2002;25(1):30-34.

45. Delamater AM, Jacobson AM, Anderson B, et al. Psychosocial therapies in diabetes: report of the psychosocial therapies working group. Diabetes Care. 2001;24(7):1286-92.

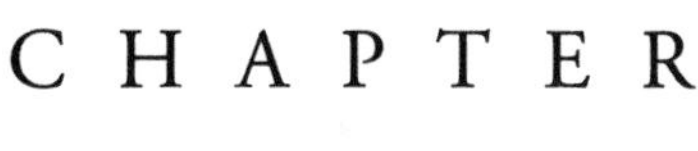

CHAPTER 35

Reducing Risks

Author

Ann L. Albright, PhD, RD

Key Concepts

- All people with diabetes should be knowledgeable about the tests, exams, and interventions that are contained within the Standards of Care, including the frequency with which they are to be performed. Inclusion and monitoring of these can help reduce risks for diabetes complications.
- Targeted, therapeutic goals are recommended for people with diabetes to reduce risks of complications. To best meet an individual's needs and to optimize health, these goals need to be individualized.
- People with diabetes should receive preventive healthcare services to maximize their health.
- To reduce their risks for diabetes complications, people with diabetes must learn and implement skills that help them develop and maintain healthy behaviors.
- A review of the approaches to dealing with barriers that can impede the process of implementing behaviors and reducing risks is valuable.

Introduction

Reducing risks, as contained in the AADE 7 Self-Care Behaviors™, means that people with diabetes implement effective risk-reduction behaviors to prevent or slow progression of diabetes complications and maximize health and quality of life.[1] The role of the diabetes or health educator is to assist the person with diabetes in understanding what risk reduction truly means. To this end, those involved in diabetes education must help those living with the disease acquire the appropriate skills, assist them in identifying and overcoming barriers to implementation, and support them in adopting preventive behaviors that will reduce risks.

The threat of complications is one of the greatest burdens that people with diabetes carry each day. People respond to this burden in many ways. Some responses facilitate the learning process and behavior change, while others may have negative effects. The person with diabetes must be actively involved in preventing complications; therefore, the educator should revisit the person's coping strategies (see chapter 34) periodically to determine if redirection would be helpful. Ongoing assessment of a person's family and community support is also important.

This chapter discusses the knowledge content areas, skills, and barriers that should be addressed when guiding people with diabetes through behavior changes that reduce their risk for complications and maximize their health. The focus is on risk factors that people have the ability to modify. Due to the broad scope of this topic, references are often made to other chapters of the book where specific risks and approaches to reducing them are discussed in more detail.

Knowledge Content Areas

To practice behaviors that minimize the risk of developing complications, people with diabetes must become knowledgeable about the Standards of Medical Care, their personal therapeutic goals, and preventive care services. It is important that this information be presented in ways that engage the person with diabetes, yet is sensitive to learning preferences, culture, language, and educational level.

Standards of Care: Diabetes

The Standards of Medical Care in Diabetes provide a comprehensive list of preventive care practices (eg, assessments, physical examinations, laboratory tests, interventions) and describe how frequently each should be recommended to all people with diabetes. The American Diabetes Association is the primary organization responsible for developing the Standards of Medical Care in Diabetes and publishes them annually as part of the Clinical Practice Recommendations.[2] These are formulated from a thorough review of the literature and rating of the scientific evidence currently available.

The Standards of Care include information on several topics, including the following: diabetes detection, diagnosis and classification of diabetes, prevention and delay of type 2 diabetes, diabetes care, prevention and management of complications, diabetes care in special populations, and diabetes care in specific settings.[2] While all of the information in the Standards of Care is valuable, the information that specifically pertains to reducing risks for diabetes complications is the focus of this chapter. Table 35.1 summarizes the Standards of Care relevant to risk reduction. Refer to the chapters in this text on self-care behaviors related to monitoring (chapter 32), healthy eating (chapter 29), being active (chapter 30), problem solving (chapter 33), and healthy coping (chapter 34) for additional information.

Glycemic Control

The results of the Diabetes Control and Complications Trial (DCCT)[3] and the UK Prospective Diabetes Study (UKPDS)[4,5] have demonstrated that intensive glycemic control is associated with decreased rates of retinopathy, nephropathy, and neuropathy. Epidemiological data have shown that a lower A1C is associated with a lower risk of myocardial infarction and cardiovascular death.[6-9]

Glycemic control is best gauged by the combination of results from self-monitoring of blood glucose (SMBG) and the results of A1C testing (see chapter 32 for more information on monitoring). The person with diabetes ought to be given information about how each of these monitoring tools can assist with diabetes management. This can be reinforced by including the person in a review of the results and how they can be used in making treatment decisions.

The frequency and timing of SMBG must be dictated by an individual's needs and goals. While there are data that demonstrate the importance of SMBG in diabetes self-management, the available studies used multifactorial interventions, which make it difficult to provide evidence to support a specific frequency or timing of SMBG.[3-5] The Standards of Care recommend the following:[2]

- People with type 1 diabetes and pregnant women taking insulin should perform SMBG 3 or more times daily.
- The optimal frequency of SMBG for those with type 2 diabetes taking oral agents is not known, but monitoring should be done frequently enough to help patients meet their treatment goals.
- Those with type 2 diabetes who use insulin should perform SMBG more frequently than those who do not use insulin.
- At this time, there are insufficient data to make recommendations about how often those with type 2 diabetes who are treated by medical nutrition therapy and physical activity ought to be using SMBG.
- Having people with diabetes monitor postprandial blood glucose should definitely be considered, especially when A1C goals are not being met even though preprandial blood glucoses are considered within the target range.[2,10] Postprandial SMBG should be done 1 to 2 hours after the start of the meal, as this is generally considered the peak glucose level.[2,11]

A1C testing should be conducted at least twice a year in people who are meeting treatment goals and quarterly in those whose therapy has changed or who are not meeting glycemic goals.[2]

TABLE 35.1 Summary of Standards of Care

Test/Exam	*Frequency*
Self-Monitoring of Blood Glucose	*Type 1 diabetes and pregnant women taking insulin:* 3 or more times per day *Type 2 diabetes:* as needed to meet treatment goals
A1C	At least twice per year if at goal Quarterly if treatment changes or not meeting goals
Weight	Each regular diabetes visit
Blood Pressure	Each regular diabetes visit
Lipids	Yearly (less frequently if normal)
Microalbumin	Yearly
Dilated Eye Exam	Yearly
Comprehensive Foot Exam	Yearly (more often if high-risk foot conditions)
Medical Nutrition Therapy	As needed to meet treatment goals
Physical Activity Plan	As needed to meet treatment goals
Immunizations	Flu annually Pneumonia at least once
Dental Care	At least twice per year

Source: Adapted from American Diabetes Association. Standards of medical care in diabetes, 2006. Diabetes Care. 2006;29suppl: S4-42.

Preventing Complications

Standards of care are important, but therapeutic goals must be determined specifically for and in collaboration with each individual.

Medical Nutrition Therapy

Medical nutrition therapy (MNT) is a key component of diabetes management and one that can require significant time and attention (see chapters 13 and 29 for more information on MNT and self-care behaviors related to healthy eating). Food is not only a means of nourishing the body and providing fuel, but also an integral part of one's personal being and culture. Food is often closely tied to celebrations, stress, and coping.

The Standards of Care recommend that people with diabetes receive MNT as needed to achieve treatment goals, preferably provided by a registered dietitian familiar with the components of diabetes MNT.[2,12] For children and adolescents with type 1 diabetes, the Standards of Care recommend that MNT be provided at diagnosis, and at least annually thereafter, by a healthcare professional experienced with the nutritional needs of growing children and adolescents and the behavioral issues that often impact their diets.[2] The Diabetes Nutrition Practice Guidelines (NPGs), developed by the Diabetes Care and Education Practice Group of the American Dietetic Association, provide information for healthcare professionals regarding the recommended process to follow when conducting MNT.[13,14] The NPGs were tested and validated by registered dietitians and are discussed further in chapter 29.

The goals of MNT that apply to all people with diabetes include the following:[2]

- Attain and maintain recommended metabolic outcomes, including glucose and A1C levels, low-density lipoprotein cholesterol (LDL-C), high-density lipoprotein cholesterol (HDL-C), triglyceride levels, blood pressure, and body weight.
- Prevent and treat chronic complications and comorbidities of diabetes. Modify nutrient intake and lifestyle as appropriate for the prevention and treatment of obesity, dyslipidemia, cardiovascular disease (CVD), hypertension, and nephropathy.
- Improve health through healthy food choices and physical activity.
- Address individual nutritional needs, taking into consideration personal and cultural preferences and lifestyle, while respecting the individual's wishes and willingness to change.

Weight Management

Overweight and obesity are strongly linked to type 2 diabetes. In addition, obesity is an independent risk factor for hypertension, hyperlipidemia, and CVD. Moderate weight loss improves glycemic control and reduces CVD risk. Consequently, weight management is an important issue for overweight or obese people with type 2 diabetes.

The Standards of Care recommend that body weight be measured at each diabetes visit.[2] Weight (in kilograms) and height (in meters) are measured to calculate body mass index (BMI). Weight loss is recommended for all overweight (BMI 25.0 to 29.9 kg/m^2) or obese (BMI greater than or equal to 30.0 kg/m^2) adults with diabetes.[2]

The primary approach for achieving weight loss is lifestyle change that includes a reduction in energy intake, an increase in physical activity, and behavioral strategies.[2] Reduction in caloric balance (500 to 1000 calories per day) results in a slow, but progressive weight loss of about 1 to 2 lb per week. Physical activity should be increased gradually, working to achieve 30 to 45 minutes of aerobic activity most days. Activity levels of 1 hour per day of moderate activity or 30 minutes of vigorous activity may be needed for long-term weight loss. Because weight loss can be difficult to achieve and maintain, the educator must work with overweight individuals in a manner that is sensitive and supportive. Emphasizing that modest weight loss is the goal is especially important.

Physical Activity

Regular physical activity provides numerous benefits to people with diabetes. It has been shown to improve glucose control, reduce cardiovascular risk factors, contribute to weight management, and improve well-being.[15,16] A regular physical activity program, adapted if complications are present, is recommended in the Standards of Care for all people with diabetes who are capable of participating.[2] See chapters 14 and 30 for additional information on physical activity.

Psychosocial Assessment and Care

People with diabetes are likely to be psychologically vulnerable at diagnosis and when their medical status changes (for example, intensification of treatment or when complications are diagnosed).[17,18] In addition, the demands of living with diabetes each day can result in "diabetes burnout" and impair a person's ability to carry out the diabetes care plan.[19] Even if individuals are equipped with accurate knowledge and sufficient skills to reduce their risks, the ability to carry out healthy behaviors can be significantly impacted by their psychological and social state.

Regarding psychosocial assessment and care, the Standards of Care recommend the following:[2]

- Psychosocial screening should include attitudes about illness, expectations for medical management and outcomes, affect or mood, general and diabetes-related quality of life, resources (financial, social, and emotional) and psychiatric history
- Screening for psychosocial problems such as depression, eating disorders, and cognitive impairment is needed when adherence to the medical regimen is poor
- Incorporating psychological treatment into routine care is preferred over waiting for identification of a specific problem or deterioration in psychological status

Refer to chapter 33 for information on problem solving and chapter 34 for information on healthy coping. Chapter 4 covers depression and eating disorders.

Standards of Care: Complications

This section discusses risk reduction and prevention and management of the following chronic complications:

- Cardiovascular disease
- Retinopathy
- Nephropathy
- Foot problems

Preventive services of importance in diabetes care, specifically for the following, are also discussed:

- Immunizations for influenza and pneumonia
- Dental care
- Prepregnancy counseling

The importance of personalizing therapeutic goals is emphasized. Blood pressure and lipid targets for children and adolescents with diabetes are summarized.

Cardiovascular Disease

CVD is the leading cause of mortality for people with diabetes.[20] Research studies support reducing cardiovascular risk factors to prevent or slow CVD. The following modifiable CVD risk factors are topics for diabetes education:

- Hypertension[21]
- Dyslipidemia[22]
- Smoking[23]
- Increased platelet adherence[24]

Blood Pressure. Hypertension is a major risk factor for cardiovascular and cerebral vascular disease as well as for microvascular complications including diabetic nephropathy and retinopathy.[2,25] Consequently, emphasis must be placed on ensuring that people with diabetes know their blood pressure values and how to use medical nutrition therapy, physical activity, and when necessary, medication to keep blood pressure at their therapeutic goals (see therapeutic goal section that follows). The Standards of Care recommend that blood pressure be measured at every routine diabetes visit.

- *Adults.* Adults with diabetes who are found to have systolic blood pressure greater than or equal to 130 mm Hg or diastolic blood pressure greater than or equal to 80 mm Hg should have blood pressure confirmed on a separate day.[2]
- *Children and Adolescents.* Hypertension in childhood is defined as an average systolic or diastolic blood pressure greater than or equal to the 95th percentile for age, sex, and height percentile measured on at least 3 separate days.[2] "High-normal" blood pressure is defined as average systolic or diastolic blood pressure greater than or equal to the 90th but less than the 95th percentile for age, sex, and height percentile measured on at least 3 separate days.[2]

Lipids. Lipid abnormalities are more common in people with type 2 diabetes than in those with type 1 or those without diabetes. Although there is less data on lipid lowering therapy in type 1 diabetes, this intervention should be considered in those with cardiovascular risk factors in addition to their diabetes.[26] Lipid management should target lowering LDL-C, raising HDL-C, and lowering triglycerides. The various lipid tests and their corresponding values should be explained to people with diabetes in terms that are easy to understand and that emphasize the importance of this matter. Instructions should be provided on MNT, physical activity, and medication, if necessary, to keep lipids at their therapeutic goals (see therapeutic goal section below).

- *Adults.* The Standards of Care recommend that adults with diabetes be tested for lipid disorders at least annually and more often if needed to achieve goals. In adults with low-risk lipid values (LDL-C less than 100 mg/dL, HDL-C greater than 50 mg/dL, and triglycerides less than 150 mg/dL), lipid assessment may be done every 2 years.[2]
- *Children and Adolescents.* The Standards of Care recommend that a fasting lipid profile be drawn for all children over 2 years of age at the time of diagnosis (after glucose control has been established) if there is a family history of hypercholesterolemia or a history of a cardiovascular event before age 55 or if family history is unknown. Otherwise, the first lipid screening should be performed at puberty (over 12 years of age). If diabetes is diagnosed in puberty, the first lipid screening should be done at diagnosis. If values are within the accepted range (LDL-C less than 100 mg/dL) for children and adolescents, a lipid profile should be repeated every 5 years. If lipids are abnormal, annual monitoring is recommended.[2,27]

Smoking Cessation. Cigarette smoking is the most important modifiable cause of premature death for those with and without diabetes. Studies of people with diabetes have repeatedly found an increased risk of morbidity and premature death associated with the development of macrovascular complications among smokers.[28] Smoking is also related to the earlier development of microvascular complications.[2]

Large randomized clinical trials, not focused specifically on people with diabetes, have shown that smoking cessation counseling is efficacious and cost-effective in reducing tobacco use.[29,30] There is no reason to believe these results do not also apply to those with diabetes. Routine assessment of tobacco use is an important part of preventing smoking or encouraging cessation. The Standards of Care recommend the following:[2]

- Advise all people with diabetes not to smoke
- Include smoking cessation counseling and other forms of treatment as a routine component of diabetes care

The educator should address the issue of smoking cessation in a nonjudgmental and supportive way. There are many programs (for example, telephone help lines for counseling) and tools (for example, gums and patches) available to assist with cessation efforts. Often several attempts are required for success with smoking cessation.

Aspirin Therapy. Aspirin therapy is recommended as both a primary[31,32] and secondary therapy to prevent cardiovascular events in people with and without diabetes. Several studies have shown a decrease in myocardial infarctions by approximately 30% and a decrease in strokes of 20% in a wide range of people with aspirin therapy.[24,33]

Recommendations in the Standards of Care for the use of aspirin include the following:[2]

- *Secondary Prevention:* Use aspirin therapy (75 to 162 mg per day) as a secondary prevention strategy in those with diabetes with a history of myocardial infarction, vascular bypass, stroke or transient ischemic attack, peripheral vascular disease, claudication, and/or angina
- *Primary Prevention:* Use aspirin therapy (75 to 162 mg per day) as a primary prevention strategy in those with type 2 diabetes or type 1 diabetes at increased cardiovascular risk, including those who are over 40 years of age or who have additional risk factors (family history of CVD, hypertension, smoking, dyslipidemia, or albuminuria)
- *Contraindications:* People with contraindications should not take aspirin, but other antiplatelet agents should be considered
- *Younger Adults and Children:* Aspirin therapy is not recommended for those under 21 years of age and has not been studied in those under 30 years of age

When reviewing medications with the person with diabetes, the educator must also ask about aspirin use.

Retinopathy

Diabetic retinopathy is considered the leading cause of new cases of blindness among adults aged 20 to 74 years.[20] The prevalence of retinopathy increases with duration of diabetes. In addition to targets for optimal glycemic and blood pressure control, the Standards of Care include the following.[2]

- *Type 1 Diabetes.* Adults with type 1 diabetes should have an initial dilated and comprehensive eye exam by an ophthalmologist or optometrist with 5 years after the onset of diabetes.
- *Type 2 Diabetes.* People with type 2 diabetes should have an initial dilated and comprehensive eye exam by an ophthalmologist or optometrist shortly after diagnosis of diabetes.
- *Follow-Up.* Subsequent examinations for those with type 1 or type 2 diabetes should be repeated annually by an ophthalmologist or optometrist who is knowledgeable and experienced in diagnosing the presence of diabetic retinopathy and is aware of its management. Less frequent exams (every 2 to 3 years) may be considered on the advice of an eye care professional when eye exams are normal. Eye exams will be required more frequently if retinopathy is progressing.

Women Planning a Pregnancy. When planning pregnancy, women with preexisting diabetes should have a comprehensive eye exam and be counseled on the risk of development and/or progression of diabetic retinopathy. Women with diabetes who become pregnant should have a comprehensive eye exam in the first trimester and close follow-up throughout pregnancy and for 1 year postpartum. This guideline does not apply to women with gestational diabetes because they are not at increased risk for diabetic retinopathy.

Children and Adolescents. For children, the first ophthalmologic exam should be obtained once the child is 10 years of age or older and has had diabetes for 3 to 5 years. After the initial exam, annual routine follow-up is generally recommended, but less frequent exams may be acceptable on the advice of an eye care professional.

The educator needs to be sure that the person with diabetes has received the necessary referral or assistance for scheduling an eye exam. The educator can help prepare the person for the eye care visit. Explaining what to expect when the eyes are dilated is important. These exams can be uncomfortable, and some individuals are reluctant to follow through with an exam for this reason. Also, the individual needs to be prepared to arrange a ride home after the exam. People can be tempted to ignore eye care, believing there are no problems because they have not noted any changes in vision. The importance of these exams to saving vision cannot be emphasized enough. Ask the individual about barriers to having an exam and work with the individual to overcome them (barriers are discussed more completely toward the end of the chapter).

Nephropathy

Diabetic nephropathy is the leading cause of end-stage renal disease (ESRD).[20] Microalbuminuria (30 to 299 mg per 24 hours) is the earliest stage of diabetic nephropathy in type 1diabetes and serves as a marker for the development of nephropathy in type 2 diabetes.[2] Microalbuminuria is also a marker of increased risk for CVD.[34,35] Those who develop macroalbuminuria (300 mg or greater per 24 hours) are at high risk for progressing to ESRD.[36,37]

In addition to optimal glycemic and blood pressure control, the other Standards of Care include the following:[2]

- Performing an annual test for the presence of microalbuminuria in individuals who have had type 1 diabetes for 5 years or more and in all individuals with type 2 diabetes, beginning at diagnosis.
- The role of annual microalbuminuria testing is less clear after the diagnosis of microalbuminuria and initiation of angiotensin-converting enzyme (ACE) inhibitor or angiotensin-receptor blockers (ARB) therapy and blood pressure control, but continued monitoring is recommended to track response to therapy and progression.
- In children, annual screening for microalbuminuria should be initiated once the child is 10 years of age and has had diabetes for 5 years.

Since people are asymptomatic throughout the early stages of diabetic nephropathy, the educator plays a key role in helping people with diabetes understand the importance of routinely getting tests to assess kidney function. Since various tests can be done to assess kidney function, the educator should be sure that individuals understand the particular test that has been prescribed.

Foot Care

Diabetes is the leading cause of nontraumatic lower limb amputations.[20] Amputation and foot ulcerations are the most common consequences of diabetic peripheral neuropathy.[2] The Standards of Care include the following:[2]

- The foot examination should include the use of Semmes-Weinstein monofilament, tuning fork, palpitation, and visual inspection.
- Educate all individuals, especially those with risk factors, including smoking or prior lower extremity complications, about the risk and prevention of foot problems and reinforce self-care behaviors (see skills section that follows).
- Perform a comprehensive foot exam annually to identify risk factors predictive of foot ulcers and amputations. Perform visual inspection of an individual's feet at each routine visit.

Many educators are responsible for performing diabetic foot exams. The educator must be appropriately trained to perform foot exams and refer to foot care specialists when appropriate.

Resources to Aid in Implementing Standards of Care

Because of the significant amount of information contained in the Standards of Care, various public health programs (ie, state and territorial-based Diabetes Prevention and Control Programs) facilitate implementation by organizing the information in user-friendly formats. Figure 35.1 is an example of one of these tools for healthcare professionals.

Therapeutic Goals

People with diabetes must understand not only the necessary tests and exams and other components in the Standards of Care, but also—and this is of utmost importance—relate these to their own personalized therapeutic goals. For example, the person with diabetes needs to know not only to get an A1C test 2 to 4 times per year; the person also must know his or her A1C target value. The American Diabetes Association[2] has developed recommended therapeutic goals for preprandial and postprandial plasma blood glucose, A1C, blood pressure, and lipids (Table 35.2). The American College of Endocrinology[38] has developed recommended therapeutic goals for preprandial and postprandial plasma blood glucose and A1C (also in Table 35.2). The variation in the goals suggested by each is the result of different interpretations of the literature and variation in expert opinion. Far too many people with diabetes are currently not at the targets recommended by either organization. Consequently, either set of therapeutic goals can serve as the targets for most people with diabetes.

Although the Association-recommended therapeutic goals are the key guide, goals must be individualized, based on the person's unique needs and capabilities. The educator must conduct a thorough assessment of needs (see chapter 25) and work with the individual and other members of the healthcare team to determine appropriate and achievable goals. Circumstances where the goals may need to be less stringent include the following:[2]

- Limited life expectancy
- Very young or older adults
- Presence of comorbid conditions that make the recommended targets unsafe

> ### *Glycemic Targets*
>
> Many people with diabetes are far from their glycemic target—this is a unique opportunity for educators to help people understand their disease and choose behaviors to achieve key targets.

BASIC GUIDELINES for DIABETES CARE

PHYSICAL AND EMOTIONAL ASSESSMENT

Blood Pressure, Weight - ***Every visit***. Blood pressure target goal <130/80 mm Hg. ***For children: Add height, normal BMI*** (body mass index) for age, plot on 2001 CDC growth charts (www.cdc.gov/growthcharts); BP <90th percentile age standard.

Foot Exam (for adults) - Thorough visual inspection ***every diabetes care visit***; pedal pulses, neurological exam yearly.

Dilated Eye Exam (by trained expert) - ***Type 1**: **Five years post diagnosis***, then ***every year***. ***Type 2**: **Shortly after diagnosis***, then ***every year***. ***Note:*** *Internal quality assurance data may be used to support less frequent testing.*

Depression - Probe for emotional/physical factors linked to depression ***yearly***; treat aggressively with counseling, medication, and/or referral.

Dental - Exams at least ***twice yearly***; Prophylaxis ***two to four times a year.***

LAB EXAM

A1C (HbA1c) - ***Quarterly,*** if treatment changes or if not meeting goals; ***One- two times/year*** if stable. Target goal <7.0% or <1% above lab norms. ***For children: Modify as necessary*** to prevent significant hypoglycemia.

Microalbuminuria (Albumin/Creatinine Ratio) - ***Type 1**: **Begin with puberty*** once the duration of diabetes is ***more than five years*** unless proteinuria has been documented. ***Type 2**: **Begin at diagnosis***, then ***every year*** unless proteinuria has been documented.

Blood Lipids (for adults) - On ***initial visit***, then ***yearly*** for adults. Target goals (mg/dL): cholesterol, triglycerides <150; LDL <100; HDL >40 for men; HDL >50 for women.

SELF-MANAGEMENT TRAINING

Management Principles and Complications - ***Initially and yearly:*** Assess knowledge of diabetes, medications, self-monitoring, acute/chronic complications, and problem-solving skills. ***Ongoing:*** Screen for problems with and barriers to self-care; assist patient to identify achievable self-care goals. ***For children: As appropriate*** for developmental stage.

Self-Glucose Monitoring - ***Type 1*****:** Typically test ***four times a day***. ***Type 2 and others**: **As needed*** to meet treatment goals.

Medical Nutrition Therapy (by trained expert) - ***Initially:*** Assess needs/condition, assist patient in setting nutrition goals. ***Ongoing:*** Assess progress toward goals, identify problem areas.

Physical Activity - ***Initially and ongoing:*** Assess and prescribe physical activity based on patient's needs/condition.

Weight Management - ***Initially and ongoing:*** Must be individualized for patient.

INTERVENTIONS

Preconception, Pregnancy, and Postpartum Counseling and Management - ***Consult*** with high-risk, multidisciplinary perinatal/neonatal programs, and providers where available (e.g., California Diabetes and Pregnancy Program "Sweet Success"). ***For adolescents: Age appropriate counseling advisable, beginning with puberty.***

Aspirin Therapy - ***(81-325 mg/day or 325 mg every other day) in adults*** as primary and secondary prevention of cardiovascular disease unless contraindicated.

Smoking Cessation - Screen, advise, assess readiness to quit, and assist at ***every diabetes care visit*** adjusting the frequency as appropriate to the patient's response. Refer to California Smokers' Helpline 1-800-NO-BUTTS

Immunizations - Influenza and pneumococcal, ***per CDC recommendations.***

FIGURE 35.1 Basic Guidelines for Diabetes Care

Source: Developed by the Diabetes Coalition of California and the California Diabetes Program, 2005/2006.

TABLE 35.2 Therapeutic Goals

	American Diabetes Association	*American College of Endocrinology*
A1C	<7.0%	<6.5%
Preprandial Capillary Plasma Glucose	90-130 mg/dL	
Peak Postprandial Capillary Plasma Glucose	<180 mg/dL	<140 mg/dL
Blood Pressure Systolic Diastolic	 <130 mm Hg <80 mm Hg	
Lipids LDL-C HDL-C Triglycerides	 <100 mg/dL *Men:* >40 mg/dL *Women:* >50 mg/dL <150 mg/dL	

Sources: American Diabetes Association. Standards of medical care in diabetes, 2006. Diabetes Care. 2006;29suppl:S4-42; American College of Endocrinology. Guidelines for glycemic control (consensus statement). Endo Pract. 2002;8suppl 1: 6-11.

TABLE 35.3 Plasma Blood Glucose and A1C Goals for Type 1 Diabetes by Age Group

Plasma blood glucose and A1C goals for type 1 diabetes			
Plasma blood glucose goal range (mg/dL)			
Values by age (years)	*Before meals*	*Bedtime/ overnight*	*A1C*
Toddlers and preschoolers (0-6)	100-180	110-200	≤8.5% (but ≥7.5%)
School age (6-12)	90-180	100-180	<6%
Adolescents and young adults (13-19)	90-130	90-150	<7.5%*
Key concepts in setting glycemic goals: • Goals should be individualized and lower goals may be reasonable based on benefit-risk assessment • Blood glucose goals should be higher than those listed above in children with frequent hypoglycemia or hypoglycemia unawareness • Postprandial blood glucose values should be measured when there is a disparity between preprandial blood glucose values and A1C levels			

*A lower goal (<7.0%) is reasonable if it can be achieved without excessive hypoglycemia.

Source: Reproduced with permission from the American Diabetes Association; American Diabetes Association. Standards of medical care in diabetes, 2006. Diabetes Care. 2005;28suppl 1:S22.

The decision to modify the therapeutic goals needs to be mutually determined by the person with diabetes and the healthcare professional.

Children and Adolescents

Blood Glucose. Glycemic control in children and adolescents with type 1 diabetes must consider the unique risks of hypoglycemia in young children. Most children younger than 6 or 7 years of age have immature counter-regulatory mechanisms, which result in a form of hypoglycemia unawareness. In addition, young children do not have the cognitive capacity to recognize and respond to hypoglycemia.[2] The A1C level attained in the "intensive" adolescent cohort in the DCCT was 1% above that achieved by adult participants.[3] The therapeutic goals for plasma blood glucose premeal and bedtime/overnight as well as A1C are listed by age in Table 35.3.[2] As in adults, postprandial SMBG is also recommended when A1C values are not reaching target despite achievement of premeal SMBG goals.

Blood Pressure. The definitions of hypertension and "high-normal" blood pressure for children were given earlier in this chapter. Information on normal blood pressure levels for age, sex, and height and methods for determinations are available online at www.nhlbi.nih.gov/health/prof/heart/hbp/hbp_ped.pdf. The therapeutic target for LDL-C in children is less than 100 mg/dL.

Preventive Care Services

In addition to the tests, exams, and interventions that are important for reducing risks for microvascular and macrovascular complications, there are also other preventive care services that people with diabetes should receive to improve their health. These include the following:

- Influenza and pneumococcal immunizations
- Dental care
- Prepregnancy counseling

Immunizations

Influenza and pneumonia are associated with high mortality and morbidity in the elderly and those with chronic diseases. These common infectious diseases are preventable. Safe and effective vaccines are available and can reduce the complications from influenza and pneumococcal disease. Influenza vaccine has been shown to reduce diabetes-related hospital admissions by as much as 79% during flu epidemics.[39]

The Centers for Disease Control and Prevention's Advisory Committee on Immunization Practices recommends influenza and pneumococcal vaccines for all individuals with diabetes.[40] The American Diabetes Association provides the following recommendations:[2]

- Annually provide an influenza vaccine to all people with diabetes 6 months of age or older.
- Provide at least 1 lifetime pneumococcal vaccine for adults with diabetes. A one-time revaccination is recommended for individuals over 64 years of age previously immunized when they were less than 65 years of age if the vaccine was administered more than 5 years ago. Other indications for repeat vaccination include nephrotic syndrome, chronic renal disease, and other immunocompromised states such as after organ transplantation.

Individuals may express a belief that the flu shot has given them the flu in the past and is something they do not really need. The educator must address these concerns and explain the benefits of getting immunizations as recommended. The Diabetes/Flu Pneumococcal Campaign by the US Centers for Disease Control and Prevention can be a resource: www.cdc.gov/diabetes/projects/cdc-flu.htm. Confirming that the person does not have any contraindications for receiving vaccine is also important.

Dental Care

Because of the frequency and severity of periodontal disease among people with diabetes, periodontal disease is considered to be a diabetes complication.[41] Oral hygiene, regular dental care, and improved metabolic control reduce the risk of periodontal disease.

People with diabetes should see a dentist every 6 months and more frequently if periodontal disease exists.[42] Periodontal disease is often asymptomatic so it is important that the educator raise this issue. During routine medical visits, people with diabetes should be assessed for signs of periodontal disease including gum redness, swelling, or bleeding, foul odor, loose teeth, and pain.[42] The importance of effective brushing and flossing should be reinforced. If patients are apprehensive about dental procedures, the educator should help them express this anxiety and reduce their fears by explaining what to expect and reinforcing the positive outcomes of dental care.

Prepregnancy Counseling

Preconception care has been shown to reduce the risk of congenital malformations. Several nonrandomized studies have compared rates of malformations in infants between mothers who participated in preconception diabetes care and women who initiated intensive diabetes management after they were already pregnant.[43-47] The preconception care programs were multidisciplinary and trained participants in diabetes self-management with MNT, intensified insulin therapy, and SMBG. In all studies, the incidence of major congenital malformations in those who participated in preconception care was much lower than the incidence in women who did not participate.

Standard care for all women with diabetes in their reproductive years with childbearing potential should include the following:[2]

- Education about the risks of malformations associated with unplanned pregnancies and poor metabolic control
- Use of effective contraception at all times, unless the patient is in good metabolic control and actively trying to conceive

Women contemplating pregnancy should be seen frequently by a multidisciplinary team experienced in managing diabetes before and during pregnancy. The goals of preconception care are as follows:[48,49]

- To integrate the patient into the management of her diabetes
- To achieve the lowest A1C test results possible without excessive hypoglycemia
- To assure effective contraception until stable and acceptable glycemia is achieved
- To identify, evaluate, and treat long-term complications of diabetes

Skills

To practice behaviors that minimize the risk of developing complications, people with diabetes must master skills that include SMBG (see chapter 32 for additional information), self-monitoring of blood pressure, self-examination of the feet, and maintaining a personal care record.

Self-Monitoring of Blood Glucose

SMBG is considered an important component of effective therapy[50] and one of the Standards of Care described earlier in this chapter. Educators must refrain from limiting their teaching about SMBG to the achievement of correctly performing fingerstick checks. People with diabetes must be taught how to use this information to make treatment decisions by monitoring their responses to food, medication, physical activity, and stressors of various types. Chapter 32 reviews this topic.

Self-Monitoring of Blood Pressure

In addition to blood pressure monitoring by a healthcare professional during each diabetes visit, some individuals may benefit by self-monitoring blood pressure. While this issue has not been specifically studied in people with diabetes, a meta-analysis found that home monitoring, or self-monitoring, of blood pressure improved blood pressure in those with essential hypertension.[51] If the healthcare professional and person with diabetes determine that this level of monitoring is important, then the individual may choose to use a home blood pressure monitor.

The educator should have the person with diabetes bring the home blood pressure monitor to a diabetes care appointment to be sure that he or she understands how to use it. Having the person perform a demonstration is a good way to assess the individual's skills and provide feedback and support.

Self-Examination of Feet and Foot Care

Lower extremity complications of diabetes result from a combination of factors including neuropathy, ischemia, trauma, ulceration, faulty wound healing, infection, and gangrene.[52,53] Careful foot care and proper patient education have been shown to reduce the amputation rate associated with diabetes by 50%.[54]

During the foot exam done by a qualified healthcare professional (a Standard of Care), the importance of the individual's foot care and self-examination can be stressed. Additionally, this is a time when the educator can assess an individual's vision and mobility to determine if these will pose difficulties in performing self-exams. If the person with diabetes has poor vision, a manual palpation may be substituted for the visual inspection. If mobility is impaired, making it difficult to reach the feet, a mirror or magnifying mirror can be used to help visualize the plantar surface and other areas of the feet. When both vision and mobility are severely impaired, a significant other may need to assist with foot inspections.[52]

Before teaching foot exam and foot care skills, the educator needs to assess the person's present knowledge, behaviors, beliefs, and abilities by finding out what the individual is currently doing for foot care and examination. The following foot exam and foot care skills should be taught to all persons with diabetes:[52]

- Look at both feet (top, bottom, and sides) and between the toes daily. This can be done when putting on or taking off socks and shoes. Look for cuts, calluses, blisters, thick or ingrown toenails, and signs of infection such as redness, swelling, or pus. Seek prompt medical attention for any problems.
- Wash and dry feet thoroughly, especially between the toes. Avoid routine foot soaks. Be sure to test the temperature of bath and shower water with an elbow before stepping in to avoid burns from hot water.
- Moisturize dry skin (except between the toes) with an emollient such as lanolin or a hand or body lotion. Be sure to avoid using lotions that contain alcohol since this can dry the skin.
- Cut toenails straight across and file the sharp corners to match the contour of the toe.
- Inspect shoes daily by feeling the inside of the shoe for torn linings, cracks, pebbles, nails, or other irregularities that may irritate the skin. Get in the habit of shaking out shoes before putting them on. Changing shoes during the day can limit repetitive local pressure.
- Avoid going barefoot or sock-footed. Wear footwear at the pool or beach and apply sunscreen to avoid burns.

Having the person with diabetes demonstrate a self-examination of the feet is important. This will allow the educator to provide positive reinforcement for those aspects that have been successfully done and point out areas that need additional attention.

Personal Care Record

A personal care record is a valuable tool for people with diabetes to keep track of their therapeutic goals and the tests and exams that are recommended in the Standards of Care. These records come in various formats and sizes. Personal preference regarding the type thought to be most user-friendly and complete should guide selection. Figure 35.2 provides an example of a personal care record. Because SMBG may be done several times per day, a separate log for SMBG is usually more practical. In addition, many blood glucose meters come with software that allows results to be downloaded to personal computers or Personal Digital Assistants. These methods may be chosen for recording blood glucose monitoring results.

The personal care record is a great way to teach people with diabetes about the Standards of Care. It provides a concise listing of the necessary tests, exams, and interventions and should include places for the person with diabetes to record his or her measured values. Educators can assist people with diabetes in keeping their personal care record up to date and using it to help them determine if they are getting all of the necessary Standards of Care and meeting treatment goals. Reviewing the personal care record is a useful way to guide this discussion in a logical and complete manner.

Diabetes Health Record

Discuss these *Basic Guidelines for Diabetes Care* with your diabetes care provider and use this to record your results. Fold to fit into your wallet.

Take charge of your diabetes!

Review Blood Sugar Records (every visit) Target (pre-meals):	Date:				
Blood Pressure (every visit) Target:	Date:				
	Value:				
Weight (every visit) Target:	Date:				
	Value:				
Foot Exam (every visit)	Date:				
A1C Blood test to measure past 3 mos. blood sugar level (every 3 months) Target:	Date:				
	Value:				
Microalbuminuria Urine kidney test (every year) Target:	Date:				
	Value:				
Dilated Eye Exam (every year)	Date:				
Blood tests to measure "fats" important to heart disease					
Cholesterol (every year) Target:	Date:				
	Value:				
Triglycerides (every year) Target:	Date:				
	Value:				
HDL / LDL (every year) Target:	Date:				
	Value:				
Flu Shots (every year)	Date:				
Pneumonia Vaccine (at least once/ask Dr.)					
Other					

Discuss these issues regularly with your health care provider to improve your diabetes management skills:

- Smoking Counseling
- Medications
- Nutrition Therapy
- Physical Activity
- Weight Management
- Complications
- Aspirin Therapy
- Hypoglycemia (low sugar)
- Hyperglycemia (high sugar)
- Sick Day Rules
- Psychosocial Issues
- Pre-pregnancy Counseling
- Pregnancy Management
- Dental Exams, twice yearly

For smoking cessation, contact California Smoker's Helpline (1-800-NOBUTTS)

Note: You may require other tests that are not listed.

Diabetes Health Record

Your Name

Diabetes Care Provider

Diabetes Care Provider Telephone

Medical Record Number

All people with diabetes need to learn diabetes self-care skills.

Take Charge of Your Diabetes!

All people with diabetes need to be actively involved in managing their diabetes. Do you know what tests you need to take care of your health and help you manage your diabetes? The *Diabetes Health Record* will help you keep track of the basic tests you need and how often you need them. It will also help you to record and remember the results of these tests.

The Diabetes Health Record is based on the *Basic Guidelines for Diabetes Care* developed by the Diabetes Coalition of California, in collaboration with the California Diabetes Program, American Diabetes Association, and the Juvenile Diabetes Research Foundation International.

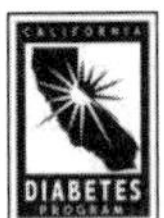

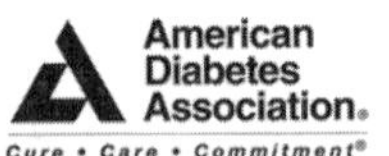

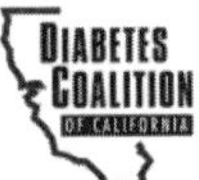

Juvenile Diabetes Research Foundation International

To order the Basic Guidelines for Diabetes Care, Diabetes Health Record (14 languages) and the *Take Charge!* training tools can be downloaded at www.caldiabetes.org

FIGURE 35.2 A Personal Care Record

Diabetes Health Record Card from the Diabetes Coalition of California and the California Diabetes Program. Can be folded to wallet size (fold in half, then in fourths).

Barriers

To successfully attain, and of equal importance, maintain risk-reduction behaviors, the educator must work with the person who has diabetes to address barriers and ways to overcome them. Barriers can be organized into 3 broad categories:[19]

- *Personal:* Includes chronic depression, physical disabilities, poor coping styles, and inaccurate health beliefs
- *Interpersonal:* Includes family conflict and lack of rapport with healthcare professionals
- *Environmental:* Includes financial constraints and other competing priorities

Many of the barriers that people with diabetes face do not have simple answers and can be disheartening for both the individual and healthcare professional. The first step toward helping people deal with barriers is to listen to their concerns in a nonjudgmental way. Sometimes a difficulty may seem overwhelming or be poorly defined if the individual has not had the chance to discuss the issue in a safe environment. Working together, the educator can assist a person in clearly defining barriers and developing an action plan to deal with the problems.[19] For more discussion regarding barriers, problem solving, and coping skills, see chapters 33 and 34.

The educator should be knowledgeable about community resources that may help people deal with such barriers as financial issues and physical disabilities. The Diabetes Prevention and Control Programs located in each state, the District of Columbia, and the 8 US territories may be able to assist educators in identifying these community resources (www.cdc.gov/diabetes/programs). Although there are gaps in services and limitations in program resources, there may be programs and services that individuals qualify for, but need assistance accessing.

Conclusion

Reducing Risks, the seventh of the AADE 7 Self-Care Behaviors™, is multifaceted and influenced by family, friends, cultural background, community, and societal pressures. As the final self-care behavior, it incorporates aspects of the preceding 6 self-care behaviors. Reducing risks involves helping people with diabetes gain knowledge and understanding about the necessary tests, exams, interventions, and achievement of therapeutic goals that can help them reduce their likelihood of developing the complications of diabetes. In addition, those living with diabetes must acquire self-care skills and develop strategies that will maximize their level of health and quality of life.

Reducing risks can be a challenging aspect of self-care behavior to address; the individual must be encouraged by the healthcare professionals on the diabetes care team to take steps to address potential problems. Yet practicing preventive behaviors may not always be a priority in the face of current life demands. The delicate balance the educator must strike falls between helping people with diabetes gain an understanding of and appreciation for the future benefits linked to preventive behaviors, while, at the same time, employing methods that do not undermine self-efficacy. The evidence is strong that following the Standards of Care and achieving therapeutic goals greatly reduces the likelihood of diabetes complications. The educator plays a vital role in partnering with the person with diabetes, family members, and the other members of the healthcare team to translate the evidence supporting risk reduction behaviors into practice.

Case in Point: Risk Reduction in a Man With Type 2 Diabetes

AJ was a 49-year-old Hispanic man who was diagnosed with type 2 diabetes 5 years earlier during a visit to the clinic for back pain. At the time of diagnosis, his weight was 179 lb, and he complained of blurry vision. In a follow-up appointment after his diabetes diagnosis, AJ and his physician discussed his therapeutic goals for A1C (<7.0%), fasting blood glucose (90-130 mg/dL), blood pressure (<130/80 mm Hg), and lipids (LDL-C <100 mg/dL, HDL-C >40 mg/dL, and triglycerides <150 mg/dL). AJ indicated he was okay with these, but he was overwhelmed by his diagnosis. Although AJ's first language was Spanish, he was fluent in English.

Current Physical Assessment

- Height: 66 in
- Weight: 182 lb
- BMI: 29.4
- BP: 132/84 mm Hg

Current Lab Values

- A1C: 8.2%
- Fasting blood glucose: 139 mg/dL
- Triglycerides: 147 mg/dL
- LDL-C: 103 mg/dL
- HDL-C: 48 mg/dL

AJ was married and had 4 adult children. He was a manager in a manufacturing plant and often felt very stressed due to the demands of his job and the financial stress he and his wife had taken on to assure their children graduated from college. AJ coped with his stress by smoking a pack of cigarettes per day and snacking on a bag of potato chips and a half-carton of dip in the evening while catching up on paperwork he brought home from the office.

His doctor started him on 500 mg of metformin twice a day. This was increased to a current dosage of 1000 mg twice daily, taken before the breakfast and evening meals. At his diagnosis, he received general nutrition and physical activity guidelines and was encouraged to lose some weight and get a dilated eye exam. AJ's physician discussed whether he needed to do self-monitoring of blood glucose (SMBG), and they decided he would since he had a hectic schedule and would feel more confident if he could check his blood glucose levels. No specific SMBG monitoring schedule was determined at that time.

AJ had been irregular in his medical visits due to his busy schedule. However, he attended a community education program where he learned more about the possible risks he might be facing for diabetes complications. This prompted him to consider changing some of his lifestyle habits. His mother and paternal grandfather had type 2 diabetes, and he worried he would suffer a future like his family members, which included kidney failure and a premature heart attack. While AJ was interested in changing some of his current habits, he was feeling overwhelmed and was not sure where to start.

Case—Part 2: Questions for Consideration

1. What were AJ's modifiable risk factors for diabetes complications?
   - Hyperglycemia as reflected in both A1C and fasting blood glucose measures
   - Overweight
   - Mild hypertension
   - Watch lipids since LDL-C is just above target
   - Smoking
   - Stress
2. Which Standards of Care were being met for AJ, and which ones needed improvement?

   While current laboratory values were available for A1C, blood pressure, lipids and weight, it was possible AJ had not been getting these tests/exams or the others as recommended in the Standards of Care since he had been irregular in his medical visits. A paper or electronic flow sheet in his medical record would allow easy monitoring to determine the frequency and values of his tests/exams in the Standards of Care. If his A1C, blood pressure, lipids, and weight were being measured as recommended, then attention should be given to microalbumin, dilated eye exam, comprehensive foot exam, immunizations, and dental care. It was also very important for AJ to meet with the registered dietitian to develop a food plan and physical activity program to help him meet realistic weight loss goals.
3. Which therapeutic goals had been met, and which ones deserved attention?

   AJ's current lab values indicated he was on target for triglycerides and HDL-C and very close to his LDL-C goal. It would be helpful to review his goals for A1C, fasting blood glucose, blood pressure, and weight. His efforts to lose 5% of his body weight (10 lb) through modifications in his food intake and an increase in his physical activity were critical first steps in helping him meet his therapeutic goals.
4. What skills did AJ need to learn or review?

   AJ would benefit from reviewing his SMBG skills and working with a diabetes educator to determine a reasonable frequency of testing. A review of his skills and a discussion about the best times to test would help him better use this information and not just randomly test. He would also benefit from learning how to inspect his feet and what signs to report to his health-care team. AJ was under a lot of stress, which impaired his ability to carry out any of the self-care behaviors necessary to reduce the risk of diabetes complications. He would benefit from learning some coping skills and stress reduction techniques (in addition to physical activity).
5. What community and educational resources would you suggest for AJ?

   AJ was fluent in English, but it was important to assess whether he preferred to receive information in Spanish or English. His language preference could impact the community and educational materials selected. Since AJ was a pack-a-day smoker, it was very important that this habit be addressed and carefully monitored. Local smoking cessation programs might be an option and a national Smoker's Helpline that referred callers to phone-based counseling cessation programs in their state (1-800-QUIT NOW). AJ should be given a health record card (Figure 35.2) so he could track his tests and exams. He also should be encouraged to continue attending community education programs since he found the one he attended helpful. He might benefit from going to the American Diabetes Association Web site (www.diabetes.org) and using the Diabetes Personal Health Decisions (PHD) to insert his information and see how lifestyle changes would help him reduce his risk for complications. Other online tools might also be of assistance since he had limited time for events or meetings.
6. What barriers was AJ facing as he worked to reduce his risk for diabetes complications and what were some suggested strategies?

   The barriers that AJ faced primarily fell in the categories of personal and environmental. Personal barriers included his use of smoking and eating high-fat snack foods late in the evening to cope with stress. These coping skills were a detriment to his health and increased his risk for diabetes complications. He would benefit from learning problem solving and coping skills that would offer a healthier alternative to his current coping strategies. Financial concerns and long work hours were environmental barriers. While these would not be easy to solve, AJ might want to see if there were any community lectures or online resources to look at time management and see if he can pick up any helpful strategies to organize his work load better. He might also benefit from talking to a financial planner to see if there were any strategies he could use to help fund his children's education.

Focus on Education: Pearls for Practice

Teaching Strategies

- **Establish the importance.** Help people with diabetes gain an appreciation for the importance of risk reduction behaviors by working in partnership with them to make these behaviors personal and meaningful. Tailor information, appealing to the individual's learning preferences, culture, language, and educational level.

- **Delivering risk information.** Use as much interactive teaching as possible, such as asking the person with diabetes to suggest specific actions he or she will take to reduce personal risk for complications and poor health. Ask individuals to demonstrate skills related to diabetes management to be sure they are performed correctly. Directly and specifically address feelings and concerns in addition to knowledge and skills acquisition. Use phrases like, "what might stop you (hold you back) from trying this?"

- **Achieve targets.** While there may be some differences in the glycemic therapeutic goals recommended by various associations and groups, too many people with diabetes are living far above any of the targets. Evidence from further studies may help elucidate this issue, but the focus should be on helping people achieve the goals.

- **Written records.** Personal care records are a valuable tool for engaging people with diabetes in risk-reducing self-care behaviors. They provide a list of the recommended tests, exams, and interventions based on the Standards of Care and help people with diabetes track their results. Encourage individuals to use a record keeping tool (such as the CDC's) that includes reminders for visits, follow-up lab testing, and immunizations and to consider keeping it in their purse of billfold for quick reference.

Messages for Patients:

- **Learn the skills.** Learn all that is needed to be a master in diabetes self-management. Knowledge alone is not enough for behavior change, but it is an important first step. Discover any barriers that can interfere with risk-reduction behaviors. Ask the healthcare team to assist in identifying gaps in information and skills. Try not to be worried or afraid of admitting the need for help.

- **It's a lot of work!** Diabetes management is a lot of work, but you and your health are worth it! Take advantage of the knowledge and recent advances in diabetes research to keep yourself healthy and reduce your risks for complications in the years to come.

- **Healthier future.** Focus on making your future a healthier one. There is no better time to begin reducing your risk for diabetes complications and living a long and healthy life than the present. Every day, month, and decade that your blood glucose, blood pressure, and blood cholesterol levels are closer to target range, you are building a healthier future.

- **Keeping records.** Work closely with your diabetes team to track blood glucose levels, blood pressure, and blood lipids. Make time for the recommended visits to associated healthcare providers and for suggested exams and immunizations. Keep a written record of the results of your diabetes tests and exams and your medications (and changes) Bring this list to each clinic visit, educational class, or urgent care visit.

References

1. Austin MA. Importance of self care behaviors in diabetes management. Diabetes Educ. In press.
2. American Diabetes Association. Standards of medical care in diabetes—2006. Diabetes Care. 2006;29suppl: S4-42.
3. The Diabetes Control and Complications Trial Research Group. The effect of intensive treatment of diabetes on the development and progression of long-term complications in insulin-dependent diabetes mellitus. N Engl J Med. 1993;329:977-86.
4. UK Prospective Diabetes Study (UKPDS) Group. Intensive blood-glucose control with sulphonylureas or insulin compared with conventional treatment and risk of complications in patients with type 2 diabetes (UKPDS 33). Lancet. 1998;352:837-53.
5. UK Prospective Diabetes Study (UKPDS) Group. Effect of intensive blood-glucose control with metformin on complications in overweight patients with type 2 diabetes (UKPDS 34). Lancet. 1998;352:854-65.
6. Diabetes Control and Complications Trial/Epidemiology of Diabetes Interventions and Complications (DCCT-EDIC) Research Group. Retinopathy and nephropathy in patients with type 1 diabetes four years after a trial of intensive therapy. N Engl J Med. 2000;3423:381-9.
7. Lawson ML, Gerstein HC, Tsui E, Zinman B. Effect of intensive therapy on early macrovascular disease in young individuals with type 1 diabetes: a systematic review and meta-analysis. Diabetes Care. 1999; 22suppl 2:B35-9.
8. Stratton IM, Adler AI, Neil HA, et al. Association of glycaemia with macrovascular and microvascular complications of type 2 diabetes (UKPDS 35): prospective observational study. BMJ. 2000;321:405-12.
9. Selvin E, Marinopoulos S, Berkenblit G, et al. Meta-analysis: glycosylated hemoglobin and cardiovascular disease in diabetes mellitus. Ann Inter Med. 2004; 141:421-31.
10. Bastyr EJ III, Stuart CA, Broddows RG, et al. Therapy focused on lowering post-prandial glucose, not fasting glucose, may be superior for lowering HbA1c. Diabetes Care. 2000; 23:1236-41.
11. American Diabetes Association. Postprandial blood glucose (consensus statement). Diabetes Care. 2001;24:775-8.
12. American Diabetes Association. Nutrition principles and recommendations in diabetes (position statement). Diabetes Care. 2003; 26suppl 1:S51-61.
13. Kulkarni K, Castle G, Gregory R, et al, for the Diabetes Care and Education Practice Group. Nutrition practice guidelines for type 1 diabetes mellitus positively affect dietitian practices and patient outcomes. J Am Diet Assoc. 1998;98:62-70.
14. Monk A, Barry B, McClain K, Weaver T, Cooper M, Franz MJ. Practice guidelines for medical nutrition therapy provided by dietitians for persons with non-insulin-dependent diabetes mellitus. J Am Diet Assoc. 1995;95:999-1006.
15. Sigal RJ, Kenny GP, Wasserman DH, Castaneda-Sceppa C. Physical activity/exercise and type 2 diabetes (technical review). Diabetes Care. 2004;27:2518-39.
16. Wasserman DH, Zinman B. Exercise in individuals with IDDM. Diabetes Care. 1994;17:924-37.
17. Rubin RR, Peyrot M. Psychological problems and interventions in diabetes: a review of the literature. Diabetes Care. 1992;15:1640-57.
18. Young-Hyman D. Psychosocial factors affecting adherence, quality of life, and well-being: helping patients cope. In: Medical Management of Type 1 Diabetes, 4th ed. Bode BW, ed. Alexandria, Va: American Diabetes Association; 2004:162-82.
19. Polonsky WH. Diabetes Burnout: What to Do When You Can't Take It Anymore. Alexandria, Va: American Diabetes Association; 1999:17-26.
20. Centers for Disease Control and Prevention. National Diabetes Fact Sheet: general information and national estimates on diabetes in the United States, 2005. Atlanta, Ga: US Department of Health and Human Services; 2005.
21. Arauz-Pacheco C, Parrott MA, Raskin P. The treatment of hypertension in adult patients with diabetes. Diabetes Care. 2002;25:134-47.
22. Haffner SM. Management of dyslipidemia in adults with diabetes. Diabetes Care. 1998;21:160-78.
23. Haire-Joshu D, Glasgow RE, Tibbs TL. Smoking and diabetes. Diabetes Care. 1999;22:1887-1989.
24. Colwell JA. Aspirin therapy in diabetes. Diabetes Care. 1997;20:1767-71.
25. UK Prospective Diabetes Study (UKPDS) Group. Tight blood pressure control and risk of macrovascular and microvascular complications in type 2 diabetes (UKPDS 38). BMJ. 1998;317:703-13.

26. Collins R, Armitage J, Parish S, Sleigh P, Peo R; Heart Protection Study Collaborative Group. MRC/BHF Heart Protection Study of cholesterol-lowering with simvastatin in 5963 people with diabetes: a randomized placebo-controlled trial. Lancet. 2003;361(9374):2005-2016.

27. The Expert Panel of Blood Cholesterol Levels in Children and Adolescents. Treatment recommendations of the National Cholesterol Education Program Report of the Expert Panel on Blood Cholesterol Levels in Children and Adolescents. Pediatrics. 1992;89:525-84.

28. American Diabetes Association. Smoking and diabetes (position statement). Diabetes Care. 2004; 27suppl 1: S74-5.

29. US Preventive Services Task Force. Counseling to prevent tobacco use. In: Guide to Clinical Preventive Services, 2nd ed. Baltimore, Md: Williams & Wilkins; 1996:597-609.

30. Fiore M, Baily W, Cohen S. Smoking Cessation: Clinical Practice Guideline Number 18. Rockville, Md: US Department of Health Services, Public Health Service, Agency for Health Care Policy and Research; 1996.

31. Hayden M, Pignone M, Phillips C, Mulrow C. Aspirin for the primary prevention of cardiovascular events: a summary of the evidence for the U.S. Preventive Services Task Force. Ann Intern Med. 2002;136:161-72.

32. US Preventive Services Task Force: aspirin for the primary prevention of cardiovascular events: recommendation and rationale. Ann Intern Med. 2002;136:157-60.

33. American Diabetes Association. Aspirin therapy in diabetes (position statement). Diabetes Care. 2004;27suppl 1:S72-3.

34. Garg JP, Bakris GL. Microalbuminuria: marker of vascular dysfunction, risk factor for cardiovascular disease. Vasc Med. 2002;7:35-43.

35. Klausen K, Borch-Johnson K, Feldt-Rasmussen B, et al. Very low levels of microalbuminuria are associated with increased risk of coronary heart disease and death independently of renal function, hypertension, and diabetes. Circulation. 2004;110:32-5.

36. Gall MA, Hougaard P, Borch-Johnson K, Parving HH. Risk factors for development of incipient and overt diabetic nephropathy in patients with non-insulin-dependent diabetes mellitus: prospective, observational study. BMJ. 1997;314:783-8.

37. Ravid M, Lang R, Rachmani R, Lishner M. Long-term renoprotective effect of angiotensin-converting enzyme inhibition in non-insulin-dependent diabetes mellitus: a 7-year follow-up study. Arch Intern Med. 1996;156:286-9.

38. American College of Endocrinology. Guidelines for glycemic control (consensus statement). Endo Pract. 2002;8suppl 1:6-11.

39. Colquhoun AJ, Nicholson KG, Botha JL, Raymond NT. Effectiveness of influenza vaccine in reducing hospital admissions in people with diabetes. Epidemiol Infect. 1997;119:335-41.

40. Prevention of pneumococcal disease: recommendations of the Advisory Committee on Immunization Practices (ACIP). MMWR Recomm Rep. 1997;46:1-24.

41. Loe H. Periodontal disease: the sixth complication of diabetes mellitus. Diabetes Care. 1993;16:329-34.

42. Hunt C. Skin and dental care. In: A Core Curriculum for Diabetes Education: Diabetes and Complications, 5th ed. Franz MJ, ed. Chicago Ill: American Association of Diabetes Educators; 2003:89-96.

43. Kitzmiller JL, Gavin LA, Gin GD, Jovanovic-Peterson L, Main EK, Zigrang WD. Preconception care of diabetes: glycemic control prevents congenital anomalies. JAMA. 1991;265:731-6.

44. Goldman JA, Dicker D, Feldberg D, Yeshaya A, Samuel N, Karp M. Pregnancy outcome in patients with insulin-dependent diabetes mellitus with preconceptional diabetic control: a comparative study. Am J Obstet Gynecol.1986;155:293-7.

45. Rosenn B, Miodovnik M, Combs CA, Khoury J, Siddiqi TA. Pre-conception management of insulin-dependent diabetes: improvement of pregnancy outcome. Obstet Gynecol.1991;77:846-9.

46. Tchobroutsky C, Vray MM, Altman JJ. Risk/benefit ratio of changing late obstetrical strategies in the management of insulin-dependent diabetic pregnancies: a comparison between 1971-1977 and 1978-1985 periods in 389 pregnancies. Diabetes Metab. 1991;17:287-94.

47. Willhoite MB, Bennert HW Jr, Palomaki GE, et al. The impact of pre-conception counseling on pregnancy outcomes: the experience of the Maine Diabetes in Pregnancy Program. Diabetes Care.1993;16:450-5.

48. Kitzmiller JL, Buchanan TA, Kjos S, Combs CA, Ratner RE. Preconception care of diabetes, congenital malformations, and spontaneous abortions. Diabetes Care. 1996;19:514-41.

49. American Diabetes Association. Preconception care of women with diabetes (position statement). Diabetes Care. 2004;27suppl1:S76-8.

50. American Diabetes Association. Self-monitoring of blood glucose. Diabetes Care. 1994;17:81-6.

51. Cappuccio FP, Kerry SM, Forbes L. Blood pressure control by home monitoring: meta-analysis of randomized trials. BMJ. 2004;329:145-51.

52. Ahroni JH. Diabetic foot care and education. In: A Core Curriculum for Diabetes Education: Diabetes and Complications, 5th ed. Franz MJ, ed. Chicago, Ill: American Association of Diabetes Educators; 2003:67-86.

53. Pecoraro RE Reiber GE, Burgess EM. Pathways to diabetic limb amputation: basis for prevention. Diabetes Care. 1990;13:513-21.

54. Edmonds ME, Blundell MP, Morris ME, Thomas EM, Cotton LT, Watkins PJ. Improved survival of the diabetic foot: the role of the specialized foot clinic. Q J Med. 1986;60:763-71.

INDEX

B

C

D

E

F

H

I

N

O

P

Q

R

S

T

U

V

W

X

Y

Z

ABOUT AADE

Purpose

Founded in 1973, AADE is a professional membership organization dedicated to promoting the professional expertise of the diabetes educator, ensuring the delivery of quality diabetes self-management training to the patient, and influencing and contributing to the future content and direction of the profession.

Membership

AADE's members are healthcare professionals who specialize in helping people with diabetes self-manage their disease. They include nurses, dietitians, pharmacists, physicians, social workers, exercise physiologists, and other members of the diabetes care team.

AADE Education and Research Foundation

Established in 1988, the foundation is dedicated to enhancing the quality of education and care for persons with diabetes by supporting activities in the areas of continuing education for health professionals, research in diabetes education, and public education about diabetes management.

Professional Development Opportunities

Annual Meeting

A four-day event that draws more than 4,000 educators, it offers the opportunity to hear experts in diabetes self-management training, participate in educational sessions and network with colleagues. The program also includes exhibits of diabetes-related products and services.

Online Courses and Audio Seminars (webinars/webcasts)

An opportunity to earn continuing education credit from home or the office. Courses cover the latest issues in diabetes self-management training and give diabetes educators the opportunity to learn new skills and sharpen existing ones.

The Diabetes Educator

A bimonthly journal (online and hard copy) that presents patient education research, lesson plan ideas, management strategies, book reviews, practical columns and self-study offerings with continuing education credit.

AADE e-FYI

A monthly newsletter providing members with relevant AADE news.

Products

AADE offers a number of resources to help today's healthcare professionals keep pace with the ever changing field of diabetes education. To order visit Online Bookstore at www.diabeteseducator.org/Products/

Awards, Grants and Scholarships

Awards and grants are given for a variety of projects, including the development of patient education tools and research in diabetes education.

For more information on AADE's membership, products, or services, please go to www.diabeteseducator.org or call 800/338-3633. Nonmembers can join the AADE mailing list by signing up online at www.diabeteseducator.org/interest.html.